DATE DUE

Demco, Inc. 38-293

CLINICAL TRANSPLANTS 2000

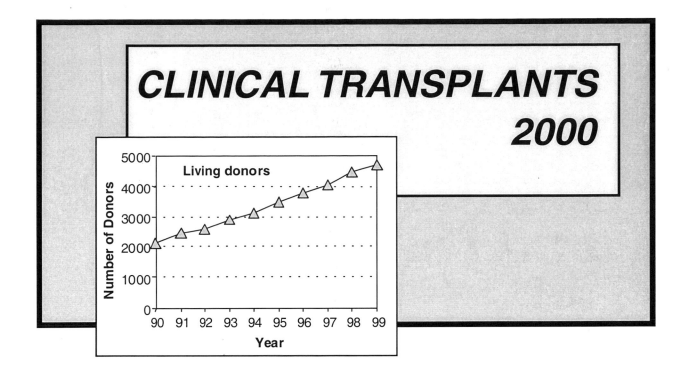

J. Michael Cecka, Ph.D.
Paul I. Terasaki, Ph.D.
Editors

Published by

UCLA Immunogenetics Center

1000 Veteran Avenue

Los Angeles, California 90095

Supported by a contract from the United States Department of Health and Human Services, Health Resources and Services Administration through a subcontract from the United Network for Organ Sharing.

Sixteenth in a series
Clinical Kidney Transplants 1985
Clinical Transplants 1986
Clinical Transplants 1987
Clinical Transplants 1988
Clinical Transplants 1989
Clinical Transplants 1990
Clinical Transplants 1991
Clinical Transplants 1992
Clinical Transplants 1993 (out of print)
Clinical Transplants 1994
Clinical Transplants 1995
Clinical Transplants 1996 (out of print)
Clinical Transplants 1997
Clinical Transplants 1998
Clinical Transplants 1999
(Most volumes still available)

Other books published by the UCLA Tissue Typing Laboratory
History of HLA
History of Transplantation: Thirty-five Recollections
Transplant Success Stories 1993
HLA 1997
HLA 1998

ISSN 0890-9016
ISBN 1-880318-09-1

UCLA Immunogenetics Center
1000 Veteran Avenue
Los Angeles, California 90095

Printed in the United States of America

PREFACE

The Millennium Edition, Clinical Transplants 2000, is our **SIXTEENTH ANNUAL SUMMARY** of the status of clinical transplantation.

To broaden our scope this year, we invited representatives of 30 countries to describe the challenges and results of **KIDNEY TRANSPLANTATION WORLD-WIDE**.

The **UNITED NETWORK FOR ORGAN SHARING (UNOS)** has provided updates on the status of transplantation in the United States from each of the organ-specific Registries. A current review of organ donation and the national waiting list have been provided in reports from the **UNOS ORGAN PROCUREMENT AND TRANSPLANTATION NETWORK**.

The **US RENAL DATA SYSTEM (USRDS)** Registry has examined the impact of transplantation on the survival of patients with kidney failure.

The **PREGNANCY REGISTRY** summarizes the results and safety of more than 2,000 pregnancies in (or fathered by) transplant recipients.

Internationally, **EUROTRANSPLANT** describes the results of their proficiency testing program for histocompatibility laboratories and the impact of testing accuracy on transplantation. The **UKTSSA** reports the results of renal transplantation in England and Ireland. The **LATIN AMERICAN TRANSPLANT REGISTRY** provides a summary of transplant activity in South America, Mexico and the Carribean.

The **SINGLE-CENTER** reports of transplant results this year include:
KIDNEY - Houston, Minnesota, Bergamo (Italy), Belfast (Ireland), Tehran (Iran), Montefiore
PANCREAS-KIDNEY - Maryland, Tennessee, Northwestern
LIVER - New York, Tennessee, Toronto, Paris, Brussels
HEART - Los Angeles
LUNG - Hannover (Germany)
BONE MARROW - City of Hope

Dr Clyde Barker, Dr James Markmann and their colleagues have neatly summarized nearly 300 articles related to transplantation and published in 2000 for our **ANNUAL REVIEW** of the transplant literature.

The **UNOS Renal Transplant Registry** studies include:
- A comparison of results of recent transplants using different immunosuppressive agents.
- A multivariate analysis of factors that influence delayed graft function and rejection.
- A comprehensive review of HLA matching effects in different patient cohorts.

The WORLDWIDE TRANSPLANT DIRECTORY

Organ	Centers	2000	Total
Kidney	588	27,424	500,545
Kidney-Pancreas	158	1,198	11,541
Pancreas	94	484	3,584
Liver	230	8,733	89,178
Heart	229	3,365	57,043
Lung	119	1,408	12,076
Bone Marrow	370	7,775	104,682

The **WORLD TRANSPLANT RECORDS** lists the longest transplant survivors, the oldest and youngest donors and recipients, and a variety of other notable or unusual transplants that are still functioning. The longest surviving grafts include a kidney that has functioned for 41 years, a liver 31 years, a heart 24 years and a lung 14 years after the transplant.

Publication Staff
We are grateful for the heroic efforts of Su-Hui Lee and Debbie Burgos who have made this volume possible. Lupita Geer also lent her considerable talents to help us meet our deadlines this year.
Editorial: Joyce Yuge, Michael Cecka
Directory: Debbie Burgos
World Records: Lupita Geer

Acknowledgements
We applaud all of those who have donated organs to extend and improve the lives of transplant recipients around the world. The transplant professionals whose work has affected so many also provide the extensive information about their patients and the results of their work that make these summaries possible. We also acknowledge Dr Elaine F Reed (Director of the new UCLA Immunogenetics Center) and Dr Jonathan Braun (Chair of Pathology) for their support of our efforts.

TABLE OF CONTENTS

Table of Contents

Chapter .... Page

TRANSPLANT CENTERS

Kidney

Pancreas-Kidney

Table of Contents

Chapter .... Page

Table of Contents

Chapter .... Page

CUMULATIVE TABLE OF CONTENTS

CENTER	PAGE											
	'88	'89	'90	'91	'92	'93	'94	'95	'96	'97	'98	'99

KIDNEY (Cont'd)

CENTER	'88	'89	'90	'91	'92	'93	'94	'95	'96	'97	'98	'99
IOWA CITY								207				
IRELAND		191										
LEUVEN, BELGIUM	91							255				
LYON, FRANCE		229										
MANCHESTER, U.K.		201								125		
MANITOBA, CANADA	159											
MARYLAND											177	
MASS. GENERAL			247									
MAYO CLINIC		267										
MIAMI		215										159
MICHIGAN												139
MILAN, ITALY							243			229		
MINNESOTA	79	253	217		227		203					
MUNICH, GERMANY	107					219						
NANTES, FRANCE			301				237	257				
NECKER, FRANCE	99											
NEW YORK										187		
OSAKA, JAPAN												
OSLO, NORWAY					207					221		
OXFORD, U.K.						233						
PHILADELPHIA					215							
PHOENIX		275										
PITTSBURGH	181	287				137	229	199				
PORTLAND				153					223			
ROME, ITALY										205		
SAN ANTONIO								233				
SAN FRANCISCO												
SINGAPORE												189
STANFORD										135		
STOCKHOLM, SWEDEN												
TAIWAN		281										
TAMPA												149
TOKYO, JAPAN	189											
TORONTO, CANADA	171										195	
UCLA			255							113		
WASHINGTON, DC			275								159	
WICHITA			265									
WISCONSIN		239	241			211	197					
YONSEI U, SEOUL					249					149		
ZURICH, SWITZERLAND									241			

CUMULATIVE CONTENTS

CHAPTER 1

The UNOS Scientific Renal Transplant Registry –2000

J. Michael Cecka

It has been 100 years since the surgical techniques for vascular anastomosis required for transplanting organs were developed and more than 60 years since the first unsuccessful attempts to transplant human kidneys between individuals were reported. But it has been less than 50 years since the first long-surviving kidney transplant was performed in Boston. As we begin the 21st Century, and a new millennium, it seems appropriate to look back briefly at what progress has been made in the relatively young field of transplantation – not by reviewing the literature, but by reviewing the results of kidney transplants over the years.

We can do this because of the unique efforts of those who have been involved in transplantation – from the pioneers (many of whom are still with us) to the complex network of transplant professionals who provide these medical miracles today. They have supported efforts to assemble their results centrally in transplant registries. There have been many different registries over the years; some now defunct, but others continuing to accrue new data while tracking the results of the transplants they recorded many years ago. The registries have provided an effective mechanism to learn from the successes and failures of others. Although no large registry can match the detailed data available to institutions about their own patients, their strength is in the enormous numbers of patients they follow, which allows more powerful statistical analyses of the many complex variables that may influence graft and patient outcomes. The results of the United Network for Organ Sharing (UNOS) organ-specific registry analyses as well as the results from the Eurotransplant, United Kingdom Transplant, and Latin American Transplant Registries make up the first several chapters of this volume. In addition, the US Renal Data System Registry of dialysis patients and the National Transplant Pregnancy Registry report other aspects of life after transplantation. These reports show what we have learned from looking at the data submitted by coordinators at many transplant centers around the world.

Publishing these data summaries and analyses in the chapters that follow is a way for us to return the favor for the hard work of reporting these data to the registries.

Kidneys were the first vascularized organs to be transplanted with success and Figure 1 summarizes the cumulative kidney transplant activity in the United States as reported to the UCLA and UNOS Registries. Through 1999, a total of approximately 135,000 cadaver kidney transplants, 53,000 living-donor kidney transplants and 8,000 kidneys transplanted in combination with other solid organs had been reported. If we include transplants that were performed during the year 2000, the total is more than 200,000 kidney transplants in the US. Of those approximately 100,000 are functioning today, 40,000 have failed and 37,000 recipients have died while being followed. These estimates are imprecise as reporting was voluntary prior to the establishment of UNOS, and

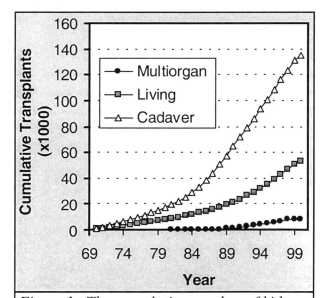

Figure 1. The cumulative number of kidney transplants performed in the United States based on data reported to the UCLA (1969-1987) and UNOS (1988-2000) Renal Transplant Registries.

Clinical Transplants 2000, Cecka and Terasaki, Eds. UCLA Immunogenetics Center, Los Angeles, California

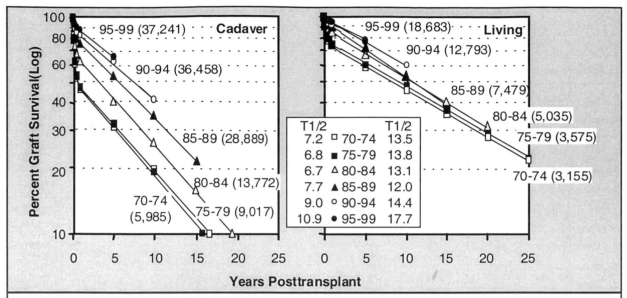

Figure 2. Graft survival rates for cadaveric and living-donor kidney transplants performed in the United States since 1970 in 5-year cohorts.

the UCLA Registry collected only about 75% of US transplants. Many patients have been lost to follow-up. However, the estimate is in line with that of the US Renal Data System Registry provided in Chapter 11. If we add the totals for kidney transplants listed in the Worldwide Transplant Center Directory at the end of this volume, the worldwide total of kidney transplants is more than 500,000. That is remarkable progress, both in the US and internationally.

The results of kidney transplants have obviously improved substantially over the years as indicated in Figure 2. Only about 5% of the 15,000 cadaver kidney transplants that were performed prior to 1980 survived 25 years (the result is below 10% on the logscale) and some of those are listed in the Worldwide Records (beginning on page 515 of this volume). The actuarial graft survival rate for transplants performed in the past 5 years is 66% at 5 years. When we project their survival to 25 years, the result suggests that only about 20% of these more recent transplants will still be functioning in 2020.

Kidneys transplanted from living donors have consistently yielded superior results compared with those of cadaver transplants. Of the 6,500 living donor transplants performed before 1980, approximately 22% survived 25 years. Of the more than 18,000 living donor transplants performed between 1995-1999, 78% will survive 5 years and projecting to 25 years, survival should be 37% in 2020. The long-term superiority of living do-

nor kidney transplants is also apparent when comparing the longest surviving kidney transplants. Of those that have survived more than 30 years listed on pages 515-528, nearly 75% were transplanted from living donors. We have attributed the higher success rates of living donor transplants to better histocompatibility when the genetically related donor and recipient share one or both HLA haplotypes. However, recent results with living-unrelated donor transplants (1) have shown that the difference is more complex and suggest that brain death itself may be an important determinant of long-term outcome (2). Therefore, we might consider that the improving graft survival rates over the years with living donor transplants show the impact of technical advances, immunosuppression, and patient management, while the larger changes in cadaver kidney graft survival rates also reflect improvements in donor selection and management and in kidney preservation.

Despite the remarkable progress shown by these figures, many challenges remain. The donor shortage – too few kidneys to meet the demand - is a growing problem that resonates through this volume of Clinical Transplants. It is a worldwide problem with as yet no clear solution. For the United States, the cadaver donor shortage, and approaches to help provide alternative donor sources are discussed at length in Chapter 6. Another serious concern lies in the long-term effects of powerful immunosuppressant drugs, which are largely unknown today. Some data on neoplasms in long-term survivors are provided in Chapter 17. Finally, there remains a significant racial disparity in access to and the outcome of renal transplantation in the US (3,4).

This chapter summarizes some of the results of renal transplants that have been reported to the UNOS Scientific Renal Transplant Registry and stratified according to risk factors identified through multivariate analyses as contributors to short- or long-term outcomes. I have presented most of the results separately for blacks and whites as the overall results of transplants are strongly influenced by the poor long-term success rates among black transplant recipients.

PATIENTS AND METHODS

The historical trends shown in Figures 1-3 were compiled from the UCLA (1969-1987) and UNOS (1988-1999) Registries. Unless otherwise indicated, multi-organ transplants were excluded from these analyses. The survival calculations were based on 55,924 transplants performed between 1995-1999 and reported to the UNOS Scientific Renal Transplant Registry through September 2000. These included 37,241 cadaver and 18,683 living donor transplants analyzed separately. All other analyses were based on UNOS Registry data from 1988-2000. Figure 5, 8-23 and Table 1 show results for recipients of cadaver donor transplants and Figures 4,6,7 and Table 1 include results for living-donor kidney transplants. Racial groupings were used as reported to UNOS without consideration as to whether the patient was Hispanic. "Other" races included Asians, American Indians, Pacific Islanders and others.

Early rejection episodes were counted as reported to UNOS whether or not they were confirmed by biopsy. Treated rejections were reported at discharge, 6 months, and one year. Delayed graft function (DGF) was defined as the need for dialysis during the first week after transplantation.

Graft survival rates were calculated as Kaplan-Meier product limit estimates using STATA software (College Station, TX). Patient deaths were considered graft failures whether or not the graft was functioning at the time of death. Graft half-lives were computed for grafts sur-

viving at one year after transplantation (5) and are expressed as the number of years before half the surviving grafts would fail. Statistical comparisons of survival curves were performed by the log-rank test and chi square analyses were used to compare groups.

RESULTS

The results are summarized in the following Figures and Table:

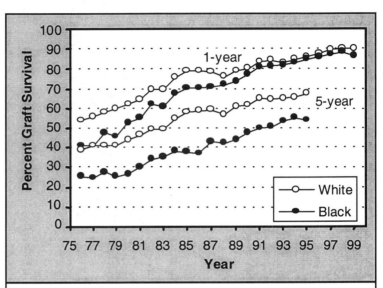

Figure 3. The annual one- and 5-year cadaver kidney graft survival rates among blacks and whites (1975-1999).

Historically, graft survival rates among black recipients have been consistently lower than among whites. The difference in one-year graft survival rates between the races declined from 10-15% in the pre-cyclosporine era (before 1985) to 2% or less since 1993. However, the 5-year graft survival rates remain significantly poorer among blacks – more than 10% lower for transplants performed in 1993-1995 (p<0.001). These graft survival disparities are not due to differences in patient survival. Blacks transplanted during 1995-1999 had an 83.5% 5-year patient survival rate compared with 85.0% for whites (p=0.846). Nevertheless, there has been some improvement in the long-term graft survival rates for blacks. The graft half-lives have improved from 5 years for transplants performed before 1991 to 7.5 years for transplants between 1996-1998.

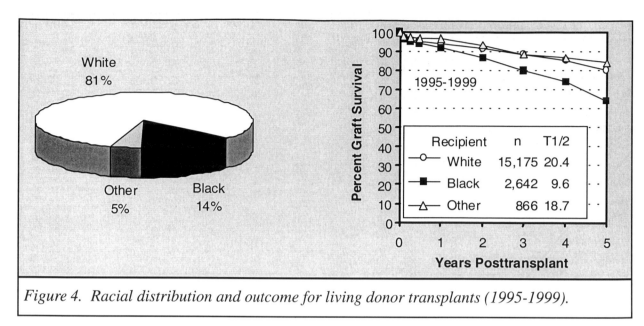

Figure 4. Racial distribution and outcome for living donor transplants (1995-1999).

Most living donor transplant recipients were white (81%). The graft survival rates were similar for whites and others who received a living donor kidney but were significantly poorer for blacks. Despite an excellent 92% success rate at one year, black recipients subsequently lost their grafts at about twice the rate of other racial and ethnic groups as indicated by the graft half-life. At 5 years, graft survival was 16-20% lower among black recipients of living donor grafts (p<0.001). The 5-year patient survival rates were 92.7%, 89.8% and 91.9% for whites, blacks and others, respectively (p=0.015).

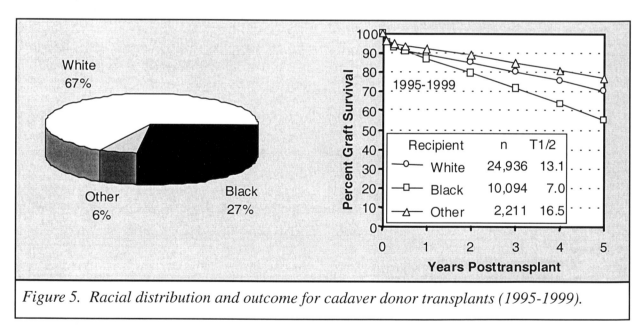

Figure 5. Racial distribution and outcome for cadaver donor transplants (1995-1999).

The racial distribution of cadaver kidney recipients was more diverse and better reflected the waiting list (Ch. 5). About two-thirds of recipients were white, 27% were black and 4% were others. Again, despite an excellent 87% one-year graft survival rate, blacks lost their grafts at a much higher rate after the first year. During this recent period, the graft survival rates for Asians and others were significantly better than for whites (p<0.001). Patient survival rates were 85.0%, 83.3% and 91.4% for whites, blacks and others, respectively, at 5 years.

Although fewer minorities than whites received living donor transplants, the donor relationships were broadly similar among the racial groups. However, a notably higher percentage of black parents received a kidney from an offspring and fewer black spouses and HLA-identical siblings donated their kidneys compared with whites and others. The higher proportion of offspring-to-parent transplants among blacks resulted in the significantly lower patient survival rate for black recipients of living donor kidneys shown in Figure 4. When offsping-to-parent grafts were excluded, patient survival rates were 93.6% for whites and 91.2 % for blacks (p=0.656).

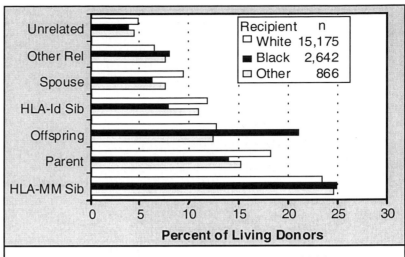

Figure 6. Living donor relationships (1995-1999).

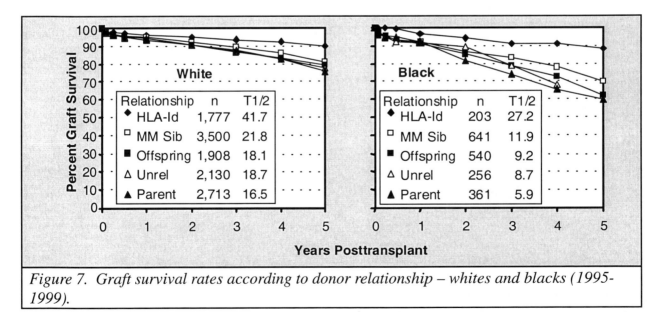

Figure 7. Graft survival rates according to donor relationship – whites and blacks (1995-1999).

The results of living donor transplants were also generally similar comparing whites and blacks. HLA-identical sibling grafts provided the highest long-term graft survival rates in each case with 88% survival at 5 years. Among whites, the results of HLA-mismatched sibling transplants were significantly better than for other living donor groups, but survival rates were nearly identical with other living donors, whether or not they were related to the recipient. Among blacks the trend was similar – a significantly higher survival rate for HLA-matched (p<0.001), and for HLA-mismatched (p=0.035) sibling transplants, but no significant graft survival differences between other HLA-mismatched living donor groups (p=0.101). The poorest survival rates were noted for recipients of parent donor transplants.

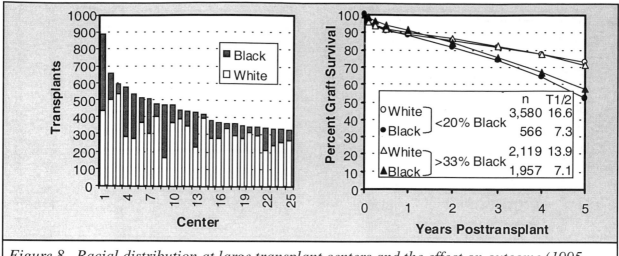

Figure 8. Racial distribution at large transplant centers and the effect on outcome (1995-1999).

One challenge to estimating the effect of race on outcomes is the striking variation in the distribution of racial groups from center to center. Among the 25 largest US transplant centers, the proportion of blacks who were transplanted ranged from 6-64%. Cadaver donor transplants from these centers were grouped if the center transplanted more than 33% blacks or less than 20%

blacks, respectively, and the graft survival rates show almost overlapping results for whites and blacks. Centers that had a larger experience with blacks also had superior results for blacks through the first posttransplant year, but thereafter, graft survival rates fell at the same rate for blacks transplanted at either center group.

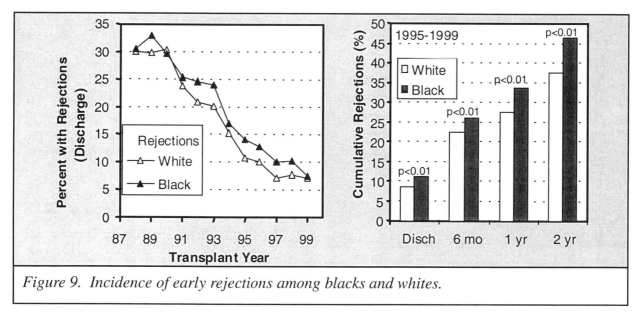

Figure 9. Incidence of early rejections among blacks and whites.

The incidence of early rejections has declined precipitously during the past 10 years. Prior to 1990, 30% of cadaver kidney recipients were treated for rejection before their hospital discharge. By 1999, fewer than 10% had early rejections. Blacks had a higher incidence of reported early rejection episodes than whites every year

except 1990. During the past 5 years about 2.5% more blacks had rejection before discharge than whites (p<0.01), but the difference increased with time after transplant so that by 2 years, acute rejections had been noted in 37% of whites compared with 46% of blacks (p<0.01).

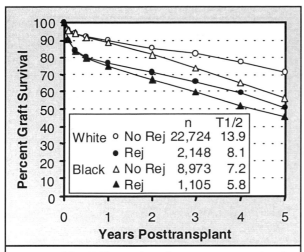

Figure 10. Effect of early rejection episodes on graft survival (1995-1999).

During the recent 5-year interval (1995-1999), 8.6% of whites and 11.0% of blacks who received a cadaveric transplant were treated for rejection prior to the hospital discharge. About 10% of patients who experienced early rejection lost their graft within the first month and by 6 months, 20% had failed. The failure rates for blacks and whites following early rejection were indistinguishable during the first posttransplant year. Between 1-5 years, blacks lost their grafts more rapidly than whites whether or not there had been a rejection prior to hospital discharge; however, early rejection was associated with a significant decrease in the graft half-life for both blacks and whites. The racial difference in long-term graft survival rates was more pronounced among those who did not experience early rejection. The 5-year graft survival rate was 15% lower for blacks than whites when there was no rejection prior to hospital discharge, compared with a 5% difference when rejection occurred early.

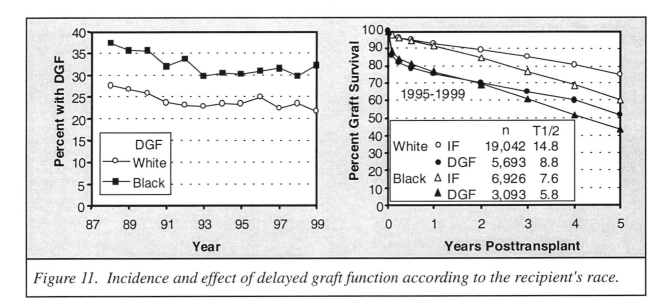

Figure 11. Incidence and effect of delayed graft function according to the recipient's race.

Blacks were more likely to experience delayed graft function (DGF) than whites each year between 1988-1999. The incidence of DGF declined by 5% in each group from 1988-1993 and has remained stable at about 23% for whites and 30% for blacks since then. In cadaveric transplants performed between 1995-1999, approximately 14% of whites and 11% of blacks lost their graft during the first posttransplant month when DGF occurred, but at one year graft survival rates were comparable for blacks and whites who had immediate function (IF) or who had delayed function. After one year blacks lost their grafts at an accelerated rate compared with whites in both groups. DGF was associated with a more rapid late graft loss rate in both blacks and whites, but the largest racial difference in graft survival (15% at 5 years) was apparent comparing those with immediate function.

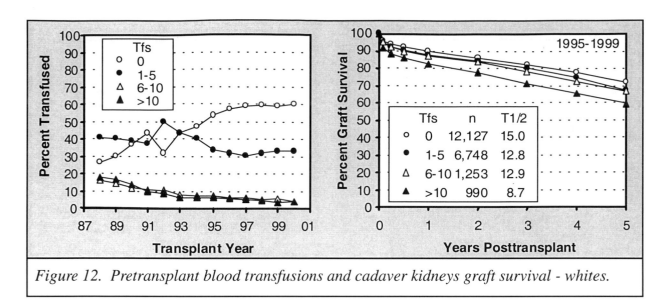

Figure 12. Pretransplant blood transfusions and cadaver kidneys graft survival - whites.

The percentage of untransfused whites who received cadaver donor transplants increased from 25% in 1988 to 60% in 1999. Concomitantly, the percentages transplanted after 6-10 or more than 10 transfusions fell from more than 15% in 1988 to less than 5% in 1999, respectively. Graft survival rates were highest among nontransfused whites and significantly poorer when the patient had received more than 10 transfusions.

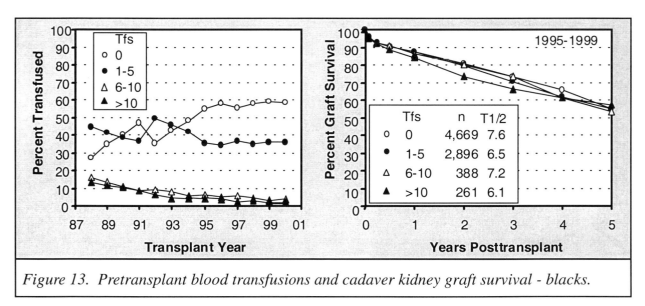

Figure 13. Pretransplant blood transfusions and cadaver kidney graft survival - blacks.

The trend toward fewer transfused patients receiving transplants was also apparent among blacks. Among black recipients, however, the role of transfusions in long-term graft survival was less apparent due to the small number of patients in the multiply transfused groups. There was no correlation between the number of pretransplant blood transfusions and the recipient's age as might be expected if patients with a longer history of disease or those who were on dialysis before erythropoeitin were disproportionately represented among the transfused groups. Even among untransfused blacks, the long-term graft failure rate was nearly double that for whites.

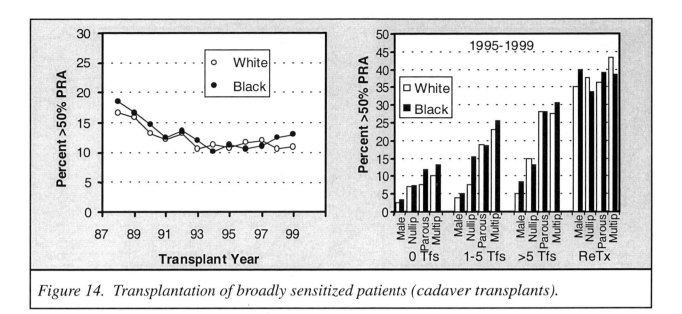

Figure 14. Transplantation of broadly sensitized patients (cadaver transplants).

The percentage of broadly sensitized (>50% PRA) patients transplanted each year declined from 16-18% in 1988 to 10-12% in 1993 and has remained at those levels since. The percentages of blacks and whites who were broadly sensitized was not significantly different.

When blacks and whites transplanted between 1995-1999 were stratified according to risks for sensitization (sex, pregnancies, transfusions and previous transplants), there was no clear pattern that suggested a higher rate of sensitization among blacks.

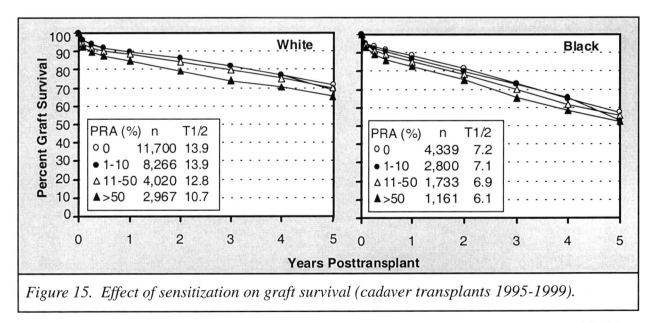

Figure 15. Effect of sensitization on graft survival (cadaver transplants 1995-1999).

Graft survival rates were not noticeably affected by low levels of sensitization, however, broadly sensitized whites and blacks (>50% PRA) had 5% lower one-year graft survival rates than their nonsensitized counterparts.

Broadly sensitized recipients had shorter graft half-lives than those who were not sensitized. The graft half-life for nonsensitized blacks was about half that for nonsensitized whites.

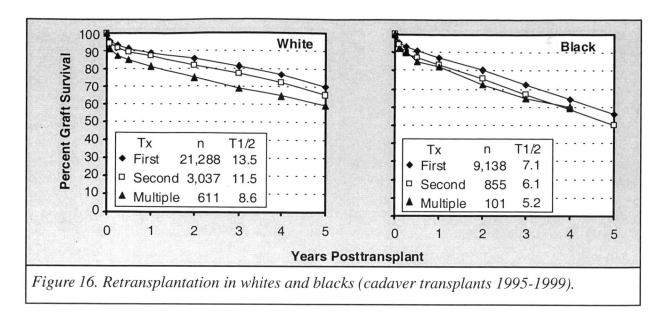

Figure 16. Retransplantation in whites and blacks (cadaver transplants 1995-1999).

A smaller percentage of blacks than whites were retransplanted (9.5% vs. 14.6%; p<0.001) during 1995-1999. The 5-year graft survival rate after retransplantation was about 5% lower for second than first transplants among both whites and blacks (p<0.001). White recipients of multiple regrafts had significantly lower regraft survival rates than those who received a second transplant (p<0.001). Very few blacks were multiply retansplanted and their regraft survival rates were also lower but did not reach statistical significance. The difference in 5-year primary graft survival rates between blacks and whites was 14%.

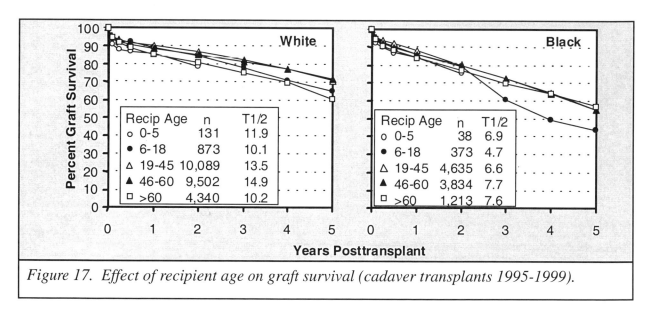

Figure 17. Effect of recipient age on graft survival (cadaver transplants 1995-1999).

The recipient age distribution among whites and blacks was similar, except that fewer older blacks were transplanted than whites (12% vs. 17%; p<0.01). The one-year graft survival rates for the youngest and oldest white recipients were 4-5% lower than those for patients in the remaining age groups. After 2 years, the graft survival rate for whites aged 6-18 began to decline and the graft half-life for this group was 10.1 years. The one-year survival rate for blacks; aged 19-45 was 88%, comparable to that for whites, however the graft half-lives were significantly lower among black recipients in each age group. The small number of blacks aged 6-18 had the poorest graft survival rates and the shortest graft half-lives.

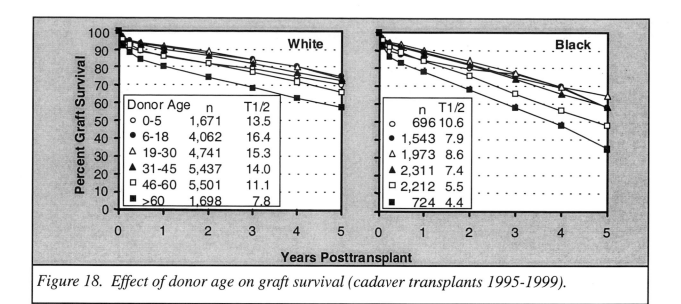

Figure 18. Effect of donor age on graft survival (cadaver transplants 1995-1999).

Older donor kidneys yielded poorer long-term graft survival rates in whites and blacks. The 5-year survival rates for kidneys from donors aged 46-60 and >60 were 66% and 57%, respectively, among whites compared with 72% when the donor was younger (p<0.001). The 5-year graft survival rates among blacks were more se-verely affected by the donor's age. Graft survival rates were 48% and 35%, respectively, when the donor was aged 46-60 and >60 compared with 64% when the donor was aged 19-30. There was no difference in the distribution of donor ages among whites and blacks.

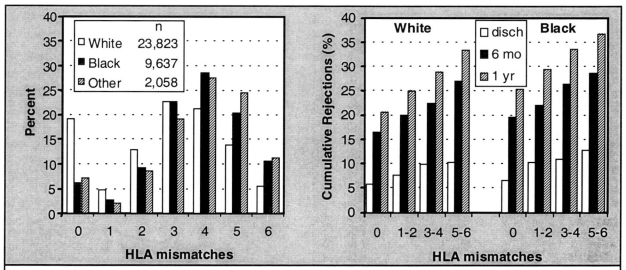

Figure 19. Distribution of HLA-matched cadaver kidneys by recipient race and the effect of HLA mismatches on rejections during the first year (1995-1999).

Nearly 20% of whites received an HLA-matched cadaver kidney during 1995-1999, compared with 6% of blacks and 7% of others. About 59% of blacks and 62% of others received kidneys with 4 or more mismatched HLA antigens compared with 40% of whites.

The cumulative incidence of treated rejection episodes increased with the number of HLA mismatches in each recipient race group. Twenty-one percent of HLA-matched whites had at least one rejection during the first year compared with 33% of those with 5-6 antigens mismatched (p<0.01). Similarly for blacks, rejections increased from 25% to 37% comparing HLA-matched with poorly matched recipients (p<0.01).

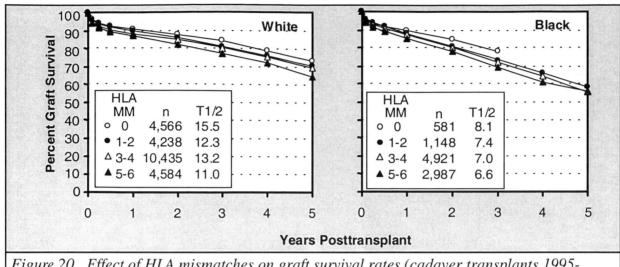

Figure 20. Effect of HLA mismatches on graft survival rates (cadaver transplants 1995-1999).

Among whites, the difference in 5-year graft survival rates associated with HLA mismatches was 9%, with a 3% difference between HLA-matched kidneys and those with 1-2 antigens mismatched and a 5% difference between the most poorly matched grafts (5-6 mismatches) and the 3-4 mismatched group. Among blacks, the results were similar with the highest survival rate and half-life for the small number of HLA-matched kidneys and the poorest results for recipients of completely mismatched grafts. After 3 years, there was a 9% survival difference between the best and worst HLA-matched grafts.

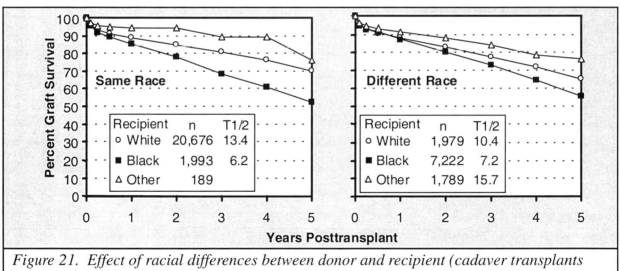

Figure 21. Effect of racial differences between donor and recipient (cadaver transplants 1995-1999).

More than 90% of whites, 76% of blacks, and 81% of others received white donor kidneys. Whites donated 87% of cadaver kidneys transplanted during this period. About 22% of blacks and 10% of others received cadaver kidneys from race-matched donors. Whites who received white kidneys had a 5-year graft survival rate of 70% versus 65% when they were transplanted from donors of a different race. Blacks who received black kidneys had a 52% 5-year graft survival rate versus 56% when the donor's race was different.

Table 1. Effect of end-stage renal disease on one-year graft survival rates (1995-1999).

	Cadaver				Living			
	White	1-yr	Black	1-yr	White	1-yr	Black	1-yr
Hypertensive Nephrosclerosis	2,378	88.7%	3,080	87.3%	1,147	94.2%	608	92.4%
Juvenile Diabetes								
Kidney Alone	2,812	89.9%	578	89.9%	1,907	94.2%	177	91.1%
Simultaneous Pancreas	3,107	90.7%	348	92.2%	23	100.0%	0	
NIDDM (adult)	2,420	86.9%	1,146	85.7%	1,015	93.1%	287	91.9%
Polycystic Kidneys	3,031	90.6%	312	89.4%	1,237	95.4%	53	94.2%
Chronic GN	1,918	89.4%	535	89.1%	1,095	96.1%	132	91.8%
Focal Sclerosis	1,183	86.6%	683	88.3%	855	93.3%	242	92.7%
Malignant Hypertension	716	84.8%	982	85.8%	299	93.2%	228	92.1%
IgA Nephropathy	836	92.7%	63	87.0%	946	95.7%	42	97.1%
Systemic Lupus	647	87.6%	486	84.8%	512	94.4%	170	90.8%
Pyelonephritis	722	89.6%	48	82.1%	620	93.5%	21	94.4%
Membranous GN	671	90.3%	204	85.0%	477	94.3%	57	94.2%
Nephritis	466	89.3%	115	83.5%	273	93.7%	32	100.0%
Adult Diabetes	406	86.5%	160	84.2%	187	91.6%	43	94.7%
Congenital OU	303	87.6%	66	88.9%	331	96.6%	27	88.7%
Alport's Syndrome	380	89.3%	32	90.1%	214	96.0%	11	100.0%
Hypoplasia	244	84.2%	72	86.6%	268	93.8%	17	100.0%
Postinfectious GN	304	88.7%	73	86.2%	174	95.6%	18	100.0%
Obstructive Uropathy	234	86.0%	52	81.5%	183	95.5%	11	100.0%
Glomerular Sclerosis	195	90.0%	66	72.0%	110	93.1%	28	91.5%
Membranoproliferative GN	166	88.4%	42	76.8%	113	92.7%	14	100.0%
Wegener's Granulomatosis	137	94.7%	9	100.0%	129	93.4%	4	100.0%
CsA Toxicity	149	77.6%	14	100.0%	93	86.4%	4	75.0%
Hemolytic Uremia	114	80.4%	16	91.7%	101	95.1%	4	66.7%
Nephrosclerosis	99	84.8%	49	86.5%	47	90.7%	9	87.5%
Membranous Nephropathy	96	90.8%	22	85.4%	61	93.1%	10	80.0%
Medullary Cystic Disease	87	95.0%	7	100.0%	68	93.5%	2	NA
Analgesic Nephropathy	77	89.4%	25	87.5%	53	87.3%	1	NA
Familial Nephopathy	90	91.6%	8	100.0%	35	100.0%	4	NA
Prune Belly	36	84.3%	12	82.5%	62	100.0%	6	100.0%
Henoch Schonlein Purpura	52	87.8%	0		51	98.0%	4	100.0%
Nephrolithiasis	58	92.1%	4	75.0%	26	96.2%	0	
Renal Cell Carcinoma	46	92.9%	9	100.0%	29	91.1%	2	NA
Goodpasture's	38	86.2%	11	63.6%	36	93.9%	0	
Amyloidosis	44	85.5%	4	66.7%	25	100.0%	4	100.0%
Scleroderma	27	76.9%	7	68.6%	29	79.3%	0	
Cortical Necrosis	28	96.4%	1	100.0%	24	95.8%	5	100.0%
Nephronophthisis	32	72.0%	7	100.0%	15	92.9%	3	33.3%
Cystinosis	28	96.4%	2	50.0%	24	100.0%	3	100.0%
Type 2 Mesangio-capillary GN	28	88.3%	12	90.9%	12	100.0%	4	NA
Oxalosis	23	91.3%	0		30	81.6%	0	
Fabry's Disease	33	89.0%	2	NA	16	93.3%	1	100.0%
NIDDM (juvenile)	24	86.2%	10	100.0%	13	100.0%	2	100.0%
Wilm's Tumor	11	100.0%	2	50.0%	33	100.0%	2	NA

Table 1 lists the primary renal diseases in descending order of overall frequency together with the incidence and one-year graft survival rates stratified by donor type and recipient race. Insulin-dependent diabetes was the most common disease among whites (including SPK transplants), but hypertension was predominant among blacks.

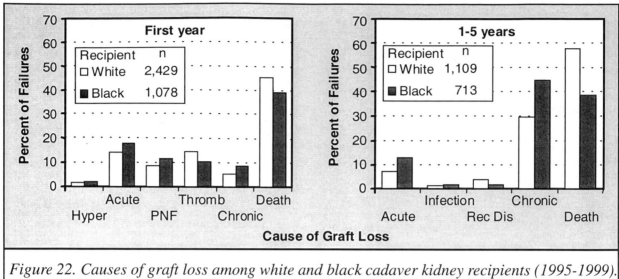

Figure 22. Causes of graft loss among white and black cadaver kidney recipients (1995-1999).

During this 5-year interval, 2,429 whites and 1,078 blacks lost their grafts within the first posttransplant year and the major cause of graft failure was death. Blacks were more likely than whites to lose their grafts to acute or chronic rejection or because of primary nonfunction, but a lower percentage of failures among blacks were due to patient death. After the first year, the major causes of graft loss were chronic rejection and death. Blacks were more likely to lose their grafts because of acute or chronic rejection and less likely to die than whites. Thus, graft losses among blacks were more often immunological, whereas whites more often died with a functioning graft.

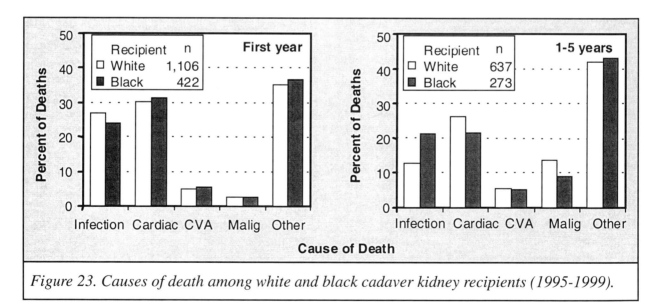

Figure 23. Causes of death among white and black cadaver kidney recipients (1995-1999).

There were 1,106 whites and 422 blacks who died within the first posttransplant year between 1995-1999 and the causes of death did not differ significantly between the races. The major causes of death within the first year were infection and cardiac disease, accounting for more than half of all deaths. After the first year, infection and cardiac deaths remained the major single causes of death, accounting for slightly less than half of the deaths. Blacks were more likely than whites to die as a result of infection after the first year, but were less likely than whites to die of cardiovascular complications or malignancies.

DISCUSSION

Racial differences in access to transplantation and in the success rates following transplantation remain important unresolved challenges in the United States (3,4). The problems are exacerbated by the high incidence of end-stage renal disease among American blacks. Although blacks comprise 13% of the US population, they account for nearly 40% of the end-stage renal disease patients on dialysis (6). At the end of October 2000, 35% of patients on the waiting list for cadaveric renal transplantation were black (Ch. 5, this volume) and during the period from 1995-1997, 27% of cadaver kidney transplant recipients were black (Fig. 5). The reasons for the serial disparities in the incidence of disease, in referrals to transplant centers, in listing for transplantation and in receiving transplants are unclear, but persist even when patients' own expectations and preferences are taken into account (7).

Once transplanted, the outcomes of renal transplantation are poorer for blacks than for others. This racial disparity in transplant outcomes is not limited to the results of renal transplants (Ch. 2, 3, this volume), however, the very high incidence of renal disease among blacks means a larger number of patients is affected. The reasons for racial differences in outcomes following renal transplantation also remain unclear despite extensive study (reviewed in 4).

Improving results for black Americans

Although graft outcomes among black recipients have been consistently poorer than for whites or other racial and ethnic groups, the picture has been changing. Figure 3 shows that the difference in one-year graft survival rates between blacks and whites diminished between 1976-1993 until there was very little disadvantage (1-2%) for black recipients compared with whites. During the same period, the difference in 5-year graft survival rates changed from 15% in 1976 to 10% in 1994. The introduction of cyclosporine in 1984 was associated with a 10% improvement in one-year graft survival rates for both whites and blacks, but the learning curve may have been extended for blacks because of racial differences in the drug's bioavailability (8). If so, narrowing the racial gap in one-year survival rates might have been delayed. Since 1992, the difference in one-year graft survival rates between whites and blacks has been 2% or less.

The incidence of treated acute rejection episodes has been consistently higher among blacks, however, with improving immunosuppression, the incidence of rejection has declined for both blacks and whites. Figure 9 shows that even during the transplant hospitalization when the patients are on the highest levels of immunosuppression and are closely monitored, blacks more often were treated for rejections than whites. During the 5 years from 1994-1999, 11.0% of blacks who received cadaver kidneys had a rejection in the hospital compared with 8.6% of whites. This higher incidence of early rejections suggests either a heightened immune response among some blacks or that immunosuppression was less effective even under the tightly controlled conditions while the patient was hospitalized.

The incidence of treated rejections was higher among blacks at least through 2 years as shown in Figure 9, and the difference between blacks and whites grew from 2.4% before the discharge to 3.5% within 6 months and to 6.0% during the first year. Blacks were more likely than whites to lose their graft to acute rejection during the first year (Fig. 22). Despite these indications of a stronger immune responsiveness in terms of the incidence of rejection and immune failures, heightened immunity was not reflected in the sensitization profiles of blacks and whites, at least not among those who were transplanted. There was very little indication that blacks became sensitized by pregnancies, transfusions or previous transplants more often than whites (Fig. 14). Since only transplanted patients were analyzed, it's possible that broad sensitization prevented more blacks than whites from receiving a transplant and the more responsive patients were not transplanted. However, a higher pretransplant sensitization rate among blacks does not readily explain the lower graft survival rates after transplantation.

The largest survival differences between blacks and whites were apparent among unsensitized, untransfused, first transplant recipients. These data suggest that rather than having innately stronger immune responses to immunization, the immune responses among blacks are less well controlled after transplantation. The higher rejection rate during the initial hospitalization indicates that even when administered at prescribed doses, immunosuppressive drugs are not completely effective, and that more blacks than whites are at least partially resistant.

Racial differences in long-term graft survival

Despite improvements in one-year graft survival rates among blacks, their long-term survival remains substantially lower than whites and the rate of graft loss after the first year in blacks is still nearly double that in whites. There has been some improvement, however, as graft half-lives improved from about 5.2-7.5 years during the past decade. The poor long-term survival rates that affect nearly one quarter of the cadaveric renal transplants performed in the US has a significant impact on overall graft survival rates. The overall 5-year graft survival rate for transplants performed during 1995-1999 was 65.8%, but the separate results for whites, blacks and others were 70.2%, 55.0% and 76.5%, respectively (Fig. 5). Thus, considering the races together masks a 20% range of 5-year graft survival rates.

Blacks were more likely than whites to experience immunological graft loss after the first year (Fig. 22). The major cause of late graft loss was chronic rejection, cited as the primary reason for 45% of graft failures in blacks. In contrast, the major cause of graft failure among whites was patient death accounting for 58% of late graft losses. Only 29% of late graft losses in whites were attributed to chronic rejection. If immunosuppression were less effective in blacks than whites in the immediate posttransplant period, chronic rejection may reflect a cumulative effect of inadequate or ineffective immunosuppression.

Among the most important issues affecting long-term graft survival is medication noncompliance. Estimates of the role of medication noncompliance in graft failures due to rejection run as high as 52% (9). Thus, the immediate cause of graft failure is rejection, but noncompliance may be a very common contributory cause. One study of patients who lost their graft to chronic allograft nephropathy revealed that as many as 35% had been noncompliant with medications (10). Noncompliance is more common among minorities, although more likely reflecting a lower socioeconomic status than a racial difference (11).

The high cost of immunosuppressive drugs may be an important contributing factor in adherence to medication doses. The annual costs range from $5,700-15,000 for standard maintenance immunosuppression, averaging more than $1,000 per month for cyclosporine + mycophenolate mofetil + prednisone or for Tacrolimus +

mycophenolate mofetil + prednisone (12). Additional drugs for infection prophylaxis, hypertension, cholesterol, and other problems add to the costs. Medicare first provided coverage for outpatient immunosuppressants to one year after renal transplantation in 1984, and extended coverage to 3 years in 1992 (12). If the cost of medication were a major determinant of compliance, one might expect these changes to be reflected in improved graft survival rates when they went into effect. Unfortunately the rapid rise in graft survival rates in 1984 (Fig.3) also correlates with the introduction of cyclosporine in the US and the 5-year graft survival rates for blacks show only a gradual improvement after 1989. Based on these results, the impact of extending coverage on long-term (5-year) graft survival rates was not apparent. Nevertheless, providing coverage for immunosuppression is important to insure that transplants do not fail for the trivial reason that the patient cannot afford the lifetime supply of drugs they will need (12).

The impact of racial differences

Analyses of registry data with large disparate groups may be confounded by the divergent long-term survival rates comparing blacks and whites. Even multivariate analyses may not effectively account for this variation, especially when the causes of late graft loss differ between the races (13). For many of the uni- and polyvariate analyses reported in this chapter, the variables have similar effects in blacks and whites, and only the shapes of the curves and the percentage of long-surviving grafts are different. However, when the races are disproportionately represented, the effects can be more complex. For example, blacks accounted for 27% of cadaver donor transplants, but only 14% of living donor grafts (Figs. 4,5). Their contribution to the half-life of cadaver transplants is greater than to the half-life of living donor transplants. A more familiar example is the effect of HLA matching on cadaver kidney graft survival. Blacks with poor long-term survival rates also receive the poorest matched kidneys whereas whites with better long-term survival rates received a much higher percentage of well-matched grafts (Fig. 18). HLA matching reduced acute rejections and improved survival in both racial groups, but the aggregate analysis would show a more pronounced effect than the separate analyses because of the skewed distribution of HLA-matched transplants.

In a few notable cases there were differential effects in blacks and whites. Young recipients (including teens) had poorer long-term survival rates overall, but the difference was striking for the small number of blacks in that age group (Fig. 16). The effect of advancing donor age was also very different among blacks and whites (Fig. 17). Black recipients of kidneys from donors over age 45 had substantially reduced graft survival rates and the 5-year graft survival rate was 35% when the donor was over age 60. Whether these differences reflect a greater susceptibility of older kidneys to immune assaults or hydrodynamic effects of posttransplant hypertension or even nephrotoxic effects of the calcineurin inhibitors is unclear. However, using older kidneys in black recipients may severely shorten the graft survival.

Graft survival rates have improved for both blacks and whites over the years. The difference in one-year graft survival rates has shrunk to less 2% during the past decade. The long-term outcomes for blacks are still poorer than for whites, but this difference is also shrinking. The racial disparity in transplant outcome may be very much reduced before its cause has been fully identified. However, the problem may still be greater than indicated by the results of these analyses. It is important to recognize that many graft failures today result from patient death with a functioning graft. It is the result we should be hoping for - a kidney transplant that lasts a lifetime. But graft failures among blacks are more often immunological, returning the patient to dialysis.

SUMMARY

During the 46 years since the first successful kidney was performed, more than 200,000 kidney transplants at United States transplant centers have been reported to the UCLA and UNOS Transplant Registries. After more than 25 years of follow-up, only 4% of cadaver donor transplants and 22% of living donor transplants performed before 1975 are still functioning. When compared with the 30% and 58% 5-year cadaveric and living donor graft survival rates, respectively, reported for kidney transplants 25 years ago, today's results of 66% and 78% are remarkably improved.

Between 1995-1999, the 5-year graft survival rates for living donor transplant recipients were 80% for whites, 64% for American blacks and 84% for Asians and others. Among recipients of cadaver kidneys the results for the same racial groups were 70%, 55% and 76%, respectively.

HLA-identical sibling transplants provided the best results in whites and blacks with 5-year graft survival rates of 90% and 88% respectively, and superior graft half-lives of 42 and 27 years. No substantial survival differences were noted among whites who received an HLA-mismatched living donor graft (5-year graft survival ranged from 76-81%). Among blacks who received HLA-mismatched living donor kidneys, 69% of sibling grafts survived 5 years compared with 60-62% of all others (p=0.035).

The racial distribution at the 25 largest US transplant centers varied from 6-64% black recipients. Graft survival rates for both blacks and whites were comparable at centers that transplanted more than 33% blacks or less than 20% blacks, suggesting that a larger experience with minority patients does not confer an advantage manifested in graft survival.

Blacks consistently had higher rates of early rejection (34% vs. 28% in the first year) and delayed graft function (31% vs. 23%) than whites. Rejection prior to discharge resulted in a decreased one-year graft survival rate from 89% to 76% for both racial groups. DGF also reduced one-year graft survival from 82% to 76% for both racial groups. However, long-term graft survival rates were 15% lower for blacks than whites when there was no rejection or when there was no DGF.

Sensitization patterns were similar comparing blacks and whites stratified according to sex, pregnancies, pretransplant transfusions, and previous transplants. There was no indication among patients transplanted between 1995-1999 for higher rates of sensitization among blacks.

Recipients over age 60 had the lowest graft survival rate among whites (60% vs. 71% for those aged 19-45; p<0.001). Among blacks, older recipients had the highest graft survival rate (57% vs. 55% for those aged 19-45; p=ns). Blacks aged 6-18 had the poorest 5-year survival rate (44%).

The donor's age was an important determinant of long-term survival in both whites and blacks. The 5-year graft survival rates fell from 74-57% when the donor age was over 60 among whites. However, the difference was more pronounced among blacks, with a 5-year survival rate of 64% when the donor was aged 19-30, 47% when the donor was aged 46-60 and 35% when the donor was over 60 (p<0.001).

Increasing numbers of HLA mismatches resulted in a significantly increased incidence of rejection episodes in both blacks and whites. More than 19% of whites received an HLA-matched graft during 1995-1999 compared with 6% of blacks. HLA matching improved 3-year graft survival by 7-8% for both whites and blacks.

Causes of graft failure were similar for blacks and whites during the first posttransplant year, however, after one year, blacks were more likely than whites to have an immunological graft loss whereas whites more often died with a functioning graft. The causes of patient death were also similar between blacks and whites during the first year, but after one year, blacks were more likely than whites to die from infection whereas whites more often died from cardiovascular disease and from malignancies.

The racial disparity in renal allograft survival rates has diminished. The graft survival difference between whites and blacks at one year is now less than 2%. The long-term survival rates have also improved for blacks but the rate of late graft loss remains nearly double that for whites.

REFERENCES

1. Gjertson DW, Cecka JM. Living unrelated donor kidney transplantation. Kidney Int 2000; 58:491.

2. Gasser M, Waaga AM, Laskowski IA, Tilney NL. Organ transplantation from brain-dead donors: its impact on short- and long-term outcome revisited. Transplant Rev 2001; 15:1.

3. Epstein AM, Ayanian JZ, Keogh JH, et al. Racial disparities in access to renal transplantation: clinically appropriate or due to underuse or overuse. N Engl J Med 2000; 343:1537.

4. Young JY, Gaston RS. Renal transplantation in black Americans. N Engl J Med 2000; 343:1545.

5. Gjertson DW, Terasaki PI. Large center variation in half-lives of kidney transplants. Transplantation 1992; 53:357.

6. US Renal Data System Annual Data Report 2000. (www.USRDS.org)

7. Ayanian JZ, Cleary PD, Weissman JS, Epstein AM. The effect of patients' preferences on racial differences in access to renal transplantation. N Engl J Med 1999; 341:1661.

8. Lindholm A, Welsh M, Alton C, Kahan BD. Demographic factors influencing cyclosporine pharmacokinetic parameters in patients with uremia: racial differences in bioavailability. Clin Pharm Ther 1992; 52:359.

9. Bergman LS, Roper L, Bow LM, Hull D, Bartus SA, Schweitzer RT. Causes of late graft failure in cadaveric renal transplantation. Transplant Proc 1993; 25:1340.

10. Gaston RS, Hudson SL, Ward M, Jones P, Macon R. Late renal allograft loss: noncompliance masquerading as chronic rejection. Transplant Proc 1999; 31:21S.

11. Schweitzer RT, Rovelli M, Palmeri D, Vossler E, Hull D, Bartus S. Noncompliance in organ transplant recipients. Transplantation 1990; 49:374.

12. Kasiske BL, Cohen D, Lucey MR, Neylan JF. Payment for immunosuppression after organ transplantation. JAMA 2000; 283:2445.

13. Gjertson DW, Dabrowska DM, Cui X, Cecka JM. Four causes of cadaveric kidney transplant failure: a competing risk analysis (submitted).

ACKNOWLEDGEMENT

I thank the many data coordinators at the kidney transplant centers who have worked hard to supply their data to the UCLA and UNOS transplant registries and who have made these analyses possible. I want to thank UNOS for providing monthly updates of the Renal Scientific Registry data they have collected. After a long and very productive association with the UNOS Scientific Registry that has been documented in the Clinical Transplants series, UCLA's contractual relationship with UNOS ended in October with the award of the new Scientific Registry contract to URREA (University Renal Research and Education Association) in Ann Arbor. However, we look forward to continuing our scientific relationship with both UNOS and URREA into the future.

CHAPTER 2

Liver Transplantation in the United States: A Report from the Organ Procurement and Transplantation Network

Carol M Smith, Darcy B. Davies, and Maureen A. McBride

Research Department, United Network for Organ Sharing, Richmond, Virginia

The United Network for Organ Sharing (UNOS), through the Organ Procurement and Transplantation Network (OPTN) maintains a database of all liver transplants performed in the United States. The data contained therein are used to investigate and report on the efficacy of liver transplantation. Details of the data collection process can be found in the 2000 Annual Report of the Scientific Registry of Transplant Recipients and the Organ Procurement and Transplantation Network (1).

This chapter describes: a) the methods used in the preparation of this report; b) the number of liver transplant centers and the number of transplants for both pediatric and adult recipients; c) the number of living donor, segmental, and multiple organ transplants; d) selected recipient and donor characteristics for pediatric and adult recipients; e) graft and patient survival rates from one to 10 years after transplantation; and f) characteristics affecting survival outcomes in both children and adults.

METHODS

The information included in this report is based on liver transplants performed between January 1, 1988, and December 31, 1999. All analyses were performed using version 8.1 of SAS (2). Percentages were calculated on totals excluding not reported or unknown cases. The Kaplan-Meier method (3) was used to estimate survival rates.

Logistic regression methods (4) were used to identify donor, recipient, and transplant characteristics that had a significant impact on graft and patient survival at 6 months after transplant. The relative impact of each characteristic on graft and patient survival for adult and pediatric patients is expressed in terms of odds ratios (OR) and a corresponding 95% confidence interval (CI). The OR is the odds of graft failure or patient death as compared to the reference category, after adjusting for the effects of all other characteristics in the model. An OR of less than 1 indicates that the characteristic was associated with reduced odds of graft failure (patient death) relative to the reference group. An OR of greater than 1 indicates that the characteristic was associated with increased odds of graft failure (patient death) relative to the reference group. The LOGISTIC procedure in SAS was used to identify the factors significant in this cohort of patients.

The Cox proportional hazards (PH) model (5) was used to identify donor, recipient, and transplant characteristics that had a significant impact on survival conditional on graft function or patient survival for the first 6 months after transplantation. The relative impact of each characteristic on graft and patient survival for adult and pediatric patients is expressed in terms of risk ratios (RR) and a corresponding 95% CI. The RR is the risk of graft failure (patient death) as compared to the reference category, after adjusting for the effects of all other characteristics in the model. An RR of less than 1 indicates that the characteristic was associated with a reduced risk of graft failure (patient death) relative to the reference group. A risk ratio of greater than 1 indicates that the characteristic was associated with an increased risk of graft failure (patient death) relative to the reference group. The PHREG procedure in SAS was used to identify the factors significant in this cohort of patients.

For both the logistic regression and proportional hazards analyses, recipient and donor factors were coded

Clinical Transplants 2000, Cecka and Terasaki, Eds. UCLA Immunogenetics Center, Los Angeles, California

such that the reference group was the largest group. When any factor was missing, it was set to the reference group or to the mean value, where appropriate. Patients with no follow-up data as well as multiple organ and heterotopic transplants were excluded from the outcomes analysis (Tables 5-8). Between 1997-1999 there were 10 transplants to recipients with unreported ages and these were excluded from all tables. Unless otherwise noted, all analyses included both primary and repeat transplants.

RESULTS

From January 1, 1988, to December 31, 1999, there were 41,070 liver transplants performed in the US. In 1988, 24% of all transplants were to pediatric recipients, but by 1999, only 11% of transplants were to children. The number of centers has doubled in the last 12 years, from 59 in 1988 to 117 in 1999 (Table 1).

Living-donor and segmental (reduced-size or split-) liver transplants have become more prevalent in recent years. Between January 1, 1997, and December 31, 1999, there were 377 living donor transplants reported, more than double the 161 living donor transplants reported in 1994-1996. The number of segmental transplants increased 43% in the same time period, from 402 to 575. Among multiple organ transplants, liver-kidney and liver-intestine were the most common (Table 2).

Recipient Characteristics

There were 41,070 liver transplants performed between January 1, 1988, and December 31, 1999. Of these, 6,129 (15%) were to pediatric recipients and 34,941 (85%) were to adult recipients. Pediatric recipients accounted for only 13% of all recipients (3,236 of 25,009) in 1994-99. Selected recipient and donor characteristics are shown in Table 3 (children) and Table 4 (adults).

Pediatric Recipients

Children less than 3 years of age accounted for half of all pediatric recipients with little variation over the years. Between 1994-99, 59% of recipients were White, 19% were Black, and another 16% were Hispanic. Among children, biliary atresia was the most prevalent liver disease; however, the percentage was down from 52% in 1988-93 to 43% in 1994-99. Pediatric recipients receiving a multiple organ transplant

Table 1. Number of centers and pediatric and adult transplants by year from 1988-1999.

Year	No. of Centers	No. of Txs.	Pediatric Txs	Adult Txs
1988	59	1,713	408	1,305
1989	66	2,201	454	1,747
1990	75	2,690	513	2,177
1991	84	2,953	501	2,452
1992	92	3,064	495	2,569
1993	95	3,440	522	2,918
1994	102	3,651	554	3,097
1995	102	3,925	496	3,429
1996	107	4,071	520	3,551
1997	108	4,174	558	3,616
1998	117	4,499	583	3,916
1999	117	4,689	525	4,164

Source: OPTN data as of December 9, 2000.

Table 2. Number of liver transplants by living donor, segmental, and multiple organ transplants.

	Year of Transplant		
	1988-93	1994-96	1997-99
All Transplants	16,061	11,647	13,362
Living Donor Transplants	107	161	377
Cadaveric Transplants	15,604	11,129	12,564
Whole	*	10,727	11,989
Split	*	129	427
Partial	*	273	148
Total Multiple Organ Transplants	350	357	421
Liver-Kidney	248	276	282
Liver-Intestine	35	58	77
Liver-Pancreas	47	2	8
Liver-Heart	3	4	11
Liver-Lung	0	4	4
Liver-Pancreas-Intestine	12	8	28
Liver-Kidney-Pancreas	3	1	1
Liver-Kidney-Heart	1	0	1
Liver-Heart-Lung	0	1	1
Liver-Kidney-Pancreas-Intestine	1	3	8

* Data not available.
Source: OPTN data as of December 9, 2000.

Table 3. Pediatric recipients — Selected recipient, donor, and matching characteristics by year of transplant.

	Total N	Total %	1988-1993 N	1988-1993 %	1994-1999 N	1994-1999 %
All Children	6,129	100.0	2,893	100.0	3,236	100.0
Recipient Age (years)						
<1	1,670	27.2	751	26.0	919	28.4
1-2	1,564	25.5	793	27.4	771	23.8
3-5	769	12.5	378	13.1	391	12.1
6-10	907	14.8	419	14.5	488	15.1
11-17	1,219	19.9	552	19.1	667	20.6
Recipient Sex						
Female	3,164	51.6	1,501	51.9	1,663	51.4
Male	2,965	48.4	1,392	48.1	1,573	48.6
Recipient Race/Ethnicity						
White	3,735	61.2	1,818	63.3	1,917	59.3
Black	1,105	18.1	508	17.7	597	18.5
Hispanic	901	14.8	391	13.6	510	15.8
Asian	174	2.9	67	2.3	107	3.3
Other	189	3.1	87	3.0	102	3.2
Unknown	25	-	22	-	3	-
Primary Liver Disease Categories*						
Non-cholestatic Cirrhosis	544	9.0	252	8.7	292	9.2
Cholestatic Liver Disease/Cirrhosis	197	3.2	71	2.5	126	4.0
Biliary Atresia	2,867	47.2	1,506	52.1	1,361	42.7
Acute Hepatic Necrosis	746	12.3	333	11.5	413	13.0
Metabolic Diseases	759	12.5	386	13.3	373	11.7
Malignant Neoplasms	164	2.7	64	2.2	100	3.1
Other	800	13.2	281	9.7	519	16.3
Unknown	52	-	0	-	52	-
Previous Transplant						
No	4,876	79.6	2,117	73.2	2,759	85.3
Yes	1,253	20.4	776	26.8	477	14.7
Multiple Organ Transplant						
No	5,853	95.5	2,825	97.6	3,028	93.6
Yes	276	4.5	68	2.4	208	6.4
Description at Time of Transplant						
Not Hospitalized	2,661	44.9	1,230	42.5	1,431	47.3
In Hospital	1,227	20.7	601	20.8	626	20.7
In ICU	777	13.1	359	12.4	418	13.8
On Life Support	1,256	21.2	703	24.3	553	18.3
Unknown	208	-	0	-	208	-
Donor Age (years)						
<1	741	12.2	438	15.2	303	9.6
1-2	1,084	17.9	576	19.9	508	16.1
3-10	1,803	29.8	908	31.4	895	28.3
11-17	654	10.8	297	10.3	357	11.3
18-34	1,106	18.3	425	14.7	681	21.5
35-49	464	7.7	166	5.7	298	9.4
50+	197	3.3	78	2.7	119	3.8
Unknown	80	-	5	-	75	-

Table 3. (Cont'd)

	Total		1988-1993		1994-1999	
	N	%	N	%	N	%
Donor Type						
Cadaveric	5,648	92.2	2,788	96.4	2,860	88.4
Living	481	7.8	105	3.6	376	11.6
Recipient/Donor Age Match						
R 0-17/D 0-17	4,282	70.8	2,219	76.8	2,063	65.3
R 0-17/D 18+	1,767	29.2	669	23.2	1,098	34.7
Unknown	80	-	5	-	75	-
Recipient/Donor Sex Match						
RF/DF	1,376	22.5	620	21.4	756	23.4
RF/DM	1,788	29.2	881	30.5	907	28.0
RM/DM	1,700	27.7	825	28.5	875	27.0
RM/DF	1,263	20.6	565	19.5	698	21.6
Unknown	2	-	2	-	0	-
Recipient/Donor Blood Type Match						
Identical	4,945	80.8	2,272	78.7	2,673	82.7
Compatible	836	13.7	417	14.4	419	13.0
Incompatible	338	5.5	197	6.8	141	4.4
Unknown	10	-	7	-	3	-

* Appendix 1 lists the individual diagnoses for all the disease categories listed here.

Source: OPTN data as of December 9, 2000. Percentages based on totals excluding unknown cases.

Table 4. Adult recipients — Selected recipient, donor, and matching characteristics by year of transplant.

	Total		1988-1993		1994-1999	
	N	%	N	%	N	%
All Adults	34,941	100.0	13,168	100.0	21,773	100.0
Recipient Age (years)						
18-29	2,267	6.5	1,167	8.9	1,100	5.1
30-44	9,817	28.1	4,164	31.6	5,653	26.0
45-54	11,794	33.8	3,959	30.1	7,835	36.0
55-64	8,810	25.2	3,233	24.6	5,577	25.6
65+	2,253	6.4	645	4.9	1,608	7.4
Recipient Sex						
Female	14,544	41.6	5,876	44.6	8,668	39.8
Male	20,397	58.4	7,292	55.4	13,105	60.2
Recipient Race/Ethnicity						
White	27,501	78.9	10,630	81.3	16,871	77.6
Black	2,319	6.7	789	6.0	1,530	7.0
Hispanic	3,247	9.3	1,015	7.8	2,232	10.3
Asian	1,083	3.1	376	2.9	707	3.3
Other	684	2.0	272	2.1	412	1.9
Unknown	107	-	86	-	21	-

Table 4. (Cont'd)

	Total		Year of Transplant 1988-1993		1994-1999	
	N	%	N	%	N	%
Primary Liver Disease Categories*						
Non-cholestatic Cirrhosis	22,545	64.9	8,009	60.8	14,536	67.3
Cholestatic Liver Disease/Cirrhosis	6,090	17.5	2,809	21.3	3,281	15.2
Biliary Atresia	94	0.3	47	0.4	47	0.2
Acute Hepatic Necrosis	2,356	6.8	843	6.4	1,513	7.0
Metabolic Diseases	1,229	3.5	480	3.6	749	3.5
Malignant Neoplasms	1,315	3.8	668	5.1	647	3.0
Other	1,120	3.2	310	2.4	810	3.8
Unknown	192	-	2	-	190	-
Previous Transplant						
No	30,305	86.7	10,645	80.8	19,660	90.3
Yes	4,636	13.3	2,523	19.2	2,113	9.7
Multiple Organ Transplant						
No	34,089	97.6	12,886	97.9	21,203	97.4
Yes	852	2.4	282	2.1	570	2.6
Description at Time of Transplant						
Not Hospitalized	18,510	54.7	6,831	51.9	11,679	56.5
In Hospital	7,447	22.0	2,874	21.9	4,573	22.1
In ICU	3,332	9.8	1,201	9.1	2,131	10.3
On Life Support	4,544	13.4	2,247	17.1	2,297	11.1
Unknown	1,108	-	15	-	1,093	-
Donor Age (years)						
0-10	734	2.1	279	2.1	455	2.1
11-17	5,229	15.0	2,240	17.0	2,989	13.8
18-34	12,930	37.1	5,809	44.2	7,121	32.8
35-49	8,747	25.1	3,085	23.5	5,662	26.1
50-65	5,898	16.9	1,562	11.9	4,336	20.0
65+	1,328	3.8	168	1.3	1,160	5.3
Unknown	75	-	25	-	50	-
Donor Type						
Cadaveric	34,777	99.5	13,166	100.0	21,611	99.3
Living	164	0.5	2	< 0.1	162	0.7
Recipient/Donor Age Match						
R 18+/D 18+	28,903	82.9	10,624	80.8	18,279	84.1
R 18+/D 0-17	5,963	17.1	2,519	19.2	3,444	15.9
Unknown	75	-	25	-	50	-
Recipient/Donor Sex Match						
RF/DF	6,574	18.8	2,552	19.4	4,022	18.5
RF/DM	7,962	22.8	3,316	25.2	4,646	21.3
RM/DM	13,681	39.2	5,182	39.4	8,499	39.0
RM/DF	6,713	19.2	2,107	16.0	4,606	21.2
Unknown	11	-	11	-	0	-
Recipient/Donor Blood Type Match						
Identical	31,296	89.7	11,690	89.0	19,606	90.1
Compatible	2,981	8.5	1,158	8.8	1,823	8.4
Incompatible	619	1.8	280	2.1	339	1.6
Unknown	45	-	40	-	5	-

* Appendix 1 lists the individual diagnoses for all the disease categories listed here.
Source: OPTN data as of December 9, 2000. Percentages based on totals excluding unknown cases.

increased from 2% in 1988-93 to 6% in 1994-99. The percentage of children not hospitalized just prior to transplant increased in 1994-99 from 1988-93 while the percentage on life support decreased during the same time period.

Among pediatric recipients, the percentage of pediatric donors decreased over time. Overall, pediatric donors made up 65% of all donors in 1994-99, down from 77% in 1988-93. The decline was especially pronounced among donors less than 3 years of age, which decreased from 35% to 26% during the same time period. Living donor transplants increased from 4% of pediatric recipients in 1988-93 to 12% in 1994-99. Recipient and donor blood type was identical in 83% of transplants between 1994-99, up from 79% of transplants between 1988-93. Incompatible blood type matches between pediatric recipients and their donors decreased from 7% in 1988-93 to 4% in 1994-99.

Adult Recipients

Adult recipients were older in 1994-99 than in 1988-93. In 1994-99, recipients aged 45 and older accounted for 69% of all recipients compared with 60% in 1988-93. Those aged 65 and older increased from 5% to 7% of all recipients. The percentage of male recipients increased from 55% in 1988-93 to 60% in 1994-99. Among adults in 1994-99, 78% of recipients were White, 7% were Black, and 10% were Hispanic. This was very different than the racial/ethnic breakdown for pediatric recipients of whom only 59% were White.

Non-cholestatic cirrhosis was the most prevalent disease category among adults, making up 61% of recipients in 1988-93 and 67% in 1994-99. The number of recipients who had had a previous transplant declined from 19% to 10% during the same time period. Adults on life support just prior to transplant decreased from 17% in 1988-93 to 11% in 1994-99.

The donor population for adult recipients was older in 1994-99 than in 1988-93. For example, donors aged 50 and older made up 13% of donors in 1988-93 and 25% in 1994-99. Approximately 16% of adults received pediatric donor livers in 1994-99, down from 19% in 1988-93. The number of living donor transplants to adult recipients increased dramatically over time, from 2 transplants in 1988-93 to 162 in 1994-99. Recipient and donor gender was matched in 19% of female recipient transplants and 39% of male recipient transplants.

Outcomes

Figure 1 shows overall one- through 10-year graft and patient survival rates following primary cadaveric liver transplants among pediatric and adult recipients. Pediatric recipients had better patient survival rates than did adults and their rates declined less over time. At one year after transplantation, both pediatric and adult patient survival was 85%. At 5 years, pediatric patient survival had declined only to 81%, while for adults it had dropped to 73%. By 10 years after transplantation, patient survival was 78% for children and 59% for adults. Although more pediatric grafts failed in the first 3 years after transplantation, adult graft survival was poorer in the long term (66% graft survival at 5 years and 51% at 10 years for adults compared with 68% at 5 years and 63% at 10 years for pediatric recipients).

Multivariate logistic regression analysis was used to identify the recipient and donor characteristics that had an impact on graft and patient survival at 6 months after transplantation. Separate models were fit for pediatric and adult recipients. Transplants performed between January 1, 1988, and December 31, 1999, were included in the analyses, excluding heterotopic and multiorgan transplants. The Cox PH model was used to determine the relative risk of graft failure or mortality at any time after the first 6 posttransplant months. In the conditional analysis, only those grafts and patients surviving the first 6 months were analyzed. Living donor

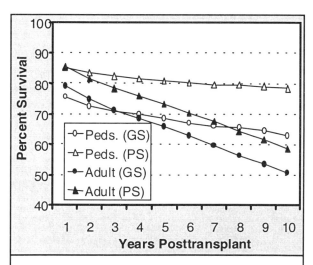

Figure 1. Graft and patient survival rates following primary cadaveric liver transplants among pediatric (n=4,108) and adult recipients (n=28,919).

Table 5. Pediatric recipients — Multivariate logistic regression of survival at 6 months after transplantation.

Risk Factor	Graft Survival (N=5,723) OR	95%CI	Patient Survival (N=5,723) OR	95% CI
Recipient Age[d] (mean age 4.8 yrs)				
linear	a		a	
quadratic	b		a	
<1 year	1.55	1.34-1.80	1.81	1.47-2.22
6 years	0.93	0.91-0.95	0.91	0.89-0.94
10 years	0.80	0.74-0.86	0.78	0.71-0.86
17 years	0.88	0.65-1.20	1.05	0.68-1.60
Recipient Female vs. Male	0.88[c]	0.77-1.00	0.80[c]	0.68-0.96
Primary Liver Disease (baseline: all but metabolic and "other" diseases-patient only)				
Metabolic disease	0.74[b]	0.60-0.91	0.68[c]	0.50-0.93
"Other" diseases	-		1.59[a]	1.23-2.05
Previous Transplant vs. Primary Transplant	2.35[a]	2.03-2.72	1.84[a]	1.46-2.33
Description at Time of Transplant (baseline: not on life support-graft, not hospitalized-patient)				
Hospitalized	-		1.56[a]	1.22-1.99
In ICU	-		1.78[a]	1.35-2.35
On life support	2.39[a]	2.06-2.77	2.74[a]	2.10-3.59
Most Recent Creatinine >2 mg/dl	1.88[a]	1.36-2.61	2.25[a]	1.47-3.46
Cold Ischemia Time[d] (mean time 9.6 hours)				
linear	c		-	
1 hour	0.88	0.79-0.98		
4 hours	0.92	0.86-0.99		
6 hours	0.95	0.90-0.99		
10 hours	1.01	1.00-1.01		
15 hours	1.08	1.01-1.16		
Donor Age[d] (mean age 13.3 yrs)				
quadratic	a		a	
1 year	1.07	1.05-1.10	1.06	1.02-1.09
10 years	1.01	1.00-1.01	1.00	1.00-1.01
20 years	1.02	1.01-1.03	1.02	1.01-1.03
35 years	1.25	1.16-1.34	1.19	1.08-1.30
Donor Race/Ethnicity				
Black vs. non-Black	1.31[b]	1.10-1.55	1.32[c]	1.04-1.68
Recipient/Donor Blood Type Match				
Incompatible vs. identical/compatible	1.37[c]	1.06-1.76	-	
Transplant Type Partial/Split Liver vs. Whole	1.47[a]	1.22-1.76	1.38[c]	1.07-1.77
Year of Transplant 1988-1993 vs. 1994-1999	1.32[a]	1.15-1.51	1.36[a]	1.13-1.64

[a] p<0.001, [b] p<0.01, [c] p<0.05
[d] Odds ratios as compared with the mean
Source: OPTN data as of December 9, 2000.

transplants were excluded from the adult analyses due to the small number of these transplants. Only factors that were significant at the p<0.05 level were retained in each of the models.

Pediatric Outcomes

The results of the logistic regression analysis can be found in Table 5. Certain factors associated with the recipient's medical condition at the time of transplant resulted in higher odds of graft failure or patient mortality at 6 months after transplantation, among them being on life support and having a recent creatinine level above 2 mg/dl. Being hospitalized or in the ICU at the time of transplant also increased the odds of patient death. Those who had received a previous transplant had increased odds of graft failure and patient mortality than those receiving their first transplant. Other factors adversely affecting the odds of pediatric graft and patient survival at 6 months were recipient less than one year old, donor age and race/ethnicity, cold ischemia time longer than the mean cold time (graft only), recipient/donor blood type match (graft only), transplant type, and year of transplant.

Having a metabolic disease decreased the odds of graft failure and patient death compared with the baseline liver diseases. Other factors associated with decreased odds of graft failure or patient death were recipient age older than one, being female, and having a cold ischemia time shorter than the mean cold time (graft survival only).

Table 6 presents the relative risk of graft failure and patient mortality among pediatric grafts and patients surviving the first 6 months after transplantation. Again, recipient medical characteristics were associated with poorer graft and patient survival, among them having malignant neoplasms, "other" liver diseases (see Appendix 1 for a list of "other" diseases), non-cholestatic cirrhosis, or acute hepatic necrosis (affecting graft survival only). Among patients who survived 6 months, having had a previous transplant more than tripled the odds of graft failure and more than doubled the odds of mortality compared with patients receiving their first transplant. This suggests that subsequent retransplants are successful in some cases. Recipients less than one year old had an increased risk of graft failure. The relationship between recipient age and mortality was non-linear, with an increased risk of patient mortality at both the youngest and oldest ages. Other factors adversely affecting graft survival were increasing donor age (graft survival only) and recipient and donor race/ethnicity. Being in the ICU at the time of transplant and younger donor age were associated with a reduced risk of graft failure.

Adult Outcomes

The logistic regression results can be found in Table 7. As with pediatric recipients, factors associated with the adult recipient's medical condition at the time of transplant resulted in higher odds of graft failure or patient mortality at 6 months after transplantation. These included having acute hepatic necrosis, malignant neoplasms, or "other" liver diseases; being in the ICU, hospitalized, or on life support at the time of transplant; and having a creatinine level above 2 mg/dl. Having received a previous transplant doubled the odds of graft failure and mortality compared with

Table 6. Pediatric recipients — Relative risk (RR) of mortality conditional on surviving 6 months after transplantation.

Characteristics	Graft Survival (N=4,041)		Patient Survival (N=4,041)	
	RR	95% CI	RR	95% CI
Recipient Age[d] (mean age 4.8 years)				
<1 year vs. 1-17 years	1.43[a]	1.17-1.75	-	
linear	-		[b]	
quadratic	-		[a]	
1 year			1.37	1.13-1.68
5 years			0.99	0.98-1.00
10 years			0.98	0.88-1.10
15 years			1.52	1.11-2.07
Recipient Race/Ethnicity				
Black vs. non-Black	1.46[a]	1.21-1.76	1.46[b]	1.11-1.93
Primary Liver Disease (baseline: acute hepatic necrosis-patient only, cholestatic liver disease/cirrhosis, biliary atresia, or metabolic diseases)				
Acute hepatic necrosis	1.52[b]	1.15-2.00	-	
Malignant neoplasms	3.82[a]	2.65-5.50	6.04[a]	3.96-9.23
Non-cholestatic cirrhosis	1.88[a]	1.46-2.41	1.50[c]	1.00-2.25
Other diseases	1.75[a]	1.35-2.27	2.12[a]	1.51-2.97
Previous Transplant vs. Primary Transplant	3.47[a]	2.90-4.15	2.24[a]	1.72-2.91
Description at Time of Transplant				
In ICU vs. non-ICU	0.77[b]	0.63-0.93	-	
Donor Age[d] (mean age 13.3 years)				
linear	[a]		-	
1 year	0.88	0.82-0.94		
10 years	0.97	0.95-0.98		
20 years	1.07	1.03-1.12		
35 years	1.26	1.11-1.43		
Donor Race/Ethnicity				
Black vs. non-Black	1.25[c]	1.01-1.55	-	

[a] p<0.001, [b] p<0.01, [c] p<0.05
[d] Odds ratios as compared with the mean
Source: OPTN data as of December 9, 2000.

Table 7. Adult recipients — Multivariate logistic regression of survival at 6 months after transplantation.

Risk Factor	Graft Survival (N=33,466)		Patient Survival (N=33,422)	
	OR	95% CI	OR	95% CI
Recipient Age[d] (mean age 48.4 years)				
linear	a		a	
20 years	0.75	0.70-0.81	0.54	0.49-0.59
35 years	0.87	0.85-0.91	0.75	0.71-0.78
50 years	1.02	1.01-1.02	1.04	1.03-1.04
65 years	1.18	1.13-1.23	1.44	1.36-1.52
Recipient Race/Ethnicity (baseline: non-Black)				
Black	-		1.21[b]	1.05-1.39
Primary Liver Disease (baseline: non-cholestatic cirrhosis, metabolic diseases)				
Acute hepatic necrosis	1.29[a]	1.16-1.44	1.19[c]	1.04-1.36
Cholestatic liver disease/cirrhosis	0.88[b]	0.82-0.95	0.70[a]	0.63-0.78
Malignant neoplasms	1.18[c]	1.03-1.36	1.30[b]	1.10-1.54
"Other" diseases	1.18[c]	1.02-1.37	1.24[c]	1.02-1.50
Previous Transplant vs. Primary Transplant	2.53[a]	2.35-2.73	2.00[a]	1.78-2.23
Description at Time of Transplant (baseline: not hospitalized)				
Hospitalized	1.23[a]	1.15-1.33	1.48[a]	1.35-1.62
In ICU	1.38[a]	1.25-1.51	1.69[a]	1.50-1.90
On life support	1.65[a]	1.49-1.83	1.83[a]	1.61-2.08
Most Recent Creatinine >2 mg/dl	1.37[a]	1.27-1.48	1.67[a]	1.52-1.84
Cold Ischemia Time[d] (mean time 9.8 hours)				
linear	a		a	
quadratic	a		c	
1 hour	0.66	0.60-0.74	0.76	0.66-0.86
4 hours	0.78	0.73-0.83	0.85	0.78-0.91
6 hours	0.86	0.83-0.89	0.90	0.86-0.94
10 hours	1.01	1.01-1.01	1.00	1.00-1.01
15 hours	1.17	1.13-1.21	1.10	1.05-1.15
Donor Age[d] (mean age 34.3 years)				
linear	a		-	
quadratic	a		a	
18 years	0.98	0.93-1.04	1.08	1.05-1.11
30 years	0.98	0.97-0.99	1.01	1.00-1.01
45 years	1.10	1.08-1.13	1.03	1.02-1.05
60 years	1.41	1.32-1.51	1.21	1.13-1.31
Donor Female and Recipient Male	1.22[a]	1.13-1.30	-	
Donor Male and Recipient Male	-		0.87[a]	0.81-0.94
Donor Race/Ethnicity (baseline: non-Black, non-Asian-graft only)				
Black	1.33[a]	1.22-1.46	1.17[b]	1.05-1.31
Asian	1.25[c]	1.00-1.56	-	
Donor Cause of Death CVA vs. All Other Causes	1.18[a]	1.10-1.27	1.20[a]	1.11-1.29
Recipient/Donor Blood Type Match (baseline: identical)				
Compatible	1.11[c]	1.01-1.22	1.22[a]	1.09-1.37
Incompatible	1.91[a]	1.59-2.29	1.43[b]	1.12-1.82
Transplant Type Partial/Split Liver vs. Whole	2.16[a]	1.66-2.81	1.48[c]	1.04-2.10
Year of Transplant 1988-1993 vs.1994-1998	1.47[a]	1.38-1.56	1.51[a]	1.40-1.63

[a] p<0.001, [b] p<0.01, [c] p<0.05, [d] Odds ratios as compared with the mean
Source: OPTN data as of December 9, 2000.

Table 8. Adult recipients — Relative risk (RR) of mortality conditional on surviving 6 months after transplantation.

Characteristics	Graft Survival (N=25,328)		Patient Survival (N=25,328)	
	RR	95% CI	RR	95% CI
Recipient Age[d] (mean age 48.4 years)				
linear	a		a	
quadratic	a		b	
20 years	0.99	0.87-1.13	0.70	0.59-0.83
35 years	0.93	0.90-0.97	0.80	0.76-0.84
50 years	1.02	1.01-1.02	1.03	1.03-1.04
65 years	1.28	1.19-1.37	1.53	1.42-1.65
Recipient Race/Ethnicity (baseline: non-Black, non-Hispanic-patient only)				
Black	1.53[a]	1.38-1.70	1.60[a]	1.42-1.80
Hispanic	-		0.88[c]	0.78-1.00
Primary Liver Disease (baseline: non-cholestatic cirrhosis)				
Acute hepatic necrosis	0.76[a]	0.66-0.87	0.73[a]	0.62-0.85
Cholestatic liver disease/cirrhosis	0.63[a]	0.58-0.68	0.56[a]	0.51-0.61
Malignant neoplasms	2.46[a]	2.22-2.73	2.90[a]	2.60-3.23
Metabolic diseases	0.68[a]	0.57-0.81	0.67[a]	0.54-0.82
"Other" diseases	0.71[b]	0.58-0.88	0.76[c]	0.60-0.96
Previous Transplant vs. Primary Transplant	2.16[a]	2.01-2.32	1.51[a]	1.37-1.66
Hospitalized (non-ICU) at Transplant vs. Not Hospitalized	1.10[b]	1.03-1.17	1.12[b]	1.04-1.20
Most Recent Creatinine >2 mg/dl	-		1.26[a]	1.14-1.38
Donor Age[d] (mean age 34.3 years)				
linear	a		a	
18 years	0.82	0.79-0.84	0.85	0.83-0.88
30 years	0.95	0.94-0.95	0.96	0.95-0.97
45 years	1.14	1.12-1.17	1.11	1.09-1.13
60 years	1.38	1.32-1.44	1.29	1.22-1.35
Donor Female and Recipient Female	0.90[b]	0.84-0.97	-	
Donor Race/Ethnicity Black vs. non-Black	1.12[c]	1.02-1.23	-	
Year of Transplant 1988-93 vs. 1994-99	1.14[a]	1.07-1.22	1.17[a]	1.09-1.25

[a] p<0.001, [b] p<0.01, [c] p<0.05, [d] Odds ratios as compared with the mean
Source: OPTN data as of December 9, 2000.

those receiving their first transplant. Recipient age had a linear relationship with graft and patient survival – the odds of graft failure and mortality increased as recipient age increased. Other factors adversely affecting the odds of adult recipient survival at 6 months were recipient race/ethnicity (patient survival only), older donor age, donor race/ethnicity, cause of donor death, recipient/donor blood type match, receiving a partial or split-liver transplant, and year of transplant.

Recipients with cholestatic liver disease/cirrhosis had reduced odds of graft failure and patient death compared with recipients with the baseline primary liver diseases. Other factors associated with a reduced odds of graft failure or mortality were younger recipient age, cold ischemia time shorter than the mean cold time, and matching a male recipient with a male donor (patient survival only).

Table 8 presents the relative risk of graft failure and mortality among adult recipients. Among patients surviving the first 6 months after transplantation with functioning grafts, having malignant neoplasms more than doubled the risk of graft failure and mortality. Other factors adversely affecting graft and patient survival were recipient and donor race/ethnicity, having a previous transplant, being hospitalized just prior to transplant, creatinine level above 2 mg/dl (patient survival only), older donor age, and year of transplant.

Among those characteristics that decreased the relative risk of graft failure and mortality were younger recipient and donor age; being an Hispanic recipient (patient survival only); having acute hepatic necrosis, cholestatic liver disease/cirrhosis, or a metabolic disease, as compared with the baseline primary liver diseases; and matching a female recipient with a female donor (graft survival only).

SUMMARY

Transplants and Centers

Between 1988-1999 the number of annual liver transplants performed in the United States more than doubled, from 1,713 to 4,689; the number of centers increased from 59 to 117. The number of living donor, segmental, and multiple organ transplants also increased over time, particularly between 1997-1999. The rate of increase in the number of centers has slowed over the last few years.

Outcomes

Survival among pediatric recipients

The one- and 10-year graft survival rates for pediatric recipients were 76% and 63%, respectively. The one- and 10-year patient survival rates were 85% and 78%. Patient survival did not decrease much after the first 2 years and graft survival stabilized after 5 years. Some of the factors associated with increased odds of graft failure and patient death at 6 months after transplantation included having a previous transplant; being hospitalized, in the ICU, or on life support at the time of transplant; a creatinine level >2 mg/dl; donor race/ethnicity; and transplant type. Factors associated with decreased odds of graft failure or patient death were recipient gender, having a metabolic disease, and a shorter than average cold ischemia time.

Among grafts, recipients surviving the first 6 months after transplantation, recipient and donor race/ethnicity, primary liver disease, and having a previous transplant were associated with a greater relative risk of graft failure and mortality. The risk of graft failure was reduced for recipients in the ICU at the time of transplant and for those receiving organs from younger donors.

Survival among adult recipients

The one- and 10-year graft survival rates among adult recipients were 79% and 51%, respectively. The one- and 10-year patient survival rates were 85% and 59%. Survival rates decreased steadily at all time points following transplantation. Some of the factors associated with increased odds of graft failure and mortality at 6 months were increasing recipient and donor age; recipient and donor race/ethnicity; primary liver disease; having a previous transplant; being hospitalized, in the ICU, or on life support at the time of transplant; longer cold ischemia time; having a nonidentical recipient/donor blood type match; transplant type; and year of transplant. Younger recipient and donor ages, having cholestatic liver disease/cirrhosis, shorter cold ischemia times, and matching male recipients with male donors were associated with decreased odds of graft failure and mortality. Many of these characteristics also affected grafts and patients surviving the first 6 months, including recipient and donor age, recipient and donor race/ethnicity, primary liver disease, previous transplant, and year of transplant.

REFERENCES

1. CM Smith, GG Beasley, Y Cheng, DB Ormond, PC Spain, Eds. 2000 Annual Report of the U.S. Scientific Registry of Transplant Recipients and the Organ Procurement and Transplantation Network. UNOS, Richmond, VA, U.S. DHHS, Rockville, MD, 2001.

2. SAS Institute, Inc., Cary, NC, 1990.

3. Kaplan, EL, Meier P. Nonparametric estimation from incomplete observations. J Am Stat Assoc 1958; 53:457.

4. Hosmer DW, Lemeshow S. In: Applied Logistic Regression. J Wiley & Sons, New York, 1989.

5. Cox DR. Regression models and life tables. J Royal Statistical Soc Series B 1972; 34:187.

ACKNOWLEDGMENTS

We extend our sincere thanks to the many liver transplant surgeons, physicians, and data coordinators in transplant programs across the country, whose timely and accurate submission of data have made these analyses possible. We also wish to thank the UNOS Clinical Data Systems, Information Technology, and Research Departments for data collection, data entry, and maintenance of the database.

Finally, we gratefully acknowledge donor families and transplant recipients, whose generosity and courage have made advances in organ transplantation possible.

Appendix 1. Primary liver disease categories and their diagnoses.

Non-Cholestatic Cirrhosis
Laennec's Cirrhosis (Alcoholic)
Laennec's Cirrhosis and Postnecrotic Cirrhosis
Cirrhosis: Postnecrotic—Type C
Cirrhosis: Cryptogenic—Idiopathic
Cirrhosis: Postnecrotic—Autoimmune, Lupoid
Cirrhosis: Postnecrotic—Type B-Hbsag+
Cirrhosis: Postnecrotic—Type Non A Non B
Cirrhosis: Postnecrotic—Type B and C
Cirrhosis: Postnecrotic—Other Specify
Cirrhosis: Drug/Indust Exposure Other Specify
Cirrhosis: Postnecrotic—Type B and D
Cirrhosis: Postnecrotic—Type A
Cirrhosis: Postnecrotic—Type D
PNC CAH

Cholestatic Liver Disease/Cirrhosis
Primary Biliary Cirrhosis (PBC)
Sec Biliary Cirrhosis: Other Specify
Sec Biliary Cirrhosis: Caroli's Disease
Sec Biliary Cirrhosis: Choledochol Cyst
Cholesatic Liver Disease: Other Specify
PSC: Other Specify
PSC: Ulcerative Colitis
PSC: No Bowel Disease
PSC: Crohn's Disease

Biliary Atresia
Biliary Atresia: Other Specify
Biliary Atresia: Extrahepatic
Biliary Atresia: Alagille's Syndrome
Biliary Atresia: Hypoplasia

Metabolic Diseases
Metdis: Alpha-1-Antitrypsin Deficiency A-1-A
Metdis: Wilson's Disease
Metdis: Hemochromatosis-Hemosiderosis
Metdis: Other Specify
Metdis: Tyrosinemia
Metdis: Primary Oxalosis/Oxaluria, Hyperoxaluria
Metdis: Glyc Stor Dis Type II (GSD-II)
Metdis: Glyc Stor Dis Type I (GSD-I)
Metdis: Hyperlipidemia-II, Homozygous Hypercholesterolemia

Malignant Neoplasms
PLM: Hepatoma—Hepatocellular Carcinoma
PLM: Hepatoma (HCC) and Cirrhosis
PLM: Cholangiocarcinoma (CH-CA)
PLM: Hepatoblastoma (HBL)
PLM: Hemangioendothelioma-Hemangiosarcoma
PLM: Other Specify
PLM: Fibrolamellar (FL-HC)
Bile Duct Cancer
Secondary Hepatic Malignancy Other Specify

Other
Other Specify
Cystic Fibrosis
Budd-Chiari Syndome
TPN/Hyperalimentation Ind Liver Disease
Neonatal Hepatitis Other Specify
Congenital Hepatic Fibrosis
Familial Cholestasis: Other Specify
Familial Cholestatis: Byler's Disease
Trauma Other Specify
Graft vs. Host Disease Secondary to Non-Liver Tx Chronic or Acute
Benign Tumor: Polycystic Liver Disease
Benign Tumor: Other Specify
Benign Tumor: Hepatic Adenoma

Acute Hepatic Necrosis
AHN: Etiology Unknown
AHN: Type B- Hbsag+
AHN: Drug Other Specify
AHN: Non-A Non-B
AHN: Type C
AHN: Type A
AHN: Other Specify
AHN: Type B and C
AHN: Type B and D
AHN: Type D
Hepatitis C: Chronic or Acute
Hepatitis B: Chronic or Acute

CHAPTER 3

Worldwide Thoracic Organ Transplantation: A Report from the UNOS/ISHLT International Registry for Thoracic Organ Transplantation

Leah E. Bennett [a], Berkeley M. Keck [a], O. Patrick Daily [a], Richard J. Novick [b], and Jeffrey D. Hosenpud [c]

[a] *United Network for Organ Sharing, Richmond, Virginia,* [b] *London Health Sciences Center, London, Ontario Canada,* [c] *St. Luke's Hospital, Milwaukee, Wisconsin*

Since October 1, 1987, the United Network for Organ Sharing (UNOS) has collected data on all thoracic organ transplants performed in the United States. Recipient demographic data, data pertaining to organ donors and histocompatibility information were collected through the national Organ Procurement and Transplantation Network (OPTN). Data related to the transplant event and subsequent follow-up were collected through the United States Scientific Registry for Organ Transplantation and the International Society for Heart and Lung Transplantation Registry (ISHLT). UNOS operates the OPTN under contract with the Division of Organ Transplantation in the United States Department of Health and Human Services. During 1994, UNOS began to operate and maintain the ISHLT International Thoracic Transplant Registry. The combined registry contains thoracic transplant cases and follow-up from the UNOS era (10/1/87-present) as well as worldwide thoracic data collected prior to the Scientific Registry.

METHODS

The information included in this report is based on thoracic organ transplant data received and entered by December 15, 2000.

All analyses were performed using version 8 of SAS (1). Frequency tabulations were performed using the FREQ procedure. The Kaplan-Meier method (2) was used to estimate survival rates; standard errors were based on Greenwood's formula (3). These calculations were obtained using the LIFETEST procedure. Multivariate analysis of the US transplant data was performed using the LOGISTIC procedure.

RESULTS

UNITED STATES REGISTRY

Number of Procedures

Since 1968 a total of 41,469 thoracic transplants was reported in the United States: 32,609 heart, 7,956 lung and 904 heart-lung transplants. Numbers of transplant procedures reflect cases reported to the registry through December 15, 2000, and are subject to change based on future data submission or correction. Table 1 shows the number of thoracic transplants by type and year from 1968-2000 and illustrates the growth of thoracic transplantation over time. The number of heart transplant operations performed in the United States reached a plateau in the mid-to-late-1990s with an apparent decrease in the number of procedures in 1999. There may also be a decline in the number of heart procedures performed in 2000 but that information is incomplete for this report. The number of lung transplants has fluctuated a bit more; even with incomplete information available for 2000, there appears to be an increase in the number of procedures from 1999-2000. Of the 7,956 lung transplants performed in the US between 1985-2000, 148 involved living donors.

Recipient and Donor Characteristics

Figures 1-4 provide a view of changes in the distribution of transplants performed for the major diagnostic categories over time for heart, heart-lung, double- and single-lung transplants. Figure 1 illustrates changes in

Clinical Transplants 2000, Cecka and Terasaki, Eds. UCLA Immunogenetics Center, Los Angeles, California

Table 1. Number of US thoracic transplants by transplant year and organ.

	Organ Transplanted			
	Heart-Lung	Heart	Lung	Total
Year	n	n	n	n
1968	0	23	0	23
1969	0	11	0	11
1970	0	10	0	10
1971	0	12	0	12
1972	0	15	0	15
1973	0	20	0	20
1974	0	17	0	17
1975	0	22	0	22
1976	0	22	0	22
1977	0	29	0	29
1978	0	49	0	49
1979	0	39	0	39
1980	0	56	0	56
1981	5	62	0	67
1982	11	111	0	122
1983	14	174	0	188
1984	19	354	0	373
1985	30	721	2	753
1986	44	1,305	0	1,349
1987	48	1,497	18	1,563
1988	74	1,676	33	1,783
1989	67	1,705	93	1,865
1990	52	2,107	203	2,362
1991	51	2,126	405	2,582
1992	48	2,171	535	2,754
1993	60	2,297	668	3,025
1994	71	2,340	723	3,134
1995	69	2,361	872	3,302
1996	39	2,346	814	3,199
1997	62	2,293	930	3,285
1998	47	2,346	864	3,257
1999	49	2,182	877	3,108
2000	44	2,110	919	3,073
	904	32,609	7,956	41,469

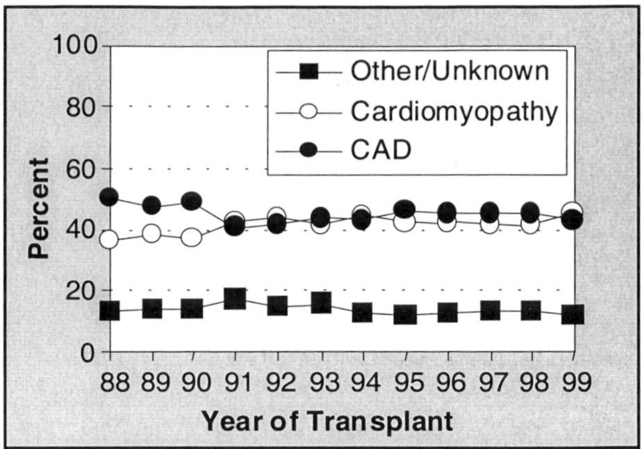

Figure 1. Primary indications for US heart transplants.

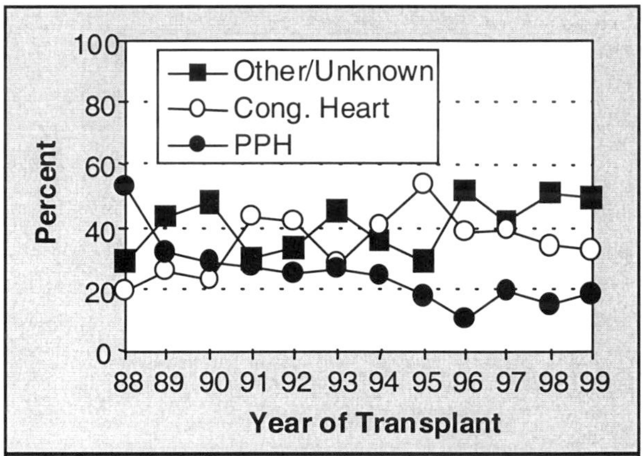

Figure 2. Primary indications for US heart-lung transplants.

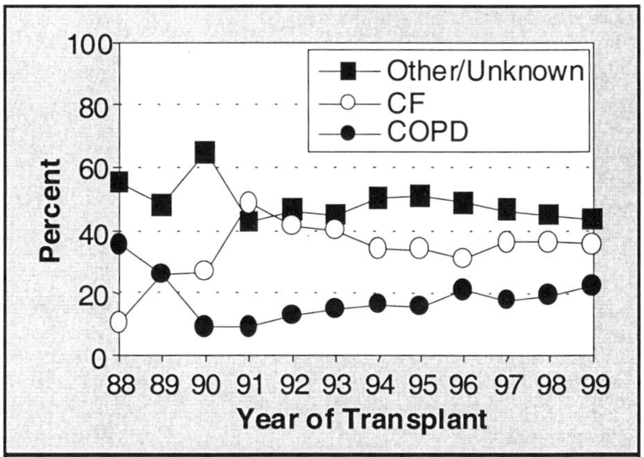

Figure 3. Primary indications for US double-lung transplants.

the percentage of heart transplants performed with a diagnosis of coronary artery disease (CAD), all cardiomyopathies and all other diagnoses over time. Although there were minor fluctuations over time in indications for heart transplantation, the percentage of cases with CAD and cardiomyopathy remained fairly stable between 1995-1998. In 1999 there appears to be a slight increase in the percentage of patients with cardiomyopathy with a concomitant decrease in both CAD and other diagnoses. While Figure 2 appears to show a changing trend

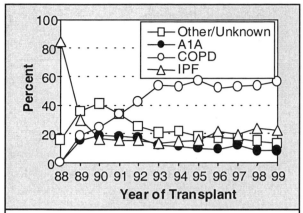

Figure 4. Primary indications for US single-lung transplants.

indications for heart-lung transplant with changes in all diagnostic groups, due to the small number of heart-lung transplant performed, it is difficult to determine a real change in diagnosis trends. The distribution of double-lung transplant diagnoses is shown in Figure 3, indicating slight annual increases in chronic obstructive pulmonary disease (COPD) between 1997-1999 and slight annual decreases in diagnoses other than COPD and cystic fibrosis (CF) since 1995. Figure 4 illustrates an annual increase between 1996-1999 in single-lung recipients with a diagnosis of COPD and an annual decrease in recipients with diagnoses other than COPD, Idiopathic Pulmonary Fibrosis (IPF) and Alpha-1-Anti-trypsin deficiency (A1A).

Table 2. Thoracic organ recipient and donor characteristics: 10/1/87-12/31/99.

	Heart-Lung		Heart		Lung			Heart-Lung		Heart		Lung	
	N	%	N	%	N	%		N	%	N	%	N	%
Recipient age group (yrs)							**Recipient condition (at transplant)**						
<1	9	1.3	1,021	3.9	44	0.6	ICU on life support	79	11.8	9,697	38	283	4.2
1-5	39	5.6	628	2.4	54	0.8	ICU no life support	35	5.2	3,380	13.3	105	1.5
6-10	19	2.7	369	1.4	79	1.1	Hospitalized	48	7.2	2,417	9.5	471	6.9
11-17	52	7.4	860	3.3	260	3.7	Not hospitalized	505	75.7	9,997	39.2	5,940	87.4
18-34	247	35.4	2,228	8.5	1,188	16.9	Not Reported	31	.	814	.	225	.
35-49	260	37.2	6,291	23.9	1,969	28							
50-64	72	10.3	13,501	51.3	3,223	45.9	**Recipient citizenship**						
65+	.	.	1,406	5.3	207	2.9	US Citizen	664	97.6	25,710	98.6	6,849	98.8
Not Reported	.	.	1	.	.	.	Non-US Citizen	16	2.4	373	1.4	82	1.2
							Not Reported	18	.	222	.	93	.
Recipient gender													
Female	401	57.4	6121	23.3	3,598	51.2	**Donor type**						
Male	297	42.6	20,184	76.7	3,426	48.8	Cadaveric	698	100	26,264	99.8	6,890	98.1
							Living	.	.	41	0.2	134	1.9
Recipient race													
White	607	87	21,412	81.4	6,310	89.9	**Donor source**						
Black	34	4.9	2,906	11.1	374	5.3	Local	482	69.1	17,546	66.7	4,152	59.1
Hispanic	33	4.7	1,326	5	234	3.3	Regional	109	15.6	4,491	17.1	1,171	16.7
Asian	15	2.1	317	1.2	47	0.7	National	107	15.3	4,174	15.9	1,674	23.8
Other	9	1.3	330	1.3	56	0.8	Non-US	.	.	94	0.4	27	0.4
Not Reported	.	.	14	.	3	.							
							Donor age group (yrs)						
Recipient blood type							<1	15	2.1	718	2.7	35	0.5
A	317	45.4	11,661	44.3	2,896	41.2	1-5	43	6.2	857	3.3	88	1.3
AB	35	5	1,352	5.1	306	4.4	6-10	36	5.2	614	2.3	152	2.2
B	75	10.7	3,278	12.5	765	10.9	11-17	182	26.1	4,247	16.2	1,277	18.2
O	271	38.8	10,014	38.1	3,057	43.5	18-34	261	37.4	11,762	44.7	3,118	44.5
							35-49	139	19.9	6,400	24.3	1,771	25.3
							50-64	20	2.9	1,644	6.3	554	7.9
							65+	2	0.3	44	0.2	11	0.2
							Not Reported	.	.	19	.	18	.

Table 2. (Cont'd)

	Heart-Lung		Heart		Lung	
	N	%	N	%	N	%
Donor gender						
Female	307	44	8,222	31.3	2,469	35.2
Male	391	56	18,081	68.7	4,555	64.8
Not Reported	.	.	2	.	.	.
Donor race						
White	534	76.6	20,511	78.2	5,359	76.7
Black	65	9.3	2,847	10.9	962	13.8
Hispanic	81	11.6	2,459	9.4	543	7.8
Asian	13	1.9	257	1	86	1.2
Other	4	0.6	155	0.6	38	0.5
Not Reported	1	.	76	.	36	.
Donor blood type						
A	278	39.8	9,749	37.1	2,534	36.1
AB	16	2.3	638	2.4	163	2.3
B	54	7.7	2,559	9.7	692	9.9
O	350	50.1	13,344	50.8	3,634	51.7
Not Reported	.	.	15	.	1	.
Donor cause of death						
Anoxia	38	5.5	1,691	6.5	262	3.9
CVA/Stroke	206	29.8	7,109	27.4	2,278	33.6
Gunshot/stab	169	24.5	5,486	21.1	1,805	26.6
Head trauma (non-MVA)	73	10.6	2,754	10.6	603	8.9
MVA	180	26	8,083	31.1	1,691	24.9
Other	25	3.6	830	3.2	144	2.1
Not Reported	7	.	352	.	241	.
Ischemia time (hours)						
0 - <1	14	2.2	483	2	73	1.2
1 - <2	78	12.3	5,562	22.6	363	5.8
2 - <3	152	24	9,036	36.7	958	15.2
3 - <4	220	34.7	6,734	27.4	1,524	24.2
4 - <6	155	24.4	2,570	10.4	2,354	37.4
6+	15	2.4	214	0.9	1,021	16.2
Not Reported	64	.	1,706	.	731	.
Gender match (donor: recipient)						
Female: Female	218	31.2	2,873	10.9	1,749	24.9
Female: Male	89	12.8	5,349	20.3	720	10.3
Male: Female	183	26.2	3,247	12.3	1,849	26.3
Male: Male	208	29.8	14,834	56.4	2,706	38.5
Not Reported	.	.	2	.	.	.
Donor-recipient ABO match level						
Identical	597	85.5	22,145	84.2	6,238	88.8
Compatible	96	13.8	4,007	15.2	737	10.5

Table 2 indicates the numbers and relative frequencies of selected recipient, donor and donor organ variables by organ type for transplants performed between October 1, 1987, and December 31, 1999. Demographic profiles of heart and lung recipients show little change from the previous year's report. Heart transplant recipients remain predominately male (76.7%), between 50-64 years of age (51.3%) and white (81.4%). Pediatric recipients (<18 years of age) received 10.9% of the reported heart transplants. Lung transplant recipients were more likely to be female (51.2%), between 50-64 years of age (45.9%) and white (89.9%). Pediatric recipients accounted for 6.2% of reported lung transplants.

Figures 5, 6 and 7 show selected donor and recipient characteristics over time. As indicated in Figure 5, the mean donor age for heart and lung transplants continues to rise with an increase from 1995-2000 of 2 years for heart and 2.9 years for lung. Figure 6 shows little change in the mean age for heart recipients between 1995-2000 ranging between 46.6-47.1 years. In 2000, the mean heart recipient age was 46.9 years. There has been an apparent increase in the mean age for lung recipients during the past 5 years, though it has not increased every year. In 1995 the mean lung recipient age was 44.2; in 2000 it was 47.2 years. The mean recipient age for heart-lung recipients is much younger than for heart and lung, with a mean of 34.4 years in 2000. Mean ischemic time, shown for each year in Figure 7, changed minimally for all organs from 1995-2000.

Outcomes

A comparison of heart, lung and heart-lung one-year patient survival by year of transplant from 1968-1999 is shown in Figure 8. One-year survival for all groups has improved dramatically over time with one-year heart transplant survival increasing from 51.2% in 1968-79 to 82.5% in 1999. Improvement in one-year lung transplant survival is indicated by a rise from 47% in 1988 to 74.8% in 1999. Heart-lung patient survival has also improved since the first cases were reported in the early 1980s with an increase from 52.6% to 60.8% in 1998. [Note that the survival for the most recent year may be artificially low due to early reports of deaths.]

Figure 9 presents a comparison of heart, lung and heart-lung 5-year patient survival rates by year of transplant. As with one-year survival, 5-year survival has improved over time with heart survival more than doubling from 28.1% in the 1968-79 era to 69.7% in 1995. Heart-

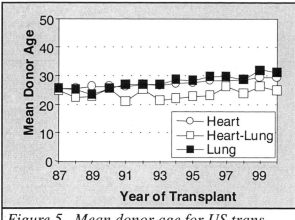

Figure 5. Mean donor age for US transplants.

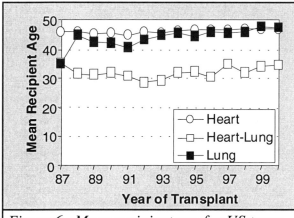

Figure 6. Mean recipient age for US transplants.

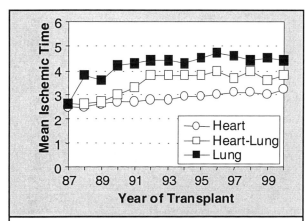

Figure 7. Mean ischemic (hrs) time for US transplants.

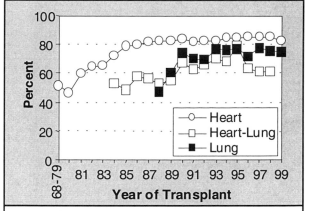

Figure 8. US thoracic transplants: one-year survival rate by organ and year of transplant.

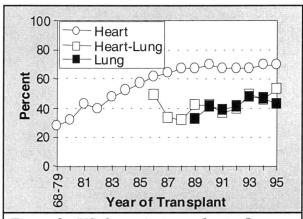

Figure 9. US thoracic transplants: 5-year survival rate by organ and year of transplant.

lung transplantation also shows a steady rise in 5-year survival rates with an increase from 32.1% in 1988 to 53.5% in 1995. The survival rates for each thoracic organ for transplants performed between 1968-1998 are shown in Figure 10. There appears to be a fairly constant decline in survival after the immediate post-operative period. The long-term patient survival rates are: 22.5% at 17 years for heart, 20.8% at 10 years for lung and 24.3% at 13 years for heart-lung recipients.

Multivariate logistic regression analysis was used to identify the donor and recipient characteristics that had an impact on patient survival following heart, lung and heart-lung transplantation for transplants performed in the United States between October 1, 1987 and September 30, 1999. The analyses were based on data entered into the UNOS computer system as of

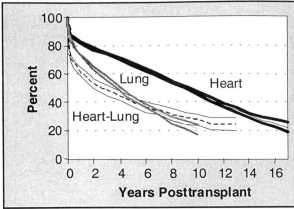

Figure 10. US thoracic ogran transplant patient survival rate (including pre-UNOS data).

December 15, 2000. Short-term survival at one-month and one-year following transplantation was analyzed for all 3 procedures. Long-term survival was examined for heart and lung transplantation using a conditional 5-year analysis. In this analysis, only those patients surviving the first year were analyzed. The conditional analysis allows us to assess factors other than those that affect survival primarily in the first year, (eg., the surgical procedure or early rejection events.) Only factors that were significant at the 0.05-level were retained in each of the models. Because the outcome in each model is mortality, an odds ratio greater than one indicates that the factor increases mortality.

Heart

The results of the heart patient survival are shown in Table 3. Consistent with the results of many other studies, patients receiving a second or subsequent transplant had a much higher likelihood of dying at all time points than patients receiving their first transplant. Several factors related to the patient's medical condition resulted in a higher odds of patient mortality at one month and at one year: the patient being in the ICU prior to transplant; requiring mechanical ventilation; or having received a VAD or balloon pump. None of these factors had an impact on the conditional 5-year survival, indicating that if even though a patient's medical condition prior to transplant reduced the probability of short-term survival, if the patient was able to survive the first year, their later survival was not adversely affected.

The only factors other than repeat transplant that had an effect in both the short- and long-term were

Table 3. Multivariate logistic regression of mortality following heart transplantation (10/1/1987-9/30/1999).

Risk Factor		Odds ratio		
		1 month (25,084)	1 year (25,084)	5 year[d] (19,636)
On ventilator		2.32[c]	2.05[c]	.
VAD implanted		2.06[c]	1.63[c]	.
On IABP		1.41[c]	1.25[b]	.
In ICU at transplant		1.16[b]	1.10[a]	.
Previous transplant		1.48[b]	2.25[c]	2.27[c]
Diagnosis:	Congenital	1.36[a]	1.55[c]	.
	Cardiomyopathy	0.55[c]	0.84[c]	.
	CAD	0.77[a]	.	1.14[b]
Donor cause of death-CVA		1.23[c]	.	.
Volume <10 transplants/year		1.44[c]	1.30[c]	.
Female recipient		1.40[c]	1.26[c]	.
Male recipient/ Female donor		1.32[c]	1.20[c]	.
Donor race	Asian	1.61[a]	1.51[b]	.
	Hispanic	.	1.14[a]	.
Recipient race	Black	.	1.37[c]	2.01[c]
	Hispanic	.	.	1.25[a]
	Other race	.	.	1.43[a]
HLA mismatch level	Linear	.	[c]	.
	0		0.73	
	2		0.84	
	4		0.97	
	6		1.11	
Year of transplant	1993-1995	0.85[b]	0.84[c]	.
	1996-1997	0.72[c]	0.71[c]	.
	1998-1999	0.78[c]	0.71[c]	.
Donor age (years)	Linear	[c]	[c]	[c]
	Quadratic	[a]	[b]	.
	0	0.98	0.92	0.73
	15	0.93	0.91	0.87
	30	1.03	1.04	1.03
	45	1.32	1.36	1.23
	60	1.97	2.05	1.46
Recipient age (years)	Linear	[c]	[c]	.
	Quadratic	[a]	[c]	[a]
	0	1.11	1.29	1.31
	15	0.93	0.98	1.13
	30	0.89	0.89	1.03
	45	0.99	0.99	1.00
	60	1.25	1.31	1.03
Ischemia time (hours)	Linear	[c]	[c]	.
	0	0.62	0.72	
	3	1.03	1.02	
	6	1.70	1.44	
	9	2.82	2.03	

[a] p < 0.05, [b] p < 0.01, [c] p < 0.001, [d] surviving ≥ 1 year
. = variable is not in model

diagnosis, donor age, recipient age and recipient race. The largest effect of donor age on survival was seen at the older ages. In the early posttransplant period, there appears to be a very slight increase in the odds of mortality for infant donors when compared with adolescents and young adults, but this effect disappears in the analysis of longer-term outcomes. As with donors, the largest impact in the short-term is seen for the oldest recipients. But the relationship of recipient age to mortality is quadratic, with an increased risk at both the youngest and oldest ages. Infants experience an increased risk in the short-term and this risk becomes even higher in the conditional long-term analysis.

Ischemia time has an impact on mortality at both one month and one year. Ischemia time has a linear relationship with mortality; the odds of mortality increase with increasing ischemia time. Other factors affecting mortality in either the short- or long-term, but not both, were transplant center volume, donor gender, recipient gender, donor race, level of HLA mismatch and donor cause of death.

Lung

As shown in Table 4, the factors having the largest impact on lung mortality in the short-term were related to either the patient's medical condition (eg., in the ICU prior to transplant) or diagnosis. At one month and one year, patients with a congenital diagnosis (including Eisenmenger's syndrome) or primary pulmonary hypertension had a greatly increased odds of mortality compared with all other diagnoses, but particularly when compared with emphysema. Patients with emphysema/COPD had decreased odds of mortality at both time points compared with those with IPF or any other diagnoses not specifically named.

Higher transplant center volume was related to lower odds of mortality at both one month and one year. Recipient gender was significant at one month and one year, with females having lower odds of mortality. Increasing level of HLA mismatch increased the odds of mortality at the 2 early time points. Increasing ischemia time increased the odds of mortality only at the one-month time point.

Heart-Lung

Due to the small numbers, multivariate analyses in Table 5 on heart-lung transplants were only performed for the one-month and one-year time points.

Table 4. Multivariate logistic regression of mortality following lung transplantation (10/1/1987-9/30/1999).

Risk Factor		Odds ratio		
		1 month (6,639)	1 year (6,639)	5 year[d] (4,468)
Double- vs. single-lung transplant		.	.	0.71[c]
In ICU and on life support at TX		4.15[c]	4.53[b]	.
In ICU and not on life support		.	1.98[b]	.
Hospitalized (not in ICU)		.	1.59[c]	.
Previous transplant		1.61[b]	1.64[c]	.
Diagnosis: Congenital		3.16[c]	2.21[c]	.
PPH		2.28[c]	1.47[c]	.
Emphysema/COPD		0.56[c]	0.55[c]	.
Transplant center volume>20/year		0.64[c]	0.80[c]	.
ABO not identical		1.29[a]	.	.
Female recipient		0.80[b]	0.86[a]	.
HLA mismatch level	Linear	[b]	[b]	.
	0	0.59	0.65	
	2	0.74	0.79	
	4	0.94	0.96	
	6	1.20	1.16	
Donor race	Black	1.30[a]	1.35[c]	.
	Hispanic	.	1.41[b]	.
Recipient race	Black	1.86[c]	1.41[b]	.
Recipient age	Linear	[a]	[c]	[a]
	Quadratic	[b]	.	[c]
	0	0.22	0.37	3.05
	15	0.46	0.51	1.53
	30	0.76	0.71	1.05
	45	1.00	0.99	1.00
	60	1.03	1.38	1.30
Donor age	Linear	.	.	[a]
	Quadratic	[b]	[c]	.
	0	1.51	1.58	0.85
	15	1.10	1.11	0.92
	30	1.00	1.00	1.01
	45	1.15	1.17	1.10
	60	1.66	1.75	1.20
Ischemia time (hours)	Linear	[a]	.	.
	0	0.76		
	3	0.91		
	6	1.10		
	9	1.32		
Transplant year	1993-1995	0.82[a]	0.88[a]	.

[a] p < 0.05, [b] p < 0.01, [c] p < 0.001, [d] surviving ≥ 1 year
. = variable is not in model

Table 5. Multivariate logistic regression of mortality following heart-lung transplantation (10/1/1987-9/30/1999).

Risk Factor		Odds ratio	
		1 month (662)	1 year (662)
On ventilator		5.49[c]	5.91[c]
Female recipient		.	0.58[b]
Recipient race	Black	.	2.20[a]
Transplant year	1993-1995	.	0.58[b]
	1996-1997	1.72[a]	.
Recipient age	Linear	[b]	.
	0		0.52
	15		0.71
	30		0.96
	45		1.31
	60		1.78

Mechanical ventilation had the largest impact on mortality. Additional factors that were significant at either time point were recipient gender, recipient race, recipient age and year of transplant. Recipient age had a linear relationship with mortality; older recipient age was associated with increased odds of mortality.

Morbidity Factors and Immunosuppression

In April 1994, the Registry began collecting information about a number of morbidity factors on thoracic follow-up forms. Data collected at one-year and 4-year follow-up periods are included in this section. Figure 11 shows rehospitalization rates during the first and fourth posttransplant years for heart recipients. The vast majority (55.7%, n=6,250) of recipients did not require hospitalization during the first year. This trend continued during the fourth year with 78.7% (n=6,522) not hospitalized. The major cause of hospitalization during the

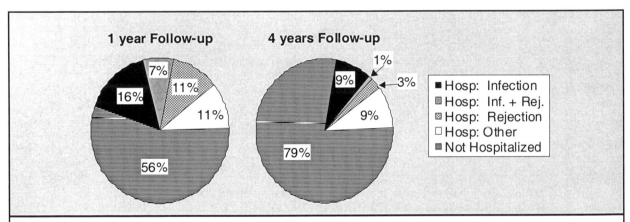

Figure 11. Rehospitalization after heart transplantation (US April 1994-Dec. 1999).

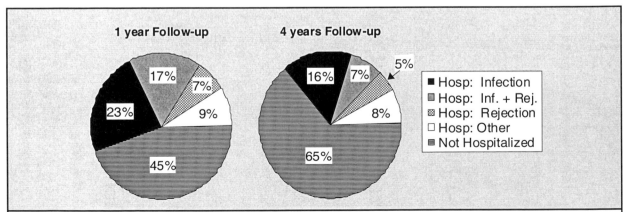

Figure 12. Rehospitalization after lung transplantation (US April 1994-Dec. 1999).

first year remains infection alone with 15.6% (n=1,754); during the fourth year the most common cause of hospitalization was for infection with or without rejection and for other reasons. Hospitalizations for rejection alone decreased from year one to year 4 from 10.9% (n=1,222) to 2.6% (n=214). Hospitalizations for both rejection and infection also decreased substantially, 6.3 points, from year one to year 4.

Figure 12 shows similar information for lung recipients. The most frequent cause of hospitalization during the first and fourth years was infection alone as indicated with 23.0% (n=896) and 16.2% (n=250) of recipients in the first and fourth posttransplant years, respectively. Hospitalizations for rejection alone decreased in percentage between the first (6.9%, n=270) and the fourth (4.5%, n=69) years. Hospitalizations for both infection and rejection decreased dramatically, from 16.8% (n=653) in year one to 7.3% (n=112) during year 4.

Table 6 provides data regarding other morbidity factors. For heart recipients, most factors were reported at similar rates in years one and 4, with coronary artery disease showing the biggest increase from 8.0% to 18.0%. Lung recipients show more variability from year one to year 4 with substantial increases in the percentage reporting hypertension (HTN), hyperlipidemia and all types of renal dysfunction combined during year 4.

Immunosuppressant usage is shown in Figures 13 and 14. At one year, there appears to be a substantially higher percentage of lung patients than heart patients on tacrolimus, azathioprine and prednisone. Conversely, at one year, the percentage of lung patients on cyclosporine and MMF is lower when compared with heart patients. The difference in usage of tacrolimus is even more dramatic at 4 years with less than 6% of heart

Table 6. Morbidity after transplantation (US April 1994-December 1999).

		Heart				Lung			
		1 year		4 year		1 year		4 year	
		N	%	N	%	N	%	N	%
1 Drug-treated	Not Reported	861		605		224		119	
hypertension	No	3,678	33.5	2,760	33.4	2,042	52.9	642	41.9
	Yes	7,317	66.5	5,500	66.6	1,820	47.1	891	58.1
2 Hyperlipidemia	Not Reported	874		649		248		132	
	No	6,656	60.6	4,706	57.3	3,403	88.7	1,281	84.3
	Yes	4,326	39.4	3,510	42.7	435	11.3	239	15.7
3 Diabetes	Not Reported	812		622		250		131	
	No diabetes	8,797	79.7	6,867	83.3	3,219	83.9	1,280	84.2
	Diabetes	2,247	20.3	1,376	16.7	617	16.1	241	15.8
4 Malignancy	Not Reported	846		660		245		128	
	No	10,604	96.3	7,544	91.9	3,653	95.1	1,443	94.7
	Yes	406	3.7	661	8.1	188	4.9	81	5.3
5 Renal	Not Reported	811		621		229		121	
dysfunction	Chronic dialysis	149	1.3	125	1.5	73	1.9	38	2.5
	Creatinine > 2.5 mg/dl	866	7.8	643	7.8	310	8	214	14
	Renal dysfunction	1,332	12.1	1,158	14	430	11.1	237	15.5
	No renal dysfunction	8,698	78.8	6,318	76.6	3,044	78.9	1,042	68.1
6 Coronary	Not Reported	1,967		1,430					
artery	No coronary artery disease	9,094	92	6,098	82				
disease	Coronary artery disease	648	6.6	1,083	14.6				
	CAD, with clin. sig. events	147	1.5	254	3.4				
7 Bronchial	Not Reported					503		240	
stricture	No bronchial stricture					3,293	91.9	1,354	95.9
	Bronchial stricture					89	2.5	19	1.3
	Bronchial stricture w/stent					201	5.6	39	2.8

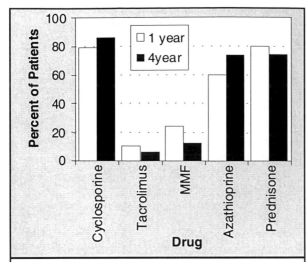

Figure 13. Heart transplant maintenance immunosuppression (US April 1994-Dec 98).

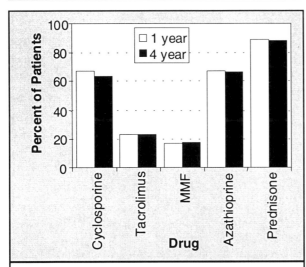

Figure 14. Lung transplant maintenance immunosuppression (US April 1994-Dec 98).

patients taking the drug as opposed to 23.7% of lung patients. While use of MMF remained stable in lung patients between years one and 4, heart patients dropped from 24.4% at year one to 12.4% at year 4.

INTERNATIONAL REGISTRY (NON-US CASES)

Number of Procedures

From January 1, 1967 to December 31, 2000, a total of 29,072 non-US cases was reported to the registry: 23,695 heart, 3,591 lung and 1,786 heart-lung

Table 7. Number of non US thoracic transplants by transplant year and organ.

	Heart-Lung	Heart	Lung	Total
Year	n	n	n	n
1967	0	1	0	1
1968	0	3	0	3
1969	0	2	0	2
1970	0	0	1	1
1971	1	2	0	3
1972	0	2	0	2
1973	0	9	0	9
1974	0	12	0	12
1975	0	11	0	11
1976	0	13	0	13
1977	0	17	0	17
1978	0	19	0	19
1979	0	20	0	20
1980	0	46	0	46
1981	0	56	0	56
1982	2	77	0	79
1983	5	150	1	156
1984	17	332	1	350
1985	54	499	2	555
1986	77	958	7	1,042
1987	111	1,208	18	1,337
1988	142	1,452	42	1,636
1989	177	1,636	93	1,906
1990	181	1,874	217	2,272
1991	172	1,993	290	2,455
1992	151	1,952	368	2,471
1993	117	1,987	418	2,522
1994	136	1,969	435	2,540
1995	136	1,863	402	2,401
1996	101	1,733	416	2,250
1997	97	1,598	376	2,071
1998	66	1,265	302	1,633
1999	43	936	202	1,181
	1,786	23,695	3,591	29,072

transplants. The growth of thoracic transplantation outside the United States over time is shown in Table 7.

As in the US, heart transplantation has declined in recent years with a decrease of 722 transplants reported to the registry from 1993-1998, though this may be due in part to the time lag in reporting. Lung transplant cases reported also appear to have declined in recent years with 116 fewer cases reported in 1998 than in 1993.

Recipient and Donor Characteristics

Frequency and percent of heart, double-lung, single-lung and heart-lung transplants by primary indication are presented in Table 8. The most frequently reported diagnoses for non-US recipients were cardiomyopathy (43.8%, n=6,981) for heart, emphysema/COPD (26.2%, n=525) for single-lung, cystic fibrosis (33.4%, n=300) for double-lung and primary pulmonary hypertension (24.8%, n=415) for heart-lung.

Numbers and relative frequencies of selected recipient, donor and donor organ variables by organ type are shown in Table 9. No significant variance from the US recipient demographic profile is noted in this analysis. Figures 15-17 illustrate mean donor age, mean recipient age and mean ischemic time change over time and indicate patterns similar to those of the US experience.

Outcomes

A comparison of heart, lung and heart-lung one-year patient survival by year of transplant from 1968-79 to 1998 is presented in Figure 18. All organs have shown steady increases in survival over time with one-year heart survival increasing from 40.2% in 1968-79 to 78.2% in 1998. One-year lung survival has improved from 54.1% in 1988 to 71.7% in 1998. Continuing this trend, heart-lung survival has increased from 51.9% in 1985 to 71.6% in 1998. There is a similar improvement in 3-year survival rates, shown in Figure 19. For heart, the survival rate has almost tripled, from 24.7% in 1968-79 to 70.9% in 1996. For lung and heart-lung, the improvement is not quite so dramatic, but nonetheless encouraging.

Figure 20 illustrates overall survival for each thoracic organ. Long-term survival is 27.8% at 11 years for heart recipients, 21.4% at 10 years for lung recipients and 20.7% at 12 years for heart-lung recipients.

Table 8. Primary indications for non-US thoracic transplants.

Organ	Primary Indication	Number	Percent
Heart-Lung	Unknown	133	.
	Cardiomyopathy	25	1.5
	Coronary Artery Disease	22	1.3
	Other	241	14.4
	Retransplant	49	2.9
	Valvular Heart Disease	6	0.4
	Congenital Heart Disease	366	21.9
	Primary Pulmonary Hypertension	415	24.8
	Cystic Fibrosis	391	23.4
	Idiopathic Pulmonary Fibrosis	56	3.3
	Alpha-1 Antitrypsin Deficiency	29	1.7
	Emphysema/COPD	74	4.4
Heart	Unknown	8,133	.
	Cardiomyopathy	6,981	43.8
	Coronary Artery Disease	6,706	42.1
	Other	498	3.1
	Retransplant	288	1.8
	Valvular Heart Disease	787	4.9
	Congenital Heart Disease	591	3.7
	Primary Pulmonary Hypertension	24	0.2
	Cystic Fibrosis	22	0.1
	Idiopathic Pulmonary Fibrosis	13	0.1
	Alpha-1 Antitrypsin Deficiency	5	0
	Emphysema/COPD	17	0.1
Single Lung	Unknown	508	.
	Cardiomyopathy	59	3
	Coronary Artery Disease	91	4.6
	Other	306	15.5
	Retransplant	52	2.6
	Valvular Heart Disease	6	0.3
	Congenital Heart Disease	48	2.4
	Primary Pulmonary Hypertension	104	5.3
	Cystic Fibrosis	128	6.5
	Idiopathic Pulmonary Fibrosis	473	24
	Alpha-1 Antitrypsin Deficiency	181	9.2
	Emphysema/COPD	525	26.6
Double Lung	Unknown	611	.
	Cardiomyopathy	10	1.1
	Coronary Artery Disease	27	3
	Other	158	17.6
	Retransplant	20	2.2
	Valvular Heart Disease	3	0.3
	Congenital Heart Disease	26	2.9
	Primary Pulmonary Hypertension	70	7.8
	Cystic Fibrosis	300	33.4
	Idiopathic Pulmonary Fibrosis	44	4.9
	Alpha-1 Antitrypsin Deficiency	93	10.4
	Emphysema/COPD	146	16.3

Table 9. Thoracic organ recipient and donor characteristics: non-US.

Organ		Hear-Lung		Heart		Lung	
		N	%	N	%	N	%
Recipient age group	<1	6	0.3	242	1	17	0.5
(years)	1-5	36	2.1	332	1.4	3	0.1
	6-10	68	4	228	1	27	0.7
	11-17	208	12.1	722	3.1	121	3.2
	18-34	740	43	2,439	10.5	846	22.4
	35-49	522	30.3	7,040	30.4	1,278	33.9
	50-64	141	8.2	11,427	49.4	1,429	37.9
	65+	0	0	695	3	50	1.3
	Not Reported	133	.	2,054	.	348	.
Recipient gender	Female	967	53.3	4,300	17.5	1,823	44.4
	Male	847	46.7	20,312	82.5	2,279	55.6
	Not Reported	40	.	567	.	17	.
Recipient blood type	A	769	45.3	10,407	49.1	1,503	47.4
	AB	82	4.8	927	4.4	148	4.7
	B	157	9.3	2,591	12.2	322	10.2
	O	688	40.6	7,253	34.2	1,198	37.8
	Not Reported	158	.	4,001	.	948	.
Donor age group (years)	<1	55	4.2	938	6.5	72	3.1
	1-5	55	4.2	183	1.3	5	0.2
	6-10	114	8.6	239	1.7	29	1.3
	11-17	309	23.4	1,576	11	243	10.5
	18-34	518	39.3	6,673	46.5	1,025	44.2
	35-49	236	17.9	3,964	27.6	706	30.4
	50-64	32	2.4	754	5.3	230	9.9
	65+	0	0	15	0.1	10	0.4
	Not Reported	535		10,837		1,799	.
Donor gender	Female	729	47.2	6,554	32.7	1,279	39.2
	Male	817	52.8	13,467	67.3	1,987	60.8
	Not Reported	308	.	5,158	.	853	.
Donor blood type	A	582	39.5	7,626	43	1,201	40.9
	AB	45	3.1	545	3.1	76	2.6
	B	106	7.2	1,784	10.1	250	8.5
	O	740	50.2	7,785	43.9	1,412	48
	Not Reported	381	.	7,439	.	1,180	.
Ischemia time (hours)	0 - <1	11	1	706	6.7	13	0.7
	1 - <2	123	11.6	2,387	22.6	57	3
	2 - <3	252	23.7	3,440	32.5	176	9.3
	3 - <4	379	35.7	2,756	26.1	387	20.3
	4 - <6	268	25.2	1,197	11.3	895	47.1
	6+	29	2.7	85	0.8	374	19.7
	Not Reported	792	.	14,608	.	2,217	.
Gender match	Female: Female	207	18.9	1,146	6.7	578	20.8
(donor: recip)	Female: Male	78	7.1	2,651	15.6	227	8.2
	Male: Female	308	28.1	1,581	9.3	552	19.8
	Male: Male	504	45.9	11,603	68.3	1,427	51.3
	Not Reported	757	.	8,198	.	1,335	.
Donor-recipient	Identical	1,302	88.5	15,565	88.5	2,539	86.7
ABO match level	Compatible	165	11.2	1,855	10.5	367	12.5
	Incompatible	4	0.3	164	0.9	22	0.8
	Not Reported	383	.	7,595	.	1,191	.

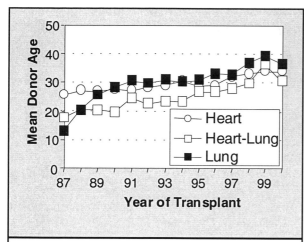

Figure 15. Mean donor age for non-US transplants.

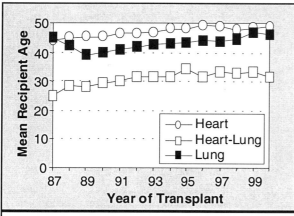

Figure 16. Mean recipient age for non-US transplants.

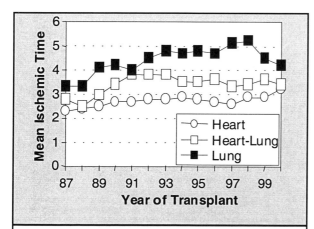

Figure 17. Mean ischemia time for non-US transplants.

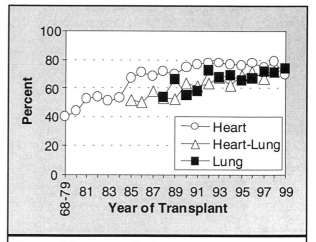

Figure 18. Non-US thoracic transplant: one-year survival rate by ogran and year of transplant.

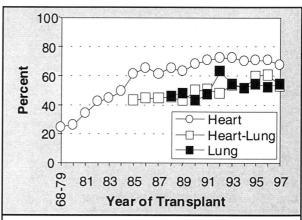

Figure 19. Non-US thoracic transplant: 3-year survival rate by ogran and year of transplant.

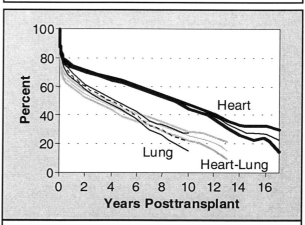

Figure 20. Thoracic organ transplant patient survival (non-US transplants).

SUMMARY

Based on data reported to the UNOS/ISHLT International Registry for Thoracic Organ Transplantation, we showed that:

1. The number of heart transplant operations performed in the United States has decreased by 164 procedures between 1998 (2,346) and 1999 (2,182). The number of lung transplants increased by 13 in 1999 to 877.

2. The most frequently reported indication for heart transplantation in the US is coronary artery disease (44.8%). For other thoracic transplants, the most frequently reported indications include cystic fibrosis (35.5%) for double lung, emphysema/COPD (49.7%) for single lung and congenital heart disease (46.6%) for heart-lung. The most frequently reported diagnoses for thoracic transplantation outside the US include cardiomyopathy (43.8%) for heart, cystic fibrosis (33.4%) for double-lung, emphysema/COPD (26.6%) for single-lung and primary pulmonary hypertension (24.8%) for heart-lung transplants.

3. US heart transplant recipients are predominately male (76.7%), between 50 and 64 years of age (51.3%) and white (81.4%). US lung transplant recipients are also predominately between 50 and 64 years of age (44.7%) and white (89.9%), but unlike heart recipients are more likely to be female (51.2%). No meaningful variance from the US recipient demographic profile is noted for the non-US recipients during the same time period.

4. Pediatric recipients (<18 years of age) received 10.9% of the reported heart transplants and 6.2% of reported lung transplants.

5. One-year survival for thoracic transplants performed in the US is 82.4% for heart, 74.1% for lung and 62.0% for heart-lung. Five-year survival for US thoracic transplants is 66.8% for heart and 43.2% for lung.

6. Long-term patient survival rates are: 22.5% at 17 years for heart, 20.8% at 10 years for lung and 24.3% at 13 years for heart-lung recipients.

7. The most important risk factor for mortality of US heart recipients at one month, one year and conditionally at 5 years after transplantation was receipt of a previous heart transplant. Significant short-term risk factors include donor age, recipient age and ischemic time. Substantial long-term risk factors include older donor age, recipient age, recipient race and diagnosis.

8. The factors having the most significant impact on lung mortality at all time points are related to either the patient's medical condition (eg., in the ICU prior to transplant, requiring mechanical ventilation) or diagnosis.

9. Mechanical ventilation, recipient race and recipient age have the largest impact on heart-lung mortality.

10. For heart and lung recipients, the major cause of hospitalization during the first year after transplantation is infection alone.

REFERENCES

1. SAS Procedures Guide, Version 8. Cary, NC, SAS Institute, Inc. 1999.

2. Kaplan EL, Meier P. Nonparametric estimation from incomplete observations. J Am Stat Assoc 1958; 53:457.

3. Kalbfleisch, JD, Prentice, RL. In: The Statistical Analysis of Failure Time Data. New York: J Wiley & Sons, 1980.

ACKNOWLEDGMENTS

We extend our sincere thanks to the many thoracic transplant surgeons, physicians and data coordinators in transplant programs throughout the world whose timely and accurate submission of data have made this analysis possible.

We also thank the members of the UNOS Scientific Advisory Committee and the ISHLT for guidance in the operation of the UNOS Thoracic Registry; Dr. Michael Kaye for collection of ISHLT data prior to April 1991; Denise Wise of the UNOS Thoracic Transplant Registry for maintaining the database; and George Beasley of the UNOS Thoracic Transplant Registry for programming support.

CHAPTER 4

Pancreas Transplant Outcomes for United States (US) Cases Reported to the United Network for Organ Sharing (UNOS) and Non-US Cases Reported to the International Pancreas Transplant Registry (IPTR) as of October, 2000

Angelika C. Gruessner and David E. R. Sutherland

International Pancreas Transplant Registry, Diabetes Institute for Immunology and Transplantation, Department of Surgery, University of Minnesota, Minneapolis, Minnesota

From December 16, 1966 to October 3, 2000, more than 15,000 pancreas transplants were reported to the International Pancreas Transplant Registry, including over 11,000 from the US and over 4,000 from outside of the US. The number tabulated by year for US and non-US cases through 1999 are shown in Figure 1. In 1999, 1,524 pancreas transplants were reported, 1,276 US (84%) and 248 non-US. Since reporting for year 2000 is not yet complete, the known cases (1,031 US and 162 non-US) are not shown on the bar graph, but those reported as of October 3, 2000 were included in the analyses when a complete record was available.

Nearly three-quarters of the pancreas transplants (73%) reported to the registries have been from the US. Since 1987, reporting to UNOS has been obligatory for US cases, while reporting to the IPTR for non-US cases is voluntary. We estimate that the number of non-US cases is at least 30% higher than illustrated.

In the following sections outcome data for non-US and US cases are given separately. Historical data are tabulated by eras since 1987 and show improvement in outcome over time. Contemporary outcomes are shown by the analyses of 1996-2000 cases.

METHODS

The methods of analysis are as previously described (1). Briefly, the statistics were calculated using SAS statistical program software package version 8.1.

Pancreas grafts were considered functioning for as long as the recipients were insulin independent, and death with a functioning graft (DWFG) was considered as a graft failure in the analyses of all cases. In some analyses, technical failure (TF) and pancreas graft primary non-function (PNF) cases were excluded (the remaining cases were considered technically successful [TS] transplants), and DWFG cases were censored at the time of death. Kidney grafts were considered functioning as long as the patients on dialysis before transplantation were dialysis-free after transplant, or as long as their posttransplant serum creatinine level was below

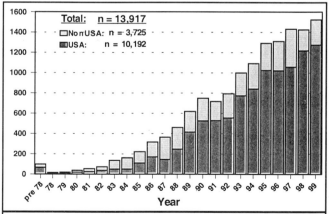

Figure 1. Annual number of US and non-US pancreas transplants reported to the IPTR, 1978-1999.

the pretransplant level in those that were not.

In univariate survival models, P values were calculated by the Wilcoxon (WC) and Log-Rank (L-R) tests and refer to the significance of the differences between the overall survival curves and not to individual time points. The WC test primarily reflects the probability that early differences are significant, while the L-R test is weighted to detect late differences. P values for univariant tests >0.05 are designated as non-significant. For P values <0.05 the actual values are given or the highest of values when both the WC and L-R were <0.05.

In addition to an analysis of outcome based on single variables, we performed logistic and Cox multivariate regression analyses using multiple variables in the models. For these analyses, a p value <0.2 was considered as noticeable.

UNITED STATES (UNOS) ANALYSES

Demographics

The total number of pancreas transplants reported to UNOS from October 1987 to October 2000 is 10,579. In 251(2%), the recipient category is unknown; of the remainder (n=10,328), 8,509 (82%) were simultaneous pancreas-kidney (SPK) transplants, 1,123 (11%) pancreas after kidney (PAK), and 554 (5%) pancreas transplants alone (PTA). The other 142 (1%) were pancreas transplants combined with at least one organ other than the kidney: 76 simultaneous pancreas-liver transplants (7 with a kidney added); 55 simultaneous pancreas-intestinal transplants (45 with a liver added, 8 with both a liver and kidney added, one with only a kidney added, and one with no other organ); and 11 simultaneous pancreas-heart transplants (6 with a kidney added). The pancreas transplants in recipients of an additional organ other than a kidney are not included in the analyses below.

Of the 10,186 pancreas transplants in the major categories (SPK, PAK, PTA), 55 (0.5%) were segmental grafts from living donors (LD). LD transplants were also not included in the analysis.

The annual number of US pancreas transplants from 1988-1999 where the major recipient category (SPK, PAK, PTA) is known is shown in Figure 2. Most have been SPK transplants, but the number of solitary transplants (PAK and PTA) has increased significantly in recent years (P=0.01). In 1999, 1,287 pancreas transplants were reported to UNOS. Of the 1,185 in which a major

recipient category was designated, 887 were SPK (75%), 209 PAK (18%), and 89 PTA (7%).

In 1999, 103 US centers did at least one pancreas transplant. Thirteen reported only one; 44 centers 2-9; 34 centers 10-19; 8 centers 20-39; 3 centers 50-75; and one reported >100 pancreas transplants in 1999. Interestingly, the annual rate of increase in number of pancreas transplants is exactly paralleled by the rate of increase in number of US centers doing pancreas transplants (Fig. 3).

The increased incidence of pancreas transplants in general has been paralleled by an increase in pancreas retransplants (Fig. 4A), but retransplantation as a proportion of total transplants has varied little between eras

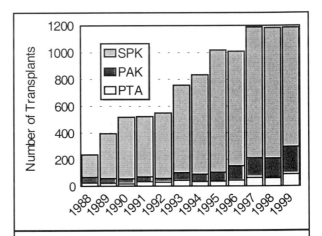

Figure 2. Annual number of US pancreas transplants in whom recipient category is known, 1988-1999.

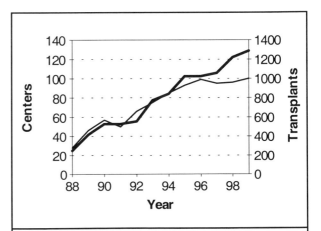

Figure 3. Annual number of US centers performing pancreas transplants (thin line) parallels the increase in annual number of transplants (thick line), 1988-2000.

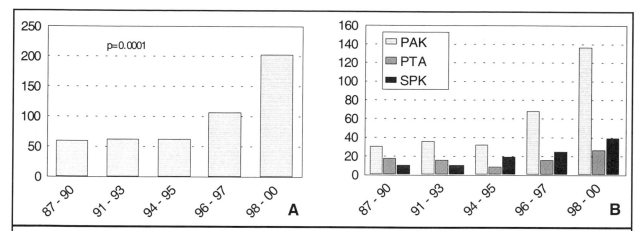

Figure 4. Number of US recipients of pancreas retransplants by era, (A) overall and (B) by recipient category, 1987-2000.

(3-6% for all categories combined). The category with the largest number of retransplants, PAK (Fig. 4B), is also the one in which the proportion of retransplants has been highest (27% for all eras combined, vs. 15% for PTA and 1% for SPK), again with little variation from era to era.

Of the 10,131 recipients of cadaver pancreas transplants in the major categories (SPK, PAK, PTA), only 49 were <21 (0.5%) years old; 8,479 were 21-45 (84%) years old, and 1,603 were >45 (16%) years old. In the SPK category (n=8,476), 33 were <21 (0.4%), 7,142 were 21-45 (84%), and 1,301 were >45 (15%) years old. In the PAK category (n=1,111), 2 were <21 (0.2%), 893 were 21-45 (80%), and 216 were >45 (19%) years old. In the PTA category (n=544), 14 were <21 (3%), 444 were 21-45 (82%), and 86 were >45 (16%) years old.

The proportion of recipients >45 years old has persistently increased (P=0.001), overall from 4% in 1988 to 26% in 2000 (Fig. 5). By category, the proportional increase from 1988-2000 was 4% to 26% for SPK; 7% to 24% for PAK; and 5% to 30% for PTA.

Since 1993, pancreas transplant recipients have been designated by reporting centers as having either Type I or Type II diabetes. The vast majority of 1994-2000 recipients were classified as Type I, but 3% were labeled Type II, and the proportion may be increasing (Fig. 6).

Pancreas duct management has evolved from being bladder drained (BD) for nearly all cases in all categories in the early eras to enterically drained (ED) for more than half of the SPKs in most recent eras and nearly half in the PAK and PTA categories. The annual number

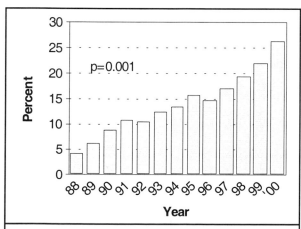

Figure 5. Annual percentage of recipients of US cadaver pancreas transplants >45 years old, 1988-2000.

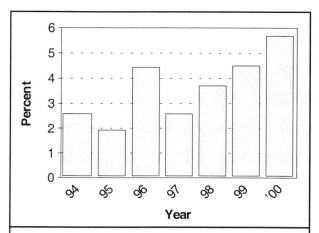

Figure 6. Annual percentage of recipients of US cadaver pancreas transplants classified as having Type II diabetes, 1994-2000.

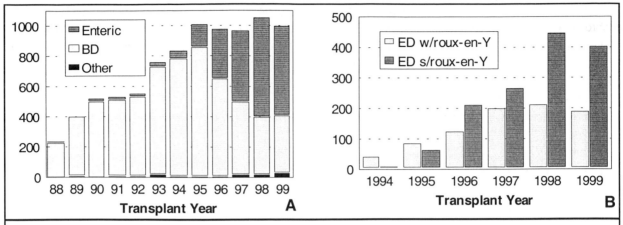

Figure 7. Annual number of US cadaver pancreas transplants (A) where duct management technique is known (1988-99), and (B) ED cases known to be done with or without a Roux-en-Y loop of recipient bowel (1994-99).

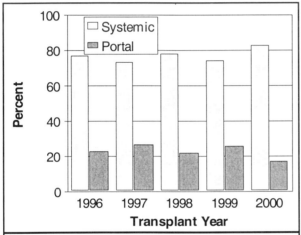

Figure 8. Annual percentage of US cadaver ED pancreas transplants managed with systemic/portal venous drainage, 1996-99.

of BD and ED pancreas transplants from 1988-1999 in which the duct management technique is known is shown in Figure 7A. At the beginning of the resurgence of ED, most were done with a Roux-en-Y limb of recipient bowel, but since 1996, most have been done without a Roux-en-Y (Fig. 7B).

In regard to management of the pancreas graft venous effluent for ED transplants, portal drainage resurged in popularity beginning in 1996 (Fig. 8). The proportion of portally drained ED transplants, however, has remained relatively constant (21% overall for 1996-2000 ED SPK cases).

The UNOS data was analyzed by eras (1987-90 vs. 1991-93 vs. 1994-95 vs. 1996-97 vs. 1998-2000) to show changes in outcome over time. The results in the last 2 eras were very similar. Thus, a separate analysis was done on 1996-2000 cases to dissect contemporary outcomes according to multiple variables.

Table 1 shows the basic demographics for cadaver (CAD) US pancreas transplants reported to UNOS from January 1, 1996 to October 3, 2000 (80% SPK, 14% PAK, 6% PTA). The PTA recipients were significantly younger than the PAK or SPK recipients. The proportion of males was higher in the SPK and PAK; the proportion of females was sig-

Table 1. Demographics. US cadaver pancreas transplants 1/1/1996-10/03/2000.

	SPK	PAK	PTA	p-value
# of Tx	4218	752	306	-
Recipient age (years)	38.7±7.6	40.1±7.2	37.5±8.7	0.0001
Male recipients	58%	58%	37%	0.001
% Minorities	10%	7%	4%	0.0001
Diabetes duration (yrs)	25±8	27±7	23±9	0.0001
% ED	55%	45%	40%	0.001
% of retransplants	2%	27%	14%	0.001
Preservation time (hr)	13±5	16±6	15±6	0.0001
Donor age (yrs)	27±12	27±12	26±12	0.460
# of HLA A,B,DR mismatches	4.4±1.3	3.7±1.4	3.6±1.5	0.0001
Waiting list time (days) 25-75%	92-415	48-363	48-310	0.0005

nificantly higher in the PTA category. Although diabetic nephropathy is more common in men, the overall incidence of diabetes is similar in both sexes (2). Thus, it is uncertain why there are more women than men in the PTA category.

The vast majority of the recipients were white (91%), but this is expected since the incidence of Type I diabetes is higher in whites than other racial groups (2). The percentage of minorities is significantly higher in the SPK than other categories of recipients. African-American individuals received 8% of the 1996-2000 pancreas transplants, slightly lower than their proportion in the general US population (12%). The percentage of minorities and especially African-Americans has increased significantly since the inception of UNOS (P=0.001). African Americans represented only 4% of pancreas transplant recipients in the 1987-90 period. Previous analyses have shown no difference in pancreas transplant outcome according to recipient race (1).

The mean duration of diabetes prior to pancreas transplantation was longest in the PAK and shortest in the PTA recipients, with SPK recipients being intermediate. The longer duration of diabetes in PAK and SPK recipients is expected because of the interval required to develop advanced nephropathy, while a PTA can be done at anytime after onset of disease.

The proportion of ED pancreas grafts was higher in the SPK than in the PAK and PTA categories. Of the ED transplants, a Roux-en-Y was used in 36% of the cases and the proportion was similar in each recipient category. The vast majority of the others were bladder drained.

The proportion of retransplants was much higher in the PAK and PTA categories than in the SPK category. Historically, the graft failure rate has been less in SPK recipients so the need for retransplantation has also been less.

The mean preservation time was significantly shorter in the SPK category. The difference probably reflects the fact that SPK transplants are locally procured, while a higher proportion of solitary pancreas transplants are shared between organ procurement organizations (OPOs).

Mean donor age was not significantly different between categories. Donors tended to be young: by quartile, the lower 25% of the donors were <18 years and the upper 25% were >36 years. Only 3% were over 50 years old. The distribution of donor age for 1996-2000 cases was no different than for previous eras.

The mean number of donor HLA-A, -B, -DR mismatches was significantly lower in the PAK and PTA categories. The emphasis on matching for solitary pancreas transplants probably reflects the fact that historically, the impact of HLA matching has been greater in these categories than in SPK recipients (1).

Waiting time for cadaver donor pancreases was significantly shorter in the PAK and PTA than in the SPK recipients. The difference reflects the availability of solitary pancreases. SPK candidates have a longer wait because of the shortage of kidneys.

Outcome by Era

From 1987-1997, there were significant improvements in outcomes in all pancreas transplant categories (Figs. 9-15), including elderly (>45 years) patients (Figs. 16-18).

SPK transplants (Fig. 9): SPK patient survival rates significantly improved in successive eras, from 89% at one year for 1987-90 cases to 95% for 1998-2000 cases (Fig. 9A). Likewise, there was a significant improvement in overall SPK pancreas graft survival rates (GSRs), from 72% at one year for 1987-90 cases to 82% for 1998-2000 cases (Fig. 9B). In addition, SPK kidney GSRs significantly improved over time, from 84% at one year for 1987-90 cases to 92% for 1997-2000 cases (Fig. 9C). The SPK kidney graft survival rates in the later eras were as high if not higher than those for kidney transplants alone as reported to UNOS (3).

The improvement in outcome was greater for ED than for BD SPK transplants over this time span, primarily because the outcome in ED cases began at a lower level (Fig. 10). For BD SPK transplants the one-year GSRs went from 74% at one year for 1987-90 cases to 85% for 1998-2000 cases (Fig. 10A); for ED SPK cases, from 39% to 81% (Fig. 10B). For BD cases the improvement in outcome was continuous from era to era, while for ED cases there was a slight decline in the GSRs from the 1996-97 to the 1998-2000 era, perhaps reflecting a learning curve as more (but less experienced) centers began using ED. For the 1996-97 era, 59% of SPK transplants were BD; for the 1998-2000 era, 63% were ED, a complete reversal in proportions.

PAK transplants (Fig. 11): PAK patient survival rates did not differ significantly over time, and were >90% at one year for each era between 1987 and 2000 (Fig. 11A). However, overall PAK pancreas GSRs improved

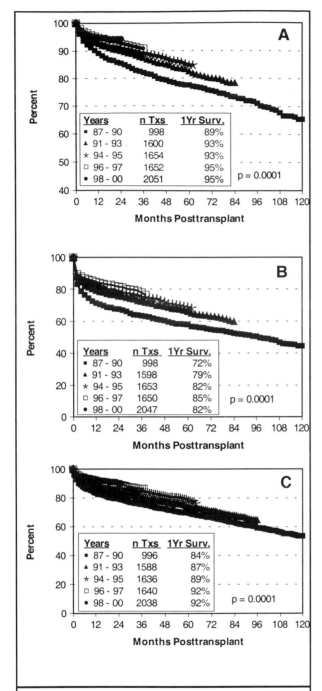

Figure 9. (A) patient survival and (B) pancreas and (C) kidney graft survival rates for US cadaver SPK transplants by era, 1987-2000.

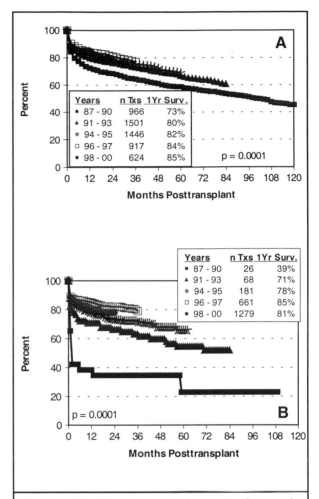

Figure 10. Pancreas graft survival rates by era for (A) BD and (B) ED US cadaver SPK transplants, 1987-2000.

significantly, going from 52% at one year for 1988-93 cases to 74% for 1997-2000 cases (Fig. 11B).

In the early eras, BD was used almost exclusively for PAK cases (Fig. 12). ED began to be used in the 1996-97 era (40% of the cases); during the 1998-2000 era, nearly half were ED. However, in each of these 2 eras, the PAK graft survival rates were higher in the BD (Fig. 12A) than in the ED (Fig. 12B) cases. With either drainage technique, PAK graft survival rates were constant in the last 2 eras.

PTA cases (Fig. 13): PTA patient survival rates did not differ significantly by era (Fig. 13A), but reached 100% at one year for the most recent era (1998-2000) (also the one with the most cases). PTA GSRs improved significantly, from 47% at one year for 1987-90 cases to 76% for 1998-2000 cases (Fig. 13B).

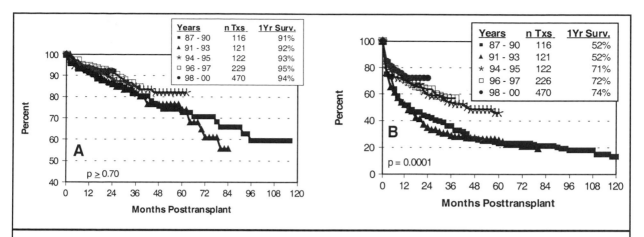

Figure 11. (A) patient and (B) pancreas graft survival rates for US cadaver PAK transplants by era, 1987-2000.

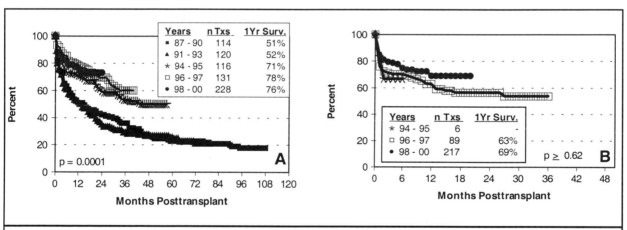

Figure 12. Pancreas graft survival rates by era for (A) BD and (B) ED US cadaver SPK transplants, 1987-2000.

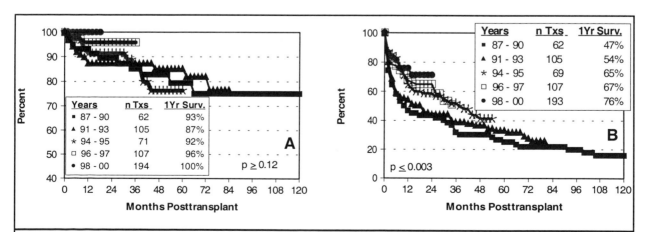

Figure 13. (A) patient and (B) pancreas graft survival rates by era for US cadaver PTA transplants, 1987-2000.

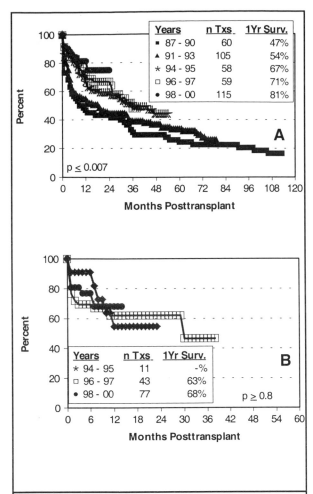

Figure 14. Pancreas graft survival rates by era for (A) BD and (B) ED US cadaver SPK transplants, 1987-2000.

As for PAK, in the early eras BD was used almost exclusively for PTA (Fig. 14). ED began to be used for a substantial proportion of the PTA cases in the 1996-97 era (42%) and the proportion has remained constant for the 1998-2000 era (40%). However, the PTA GSRs were higher in both eras with BD and continue to improve with BD (Fig. 14A), while with ED there was no significant difference between the 2 eras (Fig. 14B). Indeed, with BD the GSR for 1998-2000 PTA cases (81% at one year) was higher than for PAK cases.

Immunological graft loss rates (Fig. 15): The improvement in GSRs in all categories over time was in part due to a reduction in TF rates and in part due to a decrease in the incidence of graft losses for immunological reasons. In an analysis of TS cases in which DWFG was censored, all graft losses were considered immunological, either rejection or autoimmune recur-

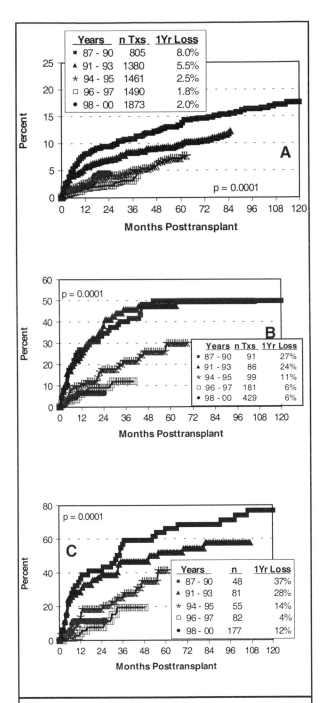

Figure 15. Immunological pancreas graft failure rates by era for US cadaver (A) SPK, (B) PAK, and (C) PTA transplants, 1987-2000.

rence of disease (Fig. 15). For SPK cases, the immunological graft loss rate went from >8% at one year for 1987-90 cases to <2% for 1996-97 and 1998-2000 cases (Fig. 15A). For PAK cases, the immunological graft loss rate went from >27% at one year for 1987-90 cases to 6% for

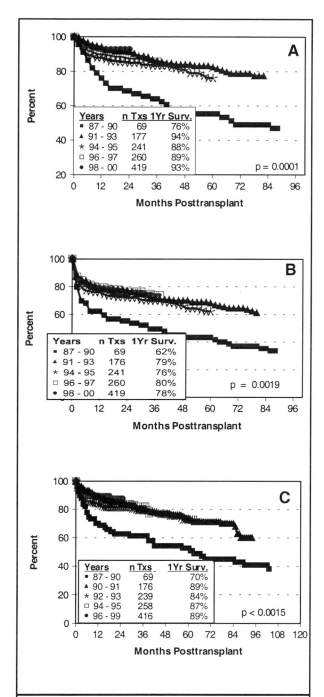

Figure 16. (A) patient survival and (B) pancreas and (C) kidney graft survival rates by era for US SPK recipients >45 years old, 1987-2000.

1996-97 and 1998-2000 cases (Fig. 15B). For PTA cases, the immunological graft loss rate went from 37% at one year for 1987-90 cases to 12% for 1998-2000 cases (Fig. 15C). In each category, the greatest decline in immunological graft loss rate occurred in 1994-95, the

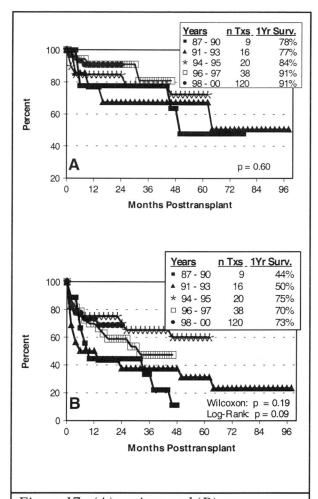

Figure 17. (A) patient and (B) pancreas graft survival rates by era for US PAK recipients >45 years old, 1987-2000.

era when tacrolimus (TAC) and mycophenolate mofetil (MMF) began to be used. The decline continued into the following era (1996-97) but not thereafter.

Decreasing impact of recipient age on outcome (Figures 16-18): The proportion of pancreas transplant recipients >45 years old has progressively increased over time, going from <5% in 1988 to >25% for 2000 cases (Fig. 5). Simultaneously, the outcome has improved in the older patients.

For SPK recipients who were >45 years old, patient (Fig. 16A), pancreas (Fig. 16B), and kidney graft (Fig. 16C) survival rates were all higher in the last 4 eras (1991-2000) than in the first era (1987-90).

In the PAK category (Fig. 17), very few recipients were >45 years old in the early eras. Although a statistically significant improvement in patient survival could not be shown, it was 91% at one year in the last 2 eras

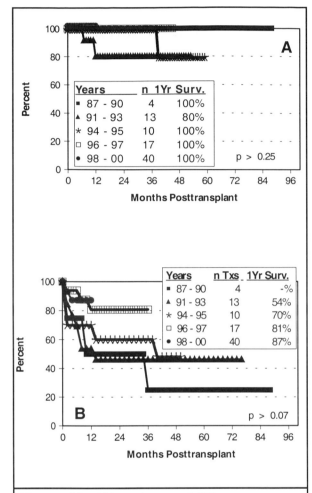

Figure 18. (A) patient and (B) pancreas graft survival rates by era for US PTA recipients >45 years old, 1987-2000.

(1996-2000) (Fig. 17A). Graft survival rates, however, have significantly improved in elderly PAK recipients (Fig. 17B).

In the PTA category (Fig. 18), again very few of the recipients were >45 years old until the last era. Patient survival rates (Fig. 18A) have been high (100% at one year in the last 3 eras), and graft survival rates (Fig. 18B) have become very high, 87% at one year for 1998-2000 elderly PTA recipients.

Pancreas Transplant Outcome for Contemporary (1996-2000) Cases

The current pancreas transplant success rates according to several variables were calculated using 1996-2000 cases (n=5,276). In each analysis, only cases with complete information were included (n=4,073).

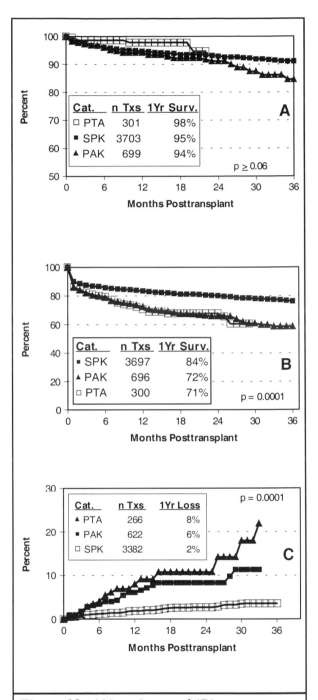

Figure 19. (A) patient and (B) pancreas graft functional survival rates and (C) pancreas graft immunological failure rates by recipient category for 1996-2000 US cadaver transplants.

Outcome by category for 1996-2000 cadaver donor pancreas transplants (Fig. 19): Patient survival rates at one year were ≥ 94% in all recipient categories (SPK, PAK, PTA), and were highest for PTA recipients

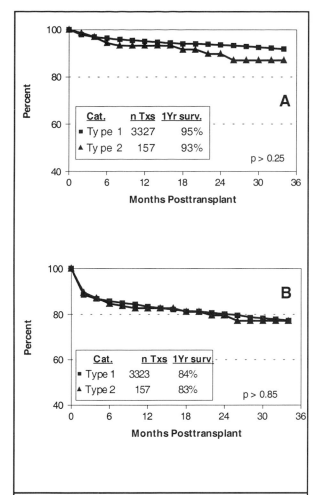

Figure 20. (A) patient and (B) pancreas graft survival rates for 1996-2000 US cadaver SPK recipients according to type of diabetes reported.

(Fig. 19A). Pancreas GSRs were significantly higher in SPK than in PAK and PTA recipients (Fig. 19B). The immunological graft loss rate was significantly lower in SPK (2% at one year) than in PAK and PTA recipients (Fig. 19C).

The differences in graft survival rates between the 3 recipient categories are greater in the overall analysis than in the subgroup of recipients of BD grafts given anti-T-cell agents for induction and tacrolimus (TAC) and mycophenolate mofetil (MMF) for maintenance immunosuppression (see subsequent section on immunosuppression).

Outcome by Diabetes Type (Fig. 20): An analysis of outcome for SPK recipients with Type I versus Type II diabetes mellitus was done for 1996-2000 cases (Fig. 20). Only 4% were designated as Type II. The age

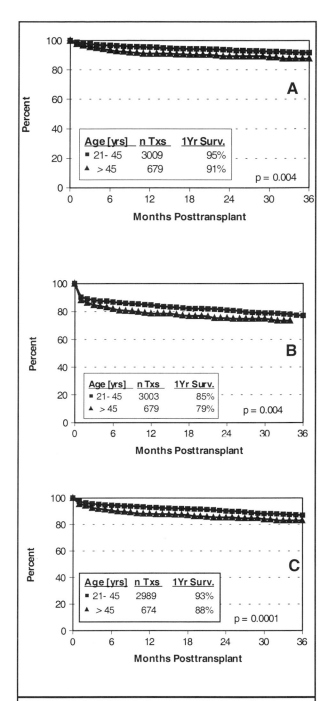

Figure 21. (A) patient survival and (B) pancreas and (C) kidney graft survival rates by recipient age for 1996-2000 US cadaver SPK transplants.

range of Type I cases was 16-69 years (mean 38±7 years) and of Type II cases was 31-59 years (mean 44±7 years) (P=0.001), consistent with the known differences in age demographics for these 2 forms of the disease (2). Patient survival rates did not differ significantly for Type I

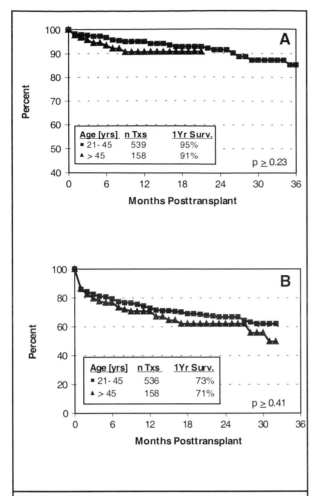

Figure 22. (A) patient and (B) pancreas graft survival rates by recipient age for 1996-2000 US cadaver PAK transplants.

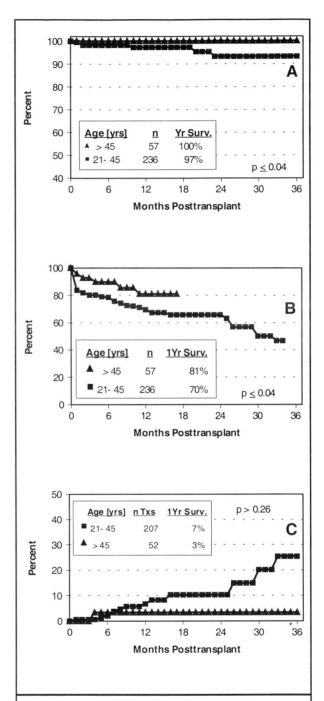

Figure 23. (A) patient survival and (B) pancreas graft functional survival rates and (C) pancreas graft immunological failure rates by recipient age for 1996-2000 US cadaver PTA transplants.

versus Type II SPK transplant recipients (Fig. 20A), nor did posttransplant insulin-independence rates (Fig. 20B).

Outcome by Recipient Age (Figures 21-23): For 1996-2000 recipients of cadaver pancreas transplants, <1% (n=27) were <21 years old; 80% were 21-45 (n=4,205); and 20% were >45 years old (n=1,044). The proportions were similar in each recipient category.

In the SPK category (Fig. 21), both patient (Fig. 21A), pancreas (Fig. 21 B) and kidney graft (21C) survival rates were significantly higher in the 21-45 year-old recipients versus older recipients, but the differences were small (4-6% at one year). The technical failure (TF) rate was 8% in the 21-45 year-old and 10% in >45 year-old recipients. The rejection loss rate for technically successful (TS) grafts were similar in the 21-45 (n=2,757) and >45 (n=613) old recipients, both 2% at one year.

In the PAK category (Fig. 22), patient (Fig. 22A) and

graft (Fig. 22B) survival rates were not significantly different for the 21-45 year-old versus older recipients. The TF rate was 10% in the 21-45 year-old and 14% in the >45 year-old recipients. The rejection loss rate for TS

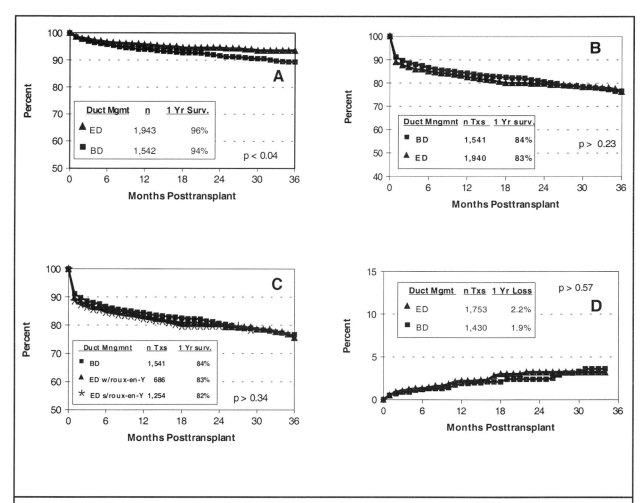

Figure 24. (A) patient survival and (B) pancreas graft functional survival rates overall, or (C) by Roux or no Roux for ED cases, and (D) pancreas graft immunological failure rates, for 1996-2000 US cadaver SPK transplants according to duct management.

grafts in the 21-45 (n=484) and >45 (n=136) year-old recipients were not significantly different, 6% and 4% at one year.

Paradoxically, in the PTA category (Fig. 23), both patient (Fig. 23A) and graft (Fig. 23B) survival rates were significantly higher in the >45 versus 21-45 year-old recipients. Both the technical failure rate (9% vs. 12%) and the immunological graft loss rate (Fig. 23C) were lower in the >45 year-old than in the younger recipients, although neither by itself was statistically significant.

Outcome by duct and vascular management (Figures 24-29): For 1996-2000, well over half of SPK (55%) and less than half of PAK (46%) and PTA (41%) cases were done with ED. Of the ED SPK cases, approximately one-fifth (21%) were portally drained. Outcome according to these variables are presented in the following subsections.

BD versus ED for 1996-2000 SPK transplants (Fig. 24): By univariate analysis, patient survival rates were slightly higher in ED than in BD SPK recipients (Fig. 24A), but pancreas GSRs (Fig. 24B) were nearly identical, with or without a Roux-en-Y (Fig. 24C). For TS SPK cases, the immunological loss rates (Fig. 24D) were low and nearly identical for ED and BD cases.

Portal versus systemic drainage for 1996-2000 ED SPK transplants (Fig. 25): Pancreas GSRs were identical for portal versus systemic drained ED SPK transplants (Fig. 25).

Kidney graft functional survival rates overall and according to duct management in SPK recipients (Fig. 26): Overall, SPK kidney grafts survival rates were 92% at one year, even higher than that calculated for diabetic recipients of cadaver kidney transplants alone in the UNOS registry (3). In regard to duct management

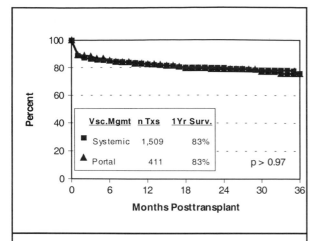

Figure 25. Pancreas graft survival rates for 1996-2000 US cadaver ED SPK according to venous vascular management.

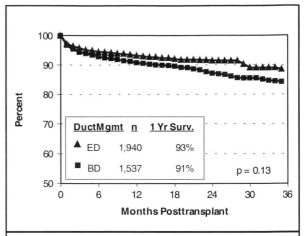

Figure 26. Kidney graft survival rates for 1996-2000 US cadaver SPK transplants according to pancreas duct management.

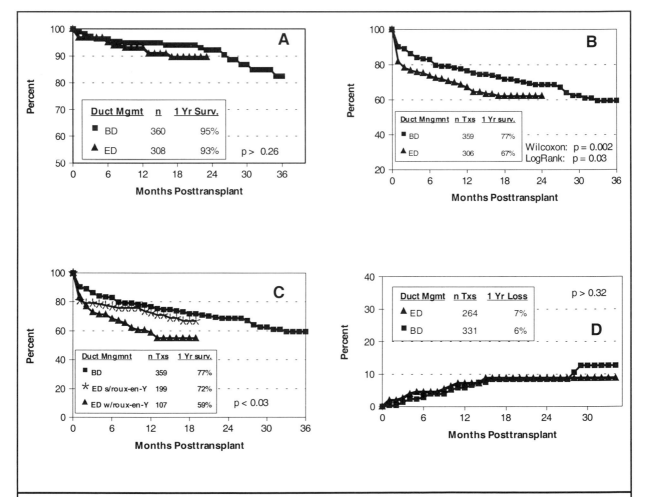

Figure 27. (A) patient survival and (B) pancreas graft functional survival rates overall, or (C) by Roux or no Roux for ED cases, and (D) pancreas graft immunological failure rates, for 1996-2000 US cadaver PAK pancreas transplants.

category, the kidney GSRs were not significantly different for ED versus BD SPK recipients (Fig. 26).

BD versus ED for 1996-2000 solitary (PAK and PTA) pancreas transplants (Figures 27 and 28): The proportion of solitary pancreas transplants done with ED has also increased in recent years, but unlike the situation for SPK transplants, the effect on outcome has not been neutral. The use of ED has not affected patient survival rates in either the PAK (Fig. 27A) or PTA (Fig. 28A) categories, but pancreas GSRs were significantly higher with BD in both the PAK (Fig. 27B) and PTA (Fig. 28B) categories. At one year, the difference was 10% in both categories. In both categories, with ED the GSRs were lower when a Roux-en-Y was used (Figures 27C and 28C), but even without a Roux-en-Y the ED GSRs were lower than those for BD.

The immunological graft failure rates were not sig-

nificantly different for ED versus BD pancreas transplants in either the PAK (Fig. 27D) or PTA (Fig. 28D) categories. The main differences in outcome between ED and BD cases in both solitary pancreas transplant categories were in the TF rates: for PAK, 8% with BD versus 12% with ED (p=0.05); and for PTA, 6% with BD versus 17% with ED (p=0.002). It is possible that some graft failures thought to be primarily technical are actually from thrombosis secondary to rejection, particularly in the solitary (PAK and PTA) ED group where neither serum creatinine nor urine amylase can be used to detect a decrease in graft function from rejection prior to secondary thrombosis. The reported thrombosis incidence for PAK cases was 9% with ED versus 5% with BD (p=0.05). In the PTA group there was a similar trend; the thrombosis incidence was 16% with ED versus 5% with BD (p=0.001). For SPK transplants the pancreas graft throm-

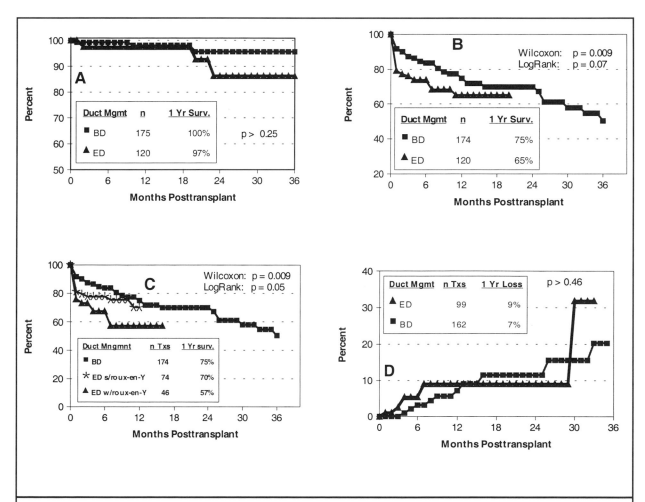

Figure 28. (A) patient survival and (B) pancreas graft functional survival rates overall, or (C) by Roux or no Roux for ED cases, and (D) pancreas graft immunological failure rates, for 1996-2000 US cadaver PTA pancreas transplants.

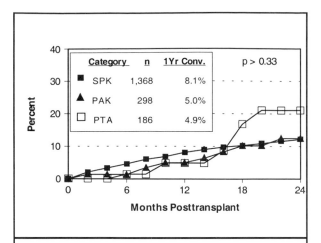

Figure 29. Conversion rate of 1996-2000 US TS cadaver BD pancreas transplants to ED by recipient category.

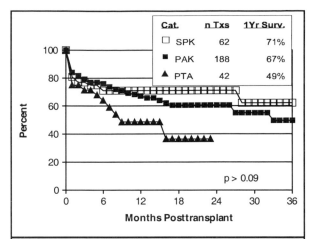

Figure 30. Pancreas retransplant cadaver graft survival rates by recipient category for 1996-2000 US cases.

bosis rates were not significantly different with ED (6%) than with BD (5%); rejection episodes (most likely involving both organs from the same donor) are easier to diagnose in SPK recipients by using serum creatinine to monitor renal allograft function.

The data show that for SPK transplants, the outcomes are similar with BD and ED (with or without portal drainage). However, for solitary pancreas transplants (PAK and PTA), the GSR with ED has not yet reached that of BD. For solitary pancreas transplants, the main advantage of ED is avoiding the chronic complications of BD that result in the need to convert some pancreas grafts to ED (Fig. 29). For 1996-2000 BD transplants, $\geq 5\%$ were converted to ED by one year and $\geq 10\%$ by 2 years, with no significant difference in conversion rates by recipient category.

Pancreas retransplants (Fig. 30): In each recipient category, pancreas GSRs were lower for retransplants than for primary transplants. Overall SPK and PAK retransplant GSRs were similar and marginally higher than the PTA retransplant GSR (Fig. 30). The influence of pancreatic graft duct management on outcome was less clear for retransplants (Fig. 31) than in the overall analyses. For SPK (Fig. 31A) and PAK (Fig. 31B) retransplants, pancreas GSRs were not significantly different for BD and ED cases, while for PTA retransplants they were significantly higher with BD (Fig. 31C).

Technical Failure Rates

The overall technical failure rate for pancreas transplants has declined significantly since the inception of

UNOS: from >15% for 1987-90 cases to 7% for 1998-2000 cases (Fig. 32A).

In the early eras, the reported technical failure (TF) rate was higher with solitary than with SPK transplants (perhaps because early rejections in the solitary graft were classified as technical). Since 1990, however, the TF rate has declined in each category in each era, and more so for solitary than SPK transplants, so that in the most recent era (1998-2000), there is no difference by category (Fig. 32B). In the SPK category (Fig. 33) the TF rate was higher for ED than BD grafts in the 1991-97 eras, the period when ED was re-introduced. However, in the latest era (1998-2000), the SPK TF rates are nearly identical for the 2 duct management techniques.

The TF rates for 1996-2000 transplants according to category and duct drainage technique are as shown in Table 2. The technical failure rate was significantly lower for BD than ED in all categories.

The TF incidence for ED cases was not significantly different for those done with versus without a Roux-en-Y loop of recipient bowel in any of the categories. In regard to ED SPK cases, overall the pancreas TF incidence was not significantly different for grafts with the venous effluent drained portally versus systemically, but was higher in the portal subgroup done without a Roux-en-Y loop of recipient bowel for exocrine drainage.

Table 3 shows the most common causes of pancreas transplant TFs by recipient category and duct management technique. Graft thrombosis predominates by far, accounting for $\geq 70\%$ of TFs in each category. Infection, pancreatitis, anastomotic leaks and bleeding

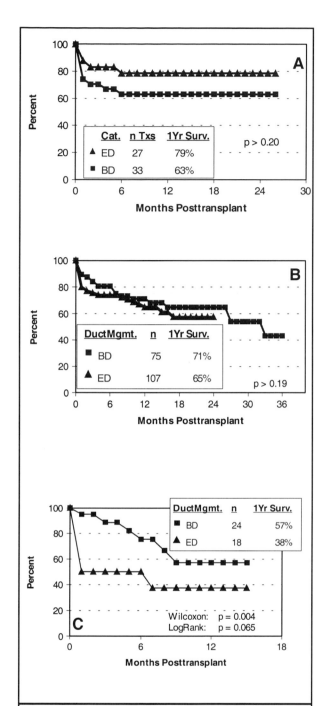

Figure 31. Pancreas retransplant graft survival rates by duct management for 1996-2000 US (A) SPK, (B) PAK and (C) PTA cases.

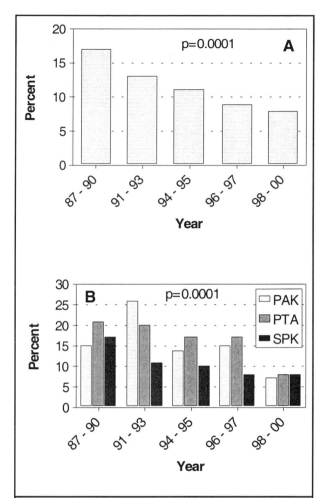

Figure 32. Technical failure rates by era, (A) overall and (B) by recipient category, for US cadaver pancreas transplants, 1987-2000.

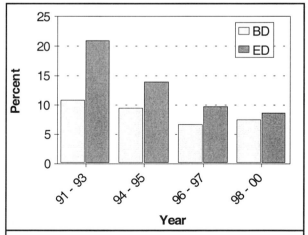

Figure 33. Technical failure rate by era and duct management for US cadaver SPK pancreas transplants, 1987-2000.

Table 2. Technical failure rate.

	BD	ED	p	ED w/Roux-en-Y	ED s/Roux-en-Y	p
SPK	6.9%	9.0%	0.030	8.0%	9.5%	0.27
(n)	(1,542)	(1,943)		(687)	(1,256)	
PAK	7.8%	12.3%	0.049	13.9%	11.5%	0.54
(n)	(360)	(308)		(108)	(200)	
PTA	6.3%	17.5%	0.02	21.7%	14.9%	0.34
(n)	(175)	(120)		(46)	(74)	
Systemic		8.9%		8.6%	9.0%	
(n)		(1,511)		(405)	(1,106)	
Portal		9.4%		7.2%	14.2%	
(n)		(412)		(278)	(134)	
p		0.71		0.49	0.05	

account for <30% of the TFs. Except for infection/pancreatitis in ED PAK recipients, the incidence of any one of these complications as a cause of graft loss was ≤1% in each category, regardless of duct management technique.

The thrombosis rate was similar for BD and ED SPK transplants, but in the PAK and PTA categories, the thrombosis rate was significantly lower with BD. Indeed, with BD the thrombosis rates were not significantly different for the SPK, PAK, and PTA categories while with ED the reported thrombosis rate was significantly higher for solitary pancreas (PAK and PTA) than for SPK transplants. Again, some early rejections may lead to early thrombosis in ED solitary pancreas transplants where the diagnosis of a rejection episode is more difficult.

Pancreas Transplant Outcome by Immunosuppressant Combinations

Nearly every possible combination of the immunosuppressants available have been used in pancreas transplant recipients. In this section, pancreas GSRs for 1996-2000 transplants are reported for SPK, PTA, or PAK recipients according to whether they were or were not given anti-T-cell agents for induction and according to which combination of TAC, CSA, MMF or Azathioprine (AZA) were used for maintenance immunosuppression (Fig. 34).

Since 1994, the predominantly used maintenance immunosuppressant combination has gone from CSA-AZA to TAC-MMF in all recipient categories (Fig. 34A). The use of anti-T-cell therapy for induction has been more variable (Fig. 34B). Since 1994, the proportion of SPK recipients given no anti-T-cell therapy has remained rather constant (~40%). The anti-CD-25 agents (Zenapax and Simulect) have been available since 1998, and in SPK recipients are now used more frequently than the other anti-T-cell agents. In solitary pancreas transplant recipients (PAK and PTA), the use of anti-T-cell agents has increased. Zenapax or Simulect has been used in nearly half of solitary pancreas transplant recipients since their introduction in 1998, but other anti-T-cell agents are currently used with equal frequency and some recipients had more than one agent for induction.

Zenapax and Simulect were considered similar, and in the analysis on outcome by agent, recipients treated with either were put into one group. Polyclonal anti-lym-

Table 3. Reasons for technical failures.

	SPK			PAK			PTA		
	BD	ED	p	BD	ED	p	BD	ED	p
Graft Thr	5.4%	6.3%	0.264	5.0%	8.8%	0.050	4.6%	15.8%	0.001
Inf/Pxitis	0.6%	1.1%	0.114	1.1%	2.9%	0.091	0.0%	0.8%	0.226
Anas leak	0.4%	0.9%	0.056	0.0%	0.7%	0.126	0.6%	0.8%	0.788
Bleed	0.3%	0.2%	0.492	0.6%	0.0%	0.190	0.0%	0.0%	−

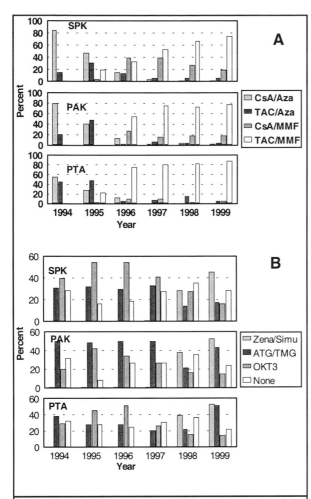

Figure 34. (A) Initial maintenance immunosuppressant and (B) anti-T-cell induction therapy agent usage by year and recipient category for US cadaver pancreas transplants, 1994-99.

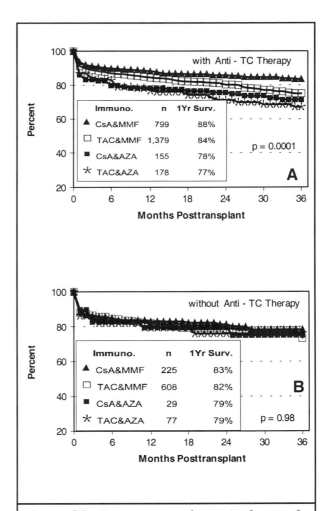

Figure 35. Pancreas graft survival rates for 1996-2000 US cadaver SPK transplants by initial maintenance immunosuppressants in recipients (A) given or (B) not given anti-T cell therapy for induction.

phocyte (ALG) or anti-thymocyte (ATG) globulins were also considered similar, and again recipients treated with either were put into one group for the analysis of outcome by agent. Recipients given more than one class of anti-T-cell agents (eg., ATG + Zenapax) (<4% of 1996-2000 cases) were not included in the analyses comparing agents, but were included in the analyses of maintenance immunosuppression divided according to whether or not induction therapy was used.

SPK outcome by immunosuppression (Fig. 35-37): Nearly three-fourths of 1996-2000 SPK recipients were given anti-T-cell agents for induction immunosuppression (Fig. 35A), while one-fourth were not (Fig. 35B). With anti-T-cell therapy, the pancreas GSRs were significantly higher in those who were given MMF than in

those given AZA, regardless which of the other 2 drugs (CSA or TAC) was used (Fig. 35A), while without anti-T-cell therapy there was no difference by maintenance immunosuppression regimen (Fig. 35B).

The largest group of SPK recipients was given anti-T-cell therapy for induction and TAC-MMF for maintenance immunosuppression (n=1,379). Within his group, the functional survival rates were similar for BD and ED grafts (Fig. 36).

In the SPK recipients given anti-T-cell therapy (regardless of maintenance regimen), the GSR was slightly higher for the subgroup given Zenapax or Simulect (Fig. 37). The higher SPK GSR in the Zenapax/Simulect subgroup was largely due to the ED subset of this SPK population. With ED (n=1,155), the one-year GSRs for

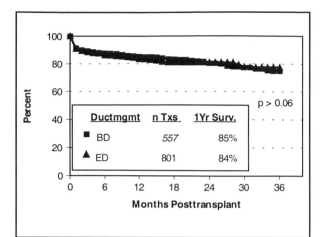

Figure 36. Pancreas graft survival rates by duct management technique for 1996-2000 US SPK recipients given anti-T-cell induction therapy and TAC-MMF for maintenance immunosuppression.

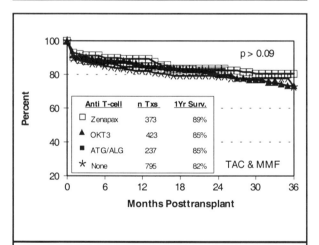

Figure 37. Pancreas graft survival rates by induction anti-T-cell agents used in 1996-2000 US SPK recipients.

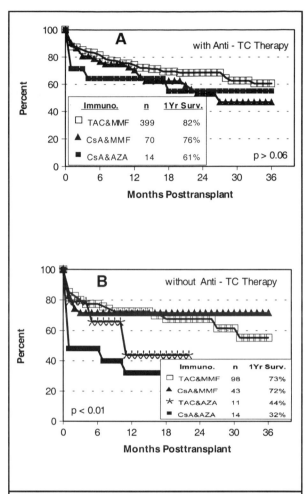

Figure 38. Pancreas graft survival rates for 1996-2000 US cadaver PAK transplants by initial maintenance immunosuppression in recipients (A) given or (B) not given anti-T cell therapy for induction.

the Zenapax/Simulect (n=271), ATG/ALG (n=107), OKT3 (n=195), and none (n=582) subgroups were 91%, 83%, 81% and 82%, respectively (P=0.13). In the BD subset (n=653), the GSRs with the corresponding induction agents were 87% (n=108), 86% (n=186), 88% (n=223) and 82% (n=200), respectively (P=NS).

PAK outcome by immunosuppression (Fig. 38 and 39): More than two-thirds of 1996-2000 PAK recipients were given anti-T-cell agents (Fig. 38A), while one-third were not (Fig. 38B). For those given anti-T-cell agents (Fig. 38A), the pancreas GSRs were highest with the TAC-MMF combination for maintenance immunosup-

pression, 82% at one year. In the PAK recipients not given the anti-T-cell induction (Fig. 38B), pancreas GSRs were similar for TAC-MMF or CSA-MMF for maintenance. Within each maintenance therapy subgroup, the pancreas GSRs were higher (P=NS) in recipients given versus those not given anti-T-cell induction.

In the PAK recipients given anti-T-cell therapy with one agent (~5% had more than one), overall the results differed little according to the agent used (Fig. 39). What differences were seen were largely attributable to the BD subset of the PAK population. With BD (n=249), the one-year GSRs for the ATG/ALG (n=67), OKT3 (n=25), Zenapax/Simulect (n=97) and none (n=60) subgroups were 84%, 82%, 68% and 79%, respectively (P=0.01). In the ED subset (n=201), the GSRs with the correspond-

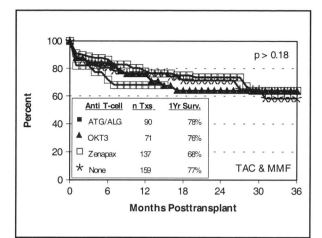

Figure 39. Pancreas graft survival rates by induction anti T-cell agents used in 1996-2000 US PAK recipients.

ing subgroups were 59% (n=23), 73% (n=46), 69% (n=140), and 74% (n=95), respectively (P=NS).

PTA outcome by immunosuppression (Fig. 40 and 41): Four-fifths of PTA recipients were given anti-T-cell agents for induction (Fig. 40A) and 20% were not (Fig. 40B). Nearly 90% of the anti-T-cell group and virtually all of the non-anti-T-cell group were given TAC-MMF for maintenance immunosuppression. The PTA GSRs in TAC-MMF treated recipients were slightly higher in those given versus not given anti-T-cell induction, 77% versus 72% at one year.

There were no significant differences in PTA GSRs overall according to the anti-T-cell agent given (Fig. 41) (~11% were given more than one agent and are not included), and this was the case in both the BD (n=113) and ED (n=88) subsets. In BD PTA recipients given Zenapax/Simulect (n=42), ATG/ALG (n=20), OKT3 (n=19) or none (n=32), one-year GSRs were 79%, 66%, 89% and 83%, respectively. In the ED PTA recipients given the corresponding induction agents, the one-year GSRs were 89% (n=10), 75% (n=4), 71% (n=28) and 68% (n=46).

Pancreas transplant outcome by category and duct management in recipients given anti-T-cell induction and TAC/MMF immunosuppression (Fig. 42): In the solitary pancreas transplant categories (PAK and PTA), the highest GSRs were associated with anti-T-cell therapy for induction and TAC-MMF for maintenance immunosuppression. In the overall analyses, the duct management technique had an impact on GSRs in the solitary pancreas transplant categories, but even with

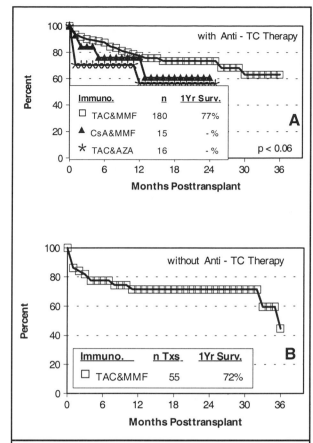

Figure 40. Pancreas graft survival rates for 1996-2000 US cadaver PTA transplants by initial maintenance immunosuppression in recipients (A) given or (B) not given anti-T cell therapy for induction.

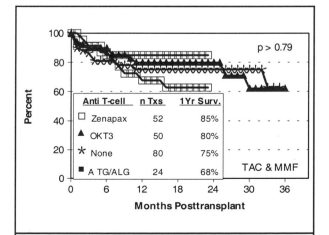

Figure 41. Pancreas graft survival rates by induction anti T-cell agents used in 1996-2000 US PTA recipients.

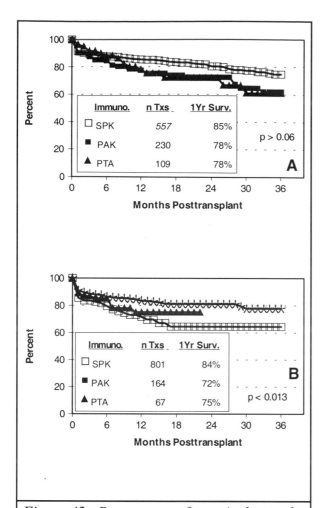

Figure 42. Pancreas graft survival rates by category for 1996-2000 US recipients of cadaver (A) BD or (B) ED transplants given anti-T cell agents for induction and TAC-MMF for initial maintenance immunosuppression.

BD, the outcome did not equal those in SPK recipients. It is possible that an improved immunosuppressive regimen could overcome these differences. Thus, GSRs were calculated in each category for the sub-groups treated with the immunosuppressive regimen that had the biggest impact in the solitary groups: anti-T-cell agents for induction and TAC-MMF for maintenance. With either BD (Fig. 42A) or ED (Fig. 42B), this regimen did not eliminate the differences in GSRs between SPK and solitary pancreas transplant recipients.

With BD (Fig. 42A), PAK and PTA GSRs were marginally significantly lower than for SPK; with ED (Fig. 42B), they were significantly lower. With this immunosuppres-

sive regimen, BD and ED SPK recipients had similar pancreas GSRs, but in PAK and PTA recipients the GSRs were still slightly higher with BD. Nevertheless, the GSRs in solitary pancreas transplant recipients were over 70% at one year, regardless of duct management technique.

Logistic and Cox Multivariate Analysis of Outcome in US Pancreas Transplants by Recipient Category

The univariate analyses presented in the preceding sections were supplemented by Cox multivariate and logistic regression analyses on 1996-2000 US cases in an attempt to calculate more precisely the impact of single variables at the same time (Table 4-7). Because of the differences in demographics and because each recipient category behaves differently, separate analyses were performed for SPK, PAK and PTA cases. Four separate analyses of relative risks (RRs) were done in each category: patient survival (Table 4); pancreas graft survival with all cases, including DWFGs as a failure, in the model (Table 5); TS pancreas graft failures for immunological reasons, with DWFGs censored (Table 6); and pancreas graft failures for technical reasons (Table 7).

Variables included in all Cox logistic regression models were: duct management; donor and recipient age (older vs. <45 years); donor cause of death (cardiovascular disease vs. traumatic causes); increasing number of HLA mismatches at each loci (A, B, and DR); preservation time (12-hour increments); recipient body mass index (BMI) above versus below 25 kg/m^2; retransplants versus primary transplants; use of anti-T-cell therapy for induction immunosuppression; and the use of TAC and MMF for initial maintenance immunosuppression. In the Tables summarizing each analysis the RRs are given for variables associated with a P value of <0.20.

Relative risks for patient survival (Table 4). In the SPK category the variable with the most significant negative effect on patient survival was recipient age, but duct management, donor cause of death (cardiovascular) and retransplantation also had an effect. Use of MMF was associated with a positive effect on SPK patient survival. In the PAK category, increasing donor age and retransplantation had significant negative effects on patient survival probabilities. In the PTA category, none of the studied risk factors had an impact on patient survival, consistent with the univariate analyses in which PTA patient survival was excellent in all subgroups.

Relative risks for pancreas graft survival (Table 5). In regard to the RR for graft loss for any reason in the SPK category, the significant factors increasing risk were donor age and donor cause of death. SPK recipient age (>45 years) and BMI (>25 Kg/m^2) modestly increased the risk for graft failure, while use of MMF reduced the risk. For PAK transplants, donor cardiovascular death and mismatching at the HLA-B locus had a negative effect on graft survival as did a high recipient BMI, while use of TAC had a positive effect. In PTA, the only variable with a negative impact on graft survival was retransplantation. Use of TAC strongly promoted PTA graft survival, and use of MMF also had a positive effect as did increasing recipient age.

Relative risks for immunological pancreas graft failure (Table 6). No variable strongly increased the RR for graft rejection in SPK recipients. MMF use was associated with a decreased risk of rejection in SPK transplants. In PAK recipients, retransplantation increased the risk of rejection loss. Older age and the use of MMF decreased the relative risk of rejection. In PTA recipients, mismatching at the B locus and retransplantation were associated with an increased risk of rejection loss, while use of anti-T-cell agents for induction or TAC for maintenance immunosuppression decreased the risk, as did increasing recipient age.

Relative risk for pancreas graft technical failure (Table 7). A logistic regression analysis assessed the RRs of several variables on TFs in each recipient category. In the SPK category, donor age >45 years and cardiovascular death increased the risk for TF, as did prolonged preservation, high BMI in the recipient, and retransplantation. Conversely, use of BD decreased the risk of TF in SPK recipients. The use of MMF decreased the RR of graft loss being classified as technical. In the

PAK category, HLA-B mismatching increased the risk for a graft outcome to be classified as a TF. Prolonged preservation also increased the TF risk in PAK recipients. The use of TAC and MMF decreased the RR of a graft loss being classified as technical. In the PTA category, only the use of TAC and MMF decreased the RR for TF. Paradoxically, MMF was associated with decreased risk for TF in all categories, as was TAC in PAK and PTA, again raising the question as to whether some graft losses classified as technical are really immunological.

Table 4. Relative risks (RR) for patient survival.

Variables	SPK		PAK		PTA	
	P	RR*	p	RR*	p	RR*
BD vs. ED	0.006	1.63	0.70	-	-	-
Donor age [45yrs]	0.71	-	0.05	3.07	0.99	-
Donor cause death	0.41	1.35	0.33	-	0.99	-
HLA MM A	0.52	-	0.27	-	0.99	-
HLA MM B	0.63	-	0.31	-	0.99	-
HLA MM DR	0.66	-	0.72	-	0.99	-
Pres. time [12hr]	0.90	-	0.44	-	0.99	-
Recipient age [45yrs]	0.0003	1.96	0.22	-	0.99	-
Retransplant	0.11	2.26	0.04	2.45	0.99	-
Anti-T-cell Therapy	0.41	-	0.75	-	0.99	-
TAC	0.37	-	0.38	-	0.99	-
MMF	0.07	0.68	0.79	-	0.99	-

*Given only if p<0.2

Table 5. Relative risks (RR) for graft survival.

Variables	SPK		PAK		PTA	
	P	RR*	p	RR*	p	RR*
BD vs. ED	0.85	-	0.21	-	-	-
Donor age [45yrs]	0.07	1.32	0.52	-	0.25	-
Donor cause death	0.002	1.42	0.003	1.83	0.61	-
HLA MM A	0.18	1.11	0.02	0.70	0.30	
HLA MM B	0.52	-	0.02	1.44	0.33	
HLA MM DR	0.53	-	0.45	-	0.47	-
Pres. time [12hr]	0.49	-	0.33	-	0.11	0.58
Recipient age [45yrs]	0.11	1.20	0.47	-	0.02	0.28
BMI [25kg/m^2]	0.19	1.14	0.10	1.37	0.64	-
Retransplant	0.11	1.72	0.34	-	0.008	2.76
Anti-T-cell Therapy	0.06	0.82	0.84	-	0.41	-
TAC	0.39	-	0.06	0.68	0.004	0.40
MMF	0.002	0.68	0.43	-	0.05	0.50

*Given only if p<0.2

Comment. Overall, the multivariate analysis showed that several factors have a variable influence on recipient and graft survival or failure probabilities for technical or immunological reasons, depending on the recipient category. Some of the findings call into question the interpretations of causes of graft failure.

NON-US ANALYSIS

Reporting of non-US pancreas transplants to the IPTR is not mandatory, and therefore the number for analysis is much less than for US cases. However, even though there is underreporting of non-US cases, the incidence of pancreas transplantation also appears to be truly lower outside of the US, including Europe (Fig. 43).

The annual number of non-US cases by recipient category reported to the IPTR between 1988-1999 is shown in Figure 44. As in the US, most of the non-US transplants are SPK, but the proportion of solitary transplants is even lower for non-US than for US. Figure 45 shows the non-US cases for which the pancreas graft duct management technique was reported. As in the US, the proportion that are ED has increased progressively and since 1998 has been >50%. Indeed, for the year 2000 cases reported (not shown), the proportion that were ED was ~75%.

SPK outcomes for 1996-2000 non-US cases are shown in Figure 46. Patient (Fig. 47A) and pancreas graft (Fig. 47B) survival rates were nearly identical with those for 1996-2000 US SPK transplants, but the kidney GSR (Fig. 47C) was inexplicably slightly lower for non-US cases. A separate analysis of European SPK transplants showed outcomes identical to that of all non-US cases, concordant with a previous comparison of outcomes in Europe and the US (4).

The number of solitary pancreas transplants reported from outside the US is very small (Fig. 48), so only a collective analysis of non-US cases is possible (Fig. 48). For the 1996-2000 non-US PAK cases (n=27) that were reported, the outcome was excellent, with a one-year patient survival rate of 100% and a pancreas GSR of 81% (vs. 72% for all US cases and 78% in the BD subset given anti-T-cell agents for induction and TAC-MMF for maintenance immunosuppression). For 1996-2000 non-US PTA cases (n=38), the patient survival rate at one year was 97%, but the GSR was only 54% at one

Table 6. Relative risks (RR) for pancreas rejection.

Variables	SPK		PAK		PTA	
	P	RR*	p	RR*	p	RR*
BD vs. ED	0.61	-	0.73	-	-	-
Donor age [45yrs]	0.97	-	0.20	-	0.99	-
Donor cause death	0.82	-	0.45	-	0.21	-
HLA MM A	0.37	-	0.30	-	0.78	-
HLA MM B	0.61	-	0.27	-	0.05	2.68
HLA MM DR	0.49	-	0.11	0.57	0.73	-
Pres. time [12hr]	0.34	-	0.68	-	0.52	-
Recipient age [45yrs]	0.38	-	0.13	0.39	0.13	0.20
Retransplant	0.69	-	0.04	2.43	0.02	4.49
Anti-T-cell Therapy	0.61	-	0.51	-	0.03	0.25
TAC	0.61	-	0.05	0.43	0.11	0.40
MMF	0.05	0.55	0.64	-	0.27	-

*Given only if p<0.2

Table 7. Relative risks (RR) for technical failures.

Variables	SPK		PAK		PTA	
	P	RR*	p	RR*	p	RR*
BD vs. ED	0.05	0.73	0.26	-	-	-
Donor age [45yrs]	0.14	1.40	0.80	-	0.30	-
Donor cause death	0.002	1.73	0.21	-	0.49	-
HLA MM A	0.10	1.23	0.02	0.60	0.58	-
HLA MM B	0.48	-	0.008	2.12	0.21	-
HLA MM DR	0.74	-	0.61	-	0.57	-
Pres. time [12hr]	0.09	1.34	0.006	2.41	0.23	-
Recipient age [45yrs]	0.84	-	0.88	-	0.61	-
BMI [25kg/m^2]	0.017	1.46	0.24	-	0.45	-
Retransplant	0.09	2.31	0.67	-	0.42	-
Anti-T-cell Therapy	0.13	0.77	0.40	-	0.76	-
TAC	0.77	-	0.09	0.55	0.04	0.27
MMF	0.009	0.59	0.14	0.50	0.02	0.21

*Given only if p<0.2

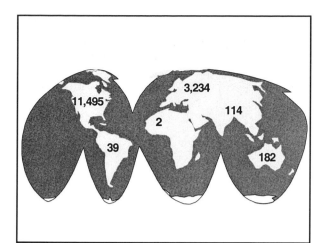

Figure 43. Number of pancreas transplants reported to the IPTR by continent from October 1987 to July 2000.

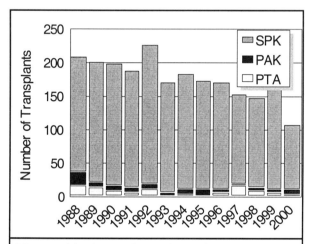

Figure 44. Annual number of non-US pancreas transplants reported to the IPTR by recipient category, 1988-99.

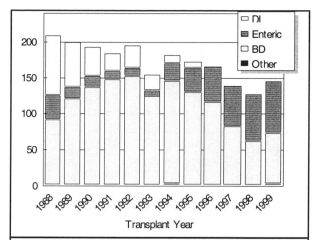

Figure 45. Annual number of non-US pancreas transplants reported to the IPTR when duct management technique is known, 1988-99.

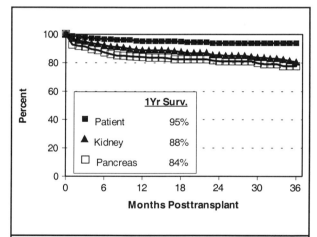

Figure 46. Patient survival and pancreas and kidney functional survival rates for non-US SPK transplants, 1996-2000.

year (vs. 71% for all US PTA cases and 78% in the BD subset given anti-T-cell agents for induction and TAC-MMF for maintenance immunosuppression [Figure 42A]).

In regard to pancreas graft duct management, there were too few non-US solitary cases for analysis. For non-US SPK transplants, a comparison of outcome by duct management was made to US SPK cases for the 1996-2000 period (Table 8). With BD, there were no significant differences between patient and pancreas graft survival rates, but again kidney graft survival rates were slightly higher for US versus non-US cases. With ED, patient and kidney graft survival rates were similar for US and non-US cases, but pancreas graft survival rates were slightly higher for non-US cases. For non-US SPK

transplants, pancreas graft survival rates were not significantly different for ED versus BD cases, while kidney graft survival rates were slightly higher for ED cases regardless of recipient location.

DISCUSSION

Pancreas transplant outcome improved dramatically in the last years of the twentieth century, but solitary pancreas transplant (PAK and PTA) GSRs are still not equivalent to those of SPK, even in anti-T-cell treated recipients given the potent immunosuppressants, TAC and MMF, for maintenance. Both the pancreas TF rates and the immunological graft failure rates have progressively

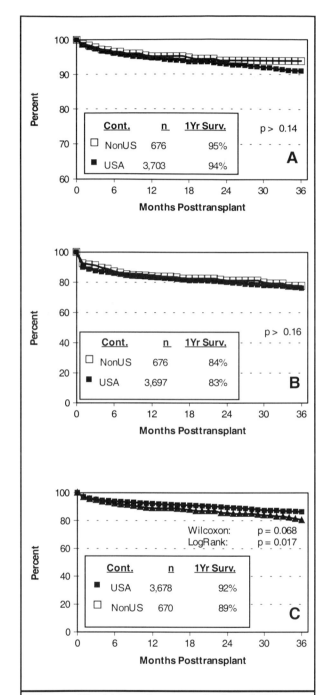

Figure 47. (A) patient survival and (B) pancreas and (C) kidney graft functional survival rates for 1996-2000 European vs. US SPK transplants.

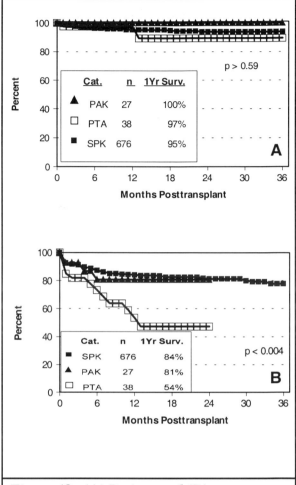

Figure 48. (A) Patient and (B) pancreas graft survival rates by recipient category for non-US cadaver transplants, 1996-2000.

declined in all recipient categories. For SPK transplants the immunological failure rate was extremely low, whether ED or BD were used. The TF rate for the last era (1998-2000) is only 7% and similar in all recipient categories.

The pancreas is the one solid organ that is not maximally utilized from the cadaver donor population, either in the US or elsewhere. Its application to SPK candidates is limited by kidney allocation, and the number of SPK transplants has plateaued. However, the number of solitary pancreas transplants is increasing annually. With the current rate of increase, the first decade of the twenty-first century should see every suitable organ utilized so the maximum number of diabetic patients can benefit from a procedure that consistently induces insulin-independence.

Table 8. Comparison of Non-US versus US one-year survival rates.

		BD		ED		p
		n	%	n	%	
Patient survival	non-US	314	96%	296	96%	NS
	US	1,536	94%	1,939	95%	p<0.03
	P	NS		NS		
Pancreas survival	non-US	314	85%	296	87%	NS
	US	1,536	85%	1,939	84%	NS
	P	NS		p=0.05		
Kidney survival	non-US	313	87%	296	91%	p=0.065
	US	1,537	91%	1,940	93%	p=0.012
	P	p=0.05		NS		

SUMMARY

As of October 2000, >15,000 pancreas transplant had been reported to the IPTR, >11,000 in the US and >4,000 outside the US. An era analysis of US cases from 1987-2000 showed a progressive improvement in outcome (p<0.04), with pancreas transplant graft survival rates (GSRs) going from 72% to 82% at one year for SPK cases, from 52% to 74% for PAK cases, and from 47% to 76% for PTA cases. The improvements were due both to decreases in technical failure (TF) rates (overall from 16% to 7%) and immunological failure rates (going from 8% to 2% for SPK, from 27% to 6% for PAK, and from 37% to 12% for PTA cases). The proportion of recipients >45 years old increased from 5% to 25%, and the improved outcomes encompassed the older patients as well. In patients >45 years old, SPK pancreas GSRs at one year increased from 62% to 78% (p<0.002). Pancreas GSRs were also similar for recipients reported to have Type 1 or Type 2 diabetes (at one year, 84% and 83%, respectively for 1996-2000 SPK transplants), the latter designated in 3% of the recipients.

Contemporary pancreas transplant outcomes were calculated separately for 1996-2000 US and non-US cases. US patient survival rates at one year were ≥94% in each recipient category, with one-year pancreas GSRs of 84% for SPK (n=3,697), 76% for PAK (n=696), and 71% for PTA (n=300) (p=0.0001). The immunological graft failure rates for 1996-2000 US SPK, PAK and PTA cases were 2%, 6%, and 8% at one year (p=0.001).

There was a progressive increase in the use of ED (as opposed to BD) for duct management, to >50% for 1996-2000 US SPK transplants. Approximately 20% of US SPK ED transplants had venous drainage via the portal system. Pancreas GSRs were not significantly different for 1996-2000 ED (n=1,940) and BD (n=1,541) US SPK transplants (83% and 84%, respectively, at one year), nor was there a difference in pancreas GSRs for systemic (n=1,509) versus portal (n=411) venous drained ED SPK transplants (83% for both at one year). Kidney GSRs were also not significantly different for ED versus BD US SPK cases, 93% versus 91% at one year (p=0.13). Duct management did matter for solitary (PAK and PTA) pancreas transplants (P≤0.07). Pancreas GSRs for PAK recipients were 77% at one year for BD (n=359) versus 67% for ED (n=306) US transplants; for PTA 75% (n=174) versus 63%. However, BD transplants were associated with a 12% conversion rate to ED by 2 years after transplantation.

Analyses of outcome by immunosuppression for US cases showed pancreas GSRs ranged from 77% to 88% at one year, but were highest in SPK recipients given anti-T-cell agents for induction and CSA-MMF for maintenance immunosuppression. For PAK and PTA recipients, those given anti-T-cell agents for induction and TAC-MMF for maintenance immunosuppression had the highest GSRs: 78% and 78%, respectively, at one year for BD pancreas transplants (vs. 85% in BD SPK recipients similarly immunosuppressed, P>0.08).

In regard to non-US cases, the overwhelming majority were in the SPK category (n=676 for 1996-2000), with a one-year pancreas GSR of 84%, not significantly different than for US cases.

In summary, pancreas transplant graft survival rates were >70% in the solitary (PAK and PTA) and >80% in SPK recipients during the last 4 years of the 20th century. These outcomes culminate a third of a century of application for the treatment of diabetes mellitus.

REFERENCES

1. Gruessner AC, Sutherland DER. Analysis of United States (US) and Non-US Pancreas Transplants as Reported to the International Pancreas Transplant Registry (IPTR) and to the United Network for Organ Sharing (UNOS). In JM Cecka, PI Terasaki, Eds. Clinical Transplants 1998. UCLA Tissue Typing Laboratory, Los Angeles, 1999: 53.

2. Harris MI. Diabetes in America, 2nd Edition, National Institutes of Health, NIH Publications No. 45-1468, Washington DC, 1995.

3. Cecka JM. The UNOS Scientific Renal Transplant Registry. In: JM Cecka, PI Terasaki, Eds. Clinical Transplants 1999. UCLA Immunogenetics Center, Los Angeles, 2000: 1.

4. Gruessner AC, Sutherland DER. Report for the International Pancreas Transplant Registry – 2000. Transplant Proc. 2001; 33 (in press).

CHAPTER 5

The OPTN Waiting List, 1988-1999

Ann M. Harper

United Network for Organ Sharing, Richmond, Virginia

The United Network for Organ Sharing (UNOS) is a tax-exempt, medical, scientific, and educational organization that operates the National Organ Procurement and Transplantation Network (OPTN) under contract to the Division of Organ Transplantation (DOT) of the Department of Health and Human Services (DHHS). UNOS maintains the organ-specific lists of all patients awaiting solid organ transplantation in the United States and operates a 24-hour Organ Center to assist in the placement of organs. The UNOS computer system (UNet[SM]) matches donors and recipients according to UNOS' allocation policies, which are developed by UNOS Committees and approved by the UNOS Board of Directors after being distributed for public comment. As part of the OPTN contract, UNOS maintains a database that includes information on every patient registered for an organ transplant since 1988, and follows each patient from listing to transplant or removal from the waiting list due to death or other reason.

This chapter provides detailed information about each organ-specific waiting list, including the number of patients waiting, percent of patients transplanted within specific time intervals after listing, and deaths while waiting for an organ transplant. Where possible, data are stratified by relevant medical and demographic characteristics, and analyses are provided in both tabular and graphical form.

METHODS

OPTN Waiting List Data

Waiting list data are entered electronically at the time the patient is registered for a transplant, usually by the personnel at the patient's transplant program. These data are updated by the listing center to reflect changes in the patient's medical urgency status and other medical factors collected on the waiting list. Because many of the variables entered into the waiting list database are used for the purposes of organ allocation, it is in the best interest of the center and the patient to provide UNOS with the most accurate data possible. Centers are required to remove patients from the waiting list in a timely manner (within 24 hours) following transplantation or death.

Registrations versus Patients

Patients may be registered on more than one organ waiting list (eg., liver and heart) or on multiple waiting lists for the same organ. A patient may also be listed more than once during year (removed and then relisted). Multiple listing (patients listed at more than one transplant center for the same organ) is allowed under current UNOS policy. For this reason, the snapshot and percent transplanted analyses are tabulated by registration rather than patient. In these analyses, the number of registrations may be slightly higher than the total number of patients registered. An analysis of the waiting list snapshot on November 30, 2000 (Table 1), shows that approximately 5% of all kidney patients were multiply listed, and no more than 3.2% of patients registered for all other organs (liver, heart, lung, pancreas, kidney-pancreas, heart-lung) were registered on more than one list. The tabulation of these data by registration rather than patient does not significantly impact the analyses, but allows each patient's data to be included wherever appropriate. Death rates are calculated on a per-patient basis.

Percent Transplanted versus Median Waiting Time

This chapter, unlike previous years', does not provide detailed information regarding median waiting times (MWT) to transplant. This is due in part to the fact that,

Table 1. Multiple Patient Listing

Organ	% of Patients Multiply Listed
Kidney	4.8
Liver	1.8
Heart	0.4
Lung	1.2
Kidney-Pancreas	3.2
Pancreas	0.9
Heart-Lung	0.5

Note: Derived from UNOS waiting list data on 10/31/00. "Multiply listed" indicates that patients are listed at more than one transplant center for the organ specified.

Calculation of Percent Transplanted

Percent transplanted data are provided for the cohort of patients added to the waiting list between January 1, 1999, and December 31, 1999. Additions to the waiting list are defined as new registrations to the waiting list during each year. The percent transplanted was computed using data from the OPTN active waiting list, waiting list removal files, and transplant data as of December 1, 2000. The percent of patients (registrations) transplanted at specific time intervals following listing (eg., 1 month, 1 year), are stratified by specific demographic and medical characteristics (eg., blood type, age, gender, medical urgency).

The percent transplanted at each time interval provides an estimate of the probability that patients with similar characteristics might be transplanted within that amount of time. The 95% confidence interval provides an indicator of the variability of the percentage; wide ranges indicate greater variability. It is extremely important to consider the confidence intervals that have been provided for each estimate. If the confidence intervals for 2 estimates overlap, then the numbers are not statistically different from one another. If there were fewer than 10 patient registrations in a subgroup who were still waiting at the time of analysis, the percent transplanted was not provided; these are denoted by 'NC'. The percent transplanted was computed using the Kaplan-Meier method (1) as contained in the LIFETEST procedure in SAS, version 8.1 (2).

as waiting times increase, it becomes more difficult to calculate the MWT for recent patient cohorts. A brief analysis of the trend in waiting times over time is shown for the cohort of patients added each year, during 1988-1999, stratified by year of entry (Fig. 1). As shown on the graph, MWTs could not be calculated for kidney patients who listed after 1997, or for lung patients who listed after 1998, because fewer than 50% of those patients had been transplanted at the time of this analysis.

In order to provide more up-to-date analyses, UNOS has begun reporting the percent of patients transplanted at specific time intervals following listing, which can be calculated for recent patient cohorts. Like MWTs, these data are most useful when stratified by medical and demographic characteristics relevant to each organ.

Stratification of Percent Transplanted

The percent of patients transplanted within specific time intervals following listing may vary greatly between individuals, transplant centers and areas of the country. These differences are caused by demographic and medical factors; for example, patients with blood type O tend to wait longer for a kidney transplant than patients with blood type AB due to a larger pool of compatible donors. For this reason, these data are most meaningful when stratified by specific medical and demographic characteristics.

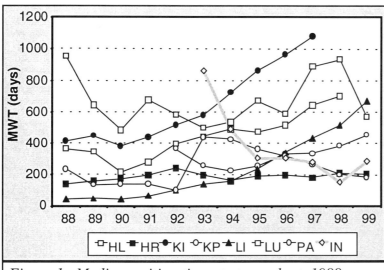

Figure 1. Median waiting times to transplant, 1988-1999.

Medical Urgency Status Codes

In addition to other demographic and medical characteristics, the waiting list snapshot and percent transplanted analyses for liver, intestine and heart are stratified by UNOS medical urgency status codes. The percent transplanted for heart-lung patients was not computed by medical urgency status due to the small number of patients involved. For kidney, kidney-pancreas, pancreas, lung, and heart-lung, patients are either in active or inactive status. Patients in inactive status are temporarily unavailable for a transplant, and do not receive offers for organs. The liver, intestine, heart, and heart-lung allocation systems use more complex status code systems, and are described in Tables 2-4.

The percent transplanted analyses for liver, intestine, and heart are provided using both the initial and final medical urgency status codes. The final status is either the status at transplant, at wait list removal, or the patient's current status if he was still waiting as of December 1, 2000. Only those status code combinations for which the final status was the same as or more urgent than the initial status were included; this encompasses the majority of cases. For example, the percent transplanted is shown for liver patients who were initially registered as Status 3 but were changed to Status 1. However, the percent transplanted is not shown for liver patients registered as Status 2B who were changed to Status 3. These data are also calculated for intervals specific to the medical urgency status, rather than at one year. For example, the percent transplanted for patients with an initial and final liver urgency status of 1 (very urgent) is provided for one week and one month after listing, while patients with an initial and final liver urgency status of 3 (least urgent) is provided for 6 months and one year.

Table 2. Liver Status Codes.

1 A patient age 18 or older with fulminant liver failure with a life expectancy of less than 7 days without a transplant; or pediatric transplant candidate less than 18 years of age in ICU due to acute or chronic liver failure, with a life expectancy of less than 7 days without a transplant. (See UNOS policies for description of fulminant liver failure.)

2A A patient in critical care unit due to chronic liver failure with a life expectancy of less than 7 days without a transplant and a long-term prognosis with a successful liver transplant equivalent to that of a patient with fulminant liver failure. Patient also has a Child-Turcotte-Pugh (CTP) score greater than or equal to 10 and meets other medical criteria. (See UNOS policies for description of CTP score and other medical criteria.)

2B A patient age 18 or older who has a CTP score greater than or equal to 10, or a CTP score greater than or equal to 7 and meets other medical criteria (see UNOS policies for description of CTP score and other medical criteria, and for pediatric medical criteria).

3 A patient who requires continuous care and, if age 18 and older, has a CTP score greater than or equal to 7.

7 Temporarily inactive.

Table 3. Intestine Status Codes

1 A patient who has liver function test abnormalities and/or no longer has vascular access through the subclavian, jugular or femoral veins for intravenous feeding, or has other medical indications that warrant intestinal organ transplantation on an urgent basis.

2 All other active registrations.

7 Temporarily inactive

Table 4. Heart and Heart-Lung Status Codes

1A Adult – A patient age 18 or older, admitted to listing hospital with at least one of the following: (a) mechanical circulatory support for acute hemodynamic decompensation; (b) mechanical circulatory support for more than 30 days with objective medical evidence of significant device-related complications; (c) mechanical ventilation, (d) continuous infusion of a single high-dose intravenous inotrope or multiple intravenous inotropes, in addition to continuous hemodynamic monitoring of left ventricular filling pressures, or (e) meets none of the criteria specified above but admitted to the listing hospital with a life expectancy without a heart transplant of less than 7 days.

Table 4. Heart and heart-lung status codes (Cont'd)

1A Pediatric —A patient under age 18 who meets at least one of the following criteria: (a) requires assistance with a ventilator; (b) requires assistance with a mechanical assist device; (c) requires assistance with a balloon pump; (d) is less than 6 months old with congenital or acquired heart disease exhibiting reactive pulmonary hypertension at greater than 50% of systemic level; (e) requires infusion of high-dose or multiple inotropes; or (f) meets none of the criteria specified above but has a life expectancy without a heart transplant of less than 14 days.

1B Adult – A patient who (a) has a left and/or right ventricular assist device implanted for more than 30 days; or (b) receives continuous infusion of intravenous inotropes.

Pediatric – A patient who (a) requires infusion of low-dose single inotropes, (b) is less than 6 months old and does not meet the criteria for Status 1A, or (c) exhibits growth failure (see UNOS policies for definition).

2 A patient of any age who does not meet the criteria for Status 1A or 1B.

7 Temporarily Inactive

Calculation of Annual Death Rates

Deaths on the waiting list for each year are reported using the ratio of the total number of waiting list deaths for the year to the number of patients "at risk" of dying on the list that year (ie., the number of patients ever waiting during the year). The formula used was:

$$\frac{\text{Total number of reported deaths during the year}}{\text{Total number of patients ever on the waiting list during the year}}$$

For example, if a total of 10,000 patients were waiting for a liver during 1999 and 1000 deaths were reported during that year, the death rate would equal 10%. This calculation includes patients who were on the list at any point during the year for any length of time.

RESULTS

Total Waiting List Registrations

The dramatic increase in the number of patients awaiting transplant is illustrated in Figure 2, which shows all patients ever on the waiting list during each year. The total registrations on the combined waiting list increased from just over 30,000 in 1988 to more than 100,000 in 1999. The number of liver registrants, now the second largest group of patients waiting, has increased nearly

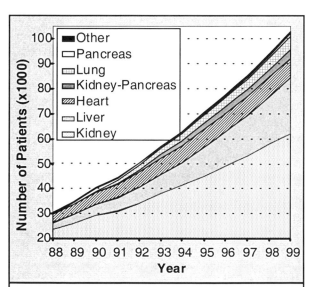

Figure 2. Total patients ever waiting, 1988-1999: all organs snapshot of the waiting list.

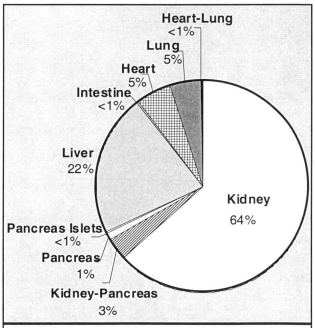

Figure 3. Composition of the combined UNOS waiting list by organ as of October 31, 2000.

9-fold since 1988. The lung waiting list showed the largest increase in registrants, growing from 148 patients in 1988 to 5,284 in 1999. The heart-lung, intestine, and pancreas islet waiting lists have been included in the "other" category, as these contribute less than 1% to the total.

The composition of the waiting list at midnight on October 31, 2000, is shown in Figure 3. There were 77,999 registrations on the UNOS combined waiting list, representing a 9.8% increase in total registrations over October 31, 1999 (71,024). The 49,456 kidney registrations represented 63.4% of all waiting list registrations. Liver registrations were the second largest group of potential candidates, with 16,731 registrations or 21.5% of total registrations; this represents a 16.6% increase in liver waiting list registrations over October 31, 1999 (14,343).

Details about the patients waiting on October 31, 2000, snapshot are presented in Tables 5-7, stratified by relevant medical and demographic characteristics. These tables can be summarized as follows:

- Patients with blood type O represented approximately 50% of registrations for all organs. Thirty percent of all registrations were of blood type A, ranging from 27.4 (kidney) to 38.0% (pancreas). Fewer than 1% of patients were listed with blood types A_1 or A_2; most of these patients were listed for a kidney.
- Approximately 18% of patients waiting for a kidney or pancreas had at least one prior transplant, while fewer than 3% of patients waiting for a kidney-pancreas, heart, heart-lung or lung had a prior transplant.
- Nearly 60% of all registrants were male, ranging from 40.3% (heart-lung) to 77.5% (heart). Approximately 60% of all registrants were white, ranging from 44.3% of kidney registrants to 85.7% of pancreas registrants. Blacks represented 25.6% of all registrants and 35.0% of all kidney registrants.
- Only 2.9% of all registrants were under the age of 18; however, 75.9% of registrants waiting for an intestine transplant and 15.7% of those waiting for a heart-lung transplant were pediatric patients.
- Only 12.7% of kidney registrations would be considered "highly sensitized" under current UNOS policy (PRA$\geq$80%), compared with 6.5% of kidney-pancreas and 5.6% of pancreas registrants. Sixty percent of kidney registrations and nearly 80% of kidney-pancreas and pancreas registrations had a current PRA level of less than 20%.

Table 5. Frequency distribution of patient characteristics based on the snapshot of the kidney, kidney-pancreas, and pancreas waiting lists on October 31, 2000.

	Kidney n	Kidney %	Kidney-Pancreas n	Kidney-Pancreas %	Pancreas n	Pancreas %
Blood Type						
O	25,964	52.5%	1,311	52.2%	456	46.3%
A	13,552	27.4%	797	31.8%	374	38.0%
A1	231	0.5%	7	0.3%	3	0.3%
A2	39	0.1%	0	0.0%	3	0.3%
B	8,410	17.0%	335	13.3%	121	12.3%
AB	1,260	2.5%	60	2.4%	27	2.7%
Previous Txs						
No	40,363	81.6%	2,472	98.5%	799	81.2%
Yes	9,093	18.4%	38	1.5%	185	18.8%
Sex						
Male	28,586	57.8%	1,417	56.5%	528	53.7%
Female	20,870	42.2%	1,093	43.5%	456	46.3%
Race/Ethnicity						
White	21,894	44.3%	1,973	78.6%	843	85.7%
Black	17,293	35.0%	333	13.3%	95	9.7%
Hispanic	6,507	13.2%	151	6.0%	33	3.4%
Asian	2,678	5.4%	29	1.2%	7	0.7%
Other	1,084	2.2%	24	1.0%	6	0.6%
Age						
0-17	628	1.3%	6	0.2%	9	0.9%
18+	48,828	98.7%	2,504	99.8%	975	99.1%
Current PRA (Panel-reactive Antibody)						
0-19	30,343	61.4%	1,929	76.9%	778	79.1%
20-79	37	13.4%	174	6.9%	70	7.1%
80+		12.7%	163	6.5%	55	5.6%
Not Rep		.5%	244	9.7%	81	8.2%
Patie						
Act			2,209	88.0%	716	72.8%
I			301	12.0%	268	27.2%
			510	100.0%	984	100.0%

Table 6. Frequency distribution of patient characteristics based on the snapshot of the heart and heart-lung waiting lists on October 31, 2000.

	Heart		Heart-Lung		Lung	
	n	%	n	%	n	%
Blood Type						
O	2,286	55.3%	119	55.1%	1,767	47.9%
A	1,325	32.0%	65	30.1%	1,349	36.6%
A1	16	0.4%	0	0.0%	0	0.0%
A2	4	0.1%	1	0.5%	1	0.0%
B	410	9.9%	19	8.8%	405	11.0%
AB	94	2.3%	12	5.6%	164	4.4%
Previous Txs						
No	4,023	97.3%	213	98.6%	3,588	97.3%
Yes	112	2.7%	3	1.4%	98	2.7%
Sex						
Male	3,203	77.5%	87	40.3%	1,494	40.5%
Female	932	22.5%	129	59.7%	2,192	59.5%
Race/Ethnicity						
White	3,239	78.3%	166	76.9%	3,098	84.0%
Black	554	13.4%	27	12.5%	354	9.6%
Hispanic	272	6.6%	18	8.3%	168	4.6%
Asian	41	1.0%	3	1.4%	38	1.0%
Other	29	0.7%	2	0.9%	28	0.8%
Age						
0-17	242	5.9%	34	15.7%	207	5.6%
18+	3,893	94.1%	182	84.3%	3,479	94.4%
Patient Status						
Active					2,555	69.3%
1A	118	2.9%	2	0.9%		
1B	398	9.6%	4	1.9%		
2	1,936	46.8%	130	60.2%		
7 / Inactive	1,683	40.7%	80	37.0%	1,131	30.7%
Total	4,135	100.0%	216	100.0%	3,686	100.0%

- Only 0.1% of liver registrants were in the most urgent medical status (Status 1); 2.9% of heart patients and 0.9% of heart-lung patients in the most urgent status (Status 1A). There are only 2 active statuses for intestine allocation, and 45% of those on the intestine waiting list were in Status 1.

Percent of Patients Transplanted

As shown in Figure 1, median waiting times (MWTs) to transplant have been increasing since 1988, and are highest for kidney, heart-lung, and lung patients. However, Figure 1 does not provide an explanation for these rising waiting times, nor does it help to identify the reasons for the differences in waiting times among those waiting for a transplant. In general, the increase in waiting times can be attributed to the growth in the waiting list relative to that of the donor supply. While the total number of registrants on the combined waiting list has more than tripled since 1988, the number of cadaver organs recovered for transplant has only increased by 74%, greatly increasing the gap between organ demand and supply. However, the continued increase in living donors (the number more than doubled since 1988), has the potential to mitigate this problem for some organs.

The reasons for the differences in waiting times between individual patients can be quite complicated, often related to each patient's specific circumstances. Tables 8-10, using percent transplanted within a specific period of time as an indicator of waiting time, are stratified by the factors that generally affect waiting time (eg., blood type, medical urgency status and PRA level).

Tables 8-10 provide estimates of the percent transplanted within one year for all patients added to the UNOS waiting list in 1999. These tables can be summarized as follows:

- Blood type is an important factor for patients waiting for a kidney transplant; patients with blood type O or B were much less likely to be transplanted within one year of listing than those with blood type A or AB. Females were as likely as males to receive a transplant within one year. A lower percentage of patients awaiting repeat transplants received a transplant than those awaiting their first transplant. Whites were more likely than other ethnic groups to receive a kidney transplant within one year. Children were much more likely to receive a transplant (37.0% vs. 18.4%; p<0.05), most likely due to preference given to children in the UNOS renal allocation system. The percentage of highly sensitized patients (PRA>80) transplanted was 14.3% compared with 20.6% (p>0.05) sensitized patients.
- Of those pa   kidney-pancreas

Table 7. *Frequency distribution of patient characteristics based on the snapshot of the liver, intestine, and heart waiting lists on October 31, 2000.*

	Liver		Intestine	
	n	%	n	%
Blood Type				
O	8,519	50.9%	64	48.1%
A	5,865	35.1%	44	
A1	40	0.2%	0	
A2	4	0.0%	0	0.0%
B	1,867	11.2%	20	15.0%
AB	436	2.6%	5	3.8%
Previous Txs				
No	15,880	94.9%	125	94.0%
Yes	851	5.1%	8	6.0%
Sex				
Male	9,610	57.4%	73	54.9%
Female	7,121	42.6%	60	45.1%
Race/Ethnicity				
White	12,531	74.9%	82	61.7%
Black	1,209	7.2%	32	24.1%
Hispanic	1,993	11.9%	16	12.0%
Asian	658	3.9%	3	2.3%
Other	340	2.0%	0	0.0%
Age				
0-17	1,012	6.0%	101	75.9%
18+	15,719	94.0%	32	24.1%
Medical Urgency Status				
1	12	0.1%	60	45.1%
2			36	27.1%
2A	50	0.3%		
2B	3,092	18.5%		
3	11,152	66.7%		
7	2,425	14.5%	37	27.8%
Total	16,731	100.0%	133	100.0%

transplant (55.0%), males (39.2), patients of "other" ethnicity (44.3%), Blacks (43.1%), and pediatric patients (54.7%) had the highest probability of receiving a transplant within one year of listing. For patients listed with an initial and final medical urgency status of 1, the percent transplanted at one week was 80%, versus 55.2% for patients with an initial and final status of 2A and 20% for patients with an initial status of 2B and a final status of 1. At 6 months, 70% of "2B:2A" patients and 63% of "3:1" patients had been transplanted. Only 6.7% of patients with an initial and final status of 3 had been transplanted at 6 months.

- Patients awaiting intestinal transplantation experienced relatively high transplant rates; ranging from 51.1% (blood type B) to 70.3% (males). Due to the small number of patients, the sample size was insufficient to calculate the percent transplanted for several categories. The percent transplanted for patients with an initial and final status of 1 was 45.9% within 6 months, versus 31.8% for 2:2 and 37.1% for 2:1.

- On the heart waiting list, patients with blood type O had the lowest probability of being transplanted, at 50.1% within one year. Patients with no previous transplant, males, Whites, and adults had similar percentage transplanted, at approximately 60%. Of patients with an initial and final medical urgency status code of 1A, just over 50% were transplanted within one month, compared with 36.6% of patients with an initial and final status of 1B and 23.3% for '1B:1A' patients. Approximately 50% of patients with an initial status of 2 and a final status of 1A or 1B were transplanted within 6 months.

- For lung candidates, the percent transplanted within one year ranged from 17.9% (Hispanics) to 32.4% (blood type AB). Patients awaiting primary transplants, females, and pediatric patients had the lowest percent transplanted at one year.

- Of heart-lung candidates, those with blood type AB had the highest percent transplanted, at 36.6%, versus 20.4% for those with blood type O. Males were not statistically different from females in terms of percent transplanted. Other comparisons could not be made due to small sample sizes.

Death Rates

More than 6,000 patients died while waiting for an organ transplant in 1999, almost 3 times more than in 1988. However, as shown in Figure 4, death rates have

transplant, patients with blood type AB were the most likely to receive a transplant (65.4% at one year). There were no statistical differences for repeat transplants, gender, or ethnicity.

- For pancreas transplant candidates, statistical differences were found only by blood type, ranging from 58.7% for patients with blood type B to 90.5% for patients with blood type AB.

- Of those waiting for a liver transplant, patients with blood type AB (60.2%), those with a previous

Table 8. Percent transplanted within one year for patients added to the kidney, pancreas, and kidney-pancreas waiting lists.

Organ	Kidney				Kidney-Pancreas				Pancreas			
		%	CI			%	CI			%	CI	
	n	Tx'd	Lower	Upper	n	Tx'd	Lower	Upper	n	Tx'd	Lower	Upper
Blood Type												
O	9,994	14.0	13.3	14.8	860	38.1	34.6	41.6	233	64.1	57.2	71.0
A	7,188	26.5	25.4	27.6	674	46.5	42.4	50.7	218	73.4	66.8	80.0
B	2,965	11.4	10.2	12.6	211	36.9	29.8	43.9	61	58.7	44.4	72.9
AB	835	43.3	39.6	47.0	63	65.4	52.4	78.4	16	90.5	73.4	100.0
Previous Txs												
No	18,031	19.6	18.9	20.2	1,762	42.0	39.5	44.5	332	68.2	62.3	74.1
Yes	2,951	15.4	14.0	16.8	46	40.8	23.6	58.0	196	68.8	61.8	75.7
Gender												
Male	12,451	19.3	18.6	20.1	1,034	43.6	40.3	46.9	265	70.2	63.9	76.5
Female	8,531	18.5	17.6	19.4	774	39.8	36.1	43.6	263	66.5	60.1	72.8
Ethnicity												
White	11,205	24.0	23.1	24.9	1,475	42.8	40.1	45.6	477	69.0	64.3	73.7
Black	5,841	13.7	12.7	14.6	214	42.5	35.4	49.6	26	NC	NC	NC
Hispanic	2,555	14.8	13.3	16.3	91	36.3	26.1	46.6	17	NC	NC	NC
Asian	996	11.6	9.5	13.7	13	NC	NC	NC	4	NC	NC	NC
Other	385	13.2	9.7	16.8	15	NC	NC	NC	4	NC	NC	
Age at Entry												
1-17	686	37.0	33.0	41.0	10	NC	NC	NC	8	NC	NC	NC
18+	20,296	18.4	17.8	19.0	1,798	42.1	39.6	44.6	520	68.7	64.2	73.2
Initial Peak PRA Level (Kidney Only)												
0	13,195	20.6	19.8	21.3								
1-79	4,464	19.5	18.3	20.8								
80 +	792	14.3	11.8	16.9								
Unknown	2,531	11.0	9.7	12.3								

Table 9. Percent transplanted within one year for patients added to the heart and liver waiting lists.

Organ	Liver				Intestine				Heart			
		%	CI			%	CI			%	CI	
	n	Tx'd	Lower	Upper	n	Tx'd	Lower	Upper	n	Tx'd	Lower	Upper
Blood Type												
O	4,986	31.4	30.0	32.9	83	67.5	53.7	81.3	1,579	50.1	47.2	53.0
A	3,873	40.7	39.0	42.5	45	59.2	37.4	81.0	1,412	68.5	65.6	71.3
B	1,270	43.3	40.2	46.3	17	51.1	19.6	82.6	409	69.4	63.8	74.9
AB	393	60.2	54.6	65.7	5	NC	NC	NC	144	83.2	75.1	90.7
Previous Txs												
No	9,638	35.9	34.9	37.0	131	62.8	50.9	74.6	3,404	60.9	59.0	62.8
Yes	884	55.0	50.9	59.1	19	NC	NC	NC	140	56.4	45.2	67.7
Gender												
Male	6,263	39.2	37.8	40.5	91	70.3	56.8	83.8	2,589	59.0	56.8	61.2
Female	4,259	34.7	33.1	36.3	59	51.7	35.5	67.8	955	65.9	62.3	69.6
Ethnicity												
White	7,955	36.9	35.7	38.1	109	67.4	54.5	80.2	2,747	59.7	57.5	61.8
Black	889	43.1	39.3	46.9	26	NC	NC	NC	502	63.0	58.0	68.1
Hispanic	1,077	36.0	32.8	39.3	9	NC	NC	NC	219	62.6	54.7	70.5
Asian	418	35.4	30.2	40.6	5	NC	NC	NC	46	NC	NC	NC

Table 9. (Cont'd)

Organ	Liver				Intestine				Heart			
	n	% Tx'd	CI Lower	Upper	n	% Tx'd	CI Lower	Upper	n	% Tx'd	CI Lower	Upper
Other	182	44.3	36.0	52.5	1	NC	NC	NC	29	NC	NC	NC
Not reported	1	NC	NC	NC	0	NC	NC	NC	1	NC	NC	NC
Age at Entry												
1-17	980	54.7	50.7	58.6	107	58.4	45.4	71.4	455	80.2	74.9	85.4
18+	9,542	35.9	34.8	36.9	43	NC	NC	NC	3,089	58.6	56.6	60.6
By Initial and Final Status*												
1:1	628	80.1	75.8	84.3	78	45.9	33.0	58.7				
1A:1A									473	51.6	46.6	56.7
1B:1A		* for liver, percent tx'd at 1 week for				* for intestine, percent tx'd at 6			215	23.3	17.5	29.1
1B:1B		statuses 1:1, 2A:2A and 2B:1, percent			months				383	36.6	31.6	41.5
2:1		tx'd at 6 months for all others			29	37.1	18.6	55.6				
2:1A									207	51.8	44.6	58.9
2:1B									367	49.1	43.9	54.4
2:2					22	31.8	10.6	53.1	1,030	26.3	23.5	29.1
2A:2A	230	55.2	48.2	62.2								
2B:1	74	20.0	10.6	29.4								
2B:2A	415	70.4	65.6	75.2					* for heart, percent tx'd at 1 month			
2B:2B	1,837	38.0	35.6	40.5					for statuses 1A:1A, 1B:1A, and			
3:1	58	63.8	50.3	77.2					1B:1B, percent tx'd at 6 months for			
3:2A	428	49.8	44.9	54.7					all others			
3:2B	1,739	21.6	19.6	23.6								
3:3	3,565	6.7	5.8	7.5								

Table 10. Percent transplanted within one year for patients added to the lung and heart-lung waiting lists.

Organ	Lung				Heart-Lung			
	n	% Tx'd	CI Lower	Upper	n	Tx'd	CI Lower	Upper
Blood Type								
O	1,009	20.0	17.2	22.8	53	20.4	7.6	33.2
A	789	24.3	20.9	27.7	34	36.6	16.6	56.6
B	273	31.2	25.0	37.5	15	NC	NC	NC
AB	86	32.4	21.4	43.4	7	NC	NC	NC
Previous Txs								
No	2,076	23.4	21.3	25.4	105	26.3	16.4	36.2
Yes	81	26.9	14.7	39.1	4	NC	NC	NC
Gender								
Male	991	27.5	24.3	30.6	47	29.6	14.6	44.5
Female	1,166	20.1	17.5	22.7	62	24.3	11.4	37.1
Race/Ethnicity								
White	1,825	24.2	22.0	26.4	83	26.0	15.1	37.0
Black	204	20.0	13.6	26.4	12	NC	NC	NC
Hispanic	90	17.9	8.9	26.8	10	NC	NC	NC
Asian	19	NC	NC	NC	3	NC	NC	NC
Other	19	NC	NC	NC	1	NC	NC	NC
Age at Entry								
1-17	215	18.8	12.2	25.4	25	NC	NC	NC
18+	1,942	23.9	21.7	26.0	84	23.1	12.7	33.5

Source: UNOS OPTN Waiting List and removal files as of December 1, 2000.

Notes: PCT represents the percentage of patients transplanted during the time period. The Lower and Upper CIs represent the 95% Confidence Interval.

N: denotes the number of new registrations during the year indicated.

NC: denotes not calculated due to small N.

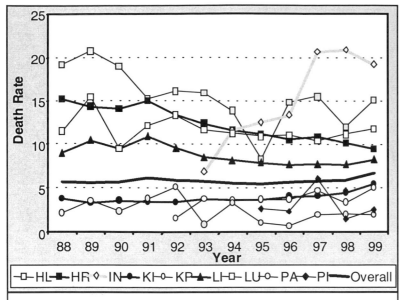

Figure 4. Annual death rates for each organ (1988-1999).

been declining for most patients awaiting life-saving organs, and have remained relatively stable for kidney, pancreas, and kidney-pancreas. Overall death rates have remained stable. In 1999, the highest death rates were for patients waiting for an intestine transplant (19.2%) followed by those waiting for a combined heart-lung transplant (15.0%). Death rates have been somewhat erratic for both of these organs because there are so few patients on these lists. Patients on the kidney and kidney-pancreas waiting lists experienced much lower death rates, most likely because of the less urgent nature of their illnesses and the availability of other treatments (dialysis and insulin). The mortality rates of kidney patients appear to be unaffected by the extreme length of their wait. Death rates for patients on the kidney waiting list have remained relatively flat, from 3.7% in 1988 to 5.4% in 1999. The trend in pancreas waiting list deaths has been erratic, although it has been stable since 1997.

DISCUSSION

As discussed in this and in previous years' chapters, the continuing increase in waiting list registrations coupled with a fairly constant donor supply has led to increasing waiting times and deaths (although not increasing death rates). The transplant community continues to grapple with issues of equity (making sure patients are treated in a similar fashion and have similar chances for transplant) versus utility (making sure the scarce supply of organs is used in the best way possible).

These questions continued to take the forefront in policy discussions during the past year. In particular, the UNOS Liver and Intestinal Transplantation Committee spent the bulk of the year discussing ways to improve the liver allocation system. The Model for End-Stage Liver Disease (MELD) scoring system, which would allow patients to be ranked based on their probability of pretransplant death within 3 months, has been examined by the liver community, and is being proposed as a replacement for the current UNOS Liver medical urgency status codes. UNOS is beginning data collection for a final validation of the MELD system prior to implementation. Ultimately, such a scoring system would incorporate posttransplant survival factors as well.

Similarly, the Thoracic Organ Transplantation Committee has proposed to replace the current thoracic medical urgency status codes with a continuous scoring system, which would attempt to balance pretransplant survival and posttransplant risk factors. The intent is to maximize the difference between pretransplant and posttransplant mortality. Thus, a patient with a high risk of pretransplant death but a good chance of posttransplant survival would most likely be ranked higher than a similar patient with a lower probability of posttransplant survival. It is anticipated that these models will be developed in 2001.

The Kidney-Pancreas Transplantation Committee, with the help of the UNOS Kidney Allocation Model (UKAM), is currently looking at ways to improve equity in renal allocation. Policies modeled thus far have analyzed the impact of mandatory sharing, paybacks, and points for HLA match and waiting time.

Committees have also discussed potential changes in organ allocation units. Most notably, the Liver Committee examined 14 policy proposals modeled by the UNOS Liver Allocation Model (ULAM) using 6 different organ allocation unit configurations, including redrawn regions, "super-regions," and combinations of OPOs, all of which increased per-million population within the sharing areas. However, the Liver Committee concluded that none of the proposals was clearly better than the others, and that the trade-offs caused by the severe organ shortage were evident in each of the proposals modeled. Additionally, it was believed that no change to organ allocation would have as significant an impact on the most medically urgent patients as the MELD system is anticipated to have, and thus further discussion related to organ allocation units has been postponed until the MELD system can be implemented and analyzed.

The "Final Rule" (3) requires that all UNOS allocation policies be reviewed in light of specific requirements, such as standardized criteria for patient listing, and the use of objective and measurable medical criteria for patient ranking. While several of these objectives have long been goals of the UNOS' Committees and Board as well, the requirements and other provisions of the Rule will to some extent provide the future context for UNOS deliberations. It is clear to those involved that the science and art of organ allocation policy will continue to evolve, and that each year will bring exciting and new challenges in improving the organ allocation system.

SUMMARY

1. On October 31, 2000, there were 77,999 registrations on the combined UNOS waiting list. Of these, 63% were awaiting kidney transplantation, and 21.5% were awaiting liver transplantation.

2. The majority of patients on the UNOS waiting list on October 31, 1999 were of blood type O (52%), White (56%) and male (58%), and awaiting their first transplant (87%).

3. Median waiting times have increased steadily for nearly every organ since 1988, especially for liver, kidney, and lung registrants.

4. In general, the percent transplanted within one year of listing is highly influenced by blood type and medical urgency. Patients awaiting heart, pancreas, and intestinal transplants experience the highest probability of receiving a transplant within one year.

5. Since 1988, death rates per patients waiting at risk have declined for most patients awaiting life-saving organs and have remained relatively stable for those awaiting a kidney transplant. Deaths are highest among intestinal patients, but appear to be declining.

UNOS OPTN WAITING LIST

REFERENCES

1. Kaplan EL, Meier P, Nonparametric estimation from incomplete observations. JASA 1958; 53:457.

2. The SAS Institute, Cary, NC.

3. 42 CFR Part 121, Organ Procurement and Transplantation Network; Final Rule (63 Federal Register 16295, at 16332, April 2, 1998).

ACKNOWLEDGMENTS

I wish to thank the staff of the UNOS Clinical Data Systems and Information Technology Departments for the data collection, entry, and maintenance of the OPTN database; the UNOS Research Department staff, and the organ procurement organizations and transplant centers for their timely and accurate submission of the data contained in this report.

UNOS DONOR REGISTRY

CHAPTER 6

Organ Donation in the United States: 1990-1999

John D. Rosendale and Maureen A. McBride

The United Network for Organ Sharing, Richmond, Virginia

The decade of the 1990s saw many changes and advances in the field of organ transplantation. As posttransplant care and survival rates continued to improve, the number of indications for which transplantation was the therapy of choice grew. While the transplant community attempts to keep up with the increasing demand for transplantable organs, the supply continues to fall far short of the need (Fig. 1). The challenge of expanding the donor pool has forced the community to look at new approaches to organ donation and to explore new sources of transplantable organs. As a result, over the past 10 years not only have organ donation rates changed, but so have the characteristics of the organ donors themselves. This chapter examines and quantifies some of the changes in the more than 51,000 cadaveric and 33,000 living donors reported between 1990-1999.

METHODS

The United Network for Organ Sharing (UNOS) administers the National Organ Procurement and Transplantation Network (OPTN) under contract to the Division of Organ Transplantation of the Department of Health and Human Services. The OPTN contract requires UNOS to collect extensive data on all organ donors in the United States. OPTN members submit donor information using the Cadaveric Donor (CDR) and Living Donor (LDR) Registration forms. The forms are reviewed for completeness and accuracy and validation reports are sent out to the organization that completed the forms, verifying the data on a monthly basis. Cadaveric and Living Donor Confirmation reports are sent out on an annual basis, verifying the number of donors and donor organs recovered. Both the CDR and LDR forms contain detailed information about the donors, including demographics and serology information. In addition, the

CDR form also includes consent information, clinical and social history and preservation techniques. UNOS began collecting donor data on October 1, 1987, and expanded the CDR form to collect more extensive data on April 1, 1994. Because many data elements were added in 1994, some cadaver donor characteristics are analyzed only from 1995 through 1999. Others are examined for 1990 through 1999. With the implementation of UNET[SM], the forms have been further expanded and will allow more in-depth analysis in the future.

A recovered cadaver donor is defined by UNOS as one from whom at least one vascularized solid organ (kidney, liver, pancreas, heart, lung, or intestine) was recovered for the purpose of organ transplantation. Cadavers from whom only hearts are recovered for heart valves or pancreata recovered for islet cells are not considered donors for the purpose of UNOS Registry analyses. An organ-specific donor is one from whom at least one of that particular organ was recovered for

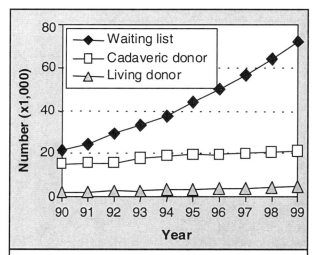

Figure 1. Total recovered organs and waiting list registrations: 1990-1999.

Clinical Transplants 2000, Cecka and Terasaki, Eds. UCLA Immunogenetics Center, Los Angeles, California

transplantation. For example, a donor from whom a heart and a kidney were recovered for the purposes of transplantation would be considered a kidney donor and a heart donor. A transplant donor is a donor from whom at least one vascularized solid organ was recovered and eventually transplanted. The statistics in this chapter are based on OPTN data as of January 4, 2000, and were calculated using version 8.1 of SAS (1). Data are subject to change based on future data submission and/or correction.

RESULTS

A patient who becomes a candidate for an organ transplant must, along with their physician, decide whether they are a candidate for a living or cadaveric organ transplant. Many factors go into this decision including the organ needed, the severity of illness, and the availability of a suitable living donor candidate. Each year the number of organ donors has increased. Figure 2 shows the number of organ donors by year categorized by donor type (living and cadaver). While the percent of all donors who were living donors has increased over the years (32% in 1990 to 45% in 1999), the largest supply of organs for transplantation in the United States still comes from cadaver donors. The following sections will concentrate on the cadaver donor.

Cadaver Donors

Overall

What is the cadaver donor potential? Estimates vary,

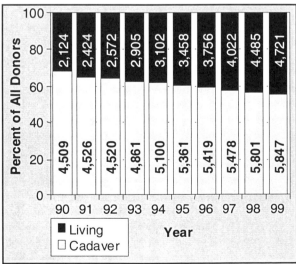

Figure 2. Cadaveric and living donors by year: 1990-1999.

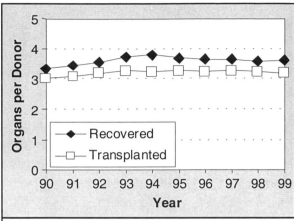

Figure 3. Organs recovered and organs transplanted per cadaveric donor recovered: 1990-1999.

but a recent study estimated the number of medically suitable organ donors to be between 12,000-15,000 annually (2). At the current rate of 3.19 organs recovered and transplanted per cadaver donor recovered (Fig. 3), this would amount to between 38,000-48,000 organs available to transplant. Of the potential donors that are identified, it is estimated that 50% of the families refuse to give consent for donation (2). Before an Organ Procurement Organization (OPO) can recover an organ from a cadaver donor, they must receive consent in order to proceed. Whether the consent comes from the next of kin, or from an advanced directive such as a living will, driver's license, or a donor card, the OPO must obtain permission to recover each organ. While we will not attempt to examine the consent issues for all potential donors, we will present data on differences in consent, recovery and transplantation of specific organs from actual donors.

In 1999, there were 5,847 cadaver donors. This number represents a 30% increase over the number of cadaver donors in 1990, but only a 0.7% increase over 1998. Preliminary numbers for 2000 show a growth rate of approximately 2-3%. Between 1990-1999, the number of organs recovered from these donors increased by 41% from 15,002 to 21,172. However, not all of the organs that are recovered are actually transplanted. Tables 1 and 2 show the number of organ-specific organ donors and the number of organs recovered and organs transplanted. The percent of recovered organs that were eventually transplanted decreased from 90% in 1990 to 85% in 1994, but has been approximately 88% since that time. Much of the increase in the recovered organs

Table 1. Number of cadaveric donors and organ-specific cadaveric donors by year: 1990-1999.

Donors	1990	1991	1992	1993	1994	1995	1996	1997	1998	1999	Total
Overall	4,509	4,526	4,520	4,861	5,100	5,361	5,419	5,478	5,801	5,847	51,422
Kidney	4,306	4,268	4,276	4,609	4,798	5,001	5,038	5,082	5,346	5,402	48,126
Liver	2,868	3,165	3,334	3,764	4,094	4,327	4,462	4,599	4,847	4,953	40,413
Pancreas	951	1,066	1,004	1,243	1,360	1,288	1,296	1,322	1,460	1,632	12,622
Heart	2,167	2,198	2,246	2,442	2,526	2,496	2,475	2,426	2,449	2,319	23,744
Lung	275	395	526	790	918	880	758	836	764	781	6,923
Intestine	6	11	21	34	62	121	48	72	78	97	550

transplanted since 1994 has been seen in pancreas, lung and intestine recovery. The number of organs recovered per donor increased each year from 1990-1994, likely due to the increase of extra-renal transplantation. Since 1994, the number has decreased slightly, which may be related to the recovery of less-than-optimal donors in response to the need to increase the donor pool. Figure 3 illustrates this trend.

Analysis of data on donors from whom at least one solid organ was recovered suggests a difference in consent requesting practices across organ types. Table 3 traces the organ recovery process of organs from cadaver donors in 1999. For the donors from whom at least one organ was recovered, the frequency with which each organ type was requested is shown. For those organs where consent was not requested, the reason for not requesting those organs is tabulated. If the request for consent was made, the percent of those who gave their consent is listed, and the reasons consent was denied are also given. For those organs for which consent was given, the percent recovered and reasons for not recovering are given. Lastly, for those organs that were recovered, the percent transplanted is listed.

The request rate for kidneys has remained steady at about 98-99% of donors from 1990-1999. The rate at which extra-renal organs are requested has risen between 1990-1999 to be at or close to the level of requests for kidneys. The largest increase was seen in lung, requests for which rose from 70% to 90%. Lungs may now be requested more often due to the increasing success of lung transplants and the growth in the number of lung programs. When consent was obtained, the recovery of lungs, livers, and pancreata increased during the period studied. In 1990, only 9% of donors from whom consent for lung donation was obtained actually resulted in a lung being recovered, as compared with 18% in 1999.

Table 2. Number of organs recovered and organs transplanted by year: 1990-1999.

		1990	1991	1992	1993	1994	1995	1996	1997	1998	1999
Kidney	Rec	8,549	8,479	8,501	9,163	9,531	9,928	10,020	10,087	10,607	10,720
	Txd	7,873	7,827	7,774	8,291	8,509	8,789	8,787	8,850	9,291	9,246
Liver	Rec	2,868	3,165	3,334	3,764	4,094	4,327	4,462	4,599	4,847	4,953
	Txd	2,645	2,894	3,011	3,380	3,571	3,859	3,976	4,036	4,350	4,439
Pancreas	Rec	951	1,066	1,004	1,243	1,360	1,288	1,296	1,322	1,460	1,632
	Txd	524	530	553	772	841	1,022	1,014	1,053	1,215	1,303
Heart	Rec	2,167	2,198	2,246	2,442	2,526	2,496	2,475	2,426	2,449	2,319
	Txd	2,134	2,166	2,202	2,349	2,400	2,421	2,370	2,351	2,392	2,245
Lung	Rec	461	684	932	1,462	1,694	1,634	1,407	1,554	1,391	1,451
	Txd	361	609	799	995	1,121	1,377	1,257	1,471	1,309	1,336
Intestine	Rec	6	11	21	34	62	121	48	72	78	97
	Txd	6	11	21	34	23	44	42	65	67	71
Total	Rec	15,002	15,603	16,038	18,108	19,267	19,794	19,708	20,060	20,832	21,172
	Txd	13,543	14,037	14,360	15,821	16,465	17,512	17,446	17,826	18,624	18,640

Table 3. Organ recovery process for cadaver donors in 1999.

	Kidney	Heart	Liver	Lung	Pancreas	Intestine
Consent requested						
Yes	98.9%	92.0%	99.3%	90.2%	88.9%	80.2%
No	1.1%	8.0%	0.7%	9.8%	11.1%	19.8%
Reason for no request						
Medical history	36.1%	13.1%	15.8%	11.4%	10.7%	3.3%
Organ quality	35.3%	13.5%	26.3%	19.2%	5.3%	5.2%
Age	18.0%	57.3%	10.5%	43.1%	70.6%	55.8%
Non-heart beating donor	0.0%	5.8%	23.7%	6.2%	5.4%	3.0%
ME/Coroner Case	0.0%	0.9%	0.0%	0.9%	0.3%	0.4%
Other	5.3%	2.6%	0.0%	11.6%	2.4%	22.9%
Not Reported	5.3%	6.8%	23.7%	7.6%	5.3%	9.4%
Consent obtained						
Yes	99.4%	94.8%	98.6%	92.5%	93.5%	83.6%
No	0.6%	5.2%	1.4%	7.5%	6.5%	16.4%
Reason consent not obtained						
Emotional	53.4%	63.1%	72.5%	56.4%	63.2%	58.1%
Cultural/Religious	1.4%	3.2%	3.8%	1.8%	2.1%	1.6%
Family conflict	8.2%	9.7%	1.3%	10.2%	9.2%	8.3%
Other	27.4%	18.6%	18.7%	18.7%	18.4%	27.2%
Not Reported	9.6%	5.4%	3.7%	12.9%	7.1%	4.8%
Recovery of consented organ took place						
Yes	93.8%	60.7%	87.9%	17.9%	39.7%	5.0%
No	6.2%	39.3%	12.1%	82.1%	60.3%	95.0%
Reason for no recovery						
Poor organ function	43.4%	46.3%	26.0%	51.6%	33.8%	19.8%
Cardiac arrest	0.3%	1.4%	1.5%	0.4%	0.7%	0.5%
Infection	0.3%	0.2%	0.3%	1.9%	0.2%	0.6%
Positive hepatitis	3.7%	4.6%	5.8%	1.8%	4.9%	3.0%
Diseased organ	3.8%	2.8%	7.6%	0.7%	2.0%	0.5%
Anatomical abnormalities	4.2%	0.7%	2.0%	0.4%	2.4%	0.8%
No recipient located	3.7%	6.4%	6.9%	4.4%	11.1%	28.8%
Donor history	12.3%	10.2%	6.0%	5.7%	12.5%	8.1%
Biopsy findings	1.1%	0.2%	14.4%	0.0%	0.3%	0.1%
Ruled out after OR evaluation	2.3%	1.6%	10.2%	1.2%	4.3%	0.2%
Trauma to organ	1.6%	0.7%	2.5%	1.3%	1.5%	0.9%
Medical examiner restricted	0.8%	1.7%	1.2%	0.9%	0.4%	0.3%
Ejection fraction <50%	0.0%	6.3%	0.0%	0.0%	0.0%	0.0%
PO_2 <200 on O_2 challenge	0.0%	0.0%	0.0%	9.1%	0.0%	0.0%
Hemodynamically unstable	0.0%	2.3%	3.8%	1.1%	2.6%	1.5%
Other	16.6%	9.6%	8.2%	8.2%	19.2%	30.4%
Not Reported	5.9%	5.0%	3.6%	11.3%	4.1%	4.5%
Organ Transplanted						
Yes	86.0%	73.1%	88.2%	77.0%	67.9%	37.0%
No	14.0%	26.9%	11.8%	23.0%	32.1%	63.0%

Pancreas and liver recovery rates also saw large increases (pancreas – from 30% to 40% of donors, and liver – from 72% to 88% of donors). Livers were requested, recovered and transplanted more often than the other extra-renal organs.

Demographics

In 1990, the typical cadaver donor was a white male with blood type O, between the ages of 18-34. This is still true in 1999, but some trends in donor characteristics have been observed. In 1999, females made up 43% of the donors as compared to 37% in 1990. The percent of donors who were minorities also rose (from 18% in 1990 to 24% in 1999). The most dramatic change was in donor age. As the need for more organs increases, the age of donors who are considered acceptable has increased. The percent of donors who were in the 18-34 year old age group dropped from 38% of all donors in 1990 to only 25% in 1999. The percent of donors who are older (50+) has been increasing over time. These trends are illustrated in Figure 4, and Table 4 shows the breakdown of recovered donors by more specific age groups from 1990-1999. While the median age in the United States general population has only increased by 3 years (from 33-36) since 1990 (3), the median age of donors has increased by 10 years (from 29-39) during the same time.

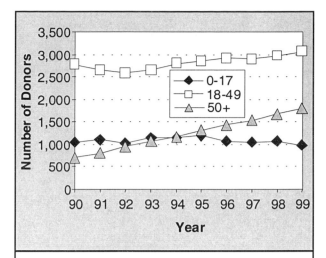

Figure 4. Cadaveric donor age over time: 1990-1999.

What is considered an acceptable age for a donor varies by organ and transplant program. While there are no definitive age ranges, an analysis of the data can provide an estimate of what most centers will accept for transplant. By looking at the inner 90% of the data (from the 5th to the 95th percentile), we eliminate many of the extreme ages that may be unacceptable to many transplant programs. Table 5 examines the inner 90% of the age data on an organ-specific basis. Since not all organs that are recovered are transplanted, the analysis is

Table 4. Age distribution of cadaver organ donors by year: 1990-1999.

	1990	1991	1992	1993	1994	1995	1996	1997	1998	1999
0-5 years	316	343	287	306	298	306	272	301	315	283
6-17 years	727	741	729	831	852	892	791	755	753	696
18-34 years	1,712	1,629	1,474	1,548	1,547	1,545	1,512	1,491	1,456	1,470
35-49 years	1,047	1,016	1,092	1,099	1,242	1,308	1,406	1,393	1,506	1,592
50-64 years	624	670	762	865	938	1,033	1,089	1,134	1,188	1,280
65+ years	83	127	176	212	223	277	349	404	492	523

Table 5. Age ranges for organ-specific cadaver transplant donors.

Transplanted	1990			1999		
	5th percentile	Median	95th percentile	5th percentile	Median	95th percentile
Kidney donors	5	28	59	7	37	64
Liver donors	2	24	53	6	37	68
Pancreas donors	11	26	48	12	23	48
Heart donors	3	25	48	4	28	53
Lung donors	12	23	46	10	29	55
US population		33			36	

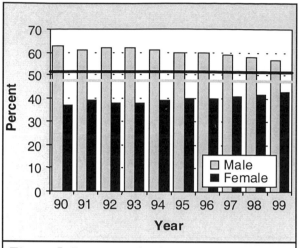

Figure 5. Donor and US population gender: 1990-1999.

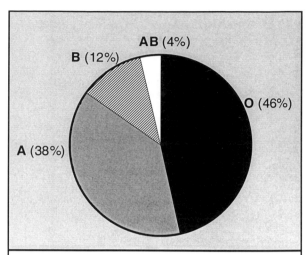

Figure 7. Blood group distribution of cadaver donors: 1999.

performed on only those organs that were actually transplanted. Analysis of transplanted organs is probably a more accurate estimate of the age ranges that most centers find to be acceptable. By comparing the numbers from 1990 and 1999, it can be observed that this acceptable range is changing over time.

The donor gender gap appears to be slowly closing. Females made up 43% of the donors in 1999 compared with only 37% in 1990. The rise has occurred during a time in which the percentage of women in the overall US population remained steady (3) (Fig. 5). Minorities have also begun to account for a larger percentage of the donors. While the number of white donors continues to increase, their proportion of the total has dropped with the increasing numbers of minority donors.

Figure 6 shows a comparison of donor population race/ethnicity between 1990-1999. There has been very little change in the distribution of blood types among donors. Figure 7 show the distribution of blood groups for donors in 1999.

On April 1, 1994, UNOS began collecting death data in 3 categories: cause of death, mechanism of death and circumstance of death. This allows a closer examination of what happened to the donor at the time of death. An analysis of the data from 1995-1999 performed on an organ-specific basis highlights some differences in causes of death. Kidney and liver donors were much more likely to die of natural causes than were pancreas, heart, lung, and intestine donors. In contrast, pancreas, heart, and lung donors were much more likely to have

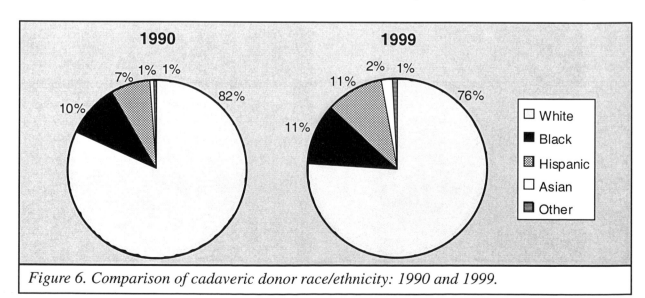

Figure 6. Comparison of cadaveric donor race/ethnicity: 1990 and 1999.

Table 6. Cause, mechanism and circumstance of death by organ type: 1995-1999.

	All donors	Kidney donors	Liver donors	Pancreas donors	Heart donors	Lung donors	Intestine donors
Cause of death	%	%	%	%	%	%	%
Anoxia	10.2	9.4	9.2	7.1	8.5	5.4	18.8
Cerebrovascular/stroke	40.6	40.1	40.1	26.6	27.0	32.3	17.1
Head trauma	44.1	45.5	45.6	61.3	59.5	57.3	54.1
Other/unknown	5.1	5.0	5.1	5.0	5.0	5.0	10.0
Mechansim of death	%	%	%	%	%	%	%
Blunt Injury	29.2	30.3	30.0	38.4	38.7	32.7	37.7
Gunshot/stab	12.5	12.9	13.3	20.2	18.1	21.9	9.6
Intracranial hemorrhage/stroke	42.7	42.3	42.3	28.7	29.6	34.2	21.9
None (natural causes)	3.7	3.4	3.5	3.3	4.2	3.9	12.0
Asphyxiation	2.6	2.5	2.5	2.4	2.8	1.5	4.3
Cardiovascular	4.2	3.9	3.8	2.6	1.9	1.6	4.6
Other/unknown	5.1	4.7	4.6	4.4	4.7	4.2	9.9
Circumstance of death	%	%	%	%	%	%	%
Homicide	6.2	6.3	6.4	9.3	8.5	9.9	5.5
Motor vehicle accident	24.3	25.3	25.2	33.7	32.8	27.8	27.4
None (natural causes)	48.9	47.7	47.6	33.2	35.0	37.8	38.5
Accident (non-motor vehicle)	8.9	8.9	8.8	8.0	8.5	8.3	11.3
Suicide	8.5	8.8	8.9	13.1	12.1	13.4	6.3
Other/unknown	3.2	3.0	3.1	2.7	3.1	2.8	11.0

died under violent circumstances (homicide, suicide or MVA), and were more often the victim of a gunshot or stabbing (Table 6). Examining the 3 categories together gives a more in-depth view of the death of the donor. Table 7 shows the top 5 combinations of cause, mechanism and circumstance of death, for all donors, and the top combination for each organ-specific donor.

Social and Medical History

The CDR form used between April 1, 1994, and October 24, 1999, included questions about donor chemical use (cigarettes, alcohol, and drugs), and were asked in 2 parts. In each case, the first question asked if the donor ever had a history of use (cigarettes and drugs) or dependency (alcohol), and the second question asked if

Table 7. Combinations of cause, mechanism and circumstance of death: 1995-1999.

	Cause of death	Mechanism of death	Circumstance of death	% of all combinations
All donors #1	Cerebrovascular	Intracranial Hemorrhage	None (Natural causes)	35%
All donors #2	Head Trauma	Blunt Injury	MVA	21%
All donors #3	Head Trauma	Gunshot/Stab	Suicide	7%
All donors #4	Head Trauma	Gunshot/Stab	Homicide	4%
All donors #5	Head Trauma	Gunshot/Stab	Accident (Non-MVA)	4%
Kidney donors #1	Cerebrovascular	Intracranial Hemorrhage	None (Natural causes)	35%
Liver donors #1	Cerebrovascular	Intracranial Hemorrhage	None (Natural causes)	35%
Pancreas donors #1	Head Trauma	Blunt Injury	MVA	30%
Heart donors #1	Head Trauma	Blunt Injury	MVA	29%
Lung donors #1	Cerebrovascular	Intracranial Hemorrhage	None (Natural causes)	28%
Intestine donors #1	Head Trauma	Blunt Injury	MVA	24%

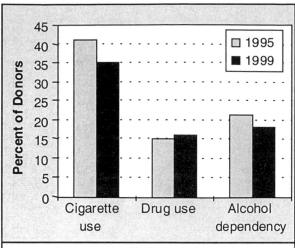

Figure 8. History of chemical use for donors: 1995 versus 1999.

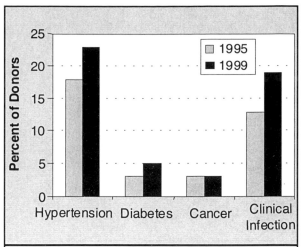

Figure 9. Medical history of cadaveric donors: 1995 versus 1999.

the donor continued to use or depend on the specified chemical. For the purpose of this analysis an answer of 'yes' to either question was counted as a history of use or dependency. Forty-five percent of the donors recovered in 1999 were reported to have had some history of chemical use or dependence (cigarette, drug or alcohol). Even with the expanding of the donor pool, the percent of donors who had a history of cigarette use or a history of alcohol dependency declined between 1995-1999 (41% to 35% and 21% to 18%, respectively). The proportion of donors who had a history of drug use remained fairly steady during the same time period (about 15% for drug use) (Fig. 8).

Also included on the CDR are questions about the donor's medical history as well as medications (either given to the donor within 24 hours prior to recovery or given to the donor in preparation for organ recovery following referral to the OPO). Figure 9 displays the percentage of donors who had a history of hypertension, diabetes or cancer, or who had an infection during the hospitalization that led to donation, While a small portion suffered from cancer, nearly a quarter of the donors had a history of hypertension. Nearly all donors received some type of pretreatment medication. The percentages in Table 8 are based on donors for whom medication information was reported.

Non-heart Beating Donors

In response to the increased use of and requests for information about non-heart beating donors, UNOS added a question to the April 1, 1994 revision of the CDR

form asking if the donor was a non-heart beating donor. In this section, characteristics of non-heart beating donors are examined since 1995, the first full year for which data are available.

Between 1995-1999, 32 different OPOs recovered at least one non-heart beating donor. However, the number of OPOs that recovered non-heart beating donors decreased each year from 1995-1998 (22 in 1995; 21 in 1996; 19 in 1997; 16 in 1998). The decrease may have been related to the controversy regarding their use. 1999 saw an increase in the number of OPOs recovering these donors (19 OPOs). The total number of donors and organs recovered has shown no consistent trend. Figure 10 shows the number of donors and organs recovered and transplanted from those donors during this time period. While kidneys are the organs most often

Table 8. Percentage of donors who received medication 24 hours prior to cross-clamp or in preparation for recovery: 1995-1999.

Medications	
Anticonvulsants	12%
Antihypertensives	12%
Dobutamine	10%
Dopamine	85%
Vasodilators	9%
Steroids	50%
Thyroxine - T4	15%
Diuretics	41%
Other medication	91%

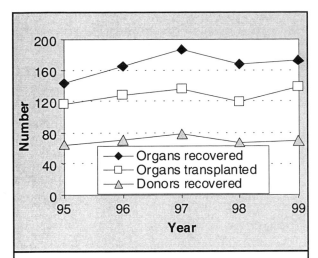

Figure 10. The number of non-heart-beating donors and organs recovered and transplanted: 1995-1999.

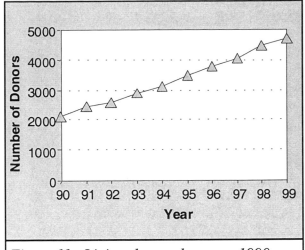

Figure 11. Living donors by year: 1990-1999.

recovered and transplanted from the non-heart beating donor, livers and pancreata are also being recovered and transplanted regularly.

Non-heart beating donors tend to be white (83%), males (64%) between the ages of 18-34 (30%), with blood type O (47%). The median age of these donors is 37, and the median age of donors from whom at least one organ was transplanted was 35. Table 9 gives a breakdown of the cause, mechanism and circumstance of death as well as the top 3 combinations of these categories for the non-heart beating donors.

Living Donors

As the shortage of organs worsens, and waiting times for cadaveric organs increases, patients and doctors are relying more on living donors as a source for organs. The number of living donors has increased every year, - increasing by a total of 122% between 1990-1999 (Fig. 11). In 1999, the number of living donors increased by over 5%, bringing the percentage of all donors who were living donors to 45%. In 1999, 4479 kidneys, 215 livers, 5 pancreata, one heart, and 26 lungs were recovered from living donors (Table 10). Occasionally, a recipient of a heart-lung combination from a cadaveric donor will donate their original heart to another recipient. This is why there are living heart donors.

Table 9. Cause, mechanism and circumstance of death for non-heartbeating donors: 1995-1999.

Cause of death	
Anoxia	27.5%
Cerebrovascular/stroke	21.2%
Head trauma	46.1%
Other/unknown	5.2%
Mechanism of death	
Blunt injury	34.7%
Gunshot/stab	12.9%
Intracranial hemorrhage/stroke	21.8%
Asphyxiation	5.4%
Cardiovascular	18.9%
None	2.3%
Other/unknown	4.0%
Circumstance of death	
Homicide	4.9%
Motor vehicle accident	27.2%
None (natural causes)	42.9%
Accident (non-motor vehicle)	11.2%
Suicide	13.8%

Combination of cause, mechanism and circumstance of death				
	Cause of death	Mechanism of death	Circumstance of death	% of all combinations
#1	Head trauma	Blunt injury	MVA	24%
#2	Cerebrovascular	Intracranial hemorrhage	None (natural causes)	19%
#3	Anoxia	Cardiovascular	None (natural causes)	12%

Table 10. Organ-specific living donors by year: 1990-1999.

	1990	1991	1992	1993	1994	1995	1996	1997	1998	1999
Kidney	2,095	2,393	2,535	2,851	3,009	3,365	3,654	3,910	4,350	4,479
Liver	14	22	33	36	60	46	56	76	86	215
Heart	12	4	1	2	3	0	1	0	0	1
Pancreas	2	1	3	2	2	7	11	6	2	5
Lung	1	4	0	14	30	45	42	33	47	26
Intestine	0	0	0	0	0	1	2	2	1	0

During 2000, UNOS began collecting more clinical information at the time of transplant and follow-up information on all living donors, but through 1999, only demographic information is available. While the majority of cadaveric donors are male, most living donors are female (57% in 1999). Living donors are most often between the ages of 35-49 (47% in 1999) with a median age of 39. The percent of living donors who are minorities has increased slightly from 24% in 1990 to 28% in 1999. Blacks and Hispanics made up 13% and 10%, respectively, of the living donors in 1999. While most living donors are genetically related to the recipient, the percentage of living donors who are not related (spouse or other unrelated) has increased from 5% in 1990 to 21% in 1999. Table 11 displays a breakdown of the demographic characteristics of the living donors recovered in 1999.

Table 11. Demographic characteristics for living donors in 1999.

	% of living donors
Relationship to recipient	
Parent	18.3%
Offspring	17.3%
Sibling	36.3%
Other relative	7.6%
Spouse (unrelated)	12.1%
Other unrelated	8.4%
Age	
0-17	0.0%
18-34	34.3%
35-49	47.1%
50+	18.6%
Race/Ethnicity	
White	72.3%
Black	13.1%
Hispanic	10.2%
Asian	2.4%
Other	2.0%
Gender	
Male	42.7%
Female	57.3%
Blood Type	
O	63.7%
A	27.3%
B	8.0%
AB	1.0%
*does not include unknown/not reported	

DISCUSSION

The growing success of transplantation continues to increase the demand for organs, yet the supply of cadaveric organs still falls far short of the need. As a result, waiting lists and waiting times are growing much longer. In an effort to meet this increased demand, more and more transplant programs are offering living donor transplantation as an alternative to cadaveric transplantation. In 1990, 2,124 people donated organs at 212 transplant centers. The number of living donors more than doubled by 1999, when 4,721 organs were donated at 236 transplant centers. In fact, living organ donation accounted for more than 50% of the kidney transplants performed at 21 centers in 1999. This trend appears to be continuing as preliminary numbers indicate that more than 5,000 people donated organs in 2000. What is sparking this dramatic increase in living organ donation? Excellent outcomes, low risk to the living donor, paired exchange kidney donation, success of adult-to-adult living liver donation, and anonymous living donation may all be part of the answer.

The very first kidney transplants involved living donors. As living donation has become a realistic option for other organs as well, a number of issues must be considered both for the donor and the recipient.

Living kidney donors. Living-related donor kidney transplants have long been documented to have superior survival rates compared with cadaver donor transplants (4). Additionally, living *unrelated* donors represent a large untapped resource of potential donors, and studies have indicated that recipients of living-unrelated kidney donor transplants also have superior outcomes compared with cadaveric kidney transplants (4,5). Postoperative mortality following living kidney donation has been calculated to be 1 in 3,000 cases, and the risk of other complications to the donor such as progressive renal failure, hypertension, and proteinuria do not appear to be increased by the donation of a healthy kidney (6). Laparoscopic donor nephrectomy has been reported to decrease post-operative surgical pain, result in shorter hospital stays and quicker recovery than standard open donor nephrectomy (7). All of these factors are leading to new living donation programs in an attempt to find suitable alternatives to cadaver donors for as many patients as possible.

Because living donation is such an appealing concept, 2 different kidney donor exchange programs have been proposed for cases where a patient has identified a living donor who would like to donate a kidney but is unable to do so because of blood type incompatibility. The first, "paired exchange," involves 2 pairs of individuals with incompatible blood types, where the potential donor of one pair would be compatible with the recipient in the other pair, and vice-versa. This is likely to be an option only for A and B blood type donor-recipient pairs; therefore, the number of transplants may be limited by the number of reciprocal pairs identified (8,9). The second program, "list-paired exchange," is a program in which the donor would provide his kidney to someone on the cadaveric waiting list in exchange for priority for the potential recipient to receive the next available kidney from the cadaveric donor pool. Both of these proposals are in the pilot phase in various regions of the US and involve complex ethical and logistical issues (10,11).

Living liver donors. The first living-related donor liver transplant occurred in November 1989. The number of living-donor liver transplants steadily increased over the subsequent 10 years, but rapidly accelerated in 1999 (Table 10). Much of this increase is due to the recent success of adult-to-adult living liver transplantation. Living liver donation in the pediatric population involved segmental transplantation, and its success spurred interest in living donation for the adult popula-

tion. However, the segment of the liver transplanted into a pediatric patient was generally deemed too small to meet the needs of an adult recipient. The right hepatic lobe is generally considered large enough for an adult recipient, but surgeons were skeptical about using this part of the liver due to the perceived risk to the donor (12). The first report of right lobe living donor liver transplantation that included a significant number of patients appeared in the literature in September 1999 (13). Reported recipient survival was approximately 88% immediately following transplant; long-term survival rates have not yet been reported.

Reports of living donor outcomes for pediatric transplantation show the overall incidence of complications ranging from 15-20% with approximately half classified as serious. There are fewer data available concerning outcomes of living donors for adult liver recipients. Reported complication rates range from 0% to greater than 50%. The most frequent complications among all living liver donors have been post-operative biliary complications. There has been very little reported mortality for living liver donors – approximately 0.13% (2 deaths in 1,500 transplants) for pediatric living donation, and 0.2% (1 death in 500 transplants) for adult living-donor liver transplant (14).

Living lung donors. Living lung transplants have been performed in the US since 1990, and living-donor lobar lung transplantation is now an acceptable alternative to cadaveric lung transplantation for selected recipients (15). The vast majority of living donor lung transplantation procedures has been performed on patients with cystic fibrosis, with favorable results (15-17). The University of Southern California has also reported successful outcome in their patients with diseases other than cystic fibrosis (18). Donor morbidity rates following surgery are apparently acceptable, and other than pain following the operation, and a 16-18% decrease in vital capacity, one center saw no other complications in donors and most returned to their usual activities (15).

Other living donors. Compared with living kidney and liver donor transplants, only a few living donor pancreas and intestine transplants have been performed, however a recent report indicated a lowered infection rate with living small bowel transplantation (19), so this field of living donor transplantation may also see an increase in the future.

A recent trend in living organ donation is the nondirected, "Good Samaritan," or stranger donor (20). This involves an individual who approaches a transplant center with the desire to donate an organ to an unknown candidate on the cadaveric waiting list. The majority of cases reported in the literature thus far involving non-directed donors have been kidney donors (21,22), but there is also at least one case of a non-directed liver donor as well (23).

As living donation becomes a larger part of nearly every transplant center's experience, the medical, social and ethical issues of live organ donation are of great interest to the entire transplant community. In order to address these issues, a national consensus conference on the living organ donor was held in June 2000. The goal of the conference was to evaluate current practices of care surrounding living donor transplantation. The conferees concluded "the person who gives consent to be a live organ donor should be competent, willing to donate, free of coercion, medically and psychosocially suitable, fully informed of the risks and benefits as a donor, and fully informed of the risks, benefits, and alternative treatment available to the recipient. The benefits to both donor and recipient must outweigh the risks associated with the donation and transplantation of the living donor organ" (11). The consensus statement was published following the meeting with the intention of providing practice guidelines for all those involved in the living donation process.

Given the low complication rate for donors and excellent results seen in recent years, we can only anticipate that living donation will continue to be further explored as an alternative to cadaveric transplantation.

SUMMARY AND ASSORTED FACTS

1. There were 5,847 cadaver and 4,721 living donors recovered in 1999, a 30% and 122% increase over those recovered in 1990.

2. The number of cadaver donors aged 50 or older has increased from 16% of all donors in 1990 to 31% of all donors in 1999.

3. The typical cadaver donor in 1999 was a white male with ABO blood type O between the ages of 18-34. In 1999, a typical living donor was a white female with ABO blood type O between the ages of 35-49.

4. Between 1990-1999, the percentage of minority donors increased for cadaver donors (18% to 24%), and for living donors (24% to 28%).

5. The number of living donors who were spouses or otherwise unrelated to the recipient increased from 5% in 1990 to 21% in 1999.

6. California (10.4%) was most often listed as the state of residence for cadaver donors, followed by Texas (7.5%) and Florida (6.8%).

7. Cadaver donors are recovered most often on Tuesdays (15.1%), followed by Wednesdays (14.6%) and Fridays (14.3%).

8. Living donors are recovered most often on Wednesdays (31.8%), followed by Tuesdays (27.5%) and Thursdays (20.9%).

9. Cadaver donors are recovered most often in August (8.8%), followed by May and October (8.7%).

10. Living donors are recovered most often in June (10.6%), followed by July (10.1%) and August (8.4%).

11. In 1999, there were 21.6 donors recovered per million population in the United States.

REFERENCES

1. SAS Procedures Guide, Version 8.1. SAS Institute, Inc., Cary, NC, 1999.

2. McNamara P and Beasley C: Determinants of Familial Consent to Organ Donation in the Hospital Setting. In: Clinical Transplants 1997. Cecka and Terasaki, Eds, UCLA Tissue Typing Laboratory, Los Angeles, California, 1998.

3. U.S. Census Bureau (1998). National Population Estimates. [On-line]. Available: http://www.census.gov/population/www/estimates/uspop.html.

4. Cecka JM. The UNOS Scientific Renal Transplant Registry. In JM Cecka, PI Terasaki,Eds. Clinical Transplants 1999. UCLA Tissue Typing Laboratory, Los Angeles, 2000; 1.

5. Gjertson DW and Cecka JM. Living unrelated donor kidney transplantation. Kidney Int 2000; 58 (2):491.

6. Tarantino A. Why should we implement living donation in renal transplantation? Clin Nephrol 2000; 53(4):55.

7. Schweitzer EJ, Wilson J, Jacobs S, et al. Increased rates of donation with laparoscopic donor nephrectomy. Ann Surg 2000; 232(3):392.

8. Delmonico FL, Stoff JS, Milford E, Harmon WE, Woodle ES. Living unrelated organ donation: an exchange proposal. Graft 1998; 1(3):119.

9. Terasaki PI, Gjertson DW, Cecka JM. Paired kidney exchange is not a solution to ABO incompatibility. Transplantation 1998; 65(2):291.

10. Ross LF, Woodle ES. Ethical issues in increasing living kidney donations by expanding kidney paired exchange programs. Transplantation 2000; 69(8):1539.

11. Delmonico FL and Authors for the Live Organ Donor Consensus Group. Consensus Statement on the Live Organ Donor. JAMA 284, 2000; 22:2919.

12. Marcos A. Right-lobe living donor liver transplantation. Liver Transp 2000; 6(6)S2:S59.

13. Marcos A, Ham JM, Fisher RA, Olzinski AT, Posner MP. Single-center analysis of the first 40 adult-to-adult living liver donor liver transplants using the right lobe. Liver Transp 2000; 6(3):296.

14. Renz JF, and Roberts JP. Long-term complications of living donor liver transplantation. Liver Transp 2000; 6(6)S2:S73.

15. Woo MS, MacLaughlin EF, Horn MV, et al. Living donor lobar lung transplantation: the pediatric experience. Pediatr Transplant 1998; 2(3):185.

16. Barbers RG. Cystic fibrosis: bilateral living lobar versus cadaveric lung transplantation. Am J Med Sci 1998; 315(3):155.

17. Shapiro BJ, Veeraraghavan S, Barbers RG. Lung transplantation for cystic fibrosis: an update and practical considerations for referring candidates. Curr Opin Pulm Med 1999; 5(6):365.

18. Starnes VA, Barr ML, Schenkel FA, et al. Experience with living-donor lobar transplantation for indications other than cystic fibrosis. J Thorac Cardiovasc Surg 1997; 144(6):917.

19. Cicalese L, Sileri P, Asolati M, Rastellini C, Abcarian H, Benedetti E. Low infectious complications in segmental living related small bowel transplantation in adults. Clin Transplant 2000; 14(6):567.

20. Spital A. Evolution of attitudes at U.S. transplant centers toward kidney donation by friends and altruistic strangers. Transplantation 2000; 69(8):1728.

21. Matas AJ, Garvey CA, Jacobs CL, Kahn JP. Nondirected living kidney donation from living donors – An opportunity to expand the donor pool. (Abstract 1119) Transplantation 2000; 69:S404.

22. Bartlett ST, Oldach D, Schimpff SC. Letter to the Editor. NEJM 2000; 343(3):1731.

23. Thomas G. Living donor liver transplant. Scarab 2000; 49(2):13.

ACKNOWLEDGEMENTS

We wish to thank the staff of the UNOS Clinical Data Systems and Information Technology Department for the data collection, entry, and maintenance of the OPTN database; the organ procurement organizations for the time and care involved in submitting data to the OPTN; and the UNOS Research Department, especially Mary D. Ellison. We also wish to thank all of the donors and their families for their precious gifts. Their generosity will not be forgotten.

CHAPTER 7

The Relevance of Proficiency Testing for Laboratories Involved in Cadaveric Organ Transplantation and Its Consequences for Graft Survival

Ilias I.N. Doxiadis [a], Marian Witvliet [a], Willem Verduyn [a], Peter de Lange, Janneke Tanke, Geziena M.Th. Schreuder [a], Guido G. Persijn [b], and Frans H.J. Claas [a]

[a]*Department of Immunohaematology and Blood Transfusion, Leiden University Medical Center and* [b]*Eurotransplant International Foundation, Leiden, THE NETHERLANDS*

It is generally considered that matching for HLA antigens is beneficial in cadaveric renal transplantation. Several national and international organizations have been established to allocate organs on the basis of HLA compatibility between donor and recipient. It is therefore important that HLA typing, screening and crossmatching in the participating centers is accurate. International histocompatibility workshops have shown that the reliability of HLA typing may vary between laboratories (1-3). In addition to HLA typing, screening patient sera for HLA specific antibodies and crossmatching are essential components of histocompatibility testing prior to transplantation. Here also accuracy and reliability must be guaranteed. Organ exchange organizations like Eurotransplant (ET), founded in 1967 by Professor J.J. van Rood (4), have established different proficiency testing schemes to improve and stabilize the reliability of the tests in the participating tissue-typing centers (TTC) (5). These programs include proficiency testing of HLA-A,-B,-DR typing, screening of sera for HLA specific antibodies and definition of the panel reactivity (termed percent PRA), crossmatching and molecular typing initially for HLA-DR and later also for HLA-A,-B. Here we report on the reliability of the results of proficiency testing within ET and the influence of accurate testing on graft survival.

PARTICIPANTS AND METHODS

The current ET proficiency testing programs include serological and molecular HLA typing, screening and crossmatching quality control exercises (QCE). All QCE are organized by the ETRL, which is located in Leiden, The Netherlands. Until 1996, all cadaver donors were routinely retyped in the Eurotransplant Reference Laboratory (ETRL).

Participants

All TTC working in the field of kidney transplantation and reporting relevant histocompatibility results to ET must participate in these proficiency tests. ET is an organ exchange organization in which 6 countries currently participate: Austria, Belgium, Germany, Luxembourg, Slovenia and The Netherlands. The TTC of Scandia Transplant and some individual non-ET laboratories in Germany also participate. In the current report, only the results of the 49 core ET TTC were analyzed.

Material

The ETRL sends out peripheral blood from healthy donors for HLA typing (8 times per year) and crossmatching; sera from multiparous women or patients for screening and definition of panel reactivity (4 sera 4 times per year); and DNA from cell lines, organ or blood donors (10 samples 2 times per year). The material sent out by regular mail is selected to mimic the situation of the daily routine of the participating TTC. Common as well as rare HLA types and easy as well as difficult sera are selected. For the screening exercises, sera from multiparous women, where the HLA type of the serum donor and the immunizing partner or children are known, are distributed. Sera containing autoantibodies have been excluded from distribution.

Reporting and Analysis of The Results

The participants are instructed to perform the respective exercises according to their usual local methods and report the results under a deadline. The data are analyzed centrally and the participants receive the results in an open manner. In essence, a 75% consensus is calculated for every typing sample. All deviations from the consensus are counted as a discrepancy.

Donor Retyping Program

Until the end of 1996, a spleen or peripheral blood sample from all the reported organ donors was sent to the ETRL (5), where typing was repeated by serology or molecular techniques. The results were reported back to the original donor-typing laboratory. In the current analysis, only the results of those TTC were included for which 10 or more retyping results per year were available. The number of TTC included varied from 29 to 31.

RESULTS

Donor Retyping Program

The reliability of HLA-A,-B typing within ET was previously reported to have increased from 64% in 1977 to

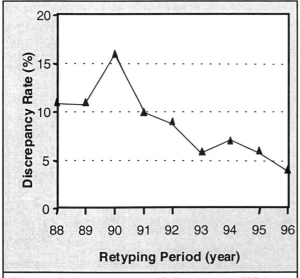

Figure 1. Percentage of discrepant HLA-A,B,DR typings of cadaveric donors in Eurotransplant between 1988-1996.

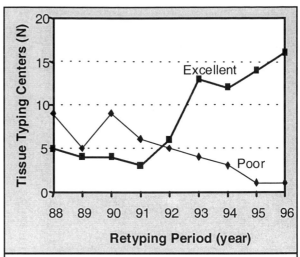

Figure 2. Increase in absolute numbers of excellent and decrease of poor performing tissue typing centers within Eurotransplant between 1988-1996.

94% in 1984. Over the same period the concordance of HLA-DR typing increased from 49% to 86% (5). Figure 1 presents the results of donor retyping for the period 1988-1996. Over this 9-year period the discrepancy rate for HLA-A,-B,-DR typing decreased from 11% in 1988 to 3.5% in 1996, the last year of the program. In Figure 2 the results are presented in a different way. The number of laboratories with a 100% (= excellent) concordance with the ETRL and those with a concordance of less than 85% (= poor) is presented. The latter number decreased with time and stabilized to a single laboratory in 1996, while the number of TTC with a 100% concordance increased gradually to 16. The introduction of molecular HLA-DR typing in 1990 contributed to the poorer results that year. The results of the donor-retyping program in 1995 showed a 2.7% higher discrepancy rate than the QCE on typing of the same period (6). This difference may be attributed to logistic problems during duty hours and to poor quality of donor typing material. Alternatively, QC typing material may be handled with special care (ie., the best technician is asked to perform the QCE).

Molecular Typing

Nine years ago the ETRL introduced a QCE on molecular typing. Initially, the participants only typed the HLA class II specificities. Later, after establishment of molecular typing for the HLA class I, these were also included in the QCE program. In view of the limited space, a short summary of the results obtained until now is presented. For the class II determinants (HLA-DR and HLA-DQ) the results of molecular typing are excellent. The few high-resolution discrepancies observed (less than 0.5%), based on the number of tested DNA samples, are usually administrative. These results are significantly better than the ones for class I typing. Here, the discrepancy rate is up to 4%, depending on the HLA type of the DNA sent. This result means that 4% of the reported typings are discordant with the consensus result. An important source of errors is the misuse of the WHO nomenclature.

Screening Patient Sera for HLA Specific Antibodies

ET patients with more than 5% PRA after exclusion of autoantibodies are considered to be immunized. Sera from these patients are distributed to all transplantation centers, which are expected to perform a crossmatch with every potential organ donor. It is the responsibility of the recipient center to perform the screening of patient sera and to define the sensitization status of the patient in a correct way. The ETRL sends out 16 sera per year to the participating TTC to test the quality of their routine screening in complement-dependent cytotoxicity tests. The mean panel size used by the participants was 58 and ranged between 41-90 HLA-typed cells.

In Figure 3 the mean PRA value reported and both the lowest and highest PRA value per individual serum reported are presented. The results are sorted on the basis of the mean value of the individual sera. In almost all instances the range was higher than 40%, and extreme cases of sera containing no HLA antibodies (0% PRA) in one TTC and more than 80% PRA in another TTC were even reported. Autoantibodies cannot contribute to these results because sera containing such antibodies are excluded from the send out. The number of cells used for the definition of the PRA value also does not contribute to this result.

Influence of Proficiency Testing

One of the most difficult tasks in the field of proficiency testing for histocompatibility testing is to show the importance of the results for clinical transplantation. It is generally accepted that matching for HLA positively influences graft survival in cadaveric renal transplantation. Therefore, we have analyzed the graft survival rates of the transplants with no HLA-A,-B,-DR mismatch (N=3,458) as reported by the donor TTC. Among those, 146 had a mismatch revealed upon retyping at the ETRL, a discrepancy rate of 4.2%. We compared the graft survival of this group to that in the group with no HLA mismatches as defined by the ETRL. The results are shown in Figure 4. A significantly lower graft survival rate was observed in the group of mismatched transplants.

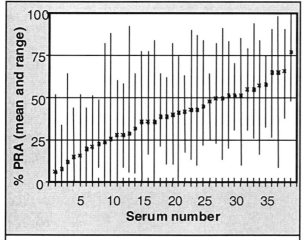

Figure 3. Variation of percentage PRA reported for individual sera during a 30-month survey of the results of screening for HLA-specific antibodies.

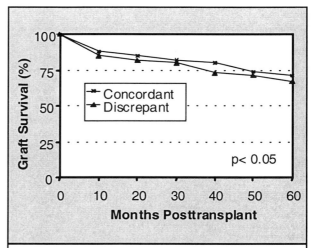

Figure 4. Graft survival in a group of reported zero-mismatched transplants, where retyping revealed a concordant or a discrepant donor typing.

DISCUSSION

Since organ exchange organizations allocate organs in a fair and open way based in part on histocompatibility between donor and recipient, QCE have to be organized to monitor the quality of tissue typing. The current results show that the quality and reliability of histocompatibility testing increased over the years. Especially in the new era of molecular typing, the HLA typing results are by far more reliable than serological typing was in the past. Typing for HLA-DR, which is used for the allocation algorithm, and HLA-DQ have reached an excellent level. This cannot yet be said for the molecular typing for HLA-A,-B. In many instances, serology is certainly more informative than molecular typing for HLA class I typing. The typing of HLA-B15 or HLA-B40 antigens by serology offers better definition than the low-resolution typing by molecular means. Furthermore, many TTC are using the current WHO nomenclature wrongly. From the organ exchange organization point of view the standard WHO nomenclature should be used as a basis for the allocation. However, when this nomenclature does not fulfill the daily routine criteria then a 'local' or organ exchange organization-specific nomenclature is often used. For example, the allele HLA-B*1522, which serologically belongs to the HLA-B35 group can be named as HLA-B35, or the allele HLA-B*4005 can be locally renamed as HLA-B50. Furthermore the allele HLA-B*5002 is actually an HLA-B45. The implementation of such 'matching determinants' (if they are used) should be clearly defined for all participating centers in order to enhance the allocation of organs. Eurotransplant is going this way in the future.

Direct evidence for the relevance of excellent quality tissue typing comes from 2 retrospective studies and from the data shown here. In 1991, retyping for HLA-DR showed a high discrepancy rate, which was associated with a lower graft survival in the wrongly typed combinations (7). True zero-mismatched transplants had the best graft survival. This was confirmed in a study within ET in 1993 (8) and once again by the current study.

The definition of panel reactivity in the sera of patients awaiting a suitable organ seems to be the most difficult part even in the new millennium. This has been illustrated by the results of the QCE presented here. The same serum screened in 49 individual TTC may lead to results varying from non-immunized to broadly sensitized. Significant discrepancies in the reported percent PRA were found in almost all cases. Therefore, we conclude that using the current procedure the PRA value is not an adequate parameter for allocation of organs. Definition of the exact specificity of the antibodies in the patient's sera is a much better alternative. The use of new techniques such as ELISA or flow cytometry may help to increase the reliability of screening in the same way as HLA-DR typing has improved by the introduction of molecular techniques.

SUMMARY

Organ exchange organizations such as Eurotransplant allocate organs on the basis of histocompatibility testing results. For this reason it is essential that all data reported by the affiliated laboratories are accurate and reliable. The Eurotransplant Reference Laboratory (ETRL) organizes proficiency testing schemes for the tissue-typing centers of the respective renal transplantation units participating in Eurotransplant. Each year, the ETRL sends out 8 peripheral blood samples of healthy blood donors for serological typing and crossmatching, 16 sera to screen for the presence and definition of HLA alloantibodies and 20 DNA samples for molecular typing to the 49 participating centers. The results are collected centrally and reported back to the participants in an open way. These exercises show that the quality of HLA typing, screening and crossmatching improved significantly over the years. In particular, the introduction of molecular typing for HLA-DR resulted in an increase of reliability. The clinical relevance of a reliable HLA typing was demonstrated in a selected group of transplants, the zero HLA-A,-B,-DR- mismatched group. After retyping the donors, 146 of the 3,458 matched transplants appeared to have a mismatch and those transplants had a significantly lower graft survival rate. A continuing problem, however, is the result of screening for panel reactive antibodies (PRA), where the percentage PRA reported for each serum varies significantly from center to center. The results indicate that the use of a PRA value for classification of patients and allocation of organs should be revisited.

REFERENCES

1. Terasaki PI, Park M, Perdue ST, Ting A. HLA testing through cell exchange. In : Kissmeyer-Nielsen F, Ed. Histocompatibility Testing 1975. Munksgaard, Copenhagen, Denmark, 1975:359.

2. Park MS, Nakat S, Omori K. Reproducibility of HLA-DR. In: Terasaki PI, Ed. Histocompatibility Testing 1980. UCLA Tissue Typing Laboratory, Los Angeles, California, 1980:161.

3. Marshall WH, Sierp G, Barhalho, Christiansen FT, Scholz S, Albert ED. Selection of a set of high-quality data for B-cell antigen analysis. In: Albert ED, Baur MP, Mayr WR, Eds. Histocompatibility Testing 1984. Springer-Verlag, New York, 1984:69.

4. Van Rood JJ. A proposal for international cooperation in organ transplantation: Eurotransplant. In: Curtoni ES, Mattiuz PL, Tosi RM, Eds. Histocompatibility Testing 1967. Munksgaard, Copenhagen, Denmark, 1967:451.

5. Schreuder GMT, Hendriks GFL, D'Amaro J, Persijn GG. An eight-year study of HLA typing proficiency in Eurotransplant. Tissue Antigens 1986; 27:131.

6. Doxiadis IIN, de Meester J, Witvliet M, Verduyn W, GMT Schreuder, FHJ Claas. Proficiency testing in histocompatibility laboratories involved in organ transplantation. Arch Hellen Med 1999; 16:62.

7. Opelz G, Mytilineos J, Scherer S, Dunckley H, Trejaut J, Chapman J, et al. Survival of DNA HLA-DR typed and matched cadaver kidney transplants. Lancet 1991; 338:461.

8. Thorogood J, Doxiadis IIN, Schreuder GMT, van Rood JJ. Survival of serologically HLA typed and matched cadaver kidney transplants and patients: Influence of serological retyping of donors. Transplant Proc 1993; 25:3051.

ACKNOWLEDGMENTS

This study could not have been performed without the generous support and continuous efforts of all the transplant centers, their tissue-typing laboratories, and the staff from donor hospitals collaborating in the frame of Eurotransplant. This work was supported in part by the JA Cohen Institute for Radiopathology and Radioprotection (IRS) the Eurotransplant International Foundation, and the Dutch National Reference Center for Histocompatibility.

CHAPTER 8

Renal Transplantation in the UK and Republic of Ireland

Rachel J. Johnson, Mark A. Belger, J. Douglas Briggs, Susan V. Fuggle, and Peter J. Morris

on behalf of the UK Transplant Kidney and Pancreas Advisory Group, UK Transplant, Bristol, UNITED KINGDOM

An analysis of the UK and Republic of Ireland Renal Transplant Database for the years 1990-1998 has recently been completed. Three aspects of the analysis have been included in this report. These are outcome following adult renal transplantation (1990-1997), changes in donor and recipient ages and changes in HLA antigen matching (1990-1998).

Analysis of Renal Transplant Outcome

Analysis of outcome was based on 5-year transplant survival of cadaver renal transplants in adult recipients (aged 18 years and over) carried out in the years 1990-1997. For the UK and Republic of Ireland as a whole, 91% of one-year follow-up information and 77% of due 5-year follow-up data were available at the time of this analysis. In order to complete the analysis on a robust dataset, a 90% threshold for due 5-year follow-up was set for each centre and data from 6 centres were excluded on this basis. Multi-organ transplants and transplants from asystolic donors were also excluded. The remaining information from 5,963 first transplants and 1,078 regrafts performed in 19 centres were included in this analysis.

Statistical Analysis

Outcome was based on transplant survival, treating both failure of the graft with a return to dialysis and death of the recipient as an event (failure). This differs from our definition of graft survival, where death with a functioning graft is treated not as an outcome event, but as a censored survival time. Where no event was recorded, the transplant survival time was censored at the date of last known function.

To analyse the combined effect of a number of factors, Cox's proportional hazards regression models were fitted. All the models included stratification by centre to allow for inherent differences between centres. In addition to 5-year transplant survival, possible changes in the effects of factors over time after transplantation were analysed through the modelling of distinct posttransplant epochs: 0-3 months, 3 months to 3 years and after 3 years. Each epoch contained approximately equal numbers of transplant failures. Log cumulative hazard plots showed no evidence of non-proportional hazards within each epoch and a Cox regression model was fitted for each.

Results are presented in terms of estimated relative risks of transplant failure between groups of individuals, compared with that of a baseline group. A relative risk of greater than 1.0 indicates an increased risk of transplant failure compared with the baseline group, while a relative risk less than 1.0 indicates a decreased risk. The 95% confidence intervals were calculated for each relative risk. Kaplan-Meier survival curves are used to illustrate the effects of significant factors identified in the multifactorial analysis. Associated p values were derived from a univariate log-rank test using a 5% level of significance.

RESULTS

Information from the 5,963 first transplants and 1,078 regrafts were analysed separately with transplant survival times censored at 5 years. One-year transplant survival was 83% (95% confidence interval (CI) 82-84%) for first grafts, 84% (95% CI 82-86%) for second grafts and 75% (95% CI 69-82%) for third and subsequent

---

Table 1. *Multifactorial analysis of 5-year transplant survival of adult cadaver kidney only transplants in the UK and Republic of Ireland, 1990 – 1997.*

Factor	Level (baseline)	No.	First grafts Relative Risk	95% CI	p	No.	Regrafts Relative Risk	95% CI	p
Graft year									
	(1990-1992)	2,330	1.00	–	–	438	1.00	–	–
	1993-1995	2,265	0.90*	0.81 – 1.00	0.04	413	0.89	0.70 – 1.13	0.3
	1996-1997	1,368	0.84*	0.73 – 0.97	0.02	227	0.77	0.54 – 1.09	0.1
Recipient age (years)									
	(18-34)	1,391	1.00	–	–	391	1.00	–	–
	35-49	1,936	0.94	0.82 – 1.08	0.4	408	0.92	0.70 – 1.20	0.5
	50-59	1,532	1.11	0.97 – 1.29	0.1	197	1.11	0.81 – 1.52	0.5
	60+	1,104	1.67*	1.44 – 1.92	0.0001	82	1.26	0.82 – 1.93	0.3
Donor age (years)									
	0-10	92	1.26	0.84 – 1.88	0.3	15	1.51	0.59 – 3.85	0.4
	11-17	361	1.23	0.98 – 1.54	0.08	77	1.54	0.94 – 2.55	0.09
	(18-34)	1,708	1.00	–	–	314	1.00	–	–
	35-49	1,899	1.34*	1.17 – 1.54	0.0001	340	1.92*	1.37 – 2.69	0.0001
	50-59	1,192	1.59*	1.37 – 1.85	0.0001	215	2.23*	1.55 – 3.20	0.0001
	60+	711	2.06*	1.75 – 2.43	0.0001	117	2.96*	1.99 – 4.42	0.0001
HLA matchgrade									
	(000 mismatch)	321	1.00	–	–	137	1.00	–	–
	Favourable	1,891	1.07	0.85 – 1.35	0.6	451	1.07	0.73 – 1.56	0.7
	Non-favourable	3,751	1.35*	1.07 – 1.70	0.01	490	1.36	0.93 – 2.00	0.1
Shipping									
	(Local)	3,621	1.00	–	–	556	1.00	–	–
	Exchanged	2,342	1.29*	1.16 – 1.43	0.0001	522	0.98	0.77 – 1.24	0.8
Donor cause of death									
	(Non-trauma)	4,129	1.00	–	–	753	1.00	–	–
	Trauma	1,834	0.91	0.81 – 1.03	0.1	325	0.85	0.64 – 1.12	0.3
Recipient diabetes									
	(Non-diabetic)	5,537	1.00	–	–	1,037	1.00	–	–
	Diabetic	426	1.60*	1.36 – 1.87	0.0001	41	1.13	0.63 – 2.03	0.7

* significant from baseline at 5% level

Table 2. *One- and 3-year transplant survival after first adult cadaver kidney transplant in the UK and Republic of Ireland, 1990-1997, by year of graft.*

		Transplant survival of first graft			
Graft year	No.	One year % surv	95% CI	Three years % surv	95% CI
1990-1992	2,330	82	80-84	74	72-76
1993-1995	2,265	83	82-85	76	74-77
1996-1997	1,368	85	83-86		

grafts. Five-year transplant survival results were 67% (95% CI 66-68%), 67% (95% CI 64-71%) and 62% (95% CI 55-69%) for first, second and third and subsequent grafts, respectively. The results of the multifactorial analysis can be seen in Table 1.

A significant improvement in transplant survival of first grafts has occurred over the 8 years analysed (Table 2). While there was a similar trend for regrafts, the degree of improvement was not statistically significant. When compared with the 5-year transplant survival of first graft recipients

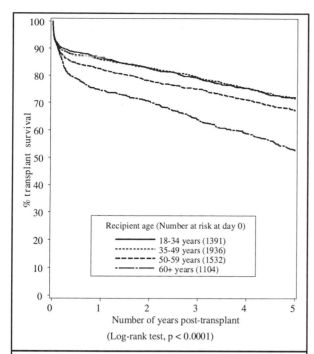

Figure 1. Five-year transplant survival after first adult cadaver kidney only transplant in the UK, 1990-1997 by recipient age.

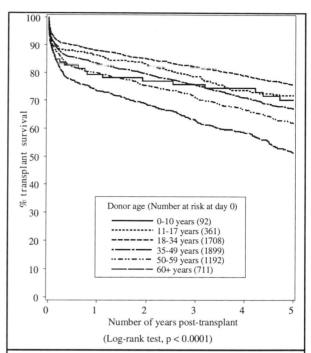

Figure 2. Five-year transplant survival after first adult cadaver kidney only transplant in the UK, 1990-1997 by donor age.

aged 18-34 years, the outcome of those aged over 60 was significantly worse due to deaths with functioning grafts (Table 1 and Fig. 1). There were 532 deaths with functioning grafts within 5 years of transplant (9%) and a further 1,218 (20%) graft failures. Only 2% of patients aged under 35 at the time of transplant were recorded as dying with a functioning graft within 5 years of the transplant compared with 8% of those aged 35-60 years and 21% of those aged over 60 years. For regraft patients there was no significant difference between those aged 18-34 years and the small number aged over 60 (8%).

The risk of transplant failure rises with increasing donor age for both first and regrafts when using kidneys from donors aged 35 years and older. Transplants from donors aged over 60 were twice as likely to fail within 5 years as those from donors aged 18-34 years. Paediatric donors (less than 18 years) were also associated with an increased risk of transplant failure compared with young adult donors. It is interesting to note that this increased risk also applied to the older paediatric donors, aged 11-17 years. The risk of using paediatric donors appeared greater for regrafts than for first grafts but the results were not statistically significant. Table 1 and Figure 2 show the effects of donor age on first grafts.

HLA-A, B and DR mismatches were analysed in 3 groups: 0A0B0DR (000) mismatches, 100, 010 and 110 mismatches and all other match grades combined. In the UK the 100, 010 and 110 HLA-A, B, DR mismatches are termed 'favourable' matches with all poorer match grades termed 'non-favourable'. In contrast to the analysis of factors affecting transplant survival in grafts carried out in the UK between 1986-1993 (1), in the period 1990-1997, there was no significant difference between the outcome of 000 and favourably matched first grafts (Table 1 and Fig. 3). The outcome of non-favourably matched first grafts was significantly poorer than that of the 000 mismatched grafts, although once again the difference was less apparent than in the 1986-1993 data. The diminishing effect of HLA matching over time can be at least partially attributed to the decreased number of poorly matched transplants. For first grafts, 10% of the non-favourable group had 2 DR antigens mismatched in the years 1990-1992, compared with only 4% in 1996-1998. The model has not taken into account the degree of sensitisation to HLA antigens or cold ischaemic time due to lack of historical data. This may, in part, explain the lack of difference in outcome between 000 and favourably matched grafts as proportionally more of the 000 mismatched grafts are exchanged for highly

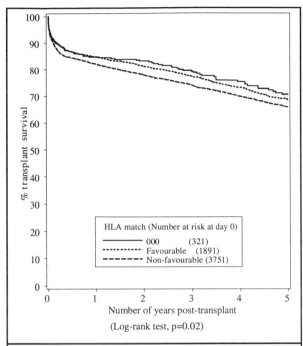

Figure 3. Five-year transplant survival after first adult cadaver kidney only transplant in the UK, 1990-1997, by HLA match.

sensitised patients. Even allowing for this, it is clear that differences in outcome relating to HLA matching are diminishing with time.

With regard to exchange of kidneys between transplant centres, inferior survival is evident for transplants involving kidneys imported from another centre. This reaches statistical significance only for first grafts (Table 1 and Fig. 4). All exchanges between centres were counted, regardless of distance. Transplants from donors who died from road traffic accidents and other trauma were associated with less risk of transplant failure than those from donors dying from other causes. This lesser risk did not reach statistical significance for either first or regrafts.

Finally, with regard to diabetes, a significantly increased risk of transplant failure was present for diabetic recipients of first kidney transplants (Table 1 and Fig. 5). To a minor extent, this increased risk was due to deaths with a functioning graft. There were too few regrafts in diabetic patients (3.8%) to analyse this group. Patients were classified as diabetic if their primary reason for transplant was given as either Type I or II diabetes.

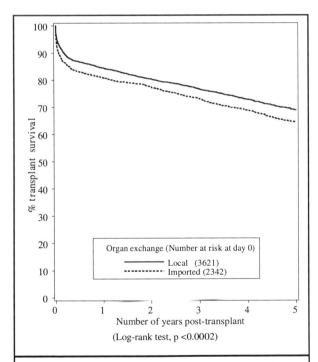

Figure 4. Five-year transplant survival after first adult cadaver kidney only transplant in the UK, 1990-1997, by organ exchange between centres.

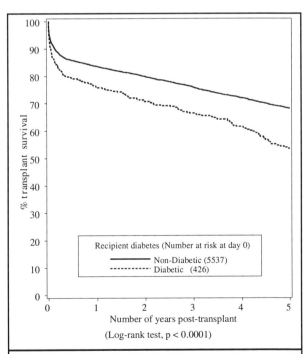

Figure 5. Five-year transplant survival after first adult cadaver kidney only transplant in the UK, 1990-1997, by recipient diabetes.

The matching between donor and recipient cytomegalovirus status (based on incomplete data), between donor and recipient blood group and between donor and recipient gender did not influence the risk of transplant failure (data not shown).

Almost half of the transplants carried out in the UK between 1990-1997 were excluded from these analyses due to the exclusion of 6 large centres on the basis of inadequate follow-up information at 5 years. In order to gauge the robustness of the results presented, the models were re-run on all transplants with follow-up information available. These analyses of 9,722 first grafts and 1,716 regrafts showed very similar results. Relative risks were comparable and one or 2 factor levels gained significance at 5% while none lost significance.

Changes in the influence of factors over the posttransplant period were investigated through analysis of distinct epochs: 0-3 months, 3 months to 3 years and beyond 3 years. Results of the epoch analysis for first cadaver renal grafts are shown in Table 3. Although there was improvement in outcome over the years studied for each of the 3 epochs, this failed to reach

Table 3. Multifactorial epoch analysis of transplant survival of first adult cadaver kidney only transplants in the UK and Republic of Ireland, 1990-1997.

Factor Level (Baseline)	<3 months Relative Risk	95% CI	No.	3 months - 3 years Relative Risk	95% CI	No.	>3 years Relative Risk	95% CI	No.
Graft year									
(1990-1992)	1.00	–	2,330	1.00	–	2,016	1.00	–	1,703
1993-1995	0.96	0.82 – 1.13	2,265	0.87	0.73 – 1.03	1,974	0.88	0.72 – 1.08	1,558
1996-1997	0.84	0.69 – 1.02	1,368	0.88	0.71 – 1.08	1,205	0.88	0.35 – 2.18	341
Recipient age (years)									
(18-34)	1.00	–	1,391	1.00	–	1,246	1.00	–	879
35-49	1.04	0.84 – 1.29	1,936	0.83	0.66 – 1.03	1,717	0.95	0.75 – 1.20	1,256
50-59	1.25*	1.00 – 1.55	1,532	1.00	0.79 – 1.26	1,324	1.12	0.88 – 1.43	914
60+	1.57*	1.25 – 1.96	1,104	1.72*	1.37 – 2.16	908	1.76*	1.36 – 2.27	553
Donor age (years)									
0-10	1.57	0.92 – 2.68	92	1.03	0.48 – 2.22	76	1.39	0.77 – 2.50	60
11-17	1.28	0.91 – 1.81	361	1.16	0.79 – 1.71	318	1.11	0.78 – 1.57	244
(18-34)	1.00	–	1,708	1.00	–	1,548	1.00	–	1,151
35-49	1.30*	1.05 – 1.61	1,899	1.39*	1.11 – 1.75	1,659	1.34*	1.07 – 1.68	1,154
50-59	1.49*	1.18 – 1.87	1,192	1.78*	1.40 – 2.27	1,019	1.61*	1.25 – 2.08	657
60+	1.91*	1.49 – 2.44	711	2.29*	1.76 – 2.97	575	2.08*	1.56 – 2.79	336
HLA matchgrade									
(000 mismatch)	1.00	–	321	1.00	–	286	1.00	–	209
Favourable	1.01	0.71 – 1.45	1,891	1.18	0.80 – 1.73	1,679	0.93	0.64 – 1.34	1,148
Non-Favourable	1.48*	1.04 – 2.10	3,751	1.36	0.93 – 1.98	3,230	1.04	0.72 – 1.49	2,245
Shipping									
(Local)	1.00	–	3,621	1.00	–	3,200	1.00	–	2,218
Exchanged	1.45*	1.24 – 1.69	2,342	1.15	0.97 – 1.37	1,995	1.17	0.98 – 1.40	1,384
Donor cause of death									
(Non-Trauma)	1.00	–	4,129	1.00	–	3,558	1.00	–	2,401
Trauma	0.89	0.74 – 1.08	1,834	0.96	0.79 – 1.17	1,637	0.96	0.79 – 1.17	1,201
Recipient diabetes									
(Non-diabetic)	1.00	–	5,537	1.00	–	4,847	1.00	–	3,369
Diabetic	1.46*	1.15 – 1.87	426	1.51*	1.16 – 1.98	348	2.60*	2.02 – 3.36	233

* significant from baseline at 5% level

UK TRANSPLANT

statistical significance. Older recipients were associated with an increased risk of transplant failure throughout the epochs. The same was true for the use of kidneys from older donors. Those from donors aged over 34 years were associated with significantly worse outcomes in each epoch compared with those from donors aged 18-34 years. Donors aged over 60 years conferred double the risk of failure in each epoch compared with the baseline group (aged 18-34 years). The increased risk associated with the youngest donor age group (1-10 years) was most evident in the first 3 months after transplantation but did not quite reach statistical significance.

With regard to HLA-A, B, DR matching, the detrimental effect of non-favourable matches was clear for the first 2 epochs (relative risks of 1.48 and 1.36, respectively), although the effect was only statistically significant in the first epoch, ie. in the first 3 months after transplantation. No significant difference existed between 000 and favourably matched grafts in any posttransplant epoch although there was a trend for the relative risk of failure to be less for 000 mismatches in the second epoch. There was a significantly detrimental effect of exchanging kidneys in the first 3 months after transplantation, but this did not extend to the 2 later epochs, while the beneficial effect of the use of kidneys from donors who died as a result of trauma did not reach statistical significance in any epoch. Finally, diabetic recipients had a significantly increased risk of transplant failure in each posttransplant epoch.

Recipient and Donor Age Matching

The changes in mean donor and recipient age for 15,419 cadaver renal transplants during the time period

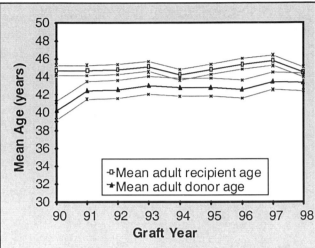

Figure 6. Mean adult donor and recipient ages (and 95% confidence intervals) for all cadaver kidney transplants in the UK and Republic of Ireland, 1990-1998.

of this analysis (1990-1998) are shown in Figure 6. Both recipient and donor ages were reported to the National Transplant Database for 99.9% of the total transplants (15,436). Although the mean recipient age in the UK increased by 5 years between 1981-1990, it has remained stable at approximately 45 years since then. The mean donor age increased from 35.6 years (s.e. 0.7) in 1981 to 42.5 years (s.e. 0.5) in 1991. As Figure 6 shows, the mean donor age since 1991 has increased at a slower rate, to 43.4 years (s.e. 0.5) in 1998.

Table 4 shows the frequency of all kidney transplants performed within different donor and recipient age groups. For two-thirds of all transplants, both donor and recipient were aged between 18-60 years. Recipients over 60 years of age accounted for 13% of transplants, while transplants in children represented 7%.

For each of the 15,419 transplants studied, the donor-recipient age difference was obtained by subtracting the donor age from the recipient age at time of transplant. In each of 5 time periods, the mean age difference was then calculated for various recipient age groups as shown in Table 5. Data for transplants in 1998 were divided into two 6-month periods. This was to reflect that in July 1998 a new allocation scheme for kid-

Table 4. Donor and recipient ages for cadaver kidney transplants in the UK and Republic of Ireland, 1990-1998.

Recipient age (years)	Donor age (years)					TOTAL	
	0-9	10-17	18-34	35-60	>60	No.	%
0-9	163	169	47	30	0	**409**	**3**
10-17	158	276	118	126	4	**682**	**4**
18-34	109	367	1,279	1,796	167	**3,718**	**24**
35-60	112	492	2,407	4,716	874	**8,601**	**56**
>60	16	78	397	1,101	417	**2,009**	**13**
TOTAL	**558**	**1,382**	**4,248**	**7,769**	**1,462**	**15,419**	
%	**4**	**9**	**28**	**50**	**9**		

neys was introduced in the UK, one of the aims of which was to minimise age differences between donor and recipient.

It is clear from Table 5 that, in general, the mean age difference for adult recipients has decreased over the period of this analysis. The main reason for this decrease is the increasing use of older donor kidneys. However, the reduction in age difference for older recipients in the second half of 1998 can be attributed in part to the increased priority for minimising age differences, which was incorporated into the new UK Kidney Allocation Scheme. It is also evident that during this 6-month period the mean age difference for childhood recipients has increased. This is due to increased access to adult organs, which the revised UK Allocation Scheme has also promoted.

Recipient and Donor HLA Matching

Of the 15,436 cadaver kidney transplants reported in the UK and Republic of Ireland for the calendar years 1990-1998, 15,163 (98.2%) had complete HLA-A, B and DR tissue-typing information available for both donor and recipient. HLA-A, -B, -DR mismatches were calculated on the basis of the antigens used for matching in the UK Allocation Scheme as defined elsewhere (1).

The proportion of 000 mismatched cadaver kidney transplants has increased from 5% to 7% over the period of the analysis (Table 6). The proportion of favourably matched transplants was 29% for the 2 earlier 3-year periods (1990-1992 and 1993-1995) but increased to 36% for the later 3 years. This was due to the introduction of the concept of favourable matching into the Kidney Allocation Scheme, which happened in January 1997. Although there has been little change in the proportion of other 0 DR-mismatched and one DR-mismatched grafts, there has been a decline in the proportion of 2

Table 5. Mean age differences (recipient - donor) for cadaver kidney transplants in the UK and Republic of Ireland, 1990-1998, by graft year.

Graft year	Recipient age (years)				
	0-9	10-17	18-34	35-59	>60
1990-1992	-6.6	-5.7	-7.4	8.7	20.9
1993-1995	-8.6	-6.3	-8.2	5.7	17.4
1996-1997	-8.7	-5.0	-9.1	5.6	18.7
1998 (Jan-Jun)	-10.6	-7.4	-8.2	3.7	20.3
1998 (Jul-Dec)	-16.0	-11.0	-7.2	3.6	14.9
OVERALL	-8.3	-6.1	-8.0	6.5	18.9

HLA-DR mismatched grafts over the 9 years from 10% of transplants in 1990-1992 to 4% in 1996-1998.

Further revisions to the National Kidney Allocation Scheme, introduced in July 1998, placed increased priority on HLA matching in that both kidneys are now offered for export to other centres when 000 mismatched patients exist in those centres but there are none locally. This has resulted in significantly more well-matched transplants in the period July-December 1998 as follows: 12% 000 mismatches, 42% favourable, 9% other 0 DR mismatches, 33% 1 DR mismatch and 4% 2 DR mismatches.

To investigate changes over time further, the mean number of HLA-A, -B and -DR mismatches were calculated for each 3-year period within the time period of the analysis both at each individual HLA-A, -B or -DR locus (0-2 mismatches) and for all 3 loci combined (total of 0-6 mismatches).

For first cadaver kidney transplants in adults, there was no change in the mean number of HLA-A and HLA-B mismatches over time, these remaining at approximately 0.92 (s.e. 0.01) and 1.02 (s.e. 0.01), respectively.

UK TRANSPLANT

Table 6. HLA-A, B, DR mismatches for cadaver kidney transplants in the UK and Republic of Ireland, 1990-1998.

HLA Matchgrade	1990-1992		1993-1995		1996-1998		TOTAL	
	No.	%	No.	%	No.	%	No.	%
000	281	5	322	6	329	7	932	6
Favourable	1,521	29	1,504	29	1,715	36	4,740	31
Other 0 DR mismatches	670	13	715	14	653	14	2,038	13
1 DR mismatch	2,188	42	2,318	45	1,878	39	6,384	42
2 DR mismatches	519	10	347	7	203	4	1,069	7

Table 7. Mean HLA-DR and total mismatches for first cadaver kidney transplants in the UK and Republic of Ireland, 1990-1998.

Graft year	Adult recipient				Pediatric recipient			
	HLA-DR mismatches		Total mismatches		HLA-DR mismatches		Total mismatches	
	Mean	S.E.	Mean	S.E.	Mean	S.E.	Mean	S.E.
1990-1992	0.62	0.01	2.58	0.02	0.81	0.04	2.93	0.08
1993-1995	0.59	0.01	2.52	0.02	0.65	0.03	2.52	0.06
1996-1998	0.49	0.01	2.45	0.02	0.60	0.04	2.60	0.07
OVERALL	**0.57**	**0.01**	**2.52**	**0.01**	**0.69**	**0.02**	**2.67**	**0.04**

The number of HLA-DR mismatches, however, has fallen from 0.62 (s.e. 0.01) in 1990-1992 to 0.49 (s.e. 0.01) in 1996-1998, with the mean number falling more rapidly in the later 3 years of the 9-year period studied. As a result, the mean number of total mismatches (HLA-A+B+DR) has fallen from 2.58 (s.e. 0.02) in 1990-1992 to 2.45 (s.e. 0.02) in 1996-1998, as seen in Table 7.

For first cadaver kidney transplants in children, as for adults, there was no change in the mean number of HLA-A and HLA-B mismatches over time but the mean number of HLA-DR mismatches has fallen from 0.81 (s.e. 0.04) in 1990-1992 to 0.60 (s.e. 0.04) in 1996-1998. As a result, the mean number of total mismatches for transplants in children has fallen from 2.93 (s.e. 0.08) in 1990-1992 to 2.60 (s.e. 0.07) in 1996-1998.

SUMMARY

Renal transplant outcome. Analysis of 5-year transplant survival in the UK showed a number of significant factors influencing outcome of adult cadaveric renal transplantation. Data from 5,963 first grafts and 1,078 regrafts carried out between 1990-1997 showed year of graft, recipient age and diabetes, donor age, kidney exchange between centres and HLA matching to influence 5-year outcome. The most important prognostic factor was donor age: the risk of transplant failure within 5 years for grafts using kidneys from donors aged 60 years and over was double that of grafts using donors aged 18-34 years. Unlike the effect of donor age, the influence of HLA matching would appear to be diminishing with time. In contrast to transplants in the 1980's, the difference in 5-year transplant survival between 000 mismatched and favourably matched (100, 010 or 110 mismatched) transplants is no longer significant. An analysis of posttransplant survival for first grafts in different epochs (0-3 months,

3 months to 3 years and beyond 3 years) showed that one factor affected only short-term outcome (exchange of kidneys between centres), whereas others affected outcome throughout the epochs (most notably donor age, recipient age and recipient diabetes).

Recipient and donor age matching. The mean recipient age in the UK and Republic of Ireland increased by 5 years between 1981-1990 but has remained at approximately 45 years since then. The mean donor age increased by 7 years to 42.5 years (s.e. 0.5) between 1981-1991 and since then has increased at a slower rate to 43.4 years (s.e. 0.5) in 1998. The mean donor-recipient age difference for more than 15,000 transplants carried out between 1990-1998 has decreased, primarily due to increasing donor age over this time. However, the introduction of a new Kidney Allocation Scheme in the UK in July 1998, part of which is aimed at minimising age differences, has increased the likelihood that recipients aged over 60 years will be allocated grafts from donors closer to their own age than previously. The new UK Kidney Allocation Scheme also gave children increased access to well-matched adult organs leading to an increased mean age difference for this group between July-December 1998.

Donor and recipient HLA matching. Modifications to the Kidney Allocation Scheme introduced in January 1997 with the aim of increasing the number of well-matched transplants has led to a rise in 000 mismatched grafts from 5% to 7% and favourably matched (100/010/110 mismatches) from 29% to 36% between 1990-1992 and 1996-1998. Over this same time the proportion of 2 DR-mismatched grafts has decreased from 10% to 4%. The revised Kidney Allocation Scheme implemented in July 1998 gave a further increase in priority to 000 mismatches, increasing the proportion of these transplants to 12% for the last half of 1998, a level which has been maintained since then.

REFERENCES

1. Morris PJ, Johnson RJ, Fuggle SV et al. Analysis of factors that affect outcome of primary cadaveric renal transplantation in the UK. Lancet 1999; 354:1147.

CHAPTER 9

Organ Transplantation in Latin America

Eduardo A. Santiago-Delpín [a] and Valter Duro García [b] for The Latin-American Transplant Collaborative Group

[a] From the Puerto Rico Transplant Program, Auxilio Mutuo Hospital and the Department of Surgery, University of Puerto Rico Medical School, San Juan, PUERTO RICO, [b]Porto Alegre, BRAZIL

Latin America has carried out kidney transplantation for more than 35 years. Argentina and Brazil were the first countries to perform dialysis and to transplant kidneys systematically in Latin America, coinciding with the early times when the northern hemisphere and Europe were embarking on their own pioneering efforts. Mexico and Colombia followed closely, then the rest of South America and subsequently Central America and the Caribbean. However, there has been a paucity of information on organ transplantation, which is not surprising since most of the studies in organ transplantation in Latin America before 1990 related to individual countries and most reports were published either in Spanish or Portuguese. Only during the past 10 years have there been systematic efforts to study solid organ transplantation in the region. Our first study reported 15,000 transplants for the period between 1970-1990 (1), and the most recent report, the eleventh, totaled 62,000-organ transplants for Latin America (2).

In the following sections, different aspects of organ donation and transplantation are analyzed and discussed, which are quite specific to the Latin America region. Although organ transplantation has been carried out in the region for almost 40 years, it was only in the last 20 years that transplantation evolved as a treatment for end-stage organ disease and that formal statistics have been kept.

METHODS

The Registry: The Registry represents the effort of members from the 2 previous Latin-American transplantation societies, the Latin-American Transplantation Society and the Pan-American Society for Dialysis and Transplantation. Both societies have joined resources, and although some publications preceded the official registry, for operational and historical purposes, they have been included as official reports. The data for each report were supplied by a voluntary Latin-American Transplant Collaborative Group (See Appendix 1), whose composition has varied through the years. Initially, data were obtained from the transplant pioneers or representatives of government. Subsequently, as the respective practices evolved, national registries and transplant societies were formed and their directors or representatives submitted the requested information. This effort helped to unify the region and was one of the seeds that gave impetus to the eventual fusion of the 2 regional transplantation societies. On March 12, 1999, a joint assembly of both societies voted for the founding of a new society comprising the members of the 2 existing societies, to represent the whole region including the Caribbean, the latter so as to include English speaking Jamaica, Barbados, the US Virgin Islands, Trinidad and other Caribbean countries involved in organ transplantation (3). A second registry on dialysis and kidney transplantation has been spearheaded and sponsored by the Latin-American Society of Nephrology and Hypertension (4). This registry, based in Uruguay, registers patients with end-stage renal disease and follows them through the different renal substitution therapies. Finally, some individual centers in the different countries report data on their patients to the international Collaborative Transplant Study (CTS) Registry in Heidelberg. Outcome data are extremely difficult to obtain from the region since most countries do not have statistics on their results through the years. The only available data are reports from individual countries where reporting results is mandatory, or where pain staking efforts are devoted to obtaining outcome results. Individual national reports as well as the data included in some of the CTS Registry reports are the only data available on graft transplant survival.

Analyses: Studies are usually conducted as polls or questionnaires. Cooperation is more than 95%. The data are collected and analyzed by the authors. Information is tabulated and the corresponding indices created for transplantation of the kidney, heart and lung, liver and pancreas. Topics studied through the years include incidence and prevalence, immunosuppression, finances, societal and governmental aspects, infections, histocompatibility, nephrology and renal diseases, trends, information regarding transplant programs (transplant surgeons, societies, training, immunology) and issues regarding allegations of organ commerce. Members of the Collaborative Transplant Group have also published related articles on topics including non-compliance, knowledge and attitudes about donation age, organ donation and procurement, organ commerce, legal aspects, living unrelated donation and two transplant textbooks, one in Spanish and one in Portuguese.

Publications: To date, there have been 11 reports collecting and analyzing transplant data and specific topics through the years. There have been 10 additional publications from the Registry regarding renal disease, histocompatibility infections, donation, organ commerce, organ shortage, and societal changes, as well as 17 articles on topics related with organ transplantation. These articles are reviewed in references 5-8.

ANALYSIS

Latin America is the name applied to a conglomerate of adjacent countries which have in common languages of Latin extraction, either Spanish or Portuguese. It includes Mexico from North America; Guatemala, Honduras, El Salvador, Nicaragua, Costa Rica, and Panamá from Central America; Colombia, Venezuela, Ecuador, Bolivia, Brazil, Perú, Paraguay, Uruguay, Argentina, and Chile from South America; the Spanish speaking islands of the Caribbean, which are Cuba, Dominican Republic, and Puerto Rico, and recently Jamaica, the US Virgin Islands, Barbados and Trinidad.

This is a vast region encompassing huge countries such as Brazil with very large populations, and tiny Caribbean islands. The extent of economic development is highly variable with agrarian-based economies in some countries co-existing with moderately industrialized neighbors. Ethnically, the population is a mixture of the initial Spanish and Portuguese settlers with the various genetically different ethnic groups that populated the different areas of this region before colonization. The Caribbean basin – the islands as well as the costal areas of Central America and South America – evidence the additional important genetic influence of the African Black. Latin-American countries are profoundly nationalistic, resisting all efforts for unification during the last 2 centuries. It is precisely this national identification of country or region which makes each population unique and which causes confusion in the United States when attempts are made to identify a common Hispanic minority. There can never be a homogeneous definition of Hispanics because culturally, at least, first and second-generation immigrants feel related to the country of origin. These differences are extremely important in the perception of death, self-image, donation and giving, culture and education, and these are important factors bearing on the organ donation pattern of the different Latin-American countries as well as the respective minorities in the United States. However, although military and political unifying initiatives have ended in failure, cultural and scientific identification is the rule, and effective efforts at unification have succeeded in the operational aspects of life, which include literature, art, sports, science and medicine. Recently various common markets have also become operational.

Resources: All countries have at least one kidney transplant program, and the number of new transplant programs is increasing rapidly (1,2). From 181 transplant programs that were performing organ transplantation in 1990, there are currently more than 350 institutions performing transplants in the area. Trained transplant surgeons provide surgical care in all countries. However, medical care and immunological follow-up rests primarily with the nephrologist. This provides continuity of care between the dialytic and posttransplant periods. The concept of "transplant program" as understood in the United States and Europe with dedicated physical facilities, offices, transplant wards, non-medical coordinators and specific transplant staff is the exception rather than the rule. The surgical transplant team usually performs organ procurement, although Argentina, Chile, Brazil, Puerto Rico and some areas in Mexico have developed dedicated organ procurement services. Ten of 18 countries have transplantation societies, 16 of 18 have nephrology societies, 10 of 18 have formal transplant registries, and there are 3 transplant journals and 3 nephrology journals. Children and small babies as well as the elderly are routinely transplanted in virtually all countries. Tissue typing and general immunology laboratories provide immunological support in 17 of 19 countries. In some Caribbean islands without transplant programs, most patients are referred to the United States, Canada, United Kingdom, Colombia, Venezuela or Jamaica.

Incidence: The incidences of end-stage cardiac and liver disease are unknown for the whole region and have not been studied systematically. However, the incidence of end-stage renal disease has been studied and has increased during the past 15 years. Initially, glomerulonephritis, hypertension, pyelonephritis and polycystic kidneys were the most frequent diseases. However, diabetes and hypertension have increased in recent years although the statistics vary for each country. Significantly, the proportion of patients reaching kidney transplantation follows a more traditional scheme with glomerulonephritis 36%, hypertension 11%, cystic disease 7% and diabetes only 4%. These are fairly uniform for the region, in spite of the rising incidence of diabetes mellitus.

Renal Transplantation Activity: Although most countries, especially those in South America, commenced renal transplantation in the 1960's, activity was slow, even piecemeal in most countries, until the mid 1970's when the numbers increased appreciably. Renal transplantation with living donors increased sharply and took precedence over cadaver transplantation. Cadaver transplantation started to increase in 1983, reflecting the wider use of cyclosporine as well as the development of supporting legal frameworks in most countries.

Our first study reported 15,000 transplants from 1970-1990 and Table 1 shows the cumulative increases thereafter. Active growth continued and currently renal transplant activity in Latin America corresponds to approximately 12% of the reported world renal transplant activity. Almost half of this activity comes from Brazil alone, followed by Mexico, Argentina, Cuba, Chile, Venezuela and Colombia, which are considered "high volume" countries. However, when the prevalence of transplantation is calculated, other countries emerge with a higher prevalence including Costa Rica, Puerto Rico,

Table 1. Cumulative total organ transplant activity in Latin America (1970-1999).

	Kidney	Heart and Heart Lung	Liver
1970-1988	15,195	45	57
1990	20,058	148	119
1991	24,080	430	236
1992	26,509	491	279
1993	29,964	643	389
1995	38,405	1,207	629
1997	46,697	1,632	1,390
1999	57,123	2,152	2,487

Table 2. The changing prevalence of kidney transplantation (living and cadaver donor) in selected Latin American countries.

	Transplants per million population[a]				
	1999	1997	1995	1991	1988
Costa Rica	21.0	25.2	18.7	—	4.1
Chile	18.9	15.9	9.6	—	9.7
Puerto Rico	14.7	10.8	10.0	10.9	8.0
Brazil	14.4	11.0	10.6	5.8	4.0
Argentina	13.8	15.4	14.5	11.6	4.0
Mexico	12.5	10.6	7.7	6.4	2.2
Uruguay	12.5	10.3	7.2	8.0	5.0
Colombia	10.4	9.3	6.9	4.6	1.4

[a] Most recent census, World Bank

LATIN AMERICA

Argentina, Brazil, Chile and Cuba. Table 2 demonstrates the increase in prevalence of kidney transplantation for the higher prevalence countries. The increase in the number of transplants per million population between 1988-1999 is evident. However, this prevalence only relates to the total number of both living- and cadaver-donor kidney transplants. Table 3 indicates a different ranking when only cadaver kidney transplantation is taken into consideration (column 5). It is evident that even with the higher volumes reported by Uruguay, Chile and Argentina, these are still below North American and European cadaver prevalence reports. In the mid 1990's there was a marked increase in the number and percentage of cadaver donors compared with living donors as shown in Table 4. Before that time, roughly two-thirds had been living donors. In the last 2 reports

Table 3. Renal transplants 1999 and updated totals[a]

	Live Donor	Cadaver Donor	Total 1999	Total Prevalence [c]	Cadaver Prevalence [d]	Approximate Total
Argentina	104	383	487	13.8 ↑	10.8	5,526
Bolivia	56	16	72	9.2	2.1	379
Brazil	1,377	999	2,376	14.4 ↑	6.1	25,239
Chile	30	235	265	18.9 ↑	16.8	3,001
Colombia	83	301	384	10.4 ↑	8.1	3,362
Costa Rica	58	16	74	21.0 ↓	4.5	1,190
Cuba	11	92	103	9.4 ↑	8.4	2,701
Dominican Rep.	23	0	23	3.0 ↑	0	160
Ecuador [b]						263+
El Salvador	26	0	26	4.5 ↑	0	197
Guatemala	20	0	20	1.8 ↓	0	177
Honduras	3	0	3	0.5	0	33
Mexico	1,081	153	1,234	12.5	1.6	10,208
Panamá	5	2	7	2.5 ↓	0.7	84
Paraguay	7	1	8	1.5	0.13	130
Perú	82	60	142	5.7	2.4	1,275
Puerto Rico	24	32	56	14.7 ↓	8.4	737
Uruguay	3	38	41	12.5 ↓	11.6	510
Venezuela	102	43	145	6.4 ↑	1.9	1,951
Totals	3,095	2,371	5,466	9.0	4.6	57,123

[a] Modified with permission from Ref 2, Elsevier Science.
[b] Data until 1997.
[c] Total transplants 1999/million inhabitants (Census of 1997 or 1998). Arrows indicate change from 1998.
[d] Total cadaver transplants 1999/million inhabitants (Census of 1997 or 1998).

there was still a preponderance of living donor transplants. Although cadaver organ transplantation prevalence and proportion are well below those of Europe and the United States, the statistics for individual countries and the trends in the past 10 years demonstrate an increase in cadaver organ transplantation. This is probably a reflection of the adoption of the "Spanish model" or modifications thereof, as well as increasing government support.

Table 3 also lists the number of renal transplants for the individual countries. Brazil and Mexico together transplanted well over 3,000 kidneys last year. The lower volume countries have lower numbers although some have a higher prevalence. Data from the smaller Caribbean islands is currently being incorporated into the registry, but personal communications with the appropriate practitioners (see Appendix) show an increased activity: Barbados 10 living donor transplants;

Jamaica 60 transplants with about 50% from cadavers; US Virgin Islands 26 living related transplants, and Trinidad 25 transplants. The total transplant prevalence for 1999 is approximately 9 per million, of which the prevalence of cadaver kidney transplantation is only 4.6.

Perhaps the most complete study on results and survival rates at selected programs was reported by Opelz (9). HLA compatibility, immunosuppressive

Table 4. Changing patterns of organ donation in Latin America (1970-1999).

	Live Donors (%)	Cadaver Donors (%)
1970-1988	71	29
1989-1992	65	35
1994-1995	49	51
1996-1997	52	48
1998-1999	57	43

induction and maintenance regimes, blood pressure, ischemic preservation time, recipient age and donor age were all factors influencing kidney graft survival in Latin America. Although the results of this CTS study were in agreement with the overall experience in Latin America, only programs in 25 cities reported to the CTS registry. Thus, the results reflect only those from the largest centers in the region.

Cardiac and Lung Transplantation: Table 5 shows thoracic organ transplantation for 1999 and the corresponding totals. Both Brazil and Argentina have well-established mature heart transplant programs and their combined activity accounts for almost 80% of heart transplantation in Latin America. However, a number of other countries have developed this activity lately, including Puerto Rico.

Liver Transplantation: Liver transplantation started piecemeal in the 1970's and increased with the introduction of cyclosporine and subsequently tacrolimus. Again, Brazil and Argentina lead in this activity (Table 6). However, other countries are gradually developing their own abdominal transplant programs. Currently, there is no published record of the regional results of either thoracic or liver transplantation.

Immunosuppression: The evolution of immunosuppressive protocols is shown in Table 7. During the period between 1985-1995, protocols were uniform throughout the region. Importantly, even though the use of cyclosporine was universal, and even though the whole region converted to the Neoral formulation quite rapidly, a significant number of patients stopped using this calcineurin inhibitor as maintenance for reasons related mainly to cost. It has been impossible to assess exactly what proportion of patients use Cyclosporine chronically or at which point they stop using the medication.

During the last 4 years, there has been modification of the induction and maintenance protocols with the gradual incorporation of tacrolimus as well as other drugs including mycophenolate mofetil and rapamycin. Biological antisera have also become entrenched in the armamentarium for induction and rejection. ATG and Thymoglobulin as well as the monoclonals OKT3, basiliximab, and daclizumab are used with increasing frequency. A caveat to be borne in mind in this type of report relates to our inability to calculate the exact number of patients or

Table 5. Thoracic organ transplants for 1999 and totals [a].

	Heart	Lung or Heart/Lung	Totals 1999	Total since Beginning
Argentina	85	21	106	633
Bolivia	0	0	0	1
Brazil	109	17	126	1,036
Chile	21	11	32	70
Colombia	0	2	2	165
Costa Rica	0	0	0	17
Cuba	2	0	2	96
Ecuador				5
Mexico	9	0	9	77
Paraguay	1	0	1	6
Perú	1	0	1	16
Puerto Rico	5	0	5	5
Uruguay	7	1	8	17
Venezuela	0	0	0	13
Totals	240	52	292	2,152

[a] Modified with permission from Ref 2, Elsevier Science.

Table 6. Abdominal organ transplants for 1999 and totals [a].

	Liver 1999	Total since beginning	Pancreas 1999	Total since Beginning
Argentina	170	760	12	24
Bolivia	3	3	0	0
Brazil	361	1,385	8[(2)]	32
Chile	32	150	0	7
Colombia	27	103	0	20
Costa Rica	3	8	0	1
Cuba	6	18	0	21[b]
Mexico	48	61	1	1
Paraguay	0	0	0	0
Perú	0	2	0	0
Uruguay	1	5	0	0
Venezuela	0	19	0	2
Totals	651	2,487	21	108

[a] Modified with permission from Ref 2, Elsevier Science.
[b] Kidney-pancreas

centers using these medications. We interpret our data as indicating only that the stated number of countries have started using the new medications, but the universality of its use cannot be ascertained with the current methods of reporting. Rather than demonstrating the universality of use, Table 7 illustrates the utilization of several new options by Latin-American transplant practitioners.

Infections: Infections in transplant recipients in Latin America, as elsewhere, are common. Fungal dermatoses and onichomycoses are highly prevalent, especially in the tropical and subtropical areas. Common infections reported include skin and nail fungi, urinary infections, prostatitis, pneumonia, upper respiratory infections, viral syndromes, gastroenteritis, cytomegalovirus, and "fever". Perhaps of more importance are the rare or more serious infections, which can be quite vexing, and at the same time tax the resources of staff and institution. Commonly reported serious infections are enumerated in Table 8.

Organ Donation: There are a number of identifiable factors that affect the meager donation pattern of most Latin-American countries. Cultural factors include the peculiar grief reaction occurring frequently upon notification of death. Typically, a highly emotional reaction occurs in which the grieving persons may even hurt themselves. During this period it is impossible to establish any type of communication with the affected members. Also, the decision-making process is frequently taken over by several members of the family – something like a "family committee" – and not necessarily by the next of kin. Thus, personal attitudes and prejudices often complicate decisions. In some countries there are differing views of death. In other countries there may be distrust of the system. All these factors compound the dynamics inherent to the decision-making process for organ donation. The result is decreased donation. So-called "administrative" factors also contribute to the meager donation pattern of Latin America. With few exceptions (currently Argentina, Chile, Venezuela, Puerto Rico, and some programs in Brazil, and Mexico) most countries lack formal organ procurement organizations as they are known in Europe and the United States. Similarly, most programs lack

Table 7. Evolution of immunosuppressive regimens.

	Induction	Maintenance	Rejection
Pre 1980	prednisone, azathioprine	prednisone, azathioprine	prednisone anti-lymphocyte sera
1985-1996	prednisone, azathioprine, cyclosporine, mono-and polyclonals	prednisone, azathioprine, cyclosporine	steroids, radiation, polyclonals and monoclonals
1997 onwards:			
steroids	18/18	18/18	18/18
cyclosporine	11/18	12/18	—
tacrolimus	6/18	7/18	8/18 (Rescue)
mycophenolate	—	11/18	7/18 (Rescue)
rapamycin	3/18	—	1/18 (Rescue)
Anti Thymocyte Globulin	4/18	—	7/18
Thymoglobulin	6/18	—	7/18
OKT3	6/18	—	14/18
basiliximab	11/18	—	—
daclizumab	3/8	—	—

Table 8. Rare or serious infections.

- *M kansasii* pneumonia
- *P carinii* pneumonia
- *M morgagnii* pneumonia
- *S stercoralis* pneumonia
- Necrotizing pneumonia
- Candida pneumonia, esophagitis, sepsis
- Nocardia pneumonia and sepsis
- Histoplasma pneumonia
- *L monocytogenes* sepsis
- Salmonella sepsis, vasculitis and aneurysms
- Amoebiasis
- *M fortuitum* sepsis
- Tuberculosis cutaneous, renal and pulmonary
- Cryptococcal meningitis
- Herpes simplex encephalitis
- Toxoplasma hepatitis
- Viral Hepatitis B, C, and non-A, non-B, non-C
- Disseminated Herpes zoster
- Cutaneous chromoblastomycosis
- Perforated appendicitis and diverticulitis
- Peritonitis
- AIDS
- Chagas
- Varicella

transplant and procurement coordinators, as well. Frequently reported administrative factors include poor hospital penetration, lack of strong national organizations, cost, difficult communication with intensive care units, meager data on potential donor pools and incomplete transplant laws.

Government Priorities and Support: One further problem suggested as a disincentive towards organ donation is the perceived lack of government support. Current governmental trends reported in the social and economic literature indicate that the important priorities for most Latin-American governments are to enhance democracy, improve education and improve infrastructure so as to become more productive and competitive in the world market. This, in turn, should result in stable economies, which would allow governments to tackle their most important priorities, namely to reduce poverty, improve social services and improve public health. Thus, transplantation would not seem to be a major priority in

this context. However, the fact that more than 60,000 transplants have been carried out in the region speaks otherwise, and suggests a major government involvement in transplantation. Indeed, government support of donation and transplantation can be surmised more indirectly than directly. It is evident in the development of legal frameworks as well as in direct financing of donation, procurement and transplantation in some countries. Transplantation is paid for in public hospitals, as is tissue typing and immunosuppression. There has been financing of education of professionals and specialists abroad, as well as the partial financing of national and regional congresses. Some public educational campaigns have been carried out with the assistance of governments. Also, some governments have helped defray the cost of their national registries. This support, even if indirect, signifies a major government involvement in organ transplantation. (Reviewed in 10,11).

SUMMARY

Organ transplantation is currently a form of treatment for end-stage organ disease in Latin America for which enthusiasm appears to be growing both in individual countries as well as in the whole region. The Latin-American Transplant Registry has been a factor in the development of communication among the different countries of the region and a focus for unification. Both renal and extra-renal organ transplantation have increased significantly during 1999 and for kidneys the activity is currently 12% of the world renal transplant statistics. Important evidence for the continuing development and maturity of transplantation in the region includes the number of new transplantation societies, the increase in the number of renal and extra-renal transplant programs, the development of national organ transplant registries, efforts towards analyzing costs and administration in

transplantation and the incorporation of new immunosuppressants. The development of cardiac transplantation in Bolivia, Cuba, Paraguay, Perú, Puerto Rico and Uruguay, intestinal transplantation in Argentina, and liver transplantation in Bolivia all reflect a marked interest in organ transplantation in the different countries. Similarly, liver and cardiac transplantation are increasing at a very fast rate. End-stage organ disease is recognized as a growing health priority and organ donation as a critical limiting factor. Governments are directly and indirectly supporting transplantation initiatives. The return of trained transplant practitioners to their countries of origin also accounts for part of the increase in activity and for the organizational aspects of transplantation. The statistics presented in this report signify increasing maturity in the transplantation activities of Latin America.

REFERENCES

1. Santiago-Delpín EA. Transplantation in Latin America. Transplant Proc 1991; 23: 1855.

2. Santiago-Delpín EA, Duro-García V. The eleventh report of the Latin American Transplant Registry: 62,000 transplants. Transplant Proc 2001; 33:1.

3. Santiago-Delpín EA, Duro-García V, Casadei D, Toledo-Pereyra L. The evolution of transplantation societies in Latin America. Transplant Proc 1999; 31: 2933.

4. Mazzuchi N, González-Martínez F, Agost-Carreño C, Duro-García V, et al. Informe de Trasplante Renal – 1999, Nefrología Latinoamericana 1999; 6:188.

5. Santiago-Delpín EA, García VD. The tenth report of the Latin American Transplant Registry. Transplant Proc 1999; 31:2937.

6. Santiago-Delpín EA. Transplantation in Latin America. Bio Medicina 1999; 2:279.

7. Santiago-Delpín EA, Duro-García V. Latin American Organ Transplant Registry. Transplant Proc 1999; 31:2232.

8. Santiago-Delpín EA, Duro-García V. Latin American Transplant Register. IMTIX-Sangstat, Lyon 1999.

9. Opelz G. Factors influencing kidney graft survival in Latin America. Transplant Proc 1999; 31:2951.

10. Santiago-Delpín EA. Societal challenges in Latin America. Ann Transplantation 1998; 3:32.

11. Santiago-Delpín EA. The organ shortage: A public health crisis, What are Latin American governments doing about it? Transplant Proc 1997; 29:3203.

Appendix I. The Latin-American Transplant Collaborative Group (1988-2000)

The following investigators and clinicians have provided data, analysis or advice for at least one of the reports or other publications from the Latin-American Transplant Registry, which has operated for at least 10 years under the combined sponsorship of the then existing representative societies, the Pan-American Society for Dialysis and Transplantation and The Latin-American Transplantation Society. Currently it is part of the "*Sociedad de Trasplante de América Latina y el Caribe*". The principal authors are extremely grateful for their participation and authorship. Countries and authors are listed alphabetically.

Argentina: César Agost Carreño, José Luis Araujo, María Bacqué, Félix Cantarovich, Domingo Casadei, Oscar López Blanco, Daniel Neustad, Jorge Rodo, Mario Turín, and Norberto Vilá

Barbados: Lowell Lewis and George Nicholson

Bolivia: Silvestre Arze, Renán Chávez, Rolando Claure Vallejo, Carlos Duchens Sánchez, and Karina Soto

Brazil: Mario Abbud-Filho, Valter Duro García, Luiz Estevam Ianhez, Alteair Jacob Mocellin, Jorge Neuman, and Emil Sabbaga

Chile: Susana Elgueta and Luis Martínez Venegas

Colombia: Mario Arbelaez

Costa Rica: Manuel Cerdas Calderón and Carlos Chaverri Montero

Cuba: José A. Copo, Adolfo Delgado Rodríguez, Raúl Herrera Valdez, and Charles Magrans Bush

Dominican Republic: Hilda La Fontaine and Nicolás Rizik

Ecuador: Rómulo Campaña Chávez, Galo Garcés Barriga, Ricardo Ortiz San Martín, and Jorge Patiño

El Salvador: Miguel Saldaña Arévalo and Benjamín Ruiz Rodas

Guatemala: Carlos Betancourt Monzón, Oscar Cordón Castañeda, Leonel De Gandarias Iriarte, and Manuel Toledo

Honduras: Plutarco Castellanos

Jamaica: Russell Lawson and Hope Russell

Mexico: Arturo Dib Kurí, Javier Castellanos, Octavio Ruiz Speare, Luis Terán, and Alejandro Treviño Becerra

Panamá: César Cuero, Manuel Díaz Tejeira, Modesto Moreno, and Elías Pérez Guardia

Paraguay: Pedro Barudí, Blanca V. Franco Acosta, and Francisco Santa Cruz

Puerto Rico: José L. Cangiano, Zulma González Caraballo, Luis Morales Otero, and Eduardo Santiago Delpín.

Perú: Walter Chanamé, Raúl Romero Torres, and Hugo Valencia Guzmán

Trinidad: M. Patrick

Uruguay: L. Curí, Francisco González, Nelson Mazzuchi, Sergio Orihuela, Dante Petrucelli, and Laura Rodríguez Juanicó

Venezuela: Jorge Domínguez and Bernardo Rodríguez Iturbe

US Virgin Islands: Clive Callender

CHAPTER 10

Report from the National Transplantation Pregnancy Registry (NTPR): Outcomes of Pregnancy after Transplantation

Vincent T. Armenti, John S. Radomski, Michael J. Moritz, Lydia Z. Philips, Carolyn H. McGrory, and Lisa A. Coscia

Department of Surgery, Thomas Jefferson University, Philadelphia, Pennsylvania

The National Transplantation Pregnancy Registry (NTPR) was established in 1991 at Thomas Jefferson University. The purpose of the registry is to study the outcomes of pregnancies in transplant recipients, including female transplant recipients who have had pregnancies after transplantation and male transplant recipients who have fathered pregnancies after transplantation. The data include long-term follow-up of parent and offspring. This report reviews data collected and analyzed by the NTPR and includes summary information collected over the first 10 years of the registry.

METHODS

The method of study includes a single page questionnaire with a consent form. The questionnaires are filled out and signed by transplant recipients who are identified by their coordinators, physicians or self-report to the registry. The consent form allows for contact with the recipient via telephone interview and for the request of medical records for both the parent and child. Periodic follow-up is obtained via phone interview with the recipient and the transplant centers. An honorarium is provided to the transplant coordinators for the initial questionnaire and for follow-up.

RESULTS

Tables 1 and 2 show the number of entries to the NTPR as of November 2000. The following sections include information on each transplanted organ for female recipients, emphasizing analyses completed this past year. A summary of all entries to the NTPR over the past 10 years follows.

Table 1. Pregnancies in female transplant recipients.

Organ	Recipient	Pregnancies	Outcomes[a]
Kidney	619	947	972
Liver	85	142	143
Liver-Kidney	3	4	5
Pancreas-Kidney	28	40	42
Heart	25	44	44
Heart-Lung	3	3	3
Lung	11	12	12
Totals	**774**	**1,192**	**1,221**

[a] Includes twins and triplets

Table 2. Pregnancies fathered by male transplant recipients.

Organ	Recipient	Fathered Pregnancies	Outcomes[a]
Kidney	476	698	708
Liver	48	57	61
Pancreas-Kidney	23	26	27
Heart	84	112	113
Heart-Lung	1	2	2
Lung	1	1	1
Totals	**633**	**896**	**912**

[a] Includes twins and triplets

Female Kidney Recipients

Table 3 compares the outcomes of female kidney recipients on Sandimmune® (CsA)-, Neoral®- and tacrolimus-based regimens. There is a higher incidence of hypertension among recipients on CsA®-based regimens but a lower incidence of diabetes when compared with those on tacrolimus. A small percentage of recipients in all immunosuppressant groups report rejection during pregnancy or in the postpartum period. Lower birthweight newborns noted in the tacrolimus-treated group may be related to differences in maternal conditions.

We sought to determine whether female kidney recipients with renal failure secondary to systemic lupus erythematosus (SLE) who had pregnancies were at greater risk than those recipients with non-SLE diagnoses (Table 4) (1). Analysis was by two-tailed independent t-test and Fisher's exact test. Maternal factors that were significantly different included hypertension during pregnancy (SLE 45.9%, non-SLE 62%; p=0.0234) and cesarean section rates (SLE 29.6%, non-SLE 53%; p=0.0053). There were no statistical differences in rejection episodes, pre-eclampsia or infections. Pregnancy outcomes including live births, mean gestational age, mean birthweight and prematurity, as well as neonatal complications, were similar between groups. From this analysis, it appeared that recipients transplanted for renal failure secondary to lupus nephritis can successfully maintain a pregnancy, with outcomes comparable to those of renal recipients with other diagnoses and no statistical differences in graft loss.

Pre-eclampsia complicates a significant percentage of pregnancies of female kidney transplant recipients. We compared pre-pregnancy factors and pregnancy outcomes in female kidney recipients on CsA-based immunosuppression, with and without the diagnosis of pre-eclampsia during their posttransplant pregnancy (Table 5). There were 193 female kidney recipients (252 pregnancy outcomes) without pre-eclampsia compared with 90 recipients (97 pregnancy outcomes) with pre-

eclampsia. Variables analyzed included graft function, mean serum creatinine before, during and after pregnancy, rejection before, during and after pregnancy, and maternal conditions during pregnancy such as hypertension, diabetes, graft dysfunction and infection, as well as newborn outcomes. Comparisons were made with a single and two-tailed Fisher's exact test and analysis of variance. Pre-pregnancy factors that were significantly greater in the pre-eclampsia group included both rejection and higher mean serum creatinine before

Table 3. Female kidney recipients.

	CsA	Neoral®	Tacrolimus
Maternal Factors			
Transplant to conception interval	3.2 yrs	4.8 yrs	2.4 yrs
Hypertension during pregnancy	63%	70 %	46%
Diabetes during pregnancy	12%	8 %	19%
Infection during pregnancy	22%	28%	32%
Rejection during pregnancy	4%	2%	15%
Pre-eclampsia	30%	24%	37%
Mean serum creatinine (mg/dL)			
Before pregnancy	1.4	1.3	1.3
During pregnancy	1.4	1.4	1.8
After pregnancy	1.6	1.5	1.7
Graft loss within 2 yrs of delivery	7%	2%	14%
Outcomes (n)[a]	**(479)**	**(92)**	**(29)**
Therapeutic abortion	8%	1%	0%
Spontaneous abortion	12%	14%	28%
Ectopic	1%	0%	0%
Stillborn	3%	1%	3%
Live birth	75%	84%	69%
Live births (n)	**(361)**	**(77)**	**(20)**
Mean gestational age	35.9 wks	35.8 wks	33.3 wks
Mean birthweight	2,491 gms	2,456 gms	2,096 gms
Premature (<37 wks)	52%	51%	63%
Low birthweight (<2,500 gms)	46%	54%	65%
Cesarean section	51%	45%	37%
Newborn complications	40%	50%	55%
Neonatal deaths n (%) (within 30 days of birth)	4 (1%)	0 (0%)	1 (5%)

[a] includes twins, triplets
CsA - Sandimmune® brand cyclosporine (313 recipients, 470 pregnancies)
Neoral® brand cyclosporine (69 recipients, 89 pregnancies)
tacrolimus (23 recipients, 28 pregnancies)

Table 4. Female kidney recipients with the diagnosis of SLE versus Non-SLE.

	SLE	Non-SLE	p value
Recipients	40	248	NS
Pregnancies	61	376	NS
Pregnancy outcomes	61	384[a]	NS
Maternal Factors			
Hypertension	45.9%	62%	0.0234
Infection	15%	22.5%	NS
Rejection	5%	3.4%	NS
Pre-eclampsia	17.8%	29.6%	NS
Live births	73.8%	75.8%	NS
Mean gestational age	36.1 wks	35.8 wks	NS
Premature (<37 wks)	42.2%	54.7%	NS
Mean birthweight	2,619 gms	2,452 gms	NS
Cesarean section	29.6%	53%	0.0053
Newborn complications	33.3%	35.7%	NS
Neonatal deaths (within 30 days of birth)	2.2% (1)	0.3% (1)	NS

NS - not significant; [a] includes multiple births

Table 5. Outcomes in female CsA kidney recipients with and without pre-eclampsia during pregnancy.

	Pre-eclampsia	No Pre-eclampsia	p value
Recipients	90	193	NS
Pregnancies	96	247	NS
Pregnancy outcomes[a]	97	252	NS
Maternal Factors			
Creatinine (mg/dL)			
Before pregnancy	1.5±0.6	1.3±0.4	0.02
During pregnancy	1.6±0.9	1.3±0.5	0.0006
After pregnancy	1.9±1.0	1.5±0.8	0.0001
Rejection episodes			
Before pregnancy	48%	33%	0.02
During pregnancy	10%	3%	0.012
After pregnancy	14%	5%	0.006
During pregnancy			
Hypertension	82%	58%	NS
Diabetes	13%	11%	NS
Graft dysfunction	16%	5%	0.003
Infections	31%	22%	NS
Live births			
Mean gestational age	34.8±3.3 wks	36.5±3.2 wks	0.0001
Mean birthweight	2,279±743 gms	2,592±747 gms	0.0006

NS - not significant; [a] includes multiple births

pregnancy (p=0.02). Newborns in the pre-eclampsia group had a lower mean gestational age (34.8 vs. 36.5 wks; p=0.0001) as well as a lower mean birthweight (2,279 vs. 2,592 gms; p=0.0006). Therefore, those female recipients with a pre-pregnancy history of rejection episodes or with an elevated creatinine before or during pregnancy may be at greater risk for pre-eclampsia, and closer surveillance in this group is warranted.

In another analysis of female pregnancies on CsA, successful outcomes have been reported regardless of the time interval from transplant to conception although the incidence of pregnancy terminations was highest in those recipients with a shorter interval (≤6 months).

To date, 5 recipients with 9 pregnancies (5 livebirths, 4 spontaneous abortions) have been entered into the registry with exposure to mycophenolate mofetil (MMF) during pregnancy, with no structural malformations reported among the liveborn. Similarly, no structural problems have been noted among the offspring of 38 fathered pregnancies with exposure to MMF at the time of conception.

Female Liver Recipients

We analyzed 136 pregnancies in 83 female liver transplant recipients resulting in 100 live births, (Table 6). Among the recipient groups, mean birthweights and gestational ages and overall maternal outcomes appear similar. One tacrolimus-treated recipient has subsequently required a postpartum kidney transplant; 2 CsA-treated recipients required hemodialysis in the postpartum period and subsequently died. Of note, there are lower incidences of hypertension and pre-eclampsia in tacrolimus-treated recipients, but a higher incidence of diabetes. Despite the differing immunosuppressive regimens, we have not yet identified specific maternal or newborn outcome differences within recipient groups. From a previous analysis, we noted that female liver recipients with biopsy-proven acute rejection during pregnancy had poorer newborn outcomes as well as an

Table 6. Pregnancy outcomes in female liver recipients.

	CsA	Neoral®	tacrolimus
Maternal Factors			
Transplant to conception interval	3.4 yrs	6.0 yrs	2.7 yrs
Hypertension during pregnancy	44%	46%	30%
Diabetes during pregnancy	2%	0%	19%
Infection during pregnancy	34%	32%	12%
Rejection during pregnancy	10%	0%	11%
Pre-eclampsia	25%	31%	12%
Graft loss within 2 yrs of delivery	9%	7%	0%
Outcomes (n)[a]	**(88)**	**(22)**	**(27)**
Therapeutic abortion	10%	0%	0%
Spontaneous abortion	16%	27%	18%
Ectopic	0%	0%	0%
Stillbirth	2%	0%	4%
Live birth	72%	73%	78%
Live births (n)	**(63)**	**(16)**	**(21)**
Mean gestational age	37 wks	37 wks	37 wks
Premature (<37 wks)	37%	38%	38%
Mean birthweight	2,686 gms	2,632 gms	2,835 gms
Low birthweight (<2,500 gms)	32%	44%	24%
Cesarean section	39%	25%	33%
Newborn complications	24%	19%	29%
Neonatal deaths	0%	0%	0%
(within 30 days of birth)			

[a] includes twins
CsA - Sandimmune® brand cyclosporine (53 recip, 87 pregnancies)
Neoral® brand cyclosporine (17 recip, 22 pregnancies)
tacrolimus (20 recip, 27 pregnancies)
Seven recipients had subsequent pregnancies on different regimens.

increased risk of recurrent rejection in the postpartum period (2).

In the NTPR liver database, there are 5 women with 6 children who reported they have breastfed (3). These 6 children ranged in gestational ages from 35-41 weeks. The birthweights range from 2,098-4,097 grams. Of these 6, 4 children were breastfed for only brief periods of time up to 2 weeks. One recipient breastfed 2 consecutive children for 6 and 8 months while administered CsA and Neoral® respectively, and these children are currently 5- and one-year-olds. To date, no adverse events have been noted in these children, who are reported to be developing well.

Investigators have taken differing views regarding the safety of breastfeeding in the transplant recipient population, especially with regard to potential drug exposure to the infant. Reports have appeared in the literature of small series of patients where breastfeeding has occurred (4-6). For some investigators, any exposure exceeds the threshold for safety, and for others, the lack of long-term effects together with the documented benefits to the infant of breastfeeding outweigh the theoretical concerns of undiscovered risk. The issue remains unresolved and some mothers have chosen to breastfeed.

Female Liver-Kidney Recipients

To date, there have been 3 female liver-kidney recipients who have had posttransplant pregnancies reported to the registry. The first delivered a healthy term infant. She had had no complications of hypertension, diabetes or rejections, but died 4.5 years postpartum of a probable accidental drug overdose with functioning grafts. The second recipient had initially received a liver only with early graft and native kidney failure, followed by a liver-kidney transplant. During pregnancy she was hypertensive but had no complications or rejections and delivered a healthy term infant. The recipient has maintained good graft function for 10 years after transplantation. The child was also doing well as of the last interview (12/4/00). A recent entry to the database reported 2 pregnancies: the first was on a CsA-based regimen with no hypertension, diabetes or complications reported, and a 37 week, 3,402 gm infant was delivered; the second pregnancy was on a Neoral®-based regimen, again with no hypertension, diabetes or rejections complicating the pregnancy, and resulted in a 39 week set of twins, 3,033 and 2,665 gms. Additional information on this entry is pending.

Female Pancreas-Kidney Recipients

We have analyzed pregnancy and graft outcomes among 6 female pancreas-kidney (P/K) recipients with postpartum graft loss (7 live births, 1 therapeutic abortion) compared with 21 recipients with no graft loss (24 live births, 3 spontaneous abortions, 2 therapeutic abortions [a twin reduction], and an ectopic [one twin])(7). These data are summarized in Table 7. Analysis was by two-tailed t-test and Fisher's exact test. Significant differences between the groups were found in mean serum creatinine level, both during pregnancy (graft loss 2.23 vs. no graft loss 1.49 mg/dL; p=0.013) and postpartum (graft loss 2.51 vs. no graft loss 1.53 mg/dL; p=0.013), and in rejection episodes during pregnancy (graft loss 3 of 8 vs. no graft loss 0 of 28; p=0.008). Three rejections were diagnosed and treated during pregnancy. One was diagnosed on biopsy during cesarean section and treated postpartum. Five recipients had graft loss within 2 years of delivery (3K, 2 P/K) with one maternal death from herpes encephalitis following P/K retransplant. One recipient had graft loss (K) at 5.4 years postpartum. The mean gestational ages were lower in the graft loss group, and there was one neonatal death in the graft loss group due to sepsis in a severely premature infant. The other 6 children in the graft loss group were healthy and developing well. Although pre-pregnancy events were not predictive, elevation of serum creatinine and rejection during pregnancy or in the postpartum period were associated with graft loss. Thus, subsequent close observation and timely intervention in the management of these patients is warranted. Table 8 summarizes the outcomes of female P/K recipients reported to date to the registry. Additional entries may help to identify pre-pregnancy factors that may be predictive of peripartum graft loss.

Female Heart Recipients and Lung Recipients

Outcomes of female heart recipients are summarized in Table 8. No graft losses were reported in the peripartum period. Five recipient deaths have occurred, all more than 2 years postpartum, attributed to (1 each): vasculopathy, atherosclerosis and cardiogenic shock, acute rejection, sepsis, and graft failure related to non-

Table 7. Pregnancy conditions comparing female P/K recipients with graft loss versus no graft loss.

	Graft Loss	No Graft Loss	p value
Mean transplant to conception interval (yrs)	2.8±2.4	3.5±2	NS
Pre-pregnancy			
Mean serum creatinine (mg/dL)	1.55±0.38	1.37±0.34	NS
Hypertension	5 (63)	16 (57)	NS
Rejection	4 (50)	23 (82)	NS
During Pregnancy			
Mean serum creatinine (mg/dL)	2.23±0.86	1.49±0.64	0.013
Hypertension	8 (100)	20 (74)	NS
Rejection	3 (38)	0	0.008
Pre-eclampsia	4 (57)	7 (44)	NS
Infections	6 (75)	13 (50)	NS
Gestational diabetes	0	0	NS
Cesarean section	6 (86)	10 (46)	NS
Post-Pregnancy Conditions			
Mean serum creatinine (mg/dL)	2.51±1.5	1.5±0.67	0.013
Hypertension	6 (75)	20 (74)	NS
Rejection	3 (38)	0	NS
NS - not significant			

compliance. Further analysis and additional experience are needed to determine whether pregnancy events impact long-term maternal survival.

Outcomes of female lung recipients are also summarized in Table 8. New entries to the registry have had more favorable outcomes than those seen in a prior report. In this recipient group, we continue to proceed cautiously with recommendations, as overall the risks appear greater than those of other organ recipients.

Children

No predominant pattern of structural malformations has been noted in the offspring of transplant recipients. Last year there was a report of a female kidney recipient with a twin pregnancy in which a neonatal death occurred due to thrombotic cardiomyopathy (8). The other twin is reported healthy and developing well. Genetic and familial conditions also need to be considered in evaluating newborn outcomes. As an example, in the heart recipient group, a recipient diagnosed with mitochondrial cardiomyopathy has had 2 children after transplantation, both recently diagnosed with the same condition.

The follow-up of children born to female kidney transplant recipients remains encouraging. One hundred and thirty-three female recipients were contacted and provided information on 175 children. In this group, 8 of the 71 children older than 5 years were diagnosed with attention deficit or hyperactivity disorder (ADD/ADHD) (11%). Two years subsequent to this survey, 114 of the 133 original recipients were recontacted for information on 147 children. From this survey, only 2 new cases of ADD/ADHD were diagnosed. Therefore, developmentally, the offspring of female kidney recipients do not appear to be adversely affected, although continued follow-up of this recipient population and their offspring is warranted. Additional issues to be addressed include effects of parental morbidity and mortality, including graft failure and retransplantation on offspring development.

A report in the literature studied aspects of cellular immunity over the first 12 months of life in 6 infants born to female kidney recipients who took CsA and methylprednisolone throughout their pregnancies (9). In these infants, total T cells were low at birth, but normalized thereafter. The expression of CD25, the alpha chain of the interleukin-2 receptor, was below the normal range or low throughout the study period. HLA-DR expression on T lymphocytes was extremely low at birth and failed to increase over 12 months. The number of total B cells was lower than normal at birth, but increased over time, while the B-cell subset bearing CD5 antigen was severely depleted during the study period. The authors concluded that continuous exposure to CsA in utero appears to impair T-, B- and natural killer cell development and/or maturation, with effects still apparent at one year. They further suggested that perhaps conventional vaccinations should be delayed in these infants. An earlier report from Pilarski, et al, noted that response to vaccination in similar children was normal (10). To date, follow-up of offspring in the NTPR has not revealed reports from parents of significant problems with immunization schedules, however further investigations are ongoing.

Table 8. Pregnancy outcomes in female recipients of other organs.

Organ (n)	Pancreas-Kidney (28)	Heart (25)	Lung (11)
Maternal Factors			
Hypertension during pregnancy	74%	48%	58%
Diabetes during pregnancy	0%	2%	17%
Infection during pregnancy	57%	14%	18%
Rejection during pregnancy	8%	24%	36%
Pre-eclampsia	33%	14%	0%
Graft loss within 2 yrs of delivery	21%	0%	46%
Outcomes (n)[a]	**(42)**	**(44)**	**(12)**
Therapeutic abortions	7%	11%	33%
Spontaneous abortion	12%	21%	8%
Ectopic	2%	2%	0%
Stillbirth	0%	0%	0%
Live births	79%	66%	58%
Live births (n)	**(33)**	**(29)**	**(7)**
Mean gestational age	35 wks	36 wks	35 wks
Premature (<37 wks)	76%	43%	57%
Mean birthweight	2,151 gms	2,696 gms	2,288 gms
Low birthweight (<2,500 gms)	61%	36%	57%
Cesarean section	52%	28%	50%
Newborn complications	55%	28%	71%
Neonatal deaths (within 30 days of birth)	3% (1)[b]	0%	0%

[a] includes twins; [b] one neonatal death due to sepsis

FDA Categories

The FDA categories of agents are summarized in Table 9. No entries as yet to the registry have been reported with exposure to Rapamune, Simulect, Gengraf, Sang-Cya or Zenapax during pregnancy.

Summary Tables

Over the past 10 years we have had reports on more than 2,000 pregnancies carried or fathered by transplant recipients. The breakdown of outcomes by immunosuppressive regimen with birthweights and percent live born are summarized in Tables 10 and 11 (Appendix). Of note, there are a few cases with no immunosuppression during pregnancy. Consistently there has been a pattern of a high incidence of prematurity and low birthweight in the newborn of female transplant recipients. Continued surveillance, as noted earlier in this paper, is warranted, certainly among female recipients' offspring for potential long-term adverse effects of immunosuppressive exposure in utero.

Table 9. Commonly used immunosuppressive drugs in transplantation.

	Animal Reproductive Data	Pregnancy Category[a]
Corticosteroids (prednisone, methylprednisolone)	Y	B
Azathioprine (Imuran®)	Y	D
Cyclosporine A (Sandimmune®, Neoral®)	Y	C
Tacrolimus, FK506 (Prograf®)	Y	C
Antithymocyte gobulin (Atgam®, ATG)	N	C
Antithymocyte gobulin (Thymoglobulin®)	N	C
Orthoclone (OKT®3)	N	C
Mycophenolate Mofetil (CellCept®)	Y	C
Gengraf™ (cyclosporine capsules USP [modified])	Y	C
SangCya™ Oral Solution	Y	C
Basiliximab (Simulect®)	Y	B
Daclizumab (Zenapax®)	N	C
Sirolimus (Rapamune®)	Y	C

[a] B = no fetal risk, no controlled studies; C = fetal risk cannot be ruled out;
D = evidence of fetal risk

A Report of Interest

Of interest in the literature was the first reported case of the use of artificial reproductive technologies in a dual transplant couple (11). A twin pregnancy resulted from in-vitro fertilization with intracytoplasmic sperm injections (IVF/ICSI) in a female liver transplant recipient whose partner was a renal transplant recipient. Healthy twin boys were delivered at 34 weeks.

SUMMARY

Safety of pregnancy in the female transplant recipient population must include consideration of 3 outcomes - mother, baby and transplanted graft. In the majority of female recipients studied, pregnancy does not appear to cause excessive or irreversible problems with graft function, if the function of the transplant organ is stable prior to pregnancy. However, a small percentage of recipients identified within each organ system may develop rejection, graft dysfunction and/or graft loss that may be related to the pregnancy and may occur unpredictably. Outcomes are not entirely similar among all organ systems, and one must consider risks on an individual organ basis.

It appears reasonable to advise female recipients to wait one or 2 years after transplantation before attempting pregnancy to insure that function of the transplanted organ is adequate and stable and also to allow for stabilization of immunosuppressive medications. Favorable outcomes, however, have occurred when recipients have become pregnant less than one year from transplant, so cases must be analyzed individually.

Immunosuppressive medications may have to be adjusted during pregnancy, and in some cases, rejections occur requiring additional immunosuppressive regimens (steroids and in several cases OKT3). Whether increasing immunosuppressive doses during pregnancy to adjust for falling levels lessens the rejection risk has never been studied prospectively.

There is concern based on animal reproductive studies that the risk of birth defects and/or spontaneous miscarriage is increased in women exposed to MMF during pregnancy. Of the 9 pregnancies reported to the registry to date, there have been no birth defects noted among 5 liveborn of female recipients exposed to MMF. Data remain limited.

For female recipients, a high incidence of low birthweight and prematurity compared to the general population has been a consistent outcome, however, there has been no specific pattern of malformation in their newborn or any apparent increase in the incidence of small-for-gestational-age newborn. Long-term follow-up of children to date by the NTPR has been encouraging.

A recent report in the literature has suggested impairment of immune function in newborn of CsA-treated mothers. Further study is needed.

Some mothers have chosen to breastfeed. The potential risk to the newborn of ingested immunosuppressives compared with the potential benefits of breastfeeding is unknown and options must be discussed with the recipient.

From earlier registry reports, recipients with deteriorating graft function, such as liver recipients with recurrent hepatitis C and/or other recipients with deteriorating graft function, appear to be at risk for worsened graft function with pregnancy.

Outcomes of male recipient fathered pregnancies have been favorable and appear to be similar to the general population, but this group has not been as well studied as female recipients. No structural problems have been noted in the 38 offspring of males on MMF at the time of conception.

Within each organ group, some female recipients have reported more than one pregnancy, sometimes on differing immunosuppressive regimens. If there is stable graft function, additional successful pregnancies are possible.

Continued entries to the registry, especially in light of newer immunosuppressives and combinations of agents, are needed to continue to provide guidelines for management.

The NTPR acknowledges the cooperation of transplant recipients and over 200 centers nationwide who have contributed their time and information to the registry. The NTPR is supported by grants from Novartis Pharmaceuticals Corp., Fujisawa Healthcare, Inc., Roche Laboratories Inc. and Wyeth-Ayerst Pharmaceuticals, Inc.

REFERENCES

1. McGrory CH, McCloskey LJ, DeHoratius RJ, et al. Pregnancy outcomes in female renal recipients: A comparison of systemic lupus erythematosus to other diagnoses. Transplantation 2000; 69:683A.

2. Armenti VT, Wilson, GA, Radomski JS, et al. Report from the National Transplantation Pregnancy Registry (NTPR): Outcomes of pregnancy after transplantation. In: JM Cecka and PI Terasaki, Eds. Clinical Transplants 1999. Los Angeles, UCLA Immunogenetics Center, 2000; 111.

3. Armenti VT, Herrine SK, Radomski JS, Moritz MJ. Pregnancy after liver transplantation. Liver Transplantation 2000; 6:671.

4. Nyberg G, Haljamae U, Frisenette-Fich C, Wennergren M, Kjellmer I. Breast-feeding during treatment with cyclosporine. Transplantation 1998; 65:253.

5. Thiru Y, Bateman DN, Coulthard MG. Drug points: Successful breast feeding while mother was taking cyclosporine. British Medical Journal 1997; 315:463.

6. Banta-Wright S. Minimizing infant exposure to and risks from medications while breast-feeding. J Perinat Neonat Nurs 1997; 11:71.

7. Wilson GA, Coscia LA, McGrory CH, et al. Post-pregnancy graft loss among female pancreas-kidney (P/K) recipients. Transplant Proc (In press).

8. Vyas S, Kumar A, Piecuch S, et al. Outcome of a twin pregnancy in a renal recipient treated with tacrolimus. Transplantation 1999; 67:490.

9. DiPaolo S, Schena A, Morrone LF, et al. Immunologic evaluation during the first year of life of infants born to cyclosporine-treated female kidney transplant recipients. Transplantation 2000; 69:2049.

10. Pilarski LM, Yacyshyn BR, Lazarovits AI. Analysis of peripheral blood lymphocyte populations and immune function from children exposed to cyclosporine or to azathioprine in utero. Transplantation 1994; 57:133.

11. Case AM, Weissman A, Sermer M, Greenblatt EM. Successful twin pregnancy in a dual-transplant couple resulting from in-vitro fertilization and intracytoplasmic sperm injection. Human Reproduction 2000; 15:626.

APPENDIX

Table 10. Female recipients by immunosuppressive regimen.

Recipient Immunosuppressive	No. of Tx recip[b]	No. of Preg[c]	No. of live births (%)	Mean birth weight (g)	Mean gestational age (wks)	No. of miscarriages (%)	No. of stillbirths (%)	No. of ectopic Preg (%)	No. of therapeutic abortions(%)
Kidney	619	947							
All C regimens	313	470	361 (75.4)	2490.5	35.9	58 (12.1)	15 (3.1)	3 (0.6)	40 (8.4)
C + A + P	232	344	271 (77.4)	2521.7	36	34 (9.7)	11 (3.1)	1 (0.3)	32 (9.1)
C + P	79	112	78 (67.8)	2321.4	35.5	23 (20)	3 (2.6)	2 (1.7)	8 (7)
C + A	6	9	7 (77.8)	2692.5	33.5	1 (11.1)	1 (11.1)	0	0
C alone	2	2	2 (100)	2253.8	33.5	0	0	0	0
All N regimens	69	89	75 (81.5)	2456.3	35.8	15 (16.3)	1 (1.1)	0	1 (1.1)
N + A + P	39	46	42 (91.3)	2538.5	36	4 (8.7)	0	0	0
N + MMF + P	2	6	3 (50)	2367.2	35.8	3 (50)	0	0	0
C/N + A + P	5	5	4 (80)	2438.1	36	0	1 (20.0)	0	0
C/N + P	1	1	1 (100)	2438.1	36	0	0	0	0
N + P	21	27	23 (76.7)	2313.5	35	6 (20)	0	0	1 (3.1)
N + A	2	2	2 (100)	2466.4	38.4	0	0	0	0
N alone	1	1	1 (100)	2296.3	37	0	0	0	0
All T regimens	23	28	20 (69)	2096.0	33.3	8 (27.6)	1 (3.4)	0	0
T + A + P	9	9	6 (66.7)	2264.2	33.8	2 (22.2)	1 (11.1)	0	0
T + MMF + P	3	3	2 (66.7)	1530.9	31.5	1 (33.3)	0	0	0
T + A	2	2	1 (50)	2395.5	33	1 (50)	0	0	0
T + P	5	8	7 (87.5)	2259.9	35.2	1 (12.5)	0	0	0
T alone	5	7	4 (57.1)	1764.8	30.8	3 (42.9)	0	0	0
Other regimens	214	360	307 (82.1)	2717.9	36.4	33 (8.8)	10 (2.7)	5 (1.3)	16 (4.3)
A+P	195	329	278 (82)	2714.6	36.4	30 (8.9)	10 (3)	5 (1.5)	16 (4.7)
P alone	15	26	23 (88.5)	2813.7	35.4	3 (11.5)	0	0	0
A alone	5	8	8 (100)	2937.1	38.3	0	0	0	0
No immunosuppression	2	2	2 (100)	2749.9	37	0	0	0	0
Liver	85	142	104 (73.2)	2715.8	36.9	26 (18.3)	3 (2.1)	0	9 (6.3)
All T regimens	20	27	21 (77.8)	2834.6	36.7	5 (18.5)	1 (3.7)	0	0
T + A + P	5	6	4 (66.7)	2374.3	36	2 (33.3)	0	0	0
T + P	13	15	12 (80)	2983.1	37.4	3 (20)	0	0	0
T alone	5	6	5 (83.3)	2846.3	35.6	0	1(16.7)	0	0
All N regimens	17	22	16 (72.7)	2631.7	37.1	6 (27.3)	0	0	0
N + A + P	7	8	7 (87.5)	2668.9	38.3	1 (12.5)	0	0	0
N + A	2	2	2 (100)	2385.6	35.9	0	0	0	0
N + P	6	9	5 (55.6)	2798.1	37.2	4 (44.4)	0	0	0
N alone	2	3	2 (66.7)	2331.8	33.5	1 (33.3)	0	0	0
All C regimens	53	87	63 (71.6)	2686.4	36.8	14 (15.9)	2 (2.3)	0	9 (10.2)
C + A + P	31	49	37 (74)	2592.7	36.8	6 (12)	2 (4)	0	5 (10)
C + A	1	1	1 (100)	4096.5	36	0	0	0	0
C + P	21	34	23 (67.7)	2734.5	36.8	8 (23.5)	0	0	3 (8.8)
C alone	2	3	2 (66.7)	3160.0	37.4	0	0	0	1 (33.3)
No Immunosuppression	2	5	4 (80)	2891.7	38.5	1 (20)	0	0	0
Unknown	1	1	0	-	-	1(100)	0	0	0

Table 10. (Cont'd)

Recipient Immunosuppressive	No. of Tx recip[b]	No. of Preg[c]	No. of live births (%)	Mean birth weight (g)	Mean gestational age (wks)	No. of miscarriages (%)	No. of stillbirths (%)	No. of ectopic Preg (%)	No. of therapeutic abortions(%)
Pancreas-kidney	28	40	33 (78.6)	2151	34.5	5 (11.9)	0	1 (2.4)	3 (7.1)
All C regimens	17	24	20 (76.9)	1973.7	34.1	2 (7.7)	0	1 (3.9)	3 (11.5)
C + A + P	12	18	14 (73.7)	1774.7	33.9	2 (10.5)	0	1 (5.3)	2 (10.5)
C + P	6	6	6 (85.7)	2438.1	34.62	0	0	0	1 (14.3)
All N regimens	8	11	8 (72.7)	2203.1	34.5	3 (27.3)	0	0	0
N + A + P	8	9	9 (77.8)	2149.3	34.5	2 (22.2)	0	0	0
N + P	1	2	1 (50)	2579.8	34	1 (50)	0	0	0
All T regimens	4	5	5 (100)	2778.3	36	0	0	0	0
T + A + P	2	2	2 (100)	2693.2	37.3	0	0	0	0
T + A	2	2	2 (100)	2338.8	34.8	0	0	0	0
T + P	1	1	1 (100)	3827.2	36	0	0	0	0
Heart	25	44	29 (65.9)	2695.5	36.6	9 (20.5)	0	1 (2.3)	5 (11.4)
All C regimens	19	37	24 (64.9)	2678.4	36.6	8 (21.6)	0	1 (2.7)	4 (10.8)
C + A + P	16	30	19(63.3)	2641.7	36	6 (20)	0	1 (3.3)	4 (13.3)
C + P	2	6	4 (66.7)	2898.7	38.8	2 (33.3)	0	0	0
C + A	1	1	1(100)	2494.8	39	0	0	0	0
N + A + P	3	3	2 (66.7)	3073.1	38	0	0	0	1 (33.3)
All T regimens	3	4	3 (75)	2579.8	36	1 (25)	0	0	0
T + A + P	2	2	1 (50)	3231.9	36	1 (50)	0	0	0
T + P	1	1	1 (100)	2012.8	39	0	0	0	0
T alone	1	1	1 (100)	2494.8	40	0	0	0	0
Heart-lung	3	3	3 (100)	2537.3	36.8	0	0	0	0
C + A + P	3	3	3 (100)	2537.3	36.8	0	0	0	0
Lung	11	12	7 (58.3)	2287.8	34.6	1 (8.3)	0	0	4 (33.3)
All C regimens	6	7	3 (42.9)	2664.9	36.2	0	0	0	4 (57.1)
C + A + P	5	6	2 (33.3)	2664.9	38.5	0	0	0	4 (66.7)
C + P	1	1	1 (100)	2664.9	31.5	0	0	0	0
N + A + P	1	1	1 (100)	1077.3	30	0	0	0	0
All T regimens	4	4	3 (75)	1912.2	33	1 (25)	0	0	0
T + A + P	3	3	2 (66.7)	2663.4	37	1 (33.3)	0	0	0
T alone	1	1	1 (100)	1615.9	30	0	0	0	0
Liver-kidney	3	4	5 (100)	3018	38.1	0	0	0	0
All C regimens	2	2	2 (100)	2993.7	38	0	0	0	0
C + A + P	1	1	1 (100)	2664.9	38	0	0	0	0
C + P	1	1	1 (100)	3322.6	38	0	0	0	0
C + A	1	1	1 (100)	3401.9	37	0	0	0	0
N + A	1	1	2 (100)	2849.1	38.5	0	0	0	0
Totals	774	1192							

[a] C - Sandimmune®, A - azathioprine, P - prednisone, N - Neoral®, MMF - mycophenolate mofetil, C/N - Sandimmune® switched to Neoral® during pregnancy, T - tacrolimus; [b] Some recipients were maintained on different immunosuppressive regimens during subsequent pregnancies; [c] Some pregnancies resulted in multiple outcomes

Table 11. *Male recipient fathered pregnancies by immunosuppressive regimen.*

Recipient Immunosuppressive	No. of Tx recip[b]	No. of Preg[c]	No. of live births (%)	Mean birth weight (g)	Mean gestational age (wks)	No. of miscarriages (%)	No. of stillbirths (%)	No. of ectopic Preg (%)	No. of therapeutic abortions(%)
Kidney	476	698	658 (92.9)	3354.3	39.1	38 (5.4)	7 (1)	1 (0.1)	4 (0.6)
All C regimens	313	431	405 (92.9)	3353.2	39.1	23 (5.3)	5 (1.2)	1 (0.2)	2 (0.5)
C + A + P	208	279	264 (93.3)	3397.5	39.3	14 (5)	3 (1.1)	1 (0.4)	1 (0.4)
C + MMF + P	3	3	3 (100)	3364.1	39.5	0	0	0	0
C + P	98	131	122 (92.4)	3244.1	38.8	7 (5.3)	2 (1.5)	0	1 (0.8)
C + A	7	7	7 (100)	3332.7	39.4	0	0	0	0
C alone	10	15	13 (86.7)	3595.6	39.6	2 (13.3)	0	0	0
All N regimens	40	43	44 (97.8)	3215.3	38	1 (2.2)	0	0	0
N + A + P	15	17	16 (94.1)	3356.3	38.6	1 (5.9)	0	0	0
N + MMF + P	17	18	18 (100)	3249.2	38.4	0	0	0	0
N + MMF	1	1	1 (100)	2324.7	36	0	0	0	0
N + A	1	1	1 (100)	3260.2	39	0	0	0	0
N + P	7	7	7 (100)	2951.5	36.4	0	0	0	0
All T regimens	13	14	14 (87.5)	2980.8	37.8	2 (12.5)	0	0	0
T + A + P	1	1	1 (100)	2438.1	36	0	0	0	0
T + MMF + P	3	3	3 (100)	3647.6	39.5	0	0	0	0
T + MMF	1	1	1 (100)	3827.2	43	0	0	0	0
T + P	7	8	7 (87.5)	2851.2	36.7	1 (12.5)	0	0	0
T alone	1	3	2 (66.7)	2282.1	37	1 (33.3)	0	0	0
Other regimens									
A+P	103	169	158 (92.9)	3414.7	39.4	9 (5.3)	2 (1.2)	0	1 (0.6)
MMF + P	2	2	2 (100)	3798.9	37.5	0	0	0	0
P alone	14	19	19 (100)	3380.3	38.8	0	0	0	0
A alone	1	1	1 (100)	4309.1	41	0	0	0	0
No immunosuppression	9	10	10 (100)	3432.4	38.3	0	0	0	0
Liver	48	57	58 (95.1)	3321.4	39.1	3 (4.9)	0	0	0
All T regimens	8	10	13 (100)	3020.3	38.3	0	0	0	0
T + A + P	5	6	6 (100)	3179.9	39.6	0	0	0	0
T + P	2	2	2 (100)	3444.5	39.5	0	0	0	0
T alone	2	3	5 (100)	2659.2	36.3	0	0	0	0
All N regimens	8	8	7 (87.5)	3773.7	40.6	1 (12.5)	0	0	0
N + A + P	2	2	2 (100)	3841.4	39.8	0	0	0	0
N + MMF + P	3	3	2 (66.7)	3968.9	41	1 (33.3)	0	0	0
N + P	3	3	3 (100)	3598.5	41	0	0	0	0
All C regimens	32	38	37 (94.9)	3351.8	39.2	2 (5.1)	0	0	0
C + A + P	21	26	24 (92.3)	3325.2	38.5	2 (7.7)	0	0	0
C + A	2	2	2 (100)	3742.1	39.5	0	0	0	0
C + P	8	9	10 (100)	3383.5	38.5	0	0	0	0
C alone	1	1	1 (100)	2891.7	40	0	0	0	0
Other regimens									
P alone	1	1	1 (100)	2948.4	38	0	0	0	0

Table 11 (Cont'd)

Recipient Immunosuppressive	No. of Tx recip[b]	No. of Preg[c]	No. of live births (%)	Mean birth weight (g)	Mean gestational age (wks)	No. of miscarriages (%)	No. of stillbirths (%)	No. of ectopic Preg (%)	No. of therapeutic abortions(%)
Pancreas-kidney	23	26	25 (92.6)	3175.7	38.3	2 (7.4)	0	0	0
All C regimens	13	16	14 (87.5)	3245.1	39	2 (12.5)	0	0	0
C + A + P	10	13	11 (78.6)	3229.5	38.9	3 (21.4)	0	0	0
C + MMF + P	1	1	1 (100)	3061.7	40	0	0	0	0
C + P	2	2	2 (100)	3430.3	39	0	0	0	0
All N regimens	4	4	4 (100)	2388.4	34.3	0	0	0	0
N + A + P	1	1	1 (100)	2438.1	36	0	0	0	0
N + MMF + P	1	1	1 (100)	3231.8	38.5	0	0	0	0
N + P	2	2	2 (100)	1941.9	31.3	0	0	0	0
All T regimens	5	5	5 (100)	3492.7	39	0	0	0	0
T + MMF + P	3	3	3 (100)	3359.4	37.5	0	0	0	0
T + P	2	2	2 (100)	3940.6	40.5	0	0	0	0
Heart	84	112	100 (88.5)	3443	39.1	9 (8)	1 (0.9)	0	3 (2.7)
All C regimens	74	99	88 (88)	3441.2	39	8 (8)	1 (1)	0	3 (3)
C + A + P	54	72	64 (87.7)	3385	39	5 (6.9)	1 (1.4)	0	3 (4.1)
C + MMF + P	1	1	1 (100)	4025.6	41	0	0	0	0
C + P	18	19	18 (94.7)	3427.9	39	1 (5.3)	0	0	0
C + A	6	7	5 (71.4)	3900.9	38.4	2 (29.6)	0	0	0
All N regimens	7	8	7 (87.5)	3361	39.4	1 (12.5)	0	0	0
N + A + P	5	5	5 (100)	3379.3	39.6	0	0	0	0
N + A	2	3	2 (66.7)	3315.5	39	1 (33.3)	0	0	0
All T regimens	3	4	4 (100)	3579.1	40.6	0	0	0	0
T + A + P	1	1	1 (100)	3402	40	0	0	0	0
T + MMF + P	1	1	1 (100)	3317	38.5	0	0	0	0
T + P	1	2	2 (100)	3799	42	0	0	0	0
Heart-lung									
C + A + P	1	2	2 (100)	3912.2	38.5	0	0	0	0
Lung									
N + A + P	1	1	1 (100)	3572	40	0	0	0	0
Totals	633	896							

[a] C - Sandimmune®, A - azathioprine, P - prednisone, N - Neoral®, MMF - mycophenolate mofetil, C/N - Sandimmune® switched to Neoral® during pregnancy, T - tacrolimus; [b] Some recipients were maintained on different immunosuppressive regimens when they fathered subsequent pregnancies; [c] Some pregnancies resulted in multiple outcomes

USRDS

CHAPTER 11

The Impact of Transplantation on Survival with Kidney Failure

Bertram L. Kasiske, Jon Snyder, Arthur Matas, and Allan Collins

For the United States Renal Data System, The United States Renal Data System Coordinating Center, Minneapolis, Minnesota

There is good news and bad news in the numbers of patients needing treatment for end-stage kidney disease (ESKD) in the United States. The bad news is that the total number of patients with ESKD continues to increase. The good news is that the rate of growth in this number appears to be slowing. However, the decline in the rate of growth is not enough to allow transplantation to keep pace with the growth in the number of ESKD patients, at least in the foreseeable future. This is indeed bad news, since the favorable impact of transplantation on the overall mortality of ESKD patients will continue to be limited by the current shortage of donor kidneys and the inability of transplantation to keep up with the growth in the number of patients with ESKD.

Mortality is declining both for patients treated with dialysis and for patients receiving a kidney transplant. However, a recent analysis of United States Renal Data System (USRDS) data demonstrated that the mortality after transplantation is substantially less than the mortality of comparable patients on the transplant waiting list (1). This was true for patients in every category, specifically for men, women, young, old, diabetic and non-diabetic. Thus, renal transplantation remains the treatment of choice for patients with ESKD. Unfortunately, the full potential for the beneficial effects of transplantation on survival with ESKD in the United States has been limited by the shortage of donor kidneys. In addition, a growing number of transplant patients who reject their kidneys become candidates for second, third, or even fourth transplants, and thereby increase the demand for the limited number of available organs. Thus, efforts to improve the survival of ESKD patients should be directed both to increasing the number of kidney donors and to decreasing the number of patients who lose their grafts to rejection.

Growth in the Number of Patients with End-Stage Kidney Disease

Both the incidence and the prevalence of ESKD have been growing, although the rate of growth appears to be slowing in recent years (Fig. 1). Calculations based on

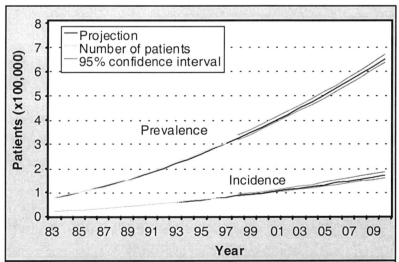

Figure 1. The number of incident and point prevalent patients with end-stage kidney disease in the United States projected to 2010. The projections use actual data from 1982-1997 and project future trends using changes in these data. Data are from the USRDS 2000 Annual Data Report (Figure 1.3).

Clinical Transplants 2000, Cecka and Terasaki, Eds. UCLA Immunogenetics Center, Los Angeles, California

the changes in the numbers of new patients (incidence) in the USRDS between 1982-1997 lead to projections that between 1998 and 2010 the incidence in ESKD will almost double, growing from approximately 87,000 per year to 173,000 per year (Fig. 1) (2). The growth in the incidence of ESKD is different in different patient groups. For example, between 1990-1998, the annual incidence of ESKD increased 80.0% overall (from 48,013 to 86,438 patients per year). The increase in incidence over this period was 26.1% (from 958 to 1,208) for ages 0-19 years, 38.8% (from 9,571 to 13,284) for ages 20-44 years, 86.1% (from 16,259 to 30,266) for ages 45-64 years, and 96.4% (from 21,225 to 41,680) for ages 65 years and over. The increase in incidence between 1990-1998 was 143.7% (from 14,313 to 34,874) for kidney disease from diabetes, 47.7% (from 12,373 to 18,273) for kidney disease attributed to hypertension, 46.9% (from 1,533 to 2,252) for cystic kidney disease, and 125.1% (from 3,157 to 7,107) for "other" kidney diseases (2). Thus, the increase in the incidence of ESKD varies by age and cause of kidney disease, but is high in all patient groups.

The prevalence – the number of ESKD patients at the end of each calendar year – will grow even faster than the incidence, more than doubling from 326,000 patients in 1998 to 661,000 patients in 2010 (Fig. 1). At the end of 1998, 64.0% of the patients in the USRDS were being treated with hemodialysis (n=196,803), 7.3% (22,605) were being treated with peritoneal dialysis, while 28.7% (88,311) had a functioning kidney transplant. Although the total numbers of prevalent patients has continued to increase, growth in the numbers of patients slowed when the growth in the period from 1990-1994 is compared with growth in the period from 1994-1998.

The growth in the number of prevalent hemodialysis patients slowed from 9.1% in the period 1990-1994 to 7.0% in the period 1994-1998. Of the prevalent patients in 1998, 38.0% had ESKD caused by diabetes, 24.8% hypertension, 13.6% glomerulonephritis, 3.1% cystic disease, and 20.5% were other/unknown. The relative rate of growth in prevalence (in the period 1990-1994 compared with the period 1994-1998) slowed less for patients with ESKD caused by diabetes (from 13.8% to 11.5%) compared with hypertension (9.6% to 3.0%), glomerulonephritis (4.4% to 2.2%) and cystic kidney diseases (4.1% to 1.6%). Changes in the year-end prevalence of ESKD in 1990-1994 compared with 1994-1998

were similar for Caucasians (8.3% to 7.1%), African Americans (9.7% to 6.7%), men (9.1% to 7.3%) and women (9.1% to 6.8%). In the period 1990-1994 the year-end prevalence of peritoneal dialysis patients increased by 10.0%, while in 1994-1998 there was a -3.2% decline. This decline occurred among all categories of patients (by cause of kidney disease, race, and gender). However patients 0-19 years old had an increase of 2.5% in 1990-1994 compared with a similar increase of 2.0% in 1994-1998.

The growth in the number of prevalent transplant patients slowed from 9.5% in the period 1990-1994 to 7.4% in the period 1994-1998. Of the prevalent patients in 1998, 19.8% had ESKD caused by diabetes, 12.1% hypertension, 28.5% glomerulonephritis, 10.7% cystic disease, and 29.1% were other/unknown. Changes in year-end prevalence of patients with a functioning kidney transplant over the period 1990-1994 compared with 1994-1998 were similar for patients with ESKD caused by diabetes (from 11.8% to 8.3%), hypertension (10.3% to 7.3%), glomerulonephritis (8.1% to 5.9%) and cystic kidney diseases (10.6% to 8.4%). Changes in the year-end prevalence of patients with a functioning kidney transplant were also similar for Caucasians (9.0% to 6.8%), African Americans (11.0% to 9.4%), men (9.2% to 7.3%) and women (10.0% to 7.7%).

Thus, the changes in the rate of growth of the number of prevalent hemodialysis patients have been similar to changes in the rate of growth of the number of kidney transplant patients, and projections indicate that these trends will continue (Fig. 1). Peritoneal dialysis will play an increasingly smaller role, except for pediatric-aged patients. Trends are similar across all categories of patients, with the exception of patients with ESKD caused by diabetes, where the slowing in the rate of growth has been less in the hemodialysis compared with the transplant population. This likely reflects the co-morbidity associated with diabetes and the fact that a relatively greater proportion of diabetic patients who had more co-morbid conditions were not considered to be transplant candidates. In addition to the fact that there were relatively fewer diabetic kidney transplant recipients at the end of 1998 (compared with hemodialysis and peritoneal dialysis) there was also less co-morbidity among the kidney transplant population compared with the dialysis population (Fig. 2).

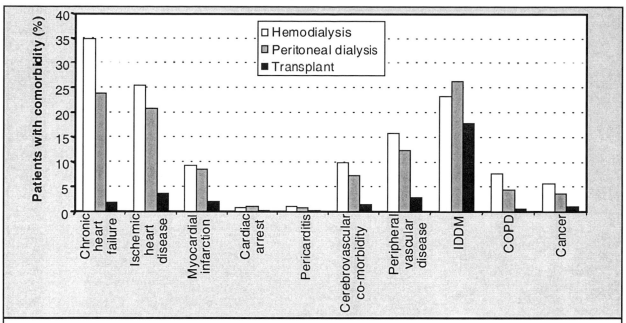

Figure 2. Reported comorbidity at initiation of hemodialysis, peritoneal dialysis, or renal transplantation in 1998. (IDDM = Insulin dependent diabetes mellitus; COPD = Chronic obstructive pulmonary disease.) Data are from the USRDS 2000 Annual Data Report (Figure 2.13).

Growth in the Number of New Kidney Transplants

The number of new (incident) transplants has grown over the past decade, but not fast enough to keep pace with the number of new patients with ESKD. The number of cadaveric transplants performed every year increased

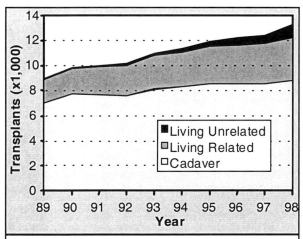

Figure 3. Trends in the numbers of new transplants by donor source from 1988-1998. Data are from the USRDS Annual Facility Survey in the USRDS 2000 Annual Data Report (Table F.1).

24.9% (from 7,006 to 8,752) between 1989-1998 (Fig. 3). During this same period the annual number of living-related transplants performed increased 89.4% (from 1,823 to 3,453) while the number of living unrelated transplants performed increased almost 15-fold, or 1,424% (from 70 to 1,067). Thus, the increase in the rate of new transplants performed over the past few years has been most marked for living-unrelated transplants. Indeed the rate of growth in the number of cadaveric transplants slowed from 7.9% over the four-year period from 1990-1994 compared with an increase of only 5.3% between 1994-1998. The rate of growth in living-related transplants was 36.8% between 1990-1994 compared with 26.1% between 1994-1998, while the rate of growth in the number of living-unrelated transplants was 191% between 1990-1994 compared with 307% between 1994-1998.

In the period 1990-1994 the overall number of new transplants increased 15.5%, while between 1994-1998 there was a 17.3% increase in the number of transplants performed. These increases in the number of transplants have not kept pace with the increases in the total numbers of new ESKD patients, which were 48,013 in 1990, 75,019 in 1994, and 84,438 in 1998. As a result, the number of patients waiting for a kidney transplant has

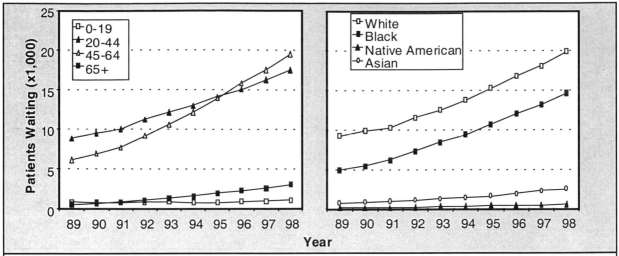

Figure 4. Growth in the cadaveric renal transplant waiting list by age (left) and race (right). Data are from the USRDS 2000 Annual Data Report (Figures 7.20 and 7.22).

also grown (Fig. 4). Unfortunately, the growth in the waiting list has been greater for racial minorities than for Caucasians (Fig. 4).

It is also unfortunate that the proportion of younger ESKD patients who ever received a kidney transplant has declined (Fig. 5). Thus, for patients 0-19 years old, the proportion who had ever received a kidney transplant declined from 77.8% to 73.4% between 1989-1998, while the proportion of 20-44 year old patients who had ever received a kidney transplant declined from 61.7%

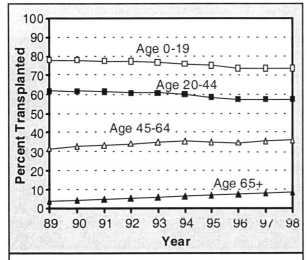

Figure 5. Ratios of ESKD patients ever transplanted, by age on December 31st of the year of transplant. Data are from the USRDS 2000 Annual Data Report (Table F.24).

to 57.2%. On the other hand, the proportion of patients age 45-64 years who had ever received a kidney transplant increased from 31.5% to 36.2%, while the proportion over age 64 who ever received a transplant increased from to 3.7% to 8.4%.

The shortage of kidneys and the resulting growth in the waiting list has not been helped by the need for repeat transplants. Fortunately, the number of patients needing a second, third, fourth or even fifth transplant has been relatively constant (Fig. 6). In 1989 there were 924 repeat cadaveric transplants compared with 5,865 first cadaveric transplants, while in 1998 there were 1,060 repeat transplants (a 14.7% increase) compared with 7,718 first cadaveric transplants (a 31.6% increase). In 1989 there were only 106 repeat living donor transplants compared with 1,717 first living donor transplants, while in 1998 there were 318 repeat living donor transplants compared with 3,620 first living donor transplants.

Declining Mortality from Kidney Failure

There has been an improvement in survival for all ESKD patients, despite an increase in co-morbidity at the time of initiation of therapy (Table 1). The improvement in survival has been most dramatic for patients treated with dialysis, but survival on dialysis remains much lower than survival after transplantation (Fig. 7). For example, one-year survival for dialysis patients (excluding the first 90 days) increased from 75.6% in 1989 to 83.4% in 1997. Over this same time period, one-year

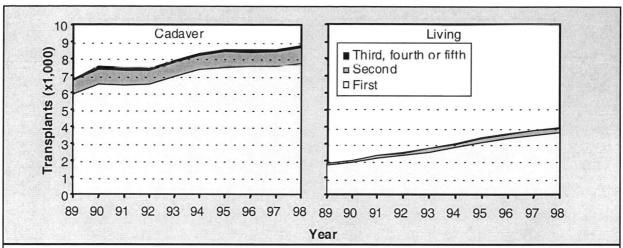

Figure 6. Number of repeat cadaveric donor transplants and living donor transplants. Data are from the USRDS 2000 Annual Data Report (Table F.3).

patient survival (including the first 90 days) improved from 93.2% to 95.8% for first cadaveric renal transplants. One-year patient survival improved from 96.7% to 97.7%

Table 1. The recent decline in co-morbidity from 1995-1998 (years for which data were collected in a similar fashion). Data are from the USRDS 2000 Annual Data Report (Figure 2.10).

	1995	1998
Chronic heart failure	31.4	33.4
Ischemic heart disease	21.9	24.6
Acute myocardial infarction	8.7	9.1
Cardiac arrest	1.1	0.8
Arrythmia	5.5	6.0
Pericarditis	1.6	0.9
CVA/TIA	8.2	9.5
Peripheral vascular disease	14.2	15.2
Hypertension	67.4	73.9
DM P/C	36.3	40.9
IDDM	22.3	23.5
Chr obstructive pulmonary disease	6.8	7.3
Smoker	5.9	5.0
Cancer	4.8	5.4
Alcohol	1.8	1.4
Drugs	1.1	1.0
AIDS	0.6	0.4
HIV	0.9	0.7
Ambulate	5.5	4.4
Transfer	1.9	1.6

for first living donor transplant recipients. The improvements in 5-year patient survival for patients beginning dialysis or receiving a transplant in 1989-1993 were relatively modest. The 5-year survival for dialysis patients improved from 25.3% to 29.5% for patients initiating therapy in 1989 compared with 1993 (Fig. 7). The 5-year survival for first cadaveric renal transplant recipients improved from 79.3% to 82.2% for patients initiating therapy in 1989 compared with 1993, while in this same time period the 5-year survival for first living donor transplant recipients went from 87.3% to 87.4%.

Relative Survival Advantage of Renal Transplantation Compared with Dialysis

The interpretation of comparisons between survival of dialysis and transplant patients is limited by the fact that transplant patients are selected to minimize the anticipated risk for surgery and immunosuppression. Therefore, transplant patients have less co-morbidity than dialysis patients (Fig. 2). Recently, the growth in the cadaveric renal transplant waiting list has made it possible to compare the survival of transplant patients with the survival of dialysis patients on the cadaveric transplant waiting list. Wolfe and co-workers reported that mortality for renal transplant recipients was reduced compared with that of patients placed on the waiting list but not transplanted (1). In the following analysis we assumed that patients placed on the transplant waiting list were considered by their physicians to be candidates for renal transplantation. We then compared survival of pa-

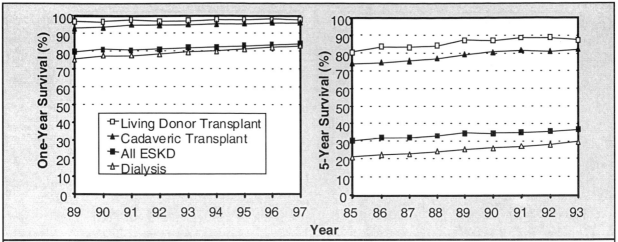

Figure 7. Changes in one-year and 5-year patient survival rates adjusted for age, gender, race and cause of kidney failure. Data are from the USRDS 2000 Annual Data Report (Tables I.26, I.28, I.34, I.36, I.42, and I.44).

tients who actually received a transplant with that of patients who did not. Although there may still be bias in the selection of patients for transplantation (bias that is not accurately reflected by placement on the waiting list) this comparison between transplant and dialysis mortality is likely to be the least biased comparison that is possible using retrospective data.

In this analysis we included patients who began maintenance dialysis for ESKD between 1993-1998, and who were subsequently listed with the United Network for Organ Sharing (UNOS) for a cadaver kidney transplant. We included only patients whose ESKD treatment was covered by Medicare (primary or secondary payer). We excluded patients who underwent transplantation before needing maintenance dialysis (pre-emptive transplants), as well as patients who had a prior transplant. We also excluded multiple listings, and included only the earliest listing on the UNOS waiting list.

The USRDS database consists of data collected by the Health Care Financing Administration (HCFA) as well as data from UNOS. Dates of placement on the transplant waiting list were determined directly from the UNOS waiting-list file. The HCFA data includes information collected using the HCFA Medical Evidence Form #2728. Prior to April 1995, this form was completed for all patients who were diagnosed with ESKD and who were filing for Medicare benefits. These data included the date of ESKD onset, age, race, gender and cause of renal disease. Starting in April 1995, the form was expanded and was required for all patients receiving treatment in

any dialysis (or transplant) facility. The revised form includes data on employment status and insurance status.

We carried out multivariate, Cox proportional hazards analysis using transplantation and allograft failure as time-dependent covariates. We performed this analysis without censoring patients at the time they were removed from the waiting list ("intent-to-transplant"). Results were considered significant for p<0.05. Analyses were carried out using SAS software version 8.1 (Cary, NC).

There were 47,713 patients included in this analysis. Patients with missing data, including missing information for risk factors (covariates) were excluded. There were 6,305 that died after placement on the waiting list and during the time of follow-up. Several independent risk factors for death after placement on the transplant waiting list were identified (Table 2). The risk of death was 53% (95% confidence interval 50-56%) lower for patients after transplantation compared with patients who did not receive a transplant, even after adjusting for multiple other risk factors. This reduction in the risk of death after transplantation is similar to the 38-58% reduction previously reported by Wolfe and co-workers (1). In the present analysis there were a number of other risk factors for mortality after placement on the transplant waiting list that were independent of the reduced mortality risk associated with transplantation.

It has previously been reported that mortality is high for patients with a failed renal allograft (3,4). However,

Table 2. *Independent risk factors for mortality in patients placed on the United Network for Organ Sharing kidney transplant waiting list.* *

Patient Characteristic	Relative Risk (95% C.I.)	Chi-Square	P-Value
Transplant status (vs. never transplanted):			
Transplanted	0.470 (0.441-0.501)	547.2	<0.0001
Transplanted then failed transplant	0.958 (0.860-1.068)	0.6	0.4398
Time from ESKD to waiting list (months)	1.016 (1.013-1.019)	130.9	<0.0001
Gender (vs. female):			
Male	0.996 (0.947-1.048)	0.0	0.8860
Race (vs. white):			
Black	0.742 (0.699-0.786)	100.0	<0.0001
Other	0.598 (0.532-0.672)	74.7	<0.0001
Age (vs. 46-60 years):			
<18 years	0.431 (0.326-0.569)	35.1	<0.0001
18-45 years	0.611 (0.576-0.648)	271.5	<0.0001
>60 years	1.487 (1.392-1.588)	139.0	<0.0001
Cause of ESKD (vs. glomerulonephritis):			
Diabetes	2.527 (2.339-2.731)	548.5	<0.0001
Hypertension	1.382 (1.264-1.515)	49.7	<0.0001
Polycystic kidney disease	0.913 (0.793-1.053)	1.6	0.2110
Other causes	1.382 (1.254-1.522)	42.8	<0.0001
Employment status (vs. working full time):			
Not working	1.378 (1.235-1.538)	32.7	<0.0001
Retired	1.176 (0.999-1.384)	3.8	0.0514
Unknown	1.259 (1.004-1.580)	4.0	0.0463
Health insurance status (vs. Medicare):			
Non-Medicare	0.850 (0.764-0.946)	8.9	0.0029
No coverage	0.643 (0.531-0777)	20.7	<0.0001
Coverage unknown	0.920 (0.736-1.149)	0.5	0.4616

*Cox proportional hazards analysis results. Abbreviations: C.I., confidence interval; ESKD, end-stage kidney disease. N=47,713 with 6,305 deaths and 41,408 censored

in the present analysis that adjusted for several covariates, there was no difference in mortality attributable to allograft failure per se. It seems unlikely that the lack of a detrimental effect of allograft failure on survival in the present analysis is due to differences in the patient populations studied. The present analysis was limited to patients who were candidates for renal transplantation. Dialysis patients in this population, therefore, might be expected to have better survival than an unselected dialysis population, and this might be expected to worsen the risk of allograft failure compared with the dialysis population that never received a transplant.

The time from the development of ESKD to place-ment on the UNOS cadaveric transplant waiting list was associated with an increased risk of death. Specifically, each month of time before placement on the waiting list increased the risk of death by 1.6% (1.3-1.9%). Others have reported that late referral for dialysis is associated with an increase in short-term morbidity, but not mortality (5). However, few studies have reported an increase in mortality associated with late referral for treatment of ESKD. It has been reported that longer waiting times for a kidney transplant are associated with increased mortality and decreased death-censored graft survival after kidney transplantation (6). It is possible, however, that this and the present result represent selection bias; the increased waiting time of those with higher mortality may be the result of pre-existing co-morbidity that delays placement on the transplant waiting list and/or transplantation.

Gender had no effect on mortality after placement on the transplant waiting list (Table 2). This is in contrast to some previous reports that mortality is higher in men than women on renal replacement therapy (7,8). This reported difference in mortality has been attributed to a higher incidence of cardiovascular disease and malignancy among men compared with women (7). It is possible that by limiting the analysis to more comparable patients who were felt to be suitable candidates for renal transplantation, we removed differences in risk and thereby removed differences in mortality attributable to gender in the present analysis.

In the present analysis race had a major effect on survival. Compared with Caucasians, African Americans were 26% (21-30%) less likely to die after being placed on the transplant waiting list. It has often been reported that African Americans have a survival advantage on maintenance dialysis compared with Caucasians matched for age, gender and cause of renal disease (7-9). The lower mortality for African Americans has been attributed to reduced cardiovascular disease, less frequent withdrawal from dialysis, and a reduced rate of fatal infections (7). In the present analysis other racial minorities had a similar survival advantage compared with Caucasians. This is in keeping with the results of a previous study from Canada, where Southeast Asians and South Asians had lower mortality than Caucasians on maintenance dialysis (9). Reasons for these racial differences in survival with ESKD are not evident.

Compared with patients with ESKD from glomerulonephritis, ESKD caused by diabetes and hypertension were associated with increased mortality (Table 2). It is likely that these 2 diagnoses were associated with greater co-morbidity from cardiovascular disease. On the other hand, patients with ESKD from polycystic kidney disease had similar survival as patients with glomerulonephritis. Differences in socioeconomic factors were also associated with mortality. Not surprisingly, patients who were not working had a higher mortality compared with patients who were working (Table 2). This likely reflects the fact that patients with more co-morbidity were less able to work. Compared with patients who relied on Medicare for their primary coverage, those who had some other form of insurance coverage also had reduced mortality.

SUMMARY

Although the growth in the incidence and prevalence of ESKD has slowed, there will nevertheless be a substantial increase in the number of patients over the next decade. Indeed, between 1998 and 2010 there will be a doubling in the number of patients in the United States treated with renal replacement therapy. There has also been an increase in the number of new transplants carried out every year. Much of the growth in the number of new transplants has been from the growth in living-unrelated donor transplants. Unfortunately, the rate of increase in the number of new transplants has not been enough to keep pace with the growing number of ESKD patients. As a result, the number of patients on the transplant waiting list continues to increase. The inability to offer more ESKD patients transplantation is unfortunate, since transplantation is associated with improved survival. Indeed, analyses of comparable patients who are placed on the transplant waiting list suggest that transplantation reduces the risk of death by roughly 50%. Thus, it is likely that the overall survival of patients with ESKD will improve if a greater proportion of patients receive transplants in a timely manner. Reducing allograft rejection and the need for repeat transplants may help reduce the demand for donor kidneys. However, this is unlikely to have a major effect on the organ shortage, since the number of repeat transplants has been relatively small (and constant) over the past decade. Thus, only if more cadaveric and living-donor kidneys are made available will more ESKD patients enjoy the improved survival of kidney transplantation.

REFERENCES

1. Wolfe RA, Ashby VB, Milford EL, et al. Comparison of mortality in all patients on dialysis, patients on dialysis awaiting transplantation, and recipients of a first cadaveric transplant. N Engl J Med 1999; 341:1725.

2. United States Renal Data System. USRDS 2000 Annual Data Report. Bethesda, MD: The National Institutes of Health, National Institute of Diabetes and Digestive and Kidney Diseases, 2000.

3. Cattran DC, Fenton SS. Contemporary management of renal failure: outcome of the failed allograft recipient. Kidney Int Suppl 1993; 41:S36.

4. Ojo A, Wolfe RA, Agodoa LY et al. Prognosis after primary renal transplant failure and the beneficial effects of repeat transplantation: multivariate analyses from the United States Renal Data System. Transplantation 1998; 66:1651.

5. Roubicek C, Brunet P, Huiart L et al. Timing of nephrology referral: Influence on mortality and morbidity. Am J Kidney Dis 2000; 36:35.

6. Meier-Kriesche HU, Port FK, Ojo AO, et al. Effect of waiting time on renal transplant outcome. Kidney Int 2000; 58:1311.

7. Bloembergen WE, Port FK, Mauger EA, Wolfe RA. Causes of death in dialysis patients: racial and gender differences. J Am Soc Nephrol 1994; 5:1231.

8. Sehgal AR. Outcomes of renal replacement therapy among blacks and women. Am J Kidney Dis 2000; 35:S148.

9. Pei YP, Greenwood CM, Chery AL, Wu GG. Racial differences in survival of patients on dialysis. Kidney Int 2000; 58:1293.

CHAPTER 12

The Development of Sirolimus: The University of Texas – Houston Experience

Barry D. Kahan, Stanislaw M. Stepkowski, Kimberly L. Napoli, Steven M. Katz, Richard J. Knight, and Charles Van Buren

Division of Immunology and Organ Transplantation, Department of Surgery, The University of Texas Medical School at Houston, Houston, Texas

Sirolimus (Rapamycin, Rapamune®, Wyeth-Ayerst, Radnor, PA) is a macrocyclic lactone produced by *Streptomyces hygroscopicus,* an actinomycete isolated from the soil of the Vai Atari region in Rapa Nui (Easter Island). This article describes the development of this drug from preclinical experiments to ongoing Phase IV open-label clinical trials by The University of Texas–Houston transplant team.

Sirolimus shows great promise as an immunosuppressive agent primarily because of its unique mechanism of action to blockade the multifunctional kinase, mammalian target of rapamycin (mTOR). This enzyme mediates steps in both the activation of the costimulatory pathway during the G_0 to G_1 transition and in the signal transduction cascades following cytokine reception during the G_1 phase of T cell activation for signal transduction driven by cytokines (1,2). The former effect is due to the role of mTOR to activate inhibitory factor kappa kinase, which generates the c-Rel transcription factors of the NF-kB complex (3) and possibly also modulates protein kinase C activity (4). This inhibition of the Signal 2 pathway complements the actions of calcineurin antagonists (CNAs) on the Signal 1 antigen-driven cascade (5). The actions of sirolimus to interrupt the G_1 build-up after cytokine Signal 3 reception enhance the action of monoclonal antibodies that blockade the interleukin-2 receptor (anti-IL-2R mAbs). These sequential drug effects form the cytokine paradigm (6) that we have proposed as a strategy for selective immunosuppression of adaptive

immune responses and exploited in the clinical development of sirolimus described briefly herein and in detail elsewhere (7) (Fig. 1).

Preclinical Studies

Synergy with cyclosporine (CsA). After initial experiments suggested its immunosuppressive effects in animal models (8,9), we documented that sirolimus interacts in synergistic fashion with CsA using the median effect analysis (10). Based on inhibition of *in vitro* human lymphocyte proliferation (11) and prolongation of rat heart, kidney, small bowel, and pancreatic allograft survival, we documented remarkable synergy (12). The combination index (CI) values were 0.01, where CI=1.0 represents an additive interaction; <1.0, a synergistic interaction; and >1.0, an antagonistic interaction (13). In contrast, our prior studies showed that other immunosuppressive drugs—mycophenolic acid, azathioprine (Aza), and mizorbine act additively, and tacrolimus,

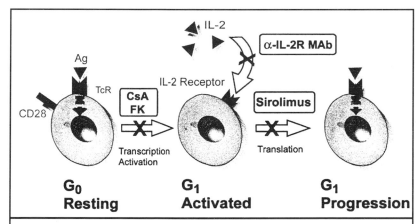

Figure 1. The cytokine paradigm: Sites of drug action at serial steps in T cell activation.

antagonistically with CsA (14).

The immunosuppressive benefits of sirolimus added to a CsA regimen were also documented in the highly immunoresponsive, mongrel canine heterotopic renal transplant model (15). In contrast to the abrupt allograft rejection displayed by untreated control animals and the only modest effect of CsA to blunt this response, addition of sirolimus (0.05 mg/kg/day) to a CsA-based regimen contributed significant prolongation with a mean survival time (MST) of 83.7±57.4 days.

Having determined that sirolimus provided prophylaxis of acute allograft rejection, we investigated its effectiveness to block ongoing rat heart allograft rejection by delaying inception of therapy until 4 days after transplantation, a time when there was histopathologic evidence of moderate cellular infiltration. Administration of 0.8 mg/kg sirolimus on posttransplant day 4 increased the MST of Buffalo (BUF; RT-1^b) cardiac allografts in Wistar-Furth (WF; RT-1^u) recipients from 6.5±0.5 to 61±6.4 days (p=0.001). When therapy was postponed to a time just before cessation of the heartbeat, there was a less prominent effect (MST=48.2±29.8; p=0.005) (16). Thus sirolimus therapy interrupts both the afferent and efferent limbs of allograft rejection.

To dissect immune vectors, we transferred spleen and lymph node T cells versus serum isolated on day 40 postgrafting from animals treated only with sirolimus into lightly irradiated (6 Gray, whole body) secondary syngeneic WF recipients. Although the cells did not have an effect, 3 mL of sera did extend BUF heart transplant survival in immunologically specific fashion. The effect, which occurred in the absence or presence of CsA, was mediated by an IgG$_{2b}$ fraction, suggesting that, in addition to its blockade of T cell maturation, sirolimus prevents isotype switching from non-cytotoxic to cytotoxic antibodies (17,18).

Pharmacokinetic interactions. We identified 2 components of the CsA/sirolimus interaction in the rat model: the pharmacodynamic component due to the complementary mechanisms of action of the 2 drugs, and a pharmacokinetic component that mutually increases their concentrations due to competition between sirolimus and CsA for metabolism by the cytochrome (CYP) P450 3A4 system and for transport by p-glycoprotein (pGP).

Using a rat model we determined that concomitant administration of sirolimus and CsA by the oral route more than the continuous intravenous infusion (CIVI) route increased the whole blood trough concentrations (Cmin$_{ss}$) of both drugs (19), due to a 2-fold increase in bioavailability and to mutual inhibition of hepatic metabolism (20), based upon analysis of microsomal activities *in vivo*. Using pure enzyme, we showed dose-dependent inhibition by addition of sirolimus *in vitro* to block the actions of human CYP P450 3A4 to transform CsA to multiple metabolites (21).

Further, we showed that concomitant administration of the drugs for 14 days either by the oral or by the CIVI route leads to drug accumulation in nonlinear fashion long after whole blood depots are saturated (22). Sirolimus depots were discovered in tissue samples from kidney, liver, intestine, muscle, and testes. CYP P450 3A4 is an important biotransformation enzyme not only in the intestine and liver, but also in the kidney, an organ of especial interest because sirolimus seems to augment the nephrotoxicity produced by the CNA antagonists, CsA and tacrolimus. These findings suggested that this apparent effect of sirolimus is due to a pharmacokinetic interaction that increases CsA tissue levels. While initial studies documented that sirolimus does not reduce either glomerular filtration rates (GFR) or renal blood flow (23), an initial report suggested that high doses of sirolimus potentiated the nephrotoxic effects of CsA in salt-depleted rats, a putative model of drug effects in man (24). We postulated that the adverse effect was due to a pharmacokinetic interaction. Our recent studies in salt-depleted rats, using both drug concentration measurements and renal function estimates, demonstrated that the glomerular dysfunction is primarily due to a pharmacokinetic interaction whereby sirolimus greatly augments renal tissue CsA concentrations disproportionately to the increase in whole blood drug levels (25). These findings demanded that analysis of drug interactions be based upon drug concentrations, not merely drug doses, in an attempt to account for pharmacokinetic interactions.

Pharmacokinetic Studies in Humans

Because sirolimus biotransformation depends on the CYP 3A4 system (26), one would anticipate marked inter-individual variation in dose-adjusted concentrations, as well as extensive drug-drug interactions. To measure drug levels, we developed a high-performance liquid chromatography assay using ultraviolet detection (LC/UV; 278 nm wavelength) (27). The utility of the method was confirmed by Svensson et al (28). Sirolimus parent compound is detected in whole blood with a sensitivity of 1.0 mg/L, a linearity over the 1.0-50 mg/L range, and an inter-day coefficient of variation (%CV) of 5.6-17%. Comparison of the concentrations in 385 samples measured by LC with detection by UV (LC/UV) versus the more sensitive yet highly cumbersome dual mass spectrometry assay (LC/MS/MS) demonstrated a correlation coefficient of 0.943, a regression line slope of 1.024, and a standard error of estimate of 2.87% (29). There was no bias; that is, no measurement was consistently higher than another. We have employed LC/UV for routine therapeutic drug monitoring of sirolimus in transplant patients (30) since it is more readily available than the LC/MS/MS methodology.

Pharmacokinetic analyses of whole blood concentrations were performed during a Phase I double-blind, placebo-controlled study in 40 stable renal transplant patients (31) using administration of a 2-week course of ascending oral doses of sirolimus (0.5, 1.0, 2.0, 3.0, 5.0, 7.0 mg/m²/12 hours). The time to peak concentration (t_{max}) was 1.4±1.2 hours, and the correlation between $Cmin_{ss}$ (trough concentrations) to the area under the concentration-time curve (AUC) was robust (r^2=0.92) (32). Because of the long drug half-life ($t_{1/2}$) of 62±12 hr, once-daily administration was believed to represent a superior dosing schedule to twice daily. The 4.5-fold variation in clearance rates (90-416 mL/h/kg) confirmed the presence of appreciable inter-patient variability. Further, based on the delay in achieving steady state after administration of a constant dose, we calculated that a loading dose of 2.56±0.70 times the maintenance dose would be required to shorten the time to achieve steady-state concentrations (32).

Sirolimus is a "critical-dose" drug (30): its concentrations display wide inter- and intra-patient variability that does not correlate with either dose or demographic features, including ethnicity, gender, age, or body mass index. Adverse reactions—increased triglyceride levels or reduced hemoglobin, leukocyte, and platelet counts—correlate with $Cmin_{ss}$ values >15 ng/mL (33). Conversely, $Cmin_{ss}$ values >5 ng/mL show an 89.5% predictive value for freedom from acute rejection episodes (30), yielding a therapeutic window of 5-15 ng/mL for sirolimus $Cmin_{ss}$ when administered in combination with CsA. Ongoing studies have failed to define a lower limit of CsA exposure. In the presence of adequate sirolimus exposure (5-15 ng/mL), reduction of CsA doses by 75% seems to be effective: namely, twice-daily doses initially of 100-150 mg and during the maintenance period of 50 mg

CsA microemulsion formulation (ME; Neoral®, Novartis, Basel, Switzerland).

Using one-month periods of crossover treatment, simultaneous administration of CsA-ME increased sirolimus AUC by 50%, compared with the AUC after a 4-hour-spaced interval, but sirolimus did not appear to alter CsA exposure (34). However, maintenance therapy with the drug combination in Phase III trials subsequently showed that patients receiving sirolimus required lower doses of the ME formulation to achieve similar target CsA concentrations (35). In contrast, the oil-based formulation Sandimmune® (Novartis, Basel, Switzerland) does not seem to augment sirolimus bioavailability.

Based on these pharmacokinetic studies we recommend high (10-15 mg) initial doses of sirolimus to achieve tissue loading. Because sirolimus displays a long $t_{1/2}$ and extensive tissue distribution and because steady-state concentrations are not achieved before 5 days of therapy with a constant dose, we believe that daily concentration monitoring is neither necessary nor useful. $Cmin_{ss}$ values should be monitored on a weekly basis for the first month and biweekly the following month, targeting a 5-15 ng/mL range when sirolimus is used concomitantly with CsA at initial CsA $Cmin_{ss}$ concentrations ≈100-150 ng/mL, tapering to $Cmin_{ss}$ ≈25-50 ng/mL by 6 months (36).

Phase I and II Tolerability and Efficacy Studies at The University of Texas–Houston

After our attempt to use intravenous delivery of sirolimus was aborted due to a formulation problem, we performed the single-center, Phase I study described above employing an oral liquid formulation. Using a double-blind, randomized design to examine the side effect profile, twice daily ascending doses totaling 1-13 mg/m² sirolimus (n=30) versus placebo (n=13) were added for a 2-week treatment period to the stable CsA/Prednisone (Pred) regimen in quiescent renal transplant patients (31). We documented a dose-dependent reduction in mean platelet number and a small decrease in leukocyte count accompanied by increased values of serum cholesterol and triglycerides. No changes were observed in GFR, blood pressure, or liver function test results.

Since the next trial—an open-label, single-center, Phase I/IIA study—represented the drug's first administration to humans, we used sirolimus in combination with full therapeutic doses of CsA/Pred in mismatched living-donor renal transplant recipients (33). The initial group of 20 patients was divided into 5 cohorts of ascending doses of sirolimus (0.5, 1.0, 2.0, 3.0, or 5.0 mg/m^2/day), each cohort including 4 patients. The only patient who experienced an acute rejection episode among these 20 subjects was an African-American male recipient of a spousal graft who was treated with the lowest dose of sirolimus. Because of this low acute rejection rate (1/20, 5%) and because of the concern about the possibility of excessive immunosuppression, we began to withdraw steroids from the treatment regimens as early as 5 months after the final patient had been entered. None of the patients experienced a rebound acute rejection episode. To assess the possibility of early steroid withdrawal, 2 additional cohorts of 10 patients each were treated with 7 mg/m^2/day sirolimus in addition to CsA with either a one-week or a one-month course of Pred. Only one rejection episode occurred in each cohort. Thus, among the 40 patients in this trial, there were 3 rejection episodes (2 of which occurred among patients not receiving steroids), an overall 7.5% incidence of acute rejection episodes. Because this outcome was significantly better than the 32% acute rejection rate observed in an immediately precedent, demographically similar CsA/Pred cohort (p=0.0006), these results demonstrated the therapeutic benefit of sirolimus and suggested strongly that this regimen permits early withdrawal of steroids.

The multicenter Phase IIB trial. To test the hypothesis that CsA and sirolimus act synergistically, the effects of full versus reduced doses of Sandimmune were examined among 149 recipients of primary mismatched cadaveric or living-unrelated donor renal allografts enrolled in a single-blind study (37). The 6 randomization groups included 3 arms treated with full and 3 with reduced levels of CsA exposure in addition to either 1, 3, or 5 mg/m^2/day sirolimus. The 8.5% incidence of biopsy-proven acute rejection episodes within the first 6 months posttransplant among non–African-American patients treated with full or reduced CsA exposure in the presence of sirolimus was significantly lower than the 32.0% among the control group patients receiving full exposure to CsA/Pred and no sirolimus.

The US Phase III Pivotal Clinical Trial

Design. The pivotal US Phase III clinical trial was conducted at 38 centers in the United States between June 1996 and September 1997. The double-blind, double-dummy protocol enrolled 719 recipients of primary cadaveric, living-unrelated, or living-related (excluding HLA-identical) donor renal allografts (35). Within the overall study, 75 patients were enrolled at our center. The randomization scheme included 2 patients receiving 2 mg/day sirolimus, 2 patients receiving 5 mg/day sirolimus versus one patient who was treated with Aza (2-3 mg/kg/day), which represented the standard of care at most centers when the study began. Because the comparator was Aza, it was necessary to stipulate an immunosuppressive regimen using full exposures to CsA and Pred to protect the control group. The treatment groups were stratified by individual center and by ethnicity (African-American vs. other ethnic groups), since this demographic factor represents an important determinant of outcome in the United States (38).

Because the previous Phase IIB multicenter study revealed an 18% overall 6-month efficacy failure rate (37) among all ethnic groups (Caucasian, African-American, Hispanic, Asian, etc.) treated with sirolimus/CsA/Pred, sample size calculations for groups of unequal size using the method of Fleiss (39) with a Bonferroni adjustment α level of 0.025 and a 90% power for 2 pair-wise comparisons (sirolimus 2 mg/day or sirolimus 5 mg/day vs. Aza) predicted that 234 patients were required in each sirolimus arm and 117 patients in the Aza arm to demonstrate a significant difference from the anticipated 35% acute rejection rate in the CsA/Aza/Pred arm.

The US protocol stipulated that the renal transplant must display function and that the first dose of CsA-ME (9-12 mg/kg/day) be administered within 48 hours of transplantation. Thereafter, CsA doses were adjusted to maintain whole blood Cmin$_{ss}$ levels of 200-350 ng/mL during the first month, 200-300 mg/mL during the second month, and 150-250 ng/mL thereafter, as measured using a fluorescence polarization immunoassay (the specific anti-CsA monoclonal antibody; TDx®, Abbott Diagnostics, Abbott Park, IL) (40). To minimize pharmacokinetic interactions (34), the study drugs—Aza/placebo or placebo/sirolimus—were administered 4 hours after the morning dose of CsA. The steroid regimen was standardized with a maximum of 500 mg methylprednisolone administered intravenously on the day of transplant surgery, and oral Pred doses subsequently tapered to 30 mg/day by day 6, 10 mg/day by month 6, and 5-10 mg/day thereafter. Investigators were able to discontinue patients from the study if they deemed graft function to be inadequate; if they wished to use antibody

Table 1. *Phase III clinical trial patient characteristics: Houston Center data versus all US centers.*

	Treatment Group					
	Houston center			Overall trial[a]		
	Sirolimus	Sirolimus	Aza	Sirolimus	Sirolimus	Aza
	2 mg/day	5 mg/day		2 mg/day	5 mg/day	
Feature	(n=29)	(n=30)	(n=16)	(n=284)	(n=274)	(n=161)
Ethnicity, n (%)						
Caucasian	9 (31)	10 (33)	10(63)	160 (56)	154 (56)	92 (57)
African-American	6 (21)	6 (20)	4(25)	63 (22)	62 (23)	41 (25)
Hispanic	12 (41)	13 (43)	2(13)	48 (17)	42 (15)	15 (9)
Asian	2 (7)	1 (3)	0	7 (2)	10 (4)	10 (6)
Other	0	0	0	6 (2)	6 (2)	3 (2)
Donor source, n (%)						
Cadaveric	20 (69)	19 (63)	13(81)	180 (63)	167 (61)	119 (74)
Living-unrelated	6 (21)	10 (33)	3(19)	18 (6)	24 (9)	9 (6)
Living-related	3 (10)	1 (3)	0	86 (30)	83 (30)	33 (20)

[a] Data described in ref. 35

induction therapy; if they suspected that an important adverse reaction was caused by the study drug; or if they believed that the blinded regimen produced efficacy failure requiring addition or substitution of other immunosuppressive agents, such as antilymphocyte sera, tacrolimus, and/or mycophenolate mofetil (MMF).

Efficacy endpoints. In clinical trials of immunosuppressive agents, the primary endpoint of efficacy failure is defined as the composite parameter, including graft loss, death, the first occurrence of a biopsy-confirmed acute rejection episode, or lost to follow-up within 6 months after transplantation. Graft loss is defined as death, transplant nephrectomy, or the need to institute continuous dialysis for more than 56 days. Patients who had clinical symptoms and/or laboratory findings suggesting an acute rejection episode were mandated to undergo a transplant biopsy, which was graded by a local pathologist using the Banff 1993 criteria. The few patients treated for acute rejection without a biopsy in the US trial were equally distributed among the treatment groups.

Our experience with 75 enrolled patients reflected the overall Phase III US pivotal trial results in the distribution of donor source (Table 1), but our study population included a greater proportion of Hispanic compared with Caucasian patients, a characteristic feature of our Texas candidate group compared with other US centers.

The major component of the efficacy failure rates was the incidence of biopsy-confirmed acute rejection episodes. The 6-/12-month rates for the Houston center versus the overall trial for the Aza arm (31.2%/29.8% vs. 37.5%/31.1%) were uniformly higher than those among patients treated with the sirolimus 2 mg/day regimen, namely, 17.2%/16.9% (p=0.002) versus 20.6%/21.8% (p<0.001), or with sirolimus 5 mg/day 6.7%/12.0% (p=0.004) versus 6.7%/14.6% (p=0.016), respectively. Thus the rates of acute rejection episodes were lower for patients in the sirolimus 5 mg/day group among the Houston cohort compared with the overall US experience, a finding also confirmed for both living and cadaveric donor allografts (Table 2). We ascribe this finding to the lower number of discontinuations with a greater fraction of randomized patients continuing sirolimus treatment.

The corresponding one-year patient and graft survival rates in the Houston center were similar among sirolimus 2 mg/day, sirolimus 5 mg/day, and Aza groups: 100%, 94.0%, and 94.0% and 94.0%, 90.0%, and 87.5%, respectively, versus the overall trial results: 97.2%, 96.0%, and 98.1% and 94.4%, 94.4%, and 93.8%, respectively (Table 3).

Among the secondary endpoints, the overall trial demonstrated that sirolimus groups showed a delay in the time to, a decreased incidence of moderate and

Table 2. Phase III clinical trial rates of biopsy-confirmed acute rejection episodes: Houston center data versus all US centers.

Acute rejection rate	Number of patients (%)					
	Sirolimus 2 mg/day		Sirolimus 5 mg/day		Aza	
	Houston	Overall Phase III[a]	Houston	Overall Phase III[a]	Houston	Overall Phase III[a]
Overall						
6 months	5/29 (17.2)	48/284 (16.9)	2/30 (6.7)	33/274 (12.0)	5/16 (31.2)	48/161 (29.8)
12 months	6/29 (20.6)	62/284 (21.8)	2/30 (6.7)	40/274 (14.6)	6/16 (37.5)	50/161 (31.1)
Donor source						
6 months						
Living	1/9 (11.1)	13/104 (12.5)	1/11 (9.1)	13/107 (12.1)	2/3 (66.7)	18/42 (42.9)
Cadaver	4/20 (20.0)	35/180 (19.4)	1/19 (5.3)	20/167 (12.0)	3/13 (23.1)	30/119 (25.2)
12 months						
Living	1/9 (11.1)	17/104 (16.3)	1/11 (9.1)	15/107 (14.0)	2/3 (66.7)	18/42 (42.9)
Cadaver	5/20 (25.0)	45/180 (25.0)	1/19 (5.3)	25/167 (15.0)	4/13 (30.8)	32/119 (26.9)

[a] Data described in ref. 35

Table 3. Phase III clinical trial one-year patient death and survival rates and graft losses and survival rates: Houston center data versus all US centers.

	Number (%) in each treatment group					
	Sirolimus 2 mg/day		Sirolimus 5 mg/day		Aza	
	Houston	Overall Phase III[a]	Houston	Overall Phase III[a]	Houston	Overall Phase III[a]
	(n=29)	(n=284)	(n=30)	(n=274)	(n=16)	(n=161)
Deaths						
Infection	0	5 (1.8)	0	2 (0.7)[b]	0	1 (0.6)[b]
Cardiac event	0	0	1 (3)	7 (2.6)[c]	1 (6)	0
Malignancy	0	1 (0.4)	0	0	0	1 (0.6)
Miscellaneous	0	2 (0.7)	1 (3)	2 (0.7)	0	1 (0.6)
Total	0	8 (2.8)	2 (6)	11 (4.0)	1 (6)	3 (1.9)
Survival rate (%)	100.0	97.2	94.0	96.0	94.0	98.1
Graft loss						
Death with functioning graft	0	7 (2.5)	2 (6.7)	8 (2.9)	1 (6)	2 (1.2)
Refractory acute rejection	0	1 (0.4)	1 (3)	6 (2.2)	1 (6)	3 (1.9)
Persistent non-function[d]	1 (3)	1 (0.4)	0	2 (0.7)	0	3 (1.9)
Renal vascular thrombosis	0	2 (0.7)	0	1 (0.4)	0	1 (0.6)
Miscellaneous	1 (3)	5 (1.8)	0	3 (1.1)	0	0
Total	2 (6)	16 (5.6)	3 (10)	20 (7.3)	2 (12.5)	9 (5.6)
Survival rate (%)	94.0	94.4	90.0	92.7	87.5	94.4

[a] Data described in ref. 35.

[b] 1 patient in the sirolimus 5 mg/day group and 1 patient in the Aza group received allografts from the same donor, later determined to have been infected with vancomycin-resistant *Enterococcus*.

[c] 2 patients with acute myocardial infarction (MI) and 5 patients with cardiac arrest. Only 1 of the 7 patients was of African-American ethnicity.

[d] Attributed by the investigators to either acute tubular necrosis or primary non-function.

severe histologic grades of, and a lower percentage of patients requiring antibody treatment for the first acute rejection episode (35). The incidences of infection and malignancy were similar among all groups. The rates of infections, including those due to sepsis, cytomegalovirus (CMV), Epstein-Barr virus, as well as herpes zoster, and those in various sites, including lungs, wound, or urinary tract, were similar across the treatment arms, except for an increased incidence of mucosal lesions (presumed to be caused by herpes simplex virus) among patients in the sirolimus 5 mg/day group (p<0.001).

None of the 4 patients who displayed lymphoma 12 months after transplantation were from the Houston cohort: one patient in the sirolimus 2 mg/day group in the overall trial died due to a central nervous system lymphoma, and 2 patients receiving sirolimus 5 mg/day discontinued study medication either 9 days before or 9 days following the diagnosis of posttransplant lymphoproliferative disease (PTLD). One patient in the Aza group received an alternate immunosuppressive regimen with CD3 mAb, MMF, and tacrolimus before and at the time of diagnosis of PTLD. The overall incidences of malignancies (other than lymphoma/PTLD) were also similar among the treatment arms (35).

Discontinuations. The number of treatment-emergent adverse events leading to study drug discontinuation were equally distributed among the 3 regimens (p=0.247) in both the overall trial and in the Houston experience. While the major cause for discontinuation among the Aza cohort in the overall trial was efficacy failure, sirolimus patients were withdrawn for various reasons, including putative acute tubular necrosis, CsA toxicity, elevated mean serum creatinine (SCr) values, arthralgia, nausea, thrombocytopenia, hemolytic uremic syndrome, abnormal liver function tests, hyperlipidemia, and hypercholesteremia (35). As the consort analysis of the overall US Phase III multicenter trial shows, among the 558 patients randomized to receive sirolimus, 364 (65%) remained on therapy at 6 months, and 292 (52%) remained on therapy at 12 months (Fig. 2). The rate of discontinuation from study medication during the first 6 months was greater among patients in the Aza arm (55% remaining the study). At the Houston center, the rates of discontinuation at 6 and 12 months were far lower, particularly at 12 months. Among the 29 patients randomized into the 2 mg/day sirolimus group, at 6 months 5 (17.0%) patients were discontinued. The reasons for cessation included

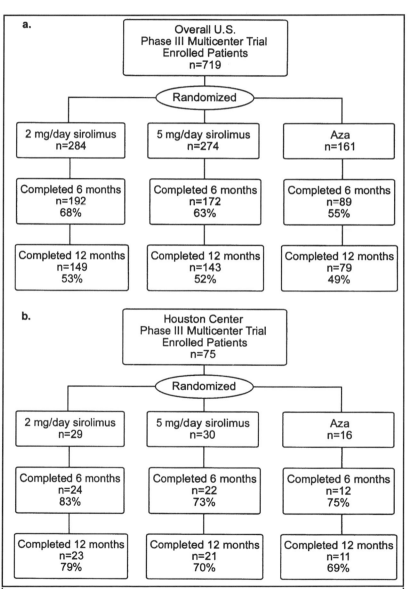

Figure 2. Consort diagrams of the enrollment and progress of patients in the pivotal multicenter Phase III clinical trial. Panel a. The entire US multicenter Phase III trial. Panel b. The Houston center cohort within the trial.

steroid-resistant acute rejection (n=3), primary graft nonfunction (n=1), and tuberculosis (n=1). Among the 30 patients randomized into the 5 mg/day group, at 6 months, 8 (27.0%) were discontinued from the trial: 4 because of patient preference, one patient experienced hemolytic uremic syndrome, one rejected the graft, one patient died, and one because of infection. Lastly, among the 16 in the Aza group, 4 patients (25%) were discontinued, all of whom had suffered acute rejection episodes. At 6 months, 83% of patients in the 2 mg sirolimus group and 73% of the 5 mg sirolimus arm remained in the trial. At 12 months, 23 (79.3%) of the 2 mg/day group, 70.0% of the 5 mg/day group, and 68.8% of the Aza group remained in the study compared with the overall trial completion rates of 52.5%, 52.2%, and 49.1%, differences that achieve statistical significance; namely, p=0.004, p=0.047, and p=0.107, respectively.

Adverse effects. The mean SCr values in the overall trial were significantly higher for both sirolimus arms compared with the Aza (p<0.001) cohort at 6 and 12 months. Interestingly, in the Houston experience the mean SCr value was significantly different only at 6 months and only in the 2 mg sirolimus arm versus Aza (1.63 vs. 1.31, p=0.04); the values for the 5 mg/day cohort were similar to those for Aza throughout. The mean values of the calculated creatinine (Cr) clearance were lower among patients in the 2 mg/day (p<0.01) and in the 5 mg/day (p<0.001) sirolimus groups in the multicenter trial (35). However, in the Houston cohort, the mean calculated Cr clearance values were no different between the sirolimus 2 mg/day and Aza arms, although they were significantly higher among the sirolimus 5 mg/day groups at 6 and 12 months (Table 4).

Since there is considerable evidence that sirolimus itself has either no effect or, at most, a modest renal tubular effect in rats, and since studies in salt-deprived animals suggested a noticeable impact of drug concentrations on kidney tissue, it seems possible that the increased SCr values observed in this trial were due to the concomitant administration of and pharmacokinetic interaction with CsA. In fact, patients treated with sirolimus/Aza/Pred displayed better renal function at 12 months than those treated with CsA/Aza/Pred (41). Indeed, the pharmacokinetic interaction may have been underestimated by the CsA $Cmin_{ss}$ values, which correlate poorly with overall drug exposure as estimated by measurements of AUC (42).

Among all US centers, mean fasting serum cholesterol and triglyceride levels increased from baseline in all groups, but to a greater extent among sirolimus versus Aza-treated patients. At 6 but not at 12 months, the mean cholesterol and triglyceride values were significantly higher among patients in the sirolimus versus Aza groups. Although at 6 months the number of patients with serum cholesterol values >240 mg/dL was greater among members of the sirolimus 2 mg/day (62%) and 5 mg/day (66.6%) versus the Aza (37.8%) groups, only 3 patients (all in the sirolimus 5 mg/day group) had to be discontinued from the study due to this side effect (35).

Similarly, within 6 months more patients in the entire US trial who were treated with sirolimus 2 mg/day (19.4%) or sirolimus 5 mg/day (19.8%) experienced moderately elevated triglyceride levels (400-1,000 mg/dL) versus the Aza group (2.3%). One patient in the sirolimus 2 mg/day and 3 in the sirolimus 5 mg/day group showed triglyceride levels >1,000 mg/dL, but pancreatitis, the major complication of hypertriglyceridemia, was observed in similar incidences among the treatment groups (3

Table 4. Houston center: effect of 2 and 5 mg sirolimus versus Aza on 3-, 6-, and 12-month serum creatinine (SCr) and calculated Cr clearance values.

Mean value	3 months			6 months			12 months		
	Sirolimus	Aza	p[a]	Sirolimus	Aza	p[a]	Sirolimus	Aza	p[a]
Sirolimus 2 mg/day									
SCr	3.59	3.47	0.86	1.63	1.31	0.04	1.81	1.48	0.35
Cr clearance	58.00	52.86	0.49	79.29	86.49	0.76	78.11	81.40	0.95
Sirolimus 5 mg/day									
SCr	3.16	3.47	0.57	1.63	1.31	0.09	2.03	1.48	0.06
Cr clearance	46.30	52.87	0.13	59.78	86.49	0.00	48.33	81.40	0.00
[a] Calculated by analysis of variance (ANOVA)									

Table 5. Houston center: effect of 2 and 5 mg sirolimus versus Aza on 3-, 6-, and 12-month cholesterol and triglyceride levels.

Mean value	3 months			6 months			12 months		
	Sirolimus	Aza	p[a]	Sirolimus	Aza	p[a]	Sirolimus	Aza	p[a]
Sirolimus 2 mg/day									
Cholesterol	250.28	239.78	0.65	286.34	235.73	0.02	264.48	232.70	0.12
Triglyceride	218.75	198.59	0.60	273.47	243.39	0.58	267.36	211.93	0.36
Sirolimus 5 mg/day									
Cholesterol	281.86	239.78	0.04	290.59	235.73	0.008	256.07	232.70	0.20
Triglyceride	282.24	198.59	0.09	296.87	243.39	0.30	280.73	211.93	0.15

[a] Calculated by analysis of variance (ANOVA)

patients in sirolimus 2 mg/day, 2 in sirolimus 5 mg/day, and 2 in the Aza group), and none of the affected patients displayed elevated triglycerides. Only one patient in the sirolimus 2 mg/day and 2 in sirolimus 5 mg/day group discontinued study medication due to hypertriglyceridemia. The need for fibrate therapy for hypertriglyceridemia was also infrequent (occurring in 8.8% of recipients in the sirolimus 2 mg/day group, 9.3% in the sirolimus 5 mg/day group, and 4.3% in the Aza group), suggesting that dietary intervention, protocol-mandated tapering of the Pred dose, and tight control of blood glucose concentrations were usually sufficient to lower triglyceride levels over time (35).

The Houston center data show a different picture (Table 5). Mean serum triglyceride values were not significantly different among the cohorts. As has been observed under CsA-steroid (43) therapy, mean serum cholesterol values were elevated at 6 months in the sirolimus 2 mg/day group and at 3 and 6 months in the sirolimus 5 mg/day group, but there were no differences from the values in the Aza patients at 12 months. The more prominent effects on cholesterol again suggest the impact of a pharmacokinetic interaction and argue that minimization of CsA exposure may mitigate these risks. Furthermore, the Houston experience suggests that vigorous therapeutic and dietary attention to hypertriglyceridemia may minimize the incidence of the disorder.

Among the sirolimus 2 mg/day group, only the mean hemoglobin values, particularly at 6 and to a lesser extent at 12 months, but not the leukocyte or platelet counts, were significantly lower than the Aza groups. Among the patients in the sirolimus 5 mg/day versus the Aza group, the mean platelet counts showed the greater decrease, which was maximal at 3 months and not significant at

one year, as previously described in our larger experience with patients in various studies (44). Also consistent with previous observations, only the sirolimus 5 mg/day group showed a significantly reduced mean leukocyte count at 3 but not 6 or 12 months (Table 6).

Single-Center Houston Phase IV Studies (Fig. 3)

Rescue therapy for refractory rejection. Because renal allograft rejection refractory to treatment with anti-lymphocyte antibodies almost always results in the loss of the graft, we conducted a single-center trial to utilize sirolimus for this indication. Our initial case report described a remarkable outcome in a woman with diabetes mellitus Type II who required hemodialysis due to ongoing refractory Grade IIB vascular rejection. Within 2 weeks after the addition of sirolimus to the regimen, she displayed reversal of clinical rejection, leading to dialysis-independence and eventually to a normal SCr value and steroid withdrawal (45).

Following this impressive result, we conducted a study to compare the efficacy of sirolimus versus MMF to salvage 36 grafts that displayed biopsy-proven refractory rejection (Banff criteria of either Grade IIB or Grade III). Patients in the demographically matched groups had all received not only pulse and/or oral recycling of steroids, but also at least one 14- to 21-day course of 5 mg/day mouse anti-human CD3 monoclonal antibody (OKT3®, Ortho, Raritan, NJ) or 15 mg/kg/day equine antilymphocyte globulin (ATGAM®, Upjohn, Kalamazoo, MI) (46).

Although the actual 12-month outcomes among the 24 patients treated with sirolimus and 12 patients with MMF added to a baseline regimen of CsA/Pred were

Table 6. Houston center: effect of 2 and 5 mg sirolimus versus Aza on 3-, 6-, and 12-month leukocyte and platelet counts and hemoglobin values.

Mean value	3 months			6 months			12 months		
	Sirolimus	Aza	p[a]	Sirolimus	Aza	p[a]	Sirolimus	Aza	p[a]
Sirolimus 2 mg/day									
Leukocytes	10.46	11.10	0.49	8.42	8.17	0.76	7.80	7.75	0.95
Platelets	215.66	227.76	0.53	234.45	249.80	0.45	223.61	238.37	0.52
Hemoglobin	3.84	3.67	0.32	4.76	4.15	0.002	5.07	4.49	0.03
Sirolimus 5 mg/day									
Leukocytes	8.34	11.10	0.01	6.83	8.17	0.09	6.63	7.75	0.15
Platelets	164.83	3.67	0.001	192.37	249.80	0.006	204.01	238.37	0.07
Hemoglobin	3.68	3.67	0.94	4.22	4.15	0.78	4.37	4.49	0.64

[a] Calculated by analysis of variance (ANOVA)

similar, sirolimus rescue therapy reversed the renal dysfunction in 96% of patients versus 67% in the MMF group (p=0.03), despite the fact that a greater percentage of patients in the sirolimus (71%) than the MMF group (50%) had experienced 2 or more episodes of acute rejection before entering the study, and 94% of patients in the sirolimus group had recurrent bouts of acute rejection within the first 6 months posttransplant versus 50% (p=0.005) in the MMF group (46). Among the patients who were reversed successfully, the rates of rebound acute rejection were similar (4% vs. 8%). Mean SCr values were slightly, though not significantly, lower among sirolimus than MMF patients at 1, 3, 6, and 12 months: namely, 2.6 versus 2.8, 2.8 versus 3.2, 3.0 versus 3.3, and 2.8 versus 3.2 mg/dL, respectively. The one-year patient and graft survival rates were also similar: namely, 88% versus 92% and 83% versus 67% for the sirolimus versus MMF groups, respectively. While the observed mortality rates were similar, the death-censored graft survival rate was higher among patients in the sirolimus group (p=0.03).

Because we assumed that patients experiencing refractory rejection require a greater degree of immunosuppression than *de novo* transplant recipients, we administered more than twice the dose and target concentrations of sirolimus than had been used in the pivotal

Phase III trial (35) as well as full exposure to CsA. While this intensified regimen may have contributed to the 3 deaths among the sirolimus-treated patients, the causes of mortality appeared to be due primarily to pre-existent cardiovascular conditions rather than infections. Further studies are needed to define concentration targets for sirolimus-based rescue regimens that optimize long-term outcomes and enhance recovery of renal function.

Use in patients of African-American ethnicity. Because this population is at increased risk of acute rejection episodes and graft loss (47), another study compared the incidences of these complications among 130 African-American renal transplant recipients treated with (n=45) versus without (n=85) sirolimus added to a concentration-controlled CsA/Pred regimen. At a complete 2-year follow-up posttransplant, African-Americans re-

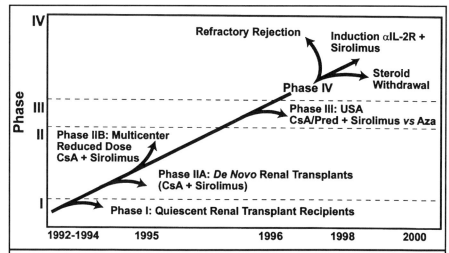

Figure 3. Timeline of the clinical development of sirolimus in Houston, including Phase I, II, III, and IV trials.

ceiving sirolimus/CsA/Pred displayed a significantly lower incidence of biopsy-proven acute rejection episodes compared with those receiving CsA/Pred alone (11.1% vs. 41.2%; p=0.004). The sirolimus/CsA/Pred cohort also experienced a higher rate of graft survival (98% vs. 84.7%; p=0.04), without apparent drug-induced toxicity or compromised patient survival (48). Our findings demonstrated that African-American renal transplant recipients benefit from the augmented immunosuppression provided by sirolimus with greater tolerability and fewer side effects.

Induction therapy. Today, as cadaveric kidneys are increasingly being obtained from marginal donors (49), delayed graft function (DGF), a condition that may be exacerbated by the intrinsic nephrotoxicity of CNAs, has become a more frequent complication. Because induction immunosuppressive therapy with antilymphocyte preparations provides only a 2-week window for recovery of renal function, and exposure to initially large amounts of CNAs may cause irreversible damage to the kidney, new regimens are needed. We conducted a single-center study to test the efficacy of the combination of sirolimus and chimeric (c-) anti-IL-2R mAbs (basiliximab, Simulect®, Novartis, Basel, Switzerland) for induction therapy in recipients of cadaveric renal transplants deemed to be at high risk for DGF.

Basiliximab adjunctive therapy had been previously shown not only to potentiate the immunosuppressive effects provided by full therapeutic doses of CsA (50-52), but also in a large randomized, double-blind US trial to promote better renal allograft function over the one-year study period than that displayed by transplants in placebo-treated patients (51). However, there are no data to suggest that treatment with c-IL-2R mAbs allows CNA dose-sparing, a limitation that possibly results from the relatively limited action of the mAbs on only IL-2 receptor-mediated events. In contrast, sirolimus has been shown to disrupt signal transduction by all cytokines. An encouraging preliminary study (53) demonstrated that 6 patients experienced 16–65-day windows of freedom from and a substantial reduction in the subsequent maintenance exposure to CNAs without the occurrence of any acute rejection episodes. Thus we undertook a pilot, nonrandomized, nonblinded, single-center trial in which we compared 3 contemporaneous cohorts for the incidence of acute rejection episodes, for patient and graft survival rates, for renal function, and for adverse reaction profiles over 12 months (54). Among patients

at high risk for DGF, 43 Group I patients induced with sirolimus/c-IL-2R mAb/Pred were treated with CsA once their SCr values had improved to ≤2.5 mg/dL. This cohort was compared with 18 Group III patients who received antilymphocyte preparations/Pred and inception of CsA after 7-14 days regardless of renal function. A third cohort of 21 Group II patients displayed immediate graft function and were treated *de novo* with CsA/c-IL-2R mAb/Pred.

As predicted, the incidence of DGF was significantly higher among patients in Groups I and III compared with Group II (p=0.02). Despite the increased incidence of DGF, the sirolimus/c-IL-2R mAb/Pred induction regimen provided the best acute rejection prophylaxis: 16% for Group I, 52% for Group II (p=0.004), and 39% for Group III (p=0.05). However, Group I patients displayed higher serum cholesterol and triglyceride values, as well as lower hemoglobin, platelet, and leukocyte values compared with the other 2 groups.

Further, fewer patients in Group I than in the other groups experienced Grade II or Grade III acute rejection episodes, and significantly fewer recipients needed treatment with additional antilymphocyte preparations (p=0.05 Group I vs. II, and p=0.03 Group I vs. III). Overall, the groups showed excellent patient survival. Although the graft survival rate in Group III was lower than that in Groups I and II, the study was not sufficiently large to draw any conclusions about the significance of possible differences.

This study however demonstrated that sirolimus and anti-IL-2R mAbs provide effective immunosuppression before inception of CNA therapy, allowing early recovery of renal allografts from ischemia/reperfusion injuries and providing freedom from the first-dose hypersensitivity or cytokine-release reactions as are seen with other antilymphocyte sera (55-57).

Steroid withdrawal. Since previous attempts at steroid withdrawal using CsA-based regimens with MMF or Aza had produced a 30-60% incidence of acute rejection episodes among renal transplant recipients within 6 months (58,59), we sought to examine the potential utility of sirolimus in this setting. During the Phase IIA trial, acute rejection episodes were experienced by 2 patients among those in whom steroids were withdrawn from a CsA/sirolimus/Pred regimen within one month versus no patients withdrawn after 5 months (33). In a prospective study to assess intermediate efficacy, we have withdrawn steroids from 124 patients leaving them on a sirolimus/

CsA regimen. Steroid withdrawal was completed between one week and more than 2 years posttransplant (mean time=437±323 days) in 49.1% Caucasian, 13.7% African-American, 28.2% Hispanic, and 9% Asian patients with a mean age of 44.5±12.4 years. The mean follow-up is presently 25 months. Following withdrawal, 95 patients (76.6%) have remained off steroids, and 5 patients experienced acute rejection episodes. An additional 24 patients required re-institution of steroid therapy for chronic rejection (4.8%), hypocorticalism (4.8%), discontinuation of sirolimus (4%), graft loss (4%), recurrent disease (1.7%), and patient preference (1.7%). A univariate regression analysis of our data suggested that cadaveric donor source, older recipient age, Asian ancestry, and lower HLA mismatch grades were associated with a reduced risk of failure of steroid withdrawal; however, multiple regression analysis showed that none of these factors was an independent predictor of success. From these results we conclude that most patients withdrawn from steroids maintain stable renal function on sirolimus/CsA therapy without steroids.

SUMMARY

The transplant team at The University of Texas–Houston has studied sirolimus from preclinical through pivotal Phase III trials to single-center Phase IV trials as we continue to refine algorithms for sirolimus therapy. The sirolimus/CsA combination produces a marked reduction in the occurrence and severity of acute allograft rejection episodes. A recently completed *post hoc* median effect analysis of drug blood concentrations displayed by patients in the 2 pivotal Phase III trials documented that the combination displays synergistic interactions. Patients in the sirolimus/CsA arms did not display an increased incidence of infectious or malignant complications. However, they did experience a range of nonimmune toxicities, including potentiation of putatively CsA-related adverse reactions, such as renal dysfunction and hypercholesterolemia, which appear to be mitigated by reduction or elimination of CsA. However, thrombocytopenia and to a lesser extent leukopenia and anemia appear to be sirolimus-related side effects. The occurrence and severity of these adverse reactions seem to be avoided or ameliorated in most patients by optimizing sirolimus exposure at concentrations (15 ng/mL or by dose reduction. Sirolimus thus appears to be a potent and unique agent for developing new immunosuppressive strategies in organ transplantation.

ABBREVIATIONS

Anti-interleukin-2 receptor (anti-IL-2R), area under the concentration-time curve (AUC), azathioprine (Aza), calcineurin antagonists (CNAs), coefficient of variation (%CV), combination index (CI), continuous intravenous infusion (CIVI), creatinine (Cr), cyclosporin (CsA), cytochrome (CYP), cytomegalovirus (CMV), delayed graft function (DGF), glomerular filtration rates (GFR), half-life ($t_{1/2}$), high-performance liquid chromatography assay with ultraviolet detection (LC/UV), high-performance liquid chromatography assay with dual mass spectrometry (LC/MS/MS), human leukocyte antigen (HLA), mammalian target of rapamycin (mTOR), mean serum creatinine (SCr), mean survival time (MST), monoclonal antibodies (mAbs), mycophenolate mofetil (MMF), p-glycoprotein (pGP), posttransplant lymphoproliferative disease (PTLD), Prednisone (Pred), time to peak concentration (t_{max}), trough concentrations ($Cmin_{ss}$).

REFERENCES

1. Abraham RT, Wiederrecht GJ. Immunopharmacology of rapamycin. Ann Rev Immunol 1996; 14:483.

2. Kahan BD. Immunosuppressive drugs: molecular and cellular mechanisms of action. In: Kahan BD, Ponticelli C, Eds. Principles and Practice of Renal Transplantation. Martin Dunitz, London, 2000:315.

3. Lai JH, Tan TH. CD28 signaling causes a sustained down-regulation of I kappa B alpha which can be prevented by the immunosuppressant rapamycin. J Biol Chem 1994; 269:30077.

4. Kimball PM, Kerman RK, Van Buren CT, Lewis RM, Katz S, Kahan BD. Cyclosporine and rapamycin affect protein kinase C induction of the intracellular activation signal, activator of DNA replication. Transplantation 1993; 55:1128.

5. Liu J, Farmer JD Jr, Lane WS, Friedman J, Weissman I, Schreiber SL. Calcineurin is a common target of cyclophilin-cyclosporin A and FKBP-FK506 complexes. Cell 1991; 66:807.

6. Hong JC, Kahan BD. Two paradigms for new immunosuppressive strategies in organ transplantation. Curr Opin Organ Transplant 1998; 3:175.

7. Kahan BD, Ponticelli C, Eds. Principles and practice of renal transplantation. Martin Dunitz, London, 2000.

8. Calne RY, Collier DS, Lim S, Pollard SG, Samaan A, White DJ, Thiru S. Rapamycin for immunosuppression in organ allografting. Lancet 1989; 2:227.

9. Morris RE, Meiser BM. Identification of a new pharmacologic action for an old compound. Med Sci Res 1989; 17:877.

10. Chou T-C, Talalay P. Quantitative analysis of dose-effect relationships: the combined effects of multiple drugs or enzyme inhibitors. Adv Enz Regul 1984; 22:27.

11. Kahan BD, Gibbons S, Tejpal N, Stepkowski SM, Chou T-C. Synergistic interactions of cyclosporine and rapamycin to inhibit immune performances of normal human peripheral blood lymphocytes in vitro. Transplantation 1991; 51:232.

12. Stepkowski SM, Chen H, Daloze P, Kahan BD. Rapamycin, a potent immunosuppressive drug for vascularized heart, kidney, and small bowel transplantation in the rat. Transplantation 1991; 51:22.

13. Stepkowski SM, Tian L, Napoli KL, Ghobrial R, Wang ME, Chou TC, Kahan BD. Synergistic mechanisms by which sirolimus and cyclosporine inhibit rat heart and kidney allograft rejection. Clin Exp Immunol 1997; 108:63.

14. Vathsala A, Goto S, Yoshimura N, Stepkowski SM, Chou TC, Kahan BD. The immunosuppressive antagonism of low doses of FK506 and cyclosporine. Transplantation 1991; 52:121.

15. Knight R, Ferraresso M, Serino F, Katz SM, Lewis R, Kahan BD. Low-dose rapamycin potentiates the effects of subtherapeutic doses of cyclosporine to prolong renal allograft survival in the mongrel canine model. Transplantation 1993; 55:947.

16. Wang ME, Stepkowski SM, Ferraresso M, Kahan BD. Evidence that rapamycin rescue therapy delays rejection of major (MHC) plus minor (non-MHC) histoincompatible heart allografts in rats. Transplantation 1992; 54:704.

17. Ferraresso M, Ghobrial R, Stepkowski SM, Kahan BD. The mechanism of unresponsiveness to allografts induced by rapamycin and rapamycin/cyclosporine treatment in rats. Transplantation 1993; 55:888.

18. Ferraresso M, Tian L, Ghobrial R, Stepkowski SM, Kahan BD. Rapamycin inhibits production of cytotoxic but not noncytotoxic antibodies and preferentially activates T helper 2 cells that mediate long-term survival of heart allografts in rats. J Immunol 1994; 153:3307.

19. Stepkowski SM, Napoli KL, Wang ME, Qu X, Chou T-C, Kahan BD. Effects of the pharmacokinetic interaction between orally administered sirolimus and cyclosporine on the synergistic prolongation of heart allograft survival in rats. Transplantation 1996; 62:986.

20. Brunner LJ, Bai S, Stepkowski SM, Napoli KL, Kahan BD. Effect of low-dose cyclosporine and sirolimus on hepatic drug metabolism in the rat. Transplantation (In press).

21. Kelly PA, Wang H, Napoli KL, Kahan BD, Strobel HW. Metabolism of cyclosporine by cytochromes P450 3A9 and 3A4. Eur J Drug Metab Pharmacokinet 1999; 24:321.

22. Napoli KL, Wang ME, Stepkowski SM, Kahan BD. Relative tissue distributions of cyclosporine and sirolimus after concomitant peroral administration to the rat: evidence for pharmacokinetic interactions. Ther Drug Monit 1998; 20:123.

23. DiJoseph JF, Sharma RN, Chang JY. The effect of rapamycin on kidney function in the Sprague-Dawley rat. Transplantation 1992; 53:507.

24. Andoh TF, Lindsley J, Franceschini N, Bennett WM. Synergistic effects of cyclosporine and rapamycin in a chronic nephrotoxicity model. Transplantation 1996; 62:311.

25. Podder H, Stepkowski SM, Napoli K, Verani RR, Chou T-C, Kahan BD. Pharmacokinetic interactions augment toxicities of sirolimus/cyclosporine combinations. J Am Soc Nephrol (in press).

26. Streit F, Christians U, Schiebel HM, et al. Sensitive and specific quantification of sirolimus (rapamycin) and its metabolites in blood of kidney graft recipients by HPLC/electrospray-mass spectrometry. Clin Chem 1996; 42:1417.

27. Napoli KL, Kahan BD. Sample clean-up and high-performance liquid chromatographic techniques for measurement of whole blood rapamycin concentrations. J Chromatogr B Biomed Appl 1994; 654:111.

28. Svensson JO, Brattström C, Säwe J. Determination of rapamycin in whole blood by HPLC. Ther Drug Monit 1997; 19:112.

29. Napoli KL, Kahan BD. Routine clinical monitoring of sirolimus (rapamycin) whole-blood concentrations by HPLC with ultraviolet detection. Clin Chem 1996; 42:1943.

30. Kahan BD, Napoli KL, Kelly PA, Podbielski J, Hussein I, Katz SM, Van Buren CT. Therapeutic drug monitoring of sirolimus: Correlations with efficacy and toxicity. Clin Transplant 2000; 14:97.

31. Murgia MG, Jordan S, Kahan BD. The side effect profile of sirolimus: A phase I study in quiescent cyclosporine-prednisone-treated renal transplant patients. Kidney Int 1996; 49:209.

32. Zimmerman J, Kahan BD. Pharmacokinetics of sirolimus in stable renal transplant patients after multiple oral dose administration. J Clin Pharmacol 1997; 37:405.

33. Kahan BD, Podbielski J, Napoli KL, Katz SM, Meier-Kriesche H-U, Van Buren CT. Immunosuppressive effects and safety of a sirolimus/cyclosporine combination regimen for renal transplantation. Transplantation 1998; 66:1040.

34. Kaplan B, Meier-Kriesche HU, Napoli KL, Kahan BD. The effects of relative timing of sirolimus and cyclosporine microemulsion formulation co-administration on the pharmacokinetics of each agent. Clin Pharmacol Ther 1998; 63:48.

35. Kahan BD, for the Rapamune U.S. Study Group. Sirolimus (Rapamune, rapamycin) is more effective than azathioprine to reduce the incidence of acute renal allograft rejection episodes when used in combination with cyclosporine and prednisone: A phase III U.S. multicenter trial. Lancet 2000; 356:194.

36. Mahalati K, Kahan BD. Clinical pharmacokinetics of sirolimus. Clin Pharmacokinet (in press).

37. Kahan BD, Julian BA, Pescovitz MD, Vanrenterghem Y, Neylan J, for the Rapamune Study Group. Sirolimus reduces the incidence of acute rejection episodes despite lower cyclosporine doses in Caucasian recipients of mismatched primary renal allografts: A phase II trial. Transplantation 1999; 68:1526.

38. Cecka MJ; Terasaki PI. The UNOS scientific renal transplant registry. In: Terasaki PI; Cecka JM, Eds. Clinical Transplants 1994; UCLA Tissue Typing Laboratory, Los Angeles 1995: 1.

39. Fleiss JL. Statistical methods for rates and proportions. 2nd Ed. Wiley, New York, 1981: 44.

40. Lindholm A, Napoli K, Rutzky L, Kahan BD. Specific monoclonal radioimmunoassay and fluorescence polarization immunoassay for trough concentration and area-under-the-curve monitoring of cyclosporine in renal transplantation. Ther Drug Monit 1992; 14:292.

41. Groth CG, Backman L, Morales JM, et al. Sirolimus (rapamycin)-based therapy in human renal transplantation: similar efficacy and different toxicity compared with cyclosporine. Sirolimus European Renal Transplant Study Group. Transplantation 1999; 67:1036.

42. Kahan BD, Grevel J. Overview: Optimization of cyclosporine therapy in renal transplantation by a pharmacokinetic strategy. Transplantation 1988; 46:631.

43. Vathsala A, Weinberg RB, Schoenberg L, et al. Lipid abnormalities in cyclosporine-prednisone-treated renal transplant recipients. Transplantation 1989; 48:37.

44. Hong JC, Kahan BD. Sirolimus-induced thrombocytopenia and leukopenia in renal transplant recipients: risk factors, incidence, progression, and management. Transplantation 2000; 69:2085.

45. Slaton JW, Kahan BD. Case report—sirolimus rescue therapy for refractory renal allograft rejection. Transplantation 1996; 61:977.

46. Hong JC, Kahan BD. Sirolimus rescue therapy for refractory rejection in renal transplantation. Transplantation (in press).

47. Cecka JM. The UNOS scientific transplant registry. In: Cecka JM; Terasaki PI, Eds. Clinical Transplants 1998. UCLA Tissue Typing Laboratory, Los Angeles, 1998; 1.

48. Podder H, Podbielski J, Hussein I, Katz SH, Van Buren CT, Kahan BD. Sirolimus improves the two-year outcome of renal allografts in African-American patients. Transpl Int (in press).

49. Shoskes DA, Cecka JM. Deleterious effects of delayed graft function in cadaveric renal transplant recipients independent of acute rejection. Transplantation 1998; 66:1697.

50. Nashan B, Moore R, Amlot P, Schmidt A-G, Abeywickrama K, Soulillou J-P. Randomised trial of basiliximab versus placebo for control of acute cellular rejection in renal allograft recipients. Lancet 1997; 350:1193.

51. Kahan BD, Rajagopalan PR, Hall ML, for the United States Simulect® Renal Study Group. Reduction of the occurrence of acute cellular rejection among renal allograft recipients treated with basiliximab, a chimeric anti-interleukin-2-receptor monoclonal antibody. Transplantation 1999; 67:276.

52. Vincenti F, Kirkman R, Light S, et al. Interleukin-2-receptor blockade with daclizumab to prevent acute rejection in renal transplantation. N Engl J Med 1998; 338:161.

53. Hong JC, Kahan BD. Use of anti-CD25 monoclonal antibody in combination with rapamycin to eliminate cyclosporine treatment during the induction phase of immunosuppression. Transplantation 1999; 68:701.

54. Hong JC, Kahan BD. A calcineurin antagonist-free induction strategy for immunosuppression in cadaveric kidney transplant recipients at high risk for delayed graft function. Transplantation (in press).

55. Norman DJ, Kahana L, Stuart Jr FP, et al. A randomized clinical trial of induction therapy with OKT3 in kidney transplantation. Transplantation 1993; 55:44.

56. Vincenti F, Grinyo J, Ramos E, et al. Can antibody prophylaxis allow sparing of other immunosuppressives? Transplant Proc 1999; 31:1246.

57. Batiuk TD, Bennett WM, Norman DJ. Cytokine nephropathy during antilymphocyte therapy. Transplant Proc 1993; 25 (2 Suppl 1):27.

58. Ahsan N, Hricik D, Matas A, et al. Prednisone withdrawal in kidney transplant recipients on cyclosporine and mycophenolate mofetil: a prospective randomized study. Steroid withdrawal study group. Transplantation 1999; 68:1865.

59. Schulak JA, Mayes JT, Moritz CE, Hricik DE. A prospective randomized trial of prednisone versus no prednisone maintenance therapy in cyclosporine-treated and azathioprine-treated renal transplant patients. Transplantation 1999; 49:327.

ACKNOWLEDGEMENT

This work was supported by a grant from the National Institute of Diabetes and Digestive Kidney Diseases (NIDDK 38016-14).

CHAPTER 13

5,000 Kidney Transplants – A Single-Center Experience

Adyr Moss, John S. Najarian, David E. R. Sutherland, William D. Payne, Rainer W.G. Gruessner, Abhinav Humar, Raja Kandaswamy, Kristen J. Gillingham, David L. Dunn, and Arthur J. Matas

Department of Surgery, University of Minnesota, Minneapolis, Minnesota

The University of Minnesota transplant program began with a living-related donor kidney transplant on June 7, 1963 (1). By the time Dr John S. Najarian arrived in mid-1967 to direct the program and to chair the Department of Surgery, about 80 kidney transplants had been done. Under Najarian's leadership, a strong commitment was made to solid organ transplantation. Special focus was on kidney transplantation for diabetic patients and for pediatric patients; the University of Minnesota was one of the first transplant centers to demonstrate encouraging results in such patients (1-7). By 1977, 1,000 kidney transplants had been done at our institution (1).

In 1990, Perez reported our experience of 3,100 kidney transplants (8). Since then, the field of solid organ transplantation has gone through several changes. Kidney transplantation was once considered primarily to improve quality of life for patients with end-stage renal disease (9,10). But now it is known to increase not only the quality of life, but also longevity (11). Maintenance immunosuppression has expanded to include tacrolimus, the microemulsion formulation of cyclosporine, mycophenolate mofetil, and rapamycin (12). New monoclonal (basiliximab and daclizumab) and polyclonal (Thymoglobulin) antibodies have also been introduced (13-15).

To analyze the impact of this ever-changing scenario on outcome, we reviewed our experience with over 5,000 kidney transplants. Importantly, although we continue to use all potential immunosuppressive drug combinations, most of our recipients have received cyclosporine (CsA)-based immunosuppression. Therefore, this review emphasizes outcome for CsA-treated recipients.

PATIENTS AND METHODS

Demographics

Between June 7, 1963, and December 31, 1998, a total of 5,069 kidney transplants were done at the University of Minnesota. Our approach to patient care, including recipient and donor selection, timing of the transplant, surgical technique, treatment of rejection, and ancillary care, has been previously described. Data on all recipients is maintained on a database in our mainframe computer. The database includes variables such as donor and recipient demographics, HLA match, cause of graft loss, and cause of death. For this review, we excluded 15 recipients whose immunosuppressive protocol was undetermined. We reviewed the outcomes of the remaining 5,054 transplants.

Recipients were grouped into 6 eras based on changes in our immunosuppressive protocols:

Era I—June 1963 through December 1967 (98 transplants were performed): Specific immunosuppressive protocols did not exist. Essentially, all recipients received prednisone (P) and azathioprine (AZA). Some received adjuvant therapy with graft irradiation, creation of a thoracic duct fistula, or actinomycin D.

Era II—January 1968 through July 1979 (1,188 transplants were performed): The routine immunosuppressive protocol (n=1,184) consisted of P, AZA, and prophylactic Minnesota antilymphocyte globulin (MALG). In addition, all patients, except for HLA-identical living-related donor (LRD) graft recipients, underwent pretransplant splenectomy. During Era II, 4 recipients followed an experimental protocol in which total body irradiation was used as the sole immunosuppressive modality.

KIDNEY – MINNESOTA

Era III—August 1979 through June 1984 (789 transplants were performed): The routine immunosuppressive protocol consisted of AZA, P, and MALG. During this period, 2 important prospective trials were initiated. In the first, 246 recipients were randomized to receive AZA, P, and MALG (n=115) or CsA and P (n=131). The CsA and P recipients had fewer rejection episodes, fewer infectious complications, and shorter hospital stays; however, they also had prolonged acute tubular necrosis, a high incidence of nephrotoxicity, and elevated creatinine levels (16). In the second trial, recipients were randomized to undergo pretransplant splenectomy or no splenectomy. Although short-term graft survival was better in the splenectomized group, we found no difference in outcome at 5 years after transplantation (17). Sixteen patients underwent total lymphoid irradiation as the sole immunosuppressive modality.

Era IV—July 1984 through September 1990 (1,006 transplants were performed): Given the outcome of our prospective randomized study, we abandoned routine pretransplant splenectomy. In addition, we began using different immunosuppressive protocols for recipients of LRD and cadaver (CAD) kidneys. LRD recipients began CsA preoperatively and were maintained on CsA, P, and AZA. CAD recipients began antibody (MALG), P, and AZA at the time of the transplant; introduction of CsA was delayed until the kidney was working well (18). For individual reasons, 37 recipients did not receive CsA.

During Era IV, we did a prospective randomized trial of MALG versus OKT3 in the sequential therapy protocol. Graft and patient survival rates were similar in both groups. The incidence of cytomegalovirus (CMV) infection was higher in the MALG group; OKT3 was associated with a higher incidence of side effects and was more expensive (19).

Era V—October 1990 through December 1995 (1,050 transplants were performed): Routine immunosuppressive protocols remained similar to those in Era IV. However, we began using ATGAM rather than MALG for induction therapy for CAD recipients. In addition, during this era, a number of clinical trials were done with new immunosuppressive agents (eg., tacrolimus, mycophenolate mofetil [MMF]).

Era VI—January 1996 through December 1998 (718 transplants were performed): As a result of clinical trials, CAD recipients began using MMF. The hallmark of this era was a more individualized approach to immunosuppression. Protocols were tailored for high- and low-

risk recipients. In addition, retrospective analyses had shown that acute rejection was the major risk factor for chronic rejection in our patient population and that the incidence of acute rejection was related to lower CsA levels; therefore, we began more aggressive attempts to maintain higher CsA levels (20). Importantly, recipients breaking through their immunosuppressive protocol with an acute rejection episode had that episode treated and then had their maintenance immunosuppression changed.

Statistical Analysis

Patient and graft survival rates for each era were calculated by actuarial techniques. Graft loss was defined by the earliest return to dialysis, by a retransplant, or by death. All causes of death were included in the analysis. All recipients were followed until December 31, 1998. P values comparing survival rates over the entire survival experience were calculated using Wilcoxon and log-rank tests, and considered statistically significant when p<0.05.

RESULTS

Demographics

Of the 5,054 transplants, 4,202 (83%) were primary and 852 (17%) were retransplants. The retransplant rate has remained stable throughout all eras. In each era, 44-57% of transplants were from living donors (Fig. 1). Throughout the years, the rate of combined kidney plus extrarenal transplants increased; for example, during Eras V and VI, more than 25% of kidney transplants were combined with another solid organ transplant.

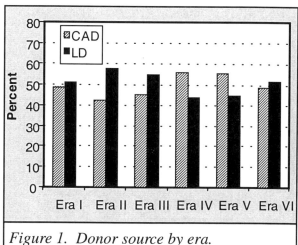

Figure 1. Donor source by era.

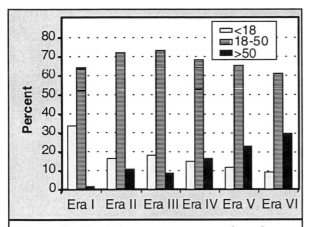

Figure 2. Recipient age at transplant by era.

Except for Era I, when most recipients were female, about 60% of our total recipients were male. Of note, the average recipient age has been increasing. This increase is due to a decrease in the number of recipients younger than 18 years and a steady increase in those older than 50 years (Fig. 2).

The primary renal disease for our adult and pediatric kidney recipients is shown in Tables 1 and 2. For our adult recipients (Table 1), diabetes mellitus was the most common cause of renal failure, affecting almost 46%, followed by glomerulonephritis (18.8%) and polycystic kidney disease (6.4%). For our pediatric recipients (Table 2), obstructive uropathy (17.0%) and congenital anomalies (16.8%) were the most common causes of renal failure, followed by glomerulonephritis (13.7%) and congenital nephrotic syndrome (9.0%).

Table 1. Primary renal diseases – adult kidney recipients.

	n	%
Diabetes	1,974	45.8
Glomerulonephritis	810	18.8
Polycystic Kidney Disease	275	6.4
Pyelonephritis	152	3.5
Posterior Urethral Valve (Obstructive Uropathy)	114	2.6
IgA Nephropathy	106	2.5
Unknown	102	2.4
SLE	84	1.9
Familial Hereditary Nephritis (Alport's Syndrome)	82	1.9
FSGS	65	1.5
Other Renal Diseases	61	1.4
Vesico-Ureteral Reflux (Nonobstructive Uropathy)	49	1.1
Congenital Anomalies	42	1.0
Goodpasture's Syndrome	32	0.7
Interstitial Nephritis	21	0.5
Medullary Cystic Disease	20	0.5
Henoch-Schoenlein Purpura	19	0.4
HUS	18	0.4

Other (<1%): Oxalosis, Fabry's Disease, Wegener's Granulomatosis, Scleroderma, Amyloidosis, Nephrolithiasis, Polyarteristis, Malignancy, Nephrocalcinosis, Toxemia of Pregnancy, Interstitial Mixed Nephrittis, Gout, Congenital Nephrotic Syndrome, Radiation Nephritis, Cortical Necrosis, Cystinosis, von Hipple-Lindau Syndrome, Alpha₁ Anti-Trypsin Deficiency

Table 2. Primary renal diseases – pediatric kidney recipients.

	n	%
Posterior Urethral Valve (Obstructive Uropathy)	125	17.0
Congenital Anomalies	124	16.8
Glomerulonephritis	101	13.7
Congenital Nephrotic Syndrome	66	9.0
FSGS	47	6.4
Other Renal Diseases	42	5.7
Medullary Cystic Disease	30	4.1
HUS	29	3.9
Pyelonephritis	24	3.3
Oxalosis	19	2.6
Polycystic Kidney Disease	18	2.4
Cortical Necrosis	16	2.2
Henoch-Schoenlein Purpura	16	2.2
Vesico-Ureteral Reflux (Nonobstructive Uropathy)	14	1.9
Familial Hereditary Nephritis (Alport's Syndrome)	14	1.9
Cystinosis	10	1.4
Unknown	10	1.4
Interstitial Mixed Nephritis	9	1.2

Other(<1%): IgA Nephropathy, Wegener's Granulomatosis, Nephrolithiasis, Interstitial Nephritis, Malignancy, Jeune Dwarf Syndrome, LES, Alpha₁ Anti-Trypsin Deficiency, Goodpasture's Syndrome

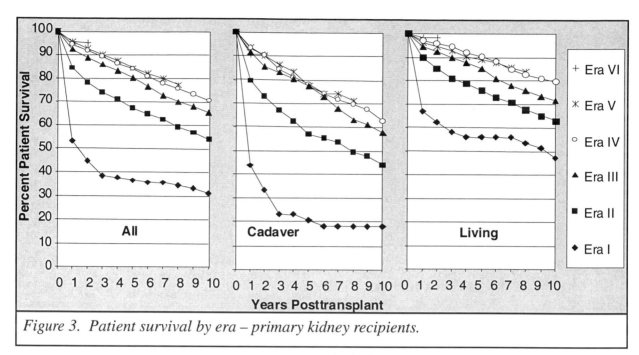

Figure 3. Patient survival by era – primary kidney recipients.

Survival

Actuarial patient survival, by era, is shown for all primary kidney recipients. For primary CAD recipients, there has been little change in survival since Era III. In contrast, for primary living donor (LD) recipients, patient survival has steadily improved (Fig. 3).

Actuarial graft survival, by era, is shown for CAD recipients. We noted a trend toward short-term improvement in each era. For primary LD recipients (Fig. 4),

both short- and long-term graft survival rates have steadily improved.

Death-censored graft survival, by era, is shown for primary CAD recipients in Figure 5. Short-term death-censored graft survival improved in each era. The one-year rate improved by 16% between Eras II and V; however, the 10-year rate improved by only 6%. For primary LD recipients, short-term death-censored graft survival also improved, as did the long-term rate (72% at 8 years in Era II vs. 86% at 8 years in Era V).

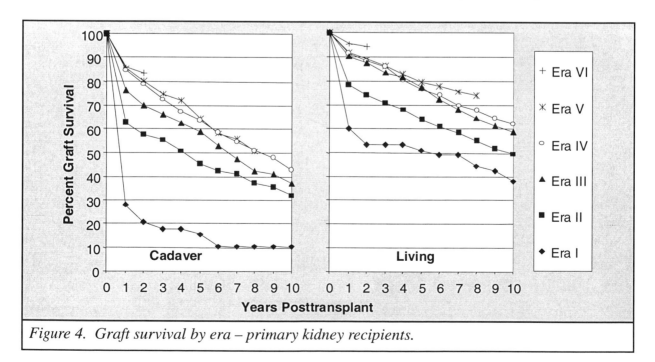

Figure 4. Graft survival by era – primary kidney recipients.

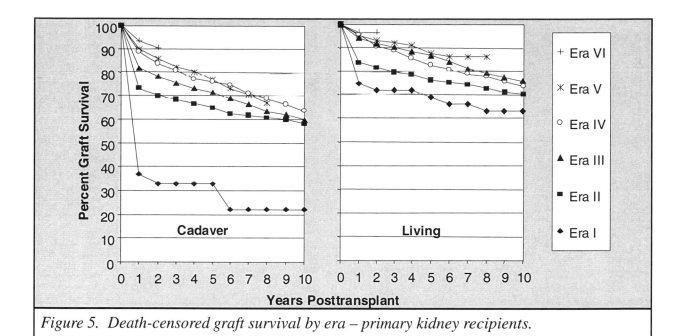

Figure 5. Death-censored graft survival by era – primary kidney recipients.

Causes of Graft Loss

Causes of graft loss in the first 5 years after transplantation for all primary kidney recipients are shown by era in Table 3. Acute rejection has become an infrequent cause of loss, and graft loss to chronic rejection is decreasing. Importantly, loss to infectious death, significant in Eras I and II, is currently much less common.

Donor Source and HLA Matching

We compared outcome, by donor source, for CsA-treated primary kidney recipients. LD recipients (for all 4 categories shown) had better patient and graft survival rates than CAD recipients (Fig. 6). We grouped CsA-treated primary LD recipients by HLA-A,-B,-DR match

(0-haplotype-match LRD, 1-haplotype-match LRD, 2-haplotype-match LRD, living unrelated donor [LURD]) and determined survival. Actuarial patient survival was similar between groups for the first 3 years after transplantation; after 3 years, 1- and 2-haplotype-match grafts were associated with better patient survival. Graft survival was best for 2-haplotype-match recipients; the other 3 groups had similar graft survival rates. Similarly, death-censored graft survival was best for 2-haplotype-match recipients (Fig. 6); the other 3 groups had similar graft survival for the first 8 years. Of concern is that at 9 and 10 years, the LURD group had somewhat worse outcomes; however, the numbers were small.

HLA-identical LD recipients had significantly less acute rejection; this translated into significantly less biopsy-proven chronic rejection (Fig. 7).

We grouped CsA-treated primary CAD recipients by HLA-A,-B,-DR mismatch (mm) (0-1 mm, 2-4 mm, 5-6 mm) and determined survival. We found no significant difference in the patient, graft, or death-censored (Fig. 8) graft survival rates for those transplanted from August 1984 through December 1998 (part of Era IV, all of V and VI). Fewer recipients with 0-1 mm had an acute rejection

Table 3. Causes of graft loss in the first 5 posttransplant years – primary kidney recipients.

	Era I	Era II	Era III	Era IV	Era V	Era VI
Acute Rejection	16%	10%	4%	4%	3%	1%
Chronic Rejection	7%	11%	7%	9%	6%	0.3%
Death with Function						
- infection	9%	8%	3%	3%	2%	1%
- cardiovascular	1%	2%	4%	2%	1%	1%
- other	14%	8%	5%	6%	8%	2%
Other	21%	7%	8%	7%	7%	4%
Functioning at 5 years	31%	55%	67%	68%	74%	91%

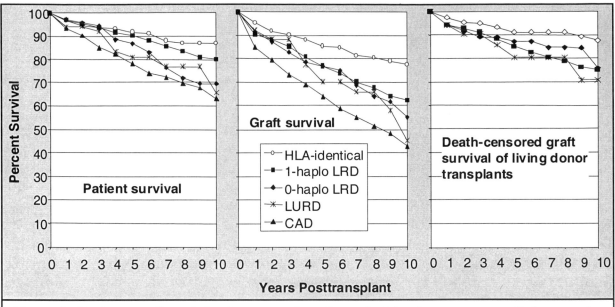

Figure 6. Patient, graft, and death-censored graft survival by donor source – CsA-treated primary kidney recipients.

episode, but the entire difference was seen in the first 6 posttransplant months. Recipients with 0-1 mm also had significantly less biopsy-proven chronic rejection (p=0.03).

Retransplantation

We analyzed the impact of retransplantation from August 1984 through December 1998 (Eras IV, V, and VI). For CsA-treated primary and retransplant (ReTx)

CAD recipients (Fig. 10), we found no difference in patient or graft survival. We found no short-term survival difference when death-censored graft survival was computed, but primary transplant recipients fared significantly better at 10 years (p=0.015). The incidence of biopsy-proven acute rejection and chronic rejection was significantly lower for primary CAD (vs. retransplant) recipients.

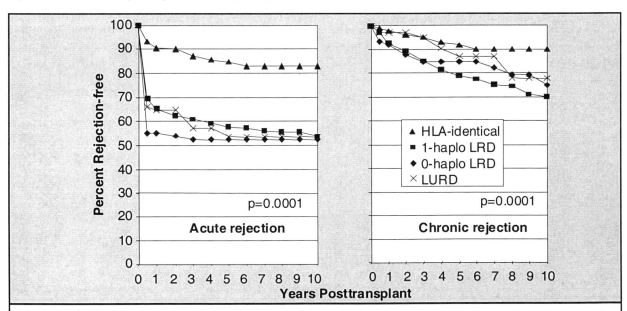

Figure 7. Time to first acute rejection and chronic rejection by LD subgroup – CSA-treated primary LD recipients, August 1984-December 1998.

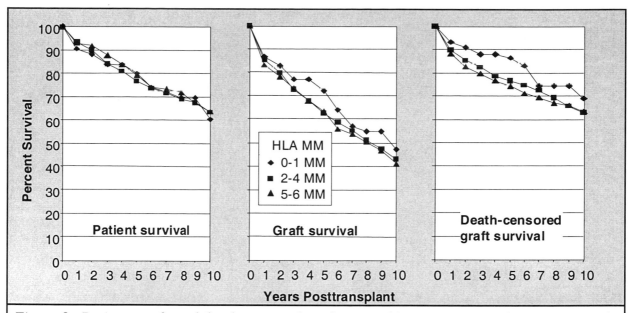

Figure 8. Patient, graft, and death-censored graft survival by HLA mismatch – CsA-treated primary CAD kidney recipients.

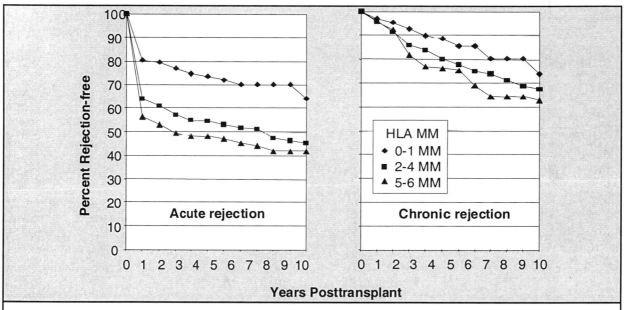

Figure 9. Time to first acute rejection and chronic rejection by HLA mismatch – CSA-treated primary CAD recipients, August 1984-December 1998.

For CsA-treated CAD retransplant recipients, HLA-A,-B,-DR mismatches had no influence on patient survival, graft survival, death-censored graft survival, or biopsy-proven acute rejection (Fig. 11). However, the incidence of chronic rejection was significantly lower for CAD retransplant recipients with a 0-1 mismatch (p<0.05).

We also compared outcome for CsA-treated primary LD and retransplant recipients. Patient survival was not significantly different between these 2 groups (Fig. 12). Graft survival and death-censored graft survival were significantly better in the primary LD group (p<0.05). Retransplantation had no impact on the incidence of biopsy-proven acute rejection or on chronic rejection.

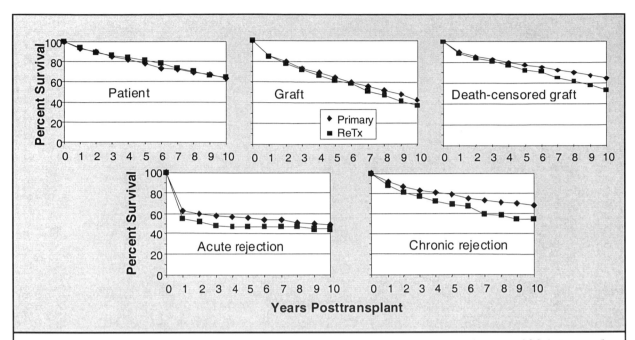

Figure 10. *CsA-treated primary CAD versus retransplant recipients, August 1984-December 1998.*

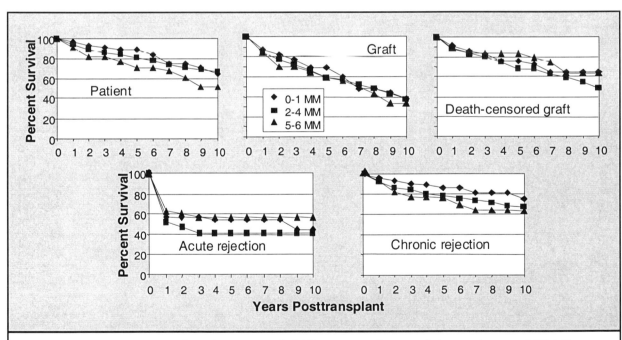

Figure 11. *HLA Mismatch – CsA-treated CAD retransplant recipients, August 1984-December 1998.*

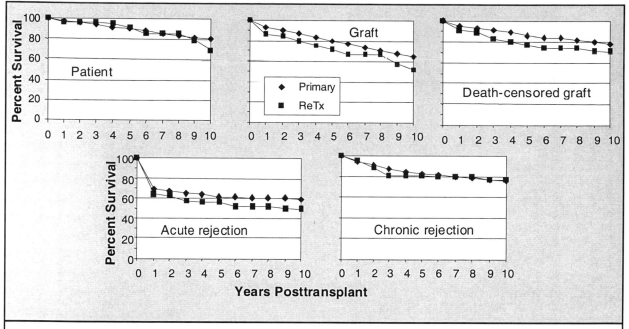

Figure 12. CsA-treated primary LD versus regraft recipients, August 1984-December 1998.

We also looked at the primary renal disease and cause of graft loss for primary and retransplant recipients. We found significant differences in primary renal disease for both CAD (Table 4) and LD (Table 5) recipients (p<.001). Of note, diseases with known worse outcome are more common in the retransplant group. The causes of graft loss for primary and retransplant recipients are shown in Table 6.

Early and Late CsA Period

The CsA period (August 1984 through December 1998) was subdivided into 2 periods: early (August 1984 through December 1995, Eras IV and V) and late (January 1996 through December 1998, Era VI).

Patient and graft survival rates for primary kidney recipients are shown in Table 7 by donor source. Better patient survival was achieved for 1-haplotype-match recipients and for HLA-identical recipients during the late CsA period. Graft survival at 2 years was better for all groups in the late CsA period.

Table 4. Primary renal disease – primary versus ReTx CAD kidney recipients, August 1984-December 1998*.

	Primary	ReTx
Hemolytic Syndrome	0.5%	2.4%
Type I Diabetes	47.0%	30.0%
Type II Diabetes	8.0%	1.0%
MPGN	2.0%	5.0%
FSGS	1.0%	5.0%
Postobstructive valves	2.5%	6.5%
CGN	4.5%	8.0%
* Only shown for diseases that differ significantly in percentage		

Table 5. Cause of graft loss – primary versus ReTx LD kidney recipients, August 1984-December 1998*.

	Primary	ReTx
Hemolytic Uremic Syndrome	1.0%	4.0%
Type I Diabetes	34.0%	21.0%
Focal Sclerosis	1.7%	3.6%
MPGN	2.9%	6.5%
CGN	5.6%	12.3%
FSGS (pediatric)	2.0%	6.0%
Postobstructive valves	6.0%	9.0%
Congenital Nephrotic Syndrome	1.6%	5.0%
Oxalosis	3.0%	2.9%
Congenital Anomalies	4.0%	7.0%
* Only shown for diseases that differ significantly in percentage		

Table 6. Cause of graft loss – primary versus ReTx recipients, August 1984-December 1998.

| | CAD | | LD | |
	Primary	ReTx	Primary	ReTx
Acute Rejection	1.7%	1.4%	1.0%	3.0%
Chronic Rejection	9.5%	15.5%	6.0%	8.0%
Recurrent Disease	0.6%	2.9%	9.0%	2.0%
Death with Function	18.0%	17.0%	9.0%	13.0%
Functioning	60.0%	53.0%	77.0%	65.0%

Table 8. Primary kidney recipients free of acute rejection by posttransplant and CsA period.

| | Early | | Late | |
	1 year	2 years	1 year	2 years
HLA-identical	89.6%	88.8%	94.4%	94.4%
1-Haplo LRD	63.0%	60.3%	72.8%	70.3%
0-Haplo LRD	49.5%	48.1%	75.6%	75.6%
LURD	55.2%	55.2%	73.6%	73.6%
CAD	57.9%	54.8%	83.8%	78.3%

Table 7. Patient and graft survival by donor and CsA period – primary kidney recipients.

| | Early | | Late | |
	1 year	2 years	1 year	2 years
Patient				
HLA-identical	96.6%	94.6%	100%	100%
1-haplo LRD	96.7%	95.4%	99.3%	99.3%
0-haplo LRD	97.1%	95.7%	95.2%	95.2%
LURD	94.1%	94.1%	96.0%	96.0%
CAD	93.2%	90.2%	90.5%	90.5%
Graft				
HLA-identical	95.2%	91.8%	95.1%	95.1%
1-haplo LRD	90.5%	88.2%	97.3%	96.1%
0-haplo LRD	91.4%	87.1%	89.8%	89.8%
LURD	92.2%	88.2%	92.3%	88.7%
CAD	84.9%	79.3%	85.7%	83.7%

Table 9. Primary kidney recipients free of chronic rejection by posttransplant and CsA period.

| | Early | | Late | |
	1 year	2 years	1 year	2 years
0-haplo LRD	89.7%	85.2%	100%	100%
1-haplo LRD	90.8%	87.7%	99.1%	95.4%
CAD	91.5%	85.4%	96.5%	92.3%
HLA-identical	97.9%	96.5%	96.8%	96.8%
LURD	95.8%	95.8%	98.0%	98.0%

The incidence of biopsy-proven acute rejection was lower during the late CsA period, irrespective of donor source or HLA mismatch (Table 8). We noted a reduction in biopsy-proven acute rejection for 0-haplotype-match LRD, LURD, and CAD recipients between the early and late periods. The incidence of chronic rejection was also lower in the late CsA period, again, irrespective of donor source or HLA mismatch (Table 9), even though the differences were less pronounced.

DISCUSSION

During the past 35 years, the Department of Surgery at the University of Minnesota has taken an active role in the development and improvement of solid organ transplantation. Our experience reflects the evolution of kidney transplantation. Our total of 5,069 kidney trans-

plants through December 1998 undoubtedly represents one of the largest single-center experiences in the world (21).

As of December 31, 1998, in the United States, patients older than 65 years comprised over 42% of the ESRD population (22). Our University of Minnesota series clearly reflects the increasing number of transplants in that age group throughout the years. The safety and efficacy of kidney transplants for that age group have been previously demonstrated (23,24).

In our series, outcome steadily improved after 1984, except for patient survival for CAD recipients. However, for LD recipients, both short- and long-term patient survival rates steadily improved, perhaps because these recipients tend to be younger and, consequently, have less comorbidity. Cardiovascular events were the most common cause of recipient death in our series.

Advances in immunobiology and immunosuppression have led to improved short-term graft survival. Unfortunately, until recently, long-term graft survival had remained essentially unchanged (25). Death with function and chronic rejection are still responsible for most late graft losses. Recent data has shown that decreasing the incidence of acute rejection (with improved immunosuppressive protocols) will, in turn, decrease the incidence of biopsy-proven chronic rejection and increase long-term graft survival (26,27).

The influence of HLA mismatch and its role in CAD kidney allocation have been the centerpiece of fierce debate for many years. Some investigators have suggested that the degree of histocompatibility among HLA-mismatched CAD recipients affected graft survival rates, by as much as 5%, at 3 years (28). Interestingly, in our series, a 0-1 mm was associated with fewer episodes of acute and biopsy-proven chronic rejection, but this decrease in rejection has not translated into improved short- or long-term graft survival. It may be that the immunosuppressive protocols we use abrogate any mismatch effect, or perhaps the number of excellent matches is too small to demonstrate an effect.

The use of LURDs is among the many strategies being implemented to expand the donor pool. Although still underused, it is the fastest growing source of kidneys in the United States (28). We previously demonstrated that, even though LURD recipients have poorer HLA mismatch and often involve older donors, their early patient and graft survival rates are similar to those of non-HLA-identical LRD recipients. And their death-censored graft survival at 8 years is similar to that for one-haplotype-match recipients. But of note, their death-censored graft survival at 9 and 10 years is lower (p=NS). Whether this finding is significant or merely an artifact of small numbers needs to be determined.

Our series confirms the efficacy of retransplantation for patients whose primary CAD kidney grafts fail. However, the incidence of acute and chronic rejection was significantly higher for our retransplant recipients compared with our primary CAD recipients. Of note, our LD retransplant recipients had significantly worse outcomes compared with our LD primary recipients. The primary renal disease was different for our primary and retransplant recipients, both LD and CAD. Diseases associated with worse outcome constituted a higher proportion of our retransplant population.

Although it has been previously suggested that HLA mismatch influences graft survival for CAD retransplant recipients (29), our series found no influence on patient, graft, or death-censored graft survival—confirming the findings from prior studies at our institution. However, in our current series, the incidence of chronic rejection was significantly lower for CAD retransplant recipients with 0-1 HLA antigens mismatched.

Our data supports the contention that an aggressive protocol to maintain calcineurin inhibitor blood levels and a more individualized approach to immunosuppression result in a better outcome. Recipients who underwent their first transplant during the late CsA period experienced overall better patient and graft survival, less biopsy-proven acute rejection, and less chronic rejection—irrespective of donor source, recipient age, or diabetes status. Longer follow-up will be necessary to further substantiate these findings.

Our analysis offered the unique opportunity to review the experience of a single institution from early in the history of clinical kidney transplantation. Patients with uremia secondary to diabetic nephropathy, once considered "pariahs of medicine" (30), now constitute half of our kidney recipients. We witnessed the evolution of clinical immunosuppression from the initial use of thoracic duct drainage and total lymphoid irradiation to the time of tailored immunosuppressive regimens with proven benefits. Newer immunosuppressive drugs continue to emerge. Steroid-free protocols are becoming common, and calcineurin inhibitors are no longer considered indispensable.

As transplantation evolves and the organ shortage worsens, the need to expand the donor pool continues. The increased use of marginal donors and the greater number of older transplant candidates demand better immunosuppressive protocols. The socioeconomic impact of graft failure, and the return of a greater number of patients to dialysis and to the waiting list, cannot be ignored. Improving long-term kidney graft survival remains a crucial goal.

KIDNEY – MINNESOTA

SUMMARY

Between 6/1963 and 12/1998, 5,069 kidney transplants were done at the University of Minnesota. Of these, about half have been living donor, half cadaver. The majority (83%) have been primary transplants. Recipients were grouped in 6 eras based on changes in our immunosuppressive protocols—6/63-12/67 (n=98); 1/68-7/79 (n=1,188); 8/79-6/84 (n=789); 7/84-9/90 (n=1,006); 10/90-12/95 (n=1,050; 1/96-12/98 (n=718)—and their outcomes were compared. Recent eras contained a higher proportion of recipients aged >50.

Since the inception of the program, there has been a steady improvement in actuarial patient survival, graft survival, and death-censored graft survival. Short-term outcome for primary and retransplant recipients has been similar; however, long-term outcome seems worse for retransplant recipients. Importantly, acute rejection and infectious death have become rare causes of graft loss. Chronic rejection and death with function (most often due to a cardiovascular event) have become the predominant causes of graft loss.

Recent changes in immunosuppressive protocols (Era VI) have included more aggressive attempts to maintain CsA levels >150 ng/ml (by HPLC) in the first 3 months and the substitution of mycophenolate mofetil for azathioprine. As a result, the incidence of acute and chronic rejection has decreased and graft survival has improved.

REFERENCES

1. Sommer BG, Sutherland DER, Kjellstrand CM, et al. 1,000 renal transplants at the University of Minnesota 1963-1977. Minn Med 1979; 62:861.

2. Sutherland DER, Gores PF, Farney AC, et al. Evolution of kidney, pancreas and islet transplantation for patients with diabetes at the University of Minnesota. Am J Surg 1993; 166:456.

3. Kjellstrand CM, Simmons RL, Goetz FC, et al. Renal transplantation in patients with insulin-dependent diabetes. Lancet 1973; 2:4.

4. Najarian JS, Kjellstrand CM, Simmons RL, et al. Renal transplantation for diabetic glomerulosclerosis. Ann Surg 1973; 178:477.

5. Najarian JS, Sutherland DER, Simmons RL, et al. Kidney transplantation for the uremic diabetic patient. Surg Gynecol Obstet 1977; 144:682.

6. Najarian JS, Simmons RL, Tallent MB, et al. Renal transplantation in infants and children. Ann Surg 1971; 174:583.

7. DeShazo CV, Simmons RL, Bernstein DM, et al. Results of renal transplantation in 100 children. Surgery 1974; 76:461.

8. Perez RV, Matas AJ, Gillingham KJ, et al. Lessons Learned and Future Hopes: Three Thousand Renal Transplants at the University of Minnesota. In: JM Cecka & PI Terasaki, Eds. Clinical Transplants 1990, Los Angeles, UCLA Tissue Typing Laboratory 1991: 217.

9. Jofre R, Lopez-Gomes J, Moreno F, et al. Changes in quality of life after renal transplantation. Am J Kidney Dis 1998; 32:93.

10. Hathaway DK, Winsett RP, Johnson C, et al. Post kidney transplant quality of life prediction models. Clin Transplantation 1998; 12:168.

11. Wolfe RA, Ashby VB, Edgar LM, et al. Comparison of mortality in all patients on dialysis, patients on dialysis awaiting transplantation, and recipients of a first cadaveric transplant. N Engl J Med 1999; 341:1725.

12. Pirsch JD, Miller J, Deierhoi MH, et al. A comparison of tacrolimus (FK506) and cyclosporine for immunosuppression after cadaveric renal transplantation. Transplantation 1997; 63:977.

13. Nashan B, Moore R, Amlot P, et al. Randomized trial of basiliximab versus placebo for control of acute cellular rejection in renal allograft recipients. Lancet 1997; 350:1193.

14. Nashan B, Light S, Hardie IR et al. Reduction of acute allograft rejection by daclizumab. Transplantation 1999; 67:110.

15. Brennan DC, Flavin K, Lowell JA, et al. A randomized, double-blinded comparison of Thymoglobulin versus Atgam for induction immunosuppressive therapy in adult renal transplant recipients. Transplantation 1999; 67:1011.

16. Ferguson RM, Rynasiewicz JJ, Sutherland DER, et al. Cyclosporine A in renal transplantation: a prospective randomized trial. Surgery 1982; 92:175.

17. Sutherland DER, Fryd DS, So SKS, et al. Long-term effect of splenectomy versus no splenectomy in renal transplant patients. Reanalysis of a randomized prospective study. Transplantation 1984; 38:619.

18. Simmons RL, Canafax DM, Fryd DS, et al. New immunosuppressive drug combinations for mismatched related and cadaveric renal transplantation. Transplant Proc 1986; 18(2 Suppl 1):76.

19. Frey DJ, Matas AJ, Gillingham KJ, et al. Sequential therapy—a prospective randomized trial of MALG versus OKT3 for prophylactic immunosuppression in cadaver renal allograft recipients. Transplantation 1992; 54:50.

20. Johnson EM, Canafax DM, Gillingham KJ, et al. Effect of early cyclosporine levels on kidney allograft rejection. Clin Transplantation 1997; 11:552.

21. Cecka JM, Terasaki PI. Worldwide Kidney Transplant Center Directory. In: JM Cecka & PI Terasaki, Eds. Clinical Transplants 1999. Los Angeles, UCLA Tissue Typing Laboratory, 2000:399.

22. Annual Data Report 1999—United States Renal Data System (USRDS), www.usrds.org

23. Benedetti E, Matas AJ, Hakim N, et al. Renal transplantation for patients 60 years or older. A single-institution experience. Ann Surg 1994; 220:445.

24. Doyle SE, Matas AJ, Gillingham K, Rosenberg ME. Predicting clinical outcome in the elderly transplant recipient. Kidney Int 2000; 57:2144.

25. Schweitzer EJ, Matas AJ, Gillingham KJ, et al. Causes of renal allograft loss. Progress in the 1980s, challenges for the 1990s. Ann Surg 1991; 214:679.

26. Matas AJ, Humar A, Payne WD, et al. Decreased acute rejection in kidney transplant recipients is associated with decreased chronic rejection. Ann Surg 1999; 230:493.

27. Hariharan S, Johnson CP, Bresnahan BA, et al. Improved graft survival after renal transplantation in the United States, 1988 to 1996. N Engl J Med 2000; 342:605.

28. Cecka JM. The UNOS Scientific Renal Transplant Registry. In: JM Cecka & PI Terasaki, Eds. Clinical Transplants 1999. Los Angeles, UCLA Tissue Typing Laboratory 2000:1.

29. Hata Y, Ozawa M, Takemoto SK, et al. HLA Matching. In: JM Cecka & PI Terasaki , Eds. Clinical Transplants 1996. Los Angeles, UCLA Tissue Typing Laboratory 1997:381.

30. Lillehei RC, Simmons RL, Najarian JS, et al. Pancreaticoduodenal allotransplantation: experimental and clinical experience. Acta Diabetol Lat 1970; 7:909.

CHAPTER 14

Fifteen-Year Experience with Pediatric Renal Transplantation at the Montefiore Medical Center

Stuart Greenstein, Jennifer Sloane, Jason Denny, Owen Prowse, John Harvey, Diane Feuerstein, Richard Schechner, Anita Principe, and Vivian Tellis

Transplant Unit, Department of Surgery, Montefiore Medical Center, and Albert Einstein College of Medicine, Bronx, New York

Renal transplantation remains the treatment of choice for children with end-stage renal disease (ESRD) (1). A retrospective review was conducted of transplants done from January 1, 1984 to October 18, 2000 at Montefiore Medical Center, the University hospital for the Albert Einstein College of Medicine. We examined factors relating to both graft and patient outcome including age, race, transplant number, donor source, pre-emptive transplantation, HLA-A,-B and -DR mismatching, immunosuppressive protocol and primary renal disease.

PATIENTS AND METHODS

Between January 1984 and October 2000, 155 renal transplants were performed in 140 children at the Montefiore Medical Center. At our institution all recipients under age 21 are considered pediatric. Recipient characteristics of patients transplanted are summarized in Table 1. The mean age at transplantation was 12.8 years (range 1-20 years), and 63.8% of patients were male and 36.2% female. The racial composition of the patient population was 68.3% Caucasian and 31.7% Black. Donor sources for the 155 renal allografts included 87 (56.1%) cadaver and 68 (43.9%) living-related donor kidneys. Primary transplants were performed in 134 children (86.4%) and retransplants were performed in 21 children (13.6%) – 5 children had previously received transplants at other centers. Pre-emptive transplantation was performed in 17 patients (11.0%). The primary diseases leading to ESRD in our patient population are shown below with the 3 most common causes being focal glomerulosclerosis (FSGS), renal hypoplasia and obstructive uropathy.

Table 1. Recipient characteristics

N	155
Sex ratio M:F	1.8:1
Not Black : Black	2.1:1
Mean Age	12.8
Proportion ≤ 7 yrs (%)	19.3%
Proportion ≥ 18 yrs (%)	25.1%
Mean Peak PRA	33.3
%Tx#>1	14%
Disease(%): FSGS	23.2%
Renal hypoplasia	18%
Obstructive uropathy	5.8%
Reflux nephropathy	5.2%
MPGN	3.2%
Alport's syndrome	3.9%
Prune-belly syndrome	2.6%
Malignant hypertension	2.6%
IgA nephropathy	1.3%
HUS	1.9%
Cystinosis	1.3%
Others	12.3%
Unknown	13.5%

Immunosuppressive Protocol

Immunosuppressive protocols were periodically adjusted in keeping with development of pharmacological and biologic agents. Choice and dosage of agents was conservative, and geared to maximize patient survival. Table 2 lists the highlights. Not shown are deliberate pretransplant blood transfusions, required during the period from January 1984 to June 1989, and abandoned after 1991.

Clinical Transplants 2000, Cecka and Terasaki, Eds. UCLA Immunogenetics Center, Los Angeles, California

Table 2. Changes in the immunosuppressive protocol from 1984 to present.

Year	Basic	Induction	Rejection
1984	P, CsA, Az	ALG standard for ATN	ALG standard for SRR
1989-93	P, CsA, Az		OKT3 for SRR FK for SRR
1993	P, CsA, Az	↓	
1996	P, CsA, Az	None	CsA switch to FK for SRR
	or P, FK for Hi Risk		or Increase FK dose
1997- present	P, FK	Il-2 blocker	↓

Legend: P- Prednisone, Az- Azathioprine, CsA- Cyclosporine, FK- Tacrolimus, M- Mycophenolate Mofetil, ALG- Anti-lymphocyte globulin, SRR- Steroid resistant rejection

Our current immunosuppressive protocol consists of steroids and tacrolimus. Solumedrol (10 mg/kg IV) is given at the time of surgery followed by prednisone (2 mg/kg/day) for the first week and tapered to a dose of 0.05 mg/kg/day by 6 months. The maximum initial dose during the first week of prednisone is 30 mg/day (for patients >30 kg). Tacrolimus dosing is 0.15 mg/kg po on call to the operating room followed by 0.3 mg/kg/day po until trough target levels are reached. The target levels in the first 2 weeks are 20-25 ng/ml followed by gradual reduction to a level of 10-15 by 3 months. Il-2 blocker induction (Basiliximab) is given at day zero and day 4 after transplantation at a dose of 12 mg/m^2.

Statistical Analysis

Patient and graft survival were determined using the cumulative log rank method with Student's t-test used to determine significance for p values. Graft loss was defined as a return to dialysis, transplant nephrectomy, retransplantation or patient death. Analyses were considered statistically significant when $p < 0.05$.

RESULTS

At the time of follow-up, 147 children were alive and 79 kidneys (primary and retransplants) were functioning. Follow-up ranged from 0-15.6 years with a mean follow-up time of 4.0 years.

Patient Survival

All patient deaths with functioning transplanted kidneys and all patient deaths within 3 months after return to dialysis were included in this calculation. Overall patient survival rates at one, 2 and 5 years were 98.0%, 96.6% and 95.8%, respectively (Fig. 1). Patient survival rates did not differ significantly according to donor source (Fig. 2). All 56 females (100%), and 76 males (93.5%) were alive at 5 years (Fig. 3). Race and retransplantation did not have a major impact upon patient survival. (Figs. 4, 5, respectively). HLA mismatching and age had no effect on patient survival.

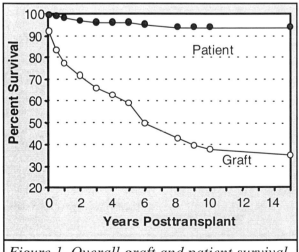

Figure 1. Overall graft and patient survival.

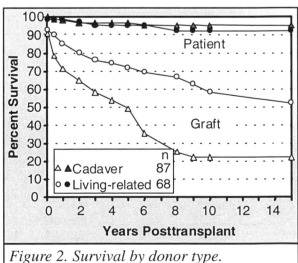

Figure 2. Survival by donor type.

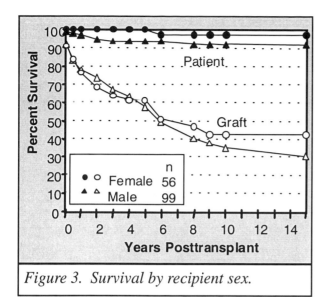

Figure 3. Survival by recipient sex.

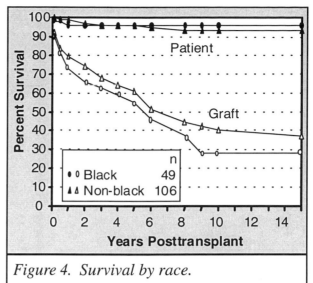

Figure 4. Survival by race.

Graft survival

With earlier years of immunosuppression, the goal of maximum patient survival implied an acceptance of increased graft loss. Overall graft survival rates at one, 2 and 5 years were 77%, 72% and 59%, respectively (Fig. 1). Graft survival for living-related donor transplants was significantly better than for cadaveric transplants at 6 years (p<0.005; Fig. 2) and was similar to that reported by other investigators (2,3). For grafts that failed, the mean time to graft failure for primary renal transplant recipients was 2.9 years. Pre-emptive transplantation had a favorable effect on graft outcome and was statistically significant (p=0.01; Fig. 6) as has been shown by others (2,4). No single primary cause of end-stage

renal disease was significantly associated with greater graft failure when assessed independently of all other causes (Fig. 7).

Effects of gender and race: Graft survival was not significantly different between the sexes (Fig. 3). This is consistent with what has been reported by our institution as well as by others for the adult population (5-7).

African-Americans constitute approximately one-third of the patients who have been transplanted at our institution; a higher percentage than reported by most centers in the United States (8). We had previously reported no difference in graft survival between Black and non-Black recipients one year after transplant in the adult population (9). This was found to be also true for the pediatric recipients (Fig. 4).

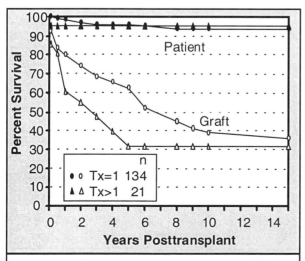

Figure 5. Survival by transplant number.

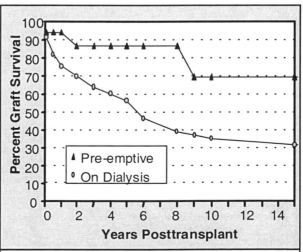

Figure 6. Graft survival by time of transplant.

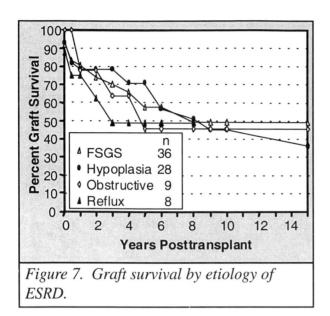

Figure 7. Graft survival by etiology of ESRD.

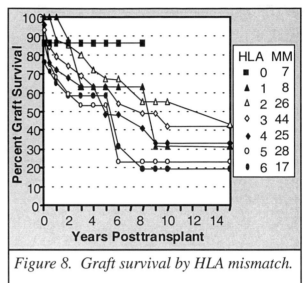

Figure 8. Graft survival by HLA mismatch.

Re-transplants: Graft survival rates were better in patients undergoing primary renal transplantation: 80%, 74% and 63% at one, 2 and 5 years, respectively. There was a difference in graft survival of approximately 19% at one year between first time and retransplanted pediatric recipients (Fig. 5). This difference increased markedly to approximately 30% by 5 years (p<0.025).

Histocompatibility mismatching: Until 1989, HLA matching was not taken into account in kidney distribution and cadaver kidneys were allocated at our institution on a "first-come, first-served" basis. Review of our data confirms other reports (10,11), that HLA mismatches play a role in graft survival. There was a greater difference in graft survival when the HLA serotypes were more disparate (5-6 mismatches vs. zero mismatch) as shown in Figure 8. When patient groups are stratified by number of mismatches, the numbers of patients at risk become too small for true statistical comparison. Differences in outcome that may result from small differences in HLA mismatches (3 vs. 4 antigens mismatched) take years to become apparent. Any possible advantage of such mismatching must be balanced against the effects on the pediatric patient of the longer time waiting to obtain the better match.

Age of recipient: Of 59 recipients 12 years of age or less at the time of transplant, 42% lost their allograft, 17% during adolescence. Ninety-six patients were 13 years of age or older and 52% lost their grafts. The 5-year graft survival rate in this group was 50% compared with 71% among patients less than 13 years of age (p=0.1). Those recipients who were less than 7 years of

age at the time of transplant had the best graft survival rates (Fig. 9). Those recipients who were between 7-12 years of age at the time of transplant had the highest rate of graft loss after 5 years with an 8-year survival rate of only 20%. Thus, whether adolescence had an impact on graft survival could not clearly be established.

Recent Experience

Figure 10 summarizes our experience based upon current immunosuppression. Patient survival for the last 39 patients (intent to treat with tacrolimus) was 97% and graft survival (combined living and cadaver donor kidneys) was 82% at one year and constant thereafter. Current management includes anti-Interleukin-2 receptor antibody for induction with tacrolimus used as

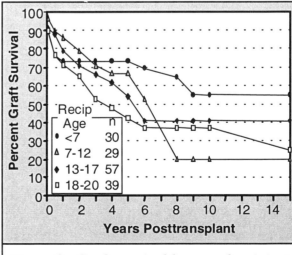

Figure 9. Graft survival by age of recipient.

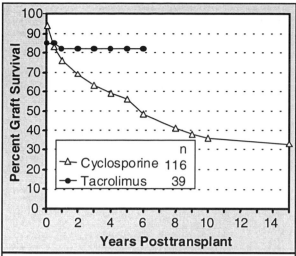

Figure 10. Graft survival by immunosuppression.

primary immunosuppression for all pediatric recipients. There is a significant difference between graft survival rates when these patients are compared with patients on cyclosporine-based immunosuppression.

DISCUSSION

One hundred forty children received 155 renal transplants over a 16-year period at our institution. Patient and graft survival rates at one, 2 and 5 years are comparable to published series (1). Unlike some series (1,4), we report a significant improvement in outcome for patients undergoing pre-emptive renal transplantation compared with those with a history of preoperative dialysis (both peritoneal and hemodialysis). There was no significant difference in graft survival according to sex, age or race of recipient. The rate of graft loss during the first postoperative year remains a concern particularly for patients receiving cadaver kidneys. As in other published series, we found significantly improved graft survival rates for patients receiving living-related donor kidneys (1,2,11,12).

Despite a large number of patients receiving living-related donor kidneys the majority of transplanted kidneys were from cadaver sources. In addition, our patient population was relatively heterogeneous. Black children accounted for 31.7% and a large proportion of the Caucasian group (68.2%) was Hispanic. The primary cause of end-stage renal disease in our population was FSGS, which is different from the majority of pediatric renal transplant series where congenital anomalies or obstructive uropathy predominate.

Although our 2- and 5-year graft survival rates are comparable to published reviews (1,2,5,11,12), our series demonstrated more than 20% of grafts were lost early (<12 months) regardless of whether they were primary or retransplants. Analyses of these cases revealed that most were lost between 0-3 months.

SUMMARY

At Montefiore Medical Center, 140 pediatric recipients have received 155 renal allografts over a 16-year period with an overall 6% mortality. Graft survival was not significantly different based upon race or sex of recipient. Graft survival was significantly better for first time transplants and the youngest recipients. Graft survival was significantly improved using Tacrolimus immunosuppression.

REFERENCES

1. Chavers BM, Matas AJ, Gillingham KJ, Schmidt WJ, Najarian JS. Pediatric renal transplants at the University of Minnesota: The cyclosporine years. In: PI Terasaki and JM Cecka, Eds. Clinical Transplants 1993, UCLA Tissue Typing Laboratory, Los Angeles, 1994; 203.

2. Tejani A, Stablein D, Fine R, Alexander S. Maintenance immunosuppression therapy and outcome of renal transplantation in North American children – a report of the North American Pediatric Renal Transplant Cooperative Study. Pediatr Nephrol 1993; 7:132.

3. Chavers BM. Causes of kidney allograft loss in a large pediatric population at a single center. Pediatr Nephrol 1994; 8:57.

4. Flom LS, Reisman EM, Donovan JH, et al. Favorable experience with pre-emptive renal transplantation in children. Pediatr Nephrol 1992; 6: 258.

5. Neugarten J, Silbiger SR. The impact of gender on renal transplantation. Transplantation 1994; 58:1145.

6. Koka P, Cecka JM. Sex and age effects in renal transplantation. In: PI Terasaki and JM Cecka, Eds. Clinical Transplants1990, UCLA Tissue Typing Laboratory, Los Angeles, 1991, 437.

7. Nyberg G, Blohme I, Norden G. Gender differences in a kidney transplant population. Nephrol Dial Transplant 1997; 12:559.

8. Schweitzer EJ, Yoon S, Fink J, et al. Mycophenolate mofetil reduces the risk of acute rejection less in African-American than in Caucasian kidney recipients. Transplantation 1998; 65:242.

9. Greenstein SM, Schechner RS, Tellis VA. Twenty-five year review of race and transplantation at a single institution. Transplant Proc 1993; 25:2448.

10. Gjertson DW. Lookup survival tables for renal transplantation. In: JM Cecka, PI Terasaki, and Eds. Clinical Transplants 1997. Los Angeles, UCLA Tissue Typing Laboratory, 1998, 337.

11. Tejani AH, Sullivan EK, Harmon WE, et al. Pediatric renal transplantation- The NAPRTCS experience. In: JM Cecka, PI Terasaki, and Eds. Clinical Transplants 1997. Los Angeles, UCLA Tissue Typing Laboratory, 1998, 87.

12. Farraresso M, Kahan BD. New immunosuppressive agents for pediatric transplantation. Pediatr Nephrol 1993; 7:567.

CHAPTER 15

The Kidney Transplant Program at the Bergamo Center

Giuseppe Remuzzi, Norberto Perico, Eliana Gotti, Piero Ruggenenti, Giovanni Rota, and Giuseppe Locatelli

Department of Immunology and Clinics of Organ Transplantation, Ospedali Riuniti di Bergamo – Mario Negri Institute for Pharmacological Research, Bergamo, ITALY

Over the last 30 years the activities of the Division of Nephrology and Dialysis at the Ospedali Riuniti di Bergamo have expanded in many directions according to the progress of medical (and particularly nephrological) sciences and technology. November 1989 marked the beginning of the kidney transplant program, which has progressively expanded during the subsequent years. At that time a fruitful and long-lasting co-operation was already established between our Clinical Division and the Negri Bergamo Laboratories of the Mario Negri Institute for Pharmacological Research in the field of renal disease progression. The experimental know-how achieved on the efficacy and toxicity of conventional and novel antirejection agents by the Negri Bergamo Laboratories, the skill of the transplant surgeons of the Pediatric Surgery Division in charge of the surgical part of the program, and the clinical expertise of the Nephrology Division allowed a joint venture to begin that resulted in the recognition of the Bergamo Kidney Transplant Program as one of the most active in Italy. By 1995, the Unit of Nephrology coordinated the activity of the Department of Immunology and Clinics of Organ Transplantation, Ospedali Riuniti - Mario Negri Institute for Pharmacological Research, Bergamo. This is an innovative public-private venture for Italy, that rests on a strict cooperation between 12 Units of the Ospedali Riuniti which had been involved in the solid organ transplant program (including kidney, heart, heart-lung, and liver) and 4 laboratories of the Mario Negri Institute with extensive experience in the field of transplant immunology and clinical pharmacology. The major efforts of the Department are directed to identify novel approaches to overcome the shortage of donor organs for transplantation; to optimize conventional antirejection therapies and search for new immunosuppressants for routine clinical application; to prevent or limit relevant complications of transplantation, such as infections and neoplasias; and to identify strategies for induction and maintenance of transplant tolerance without the need of chronic immunosuppressants.

To achieve these objectives, a peculiar and active interaction between basic science and the clinics is mandatory. This provides the basis for a rapid transfer of the most recent insights into clinical practice and should be viewed as a critical step for the most advanced improvement in the quality of healthcare and also of transplant medicine.

Here we briefly review the results obtained so far by the kidney transplant program in the Unit of Nephrology and Dialysis of the Ospedali Riuniti di Bergamo and provide information on ongoing studies and future plans of investigations.

RESULTS OF THE CLINICAL TRANSPLANT PROGRAM

From the beginning of the kidney transplant activity in 1989 through October 30, 2000, 367 transplants were performed in adult recipients. These include 357 kidney transplants from cadaver donors and 10 from living-related donors. Among them, 348 were first transplants and 19 were second transplants.

As shown in Table 1, a mean of 39.5 transplants per year were performed in the last 4 years with a male to female ratio of 2:1. The mean age at transplant was 44 years, ranging from 15-66 years.

Table 1. Kidney transplant activity at the Bergamo center in the period 1996-2000.

	1996	1997	1998	1999	2000*
Total	36	44	42	36	28
Male	29	32	29	24	16
Female	7	12	13	12	12

*Up to October 30, 2000

Table 2. Renal function in kidney transplant recipients (n=301) at 1,3,4 or >4 years after surgery, stratified according to 3 different ranges of serum creatinine concentrations.

SCr (mg/dl)	Years after Surgery			
	1	3	4	>4
<1.5	141	90	70	68
≥1.5-<3	62	45	42	35
≥3	6	5	4	4

The standard immunosuppressive therapy is based on a triple antirejection drug regimen with cyclosporine (CsA), steroids and azathioprine, substituting mycophenolate mofetil – MMF since 1997. This is the current immunosuppressive treatment protocol for recipients of a first cadaver kidney. Induction therapy with rabbit antithymocyte globulin (RATG) is limited to recipients of a second cadaver kidney and living-related transplants. When posttransplant anuria occurs, the immunosuppressive treatment protocol includes RATG, steroids, and azathioprine or MMF, temporarily avoiding CsA until urine output is restored.

Patient and Graft Survival

After 10 years of transplant activity, 94% of patients are alive. Indeed, up to now, 23 kidney transplant recipients have died. As reported in Figure 1, actuarial graft survival at 3 years (combining dialysis and death

as end-points) was 92%, and at 8 years it was 77%. Considering dialysis as a single end-point, actuarial kidney graft survival at 8 years after transplantation was 84%.

Graft Function

Most patients had a rapid recovery of graft function in the immediate posttransplant period. Posttransplant anuria was documented in 16.6%. The outcome of the kidney transplant, however, has to be evaluated in the long-term. To this end, we have examined graft function as serum creatinine in patients who reached one, 3, 4 or more than 4 years after surgery. At each of these time points patients were stratified according to 3 different ranges of serum creatinine concentration, namely <1.5 mg/dl (normal renal function), ≥1.5 to <3 mg/dl (mild to moderate renal insufficiency) and ≥3 mg/dl (severe renal insufficiency). As shown in Table 2, for each time point considered most patients were in the lowest tertile of graft function, ie. normal renal function. Very few patients had severe renal dysfunction.

Complications: Neoplasias/ Infections

Current antirejection medicines invariably reduce systemic immunity non-selectively and increase the risk of infections and cancer. Tumors of viral origin are 6.5 times commoner among transplant recipients than among the general population (1), and their frequency is estimated to increase with time. From the analysis of the first 301 transplant patients, a 5.0% incidence of neoplasia has been documented. This includes lymphoproliferative diseases, skin cancer; Kaposi's sarcoma and

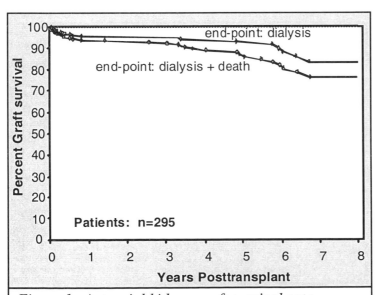

Figure 1. Actuarial kidney graft survival rate (Kaplan-Meier) considering combined end-points of dialysis and death or only return to dialysis.

less frequently hepatocarcinoma and renal carcinoma. In particular, we documented a high frequency of EBV-negative lymphoproliferative disorders developing in long-term survivors after kidney transplantation (2,3). As for skin cancer, an Italian registry-based study coordinated by the Division of Dermatology and Nephrology of the Ospedali Riuniti Bergamo has recently reported on a total of 1,329 patients who received their first kidney (1,062 subjects) or heart allograft (267 subjects) an overall incidence of nonmelanoma skin cancer of 10 cases per 1000 posttransplant person-years (95% C.I. 8.2-11.7), a value higher than that expected in the general population (4). The overall risk of developing skin cancer increased from a cumulative incidence of 5.8% after 5 posttransplant years to an incidence of 10.8% after 10 years of graft survival. After adjustment for age at transplantation and sex, no increased risk was documented among kidney compared with heart transplant recipients.

In the same transplant population, one or more infectious episodes was found in 46.5% of patients. The most common were CMV infection that accounted for 65.7% of all cases. It should be pointed out that no CMV prophylaxis is used in our center. This practice is based on the results of a retrospective analysis performed by our group some years ago on 160 kidney transplant recipients who did not undergo CMV prophylaxis (5). Of the 71 patients with clinical and/or laboratory signs of suspected CMV infection, the early CMV antigen test in peripheral blood leukocytes was positive in 35. All positive patients completely responded to gancyclovir therapy, except one, who required foscaenet treatment, whereas none of the 36 with a negative CMV antigen test developed CMV disease. These findings indicated that early treatment of CMV infection documented by a positive CMV antigen test was successful even in those patients who were not previously exposed to specific prophylaxis with antiviral drugs. This strategy avoids the need of long-term prophylaxis with potentially toxic agents.

As for other opportunistic infections occurring in our transplant patients, the incidence of *Pneumocystis carinii* (for which prophylaxis with pentamidine is routinely performed) was 1.3% and for *Nocardia* was 0.3%.

Multiorgan Transplant Program

In August 1997, a program for transplantation of dual "marginal kidneys" in the same recipient was activated.

Since then 19 double kidney transplants have been successfully performed.

Four combined heart-kidney transplants have been performed from the beginning of this program (March 1994). All the heart transplants are functioning well, but one patient lost the kidney graft 3 years after transplantation and now is on dialysis replacement therapy.

The first combined liver-kidney transplant was performed in 1999. The patient is still in good health and both grafts are functioning well. A second successful combined liver-kidney transplant has been done this year.

RESULTS OF THE RESEARCH TRANSPLANT PROGRAM

In parallel, but strictly integrated with this clinical activity, is the research transplant program that involves physicians, biologists, molecular biologists, pathologists, immunologists, chemists, pharmacologists, bio-engineers, statisticians, and research nurses from the Unit of Nephrology and Dialysis at the Ospedali Riuniti Bergamo, the Negri Bergamo Laboratories and the Clinical Research Center "Aldo e Cele Daccò" of the Mario Negri Institute. These activities are aimed to address key issues of transplant medicine - namely, the shortage of donor kidneys, the need to optimize the current antirejection therapies, the evaluation of novel immunosuppressants and identifying strategies of transplant tolerance. Here we will briefly survey all these research programs.

Tackling the Shortage of Donor Kidneys

The shortage of kidney donors is the major limitation to kidney transplantation (6). The already inadequate pool of donors is further reduced by discarding "marginal" kidneys from old donors (>60 years) or donors with a history of hypertension or diabetes, or evidence of chronic renal diseases, which are expected to fail prematurely due to a process of accelerated exhaustion of their already low functional units. In an effort to overcome the disparity between supply of cadaveric donors and demand, various strategies have emerged to expand the existing donor selection criteria. One possibility to actually enhance the kidney donor pool is not to discard those suboptimal kidneys and use both in the same recipient instead (7). In this case, the limit of using suboptimal or "marginal" kidneys would be balanced by the advantage for the patients of receiving a nephron mass larger than that provided by a single "ideal" kidney. Indeed the higher number of functioning nephrons supplied by dual marginal kidneys should theoretically slow or even prevent the activation of a sequence of events associated with progressive deterioration of graft function that ultimately leads to graft loss (8). Moreover, should one of the 2 marginal kidneys be lost due to vascular or urologic complications, the remaining kidney would still contribute to a delay in restarting renal replacement therapy with dialysis. On the other hand, a possible disadvantage of the procedure is a more prolonged and complex surgery as required by the dual kidney transplantation. Our group, in collaboration with Harvard Medical School at Boston, has established the Double Kidney Transplant Group (DKG), an international cooperative network created to address the possibility of using double transplantation of suboptimal kidneys usually discarded for the single transplant procedure. Five kidney transplant centers in Europe (Barcelona, Madrid, Bergamo, Milano, Genova) and 2 in North America (Boston, Toronto) have been involved in this multicenter study. For each case, 2 controls done at the same institution, satisfying the same inclusion criteria (informed consent, age >50 years, no previous kidney transplant, panel-reactive antibodies <50%) and receiving the same immunosuppressive protocol (steroids, cyclosporine and mycophenolate mofetil) were identified. This prospective, case-control study compared adverse events and graft outcomes in 24 recipients of 2 marginal kidneys from donors who were >60 years old or who had diabetes, hypertension, or non-nephrotic proteinuria (case) with 48 age- and gender-matched control subjects who received single ideal grafts at the same center and were given the same immunosuppressive therapy (9). Marginal kidneys with no macroscopic abnormalities were selected for the double transplant on the basis of a predefined score of histologic damage. Six-month patient and kidney survival was 100% with both procedures. The incidence (20.8%) and median (range) duration of posttransplant anuria [5 (2-12) versus 7 (2-13) days] were comparable in cases and control subjects, respectively. Time to normal serum creatinine and mean serum creatinine values at each visit were comparable as well, but with

significantly lower levels in cases compared with control subjects from month 2 to the last follow-up (1.56±0.65 vs. 1.74±0.73 mg/dl, p=0.04) (Fig. 2). Diastolic blood pressure values averaged during the entire posttransplant period were significantly lower in cases than in control subjects (83.2±11.5 vs. 85.1±12.5 mmHg, respectively, p=0.008). Donor/recipient body weight ratio was the only covariate significantly associated with the last available serum creatinine concentrations in univariate (p=0.002) and multivariate (p=0.001) analyses. Incidence of acute allograft rejections (20.8% vs. 18.8%) and of major surgical complications was comparable in the 2 groups. No renal artery or vein thrombosis was reported in either group. Hence, these findings indicate that dual transplants of marginal kidneys in the same recipient are as safe and well tolerated as single transplants and may offer an improved filtration power without exposing the recipient to the enhanced risk of delayed renal function recovery, acute allograft rejection, or major surgical complications. This novel strategy would contribute to expanding the present limited pool of cadaveric organs by giving access to kidneys not otherwise considered for transplantation. Further investigations will show whether double kidney transplantation, by providing more nephron mass, will serve to delay or prevent chronic allograft dysfunction in the long-term. To this purpose an ongoing trial, coordinated by the Nord Italia Transplant (NITp), the main

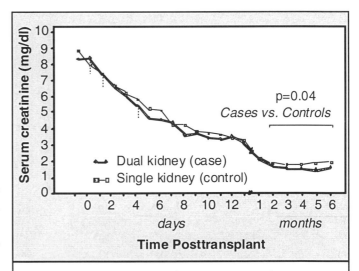

Figure 2. Time course of serum creatinine concentration in patients undergoing dual kidney transplants (cases, n=24) and in those receiving a single ideal kidney (control, n=48) from marginal donors.

organ allocation organization in northern Italy, and involving transplant centers at Bergamo, Genova, Padova, and Varese, aims to compare the long-term outcome of dual transplants of marginal kidneys and of single transplants of ideal kidneys from marginal cadaver donors over a 3-year follow-up in a controlled, prospective trial. Preliminary results after one year of 38 double marginal kidney transplants show a 94% graft survival rate compared with 91% in 568 single kidney transplants (1997-2000) from donors >50 years (Fig. 3). Moreover, better graft function (as serum creatinine) of double than single kidney transplants was found at the same time point. All patients receiving the dual kidney transplant (vs. 96% in those with single kidney) were alive one year after transplantation.

Optimization of Conventional Antirejection Therapies

One of the research activities of our center is devoted to optimize the use of conventional immunosuppressive drugs to minimize their toxicity and maximize their antirejection properties. In particular, we have focussed our attention on CsA, approaching this issue by using pharmacokinetics and more recently, by pharmacodynamic strategies.

A simplified method to evaluate daily exposure to CsA in kidney transplant patients

Historically our group has paid major attention to monitoring CsA exposure in transplant recipients, initially by setting up a specific method for measuring whole blood CsA concentration using high performance liquid chromatography and subsequently by attempting to identify simple and specific CsA pharmacokinetic parameters that could be applied to routine assessment of patients, helping to optimize the efficacy and safety of this antirejection drug (10). Indeed, given the appreciable interindividual variation both in clinical responses and in the blood drug concentration despite the same dosage regimens, major efforts have been devoted to individualize CsA regimen for rejection prophylaxis in order to minimize the toxicity and improve the risk/benefit ratio. Current methods include measurement of the 'trough' whole blood CsA concentration. However, trough level monitoring is not universally helpful, as documented by findings that some patients may experience rejection in the presence of adequate or even high blood CsA levels, whereas others may develop toxicity even when

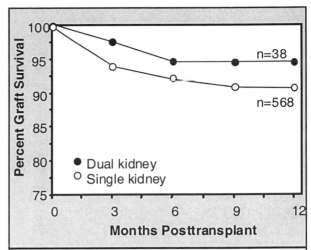

Figure 3. One-year kidney graft survival in patients undergoing dual kidney transplants from marginal donors (n=38) and in those who received a single kidney transplant from donors >50 years of age (n=568, 1997-2000).

blood trough values are low (11). More informative than the trough CsA level is the area under the concentration-time curve (AUC), calculated from the individuals' complete pharmacokinetic profile (12). Although AUC is an accurate index of patients' exposure to the drug, this approach is quite expensive and time consuming and it increases discomfort for the patients, making it rarely feasible in routine outpatient clinic monitoring. Therefore abbreviated CsA AUC profiles have been proposed. We have investigated whether a limited sampling strategy to be used in routine clinical practice reflects the actual AUC in kidney transplant patients given CsA Neoral (13). Stepwise multiple regression analysis of CsA blood levels recorded after CsA Neoral administration to 20 renal transplant patients showed the best results in AUC prediction with 3 sampling points (1.5, 8, 11 hours after Neoral dosing; r=0.992, with an associated error in AUC prediction ranging from -8.0-8.8 %). Because blood sampling at 8 and 11 hours is not practical in routine clinical practice, sample points from 0-3 hours after Neoral dosing, that is, up to the time of maximum mean blood CsA concentration plus 2 standard deviations, were considered. The best results were obtained with a 3-point strategy (0, 1, and 3 hours after Neoral dosing; error in prediction: -9.0 to 7.2%); which gave an excellent correlation between the measured and predicted AUC (r=0.989).

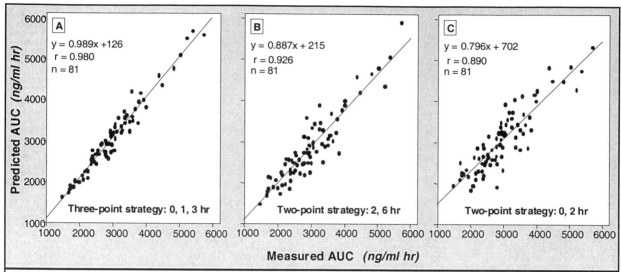

Figure 4. Correlation between measured and predicted CsA area under the time-concentration curve (AUC) using 3 different blood sampling strategies in kidney transplant recipients with stable graft function.

Others have favored a 2-time sample strategy after drug dosing (2 and 6 hours or 0 and 2 hours). Thus, we first analyzed our data according to the model equation for 2 and 6 hour time point sampling to predict AUC (14). Using this model equation, however, the AUC prediction was not as good and the correlation coefficient was numerically lower than the 3-point sampling at zero, one, and 3 hours after Neoral dosing (Fig. 4A,B) (15). The discrepancy may be the consequence of the analysis performed on different sets of data or related to differences in the analytical method employed for CsA blood determination. On the other hand, although it is substantially easier than the full kinetic analysis, the use of 2 and 6 hour time sampling remains time consuming and therefore impractical for routine clinical monitoring. We have also analyzed our CsA concentration data using the model equation of the zero and 2 hour sampling point (16). Although in this case the correlation coefficient between measured and predicted AUC was similar to that obtained with zero, one and, 3 hour points after Neoral dosing (r=0.89) (Fig. 4C), the associated error in AUC prediction was wider (from -31.5-50%) (15). When one compares 2 methods for evaluating AUC, the agreement between them is usually assessed by calculating the correlation coefficient (r). However, *r* does not measure the agreement, but rather the strength of a relationship between 2 variables. Actually, the correlation depends on the range of values considered for the analysis, and data with quite high correlation may be in poor agreement (17). Thus, given the large range of agreement, expressed by the wide error in prediction of the zero and 2 hour point strategy, this abbreviated estimation of AUC seems less reliable than the 3-point sampling approach. The possibility of estimating the CsA AUC within a reasonable percentage of error (less than 10%) by using only 3 very early blood samples after Neoral dosing has opened a new way for a more accurate monitoring of drug therapy and patient exposure to CsA with minimum effort. Monitoring of CsA dosing by abbreviated AUC is now part of our routine approach to kidney transplant patients. We believe that individualizing CsA dosing with this simplified pharmacokinetic strategy can help to maximize the antirejection effect of CsA and minimize the risk of side effects.

Monitoring of CsA immunosuppressive activity by measuring calcineurin activity

To improve monitoring of CsA immunosuppressive activity further, we reasoned that a pharmacodynamic approach could be better than a pharmacokinetic one. Thus, in recent years our efforts have been devoted to evaluating the activity of calcineurin (CN), the target enzyme of CsA, as a way to optimize CsA dosing (18). We have measured CN activity in whole blood in an attempt to overcome the high variability of results previously obtained with the peripheral blood mononuclear cells (PBMC) matrix (19). We also explored a possible in vitro relationship between CsA concentration and CN inhibition in whole blood. Finally we assessed whether CsA blood trough level correlates with whole blood CN activity in 9 kidney transplant recipients on maintenance immuno-suppression with CsA. In 14 healthy subjects, the coefficient of variation of CN activity measured in whole blood (25%) was significantly lower than that in PBMC (110%). After ex-vivo incubation of whole blood from healthy subjects with increasing concentrations of CsA (50-1000 ng/ml for 1 hr), a concentration-dependent inhibition of CN activity was found, comparable to that in PBMC. Moreover, in 9 kidney transplant recipients no relationship was found between CsA pharmacokinetic parameters and CN activity at time zero (Fig. 5). However, a highly significant correlation was found between the area under the CN activity-time curve (AUA_{0-12h}), which represents the extent of the CN daily inhibition, and CN activity at time zero and at 12 hours after dosing (r=0.75 p<0.01; r=0.95, p<0.01). Thus, measuring CN activity in whole blood samples is a reliable and reproducible method. In kidney transplant recipients CsA trough levels do not predict baseline CN activity. Moreover, a single CN activity monitoring at baseline or 12 hours after CsA dosing is a useful surrogate for the daily inhibition of enzyme by CsA and therefore could be a reliable index to optimize CsA dosing. However, further work is needed to simplify the proposed method before it can be used for a routine monitoring of transplant patients.

New Immunosuppressants for Routine Clinical Application: The Case of Mycophenolate Mofetil

The continuing search for more selective and specific agents has become a priority in the past decade. Some of these compounds have now entered routine clinical practice. We participated in the clinical development of mycophenolate mofetil (MMF) through the tricontinental double-blind, multicenter trial (20), which compared the efficacy and safety of MMF and azathioprine within a standard immunosuppressive regimen for patients receiving a first or second cadaver renal graft. Since that time MMF has become part of the conventional immmunosuppressive regimen in combination with CsA Neoral and steroids. Our center is currently involved in 2 lines of research in the field of MMF.

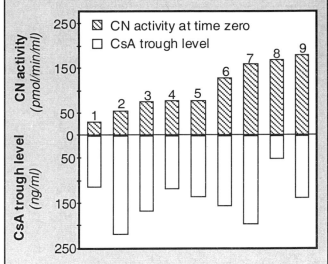

Figure 5. Lack of correlation between inhibition of whole blood calcineurin (CN) activity at baseline and CsA trough levels in 9 kidney transplant recipients.

Co-ordination of a prospective multicenter randomized trial of steroid sparing in kidney transplant recipients given MMF

Concern over potential side effects has led some investigators to suggest that discontinuation of one or more drugs from the triple-drug maintenance therapy may be advantageous in patients with stable graft function after the early posttransplant period (when the risk of rejection is highest). Since the use of steroids has been associated with multiple side effects, withdrawing patients from steroid therapy has been attempted. The introduction of potent immunosuppressants like MMF may facilitate discontinuation of corticosteroids. This led us to design a multicenter, randomized, Italian/European clinical trial with the general aim of evaluating the possibility of steroid discontinuation at 6 months after transplantation in kidney transplant recipients given MMF or azathioprine as a part of their immunosuppression therapy. It is called the Mycophenolate Steroid Sparing (MY.S.S Study,). The trial is coordinated by our Nephrology Unit at the Ospedali Riuniti di Bergamo and by the Laboratory of Biostatistics of the Clinical Research Center "Aldo e Cele Daccò" of the Mario Negri Institute. The study consists of 2 phases: the primary aim of phase 1 is to prove that the incidence of acute rejection episodes in cadaveric kidney allograft recipients given MMF in conjunction with Neoral and steroids is reduced compared with those on a triple immunosuppressive regimen with azathioprine, Neoral and steroid during the first 6 months; the primary aim of phase 2 is to compare the steroid sparing potential of an MMF-based regimen with that of an azathioprine-based therapy by evaluating the proportion of patients in each group who experience one or more acute rejection episodes during tapering and after dis-continuation of corticosteroids starting 6 months after transplantation. According to sample size estimation, 386 first cadaveric kidney transplant recipients are expected to be enrolled. Preparation of casebooks and a database, monitoring of the study and data analysis is centralized at the Clinical Research Center "Aldo e Cele Daccò". As shown in Figure 6, 9 Italian transplant centers and 2 European centers are currently participating to the study. Up to now 325 patients have been randomized.

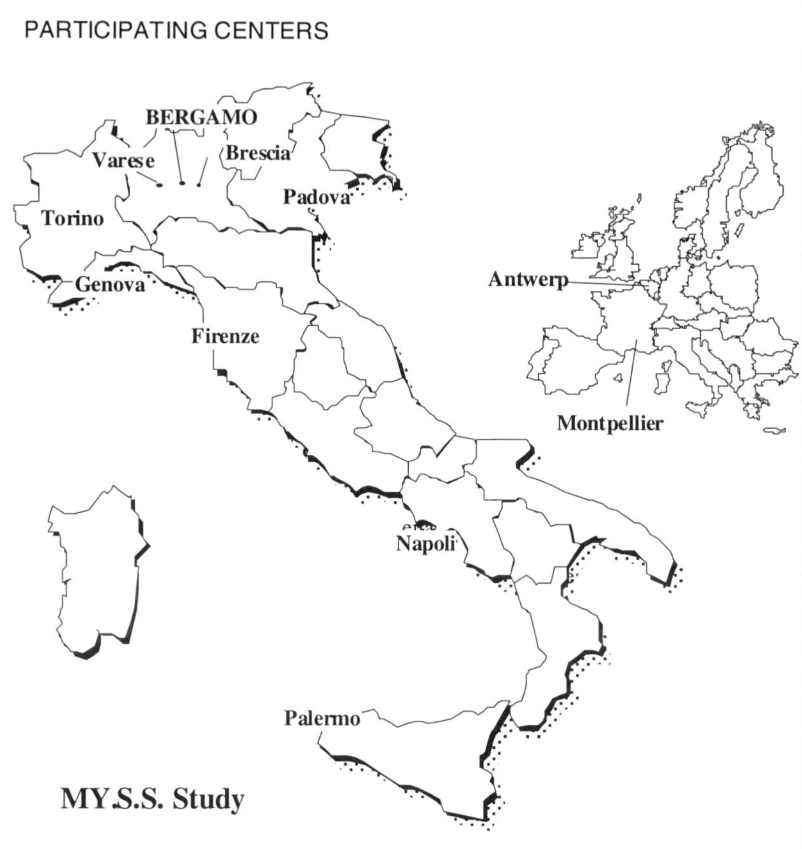

Figure 6. Transplant centers in Italy and other European countries participating in the Mycophenolate Steroid Sparing (MY.S.S.) study.

Pharmacokinetics to optimize mycophenolate mofetil dosing in kidney transplant recipients

As in all transplant centers worldwide, we are currently using MMF in a fixed daily dose of 2 g as a part of a combination regimen with Neoral and steroids. In individual patients, MMF dosing is reduced empirically only when gastrointestinal events, leukopenia/thrombocytopenia or other side effects occur. But this leaves us with the open question of whether the patient is still properly immunosuppressed to avoid graft rejection. Thus, we thought that therapeutic drug monitoring should be also applied to MMF as it is currently performed with CsA in order to optimize immuno-suppression and minimize potential toxic effects. Therefore we have set up an HPLC method for measuring plasma mycophenolic acid (MPA), the active molecule of the prodrug MMF, and examined the possibility of optimizing MMF dosing by drug pharmacokinetic monitoring in 46 stable kidney transplant recipients (21). MPA plasma concentration profiles were measured 6-9

months after transplantation and compared with routine laboratory analysis tests. Since MPA is extensively bound to serum albumin and only the free fraction is pharmacologically active, in a subgroup of 23 patients free plasma MPA was also determined. Despite a comparable MMF dose, a large interindividual variability both in MPA area under the curve (AUC) from 0-12 hours (range 10-99 µg/ml.h) and in trough levels (range 0.24-7.04 µg/ml) was found. As shown in Figure 7, patients with AUC >40 µg/ml.h showed better renal function than patients with lower AUC (creatinine clearance 85.7±23.2 vs. 64.5±17.5 ml/min), despite having no differences in CsA dose, CsA AUC and blood CsA trough level. The percentage of free plasma but not total MPA correlated with the risk of toxicity (anemia and leukopenia). These findings would suggest the need of routine therapeutic drug monitoring for MMF also to optimize drug dosing and to assess the risk/benefit associated with a target drug concentration in individual kidney transplant recipients.

The Problem of Chronic Allograft Nephropathy

The past 20 years have seen substantial refinements in our ability to control acute rejection through more effective immunosuppressive regimens, but these improvements have had little impact on the rate of decline of long-functioning grafts. The leading cause of the gradual deterioration of renal function in kidney transplant recipients is an ill-defined process termed "chronic allograft nephropathy", which accounts for the fact that the half-life of allografts has remained quite constant, although short-term results of organ survival have improved significantly. In this area of transplant medicine our interest has been focussed on the contribution of CsA nephrotoxicity and, more recently, on that of posttransplant artery stenosis to progressive graft function deterioration.

Nature and mediators of renal lesions in kidney transpant patients given CsA for more than one year

In the past we have worked aggressively to clarify the mechanisms and mediators of acute and chronic CsA nephrotoxicity using experimental animal models (22). This know-how has been translated into the clinics, first in heart transplant patients and subsequently in kidney transplant recipients. As a part of a clinical trial in kidney transplant recipients on triple immunosuppressive

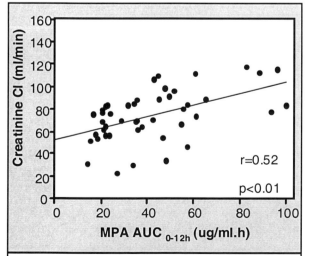

Figure 7. Relationship between plasma mycophenolic acid (MPA) AUC_{0-12h} and creatinine clearance values in kidney transplant recipients (n=46).

therapy (CsA, azathioprine, and steroid), which includes protocol renal biopsies, we enrolled 22 patients between 12-24 months after transplantation in a study in which they underwent renal hemodynamic evaluation by measuring glomerular filtration rate and renal plasma flow by plasma clearance of unlabeled iohexol and renal clearance of para-aminohippuric acid, respectively (23). In parallel, the CsA pharmacokinetic profile was also determined. A week later, a protocol biopsy of the kidney graft was performed. Light microscopy examination and localization of endothelin-1, RANTES, monocyte chemoattractant protein-1 (MCP-1) gene expression by in situ hybridization in the graft specimens were evaluated and related to the pattern of histologic lesions. Ten out of 22 kidney transplant recipients who underwent the protocol biopsy had CsA nephrotoxicity, 8 had chronic rejection, and 4 had no lesions at histological examination. The total daily exposure to CsA was higher in patients with CsA nephrotoxicity than in those with chronic rejection or no lesions at biopsy. Renal function was better preserved in the CsA toxicity group compared with the chronic rejection group, despite some degree of renal hypoperfusion. Tubular atrophy and stripped interstitial fibrosis were found in all patients with light microscopy evidence of CsA nephrotoxicity, whereas glomerular and arteriolar lesions were less frequent. Intense staining for endothelin-1, RANTES, and MCP-1 mRNAs selectively localized at tubular epithelial cells was found in biopsies taken from patients with CsA nephrotoxicity, but not in the chronic graft rejection group, whose tubuli had only minimal staining for RANTES mRNA on a few occasions (Fig. 8). Thus, long-term CsA administration to kidney allograft recipients leads to tubulointerstitial injury independently of its vascular effect. We proposed a possible contribution to the development of interstitial fibrosis of inflammatory and growth factors released by tubular cells in which CsA accumulates. Further research should clarify this potential mechanism of CsA-induced chronic nephrotoxicity and may disclose possible strategies for new medical treatments.

Posttransplant renal artery stenosis

Percutaneous transluminal angioplasty and stenting is our current approach to treat posttransplant renal artery stenosis. We have recently examined the impact of this procedure on renal function recovery and the value of Doppler ultrasound scanning to monitor these changes. In 8 consecutive renal transplant patients with renal graft

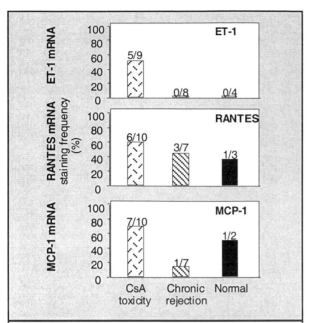

Figure 8. Frequency of positive tubular staining for endothelin-1 (ET-1), RANTES (regulated upon activation, normal T cell expressed and secreted), and monocyte chemoattractant protein-1 (MCP-1) mRNAs in kidney allograft biopsies from kidney transplant recipients with biopsy-proven CsA toxicity, chronic rejection or normal tissue pattern. Staining was considered positive when the score staining intensity was >1 in 2 or more tubuli. The numbers indicate positive staining/total biopsies analyzed.

artery stenosis, we evaluated blood pressure, body weight and anatomical, functional and Doppler ultrasound parameters before and one month after renal artery transluminal angioplasty and stenting (24). At both time points, glomerular filtration rate and renal plasma flow were measured by inulin and p-aminohippuric acid renal clearances and glomerular size-selective function was assessed by the fractional clearances of neutral dextran macromolecules. Correction of renal artery stenosis by normalizing renal vascular resistances fully restored kidney perfusion, decreased arterial blood pressure, relieved water and sodium retention, restored an almost laminar arterial blood flow and normalized vascular shear stress without appreciable effects on glomerular barrier size-selective function and proteinuria. Pre- and post-angioplasty renal resistance indices and peak systolic blood velocity estimated by Doppler ultrasounds were significantly correlated with the effective renal plasma flow and the blood velocity calculated at the site of stenosis. All patients were discharged without sequelae one or 2 days after angioplasty. We conclude from this study that percutaneous angioplasty and stenting is a safe and effective procedure to normalize the functional changes sustained by hemodynamically significant artery stenosis after renal transplantation. Moreover, we believe that Doppler ultrasound scanning is a useful, reliable, non-invasive tool to predict the severity of stenosis and to monitor the renal functional response to artery revascularization.

From Bench to Bedside

Thanks to the long-lasting cooperation with the Negri Bergamo Laboratories, we still have an active program in experimental animals to investigate the most challenging strategies for transplant tolerance and transplant gene therapy, beside addressing some issues related to the immunological barrier of xenotransplantation (25), as briefly summarized below.

Strategies for transplant tolerance

In the past our group has documented that intrathymic injection of donor cells in MHC incompatible rat recipients allowed the development of a state of donor-specific unresponsiveness to a subsequent kidney graft from the same donor (26). With this background, we recently studied the effect of pretransplant infusion of donor peripheral blood leukocytes on long-term outcome in kidney allograft in rats (27). A short course of CsA (which per se is unable to prolong graft survival), started the same day of donor Brown-Norway (BN) rat leukocyte infusion into Lewis rat recipients, prolonged the survival of a BN kidney transplant, but not of a third party graft. Some animals even developed tolerance. The possibility exists that upon systemic infusion, donor mononuclear cells and hematopoietic precursor cells migrate to the thymus and become capable of negatively selecting newly developing T cells. Eventually the peripheral T-cell components would be devoid of alloreactive cell population. The tolerance potential of such a regimen is a further step toward the ultimate goal of inducing donor-specific tolerance while leaving the response to third party antigens intact.

Intragraft gene transfer to prolong graft survival and induce donor-specific tolerance

We have recently achieved prolonged allograft survival in rats by adenovirus-mediated transduction of the cold-preserved kidney with sequences encoding CTLA4Ig, a recombinant fusion protein that blocks T-cell activation (28). Pending appropriate large animal testing, ex-vivo genetic manipulation of the organ before surgery may represent a major step forward in human transplant medicine.

Xenotransplantation

In 'in-vitro' studies we have found that human serum - as a source of xenoreactive natural antibodies and complement - markedly enhanced the adhesion of human leukocytes to porcine aortic endothelial cells in culture under dynamic flow conditions when compared with porcine serum and promoted transmigration through the porcine endothelium (29). The mechanisms involved in leukocyte adhesion imply a complex interplay of molecular signaling, including NF-kB, that alter gene expression in endothelial cells. Findings that xenogeneic serum promotes leukocyte-endothelium interaction possibly through NF-kB activation might be relevant for designing future therapeutic strategies aimed at prolonging xenograft survival.

SUMMARY

The kidney transplant program at the Ospedali Riuniti of Bergamo, Italy was established in 1989. Since its inception, 367 patients have been transplanted, including 357 kidney transplants from cadaveric donors and 10 from living-related donors. Overall 8-year patient and graft survival rates were 94% and 77%, respectively. By 1995 our unit co-ordinated the activity of the Department of Immunology and Clinics of Organ Transplantation, Ospedali Riuniti - Mario Negri Institute for Pharmacological Research, Bergamo.

The dual "marginal" kidney transplant program in the same recipient was launched in August 1997, as a part of an international cooperative network which established the "Double Kidney Transplant Group" (DKG). To date, 19 dual kidney transplants have been successfully performed in our center. Four combined heart-kidney transplants and 2 combined liver-kidney transplants have also been performed.

During the past 4 years several studies involving conventional antirejection drugs were carried out, particularly focussing our attention on cyclosporine (CsA) through pharmacokinetic and pharmacodynamic approaches: 1) a simplified method to evaluate daily exposure to CsA has been set up; 2) the monitoring of calcineurin activity in whole blood samples was evaluated as a way to optimize CsA dosing.

As for the new immunosuppressants, studies are ongoing with mycophenolate mofetil (MMF). We are co-ordinating a prospective multicenter randomized trial of steroid sparing in kidney transplant recipients given MMF or azathioprine as a part of their immuno-suppression therapy (MY.S.S. study). This involves 9 Italian transplant centers and 2 European centers. Up to now 325 patients have been randomized. Moreover we have set up an HPLC method for measuring plasma mycophenolic acid (MPA), and examined the possibility of optimizing MMF dosing by drug pharmacokinetic monitoring.

Further studies have been addressed to chronic allograft nephropathy. The nature and mediators of renal lesions in kidney transplant patients given CsA have been explored taking into account the gene expression of endothelin-1, RANTES and MCP-1 in graft specimens from patients who had evidence of CsA nephrotoxicity, chronic rejection, or no lesions at histological examination.

The impact of percutaneous transluminal angioplasty and stenting of posttransplant renal artery stenosis on renal function recovery was also recently examined. From this study we conclude that the procedure is safe and effective to normalize the functional changes sustained by hemodynamically significant artery stenosis. Moreover, Doppler ultrasound scanning is an useful, reliable, non-invasive tool to monitor the renal function response to artery revascularization.

Thanks to the long-lasting co-operation with the

Negri Bergamo Laboratories, we had in the past and still have an active program in experimental animals to investigate strategies for transplant tolerance and transplant gene therapy, besides addressing some issues related to the immunological barrier of xenotransplantation.

REFERENCES

1. London NJ, Farmery SM, Will EJ, Davison AM, Lodge JPA. Risk of neoplasia in renal transplant patients. Lancet 1995; 346: 403.

2. Dotti GP, Fiocchi R, Motta T, et al. High frequency of EBV-negative lymphoproliferative disorders developing in long term survivors after heart, kidney, and liver transplant. Transplantation 2000; (in press)

3. Gotti E, Remuzzi G. Posttransplant Kaposi's sarcoma. J Am Soc Nephrol 1997; 8: 130.

4. Naldi L, Belloni A, Lovati S, et al. Risk of nonmelanoma skin cancer in Italian organ transplant recipients. A registry-based study. Transplantation 2000; (in press)

5. Gotti E, Suter F, Baruzzo S, Perani V, Moioli F, Remuzzi G. Early ganciclovir therapy effectively controls viremia and avoids the need for cytomegalovirus (CMV) prophylaxis in renal transplant patients with cytomegalovirus antigenemia. Clin Transplant 1996; 10: 550.

6. Gridelli B, Remuzzi G. Strategies for making more organs available for transplantation. N Engl J Med 2000; 343: 404.

7. Remuzzi G, Ruggenenti P. Renal transplantation: single or dual for donors aging ≥60 years? Transplantation 2000; 69: 2000.

8. Remuzzi G, Perico N. Protecting single-kidney allograft from long-term functional deterioration. J Am Soc Nephrol 1998; 9: 1321.

9. Remuzzi G, Grinyo J, Ruggenenti P, et al. Early experience with dual kidney transplantation in adults using expanded donor criteria. J Am Soc Nephrol 1999; 10: 2591.

10. Perico N, Remuzzi G. Prevention of transplant rejection. Current treatment guidelines and future developments. Drugs 1997; 54: 533.

11. Kahan BD, Grevel J. Optimization of cyclosporine therapy in renal transplantation by a pharmacokinetic strategy. Transplantation 1988; 46: 631.

12. Grevel J, Welsh MS, Kahan BD. Cyclosporine monitoring in renal transplantation. Area under the curve is superior to trough level monitoring. Ther Drug Monit 1989; 11: 246.

13. Gaspari F, Anedda MF, Signorini O, Remuzzi G, Perico N. Prediction of cyclosporine area under the curve using a three-point sampling strategy after Neoral administration. J Am Soc Nephrol 1997; 8: 647.

14. Amante AJ, Kahan BD. Abbreviated AUC strategy for monitoring cyclosporine microemulsion therapy in the immediate posttransplant period. Transplant Proc 1996; 28: 2162.

15. Gaspari F, Perico N, Signorini O, Caruso R, Remuzzi G. Abbreviated kinetic profiles in area-under-the-curve monitoring of cyclosporine therapy. Kidney Int 1998; 54: 2146.

16. Keown P, Landsberg D, Halloran P, et al. A randomized, prospective multicenter pharmacoepidemiologic study of cyclosporine microemulsion in stable renal graft recipients. Report of the Canadian Neoral Transplantation Study Group. Transplantation 1996; 62: 1744.

17. Bland JM, Altman DG. Statistical methods for assessing agreement between two methods of clinical measurement. Lancet 1986; 1: 307.

18. Piccinini G, Gaspari F, Signorini O, Remuzzi G, Perico N. Recovery of blood mononuclear cell calcineurin activity segregates two populations of renal transplant patients with different sensitivities to cyclosporine inhibition. Transplantation 1996; 61: 1526.

19. Caruso R, Gaspari F, Perico N, Remuzzi G. In renal transplant recipients baseline calcineurin activity is not predicted by CsA trough levels. J Am Soc Nephrol 2000; 11: 682A.(Abstract)

20. Tricontinental Mycophenolate Mofetil Renal Transplantation Study Group. A blinded, randomized clinical trial of mycophenolate mofetil for the prevention of acute rejection in cadaveric renal transplantation. Transplantation 1996; 61: 1029.

21. Cattaneo D, Perico N, Gotti E, Remuzzi G, Gaspari F. Pharmacokinetic and trough concentrations help optimizing mycophenolate mofetil dosing in kidney transplant patients. J Am Soc Nephrol 2000; 11: 682A.(Abstract)

22. Remuzzi G, Perico N. Cyclosporine-induced renal dysfunction in experimental animals and humans. Kidney Int 1995; 48 (suppl 52): S70.

23. Benigni A, Bruzzi I, Mister M, et al. Nature and mediators of renal lesions in kidney transplant patients given cyclosporine for more than one year. Kidney Int 1999; 55: 674.

24. Mosconi L, Fasolini G, Bruno S, et al. Doppler ultrasounds (DU) reliably predict pre- and post-stenting renal hemodynamics in posttransplant artery stenosis. J Am Soc Nephrol 2000; 11: 723A.(Abstract)

25. Remuzzi G. Cellular basis of long-term organ transplant acceptance: pivotal role of intrathymic clonal deletion and thymic dependence of bone marrow microchimerism-associated tolerance. Am J Kidney Dis 1998; 31: 197.

26. Remuzzi G, Rossini M, Imberti O, Perico N. Kidney graft survival in rats without immunosuppressants after intrathymic glomerular transplantation. Lancet 1991; 337: 750.

27. Noris M, Azzollini N, Mister M, et al. Peripheral donor leukocytes prolong survival of rat renal allografts. Kidney Int 1999; 56: 1101.

28. Tomasoni S, Azzollini N, Casiraghi F, Capogrossi M, Remuzzi G, Benigni A. CTLA4Ig gene transfer prolongs survival and induces donor-specific tolerance in a rat renal allograft. J Am Soc Nephrol 2000; 11: 747.

29. Morigi M, Zoja C, Colleoni S, et al. Xenogeneic serum promotes leukocyte-endothelium interaction under flow through two temporally distinct pathways: role of complement and nuclear factor -kB. J Am Soc Nephrol 1999; 10: 2197.

ACKNOWLEDGEMENTS

We thank Professor Girolamo Sirchia and his collaborators for providing the data given in Figure 3. Most of the merit of these results goes to the nurses of the Department, specifically the ones working in the Pediatric Surgery Unit and the Unit of Nephrology and Dialysis, of the Ospedali Riuniti di Bergamo.

CHAPTER 16

One Thousand Renal Transplants at Belfast City Hospital: Post-Graft Neoplasia 1968-1999, Comparing Azathioprine Only with Cyclosporin-Based Regimes in a Single Centre

Mary G. McGeown [a], James F. Douglas [b], and Derek Middleton [c]

[a]Department of Medicine, The Queen's University of Belfast, [b]Department of Nephrology and [c]N Ireland Histocompatibility and Immunogenetics Laboratory, Belfast City Hospital, Belfast, NORTHERN IRELAND

From 1968-1998, 1,000 renal transplants were carried out on 868 patients at Belfast City Hospital. All patients prior to 1986 received azathioprine only (with low-dose steroids) as long-term immunosuppression (the A regime). From 1986 onward the C regime, based on cyclosporin (CSA), although often including some azathioprine as well as low-dose steroids and other drugs, began to appear. By 1989, it had become the dominant regime, prescribed for 87% of new recipients compared with 9% in 1986. Both A- and C-regime patients experienced the increased tumour incidence associated with long-term immunosuppression. The distinct nature of the regimes gave the opportunity to compare trends in neoplasia between them. Although the population studied was small, the quality of data (867 out of 868 patients were available for follow-up) was a compensatory factor.

PATIENTS AND METHODS

Clinical information was collected from case notes and follow-up charts; the renal unit computer, updating from 1985, material assembled manually since 1965 (MG McGeown); computer records of the Northern Ireland tissue typing laboratory; correspondence, in some cases, with colleagues in the United Kingdom and elsewhere; and copies of death certificates in 5 cases where hospital records were missing.

Information available included: full clinical details; underlying diagnoses; evidence of pretransplant neoplasia; the dates, numbers and durations of transplants; the type, duration and doses of immunosuppressive agents; and full blood group and tissue typing data for both donor and recipient. Dates and diagnoses of neoplasia, results of treatment and follow-up, with patient outcome, including causes of death up to 31 December 1999, were also included.

Of 102 tumours diagnosed, 96 (94%) were based on histopathology. One was based on radiological evidence of metastases combined with positive cytology. Four (3.9%) were based on clinical and radiological evidence of metastatic disease and one was accepted on the basis of the consultant's clinical report.

Causes of death were compiled from case notes, computerised records, correspondence and death certificates, as appropriate. Information was available for all deaths. These frequently occurred suddenly at home, without the exact cause being clear. Some of these deaths could have involved neoplasia or its complications. However, in all such cases, the certified cause of death has been accepted for the purpose of this study.

Immunosuppression Regimes

Three distinct maintenance groups emerged.

Azathioprine (A regime). This consisted of azathioprine plus low-dose steroids, without the addition of CSA at any time (apart from occasional brief use during terminal graft failure). Two patients who developed neoplasia and later changed to CSA for second transplants were classified as A regime because both tumours occurred during the currency of the first transplant, when only azathioprine was being used.

Cyclosporin (C Regime). For all C-regime patients, CSA had been used in significant doses as the basis of maintenance immunosuppression. Over 90% had taken it from the time of first graft function. Most, in accordance with the unit's policy of initial triple therapy, had also taken azathioprine. This was usually withdrawn within a few months of graft function, although some patients continued indefinitely on a combined regime. Others, having started out on the A regime, switched to CSA, mainly as rescue therapy, within 6 months of transplant or later, while a few, having been established on CSA, later transferred back to azathioporine, the chief indication being CSA toxicity. All these patients were classified as C regime. However, out of all those whose early treatment included CSA and who later developed tumours, only 2 had received a total azathioprine dose of more than 15,000 mgs. From 1997 onward, selected patients (in addition to receiving CSA) were also treated with tacrolimus or mycophenolate at varying times. There were 2 cases of early neoplasia in this group.

Between 1995-1996, almost all C-regime patients changed from CSA Sandimmune (suspension) to CSA Neoral (emulsion). Neoral is better absorbed than Sandimmune and more bioavailable. The incidence of neoplasia subsequent to the change was recorded.

A-C Conversion. Thirty-five patients converted from A to C regimes after spending significant periods on the former therapy (mean 10.5 years, range 2-15 years). The reasons for converting were:second and subsequent transplants (n= 20); steroid-reducing policies (n= 5); attempts to stabilise or rescue poorly functioning grafts (n= 5); and azathioprine complications such as leucopenia (n= 4). In one case, the reason for changing was unclear. For some purposes it was possible to assign these converting patients to both groups. However, their experience after changing therapy was also of interest. Therefore, the incidence of tumours occurring in such patients after the point of A-C conversion was compared with the incidence of tumours occurring in a general group of non-converting A-regime patients (215 in total) who had all already achieved a similar length of graft survival to the converters without any evidence of neoplasia. In effect, in order to equate the position of these controls to that of the converters, their start line for further tumour screening was moved to 10.5 years after transplantation.

Steroids and Other Immunosuppression

Low-dose maintenance steroids were used for both groups. In general, long-term doses were lower for C-regime patients and, in a significant minority, steroids were withdrawn completely. The standard treatment for acute rejection was a short course of high-dose steroids given orally or in pulses. This was the same for both A and C regimes. Resistant acute rejection in A-regime patients was treated mainly with further steroid courses. Actinomycin, increased doses of azathioprine, local irradiation and plasmapheresis were also used occasionally. Very few patients received ATG. C-regime patients were less prone to resistant rejection. None received plasmapheresis. ATG was widely used. A few more recent cases were also treated with mycophenolate, tacrolimus and genetically modified monoclonal antibodies in various combinations. Tacrolimus (first used in 1997) was implicated in 2 cases of early tumour (1 PTLD and 1 metastatic case).

Pretransplant immunosuppression was used occasionally for appropriate indications, such as vasculitis, lupus nephropathy, proliferative glomerulonephritis, etc. Among patients who developed neoplasia, one (A regime) had undergone prior (inadvertent) splenectomy and 2 (both A regime) had previously been treated with cyclophosphamide (for vasculitis and proliferative glomerulonephritis, respectively).

Comparison of Azathioprine and CSA Doses

Forty of 56 (72%) A-regime and 21 of 30 (70%) C-regime patients' notes provided full data on immunosuppressive doses from transplantation to tumour diagnosis. For these patients, total immunosuppressive dose up to the time of tumour diagnosis was calculated as mg/kg and mg/kg/day. To analyse the relationship of total dosage to the incidence of neoplasia, controls were allocated to each tumour case from among patients on the same form of therapy, matched as far as possible for age, sex and duration of therapy up to the time of tumour. These controls had not developed any form of neoplasia on immunosuppression during the period of study and did not do so later. The allocations were random, with no prior knowledge of the dose actually prescribed to each control. The dose ratios between tumour patients and their controls were measured.

RESULTS

Table 1 shows the overall posttransplant tumour data. C-regime patients were, on average, older at transplant than A-regime patients, with a wider age scatter, although ages at the time of tumour diagnosis were similar. The C regime also included patients with a wider range of diagnoses and ancillary diseases. These differences reflect changes in practice brought about by greater clinical experience and gradual expansion of dialysis and transplantation facilities over the period of this study. One patient who was transplanted at the Belfast City Hospital has been excluded from the figures. He left Belfast for Libya after the failure of his second, living related graft at 127 days and no further information could be obtained. Table 2 outlines the overall tumour incidence. The list includes 3 tumours - one carcinoid lesion, one phaeochromocytoma (both A regime) and one pituitary adenoma (C regime) - which were

Table 1. Basic tumour data.

	All	A regime	C regime
Patients	868	408	460
Era	1968-99	1968-86	1987-99
Tumours	103	62	41
Mean follow-up (years)	10.2	12.6	5.7
Range	1-31	2-31	1-13
Mean age at transplant (years)	43	38	48
Range	3-76	6-71	3-76
Mean age at tumour (years)	53	55	51
Range	5-77	32-74	5-77
Mortality (% tumours)	41 (40.2)	28 (44.4)	13 (33.3)
As % of all patients at risk	4.7	6.8	2.9
As % of tumours other than skin	81.2	78.8	61.9

Table 2. Detailed posttransplant tumour data.

	ALL			A regime		C regime	
	Number	% of patients	% of tumours	Number	(%)	Number	(%)
Patients	86			56		30	
Tumours	103	11.9		62	15.2	31	7.5
SCC	32	36.0	31.1	20	32.3	5	16.1
BCC	16	18.0	15.5	8	129.0	6	19.4
PTLD	11	12.4	10.7	4	6.5	7	22.6
GI	9	10.1	8.7	8	12.9	1	3.2
Breast	5	5.6	4.9	5	8.1	-	-
ENT	5	5.6	4.9	2	3.2	2	6.4
Lung	4	4.5	3.9	2	3.2	2	6.4
Ovary	3	3.4	2.9	2	3.2	1	3.2
Metastatic	3	3.4	2.9	-	-	4	12.9
Kidneys	3	3.4	2.9	2	3.2	1	3.2
Uterus	2		1.9	2	3.2	-	
Teratoma	2		1.9	1	1.6	-	
Leukaemia	1		1.0	1	1.6	-	
Myeloma	1		1.0	1	1.6	-	
Prostate	1		1.0	1	1.6	-	
Vulva	1		1.0	1	1.6	-	
Carcinoid	1		1.0	1	1.6	-	
Phaeochromocytoma	1		1.0	1	1.6	-	
Haemangioblastoma	1		1.0	-	1.6	1	3.2
Pituitary Adenoma	1		1.0	-		1	3.2

SCC: squamous cell carcinoma of skin (excluding recurrences), BCC: basal cell carcinoma, PTLD: posttransplant lymphoproliferative disease, GI: gastrointestinal, ENT: ear, nose or throat cancer

Table 3. *Tumours in multiple graft recipients.*

	All	A regime	C regime
Patients	11	5	6
Transplants	15	8	7
Mean age at transplant	40	43	38
Ca: SCC	8	3	5
BCC	3	2	1
Other	4	3	1
Total	15	8	7
Time to tumour: days	5,029	4,620	5,490
(years)	(13.8)	(12.6)	(15.0)
Time at risk: days	6,788	33,040	41,631
(years)	(18.6)	(90.5)	(114.1)
Deaths	3	2	1

Table 5. *Late conversion, A to C regime: reasons.*

	All	Tumours
Second transplant	16	1
Third transplant	3	2
Fourth transplant	1	1
Azathioprine problems	4	1
Steroid sparing	5	2
Graft nephropathy	5	2
Unclear	1	

histologically benign, but dangerous because of their site or potential for local spread. One fatal "tumour" was eventually diagnosed as a cerebellar haemangioblastoma in a patient with pre-existing renal carcinoma and evidence of Von Hippel -Lindau disease. She had received a single azathioprine dose prior to removal of the graft for uncontrollable bleeding during the transplant operation. Table 3 shows the incidence of tumours in multiple graft recipients. There was no significant difference between A and C regime cases. Tables 4 and 5 show the tumour incidence among patients who made a late conversion from A to C regimes with their reasons for changing. When compared with the bulk of patients who did not change, there was no significant difference in the survival of these patients or of their grafts. However, late change in immunosuppression did lead to a significant increase in subsequent incidence and recurrence of squamous carcinoma, chiefly of the skin. Table 6 shows the outcome for patients with neoplasia existing before transplant. Three of this group developed post-graft neoplasia, 2 clearly being recurrences and one a new malignancy. Table 7 shows the distribution and severity of carcinoma of the skin, recurrences being here regarded

as evidence of tumour aggression rather than as new lesions. Two patients (both on the A regime) died of skin carcinoma. One developed the lesion after 25 years on therapy and the other after emigrating to Australia. Late converters from the A to the C regime produced particularly aggressive lesions with no skin tumour death to date, although one patient developed ultimately fatal squamous carcinoma of the oral cavity

Table 6. *Pretransplant neoplasias.*

	All	A regime	C regime
Number	9	5	4
Age	50.8	52.0	49.3
Tumours:			
GU	4	1	3
Breast	3	2	1
Teratoma	1	1	-
AML	1	-	1
Posttransplant neoplasia:			
Recurrence	2	2	-
Other	1	-	1
Time to tumour (years)	5.1	5.9	3.5
Time at risk (years)	4.8	6.8	7.3
Deaths	2	2	-

AML: acute myelocytic leukaemia

Table 4. *Effect on neoplasia of conversion (A to C regime) after long-term A regime therapy.*

	Number	Mean time on A regime (yrs)	Neoplasia post conversion (%)	N (3 yrs)	N (5 yrs)	Total	SCC	Other
Converted	35	10.5	9 (26%)	8	9	14 (40%)	12*	2
Non-converted	215	10.5	26 (12%)	16	20	30 (14%)	14	16

* including 5 recurrences. Differences significant (p<0.001) for patient and tumour numbers

Table 7. Numbers and recurrence rates of squamous skin cancer.

	All	A regime	C regime	A-C Converters
Number	32	20	5	7
Recurrence:				
None	24 (75%)	15 (75%)	5 (100%)	3 (43%)
1	4	2	-	2
2	1	1	-	1
3 or more	3	2	-	2

Table 8. Squamous and squamous epithelial tumours after transplantation.

	All	A regime	C regime
Numbers	36	23	13
Mean age at tumour	55	57	55
Mean time after graft (years)	12.3	12.6	2.6

after conversion. Table 8 shows the mean time from transplant to squamous epithelial tumour. Table 9 compares the 5-year incidence of post-graft neoplasia for A and C regimes. It was significantly higher in C-regime patients – 34 (12.7%) of 268 patients at risk for 5 years compared with 15 of 335 (4.5%) A-regime patients (p< 0.001; see also Fig. 1 and Table 10). For the period 0-5 years after transplantation, the approximate tumour incidence rate for the C regime was 18.8 per 1,000 patient years (95% CI: 13.0, 26.3), compared with 7.7 (95% CI: 4.3, 12.6) for the A regime, a relative incidence for the C regime of 2.45 (95% CI: 13.0, 26.3). Figure 2 shows the cumulative incidence of tumours up to the end of 1999. The linear increase in A-regime neoplasia up to 30 years after transplantation reflects the long-term survival figures for patients on the Belfast azathioprine and low-dose steroid regime, which have already been reported (2). Figure 3 compares the cumulative incidence of neoplasia for Neoral (CSA emulsion), Sandimmune (the original CSA suspension) and azathioprine. Neoral was associated with more early tumours than its less well-absorbed predecessor was. The significance of this finding is unclear, since there was considerable variation in overall immunosuppressive histories. Table 11 shows the total doses of azathioprine or CSA (as mg/kg and mg/kg/day) prescribed for patients who developed neoplasia after transplantation up to the time when malignancy was diagnosed and compares them to the doses prescribed for tumour-free controls. No differences were seen in the A regime, but C-regime tumour patients had taken significantly greater doses of CSA than their controls [5,764 vs. 3,887 mg/kg (p= 0.026) and 4.47 vs. 3.42 mg/kg/day (p=0.014)].

Table 9. Cumulative incidence of all posttransplant tumours within 5 years of starting therapy.

	All therapies		A regime		C regime	
	Total	As % at risk	Total	As % at risk	Total	As % at risk
Numbers	603		335		268	
Cumulative tumours to 5 years	49		15	4.5*	34	12.7*
SCC	12	2	2	0.6	10	3.7
BCC	10	1.7	3	0.9	7	2.6
PTLD	10	1.7	4	1.2	6	2.2
GI	3	0.5	2	0.6	1	0.4
Other	14	2.3	4	1.2	10	3.7
Mortality:		3.6		3.0		4.5
(a) number	22		10		12	
(b) as % tumours	45%		67%		35%	

*p<0.001

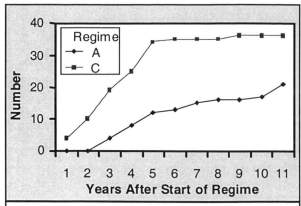

Figure 1. Early posttransplant neoplasms - cumulative incidence on A and C regimes.

Table 10. Numbers at risk of neoplasia posttransplant – A and C regimes.

| | | At risk for | |
	Number*	5 years	≥10 years
A Regime	448	335 (75%)	242 (54%)
C Regime	455	268 (61%)	63 (13%)

* Converters from A to C regime (N=35) included as at risk in each group from date of starting the relevant regime (see Fig. 1).

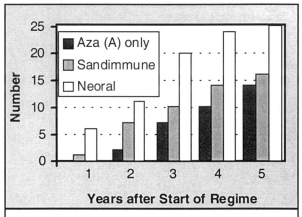

Figure 3. Posttransplant neoplasms: Neoral and Sandimmune compared with Azathioprine.

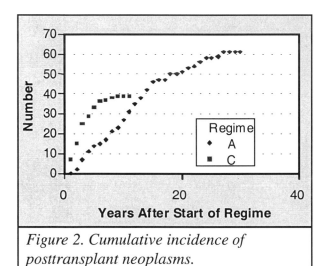

Figure 2. Cumulative incidence of posttransplant neoplasms.

DISCUSSION

This study of posttransplant neoplasia in Northern Ireland deals with much smaller numbers than have been reported by the Cincinnati Tumour Registry and the United Network for Organ Sharing (UNOS), which together hold records for more than 16,000 kidney transplants (2). But it is of interest because of its relatively complete data and the opportunity it provides to compare the effects of different immunosuppressive regimes on posttransplant neoplasia within a single centre. It is important to note that all recipients were on the A regime before 1987. After that date, C-regime

cases steadily increased until, by 1989, the great majority of new patients were receiving CSA. As a result, few C-regime patients (13%) had data extending beyond 10 years compared with A-regime patients, of whom 54% were available for study beyond the 10-year point and who also provided significant numbers (13.5% of the total) for analysis at 20 years or more. Thus, while the

Table 11. Total Doses : Tumour cases (A and C regimes) compared with controls.

| | A regime | | C regime | | Paired |
	Tumours	Controls	Tumours	Controls	T test
Numbers	40	40	21	21	
Dose (mg/kg)	6,655	6,936	5,764	3,887	p=0.026
Tumour/control	0.97		1.33		
Dose (mg/kg/day)	1.82	2.05	4.47	3.42	p=0.014
Tumour/control	0.89		1.31		

numbers allow satisfactory comparisons to be made between A and C regimes for up to 10 years, the later trends overwhelmingly reflect the experience of A-regime recipients only.

The overall tumour incidence (11.8%) is comparable to that in other studies (3,4), but the mean time to tumour (9 years) for all cases significantly exceeds the 5 years reported elsewhere (2). A possible explanation is the contribution to the total made by late tumours in A-regime patients. These continued to accumulate steadily for up to 30 years after transplantation, in keeping with the long-term survival figures reported for this group (1). In particular (and in agreement with other studies), skin and squamous epithelial cancers rose linearly. This explains the high mean time to squamous tumour diagnosis (151 months) and BCC (106 months) noted for A-regime patients, compared with the average of 69 months for epithelial cell tumours quoted elsewhere (3,4). When squamous carcinoma is excluded, the overall tumour rate in A-regime patients surviving 10 years or more after transplantation declines to 6.9% (see Table 9). In spite of evidence that the cumulative incidence of cancer continues to grow in the late posttransplant period (3), the A-regime group had a comparatively low incidence of renal (0.5%), uterine (0.7%) and vulval (0.2%) carcinoma. Overall PTLD incidence was also relatively low (1% of patients at risk and 6.3% of recorded tumours). ATG/ALG was rarely used and the mean dose of azathioprine in tumour cases and controls was less than 2 mg/kg/day. Although the risk of neoplasia persists, fairly good long-term graft survival on this regime has been achieved. Total azathioprine doses have been modest with little or no supplementary immunosuppression other than low-dose steroids and there appears to be some hope of long-term tumour containment.

For the C regime, the situation is more disturbing. The cumulative tumor incidence within 5 years of starting CSA (see Tables 9,11, Fig. 1) is significantly greater than for the A regime (p<0.001), particularly when expressed as a percentage of those at risk for 5 years (12.7% vs. 4.5%) and as a relative incidence rate per 1000 patient years (2.4). There is a higher representation of PTLD in the C than in the A regime (1.5% of patients at risk and 17.9% of recorded tumours), with an earlier onset. At least 3 such cases involved young patients who had been EBV-negative before transplant. The shorter mean time to tumour for C-regime patients (3.4 years) than for those on the A regime (12.4 years) is

misleading to some extent. Since only 13% of the C-regime patients have been at risk for more than 10 years, their later tumour experience has yet to contribute to this mean time. In the case of long surviving A-regime patients, 54% have been at risk for more than 10 years, and over 13% for more than 20 years with a continuing accumulation of late neoplasia. For the same reason, the apparent slowing of the cumulative neoplasia rate for the C-regime patients after 10 years (Figs. 1 and 2) is not significant. In fact, the true concern must be that, with longer follow-up, the increased relative incidence of the first 5 years, shown by the steeper slope of early tumour accumulation in Figures 1 and 2, will persist into later periods.

Dosage data (available for over 70% of cases) reveal significantly higher CSA doses for C-regime tumour cases than for randomly matched C-regime controls who remained tumour free. No such difference is seen between A-regime tumour cases and their similarly selected controls. Those who developed neoplasia on the C regime had received a mean total CSA dose of 4.47 mg/kg/day, while their controls had taken a mean of 3.42 mg/kg/day without increased graft loss. This suggests that the C regime, although helping early graft survival by reducing acute rejection episodes and steroid requirements, has led to greater maintenance doses of CSA than are necessary for good graft survival, increasing the risk of neoplasia without any compensatory clinical gain. There seems to be a clear indication for a more cautious approach to the challenge of long-term immunosuppression.

The use of CSA emulsion (Neoral), whenever introduced, is seen to be followed by an increase in early tumours (24 within 3 years compared with 10 and 3, respectively, at a similar point for patients on Sandimmune and the A regime). These findings refer to the time of starting the drug rather than to the time of transplant, but suggest that Neoral's improved bioavailability may also increase its neoplastic potential.

There appears to have been a particular risk associated with late conversion from the A to the C regime (this was undertaken by 35 long-surviving patients for various reasons). Within 5 years of switching, 9 patients (25.7%) had developed tumours, 8 being squamous carcinoma (including one fatal case of oral neoplasia). There were 5 recurrences of tumour (4 aggressive). This contrasts with a 12% incidence of neoplasia among the 215 comparable long-standing

A-regime patients who did not convert to the C regime. It should be noted that such conversions obtained no obvious benefit for the patients concerned in terms of graft survival, etc, to compensate for the change. Most (93%) of the tumours related to conversion were of skin or squamous epithelium, compared with only 50% of tumours in non-converted cases. Although this finding appears initially surprising, it probably could have been predicted. Metabolites of azathioprine tend to sensitise skin to the effects of ultra-violet light (5), contributing to the late increase of squamous carcinoma on this regime. CSA has been shown to promote tumour growth when given alone, both in animal models (mainly by excess production of TGF beta) and in vitro, where its administration results in invasiveness of non-transformed cells in association with striking morphological changes (6). Both of these changes could be prevented by giving antibodies to TGF beta. Thus, in the converted cases in this study, CSA appears to have added co-carcinogenic support to a known carcinogen.

This survey is likely to influence practice in the Belfast Unit. It points to the importance of dose reduction in well-functioning grafts. C-regime controls on lower doses retained adequate graft function and remained tumour-free. Thus, it seems that doses of 3.5 mg/kg/day or less may cause significantly fewer tumours than higher doses. The reduction of CSA-induced graft nephrotoxicity may be an added bonus of such an approach. The study also highlights the dangers of converting to CSA in stable, longstanding A-regime patients. When this becomes necessary for any reason, the importance of reduced dosing should be recognised. There is some evidence that the long-term use of azathioprine, although associated with a cumulative risk of skin carcinoma, may not otherwise lead to an intolerable tumour burden. However, there is a need for better tumour screening. Regular ultrasound scanning of graft and native kidneys, yearly gynaecological assessment and early investigation of hepato-biliary or ENT disorders are obviously important.

The risk of EBV infection, especially in younger graft recipients, should be taken more seriously. No EBV-positive donors should be used for EBV-negative recipients and all measures, including immunisation if it becomes available, should be taken to render patients EBV-positive before transplantation. Fortunately, there is some evidence that early diagnosis of PTLD, with appropriate reduction in CSA (or other calcineurin inhibitor) doses, is associated with improving results for these lesions (7,8). Similar arguments may well apply to the relationship between posttransplant Kaposi's sarcoma and its association with human herpes virus (9).

The dominance of skin and squamous epithelial carcinoma in post-graft neoplasia is demonstrated for all types of patients. Obsessive dermatological review and the avoidance of all dangerous co-carcinogenic influences (particularly ultra-violet light) are minimum precautions. The value in immune surveillance of associated CD4 lymphopenia seems likely to increase (10). It remains to be seen whether azathioprine's bad reputation in this regard can be bettered by newer agents such as mycophenolate or rapamicin.

There already exists impressive evidence that posttransplant neoplasia is related to total immunosuppressive dose (11). The present study also relates neoplasia to measurable differences in total CSA doses for patients within a single centre who have been otherwise selected and treated in a similar manner. It confirms that low-dose strategies are compatible with good long-term survival and reduced tumour risk. Even before transplant, renal failure predisposes to neoplasia (12). Since immunosuppression greatly increases that risk, the need for minimally carcinogenic anti-rejection policies is obvious. Azathioprine has been implicated in much post-graft neoplasia (11). However, its early record is less sinister than that of CSA and it may also prove less harmful in the long run. The ultimate goal of transplantation - preservation of the graft without danger to the recipient - has yet to be achieved. Much transplant literature emphasises ways of improving graft survival. However, the long-term danger of neoplasia remains real and may even be increasing with current therapies. The welfare of our patients demands equally rigorous attention to the detection, diagnosis and early treatment of these life-threatening lesions.

SUMMARY

From 1968-1999, 868 recipients of 1,000 renal transplants were followed up for neoplasia. Altogether, 102 tumours were diagnosed in 94 patients (11.8% incidence). Eighty-seven occurred among 750 single and 15 occurred among 118 multiple graft recipients. Three of 11 patients with pre-existing tumour developed posttransplant neoplasia, either new or recurrent. The most frequently seen posttransplant neoplasms were squamous carcinoma of skin, basal cell carcinoma (BCC), posttransplant lymphoproliferative disease (PTLD) and gastro-intestinal (GI) cancer. Forty-one tumour-related deaths occurred (44% mortality). Patients on CSA (C) regimes had a greater cumulative incidence of tumour after transplantation than those on azathioprine and low-dose prednisolone alone (A regime) had – 12.7% (34 of 268) vs. 4.5% (15 of 335) of those at risk up to 5 years (relative increased rate of incidence 2.4) with more early cases of PTLD. C-regime patients who developed neoplasia had been prescribed significantly higher CSA doses than tumour-free controls (4.5 vs. 3.4 mg/kg/day; p=0.014). Patients who made a late conversion from the A to the C regime subsequently developed more neoplasms than non-converted controls (25.7% vs. 12%), mainly due to early and often aggressive squamous carcinoma. Transplant survival figures were similar for both A- and C-regime groups. These findings suggest that current CSA doses are higher than are necessary for optimal graft survival and thus increase the risk of early neoplasia without any compensatory advantage. A dose reduction of CSA to less than 3.5 mg/kg/day in long-surviving, stable graft recipients should reduce tumour risk without imperilling function. Late conversion from the A to the C regime should be avoided where possible and CSA doses in this situation kept to a minimum.

REFERENCES

1. McGeown MG and Craig WJC. Results of renal transplantation five to twenty-six years after surgery, using azathioprine and low dose prednisolone as sole immunosuppression. In: Clinical Transplants 1996, JM Cecka and PI Terasaki, Eds. UCLA Tissue Typing Lab. Los Angeles 1997:265.

2. Kauffmann HM. Recent data on immunosuppression regimes. The Israel Penn Symposium on Malignancies in Transplantation, Eighteenth International Congress of the Transplantation Society, Rome, August 2000. Book of Abstracts, 358: 102.

3. Danpanich E, Kasiske BL. Risk factors for cancer in renal transplant recipients. Transplantation 1999; 68:1859.

4. Penn I. The changing patterns of posttransplant malignancies. Transplant Proc 1991; 232:1101.

5. Stewart T, Tsai SC, Grayson H, et al. Incidence of denovo breast cancer in women chemically immunosuppressed after organ transplantation. Lancet 1995; 346:796.

6. Hojo M, Morimoto T, Maluccio M, et al. Cyclosporin induces cancer progression by a cell-autonomous mechanism. Nature 1999; 397:530.

7. Penn I. Cancers complicating organ transplantation. N Engl J Med 1990; 323:1767.

8. Opelz G, Henderson R. Incidence of non-Hodgkins lymphoma in kidney and heart transplant recipients. Lancet 1993; 342:1514.

9. Penn I. Sarcomas in organ transplant recipients. Transplantation 1995; 60:1485.

10. Ducloix D, Carron P-L, Rebibou J-M, et al. CD4 lymphocytopenia as a risk factor for skin cancers in renal transplant recipients. Transplantation 1998; 65:1270.

11. Penn I. Cancers in Cyclosporin-treated V Azathioprine-treated patients. Transplant Proc 1996; 28:876.

12. Maisonneuve P, Agodoa L, Gellert R, et al. Cancer in patients on dialysis for end-stage renal disease: an international study. Lancet 1999; 354:93.

ACKNOWLEDGEMENTS

Mr. WJC Craig, Department of Nephrology, Belfast City Hospital, for essential help in retrieving and analysing material from the department's computer files.

Dr. GW Cran, Department of Epidemiology, The Queen's University of Belfast, for statistical advice.

Mrs. A Cunningham, Medical Records Department, Belfast City Hospital, for help in retrieving records.

Dr. D Fogarty, Consultant Nephrologist, Antrim Area Hospital, for advice on data analysis.

Dr. CM Hill, Department of Histopathology, Royal Victoria Hospital, Belfast, for confirmation of, and advice on, tumour diagnosis.

Dr. JC McMillan, Consultant Dermatologist, Belfast City Hospital, for advice on skin cancer, as well as for successfully undertaking the treatment of many cases.

Dr. PT McNamee, Consultant Nephrologist, Belfast City Hospital, for help in retrieval and analysis of data.

Dr. MG O'Connor, Consultant Paediatric Nephrologist, Royal Belfast Hospital for Sick Children, for help with data on paediatric cases.

Mrs. L Trouton, Research Secretary, Department of Nephrology, Belfast City Hospital, for essential help in collecting and interpreting patient records.

CHAPTER 17

Results of Renal Transplantation of the Hashemi Nejad Kidney Hospital - Tehran

Ahad J. Ghods, Shahrzad Ossareh, and Shekoufeh Savaj

Transplantation Unit, Hashemi Nejad Kidney Hospital
Iran University of Medical Sciences, Tehran, IRAN

The first chronic hemodialysis unit was established and the first renal transplantation was performed in Iran in 1967. Between 1967-1988 the number of patients on dialysis steadily increased but the renal transplantation program of the country severely lagged in growth in comparison with hemodialysis. In 1988, a controlled living-unrelated donor (LURD) renal transplantation program was adopted. As a result, more than 9,500 renal transplants were performed through the end of 1999 and Iran's renal transplant waiting list was eliminated.

In this chapter we review the history of renal transplantation in Iran from 1967-1999, describe the characteristics of our LURD renal transplantation program and report the results of 1,350 consecutive renal transplants from living related donors (LRD) and LURDs that have been carried out in our center. Finally, we discuss the necessity for and the ethical issues involved with our LURD renal transplantation program.

History of Renal Transplantation in Iran (1967-1999)

The first renal transplant in Iran was carried out in 1967 (1). The growth of the renal transplant program was severely delayed compared with the growth of hemodialysis until 1988 (2). Only about 100 renal transplants were performed between 1967-1985 and more than 400 patients traveled abroad using government funds to receive a renal transplant. The majority of these transplants were performed in the United Kingdom from LRDs (3).

In 1985 the high expense of renal transplantation abroad prompted our health authorities to foster renal transplantation in Iran. Two renal transplant teams were organized between 1985-1987 and 274 LRD renal transplants were performed.

Because a large number of dialysis patients who had no potential LRD needed renal transplantation and no cadaveric organ donation program had been established nor seemed likely to become a reality in the near future, a controlled renal LURD transplantation program was adopted in 1988 (4). As a result, the number of renal transplant teams gradually increased from 2 to 26 (14 in Tehran and 12 in the provinces) by the end of 1999 and 9,535 renal transplants (2,295 LRD, 7,182 LURD and 58 cadaveric) were performed. In 1999, the renal transplant waiting list of the country was eliminated. Figure 1 shows the number of renal transplants performed

KIDNEY — IRAN

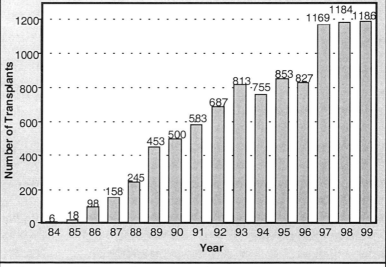

Figure 1. The number of renal transplants performed in Iran from 1984-1999.

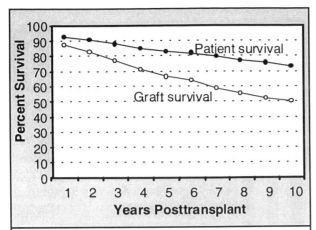

Figure 5. Overall patient and graft survival rates of renal transplant recipients in Hashemi Nejad Hospital, Tehran; 1986-1999.

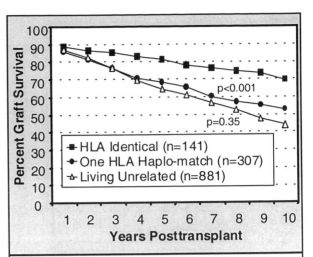

Figure 7. Graft survival rates in HLA identical, one HLA haplotype-match and living- unrelated renal transplants in Hashemi Nejad Hospital, Tehran; 1986-1999.

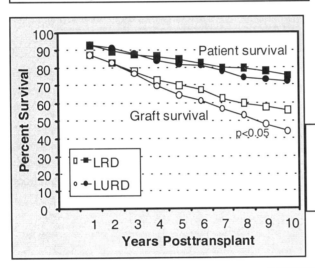

Figure 6. Patient and graft survival rates in living-related (LRD) and living-unrelated (LURD) renal transplantation in Hashemi Nejad Hospital, Tehran; 1986-1999.

and LURD transplants (p=0.35).

Two hundred twenty-seven patients died during this period. The most common cause of patient death was infection 52%, followed by cardiovascular events 29.5% (Fig. 8).

Twenty-six malignancies were diagnosed in our patients with an overall incidence of 1.9%. Eighteen cases occurred in males (M) and 8 in females (F) with an M to F ratio of 9: 4. The most common malignancy was lymphoma (7M, 1F) followed by Kaposi's sarcoma (5M, 1F), skin cancer (3 M, including 2 squamous cell carcinomas and one basal cell carcinoma), pancreatic cancer (2F, 1M), lung cancer (2M), liposarcoma (1F), adrenal cancer (1F), thyroid cancer (1F), and meningioma (1F).

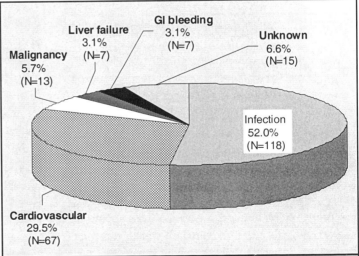

Figure 8. Causes of patient death in renal transplant recipients in Hashemi Nejad Hospital, Tehran; 1986-1999.

DISCUSSION

The short- and long-term results of renal transplants from our unit are comparable to the results of several other renal transplant centers (5-6). As we have previously reported, the graft survival rates of our LURD transplants are also similar to the results of our parental and one HLA-haplotype matched LRD transplants (7). The United Network for Organ Sharing (UNOS) Transplant Registry and some individual transplant centers have reported higher results with LURD transplants (8-11). We believe that the following factors have decreased our renal transplant patient and graft survival rates:

1. Due to a limited health care budget and lack of administrative expertise in our health authorities, all renal transplant units (including our unit) are insufficiently equipped. Some patient deaths and graft losses could have been prevented resulting in better patient and graft survival rates if our transplant unit was not deficient with respect to laboratory facilities, scientific consulting staff and pharmaceuticals, including necessary antibiotics.

2. Many dialysis patients from small towns and rural areas are referred to our center for renal transplantation. After transplantation these patients have to return home where optimal long-term posttransplant care is difficult to achieve. With a high prevalence of infection and a lack of skilled physicians in their hometowns, the patient deaths and graft losses have understandably been higher in this population of our transplant recipients.

3. Posttransplant complications and delayed graft function were more common in the early years of our transplant program. The frequency of posttransplant complications and early graft losses has gradually decreased (there is a center effect) as the experience of our transplant teams has improved (12,13).

As we have previously reported, the most common neoplasia in our renal transplant recipients is lymphoma. This finding is also different from the experience of other transplant units in the region (14).

The Necessity of and Ethical Issues Involved in Our LURD Renal Transplantation Program

Iran is an Islamic country with a long history and an ancient culture. According to Iranians' religion and culture, the human body should be venerated and declaration of death does not lessen its sanctity. On the other hand, cadaveric organ donation for saving a human life cannot be regarded as an act of disrespect in Islam because Muslims have been asked to be compassionate to every human being. In the last 10 years several decrees from top Islamic leaders of the country allowing cadaveric organ donation have been obtained and recently legislation for acceptance of brain death and cadaveric organ transplantation has passed our parliament (in April 2000). However, due to strong cultural barriers, we expect that cadaveric renal transplantation will begin in Iran on a very limited scale in the coming years. Thus, only a small proportion of ESRD patients will benefit from cadaver organ transplantation in the next few years.

Developing countries often must make adjustments when new technologies are introduced from Western or technologically advanced countries in order to integrate the changes into the existing culture and socioeconomic conditions. For example, the use of antibiotics and vaccination against infectious diseases has decreased children's mortality in Western countries while appropriate family planning has prevented significant population growth. In contrast, in some Asian countries with old traditions of having more children and more boys and where the importance of family planning was not well understood, the introduction of vaccination and antibiotics has resulted in severe population growth and its related socioeconomic problems. In China strict enforcement of family planning regulation and a one child family policy was adopted in 1979 to stop the population explosion (15). This one child family policy, which might be condemned by Western ethical standards, especially due to the uglier aspects of female infanticide or sex-selective abortions, had to be adopted in China for its very important role in preventing severe population growth.

Western dialysis and organ transplantation technologies have also reached developing countries. Iran is an oil producing country, yet has a limited health care budget and a high prevalence of infectious diseases and malnutrition. It also has a rich cultural and religious heritage. Starting an organ transplantation program according to Western models has not been feasible or justifiable. Hemodialysis is a costly life-saving modality, which has been increasingly used without any patient selection criteria. This has placed a great burden on our limited financial resources. To reduce the demand for dialysis and to serve the large number of patients needing renal transplants, we adopted a controlled LURD renal transplantation program. Cadaver donors were not available and many patients had no suitable relatives who were willing to donate.

Unfortunately much of the world's experience with LURD renal transplantation is from centers that have approached it with little regard for ethical standards. Prior to 1995, several thousand uncontrolled commercial renal transplants were performed in India each year. According to Professor Chugh (16), almost all of these were done in private backstreet clinics with incomplete donor and recipient evaluation and resulted in a high incidence of surgical complications and transmission of HIV and hepatitis infections. The kidneys were sold by middlemen to wealthy patients who came not only from India but also from overseas.

In China, kidneys from executed prisoners have been used on a large scale for renal transplantation of patients from China and foreign countries. Organ procurements have been done under uncertain conditions often without obtaining appropriate consent from the prisoner or his family (17).

In response to the commercial transplants, transplants from executed prisoners and sporadic news media reports of an organ "Mafia", the Transplantation Society and the World Health Organization have condemned paid LURD transplantation. The LURD renal transplantation program in Iran involves paid organ donation, but the transplant teams and the Iranian Society of Organ Transplantation strictly enforce the ethical aspects. The program is very different from LURD transplantation carried out elsewhere.

In a cultural sense, the LURD renal transplantation in Iran might be compared with breast feeding of unrelated infants by wet nurses, which was a common practice until several decades ago. Before the introduction of condensed and dehydrated milk, some women would breast feed unrelated infants whose mothers had died or who had no breast milk. Wet nursing was a paid donation and was usually from lower to higher socioeconomic classes. Not only was the practice ethically accepted, but in Islamic religion wetnursing was so encouraged and admired that unrelated infants breastfed by one woman were considered as siblings. When the transplant teams and the national transplantation societies ensure the ethics of LURD transplantation, this approach can be used effectively in developing countries to supplement to their limited scale cadaveric

renal transplantation.

One argument against paid LURD renal transplantation is that wealthy patients will be transplanted and poor patients will be denied. In Iran's LURD renal transplantation program, all donors receive a defined government award and most donors also receive a rewarding gift from the recipient. The amount of the gift or payment for an LURD kidney has been controlled within a range by DATPA so that poor patients have also been able to afford transplantation. We previously conducted a study on 500 renal transplant recipients and their LURDs to see which socioeconomic classes are being transplanted more from LURDs (18). In this study 6.0% of LURDs were illiterate, 24.4% had elementary school, 63.4% high school and 6.2% university training. These same education levels in their 500 recipients were 18.0%, 20.0%, 50.8% and 11.2%, respectively. All 500 LURD and their recipients were also grouped according to whether they were poor, rich or middle class. The results showed that 84.0% of LURDs were poor and 16.0% were middle class. Of the 500 LURD transplant recipients, 50.4% were poor, 13.4% were rich and 36.2% were from the middle socioeconomic class. So more than 50% of LURD kidneys were transplanted to patients from the poor socioeconomic class (Fig. 9).

Another argument against paid LURD renal transplantation is that it will have an adverse effect on the development of a cadaveric organ transplantation program especially in developing countries and that it may also inhibit LRDs. LURD renal transplantation in Iran definitely had some, but not much of an inhibitory effect

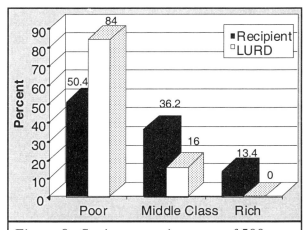

Figure 9. Socioeconomic status of 500 transplant recipients and their 500 living unrelated donors

on the development of cadaveric organ transplantation. Against the strong cultural barriers that exist in Iran, it would have required many years to perform a number of cadaveric renal transplants comparable to what we have already accomplished with the LURDs. We performed only LRD renal transplants until 1988, when we adopted LURD renal transplantation for patients who had no LRD or whose potential donors were reluctant to donate. The superior results of LRD compared with LURD renal transplantation and the very minimal risk to the donor has always been emphasized to these patients and their families. In spite of this approach, the ratio of LURD to LRD renal transplants has increased steadily since 1988. In one study we found that 81% of our LURD renal transplant recipients had a potential LRD (19). The LRD was not used in these cases for cultural reasons, because the LRD was reluctant to donate or because of the availability of LURD renal transplantation. With a well-controlled LURD renal transplantation program in place, it may be more ethical to perform a paid renal transplant from a volunteer LURD than from a LRD or spouse under family pressure or with some coercion. It is noteworthy that we have seen rewarded gifting or paid kidney donation in LRD renal transplants, as well.

SUMMARY

The first renal transplant in Iran was carried out in 1967. The renal transplant program severely lagged behind hemodialysis in growth until 1988. In 1988, a controlled LURD renal transplant program was adopted to provide kidneys for the large number of dialysis patients needing a renal transplant. There was no cadaveric donor transplant program. By the end of 1999, a total of 9,535 renal transplants were performed and the renal transplant waiting list of the country had been eliminated.

In Iran's LURD renal transplant program, the Dialysis and Transplant Patients Association introduces the volunteer LURD to the recipient and the transplant team. There are no middlemen and no incentives for transplant teams. The government pays all of the hospital expenses for transplantation. Many poor patients are able to afford LURD transplantation and more than 50% of our LURD transplant recipients are from the poor socioeconomic class. Ethical issues within the program are under the strict observation of the transplant teams and the Iranian Society for Organ Transplantation.

We have noted that many LURD transplant recipients had a potential LRD who did not donate for cultural reasons or who was reluctant to donate. In the presence of a controlled LURD renal transplant program, we feel it is more ethical to perform a paid renal transplant from volunteer LURD than a renal transplant from an LRD who may be under family pressure or coerced.

The patient and graft survival rates reported from our unit are comparable to the results of renal transplants reported from centers of some other countries. Some patient deaths and graft losses could have been prevented if our transplant units were not deficient with respect to laboratory facilities and access to pharmaceutical agents.

In April 2000, legislation recognizing brain death and cadaveric organ transplantation passed our parliament. Strong cultural barriers may limit the scale of cadaver donor transplantation in the coming years and we expect the programs will grow slowly. In the meantime, the LURD renal transplant program continues to serve the needs of many ESRD patients in Iran today and has allowed us to adapt this life-saving technology to our culture.

REFERENCES

1. Ghods AJ, Abdi E. Dialysis and renal transplantation in Iran. In: MA Haberal, Ed. Chronic Renal Failure and Transplantation. Ankara, Semith Offset. 1987; 103.

2. Ghods AJ, Taghavi M, Fazel I. Dialysis and Renal Transplantation in Iran - 1988. In : MA Haberal, Ed. Recent Advances in Nephrology and Transplantation. Ankara, Pelin Offset. 1990; 49.

3. Ghods AJ. Long - term results of renal transplantation in 104 Iranian patients transplanted abroad. Acta Medica Iranica 1994; 32:51.

4. Ghods AJ, Prooshani F, Ghahramani N, Nobakht A. Renal Transplantation in Iran. In : K S Chugh, Ed. Asian Nephrology. New Delhi, Oxford University Press 1994; 701.

5. Sesso R, Josephson MA, Ancao MS, et al. A retrospective study of kidney transplant recipients from living unrelated donors. J Am Soc Nephrol 1998; 9:684.

6. Velidedeoglu E, Bilgin N, Haberal M. Is it worth it to use kidneys between spouses? Transplant Proc 1993; 25:2185.

7. Ghods AJ, Khosravani P. Survival rates of parental donor renal allografts are similar to living unrelated donor grafts: Is it due to inadequate nephron supply? Transplant Proc 1997; 29:2767.

8. Terasaki PI, Cecka JM, Gjertson DW, et al. High survival rates of kidney transplants from spousal and living unrelated donors. N Engl J Med 1995; 333:333.

9. Gjertson DW. Cecka JM. Living unrelated donor kidney transplantation. Kidney Int 2000; 58:491.

10. Alfani D, Berloco P, Bruzzone P, et al. Kidney transplantation from unrelated donors: Ten – year experience. Transplant Proc 1996; 28:3455.

11. Park K, Kim SI, Kim YS, et al. Results of kidney transplantation from 1979 to 1997 at Yonsei University. In: JM Cecka and PI Terasaki, Eds. Clinical Transplants 1997. Los Angeles, UCLA Tissue Typing Laboratory, 1998; 149.

12. Ghods AJ, Fazel I, Nikbin B, et al. Results of 319 consecutive renal transplants from living related and living unrelated donors. In : Abouna GM, Kumar MSA, White AG, Eds. Organ Transplantation 1990. Netherlands, Kluwer Academic Publishers. 1991; 247.

13. Ghods AJ, Khosravani P. Effect of first day graft nonfunction on the short - and long - term graft survival rates in living related and living unrelated donor renal transplants. Transplant Proc 1997; 29:2773.

14. Ghods AJ, Ossareh S. Lymphoma - The most common neoplasia in renal transplant recipients. Transplant Proc 2000; 32:585.

15. Hesketh T, Zhu WX. The one child family policy: the good, the bad, and the ugly. Brit Med J 1997; 314:1685.

16. Chugh KS, Jha V. Commerce in transplantation in Third World countries. Kidney Int 1996; 49:1181.

17. Briggs JD. The use of organs from executed prisoners in China. Nephrol Dial Transplant 1996; 11:238.

18. Ghods AJ, Ossareh S, Khosravani P. Comparison of some socioeconomic characteristics of donors and recipients in a controlled living unrelated donor renal transplantation program. Transplant Proc 2001 (in press).

19. Ghods AJ, Savaj S, Khosravani P. Adverse effect of a controlled living unrelated donor renal transplant program on living related and cadaveric kidney donation. Transplant Proc 2000; 32:541.

ACKNOWLEDGMENTS

Transplantation is a team effort and the credit for any success should go to all members of that team. The author wishes to gratefully acknowledge the contribution of the following members of the transplant team : Dr. F. Prooshani, Dr. H. Nejad Gashti, Dr. E. Abdi and Dr. S. Aris. Without their dedicated efforts this work would not have been possible. My special note of thanks to Dr. S. Abedi Azar and to P. Khosravani R.N. for their sincere efforts in collection of data and to Miss L. Lak for her assistance in the preparation of the manuscript.

CHAPTER 18

Simultaneous Pancreas-Kidney (SPK) and Pancreas Living-Donor Kidney (SPLK) Transplantation at the University of Maryland

Benjamin Philosophe, Alan C. Farney, Eugene J. Schweitzer, John O. Colonna, Bruce E. Jarrell, Clarence E. Foster III, Anne M. Wiland, and Stephen T. Bartlett

The Joseph and Corrine Schwartz Division of Transplantation, Department of Surgery, University of Maryland Medical Center, Baltimore, Maryland

Over the past few years, we have witnessed a significant improvement in pancreas graft survival due to better immunosuppression and due to technical advances, which have increased the popularity of this operation by eliminating some of the problematic side effects of the transplant. The success rate of pancreas transplants has increased so significantly that the procedure has been endorsed by the American Diabetes Association as an accepted treatment for patients with Type 1 diabetes and end-stage renal disease (ESRD) (1). In 1998, more than 1,200 pancreas transplants were performed in the United States, a 15% increase from the previous year (2).

In 1991, the pancreas transplant program was initiated at the University of Maryland. Initially, the program was dedicated to establishing the standard simultaneous pancreas and kidney (SPK) transplant technique with the lowest possible morbidity. As the program evolved, solitary pancreas transplantation (PA) has improved to the point where graft survival is now comparable to that for SPK transplants. Through January 2000, 434 pancreas transplants have been performed (Fig. 1). This includes 204 SPK transplants for patients with ESRD and Type 1 diabetes mellitus, 124 pancreas after kidney (PAK) transplants for patients with Type 1 diabetes mellitus and a prior successful kidney transplant, 68 pancreas transplants alone (PTA), and 38 simultaneous cadaveric pancreas and living-donor kidney (SPLK) transplants.

The evolution of laparoscopic living donor nephrectomy and its influence on pancreas transplantation. Live-donor renal transplantation continues to be an underutilized resource that can substantially reduce waiting times and provide survival benefits. Resistance to living kidney donation can be attributed to concerns by the donors regarding the operation, the necessary hospital stay, a prolonged recuperative period, and the financial feasibility. Laparoscopic nephrectomy for neoplasms has proven to reduce post-operative pain, hospital length of stay, and convalescent time compared with the open approach (3). This has provided the rationale for the development of minimally invasive donor nephrectomy. Laparoscopic

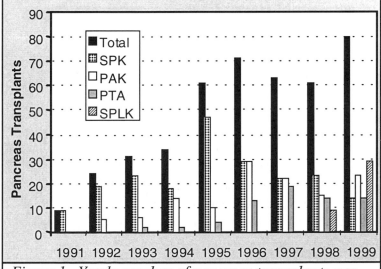

Figure 1. *Yearly number of pancreas transplants performed at the University of Maryland.*

live donor nephrectomy has been performed at the University of Maryland since March 1996. The morbidity and mortality is comparable to that of open donor nephrectomy, but with substantial improvements in donor recovery (4). The sum of these improvements has resulted in a significant increase in acceptance of the donor operation, resulting in an expanded pool of potential kidney donors.

In contrast, the slower development of pancreas transplantation in the United States has provided a relatively large number of pancreases available for transplantation through national sharing. The heavy reliance on living-donor renal transplants to alleviate the cadaveric donor shortage has also resulted in the development of strategies to reduce significantly the waiting time required for Type 1 diabetics with renal failure to receive both kidney and pancreas transplants. To date, 681 living-donor renal transplants were performed in our institution and 108 of those received pancreas transplants either 3-6 months following the renal transplant, or simultaneously as SPLK.

Simultaneous cadaver pancreas-living-donor kidney transplantation (SPLK). In the past, Type 1 diabetics with ESRD who had a living donor had to choose between one of 3 options. Option 1 was to reject living kidney donation and wait for a cadaver SPK. The recipient's insurance carrier sometimes mandates this choice. Option 2 was to receive a living-donor kidney transplant alone and accept life as a diabetic. Option 3 was to have a living-donor kidney transplant and then have a PAK procedure, usually 3-6 months later. We hypothesized that a living-donor kidney and cadaver pancreas transplant could be performed together safely, thereby avoiding a second operation and its associated morbidity (5). Our results after 46 cases have yielded one-year pancreas and kidney graft survival rates of 91% and 97%, respectively, and a patient survival of 97% (Fig. 2). Moreover, the waiting time for SPLK is substantially less than for cadaver SPK. Finally, the cost of SPLK has been less than the combined cost of living-donor kidney and PAK transplantation as separate procedures.

PATIENTS AND METHODS

Patient Selection

Pancreas transplantation has been reserved for patients with Type 1 diabetes. Adult onset, obesity, ab-

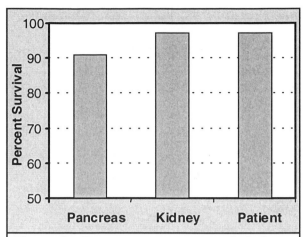

Figure 2. One-year pancreas graft, kidney graft and patient survival for SPLK transplants (n=46)

sence of a history of ketoacidosis, periods of insulin independence or extraordinary insulin requirements may suggest a diagnosis of Type 2 diabetes. Diagnostic uncertainty is resolved by the administration of a 100g oral glucose challenge, followed one hour later by simultaneous measurement of a blood C-peptide and glucose. A Type 1 diabetic will have undetectable C-peptide levels despite maximal stimulation of the pancreas with simultaneously elevated blood glucose. Conversely, a Type 2 diabetic will have blood insulin levels that are normal or elevated as a result of insulin resistance.

The majority of patients evaluated for pancreas transplantation have ESRD. Thus, the patients are either on dialysis, approaching dialysis or have had a successful kidney transplant. In addition to ESRD, most patients have other secondary complications of diabetes including retinopathy, neuropathy, autonomic neuropathy, gastroparesis, and evidence of accelerated atherosclerosis. The evidence clearly shows that pancreas transplantation prevents recurrent diabetic nephropathy in transplanted kidneys (6). This fact alone, combined with the marked improvement in quality of life achieved with a successful pancreas transplant strongly supports pancreas transplantation either simultaneously, or after a kidney transplant in the Type 1 diabetic with renal failure. It is rare to have ESRD as an isolated secondary complication of diabetes. Thus, the vast majority of candidates have varying degrees of other secondary complications that will be arrested or reversed with pancreas transplantation.

Postoperative Care of the Pancreas Transplant Patient

The post operative care, including the immunosuppressive strategy, has evolved over the past few years. At the University of Maryland, all patients receive prophylactic intravenous antibiotics. Currently, piperacillin/ tazobactam is administered pre-operatively and for at least 2 days following the pancreas transplant. Modifications are made if the patients are penicillin allergic. All recipients, regardless of their cytomegalovirus (CMV) match, receive intravenous gancyclovir for CMV prophylaxis until the patient is able to tolerate oral feeding, at which point oral gancyclovir is administered for 14 weeks following transplantation.

Since 1998, we have implemented a protocol of low-dose anticoagulation in recipients of solitary pancreas transplants (PAK and PTA) and in pre-uremic SPK or SPLK recipients. Intravenous heparin is administered at a dose of 300 U/hr immediately following surgery and, over the next 24 hours, is increased to 500 U/hr. Heparin is maintained at this dose and the serum hematocrit, platelet count, prothrombin time (PT) and partial thromboplastin time (PTT) are monitored serially, although we do not attempt to attain a therapeutic PTT.

Diagnosis of Rejection

Diagnosis of rejection following pancreas transplants is initiated by any of the following indicators: 1) hyperamylasemia, 2) hyperlipasemia, 3) unexplained hyperglycemia, or 4) unexplained fever or allograft tenderness. In SPK or SPLK recipients, a 20% rise in serum creatinine or a failure of the serum creatinine to fall to an appropriate level were signs of rejection that prompted a percutaneous biopsy. After the technique of ultrasound-guided percutaneous pancreas biopsy (PPB) was established (7), it was used routinely in all cases of suspected pancreas rejection. The PPB is performed with an 18-gauge automated biopsy needle, utilizing color-flow duplex ultrasound to identify the tail of the pancreas in an area free of overlying bowel and clear of the splenic artery and vein. Occasionally, poor visualization due to over-

lying loops of bowel may necessitate further attempts with CT or laparoscopy. In patients with chronic rejection, fibrotic changes resulting in a small, shrunken pancreas may require laparotomy to obtain an adequate tissue sample. Interpretation of pancreatic biopsies is based on the scheme listed in Table 1, which was developed by our pathologists (8).

Outpatient Follow-up of the Pancreas Transplant Recipient

Outpatient management of the pancreas transplant recipient varies little from that of the kidney transplant patient. Routine clinical follow-up, serial laboratory studies and immunosuppressive drug monitoring are the focal point of outpatient management.

Immunosuppression

The International Pancreas Transplant Registry (IPTR) data shows that 75% of pancreas transplant centers utilize anti-lymphocyte induction therapy. At the University of Maryland, post operative anti-lymphocyte antibody is administered as immune induction for nearly all pancreas transplants. ATGAM doses were adjusted daily to achieve less than 50 CD3+ lymphocytes per cubic millimeter, and OKT3 was adjusted to keep CD3+ cells less than 5% of the total lymphocyte count. Currently, Thymoglobulin is preferentially used, given its efficacy

Table 1. Histologic classification system for acute pancreas allograft rejection.

Grade	Class	Histology
0	Normal	Normal pancreas histology
1	Borderline	Changes consisting of rare lymphocytic septal infiltrates while the acinar parenchyma is free of inflammation
2	Mild	Mixed inflammatory septal infiltrates with focal involvement of acinar parenchyma. Ductal inflammation and /or venulitis are often seen.
3	Moderate	Septal inflammation with multifocal involvement of acinar parenchyma associated with single cell injury, such as vacuolization, necrosis, or apoptosis.
4	Moderate with vascular rejection	Moderate rejection with arterial endothelitis or vasculitis.
5	Severe	Extensive inflammatory infiltrates with confluent acinar necrosis.

and apparent fewer cytokine release symptoms. Like ATGAM, it is adjusted daily to achieve less than 50 CD3+ lymphocytes per cubic millimeter.

Mycophenolate mofetil (Cellcept®, Hoffman La Roche Pharmaceuticals) has proven to be superior to azathioprine thereby replacing it in virtually all solid organ transplantation. Mycophenolate mofetil is combined with one of the calcineurin inhibitors, either tacrolimus or cyclosporine. While there is no clear advantage of one calcineurin inhibitor for SPK transplants, the results for solitary pancreas transplants with cyclosporine have been poor. Therefore, tacrolimus-based therapy became our standard in 1995 except in those few circumstances in which Neoral® was used for tacrolimus intolerance (less than 5% of cases).

The role of the newer cell cycle inhibitor, sirolimus, has not been established in pancreas transplantation, but its success in islet and kidney transplantation predicts that it will have a significant role in pancreas transplant management, at least as a replacement for those patients experiencing unacceptable toxicity with the standard agents.

Our induction therapy for low-risk SPK and SPLK now consists of the chimeric anti-IL-2 receptor antibody, basiliximab (Simulect®, Novartis Pharmaceuticals), tacrolimus, mycophenolate mofetil and steroids. Our current maintenance immunosuppression is equivalent for all types of pancreas transplants, and generally includes tacrolimus, mycophenolate mofetil, and a tapering regimen of steroids.

Current Techniques: Venous Reconstruction

Portal venous (PV) drainage, a more physiologic method that eliminates hyperinsulinemia, is gaining interest among pancreas transplant centers. Following the initial description by Calne in 1984, PV drainage of pancreas allografts underwent several technical modifications (11,12). The current technique of PV drainage used in most centers is based on the technique described by Shokouh-Amiri, et al. (13). Although follow-up is limited, several centers, including ours, have shown excellent graft survival rates and a reduced number of surgical complications with PV drainage (7,9,14). Portal venous drainage remains our preferred technique for reasons discussed below. In this technique, an end-to-side anastomosis between the portal vein and the SMV is performed. The technique of SV drainage involves anasto-

mosis of the donor portal vein to the recipient iliac vein or vena cava.

In addition to its potential physiological advantages, PV drainage may be technically easier to perform in comparison to SV drainage procedure. Complete mobilization of the iliac vein can be time consuming and technically challenging, particularly in a deep pelvis. With PV drainage, a large tributary of the SMV can be isolated quickly and the anastomosis is generally performed in a well-exposed area of the operative field.

RESULTS

The Impact of PV Drainage on Graft Survival and Rejection

It has long been hypothesized that PV drainage of pancreas allografts should offer physiologic benefits. The prevention of hyperinsulinemia and improvement in lipoprotein profiles in patients receiving portal-drained pancreas allografts have been well documented (10, 15). The improvement in physiologic profiles has been supplemented with lower rejection rates in portal-drained pancreas transplants resulting in significantly higher graft survival rates since the routine use of this technique. We have shown that pancreas allografts drained into the portal vein, irrespective of whether a kidney was co-transplanted, had a significantly lower incidence of acute rejection compared with allografts that were drained systemically into the iliac vein (16). With the introduction of mycophenolate mofetil and tacrolimus, allograft survival and rejection rates for both renal and pancreas transplants have significantly improved. In our institution, multivariate analysis of variables affecting graft survival and rejection following pancreas transplantation since 1991 revealed that tacrolimus and mycophenolate mofetil

Table 2. Multivariate analysis of variables affecting graft survival and rejection in all pancreas transplants.

Variable	Graft survival		Rejection-free	
	p value	R.R.	p value	R.R.
Type	0.62		0.64	
HLA MM	0.16		0.19	
AB MM	0.21		0.68	
DR MM	0.68		0.69	
FK-506	0.009	0.25	0.02	0.51
MMF	0.06		0.03	0.53

are the only variables with a significant positive impact (Table 2). HLA antigen matching has had no effect on either survival or rejection (manuscript submitted). With these factors in mind, it was important to assess the immunological impact of portal drainage within a period when the immunosuppressive protocol had not varied. Figure 3, therefore, depicts the Kaplan-Meier graft survival for portal and systemically drained pancreas transplants during this period. The higher graft survival was also seen for each type of pancreas transplant. Figure 4 depicts the one-year graft survival for SPK, PAK and PTA.

In addition to improved patient and graft survival, there appear to be immunologic benefits. A lower overall rejection rate with PV drainage compared with systemic venous drainage for SPK transplants is seen in Figure 5. The 36-month rejection rate for SPK is 9% for PV and 45% for SV (p=0.0002).

In our analysis of SPK transplants, a similar difference in kidney rejection rates was noted between systemic and PV drainage of pancreas transplants. At 36 months, there was a 17% difference in rejection rates (43% for SV vs. 26% for PV; p=0.002) (Fig. 6). The introduction of peripancreatic nodal tissue in the portal vein could theoretically induce an immunomodulatory response in the host liver, which can have a protective effect on both organs from the same donor. This is an interesting, albeit unproven concept that is the basis of future investigation.

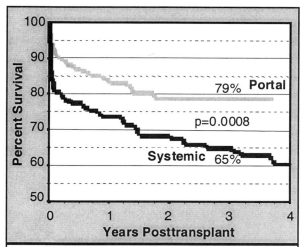

Figure 3. Overall graft survival following pancreas transplantation.

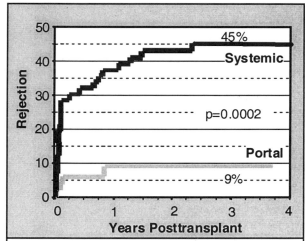

Figure 5. Cumulative rate of at least one rejection episode following SPK pancreas transplantation.

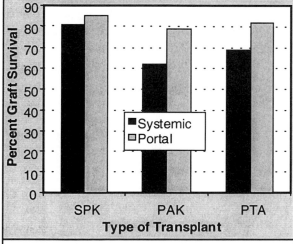

Figure 4. One-year pancreas graft survival for SPK, PAK and PTA.

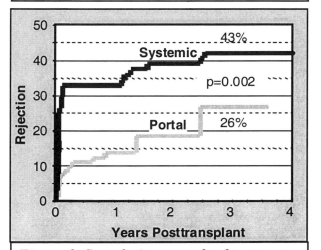

Figure 6. Cumulative rate of at least one rejection episode of kidneys following SPK transplantation.

SUMMARY

The evolution of enteric and portal venous drainage, better immunosuppression, and better patient care has elevated pancreas transplantation with dramatically improved results. At our center, long-term graft survival and rejection has significantly improved with portal venous drainage, which has become our gold standard. This improvement is exemplified by the excellent one-year patient and graft survival rates for SPLK transplants. SPLK has proven to be an ideal approach in uremic Type 1 diabetic patients with living donors and should become the procedure of choice for that population. Moreover, the improved monitoring of rejection has allowed a similar success of pancreas transplantation alone in non-uremic patients with brittle diabetes.

The treatment of diabetes mellitus has room for great improvement, however, and there is no question that islet transplantation, xenotransplantation, and the pursuit of immunologic tolerance will play an extremely important role in that endeavor.

REFERENCES

1. American Diabetes Association Position statement. Pancreas transplantation for patients with diabetes mellitus. Diabetes Care 1993; 16:21.

2. 1998 Annual Report of the U.S. Scientific Registry of Transplant Recipients and the Organ Procurement and Transplantation Network-Transplant Data: 1988-1998. UNOS, Richmond, VA and the Division of Transplantation,Bureau of Health Resources and Services Administration, U.S. Department of Health and Human Services, Rockville, MD, 1996.

3. Kavoussi LR, Kerbl K, Capelouto CC, McDougal EM, Clayman RV. Laparoscopic nephrectomy for renal neoplasms. Urology 1993; 42:603.

4. Flower JL, Jacobs S, Cho E, et al. Comparison of open and laparoscopic live donor nephrectomy. Ann Surg 1997; 226:483

5. Farney AC, Cho E, Schweitzer EJ, et al. Simultaneous cadaver pancreas living-donor kidney transplantation (SPLK): A new approach for the Type 1 diabetic uremic patient. Ann Surg 2000; 232: 696.

6. Fioretto P, Steffes MW, Sutherland DE, Goetz FC, Mauer M. Reversal of lesions of diabetic nephropathy after pancreas transplantation. N Engl J Med 1998; 339:69.

7. Bartlett ST, Schweitzer EJ, Johnson L, et al. Equivalent success of simultaneous pancreas kidney and solitary pancreas transplantation: A prospective trial of tacrolimus immunosuppression with percutaneous biopsy. Ann Surg 1996; 224:440.

8. Drachenberg CB, Papadimetriou JC, Klassen DK, Bartlett ST. Histologic grading of pancreas acute allograft rejection in percutaneous needle biopsies. Transplant Proc 1996; 28:512.

9. Di Carlo V, Castoldi R, Cristallo M, et al. Techniques of pancreas transplantation through the world: an IPITA Center survey. Transplant Proc 1998; 30:231.

10. Hughes TA, Gaber AO, Amiri HS, et al. Kidney-pancreas transplantation. The effect of portal versus systemic venous drainage of the pancreas on the lipoprotein composition. Transplantation 1995; 60:1406.

11. Calne RY. Paratopic segmental pancreas grafting: a technique with portal venous drainage. Lancet 1984; 1:595.

12. Rosenlof LK, Earnhardt RC, Pruett TL, Stevenson WC, Douglas MT, Cornett GC, Hanks JB. Pancreas transplantation. An initial experience with systemic and portal drainage of pancreatic allografts. Ann Surg 1992; 215:586.

13. Shokouh-Amiri MH, Gaber AO, Gaber LW, Jensen SL, Hughes TA, Elmer D, Britt LG. Pancreas transplantation with portal venous drainage and enteric exocrine diversion: a new technique. Transplant Proc 1992; 24:776.

14. Stratta RJ, Gaber AO, Shokouh-Amiri MH, Reddy KS, Egidi MF, Grewal HP, Gaber LW. A prospective comparison of systemic-bladder versus portal-enteric drainage in vascularized pancreas transplantation. Surgery 2000; 127:217.

15. Gaber AO, Shokouh-Amiri H, Hathaway DK, Hammontree L, Kitabchi AE, Gaber LW, Saad MF, Britt LG. Results of pancreas transplantation with portal venous and enteric drainage. Ann Surg 1995; 221:613.

16. Philosophe B, Farney AC, Schweitzer EJ, et al. The superiority of portal venous drainage over systemic venous drainage in pancreas transplantation. Ann Surg; (in press).

CHAPTER 19

Portal-Enteric Pancreas Transplantation at the University of Tennessee, Memphis

Robert J. Stratta, M. Hosein Shokouh-Amiri, M. Francesca Egidi, Hani P. Grewal, A.T. Kizilisik, Donna K. Hathaway, Lillian W. Gaber, and A. Osama Gaber

Departments of Surgery (Divison of Transplantation), Medicine, Nursing, and Pathology
University of Tennessee Memphis, Memphis, Tennessee

Vascularized pancreas transplantation (PTX) was first developed as a means to re-establish endogenous insulin secretion responsive to normal feedback controls. PTX is currently the only available form of auto-regulating total endocrine replacement therapy that reliably establishes an insulin-independent euglycemic state and normal glucose homeostasis resulting in the successful treatment of diabetes mellitus. With improvements in organ retrieval and preservation technology, refinements in diagnostic technology and surgical techniques, advances in clinical immunosuppression and anti-microbial prophylaxis, and experience in donor and recipient selection, success rates for PTX have steadily increased. From 1966 through July 2000, more than 14,000 PTXs were performed worldwide and reported to the International Pancreas Transplant Registry (IPTR) (1). In the United States, more than 1,200 PTXs are performed annually, with 83% being simultaneous kidney-PTXs (SKPTs). The current one-year actuarial patient, kidney, and pancreas (with complete insulin independence) graft survival rates after SKPT are 95%, 92% and 84%, respectively (1). Solitary PTXs comprise the remaining activity, including either sequential pancreas after kidney transplants (PAKT, 12%) or PTX alone (PA, 5%). The current one-year actuarial pancreas graft survival rates are 73% for PAKT and 70% for PA (1). With the advent of Medicare coverage, SKPT and PAKT have become accepted as preferred treatment options in selected patients with insulin-dependent diabetes mellitus (IDDM) and advanced nephropathy.

According to IPTR data, most PTXs are performed with systemic venous delivery of insulin and either bladder (systemic-bladder [S-B]) or enteric (systemic-enteric [S-E])drainage of the exocrine secretions (2). From 1988 through 1995, more than 90% of PTX procedures were performed by the standard technique of S-B drainage using a duodenal segment conduit. Although well tolerated in most PTX recipients, S-B drainage was associated with a finite and troublesome rate of unique metabolic and urologic complications resulting from altered physiology. When these complications became persistent or refractory, conversion from bladder to enteric drainage (enteric conversion) was often necessary and successful (3). Because of a favorable experience with enteric conversion, coupled with advances in preservation, donor selection, and immunosuppression that placed the duodenal segment at a lower risk for ischemic or immunologic injury, a resurgence of interest occurred in primary enteric drainage in an effort to avoid the complications of bladder drainage.

Since 1995, the number of PTX procedures performed with primary enteric drainage has steadily increased, accounting for 60% of cases in 1999 (1). In the last few years, the results of SKPT with enteric drainage have improved and are now comparable to SKPT with bladder drainage (2). Despite an evolution in surgical techniques, the majority of PTXs with enteric drainage are performed with systemic venous delivery of insulin, resulting in peripheral hyperinsulinemia. In the non-transplant setting, chronic hyperinsulinemia has been associated with insulin resistance, dyslipidemia, accelerated atherosclerosis, and macroangiopathy. To improve the physiology of PTX, a new surgical technique was developed at our center, combining portal venous delivery of insulin with enteric drainage of the exocrine secretions (portal-enteric [P-E]) (4-6). In a recent survey of surgical techniques among PTX centers, 7 reported experience with the P-E technique, of which 5 used a diverting Roux limb (7). Table 1 provides a list of centers that have reported experience in PTX with P-E drainage. Many of these centers have adopted the P-E technique as their preferred method of PTX. However, the proportion of cases with P-E drainage has remained low and represents only 15-20% of enteric-drained PTXs (1,2). In the most recent IPTR analysis including PTXs performed between 1996-1999, the one-year pancreas graft survival rates were similar for P-E versus S-E drainage, 83% and 84%, respectively (2)

Whole organ PTX using the P-E technique was first described clinically by our group in 1992 (4) and was based on experimental work by Shokouh-Amiri, et al, in a porcine model (8-10). This new technique employed a tributary of the superior mesenteric vein to re-establish portal venous drainage and differed substantially from other initial reports of whole organ PTX with portal venous drainage. We have previously reported our initial experience with P-E drainage, including both retrospective and prospective comparisons to control groups of patients who underwent SKPT with either S-B or S-E drainage (6,11-15). We have also reported our initial experience in solitary PTX with P-E drainage, including a retrospective comparison to a control group of solitary PTX recipients with S-B drainage (16). Herein we report the chronology of our 10-year single-center experience with 126 PTXs with P-E drainage spanning different immunosuppressive eras.

PROGRAM OVERVIEW

The University of Tennessee (UT) Memphis PTX program began in 1989 (Fig. 1). Between April 1989 and September 1990, 24 consecutive SKPTs were performed with S-B drainage (Fig. 2). The first SKPT with P-E drainage was performed in October 1990, and this patient continues to enjoy excellent dual allograft function more than 10 years later. Also in 1990, the first solitary PTXs were performed at our program including both sequential PAKT and PA (Fig. 1).

From October 1990 through December 1994, we performed 42 SKPTs, including 26 with P-E and 16 with S-B drainage (Fig. 2) (11). During the same interval, 18 solitary PTXs were performed with S-B drainage, including 13 PA and 5 PAKT

Table 1. Recent experience in pancreas transplantation with P-E drainage.	
Center	# Cases
UT Memphis	>100
University of Chicago	>100
University of Maryland	>100
Lyon, France	>20
Toronto	>20
Louisiana State University	>15
University of Virginia	>10
Duke University	>10
University of Massachusetts	>10
Northwestern University	>5

(Fig. 1). In 1995 and 1996, 42 consecutive PTXs (29 SKPT, 9 PAKT, 4 PA) were performed exclusively with P-E drainage (Fig. 2). From February 1997 through March 1998, we compared 32 consecutive PTXs performed with either S-B or P-E drainage (12). From April 1998 through May 2000, 54 consecutive SKPT recipients were entered into a prospective study of S-E versus P-E drainage at our center (Fig. 2) (14). From 1989 through 2000, we performed a total of 276 PTXs, including 153 with P-E, 76 with S-B, and 47 with S-E drainage (Fig. 3). This overall experience accumulated over a decade includes 196 SKPTs, 43 PA, and 37 PAKTs (Fig. 4). The UT Memphis PTX program is currently one of the 7 largest centers in the United States and recently became the thirteenth center worldwide to perform 250 PTXs. Through

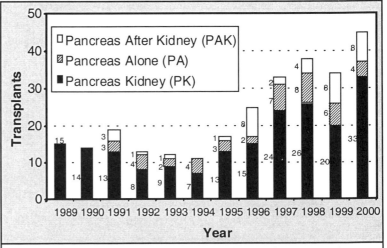

Figure 1. UT Memphis Pancreas Transplant experience by year according to type of transplant.

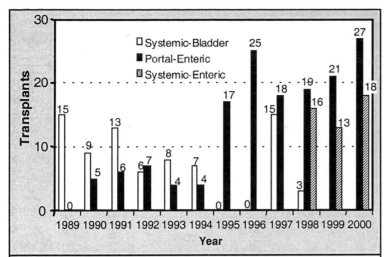

Figure 2. UT Memphis Pancreas Transplant experience by year according to technique of transplant.

1999, we have one of the largest single-center experiences with the P-E technique, including 126 PTXs (90 SKPT, 18 PAKT, 18 PA) with P-E drainage (Fig. 5). This report represents a case series and our collective experience with the P-E technique.

Organ Procurement, Preservation, and Preparation

Donor selection and organ procurement were recognized to be of paramount importance to the success of the new procedure. Most heart-beating donors who have been declared brain dead and are appropriate for kidney, heart, lung, and liver donation are also suitable for pancreas donation (Table 2). In general, ideal pancreas donors range in age from 10-40 years and range in weight from 30-80 kg.

The pancreas and/or kidney were procured from heart-beating cadaveric donors in conjunction with multiple organ retrieval using standardized techniques. We believe that combined liver, kidney, and whole organ pancreaticoduodenal retrieval can be safely performed in virtually all donors regardless of vascular anatomy. Whole organ pancreaticoduodenosplenectomy was performed by an en-bloc technique. In cases in which a replaced or accessory hepatic artery originated from the superior mesenteric artery, we were either able to dissect the superior mesenteric artery in situ to include the accessory hepatic artery with the liver or alternatively (and preferentially) performed combined en-bloc hepatico-pancreatico-duodenosplenectomy followed by back table ex-vivo separation of the liver and pancreas. University

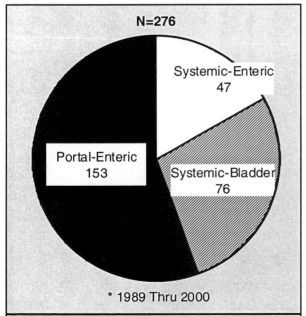

Figure 3. Total number of pancreas transplants at UT Memphis according to technique.

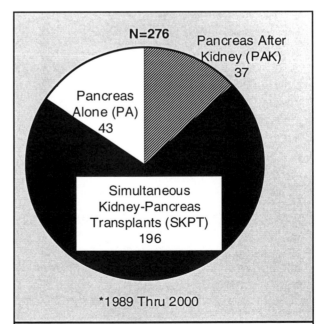

Figure 4. Total number of pancreas transplants at UT Memphis according to recipient category.

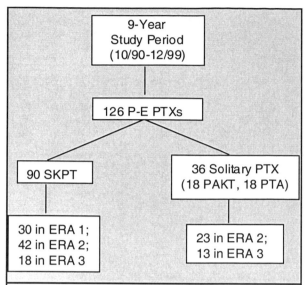

9-Year
Study Period
(10/90-12/99)

126 P-E PTXs

90 SKPT

36 Solitary PTX
(18 PAKT, 18 PTA)

30 in ERA 1;
42 in ERA 2;
18 in ERA 3

23 in ERA 2;
13 in ERA 3

Figure 5. Overall experience in pancreas transplantation with portal-enteric drainage spanning different immunosuppressive eras.

of Wisconsin (UW) solution was used for both in-situ flush and preservation of all organs under cold storage conditions. Cold ischemia was kept to a minimum and pancreas preservation times were below 24 hours in all cases and below 12 hours in about 1/3 of cases. The mean pancreas cold ischemia time was 13 hours. In a retrospective analysis of our data, we found that steroid administration to the donor resulted in a significant reduction in post-reperfusion pancreatitis (17). In the same analysis, we demonstrated that post-reperfusion pancreatitis increased significantly when cold ischemia exceeded 12 hours. Moreover, by using calcium channel blockers in the early post-operative period, we were able to significantly decrease the incidence of posttransplant pancreatitis (17). Because of these observations, whenever possible, we limit preservation times, administer steroids to the donor and give calcium channel blockers to the recipient.

Recipient Selection and Pretransplant Evaluation

Indications for PTX at UT Memphis include the presence of IDDM (Type 1 or Type 2) and the predicted abilities to tolerate the operative procedure, the requisite immunosuppression after transplantation, and possible associated complications (Table 3) (13,18). Patient selection is aided by a comprehensive medical evaluation before transplantation (Table 4) performed by a

Table 2. Cadaver pancreas organ donation.

I. Indications
 A. Declaration of brain death
 B. Informed consent
 C. Age 6-55 years (ideal 10-40)
 D. Weight 30-100 kg (ideal 30-80)
 E. Hemodynamic stability with adequate perfusion and oxygenation
 F. Normal glycosylated hemoglobin level (only needed in cases of severe hyperglycemia, extreme obesity, or positive family history of diabetes)
 G. Absence of infectious or transmissible diseases (ie.- tuberculosis, syphilis, hepatitis, AIDS)
 H. Negative serology (HIV; hepatitis B and C)
 I. Absence of malignancy (unless skin or low-grade brain cancer)
 J. Absence of pancreatic disease

II. Contraindications:
 A. History of diabetes mellitus (Type 1, 2 or gestational)
 B. Previous pancreatic surgery
 C. Moderate to severe pancreatic trauma
 D. Pancreatitis (active acute or chronic)
 E. Significant intra-abdominal contamination
 F. Major (active) infection
 G. Chronic alcohol abuse
 H. Recent history of intravenous drug abuse
 I. Recent history of homosexuality
 J. Prolonged hypotension or hypoxemia with evidence for significant end-organ (kidney, liver) damage
 K. Severe atherosclerosis
 L. Inexperienced retrieval team
 M. Severe fatty infiltration
 N. Severe pancreatic edema
 O. Severe obesity (>150% ideal body weight)

III. Risk Factors:
 A. Massive transfusions
 B. Prior splenectomy
 C. Mild to moderate obesity (<150% ideal body weight)
 D. Aberrant hepatic artery anatomy
 E. Positive VDRL/RPR serology
 F. Prolonged length of hospital stay
 G. Donor age above 45 years
 H. Cardiovascular or cerebrovascular cause of brain death
 I. Mild to moderate fatty infiltration
 J. Mild to moderate pancreatic edema
 K. Donor instability
 L. Mild pancreatic trauma
 M. Mild to moderate atherosclerosis

HIV: Human Immunodeficiency Virus
AIDS: Acquired Immunodeficiency Syndrome
VDRL: Venereal Disease Research Laboratory
RPR: Rapid Plasma Reagin

Table 3. Indications for pancreas transplantation: Eligibility guidelines

I. Medical Necessity
   A. Presence of insulin-treated diabetes mellitus:
      1. Documentation of insulin dose
      2. Type 1 or 2 diabetes
   B. Ability to withstand surgery and immunosuppression (as assessed by pretransplant medical evaluation):
      1. Adequate cardiopulmonary function (Cardiac stress testing ± coronary angiography to rule out significant coronary artery disease or other cardiac contraindications. Patients with significant coronary artery disease should have it corrected pretransplant)
      2. Absence of other organ system failure (other than kidney)
   C. Emotional and sociopsychological suitability
   D. Presence of well-defined diabetic complications (any 2):
      1. Proliferative retinopathy
      2. Nephropathy (hypertension, proteinuria, or decline in GFR)
      3. Symptomatic peripheral or autonomic neuropathy
      4. Microangiopathy
      5. Accelerated atherosclerosis (macroangiopathy)
      6. Glucose hyperlability, insulin resistance, or hypoglycemia unawareness with a significant impairment in quality of life
   E. Absence of any contraindications
   F. Financial resources
II. Type of pancreas transplant
   A. Specific entry criteria based on degree of nephropathy:
      1. Simultaneous kidney-pancreas transplant: creatinine clearance below 30 ml/min
      2. Sequential pancreas after kidney transplant: creatinine clearance ≥40 ml/min (on calcineurin inhibitor)
      3. Pancreas transplant alone: creatinine clearance above 60 ml/min
   B. Primary determinants for recipient selection are the presence of diabetic complications, degree of nephropathy, and cardiovascular risk

GFR: Glomerular Filtration Rate

PANCREAS – MEMPHIS, TENNESSEE

---

multi-disciplinary team that confirms the diagnosis of IDDM, determines the patient's ability to withstand the operative procedure, establishes the absences of any exclusion criteria (Table 5), and documents end-organ complications for future tracking after transplantation (13,18). The primary determinants for recipient selection are the presence of diabetic complications, degree of nephropathy, and cardiovascular risk (Table 3) (18).

We believe that SKPT should be at least considered in all IDDM patients with advanced nephropathy, defined as those who are dialysis dependent or dialysis imminent with a creatinine clearance less than 30 ml/min or failure of a previous kidney transplant. In our experience, about two-thirds of diabetic patients screened are actually accepted for SKPT. In contrast to some centers, we do not regard blindness, history of major

amputation, or history of cardiac disease as absolute contraindications for SKPT. With increasing experience in PTX, previous absolute contraindications have become relative contraindications, and relative contraindications have become risk factors for a successful outcome. Inclusion and exclusion criteria for PTX are listed in Tables 3 and 5.

Selection criteria for solitary PTX are based on the presence of early diabetic complications associated with either hypoglycemia unawareness or exogenous insulin failure with hyperlabile diabetes and a significant impairment in quality of life (13,18). Diabetic patients with a creatinine clearance above 60 ml/min and evidence of overt diabetic complications or unawareness of hypoglycemic symptoms are potential candidates for PA (Table 3). Diabetic patients that have previously received

Table 4. Evaluation of the pancreas transplant candidate.

I. Interviews and Consults
    A. History and physical examination by nephrologist, endocrinologist and transplant surgeon
    B. Ophthalmology evaluation including visual acuity, fluorescein angiography, retinal fundus photography with retinopathy score and slit-lamp examination
    C. Transplant coordinator and medical social worker interview including completion of quality of life questionnaire
    D. Gynecology consultation for all females (pelvic examination with Pap smear)
    E. Dental evaluation
    F. When indicated, additional evaluations may be required by orthopedic surgery, podiatry, psychology, psychiatry, neurology or gastroenterology

II. Cardiovascular, Respiratory, and Peripheral Vascular Evaluations
    A. Standard testing includes orthostatic vital signs, 12 lead electrocardiogram, chest radiograph, echocardiography, and exercise treadmill, stress thallium, or dobutamine stress echocardiography
    B. Additional studies may include arterial blood gases, 24-hour Holter monitoring, autonomic and peripheral vasomotor reflexes, Doppler arterial studies, ankle/brachial index, transcutaneous oxygen monitoring, plethysmography, carotid Doppler examination, aortography with run-off, or pulmonary function tests as indicated
    C. Cardiology consultation with or without coronary angiography as indicated

III. Metabolic and Endocrine Evaluation
    A. Standard testing includes fasting blood glucose, glycohemoglobin, and fasting lipid panel (cholesterol, triglycerides and HDL-cholesterol)
    B. Fasting and stimulated C-peptide levels are used to assess type of diabetes if needed
    C. Additional studies may include oral or intravenous glucose challenge, anti-insulin and islet cell antibodies, proinsulin level, and lipoprotein profile

IV. Genitourinary/Renal Evaluation
    A. Standard testing includes electrolytes, blood urea nitrogen, serum creatinine, urinalysis with culture, and 24-hour urine for protein and creatinine clearance
    B. Voiding cystourethrogram and urodynamics when indicated
    C. Radiometric glomerular filtration rate if needed
    D. In addition, kidney biopsy, or evaluation of erectile dysfunction may be indicated
    E. Calcineurin inhibitor challenge test when indicated
    F. Hormonal profiles as indicated

V. Serology and Immunology Evaluation
    A. ABO blood type and HLA tissue type
    B. Cytotoxic antibodies
    C. Viral titers (Epstein Barr Virus, Herpes Simplex Virus, Varicella-Zoster virus, Human Immunodeficiency Virus, Hepatitis B virus, Hepatitis C virus, and Cytomegalovirus); PCR quantitation when indicated
    D. VDRL/FTA test for syphilis

VI. Other Laboratory Tests
    A. Complete blood count with differential and platelets, prothrombin time, partial thromboplastin time, chemistry profile, amylase, lipase
    B. Abdominal ultrasound of kidneys and gallbladder
    C. Mammography in females over 35 years
    D. Hemoccult x 3; contrast studies or endoscopy when indicated
    E. When indicated, nerve conduction studies, gastric emptying scan, electromyography
    G. Hypercoagulable work-up (when indicated)

HDL: High Density Lipoprotein
PCR: Polymerase Chain Reaction
VDRL: Venereal Disease Research Laboratory
FTA: Fluorescent Treponemal Antibody

Table 5. Absolute and relative contraindications and risk factors for pancreas transplantation.

I. Absolute Contraindications
   A. Insufficient cardiovascular reserve; one or more of the following:
      1. Coronary angiographic evidence of significant non-correctable or untreatable coronary artery disease
      2. Recent myocardial infarction
      3. Ejection fraction below 30%
   B. Active infection
   C. History of malignancy diagnosed within past 3 years (excluding non-melanoma skin cancer)
   D. Positive HIV serology
   E. Positive Hepatitis B surface antigen serology
   F. Active, untreated peptic ulcer disease
   G. Ongoing substance abuse (drug or alcohol)
   H. Major ongoing psychiatric illness
   I. Recent history of non-compliance
   J. Inability to provide informed consent
   K. Any systemic illness that would severely limit life expectancy or compromise recovery
   L. Significant, irreversible hepatic or pulmonary dysfunction
   M. Positive crossmatch
II. Relative Contraindications
   A. Age less than 18 or greater than 65 years
   B. Recent retinal hemorrhage
   C. Symptomatic cerebrovascular or peripheral vascular disease
   D. Absence of appropriate social support network
   E. Extreme obesity (greater than 150% ideal body weight)
   F. Active smoking
   G. Severe aorto-iliac vascular disease
III. Risk Factors
   A. History of myocardial infarction, congestive heart failure, previous open heart surgery, or cardiac intervention
   B. History of major amputation or peripheral bypass graft
   C. History of cerebrovascular event or carotid endarterectomy
   D. History of hypercoagulable syndrome

HIV: Human Immunodeficiency Virus

assessed carefully because significant (and silent) coronary artery disease is not uncommon in this population (19). The cardiac evaluation consists of a noninvasive functional assessment such as an exercise or pharmacologic stress test in addition to echocardiography (18). Coronary angiography is reserved for specific indications such as age over 45 years, diabetes for more than 25 years, a smoking history, longstanding hypertension, previous major amputation due to peripheral vascular disease, history of cerebrovascular disease, or cases in which the history, physical examination, or noninvasive cardiac studies reveal an abnormality. A history of previous myocardial infarction, angioplasty, stenting, or coronary artery bypass grafting is not necessarily a contraindication for PTX. We have found that pharmacologic stress cardiac imaging is an excellent screening tool, with only about one-third of our evaluants undergoing coronary angiography. However, sudden cardiac death, in the absence of significant structural heart disease, continues to be a major cause of mortality after PTX (20). For this reason, cardiac autonomic function is currently measured by 2 methods; laboratory evoked cardiovascular tests and 24-hour heart rate variability measurements (19-21). These methods are able to detect alterations in autonomic function prior to the onset of disabling symptoms.

Because of the impact that PTX has on quality of life, we are conducting comprehensive, prospective studies examining quality of life changes in this patient population (22-26). The dramatic increase in posttransplant patient and graft survival rates over the last decade has resulted in great interest in quality of life. This is of particular importance for those patients with ESRD and IDDM who not only have symptoms associated with uremia, but complications related to longstanding diabetes. Quality of life is a multi-dimensional construct reflecting an individual's perception of health, well-being, and happiness. Since 1990, UT Memphis has included 3 measurements of quality of life in order to capture as many dimensions as possible. Functional disability is measured by the Sickness Impact Profile (SIP), while a more

a renal allograft, whether from a living or a cadaver donor, are considered potential candidates for PAKT if the creatinine clearance is above 40 ml/min on either cyclosporine (CYA) or tacrolimus (TAC) immunosuppression (Table 3).

The cardiac status of each candidate must be

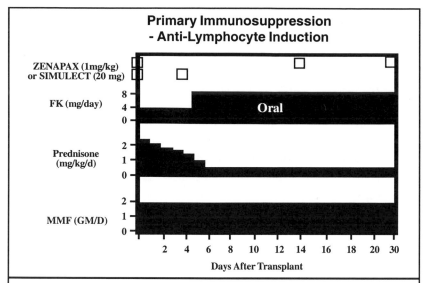

Primary Immunosuppression - Anti-Lymphocyte Induction

Figure 7. Regimen of immunosuppression in Era 3 with selective use of monoclonal antibodies directed against the interleukin-2 receptor (IL2R) as induction therapy. Maintenance immunosuppression was triple therapy with tacrolimus (FK), mycophenolate mofetil (MMF) and steroids.

allograft histopathology (27,31). Renal allograft rejection was suggested by an unexplained rise in serum creatinine of 0.3 mg/dl or greater and confirmed by ultrasound-guided percutaneous biopsy. Because of our concern regarding the ability to diagnose rejection after enteric drainage, we developed a safe outpatient technique of percutaneous pancreas allograft biopsy (27). Pancreas allograft rejection was suggested by an unexplained elevation in serum amylase, lipase, or glucose and confirmed by ultrasound-guided percutaneous biopsy (27,31). Mild renal allograft rejection was treated with intravenous methylprednisolone 500-1,000 mg/day for 3 doses. Anti-lymphocyte therapy with OKT3, ATGAM, or Thymoglobulin for 5-10 days was used as the initial treatment for moderate or severe renal allograft rejection or for any pancreas allograft rejection. Steroid-resistant mild renal allograft rejection was also treated with anti-lymphocyte therapy.

Long-term Follow-up and Statistical Analysis

Long-term posttransplant follow-up is designed to document changes in metabolic and target organ function that could be attributed to the pancreas allograft. To achieve this goal, all pretransplant evaluations were replicated at regular posttransplant intervals. All tests are performed not only for the pancreas recipients but also on a comparable group of diabetic patients who only receive a kidney allograft. This enables us to consider the influence that correction of uremia alone might have on the secondary complications of diabetes.

Data are reported as mean and range. Renal allograft loss was defined as death with function, transplant nephrectomy, return to dialysis or to the pretransplant serum creatinine level. Pancreas graft loss was defined as death with function, transplant pancreatectomy, or the need for daily scheduled insulin therapy.

RESULTS

S-B Versus P-E Drainage

In 1998, we reported our initial experience with 30 SKPTs receiving TAC, MMF, and steroids without ALI (32). Eighteen patients underwent PTX with P-E and 12 with S-B drainage. All patients experienced immediate function of both kidney and pancreas grafts. One-year actuarial patient, kidney, and pancreas graft survival rates were 93%, 93%, and 90%, respectively. Nine patients (30%) had a total of 13 rejection episodes (12 biopsy-proven), including 4 within 2 weeks, 6 between 2 weeks and 3 months, and 3 more than 3 months after SKPT. Three rejection episodes were treated with steroids alone while 10 were treated with anti-lymphocyte therapy (5 OKT3 and 5 ATGAM). A total of 7 patients (23%) received anti-lymphocyte therapy. Three patients (10%) had more than one rejection episode. Two pancreas grafts (7%) and one kidney graft (3%) were lost from rejection. Four patients (13%) developed CMV infection, but none had tissue-invasive CMV disease. At present, 22 patients with excellent dual graft function (81%) remain on triple immunosuppression with TAC, MMF and prednisone. In this study, the death-censored kidney and pancreas graft survival rates were 96% and 93%, respectively. The preliminary results of this study suggested that TAC, MMF and steroid immunosuppression without ALI is safe and effective after SKPT.

In 2000, Lo, et al, studied long-term outcomes in 45

Table 7. Patient characteristics.

	Portal-Enteric (All)	Portal-Enteric (CsA subgroup)	Systemic-Bladder	P*
Number of patients	26	14	19	
Duration of follow-up (years)	5.9 ± 2.0	6.3 ± 0.8	7.8 ± 2.8	
Demographics				
Mean Age (years)	37 ± 7	35 ± 1	39 ± 6	NS
Male	15 (58%)	6 (43%)	8 (42%)	NS
African-American	1 (4%)	1 (7%)	2 (11%)	NS
Caucasian	25 (96%)	13 (93%)	17 (89%)	NS
Pre-transplant characteristics				
Dialysis				
Pretransplant dialysis (months)	15 ± 11	12 ± 7	32 ± 64	0.12
Hemodialysis	7 (25%)	3 (22%)	9 (46%)	NS
Peritoneal dialysis	9 (35%)	3 (22%)	6 (33%)	NS
Dialysis independent	10 (40%)	8 (56%)	4 (21%)	NS
Hemoglobin A_1C (%)pretransplant	8.2 ± 1.6	7.4 ± 1.6	7.1 ± 1.0	NS
Insulin requirement per 24 hours (units)	42 ± 17	42 ± 18	45 ± 28	NS
Diabetic Complications				
Coronary artery disease	5 (19%)	4 (29%)	2 (11%)	NS
Cerebrovascular disease	3 (12%)	1 (7%)	0 (0%)	NS
Peripheral vascular disease	11 (42%)	3 (21%)	6 (29%)	NS
Retinopathy	17 (65%)	8 (57%)	11 (56%)	NS
Legally blind	3 (11%)	2 (14%)	0 (0%)	
Immunosuppression				
OKT3 Induction	26 (100%)	14 (100%)	19 (100%)	
Tacrolimus	12 (48%)	0 (0%)	0 (0%)	
Cyclosporine (Sandimmune)	15 (52%)	14 (100%)	19 (100%)	
Azathioprine	26 (100%)	14 (100%)	19 (100%)	
Prednisone	26 (100%)	14 (100%)	19 (100%)	

*Comparing P-E (n=26) vs S-B (n=19)

SKPT recipients at our center, including 26 with P-E and 19 with S-B drainage (37). All patients were alive with functioning kidney and pancreas grafts at one year after SKPT and had a minimum follow-up of 3.5 years (mean 5.9 years). Demographic, immunologic, and transplant characteristics were similar between the P-E and S-B groups (Table 7). All patients received OKT3 for induction, and Azathioprine and prednisone as maintenance immunosuppression. In the P-E group, 48% of the patients received TAC and 52% received CYA-Sandimmune-based therapy. In the S-B group, all of the patients received CYA, but 10% of the patients were switched to TAC at a mean of 2 years after transplantation. At 5 years, there were no differences in the actual patient, kidney, and pancreas graft survival rates between the P-E and S-B groups; 92% versus 84%, 81% versus 79%, and 88% versus 74%, respectively (P=NS) (Table 8). The 10-year actuarial patient, kidney, and pancreas graft survival rates in the P-E group were 74%, 50%, and 53%, respectively, compared with 37%, 31%, and 32%, in the S-B group, respectively.

During the first posttransplant year, patients in the S-B group had more readmissions, including more readmissions for urinary tract infections and dehydration. Renal and pancreas functions remained stable and comparable between the 2 groups. Patients in the S-B group received fewer anti-hypertensive agents than patients in the P-E group. At 5 years, patients in the P-E group

Table 8. Results.

	Portal-Enteric (All)	Portal-Enteric (CsA subgroup)	Systemic-Bladder	*P**
Number of patients	26	14	19	
5-Year Actual Survival				
Patient Survival	92%	93%	84%	NS
Kidney Graft Survival	81%	79%	79%	NS
Pancreas Graft Survival	88%	85%	74%	NS
10-Year Actuarial Survival				
Patient Survival	74%	74%	37%	0.43
Kidney Graft Survival	50%	33%	31%	0.04
Pancreas Graft Survival	53%	56%	32%	0.09
Hospitalization				
During the first year				
Number of re-admissions/patient	1.7	3.3	3.2	0.03
Duration of hospital re-admission	7 days	4 days	4 days	0.09
Reasons for re-admission				
Infection	29%	29%	32%	NS
(Urinary Tract Infection)	(11%)	(7%)	(32%)	0.09
Rejection	13%	21%	11%	NS
Elective Surgery	11%	21%	13%	NS
Dehydration	7%	7%	16%	<0.01
Renal and Pancreas functions at 5 years				
Serum Creatinine (mg/dL)	1.6 ± 0.6	1.6 ± 0.6	1.9 ± 0.8	NS
Hemoglobin A1C (%)	6.0 ± 0.9	5.7 ± 0.5	5.6 ± 0.7	NS
Cardiovascular endpoints at 5 years				
Total Cholesterol (mg/dL)	199	192	192	NS
Systolic blood pressure (mm Hg)	137	137	135	NS
Number of anti-hypertensive agents/patient	1.7	1.4	1.0	NS
Weight (Kg)				
Pre-transplant	68 ± 14	65 ± 14	68 ± 12	NS
At 5 years post-transplant	66 ± 17	67 ± 19	$74 \pm 15^{**}$	NS

* Comparing P-E (n=26) vs S-B (n=19)

** In S-B group, the posttransplant weight change was significant when compared with pretransplant values; p=0.03.

experienced a slight decline in body weight. In contrast, patients in the S-B group had a significant increase in weight over time. At 3 years, 53% of the patients in the S-B group reported no activity limitation compared with 76% in the P-E group (P=0.11). Irrespective of surgical technique, more patients reported no activity limitations after transplantation than before their transplant. Improved quality of life was reported in all but one of the scales, with many dimensions showing a significant improvement. At the end of follow-up, stabilization in microvascular complications including retinopathy, peripheral neuropathy, and autonomic function were reported in both groups of patients. The results of this study suggested trends toward better patient and graft survival, fewer metabolic complications, less morbidity, and improved quality of life in the P-E group when compared with the S-B group long term.

S-E Versus P-E Drainage

As the number of PTXs with enteric drainage has

Table 9. Demographic and transplant characteristics.

	S-E: (n=27)	P-E: (n=27)
Age (years)	40.6 (27-57)	39.2 (26-58)
Gender:		
Male	19 (70%)	16 (59%)
Female	8 (30%)	11 (41%)
Weight (kg)	73.9 (45-103)	73.3 (49-95)
Race:		
Caucasian	22 (81%)	18 (67%)
African-American	4 (15%)	9 (33%)
Asian	1 (4%)	0
Pre-Transplant Dialysis: #	21 (78%)	18 (67%)
Duration (months)	16 (5-36)	13 (1-46)
Peritoneal Dialysis	7 (26%)	10 (37%)
Hemodialysis	14 (52%)	8 (30%)
None	6 (22%)	9 (33%)
Hepatitis C Positive	2 (7%)	1 (4%)
Years of Diabetes	24 (4-50)	23.2 (9-46)
Type 2 Diabetes	4 (15%)	2 (7%)
Daily Insulin Dose (U/day)	38 (15-80)	44 (15-80)
Prior Kidney Transplant	2 (7%)	3 (11%)
PRA >10%	2 (7%)	2 (7%)
HLA-Match: ABDR	1.4 (0-4)	1.4 (0-4)
HLA-Mismatch	4.6 (2-6)	4.6 (2-6)
CMV D+/R-	7 (26%)	5 (19%)
Cold Ischemia (hours):		
Kidney	14.3 (8-23)	15.1 (9.5-2.6)
Pancreas	14.2 (7.5-22.5)	15.3 (10.5-23)
Waiting Time (months)	2.8 (0.1-7)	3 (0.25-8.5)
Immunosuppression; FK, MMF, steroids +:		
No Antibody Induction	17 (63%)	12 (44%)
Daclizumab	6 (22%)	8 (30%)
Basiliximab	4 (15%)	5 (19%)
Thymoglobulin	0	2 (7%)

Mean (Range), P=NS
D: Donor, R: Recipient, FK: Tacrolimus,
MMF: Mycophenolate Mofetil, CMV: Cytomegalovirus
PRA: Panel Reactive Antibody
HLA: Human Leukocyte Antigen

Table 10. Results.

	S-E: (n=27)	P-E: (n=27)
Patient Survival	25 (93%)	26 (96%)
Graft Survival: Kidney	25 (93%)	25 (93%)
Pancreas	20 (74%)	23 (85%)
Follow-up (months)	17.4 (5-30)	17 (5-29)
ATN (post-op dialysis)	1 (4%)	2 (7%)
Early Technical Problems	3 (11%)	2 (7%)
Initial Hospital Stay (days)	12.4 (7-30)	12.8 (7-38)
Initial Hospital Charges ($)	102,255	105,789
Re-admissions	2.8 (0-10)	2.2 (0-10)
No Re-admissions	8 (30%)	5 (19%)
Acute Rejection	9 (33%)	9 (33%)
Anti-T Cell Therapy	4 (15%)	6 (22%)
Immunologic Pancreas		
Graft Loss	3 (11%)	1 (4%)
Early Relaparotomy		
(<3 months)	8 (30%)	7 (26%)
Pancreas Thrombosis	2 (7%)	1 (4%)
Major Infection	14 (52%)	14 (52%)
CMV Infection	1 (4%)	1 (4%)
Intra-Abdominal Infection	7 (26%)	3 (11%)
Total Hospital Days	33 (9-160)	24 (8-92)
Event-Free Survival (No Rejection,		
Graft Loss, or Death)	15 (56%)	16 (59%)

Mean (Range), P=NS

steadily increased, we decided to compare SKPT with S-E versus P-E drainage in a prospective fashion with standardized immunosuppression (14). During a 26-month period from April 1998 through May 2000, 54 consecutive SKPT recipients were entered into a prospective study of S-E (n=27) vs. P-E (n= 27) drainage. The technique to be performed was chosen before the transplant with selection determined by an alternating methodology. The 2 groups were well matched for most donor and recipient demographic, immunologic, and transplant characteristics (Table 9). The racial distribution differed slightly, with African-American patients representing 15% of the S-E and 33% of the P-E group. With regard to immunosuppression, 63% of S-E and 44% of P-E patients were managed with no antibody induction. The remaining S-E patients received either Daclizumab or Basiliximab induction, while the P-E patients received Daclizumab, Basiliximab, or Thymoglobulin in 2 patients with acute tubular necrosis (ATN). Maintenance immunosuppression in both groups consisted of TAC, MMF, and steroids.

Results are depicted in Table 10. Patient survival rates were 93% S-E versus 96% P-E, while kidney graft survival rates were 93% in both groups. PTX survival (complete insulin independence) was 74% after S-E versus 85% after P-E drainage, with a mean follow-up of 17 months. All but 3 of the 54 transplanted renal allografts had immediate function. ATN, defined as the need for dialysis in the first week after transplant, occurred in one patient after S-E and 2 patients after P-E drainage. All 3 of these kidneys eventually functioned. All 54 transplanted pancreas allografts had initial function, although 3 were subsequently lost to thrombosis in the first week after transplant. The incidence of allograft pancreatitis, early leaks, and other technical problems related to the pancreas allograft were similar between groups.

The mean length of initial hospital stay was 12.4 days in the S-E and 12.8 days in the P-E groups, respectively. Mean initial hospital charges were comparable between groups. The S-E group was characterized by a slight increase in the number of readmissions (mean 2.8 S-E vs. 2.2 P-E; P=NS) and total hospital days (mean 33 days S-E vs. 24 days P-E; P=NS). The incidence of acute rejection was similar (33%) in both groups, with immunologic pancreas graft loss occurring in 3 S-E patients versus one P-E patient. The incidence of major infection was 52% in both groups, with one CMV infection (4%) in each group. The incidence of intra-abdominal infection was slightly higher in the S-E group (26% S-E vs. 11% P-E; P=NS). However, the early relaparotomy rate was similar between groups (30% S-E vs. 26% P-E). The composite endpoint of no rejection, graft loss, or death was attained by 56% of S-E and 59% of P-E patients (Table 10). These results suggested that SKPT with S-E or P-E drainage could be performed with comparable short-term outcomes.

Overall Results

From October 1990 through December 1999, we performed 126 PTXs with P-E drainage (Fig. 5), including 90 SKPTs and 36 solitary PTXs (18 PAKT, 18 PA) (38). The P-E group included 69 male and 57 female patients with a mean age of 39 years (Table 11). The mean duration of pretransplant diabetes was 24 years (range 8-50). The majority of recipients were Caucasian, although 15 (12%) were African-American recipients. A total of 13 patients (10%) underwent pancreas re-transplantation with the P-E technique. The majority of patients had poor HLA matching (mean 1.4, range 0-5), and the mean pancreas cold ischemia was 13 hours (range 6-23). Minimum follow-up was 11 months (mean 4.6 years).

Table 11. Demographic and transplant characteristics.	
N	126
Age (Years)	39 (Range 19-56)
Gender: Female	57 (45%)
Male	69 (55%)
Race: Caucasian	111 (88%)
African-American	15 (12%)
Years of Diabetes	24 (Range 8-50)
Transplant Type: SKPT	90 (72%)
PAKT	18 (14%)
PA	18 (14%)
Prior PTX	13 (10%)
HLA-Match: ABDR	1.4 (Range 0-5)
Pancreas Cold Ischemia (Hrs)	13 (Range 6-23)
Mean (Range)	
HLA: Human Leukocyte Antigen	

Thirty patients underwent SKPT with P-E drainage in Era 1 and were compared with 42 SKPTs performed in Era 2 and 18 in Era 3 (Table 6). The patients in Era 1 were managed with CYA while those in Eras 2 and 3 received TAC/MMF. We also compared 23 solitary PTXs (11 PAKT, 12 PA) performed in Era 2 with 13 (7 PAKT, 6 PA) performed in Era 3 (Fig. 5). One-year patient survival rates after SKPT (Fig. 8) were 77% in Era 1, 93% in Era 2, and 100% in Era 3 (P=0.03). The one-year kidney graft survival rates were 77% in Era 1, 93% in Era 2, and 94% in Era 3 (P=0.08). The one-year pancreas graft survival rates after SKPT (Fig. 8) were 60% in Era 1, and 83% both in Eras 2 and 3 (P=0.06). The most common causes of kidney graft loss were death with function and chronic rejection (Table 12). The overall incidence of kidney graft loss decreased from 56% in Era 1 to 23% in Era 2 to 11% in Era 3 (P<0.001). The most common causes of pancreas graft loss were thrombosis, death with function, chronic rejection, and infection (Table 13). The overall incidence of pancreas graft loss decreased from 60% in Era 1 to 31% in Era 2 to 22% in Era 3 (P<0.001).

The incidences of rejection (63% vs. 33% vs. 39%; P<0.001) and major infection (60% vs. 43% vs. 44%; P=NS) after SKPT were decreased in each successive era (Fig. 9). The rates of thrombosis (20% vs. 7% vs. 6%; P<0.001) and early relaparotomy (47% vs. 31% vs. 33%; P=NS) after SKPT were also decreased in each consecutive era (Fig. 10).

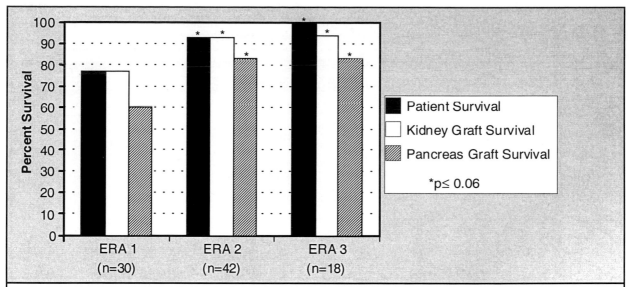

Figure 8. One-year patient and graft survival rates after SKPT according to immunosuppressive era.

Table 12. Results (SKPT).

	Era 1 (n=30)	Era 2 (n=42)	Era 3 (n=18)	P Value
One-year survival:				
Patient	23 (77%)	39 (93%)	18 (100%)	0.03
Kidney	23 (77%)	39 (93%)	17 (94%)	0.08
Pancreas	18 (60%)	35 (83%)	15 (83%)	0.06
Acute rejection	19 (63%)	14 (33%)	7 (39%)	< 0.001
Major infection	18 (60%)	18 (43%)	8 (44%)	NS
Thrombosis	6 (20%)	3 (7%)	1 (6%)	< 0.001
Relaparotomy	14 (47%)	13 (31%)	6 (33%)	NS
Overall graft loss:				
Kidney	17 (56%)	10 (23%)	2 (11%)	< 0.001
Pancreas	18 (60%)	13 (31%)	4 (22%)	< 0.001
Causes of kidney graft loss:				
DWFG	7 (23%)	5 (12%)	1 (5.5%)	< 0.001
Chronic rejection	4 (13%)	3 (7%)	1 (5.5%)	NS
Infection	2 (7%)	1 (2%)	0	NS
Acute rejection	1 (3%)	0	0	NS
PTLD	2 (7%)	1 (2%)	0	NS
Thrombosis	1 (3%)	0	0	NS
Causes of pancreas graft loss:				
Thrombosis	6 (20%)	3 (7%)	1 (5.5%)	< 0.001
DWFG	5 (17%)	2 (5%)	1 (5.5%)	< 0.001
Chronic rejection	1 (3%)	5 (12%)	1 (5.5%)	NS
Infection	3 (10%)	1 (2%)	1 (5.5%)	NS
PTLD	2 (7%)	1 (2%)	0	NS
Acute rejection	1 (3%)	1 (2%)	0	NS

DWFG: Death with functioning graft
PTLD: Posttransplant lymphoproliferative disease

The one-year patient survival rates after solitary PTX were both 100% in Eras 2 and 3, while the corresponding pancreas graft survival rates were 61% and 69%, respectively (Table 13). The most common causes of graft loss after solitary PTX were thrombosis and chronic rejection. The overall incidence of pancreas graft loss after solitary PTX decreased from 70% in Era 2 to 31% in Era 3 (P=0.02). The rates of acute rejection (57% vs. 38%), major infection (35% vs. 31%), thrombosis (22% vs. 15%), and relaparotomy (43% vs. 38%) after solitary PTX were all slightly improved in Era 3 compared with Era 2 (P=NS). This overall experience demonstrates that SKPT and solitary PTX with P-E drainage can be performed with improving outcomes. Increasing experience with the P-E technique coupled with advances in immunosuppression are associated with: (1) increasing patient, kidney, and pancreas graft survival rates; (2) less medical morbidity with a decreasing incidence of acute rejection and major infection; and (3) reduced surgical complications including decreasing rates of thrombosis and relaparotomy. The P-E technique does not appear to incur any additional or unique risks, and can be performed with results comparable to the other standard techniques of PTX. We believe that this technique should be included in the repertoire of PTX, because it offers potential physiologic, metabolic, and immunologic advantages over the other techniques currently available.

Metabolic, Physiologic, Quality of Life, and Long-term Outcomes

With the improving short-term success of PTX, long-term prognosis after the first year is excellent and at least provides the potential for stabilization of diabetic complications. We retrospectively reviewed remote SKPT recipients with P-E drainage; 26 patients (65%) were alive with functioning grafts one year after SKPT and were followed for a minimum of 3 years (mean 5 years) (39). Hospital admissions decreased significantly from a mean of 2.4 admissions per patient in the first year to 0.6 by year 4. Mean systolic blood pressure and diastolic blood pressure fell to 132 mm Hg (P=0.02) and 80 mm Hg (P=0.02) at one year after SKPT, respectively, and remained stable thereafter. The daily mean Prednisone dose decreased by 23% at 3 years, but CYA and TAC doses remained stable. Patients showed a gain in weight from a mean of 68.2 kg at SKPT to 77.3 kg at year 4 (P=0.02). Fasting serum glucose fell to 85 mg/dl at year one (P<0.01) and remained stable thereafter. Glycosylated hemoglobin levels decreased to 6.0% at one-year after SKPT (P<0.05) and 5.8% at year 4. Serum creatinine was 1.6 mg/dl at year one and 1.8 mg/dl at year 4 (P= NS). Total cholesterol remained stable over 4 years

(mean 206 mg/dl, HDL >50) but mean triglycerides decreased over time from 224-182 mg/dl at year 4. At one year after transplantation, improvements in most diabetic complications were noted. No activity limitations were reported in 80% of patients at one year after SKPT compared with 23% before transplant. Four quality-of-life

Table 13. Results (Solitary PTX).

	Era 2 (n=23)	Era 3 (n=13)	P Value
PAKT	11 (48%)	7 (54%)	NS
PA	12 (52%)	6 (46%)	NS
One-year survival:			
Patient	23 (100%)	13 (100%)	NS
Pancreas	14 (61%)	9 (69%)	NS
Acute rejection	13 (57%)	5 (38%)	NS
Major infection	8 (35%)	4 (31%)	NS
Thrombosis	5 (22%)	2 (15%)	NS
Relaparotomy	10 (43%)	5 (38%)	NS
Overall pancreas graft loss	16 (70%)	4 (31%)	0.02
Causes of graft loss:			
Thrombosis	5 (22%)	2 (15%)	NS
Chronic rejection	4 (17%)	2 (15%)	NS
Infection/PTLD	3 (13%)	0	NS
Acute rejection	2 (9%)	0	NS
Primary non-function	1 (4%)	0	NS
DWFG	1 (4%)	0	NS

DWFG: Death with functioning graft
PTLD: Posttransplant lymphoproliferative disease

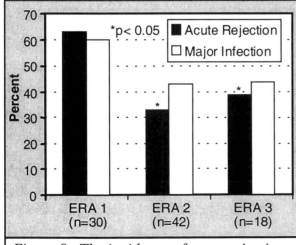

Figure 9. The incidence of acute rejection in Eras 1, 2 and 3.

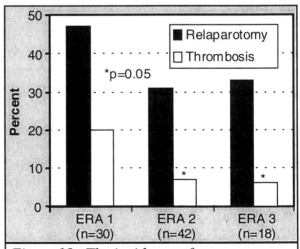

Figure 10. The incidence of pancreas allograft thrombosis in Eras 1, 2 and 3.

surveys that provided 29 scores were completed 6-24 months (mean 18 months) after SKPT. Improved quality of life was reported in all but one of the scales. Actual patient, kidney, and pancreas graft survival rates were 92%, 81%, and 89%, respectively. These results demonstrated that SKPT with P-E drainage is a safe and effective method to treat advanced diabetic nephropathy and is associated with decreasing morbidity, improving rehabilitation and quality of life, and stable metabolic function over time.

In addition to correcting dysmetabolism and freeing the patient from exogenous insulin therapy, data are emerging on the course of secondary diabetic complications after PTX. Besides our work on procedure development and describing the diagnosis of rejection and management strategies, members of our group have published significant work regarding various physiologic, metabolic, and quality-of-life outcomes (19-26).

We demonstrated a decline in the incidence of rejection and graft loss to rejection with P-E drainage in the CYA era (35). This has led to significant interest in research related to portal antigen delivery and its effect on tolerance. In addition to describing utilization of intravenous glucose tolerance as a non-invasive marker for rejection (36), we examined determinants of altered glucose tolerance with TAC immunosuppression in P-E recipients (40). In 1995, Hughes, et al, analyzed lipoprotein profiles in 31 SKPT recipients at our center, including 20 with S-B and 11 with P-E drainage (41). By 6 and 12 months after PTX, patients with P-E drainage experienced a significant improvement in lipoprotein profiles and particle composition that was not seen in patients with S-B drainage. This data was further supported by our collaborative work with Bagdade, et al (42). Also in 1995, El-Gebely, et al, analyzed renal function 2 years after transplant in SKPT and diabetic KTA recipients at our center (43). The KTA recipients experienced a mild but significant deterioration in the serum creatinine coincident with the development of microalbuminuria after 2 years, findings that were not observed in SKPT patients despite significantly higher CYA levels in the latter.

In a study of 28 SKPT and 20 KTA recipients with IDDM, Nymann, et al, from our group reported improvements in motor nerve conduction and sensory nerve amplitude that were exclusive to the SKPT group (44). Although we noted a transitory, beneficial effect of reversal of uremia by KTA on motor nerve conduction in the first 12 months after transplant, only SKPT recipients continued to experience improvement in nerve conduction over time.

Chronic hyperglycemia has been associated with depressed myocardial contractility independent of the effects of hypertension, coronary disease, or renal function. Gaber, et al, compared echocardiographic parameters in 20 SKPT, 2 PAKT, and 11 diabetic KTA recipients at 6 and 12 months follow-up (45). In the KTA group, systolic function improved at 6 months and remained stable thereafter. In comparison, a significant improvement in all echocardiographic measures (systolic function, diastolic function, left ventricular geometry) occurred at 6 and 12 months after SKPT. Moreover, the improvements that occurred in all echocardiographic measures represented a restoration of normal cardiac function in most SKPT recipients. A follow-up study from our group by Wicks, et al, documented sustained improvements in cardiac function at 24 months after SKPT (46).

Autonomic neuropathy is one consequence of IDDM that has been associated with severe morbidity and mortality (19-26). Both uremia and diabetes cause autonomic dysfunction leading to symptoms that can greatly compromise quality of life (19-22). Autonomic function is currently measured by 2 methods at our center; laboratory evoked cardiovascular tests and 24-hour rate variability measurement. The evoked cardiovascular tests, which include change in heart rate with deep respiration and Valsalva ratio, are performed in a temperature controlled laboratory equipped with computer, data acquisition, and analysis systems to obtain heart rate and blood pressure responsiveness to postural and respiratory maneuvers. Heart rate variability is measured by 24-hour Holter monitoring, with oscillations in R-R intervals examined in both time and frequency domains. Two of the 3 time domains reflect circadian rhythmicity, with one of these domains being closely associated with cardiac death. The remaining time domain reflects vagal function and is virtually independent of circadian rhythm. The frequency domains estimate parasympathetic and sympathetic control of the variations in the R-R intervals. We have had the unique opportunity to examine the association between quality of life and biologic outcomes longitudinally as well as constructing study designs to determine the degree to which these constructs are correlated and the relative contribution of biologic outcomes to overall quality of life (22-26).

Gaber, et al, compared autonomic function in SKPT versus diabetic KTA recipients at 6 and 12 months follow-up (25). Several parameters were tested to generate an autonomic index or composite autonomic score. These parameters included tests of vasomotor function (total capillary pulse amplitude, reflex vasoconstriction, postural adjustment ratio), cardiorespiratory reflexes, and gastric function. We noted an improvement in nearly all of these autonomic parameters after SKPT versus KTA, although the differences were not always significant. In the one parameter that did not change (R-R respiratory interval variation), stabilization occurred after SKPT whereas continued progression occurred after KTA.

Hathaway, et al, from our group demonstrated improvement in the Valsalva ratio but not in the electrocardiographically derived R-R interval respiratory variation after PTX (22). In spite of the improvement in cardiac autonomic function following SKPT, sudden cardiac death continues to be a concern in this population. We evaluated 5 otherwise healthy diabetic transplant recipients (3 SKPT, 2 KTA) who experienced sudden cardiac death and compared their laboratory evoked cardiac autonomic responses with those in a group of surviving diabetic transplant recipients (n=26) (20). Autonomic function was also compared with the patients with diabetes who had sudden cardiac death prior to receiving a transplant (n=5). Of those patients who died while waiting, 4 of the 5 had extremely compromised Valsalva ratios. Sixteen surviving diabetic patients showed improvement in the Valsalva ratio from before to after transplant. Patients with transplants who experienced sudden cardiac death demonstrated no improvement in the Valsalva ratio. While the study could not categorically state that impaired Valsalva ratio was indicative of a poor transplant outcome, it did suggest that an abnormal Valsalva ratio might become a marker for patients who could be at potential risk for sudden cardiac death, particularly in the absence of improvement after successful transplantation.

We also analyzed laboratory evoked cardiovascular responses as well as 24-hour heart rate variability in non-diabetic and diabetic KTA and SKPT recipients (21,26). The non-diabetic KTA recipients displayed the least improvement in heart rate variability, however, their values were not as severely compromised pretransplant and therefore we were unable to show much improvement. By 12 months after transplant, most measures of heart rate variability for the non-diabetic KTA recipients had, in fact, reached values that approached those seen in healthy adults. Although the number of diabetic KTA recipients was small, it is interesting to note that the heart

rate variability actually continued to decline somewhat in this group. This is in contrast to SKPT recipients who, following a slight decline in some measures at 6 months, showed improvement in heart rate variability at 12 months. Exercise has been associated with improved heart rate variability in a normal male population. We were able to demonstrate that those patients with diabetes who exercised regularly had significantly better heart rate variability than non-exercising diabetic individuals. This finding led us to initiate a prospective study of exercise on heart rate variability in both diabetic and non-diabetic KTA and SKPT recipients.

Improvement in quality of life is one of the major goals of PTX. Current data documents the presence of poor overall quality of life in patients with diabetes as compared with their non-diabetic counterparts. It is interesting to note that the baseline quality of life reported for our more recent diabetic patients has generally improved from previous reports (22-26). We could only surmise that advances in medical care (erythropoietin) and/or earlier transplant referral may have influenced this outcome. When comparing SKPT to non-diabetic KTA recipients, patients with pretransplant diabetes had a poorer quality of life in 2 of 5 measures, primarily reflecting greater physical dysfunction and a less positive view of their overall health. Following transplantation, quality of life improved in 4 of the 5 categories for both groups. However, at 24 months, a lingering disparity was still noted between diabetic KTA and SKPT recipients with respect to physical function and overall health perspective.

Numerous studies have demonstrated that a successful SKPT results in improvements in physical function, activities and daily living, energy level, mobility, vocational rehabilitation, social well-being, communication, role function, health perception, health-image, pyschologic function, future expectations, sense of well-being, overall satisfaction, diet flexibility, diabetes-related concerns, time to manage health, health impact on family, and autonomy (23,24). The major benefits of PTX are an enhanced quality of life characterized by the following: 1) rehabilitation to "normal" living with physical, social, and psychological well-being with near normal activities and daily living and a self perception of normality; 2) global improvement in quality of life with the perception of being healthy and having control over one's destiny; and 3) fewer restrictions and enhanced capacities leading to an improved sense of well-being and independence. Freedom from daily insulin injections and blood glucose monitoring are important advantages in patients with a successful PTX. Although the long-term commitment to immunosuppression is the major trade-off, most patients with diabetes find the transition of transplantation easier than continued insulin therapy because of an improved sense of well-being with fewer dietary and activity restrictions. With the increasing short- and long-term success of PTX, the emphasis has shifted from survival outcomes to health-related quality of life.

Because transplant recipients are living longer, interest in long-term quality-of-life outcomes is emerging. Given the projection that many recipients will live well into the second decade following transplantation, it is important to know that some forms of neuropathy continue to demonstrate improvements in these later years, that neuropathy is associated with mortality as well as quality of life in the transplant population (22-26), and that some interventions may be available to improve neuropathy in the long term. Therefore, it seems apparent that well-designed, longitudinal studies are needed not only to assess quantity but quality of life as well as physiologic function.

SUMMARY

The UT Memphis group has made a number of important contributions to the field of PTX, including: 1) pioneering studies on the effects of PTX on autonomic neuropathy, 2) comprehensive reports dealing with quality of life after PTX, 3) seminal studies on the metabolic effects of PTX with portal venous delivery of insulin, 4) refining and perfecting a novel technique of PTX with portal venous drainage of insulin and primary enteric drainage of the exocrine secretions, 5) describing a safe outpatient percutaneous technique of pancreas allograft biopsy, 6) developing the use of glucose tolerance for rejection surveillance, and 7) managing PTX patients with biopsy-directed immuno-suppression and no anti-lymphocyte induction therapy.

The P-E technique has the potential to become the standard of care in the near future because it is more physiologic, normalizes carbohydrate and lipid metabolism, and minimizes complications attributed to the transplant procedure. In addition, we have been actively involved in studying new immunosuppressive regimens in order to improve and simplify the care of the PTX recipient. We believe that PTX will remain an important treatment option for IDDM until other strategies are developed that can provide equal glycemic control with less or no immunosuppression and less overall morbidity.

PANCREAS – MEMPHIS, TENNESSEE

ABBREVIATIONS:

ALI:	Anti-lymphocyte Induction
ATN:	Acute Tubular Necrosis
CMV:	Cytomegalovirus
CYA:	Cyclosporine
ESRD:	End Stage Renal Disease
HIV:	Human Immunodeficiency Virus
HLA:	Human Leukocyte Antigen
IDDM:	Insulin Dependent Diabetes Mellitus
IPTR:	International Pancreas Transplant Registry
KTA:	Kidney Transplant Alone
MMF:	Mycophenolate Mofetil

PA:	Pancreas Alone
PAKT:	Pancreas After Kidney Transplant
P-E:	Portal-Enteric
PRA:	Panel Reactive Antibody
PTX:	Pancreas Transplant
S-B:	Systemic-Bladder
S-E:	Systemic-Enteric
SKPT:	Simultaneous Kidney-Pancreas Transplant
TAC:	Tacrolimus
UNOS:	United Network for Organ Sharing
UT:	University of Tennessee

REFERENCES

1. Sutherland DER, Gruessner AC. International Pancreas Transplant Registry Update. IPTR Newsletter 2000; 12:1.

2. Gruessner AC, Sutherland DER. Analyses of pancreas transplant outcomes for United States cases reported to the United Network for Organ Sharing (UNOS) and non-US cases reported to the International Pancreas Transplant Registry (IPTR). In: JM Cecka, PI Terasaki, Eds. Clinical Transplants 1999. Los Angeles, UCLA Immunogenetics Center, 2000; 51.

3. Sindhi R, Stratta RJ, Lowell JA, et al. Experience with enteric conversion after pancreas transplantation with bladder drainage. J Am Coll Surg 1997; 184:281.

4. Shokouh-Amiri MH, Gaber AO, Gaber LW, et al. Pancreas transplantation with portal venous drainage and enteric exocrine diversion: A new technique. Transplant Proc 1992; 24:776.

5. Gaber AO, Shokouh-Amiri H, Grewal HP, Britt LG. A technique for portal pancreatic transplantation with enteric drainage. Surg Gynecol Obstet 1993; 177:417.

6. Gaber AO, Shokouh-Amiri H, Hathaway DK, et al. Pancreas transplantation with portal venous and enteric drainage eliminates hyperinsulinemia and reduces post-operative complications. Transplant Proc 1993; 25:1176.

7. Di Carlo V, Castoldi R, Cristallo M, et al. Techniques of pancreas transplantation through the world: An IPITA center survey. Transplant Proc 1998; 30:231.

8. Shokouh-Amiri MH, Rahimi-Saber S, Andersen AJ. Segmental pancreatic autotransplantation in the pig. Transplantation 1989; 47:42.

9. Shokouh-Amiri MH, Falholt K, Holst JJ, et al. Pancreas endocrine function in pigs after segmental pancreas autotransplantation with either systemic or portal venous drainage. Transplant Proc 1992; 24:799.

10. Shokouh-Amiri MH, Rahimi-Saber S, Anderson HO, Jensen SL. Pancreas autotransplantation in pig with systemic or portal venous drainage: Effect on the endocrine pancreatic function after transplantation. Transplantation 1996; 61:1004.

11. Gaber AO, Shokouh-Amiri MH, Hathaway DK, et al. Results of pancreas transplantation with portal venous and enteric drainage. Ann Surg 1995; 221:613.

12. Stratta RJ, Gaber AO, Shokouh-Amiri MH, et al. A prospective comparison of systemic-bladder versus portal-enteric drainage in vascularized pancreas transplantation. Surgery 2000; 127:217.

13. Stratta RJ, Gaber AO, Shokouh-Amiri MH, et al. Experience with portal-enteric pancreas transplant at the University of Tennessee-Memphis. In: JM Cecka, PI Terasaki, Eds. Clinical Transplants 1998. Los Angeles, UCLA Tissue Typing Laboratory, 1999; 239.

14. Stratta RJ, Shokouh-Amiri MH, Egidi MF, et al. Simultaneous kidney-pancreas transplant with systemic-enteric versus portal-enteric drainage. Transplant Proc (in press).

15. Nymann T, Elmer DS, Shokouh-Amiri MH, Gaber AO. Improved outcome of patients with portal-enteric pancreas transplantation. Transplant Proc 1997; 29:637.

16. Eubanks JW, Shokouh-Amiri MH, Elmer D, Hathaway D, Gaber AO. Solitary pancreas transplantation using the portal-enteric technique. Transplant Proc 1998; 30:446.

17. Grewal HP, Garland L, Novak K, et al. Risk factors for post-implantation pancreatitis and pancreatic thrombosis in pancreas transplant recipients. Transplantation 1993; 56:609.

18. Stratta RJ, Taylor RJ, Gill IS. Pancreas transplantation: A managed cure approach to diabetes. Curr Prob Surgery 1996; 33:709.

19. Hathaway DK, Cashion AK, Milstead EJ, et al. Autonomic dysregulation in patients awaiting kidney transplantation. Am J Kidney Dis 1998; 32:221.

20. Hathaway DK, El-Gebely S, Cardoso S, et al. Autonomic cardiac dysfunction in diabetic transplant recipients succumbing to sudden cardiac death. Transplantation 1995; 59:634.

21. Cashion AK, Hathaway DK, Milstead EJ, Reed L, Gaber AO. Changes in patterns of 24-hour heart rate variability after kidney and kidney-pancreas transplant. Transplantation 1999; 68:1846.

22. Hathaway DK, Abell T, Cardoso S, et al. Improvement in autonomic and gastric function following pancreas-kidney versus kidney-alone transplantation and the correlation with quality of life. Transplantation 1994; 57:816.

23. Hathaway DK, Hartwig MS, Milstead J, et al. A prospective study of changes in quality of life reported by diabetic recipients of kidney-only and pancreas-kidney allografts. J Transplant Coord 1994; 4:12.

24. Hathaway DK, Hartwig MS, Crom DB, Gaber AO. Identification of quality of life outcomes distinguishing diabetic kidney-alone and pancreas-kidney recipients. Transplant Proc 1995; 27:3065.

25. Gaber AO, Hathaway DK, Abell T, et al. Improved autonomic and gastric function in pancreas-kidney versus kidney-alone transplantation contributes to quality of life. Transplant Proc 1994; 26:515.

26. Hathaway DK, Wicks MN, Cashion AK, et al. Heart rate variability and quality of life following kidney and kidney-pancreas transplantation. Transplant Proc 1999; 31:643.

27. Gaber AO, Gaber LW, Shokouh-Amiri MH, Hathaway D. Percutaneous biopsy of pancreas transplants. Transplantation 1992; 54:548.

28. Stratta RJ. Ganciclovir/acyclovir and fluconazole prophylaxis after simultaneous kidney-pancreas transplantation. Transplant Proc 1998; 30:262.

29. Somerville T, Hurst G, Alloway RR, Shokouh-Amiri MH, Gaber AO, Stratta RJ. Superior efficacy of oral ganciclovir over oral acyclovir for cytomegalovirus prophylaxis in kidney-pancreas and pancreas alone recipients. Transplant Proc 1998; 30:1546.

30. Lo A, Stratta RJ, Egidi MF, et al. Patterns of cytomegalovirus infection in simultaneous kidney-pancreas transplant recipients receiving tacrolimus, mycophenolate mofetil, and prednisone with ganciclovir prophylaxis. Transplant Infectious Disease (in press)

31. Gaber LW, Stratta RJ, Lo A, et al. Importance of surveillance biopsy monitoring in solitary pancreas transplant patients receiving tacrolimus and mycophenolate mofetil. Transplant Proc (in press).

32. Reddy KS, Stratta RJ, Shokouh-Amiri H, et al. Simultaneous kidney-pancreas transplantation without anti-lymphocyte induction. Transplantation 2000; 69:49.

33. Stratta RJ, Gaber AO, Shokouh-Amiri MH, et al. Evolution in pancreas transplantation techniques: Simultaneous kidney-pancreas transplantation using portal-enteric drainage without anti-lymphocyte induction. Ann Surg 1999; 229:701.

34. Lo A, Stratta RJ, Alloway RR, et al. Limited benefits of induction with monoclonal antibody to interleukin-2 receptor in combination with tacrolimus, mycophenolate mofetil, and steroids in simultaneous kidney-pancreas transplantation. Transplant Proc (in press).

35. Nymann T, Hathaway DK, Shokouh-Amiri MH, et al. Patterns of acute rejection in portal-enteric versus systemic-bladder pancreas-kidney transplantation. Clin Transplant 1998; 12:175.

36. Elmer DS, Hathaway DK, Abdulkarim AB, et al. Use of glucose disappearance rates (Kg) to monitor endocrine function of pancreas allografts. Clin Transplant 1998; 12:56.

37. Lo A, Stratta RJ, Hathaway DK, et al. Long-term outcomes in simultaneous kidney-pancreas transplant recipients with portal-enteric versus systemic-bladder drainage. Transplant Proc (in press).

38. Stratta RJ, Gaber AO, Shokouh-Amiri MH, et al. A 9-year experience with 125 pancreas transplants with portal-enteric drainage. Transplant Proc (in press).

39. Stratta RJ, Lo A, Hathaway DK, et al. Long-term outcome in simultaneous kidney-pancreas transplant recipients with portal-enteric drainage. Proceedings of the 7th World Congress of the International Pancreas and Islet Transplant Association (Abstract #P52); 1999:71.

40. Elmer DS, Abdulkarim AB, Fraga D, et al. Metabolic effects of FK506 (tacrolimus) versus cyclosporine in portally drained pancreas allografts. Transplant Proc 1998; 30:523.

41. Hughes TA, Gaber AO, Shokouh-Amiri H, et al. Kidney-pancreas transplantation: The effect of portal versus systemic venous drainage of the pancreas on the lipoprotein composition. Transplantation 1995; 60:1406.

42. Bagdade JD, Ritter MC, Kitabchi AE, et al. Differing effects of pancreas-kidney transplantation with systemic versus portal venous drainage on cholesterol ester transfer in IDDM subjects. Diabetes Care 1996; 19:1108.

43. El-Gebely S, Hathaway DK, Elmer DS, et al. An analysis of renal function in pancreas-kidney and diabetic kidney-alone recipients at two years following transplantation. Transplantation 1995; 59:1410.

44. Nymann T, Hathaway DK, Bertorini TE, et al. Studies of the impact of pancreas-kidney and kidney transplantation on peripheral nerve conduction in diabetic patients. Transplant Proc 1998; 30:323.

45. Gaber AO, El-Gebely S, Sugathan P, et al. Early improvement in cardiac function occurs for pancreas-kidney but not diabetic kidney-alone transplant recipients. Transplantation 1995; 59:1105.

46. Wicks MN, Hathaway DK, Shokouh-Amiri MH, et al. Sustained improvement in cardiac function 24 months following pancreas-kidney transplant. Transplant Proc 1998; 30:333.

ACKNOWLEDGEMENTS:

We gratefully acknowledge the expertise of Joyce Lariviere and Cassie Heidelberg in preparation of the manuscript.

CHAPTER 20

Pancreas Transplantation at Northwestern University

Dixon B. Kaufman, Joseph R. Leventhal, Michael D. Elliott, Lorenzo G. Gallon, Michele A. Parker, Mihai Gheorghiade, Alan J. Koffron, Mario Ferrario, Michael M. Abecassis, Jonathan P. Fryer, and Frank P. Stuart

Northwestern University Medical School, Department of Surgery, Division of Transplantation, Department of Medicine, Divisions of Nephrology and Cardiology, Chicago, Illinois

The Pancreas Transplantation Program at Northwestern University Medical School began in March 1993. Two hundred pancreas transplants have been performed through October 2000. This total includes 181 simultaneous pancreas-kidney (SPK) transplants, 12 pancreas after kidney (PAK) transplants, and 7 pancreas transplants alone (PTA). The vast majority of the program's activity is in SPK transplantation. A liberal approach has been taken in accepting patients for SPK transplantation. This is exemplified by the broad age range (15-59 years, 10% ≥45 years of age) of recipients, and evidenced by a philosophy that SPK transplantation is appropriate in patients with coronary artery disease (CAD) treated by revascularization. Nearly 25% of the SPK recipients have undergone coronary revascularization prior to transplantation.

Since the program's inception there has been a systematic approach to determine relevant clinical maneuvers that contribute to improvement in the care of the pancreas transplant recipient. Every 2 years, beginning in January, after an examination of the transplant results, a change in protocol is undertaken and studied to determine if a positive effect was achieved. In 1996, the maintenance immunosuppression was changed to the routine use of MMF/tacrolimus/prednisone; in 1998, enteric drainage of the exocrine pancreas was used; and in 2000, a prospective study of rapid corticosteroid withdrawal was undertaken. The following 4 areas are representative of these and other contributions to the care of the SPK transplant recipient:

1. Development of safe and effective immunotherapy that maximizes patient and graft survival rates and minimizes rejection episodes.

2. Analyses of surgical technique of pancreas exocrine drainage on outcome.

3. Determination of the role of SPK transplantation in patients with significant cardiovascular disease and hypertension.

4. Development of a rapid corticosteroid withdrawal protocol in SPK transplantation.

For each of the analyses of transplant outcomes, actuarial survival estimates were calculated by Kaplan-Meier life table methodology. Kidney graft failure was defined as removal, loss of function that required return to dialysis, or death with function. Pancreas graft failure was defined as removal of the graft, the loss of endocrine function requiring return to exogenous insulin therapy, or death with function.

Safe and Effective Immunotherapy

Since the pancreas transplant program started, numerous changes in the pharmacologic armamentarium of immunosuppression have occurred. Figure 1 illustrates the modifications of our approach to maintenance immunosuppression since 1993. Our group was among the first to report on the beneficial effects of combining mycophenolate mofetil (MMF) and tacrolimus as primary maintenance immunosuppression for SPK transplantation (1). We began this protocol in 1995. Figure 2 shows the most recent results of our series of SPK transplant recipients (n=118) receiving MMF/tacrolimus/prednisone maintenance immunosuppression with the longest follow-up published to date – a mean of 28 months. The current actuarial one-year patient, kidney and pancreas survival rates are 97.2%, 94.5%, and 92.9%, respectively. For comparison, the benchmark

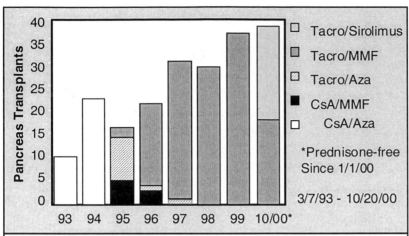

Figure 1. Number of pancreas transplants performed by year and stratified by maintenance immunosuppression protocol.

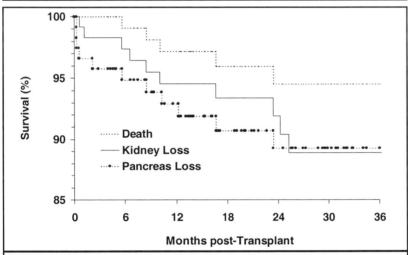

Figure 2. Actuarial 3-year patient and graft survival rates in SPK transplant recipients given MMF/tacrolimus maintenance immunosuppression.

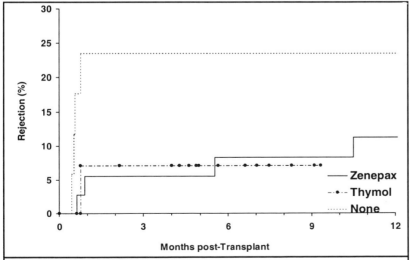

Figure 3. Acute rejection rates following SPK transplantation according to induction therapy.

actuarial one-year patient, kidney, and pancreas survival rates reported by the International Pancreas Transplant Registry (IPTR) for all US cases of SPK transplantation (1998 – 5/2000) were 95%, 92% and 83%, respectively.

We were astonished at the effectiveness of induction therapy in combination with MMF and tacrolimus in preventing acute rejection. Our rejection rates utilizing previous combinations of CsA/Aza, CsA/MMF or tacrolimus/Aza (also with induction and chronic corticosteroids) were 60-80%. The overall 6-month actuarial rejection rate using MMF/tacrolimus/ prednisone was reduced to 7-24 depending on whether induction therapy was employed. We advocate the use of induction therapy for SPK transplantation based on our experience without induction therapy compared with either T-cell depleting agents or IL-2 receptor antagonists. Figure 3 shows the specific acute rejection rates in SPK transplant recipients receiving no induction, or induction with a rabbit anti-thymocyte globulin (Thymoglobulin[®]), or an IL-2 receptor antagonist (Daclizumab, Zenepax[®]). The 6-month rejection rate among the non-induction recipients was 24% versus 7-8% with induction. Our experience showing the benefits of induction therapy was consistent with those findings reported in recent multi-center studies of the use of induction therapy in SPK transplantation (2, 3). The use of MMF/tacrolimus/prednisone has become the standard maintenance immunosuppression regimen in SPK transplantation in the US.

Surgical Technique Pertaining to Pancreas Exocrine Drainage

Avoiding complications of pancreas transplantation relates primarily to the effective control of pancreas exocrine drainage. In the past, enteric drainage was associated with high rates of infectious and technical complications. Several groups have reported good results with primary enteric drainage in SPK transplantation using CsA/MMF or tacrolimus/azathioprine immunosuppression. There is a paucity of data with primary enteric drainage in SPK transplantation in recipients receiving MMF/tacrolimus/prednisone maintenance immunosuppression that is also stratified according to the inclusion or exclusion of induction therapy. This distinction is important since the risk of severe infectious complications in the setting of enteric drainage, and the use of very potent immunosuppression, could offset the potential benefits of enteric drainage that have been previously described.

We have analyzed the role of bladder (n=50) versus enteric (n=50) exocrine drainage in 2 sequential series of SPK transplant recipients receiving MMF/ tacrolimus/ prednisone maintenance immunotherapy (4). The actuarial SPK outcomes of patient and graft survival, and rejection rates at one year were evaluated. We also examined endpoints pertaining to infectious complications and re-hospitalizations.

Table 1 shows the actuarial one-year patient, kidney, and pancreas graft functional survival rates in the bladder and enteric drainage groups. The one-year actuarial patient, kidney, and pancreas survival rates in the bladder drainage group were 98.0%, 94.0% and 94.0%, respectively. The one-year actuarial patient, kidney, and pancreas survival rates in the enteric drainage group were 96.8%, 96.8% and 89.4%, respectively. Furthermore, renal allograft function, as assessed by serum creatinine values, was found to be equivalent in the 2 groups.

There were more bacterial infections in patients who underwent bladder drainage. Urinary tract infections were frequent with 48% of the recipients treated with antibiotics for a urinary tract infection during the 6-month postoperative period. In the enteric drainage group the incidence of urinary tract infections was 37%. There were no localized or systemic fungal infections.

Table 1. One-year actuarial patient and graft survival rates in SPK transplantation according to pancreas exocrine drainage procedure and induction immunotherapy.

Group (n)	Patient	Kidney	Pancreas
All (100)	97.7%	95.5%	92.4%
Bladder (50)	98.0%	94.0%	94.0%
Enteric (50)	96.8%	96.8%	89.4%
Induction (33)	93.3%	93.3%	84.0%
Non-induction (17)	100.0%	100.0%	94.1%

The length of inpatient hospitalization for transplantation was nearly identical among recipients with bladder (8.0±3.0 days) or enteric (8.4±3.3 days) drainage of the pancreas. Table 2 shows significantly fewer readmissions among recipients with enteric drainage. The average number of readmissions per SPK transplant recipient with bladder drainage was 1.8 versus 0.9 among recipients with enteric drainage. The proportion of patients requiring re-hospitalization within the 6-month postoperative time period also favored the enteric drainage group. Seventy-two percent of SPK transplant recipients with bladder drainage required 2 or more re-hospitalizations compared with 21% of recipients with enteric drainage. The increased readmissions for recipients with bladder drainage related to more frequent episodes of hematuria and dehydration. Within the enteric drainage group, those not receiving induction therapy had a higher rate of early readmission because of more frequent episodes of early rejection.

Although much has been published extolling the virtues and vices of bladder and enteric drainage

Table 2. Initial hospitalization and readmissions following SPK transplantation.

Outcome	Drainage Bladder	Enteric
Length of transplant stay (days)	8.0±3.0	8.4±2.9
Readmissions per patient*	1.8	0.9
0-1 (%)	28%	79%
≥2 (%)	72%	21%
Average number of readmission days per patient*	10.8	5.1

*within 6-month postoperative time period

techniques, there remains no consensus. The IPTR shows that about 75% of US SPK transplant programs use enteric drainage (usually without a Roux-en-Y technique), so it remains for each program to determine the benefits and detriments of their pancreas exocrine drainage technique of choice. What we have learned is that use of the newer immunosuppressive agents has decreased the risk of rejection and this may partially explain why enteric drainage is no longer associated with a high complication rate.

SPK Transplantation in Patients with Cardiovascular Disease and Hypertension

It is established that patients with Type I diabetes and chronic renal insufficiency experience excessive morbidity and mortality due to ischemic heart disease. The great majority of patients referred for SPK transplantation do not have known CAD at the time of initial evaluation. However, a high index of suspicion is warranted since coronary angiographic studies of asymptomatic Type 1 diabetic, uremic patients being evaluated for transplantation reveal an incidence of obstructive coronary artery disease approaching 35%. The unique amalgam of concomitant pre-existing illnesses, such as cardiovascular disease, in patients referred for SPK transplantation demands that any evaluation of risk address the long-term risk of death or myocardial infarction, as most transplant candidates undergo transplantation between one and 2 years after they have been placed on the transplant waiting list.

We established an algorithm for cardiac evaluation of all of our diabetic, uremic SPK transplant candidates (Fig. 4). Patients who have no prior history of CAD (myocardial infarction,

percutaneouscoronary intervention (PCI), coronary artery bypass surgery (CABG) or documented obstructive coronary artery disease on angiography) undergo pharmacologic myocardial perfusion stress testing. We employ a dual-isotope (thallium-rest, sestamibi-stress) adenosine perfusion stress test. Vasodilator (adenosine or dipyridamole) stress testing is preferred over treadmill exercise due to the frequent inability of transplant candidates to achieve or exceed 85% of their maximal predicted heart rate during treadmill exercise. The presence of peripheral neuropathy, peripheral vascular disease, autonomic neuropathy, and general

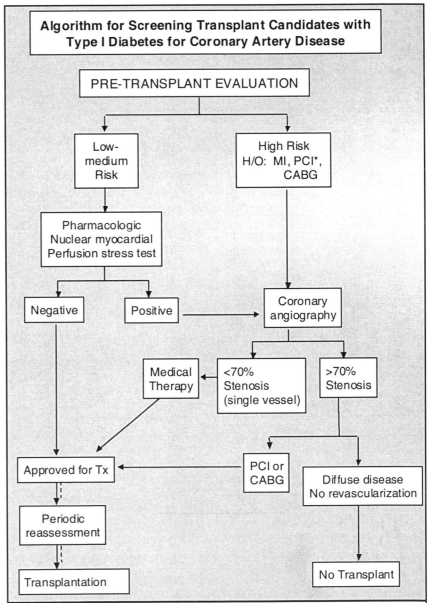

Figure 4. Algorithm for screening diabetic, uremic transplant candidates for coronary artery disease.

Table 3. *Five-year actuarial patient and graft survival rates in SPK transplantation according to coronary revascularization.*

Group (N)	Mean follow-up	Patient	Kidney	Pancreas
No revascularization (139)	35.0±25.2 mo.	87.9%	78.1%	76.6%
Revascularization (42)	30.5±26.2 mo.	88.9%	81.8%	77.9%

deconditioning are common factors that limit the utility of treadmill stress testing in this patient population. Gated SPECT imaging allows evaluation of regional and global left ventricular systolic function in addition to coronary perfusion. The presence of any ischemic or fixed perfusion defect or a calculated left ventricular ejection fraction of ≤45% would mandate diagnostic coronary angiography. For our transplant candidates who have chronic renal insufficiency not requiring dialysis, coronary angiography is performed using the biplane technique and a left ventriculogram is not performed to minimize contrast exposure and the risk of developing contrast nephropathy. Transplant candidates with a prior history of coronary artery disease are referred directly to coronary angiography.

Percutaneous or surgical revascularization is performed for all patients found to have obstructive coronary artery disease amenable to revascularization regardless of symptom status. Following successful recovery from coronary revascularization (PCI or CABG) patients proceed to transplantation. In addition to coronary revascularization, an aggressive medical treatment plan is prescribed - aspirin, lipid-lowering with a goal LDL level <100, ace-inhibitors, and beta-blockers.

CAD was a frequent finding in our patient population with diabetes and uremia being evaluated for SPK transplantation. Many groups advocate kidney transplantation alone if significant CAD is present requiring coronary revascularization. This was rarely occasioned in our group. Fewer than 5 patients, all with other medical problems such as being wheelchair bound, have been denied SPK transplantation with correctible CAD (among nearly 60 patients with coronary revasculaization either transplanted or on the waiting list). We have adopted a liberal policy based on the hypothesis that long-term outcomes following SPK transplantation will be the same in patients with coronary revascularization as in patients without CAD. To determine the risk of loss of patient or graft survival in the SPK transplant population that is associated with coronary revascularization, we have evaluated the entire series of 181 SPK transplants to determine the long-term outcomes in patients who have undergone coronary revascularization prior to SPK transplantation. Forty-two SPK transplant recipients underwent CBI or CABG prior to SPK transplantation. The method of SPK transplantation and the immunosuppression used was the same in both groups. Five-year actuarial patient and graft survival rates are shown in Table 3.

The outcomes were not statistically significant different. Among the 42 SPK transplant recipients with revascularization (mean follow-up 30.5±26.2 months) there were 2 deaths: a suicide (6 months after transplantation), and one heart failure (at 2 years). Among the 139 recipients without CAD (mean follow-up 35.0±25.2 months), 10 deaths occurred: 5 infectious (at 1.5, 2, 2.5, 7, and 8 months), 2 undetermined (4.5 and 8.5 months), one stroke (7 months), a suicide (at 1.5 years) and uremia (at 3.5 years). Cumulative cardiac event rates (eg., infarction) have been less than 3% over 5 years in both groups. Based on this experience, we conclude that SPK transplantation is appropriate in patients with CAD successfully treated by revascularization. Patients with Type I diabetes should not be denied the opportunity for pancreas transplant based on concerns of early cardiac death or premature graft loss.

The effect of successful pancreas transplantation on essential hypertension has been examined by our group and others (1, 4-7). We observed that amelioration of diabetes by pancreas transplantation has a significant beneficial effect on hypertension that was independent of the calcineurin inhibitor used for immunosuppression (7), and independent of the method (bladder vs. enteric) of pancreas exocrine drainage (4).

Table 4 shows the comparative effects of kidney alone versus SPK transplantation on control of hypertension one year after transplantation in a series of patients with Type I diabetes. In the pretransplant period, the vast majority of patients required multiple antihypertensive drugs. The mean (±SD) number of pretransplant medications in the kidney alone, SPK bladder drainage, and SPK enteric drainage groups were 2.3±1.1, 2.5±1.1, and 2.5±1.2, respectively. One year after transplantation, the mean number of medications to control hypertension in the kidney alone, SPK bladder drainage, and SPK enteric drainage groups were 2.0±1.3,

0.8±1.0, and 0.6±1.0, respectively. Importantly, the proportion of patients no longer requiring antihypertensives one year following SPK transplantation was 69% in the bladder drainage group and 67% in the enteric drainage group. The surgical method of exocrine pancreas drainage did not influence the response rate. The results are consistent with the hypothesis that improvement in hypertension following successful pancreas transplantation is secondary to achieving normoglycemia. This would support the findings by others that significant improvement in blood pressure control occurs with improved metabolic control of diabetes (8).

Rapid Corticosteroid Withdrawal Protocol in SPK Transplantation

Our most recent interest is the development of a very rapid corticosteroid withdrawal protocol in SPK transplant recipients. The rationale for rapidly withdrawing steroids is to eliminate the side-effects such as cosmetic problems, weight gain, posttransplant diabetes, hypertension, hyperlipidemia, bone disease, cataracts, etc. This approach is an extension of the rapid steroid withdrawal that has been successfully applied in our kidney-alone transplant population (9). Described below is our early experience with a prospective study of rapid (6 days) corticosteroid withdrawal in 32 consecutive SPK transplant recipients receiving either MMF/tacrolimus (n=15) or sirolimus/tacrolimus (n=17) each combined with anti-thymocyte globulin (Thymoglobulin®) induction.

We have compared the early outcomes of SPK transplantation in the rapid steroid-withdrawal group (n=32) to a control group (n=87) of SPK transplant recipients who received MMF/tacrolimus/prednisone maintenance immunosuppression with induction therapy with either equine anti-thymocyte globulin (n=50) or an IL-2 receptor antagonist (n=37). In the maintenance steroid group, transplants were performed from 7/95 – 12/99. In the rapid

steroid-withdrawal group, all transplants have been performed since 1/2000; therefore, the follow-up has been comparably short (mean time 5.0±2.4 months). The study group consisted of 32 consecutive SPK transplant recipients who received only 6 days of corticosteroids. All recipients received induction therapy with rabbit ATG (1.25 mg/kg/dose x 8 doses over 14 days). Maintenance immunotherapy consisted of either tacrolimus (target 12 hr trough concentration of 9-11 ng/ml) /MMF (target dose 3 gm/d, n=15) or tacrolimus (same target levels)/ sirolimus (4 mg/d, no levels, n=17).

The early results have been very encouraging. Table 5 shows the pertinent outcomes following SPK transplantation in the control group and in the prospectively studied steroid-withdrawal group stratified according to tacrolimus/MMF or tacrolimus/sirolimus immunosuppression. The important finding was that rapid steroid withdrawal was successful based on the excellent patient and graft survival rates and low rates of rejection. The actuarial 6-month patient, kidney and pancreas graft survival rates in the rapid steroid-withdrawal group were all 100%. Rejection has occurred

Table 4. Number of antihypertensive medications required in SPK transplant recipients with functional allografts one year or more after transplantation according to pancreatic exocrine drainage procedure.

Number of medications	Kidney-alone (n=28)		SPK Bladder Drainage (n=45)		SPK Enteric Drainage (n=46)	
	Pre-tx %	Post-tx %	Pre-tx %	Post-tx %	Pre-tx %	Post-tx %
0	4%	4%	16%	69%	2%	67%
1	19%	30%	29%	29%	20%	18%
2	37%	40%	33%	2%	32%	9%
3	33%	15%	16%	0%	26%	4%
4	7%	11%	6%	0%	20%	2%

Table 5. Six-month actuarial patient and graft survival rates and rejection rates in SPK transplantation according to steroid withdrawal therapy.

Group (n)	Patient	Kidney	Pancreas	Rejection
Steroids (87)	98.8%	96.5%	93.1%	12.7%
Steroid withdrawal (32)	100%	100%	100%	3.3%
MMF (15)	100%	100%	100%	7.3%
Sirolimus (17)	100%	100%	100%	0.0%

in only one patient for an actuarial 6-month rejection rate of 3.3%. All patients in the rapid corticosteroid withdrawal group remain off prednisone.

We observed a greater incidence of leukopenia in the rapid corticosteroid withdrawal group. At the 3-month posttransplant mark, the mean (±SD) white blood cell count (WBC) had fallen from a baseline value of 8.6±2.2K/µl to 3.8±2.2K/µl. There were no differences in platelet counts or hemoglobin levels between the 2 groups. We also performed a comparative analysis of the MMF and sirolimus subgroups within the rapid steroid withdrawal group with respect to tolerability of the agents and hematologic and lipid abnormalities. Interestingly, there were no differences in the WBC. At the 3-month mark after transplantation, the WBC in the MMF and sirolimus groups were 4.2K/µl and 3.5K/µl, respectively. However, 2 patients in the MMF group were converted to sirolimus because of leukopenia. We also observed a higher incidence of lower gastrointestinal symptoms in the MMF group that required 2 additional recipients to be converted to sirolimus. In the sirolimus group, one patient was converted to MMF because of GI intolerability. Analysis of platelet counts and lipids have not demonstrated any clinically significant differences between the MMF and sirolimus groups during this early posttransplant period.

The observation of leukopenia in the early posttransplant period was not unexpected. Corticosteroids are known to cause capillary demargination of leukocytes thereby elevating the levels of peripheral circulating cells. In recipients given chronic corticosteroids, the circulating WBC is "augmented" and the leukopenic effects of rabbit ATG induction and MMF are less apparent. The possibility that marrow suppression induced by ATG or MMF caused the leukopenia was not supported by the observation that platelet counts and hemoglobin levels were not different in recipients rapidly withdrawn from corticosteroids. The early results of rapid corticosteroid withdrawal in SPK transplant recipients using induction therapy and either tacrolimus/MMF or tacrolimus/sirolimus were very encouraging. Longer term follow-up with a greater number of patients will be required to define the role of rapid corticosteroid withdrawal and the optimal maintenance agents more clearly.

SUMMARY

The collective advances made by many groups have significantly improved the results of pancreas transplantation. We have focused on the development of safe and effective immunotherapy, including a new protocol of rapid withdrawal of corticosteroids, the analysis of surgical technique of pancreas exocrine drainage on outcome and the role of SPK transplantation in patients with significant cardiovascular disease. We have found that multi-modal immunotherapy including induction with tacrolimus-based maintenance combined with either MMF or sirolimus, with or without corticosteroids, resulted in excellent patient and graft survival rates with low rates of rejection. In this setting, enteric drainage was preferable to bladder drainage because of a lower rate of complications leading to hospital readmissions. Careful pretransplant screening for cardiovascular disease should be routinely performed for all SPK candidates. If successful coronary revascularization can be achieved, these patients can safely undergo SPK transplantation, with 5-year outcomes similar to those for recipients without coronary disease. Finally, we have observed that pancreas transplantation has an important ameliorating effect on hypertension that is independent of the method of pancreas exocrine drainage.

REFERENCES

1. Kaufman DB, Leventhal JR, Stuart J, et al. Mycophenolate mofetil and tacrolimus as primary maintenance immunosuppression in simultaneous pancreas-kidney transplantation: Initial experience in 50 consecutive cases. Transplantation 1999; 67: 586.

2. Stratta RJ, Alloway RR, Lo A, for the PIVOT Study Group. A multicenter, open-label, comparative trial of two daclizumab dosing strategies versus no antibody induction in combination with tacrolimus, mycophenolate mofetil and steroids for the prevention of acute rejection in simultaneous kidney pancreas transplant recipients: interm analysis. Transplantation (submitted).

3. Kaufman DB, Burke G, Bruce D, et al. The role of antibody induction in simultaneous pancreas kidney transplant patients receiving tacrolimus + mycophenolate mofetil immunosuppression. Transplantation 2000; 69: S206.

4. Kaufman DB, Leventhal JR, Koffron AJ, et al. Simultaneous pancreas-kidney transplantation in the mycophenolate mofetil / tacrolimus era: evolution from induction therapy with bladder drainage to non-induction therapy with enteric drainage. Surgery 2000;128: 726.

5. La Rocca E, Gobbi C, Ciurlino D, et al. Improvement of glucose/insulin metabolism reduces hypertension in insulin-dependent diabetes mellitus recipients of kidney-pancreas transplantation. Transplantation 1998; 65: 394.

6. Hricik DE, Chareander C, Knauss T, et al. Hypertension after pancreas-kidney transplantation: role of bladder versus enteric pancreatic drainage. Transplantation 2000; 70: 494.

7. Elliott MD, Kapoor A, Parker MA, et al. Improvement in hypertension in patients with diabetes mellitus after kidney/pancreas transplantation. Circulation (submitted).

8. Aoki TT, Arcangeli MA, Grecu EO, et al. Effect of chronic intermittent intravenous insulin therapy on antihypertensive medication requirements in IDDM subjects with hypertension and nephropathy. Diabetes Care 1995; 18: 1260.

9. Kaufman DB, Leventhal JR, Fryer JP, et al. Kidney transplantation without prednisone. Transplantation 2000; 69: S133.

ACKNOWLEDGEMENTS

We thank Joan Stuart and Suzanne Pellar for their invaluable assistance and expertise in database management.

CHAPTER 21

Liver Transplantation at Mount Sinai

Leona Kim-Schluger, Sander S. Florman, Gabriel Gondolesi, Sukru Emre, Patricia A. Sheiner, Thomas M. Fishbein, Myron E. Schwartz, and Charles M. Miller

The Recanati/Miller Transplantation Institute, The Mount Sinai Hospital, New York, New York

Liver transplantation at the Mount Sinai Medical Center in New York began in August 1988 with the first liver transplant performed in New York State. By the end of November 2000, 1,941 liver transplants had been performed in 1,651 patients at Mount Sinai (Fig. 1). Of these, 1,733 (89%) were performed in 1,471 adults and 208 (11%) were performed in 180 children (age <18). Overall, 1,397 patients received a single hepatic graft, 221 were transplanted twice, and 30 were transplanted 3 times. Three patients each had 4 transplants. Indications for transplantation in adults and children are presented in Table 1.

Overall patient and graft survival rates at one year are 83% and 73%, respectively, 69% and 58%, respectively, at 5 years, and 56% and 45%, respectively, at 10 years (Fig. 2). Patient and graft survival for adult and pediatric patients is shown in Figure 3.

LIVING-DONOR LIVER TRANSPLANTATION

With an active adult waiting list of more than 800 patients and a pediatric waiting list of more than 50 patients, the demand for liver grafts at our center has exponentially increased. Unfortunately, nearly 11% of the patients on our waiting list die each year while waiting for an organ. Because the number of cadaver donors in our region has remained relatively constant, we have aggressively expanded our criteria for usable donors, including older donors (1), donors with microvesicular

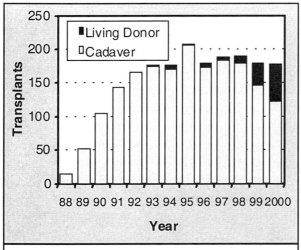

Figure 1. Annual liver transplants at Mount Sinai, 1988-2000.

Table 1. Indications for liver transplantation in adult and pediatric patients, 1988-2000.

	Adult (n=1,471)	Pediatric (n=180)
Alcoholic liver disease	14%	–
Budd-Chiari	1%	–
Hepatic failure, idiopathic	3%	11%
Autoimmune	5%	7%
HCC	1%	
Cryptogenic	9%	10%
Hepatitis B	8%	2%
Hepatitis C	35%	2%
Wilson's	1%	2%
PBC	10%	0%
PSC	6%	2%
Drug toxicity	2%	3%
Fulminant hepatitis	1%	2%
Biliary atresia	–	47%
Alagille's syndrome	–	2%
Other	4%	9%

Clinical Transplants 2000, Cecka and Terasaki, Eds. UCLA Immunogenetics Center, Los Angeles, California

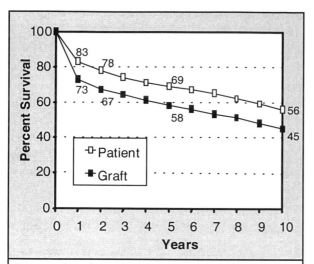

Figure 2. Overall patient and graft survival, 1988-2000.

fat (2), hepatitis C virus-positive donors (3) and hepatitis B core antibody-positive donors (4). Despite these measures, the huge discrepancy between liver supply and demand persists.

In 1993, because of the increasing shortage of cadaveric pediatric liver grafts, we initiated a living-donor liver transplant program utilizing left lateral segment grafts. Increasing experience with complex hepatic resections on our hepatobiliary service led us to apply innovative techniques, including split and reduced-size cadaveric grafts, to address the growing disparity between supply and demand. Our pediatric liver transplant

program has flourished, with reduced mortality on the waiting list and improved graft and patient survival (Fig. 4). Altogether, 208 pediatric liver transplants have been performed at Mount Sinai, using 109 whole cadaveric grafts, 28 reduced-size cadaveric grafts, 21 split cadaveric grafts and 50 living donor grafts. The youngest recipient was an 18-day-old, 1.8 kilogram neonate with liver failure secondary to neonatal hemochromatosis, who is currently doing well at home 2 years after transplantation.

Beginning in 1998, we expanded our living-donor liver transplant program to include adult recipients. Initially, left lobe grafts were used. As we gained experience, we began to utilize right lobe grafts. Through November 2000, we have performed 111 living donor transplants in 61 adults and 50 pediatric patients.

Pediatric Living-Donor Liver Transplantation

Fifty pediatric patients (30 males; 60%) have received grafts from living donors. Three received left lobe grafts; 47 received left lateral segments. Recipients ranged in age from 4 months to 17 years. Forty-eight (96%) donors were relatives; 2 were unrelated. The indications for these transplants are shown in Table 2.

Forty-one (82%) grafts had a single bile duct and 9 (18%) had 2 ducts. All biliary reconstructions were done with a Roux-Y hepaticojejunostomy. Two patients (4%) had bile leaks. The incidence of biliary strictures was

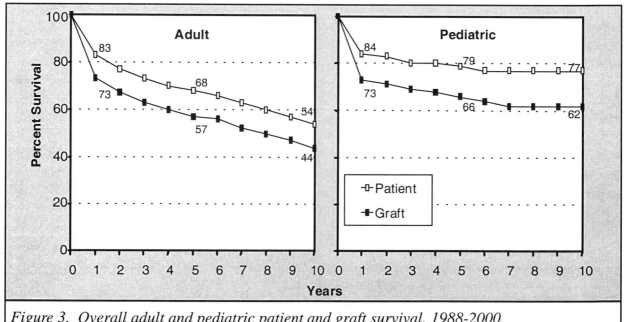

Figure 3. Overall adult and pediatric patient and graft survival, 1988-2000.

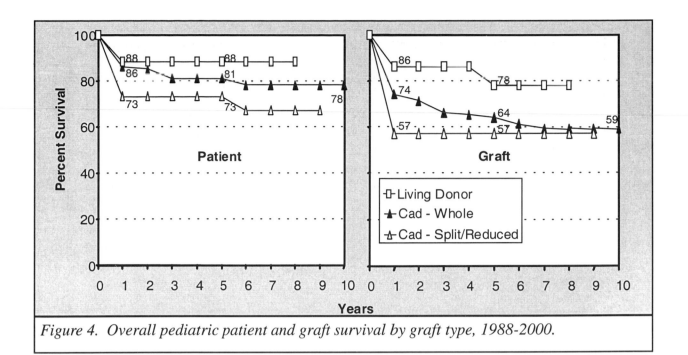

Figure 4. Overall pediatric patient and graft survival by graft type, 1988-2000.

12% (n=6) and compares very favorably to that among our pediatric recipients of cadaveric grafts (15%).

The incidence of vascular complications in our pediatric recipients was 15% after cadaveric transplants and 10% after living donor transplants. Early recognition and operative intervention salvaged all living donor grafts with vascular complications (portal vein thrombosis in 3 patients and hepatic artery thrombosis in 2 patients).

Actuarial patient and graft survival for pediatric living donor liver transplants is 86% and 84%, respectively, at one year, and 86% and 73%, respectively, at 5 years. These results are better than survival rates in pediatric recipients of whole cadaveric grafts, reduced-size and split cadaveric grafts (combined) over the same time period (Fig. 4). The better patient and graft survival among living donor recipients has several possible explanations, most important of which is the considerably shorter cold ischemic time in livers from healthy donors, resulting in no primary nonfunction. In addition, the elective nature of most living donor transplants allows for optimization of the recipient's condition in the majority of cases.

Six of our 50 pediatric living donor recipients have died. Causes of death were sepsis 1-6 months after transplantation (n=3), cerebrovascular accident one month after transplantation (n=1), posttransplant lymphoproliferative disease (n=1), and brain death (n=1) in a patient who never recovered neurologically following transplantation for fulminant hepatic failure.

There have been no donor deaths or major surgical complications. Recovery after living donation has been excellent. One donor required one unit of packed red blood cells. The average hospital stay after donation has been 5 days. All donors have returned to normal activity within 3 months.

Adult Living-Donor Liver Transplantation

The success of living-donor liver transplantation for pediatric patients and the increasing mortality rate among adults awaiting cadaveric liver transplantation were the impetus for our team to undertake adult-to-adult living donor transplantation. Initially, we used left lobe grafts,

Table 2. Indications for living donor transplantation in pediatric recipients (n=50).

Biliary atresia	55%
Fulminant hepatitis	2%
Cryptogenic	6%
Autoimmune	4%
Hepatic failure, idiopathic	13%
Acetaminophen toxicity	2%
Glycogen storage disease	4%
PBC	2%
Wilson's	2%
Other	10%

but our experience was less than optimal, mainly due to marginal graft size. Of the 9 recipients who received left lobe grafts, 4 (44%) had small-for-size syndrome. As a result, we began to use right lobe grafts, with considerably better outcomes.

We have performed 61 adult-to-adult living-donor liver transplants, using 9 left lobes and 52 right lobes. Recipients (35 males; 57%) ranged in age from 20-74 years (mean 51 years). The option of living donation was offered only to first-time recipients at UNOS Status 2B and 3. Indications for transplant are shown in Table 3. In 22 patients (36%), hepatocellular carcinoma was either the primary or secondary diagnosis. The 61 donors (40 males; 66%) ranged in age from 20-59 years (mean 39 years). Forty-five (74%) donors were relatives; 16 (26%) were unrelated.

Donor Evaluation

The intensive donor evaluation process involves a complete medical history, physical examination, laboratory tests (including blood type and viral serology), cardiology clearance when indicated, and imaging studies (including magnetic resonance imaging with hepatic volumetry, vascular reconstruction, and an assessment of steatosis). Liver biopsies are only done when specifically indicated (5). We have found that a calculated graft volume-to-recipient weight ratio (GRWR) of more than 0.8% is optimal. All donors are evaluated by social workers in an attempt to insure that donation is voluntary and that the donor has not been coerced. Psychological evaluations are obtained as needed. Each case is then presented to a multidisciplinary living donor committee. If approved, an operative approach is planned (6). One unit of autologous blood is stored prior to surgery.

Table 3. Indications for living donor transplantation in adult recipients (n=61).

Alcoholic liver disease	5%
Autoimmune hepatitis	3%
Cryptogenic	15%
Hepatitis B	8%
Hepatitis C	39%
HCC	3%
PBC	11%
PSC	8%
Other	8%

One potential donor was declined because pre-operative imaging studies showed a wandering left portal vein that crossed into his right lobe. Two other potential donors whose scans were suggestive of fatty infiltration were eventually declined when their biopsies showed greater than 40% macrovesicular steatosis. Because of the wide variability of hepatic anatomy, the operative approach in the donor must be carefully planned. The controlled parenchymal transection has been one of the keys to success with this procedure. Slight Trendelenburg position and maintenance of low central venous pressure are important factors.

Results of Adult-to-Adult Living-Donor Liver Transplants

Donors

All donors are alive. Except for blood recovered with the cell saver and one unit of autologous blood, no additional blood transfusions were required in these donors. Four donors (6.6%) had bile leaks from the cut surface of the liver in the immediate post-operative period. Three were managed conservatively with the existing drain; one required percutaneous placement of an additional drain. None required re-exploration. In addition, 2 donors (3.3%) were readmitted during the first post-operative month with clinical evidence of small bowel obstruction. One improved with conservative treatment; the other required laparoscopic lysis of adhesions. Donor recovery has been excellent, with an average hospital stay of 6 days.

Recipients

Overall one-year actuarial patient and graft survival rates for our adult living-donor liver transplant recipients are 84% and 75%, respectively (Fig. 5). Right lobe recipients had significantly better graft and patient survival, due mainly to higher GRWRs. With left lobes, the mean GRWR was 0.74%. With right lobes, the mean GRWR has been greater than 1.0%.

Eleven recipients have died, including 5 left lobe recipients and 6 right lobe recipients. Causes of death were: sepsis (n=5), cardiac arrest (n=1, on post-operative day 1), recurrent hepatocellular carcinoma (n=2; at 5 and 19 months after transplantation), mycotic aneurysm rupture after a bile leak (n=1), recurrent leiomyosarcoma (n=1, at 19 months after transplantation), and recurrent neuroendocrine tumor (n=1, at 16 months after transplantation).

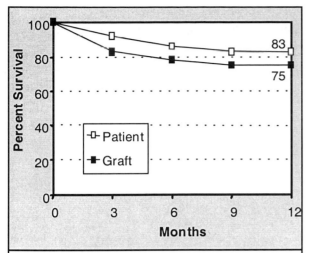

Figure 5. One-year patient and graft survival in adult living donor recipients.

When the right lobe is resected for transplantation, multiple bile ducts are often present and require reconstruction in the recipient. Among our 61 adult recipients, 30 (49%) had a single bile duct, 26 (43%) had 2 ducts, 3 (5%) had 3 ducts and 1 (1.5%) had 4 ducts (data on 1 graft is not available). The incidence of bile leak was 44.4% (n=4) among left lobe recipients and 21% (n=11) among right lobe recipients. Most leaks were small and resolved with conservative, non-operative treatment. Operative intervention was reserved for clinically significant bile leaks that did not resolve with drainage alone.

The only major vascular complications were hepatic artery thromboses, which occurred in 4 patients (6.6%). Two were left lobe recipients; both required retransplantation. The other 2 were right lobe recipients; one required retransplantation, and the other graft was salvaged. No adult recipient had portal vein thrombosis.

In November 2000, we performed the "ideal" liver transplant case – the first successful living-donor liver transplant between identical twin brothers. The recipient was a 43-year-old male with hepatitis B and hepatocellular carcinoma. The donor right lobectomy and recipient transplant procedures were uneventful. Both patients recovered without incident. Besides one bolus of Solumedrol (500mg) at reperfusion, no induction or maintenance immunosuppression was used. A liver biopsy performed on post-operative day 4 for elevated liver function tests was unremarkable, without evidence of rejection or hepatitis. Both patients are currently doing well at home.

Psychosocial Aspect of Living Donation

Little is known about the psychosocial impact of living liver donation. Published reports on living kidney donors generally indicate an improved sense of well-being and a boost in self-esteem following donation. We assessed the psychological impact of adult-to-adult liver donation. Structured questionnaires (addressing such issues as coercion, informed consent, expectations, post-operative physical and emotional experience, financial impact, sexual function and stress related to donation) were sent to our first 48 adult living donors. These donors were also asked to complete the SF-36 Health Survey, a standardized and validated multi-dimensional measure of quality of life that assesses physical and emotional well being in 8 domains. Thirty (63%) donors responded at a mean of 280±157 days after donation.

None of the donors regretted their decision to donate. Twenty-eight (93%) were back at work or school at a mean of 8.8±4.5 weeks following donation and reported no negative impact on business or social interactions. Ten (33%) reported unresolved problems with their insurers. Additionally, 10 donors found donation to be a "moderate" financial burden.

On the SF-36 survey, living donors scored higher than published US norms in 7 of 8 domains. In mental health and general health domains, living donors' scores were significantly higher than published norms. These differences were particularly significant for those donors whose recipients had no post-operative complications (7).

TRANSPLANTATION FOR HEPATOCELLULAR CARCINOMA

Liver replacement for hepatocellular carcinoma (HCC) is an important option for patients with tumors in unresectable anatomic locations, patients with multiple tumors confined to the liver, and patients who, because of liver dysfunction, would not tolerate resection. Patients with small HCCs (<5 cm single lesion or 3 lesions less than 3 cm each) do well after liver transplantation (8) and, under the current UNOS allocation system, are given priority as UNOS Status 2B. The longer these patients wait on the waiting list, however, the greater the risk of tumor progression that will effectively rule out their candidacy for cadaveric liver transplantation.

The UNOS criteria do not address the needs of patients with tumors >5 cm, for whom liver transplantation offers the potential for cure if performed in a timely fashion. In 43 patients with HCC >5 cm who underwent transplantation with multimodal adjuvant therapy (including pre-operative chemoembolization, intra-operative chemotherapy and post-operative chemotherapy), at a mean of 49 months after transplant, survival at one and 5 years was 89% and 44%, respectively. Additionally, recurrence-free survival at one and 5 years is 78% and 48%.

One of the more important uses of adult living-donor liver transplantation has been for timely transplantation of patients with HCC, and in particular, those who do not meet UNOS Status 2B criteria. Since 1998, 72 patients have been transplanted with known HCC (50 cadaveric, 22 with living donors). The mean waiting time for these cadaveric recipients was 414 days and for the living donors the mean time to transplantation was 83 days. At our center, patients with large HCCs who are candidates for liver transplantation with living donors undergo exploration at the time of transplant, to exclude the presence of extrahepatic disease. If exploration is negative, the hepatectomy proceeds and the donor operation is begun. All patients with HCC are treated with a multimodal protocol (9).

Of the 61 adult living donor transplants performed at our center, 22 (36%) patients had known HCC. Three (14%) of these patients had recurrent HCC after resection. Seventeen (77%) of these patients had tumors that exceeded UNOS 2B criteria. The early (< 3 months) non-tumor-related mortality was 14% (n=3). One patient (5%) had evidence of HCC recurrence 4 months after transplant and died one month later (10).

RECURRENT DISEASES

Most liver disease recurs after liver transplantation. The severity of recurrence and the effect on patient and graft survival, however, vary with the etiology of liver disease. Recurrent cholestatic liver diseases, such as primary sclerosing cholangitis and primary biliary cirrhosis, are usually mild, with minimal clinical significance. Recurrent hepatitis B and C can be severe and rapidly progressive, with graft loss and death within a short time after initial transplant. Since 1988, 290 (15%) liver transplants at our center have been retransplants (Table 4).

Recurrent Hepatitis C

Reflecting the national trend, the most common

indication for transplantation at Mount Sinai is for hepatitis C. Although most patients who undergo transplantation for hepatitis C do well, it has become increasingly apparent that recurrent disease can be progressive and may result in poorer long-term survival (11). Our patients have had a 44% incidence of histological recurrence and a 7% incidence of a severe form of fibrosing cholestatic hepatitis characterized by rapidly progressive graft dysfunction leading to death or retransplantation (12). The progression of recurrent hepatitis C in the allograft appears to be related to increased immunosuppression for the treatment of rejection. In particular, the use of OKT3 for severe or steroid-resistant rejection appears to increase the incidence of recurrent disease (13). Of our 515 patients transplanted for hepatitis C, 31 (6%) have required retransplantation for recurrent disease. Given the large number of patients transplanted for hepatitis C, we expect that even more patients will require retransplantation in the future. Currently, we are evaluating a number of investigational agents, including a novel hepatitis C immunoglobulin and pegylated interferon, which may have utility in the prevention of recurrent hepatitis C after transplantation.

Recurrent Autoimmune Hepatitis

Several transplant programs have reported the recurrence of autoimmune hepatitis (AIH) after transplantation, with incidences ranging from 10-30% and with a low rate of graft loss. In our own experience, of 32 patients transplanted for AIH, 24 (75%) had chronic disease and 8 (25%) had fulminant hepatitis. None of the patients transplanted for fulminant hepatitis had recurrent disease. Six patients with chronic disease had

Table 4. Indications for retransplantation, 1988-2000.

	N
Primary graft nonfunction	108
Hepatic artery thrombosis	41
Portal vein thrombosis	6
Acute rejection	18
Chronic rejection	33
Acute hepatitis B	3
Drug induced hepatic failure	2
Recurrent hepatitis C	31
Other	8

histologically proven recurrence, with 3 requiring retransplantation. Our incidence of graft loss is greater than that reported from other centers. Overall, our

results show that patients transplanted for AIH do very well, although the incidence of graft loss due to recurrent disease at 2 years was approximately 12% (14).

SUMMARY

Nearly 2000 liver transplants have been performed over the past 12 years at Mount Sinai, with a recent exponential growth in living donor surgeries. Living-donor liver transplantation has emerged as an important option for our patients with end-stage liver disease. We are only beginning to recognize fully the advantages that 'scheduled' liver transplantation can offer. In this era of severe cadaver organ shortages, living donation offers patients the option of liver replacement in a timely fashion, before life-threatening complications of hepatic failure and/or carcinoma progression prohibit transplantation.

The next era of transplantation at Mount Sinai will bring significant increases in the number of transplants performed with living donors, with projections of over 50% of the total transplants each year expected to involve living donations. We are committed to offering this option while recognizing that donor safety remains paramount and cannot be overemphasized. Proper donor and recipient selection, as well as surgical experience are imperative to success with this technically demanding procedure.

Recurrent disease after transplantation, particularly with hepatitis C, remains a challenge clinically. Further investigations into the pathogenesis of the rapid progression of recurrent hepatitis C need to be addressed. Living donor transplantation could be an important option for these patients and would allow timely transplantation and the potential for improved survival in patients with hepatocellular carcinoma.

REFERENCES

1. Emre S, Schwartz ME, Altaca G, et al. Safe use of hepatic allografts from donors older than 70 years. Transplantation 1996; 62:62.

2. Fishbein TM, Fiel MI, Emre S, et al. Use of livers with microvesicular fat safely expands the donor pool. Transplantation 1997; 64:248.

3. Torres M, Weppler D, Reddy KR, Tzakis A. Use of hepatitis C-infected donors for hepatitis C-positive recipients. Gastroenterology 1999; 117:1253.

4. Dodson SF, Bonham CA, Geller DA, et al. Prevention of de novo hepatitis B infection in recipients of hepatic allografts from anti-HBc positive donors. Transplantation 1999; 68:1058.

5. Kim-Schluger L, Abittan CS, O'Rourke M, et al. Evaluation of potential adult-to-adult living donors: routine biopsies are not indicated (abstract). Hepatology 2000; 32(4; Pt. 2):251A.

6. Schiano, TD, Kim-Schluger L, Gondolesi G, Miller CM. Adult living donor liver transplantation: the hepatologist's perspective. Hepatology 2001; 33:3.

7. Kim-Schluger L. Psychological follow-up after liver donation. NIH Workshop on living donor liver transplantation, December 4-5, 2000; Bethesda, MD: p 22.

8. Mazzaferro V, Regalia E, Doci R, et al. Liver transplantation for the treatment of small hepatocellular carcinoma in patients with cirrhosis. N Engl J Med 1996; 334:693.

9. Schwartz ME, Sung M, Mor E, et al. A multidisciplinary approach to hepatocellular carcinoma in patients with cirrhosis. J Am Coll Surg 1995; 180:596.

10. Schwartz, M. Living donor transplantation for hepatocellular carcinoma. NIH Workshop on living donor liver transplantation (oral presentation). December 4-5, 2000; Bethesda, MD.

11. Sheiner PA, Schluger LK, Emre S, et al. Retransplantation for recurrent hepatitis C. Liver Transpl Surg 1997; 3:130.

12. Schluger LK, Sheiner PA, Thung SN, et al. Severe recurrent cholestatic hepatitis C following orthotopic liver transplantation. Hepatology 1996; 23:971.

13. Sheiner PA, Schwartz ME, Schluger LK, et al. Severe or multiple rejection episodes are associated with early recurrence of hepatitis C after orthotopic liver transplantation. Hepatology 1995; 21:30.

14. Reich DJ, Fiel I, Guarrera JV, et al. Liver transplantation for autoimmune hepatitis. Hepatology 2000; 32:693.

CHAPTER 22

Eighteen Years of Experience with Adult and Pediatric Liver Transplantation at the University of Tennessee, Memphis

M. Hosein Shokouh-Amiri, Hani P. Grewal, Santiago R. Vera, Robert J. Stratta, Caroline A. Riely, Jaquelyn F. Fleckenstein, Patty Cowan, and A. Osama Gaber

Transplantation Program, University of Tennessee, Memphis, Tennessee

The goal of the liver transplantation program in Memphis is to increase access of patients with advanced liver disease to transplantation and to provide innovative new opportunities in the treatment of liver disease. Our commitment is to ensure the highest level of patient care in a fiscally responsible environment allowing our program to thrive as a community resource in the new era of health care financing.

The Liver Transplantation Program at UT Memphis was one of the first to be established in the United States in the early 1980s. The pioneering efforts of the Memphis transplant team led to the establishment and proliferation of transplantation programs in the southeastern United States. With the expansion and modernization of Hepatology services and the recruitment of new staff in the transplantation division, UT Memphis has undergone a significant recent revitalization. The new team has dedicated itself to aggressively expanding the program reach into the community and to excellence in medical care.

In the current era of rapid advancements in transplantation science and excellent national survival rates, the differentiation between programs cannot only be based on traditional outcomes (patient and graft survival) since most programs have similar overall results. Our mission is also to achieve the highest possible quality of life for our patients. Thus, besides having excellent survival outcomes, our focus on total quality of life provides a unique value to our patients. We have developed some of the most innovative quality-of-life research programs in transplantation and have decided to focus our protocols and management ideas not only on prevention of rejection and infection, but also on the prevention and outpatient management of other co-morbid conditions associated with transplantation that can compromise quality of life. We have devoted a significant amount of attention to the prevention of posttransplant osteoporosis, renal dysfunction, hypertension, left ventricular hypertrophy, weight gain, malignancies, psychological maladjustment and depression. In addition, we have emphasized rehabilitation and job training, resulting in better long-term outcomes for our patients. These innovative programs have gained recognition from the National Institutes of Health and represent a collaborative effort of several colleges at the University.

The Kidney Transplant Program at the University of Tennessee was started on April 9, 1970, and the Liver Transplant Program was established 12 years later with the first adult liver transplant performed on May 19, 1982. The first pediatric liver transplant was performed at the LeBonheur Children's Hospital on April 23, 1983. Since 1982, 358 adult and 54 pediatric patients have undergone liver transplantation at our institution. The shortage of donor organs (1), especially during the last 10 years, has been the limiting factor for wider application of liver transplantation at our center. In order to circumvent this shortage, we have been using reduced-size liver allografts in our pediatric population since 1992. Recently, we have begun performing *in-situ* splitting of suitable donor livers for transplantation of 2 recipients in order to use available organs more efficiently. Living related adult-to-adult liver transplantation is another innovative procedure that we have added to our armamentarium for handling the problem of organ shortage.

Being one of the first liver programs in the nation, our transplant program has traditionally served a large area, including Tennessee, Mississippi, Arkansas, and some parts of Missouri, Louisiana, Alabama, Kentucky, and Florida. Because of our emphasis on access, our program has provided service for all patients regardless of their funding sources. This commitment to treatment of the underprivileged patient has distinguished our efforts since the inception of this program.

Patient Selection and Indication

Through a weekly multidisciplinary group meeting of our hepatologists, transplant surgeons, anesthesiologists, interventional radiologists, social worker, and financial counselors, patients with end-stage liver disease are selected for placement on the liver transplant waiting list. Patients between 6 months and 72 years of age have been transplanted at our program. The primary indications for liver transplantation are shown in Table 1 for adult and Table 2 for pediatric patients. The majority of adult patients have had severe liver disease (Child's B, 47%; and Child's C, 33%) and the male-to-female ratio has been 61% to 39% in our adult population and 46% to 54% in children. At least 6 months of abstinence from alcohol/drug use has been a requirement in order to be considered for listing for transplantation.

All potential living-related adult donors undergo a comprehensive evaluation consisting of history, physical exam, social and psychological work-up, CT volumetry, MRA, ultrasonography, CBC, liver function tests, and serology. All potential donors meet with a donor advocate and provide informed consent under an Institutional Review Board (IRB) protocol. Not more than 25% of potential living donors under this strict algorithm have been accepted for liver donation. All potential recipients for a living-related donor liver transplant must satisfy criteria for listing on the cadaver liver transplant list and are approved by the transplant selection committee.

Results

Liver transplant activity for pediatric and adult patients at the University of Tennessee, Memphis, is shown in Figure 1. Three hundred eighty (380) liver

Table 1. Indications for adult liver transplantation.

Hepatitis C	40.0%
Hepatitis B	7.0%
Retransplant	5.7%
Primary sclerosing cholangitis	8.0%
Primary biliary cirrhosis	11.0%
Alcohol	11.0%
Fulminant hepatic failure	2.0%
Others*	15.3%

* Others: cryptogenic, autoimmune, Budd-Chiari, sarcoidosis, non-alcoholic steato hepatitis, malignancy

Table 2. Indications for pediatric liver transplantation.

Biliary atresia	50.0%
Alpha 1 anti trypsin deficiency	7.7%
Fulminant hepatic failure	12.0%
Hepatitis (C, nonA, nonB)	10.0%
Malignancy	10.0%
Others*	10.3%

* Others: histiocytosis X, choledochal cyst, primary sclerosing cholangitis, Budd Chiari syndrome, Alagille syndrome

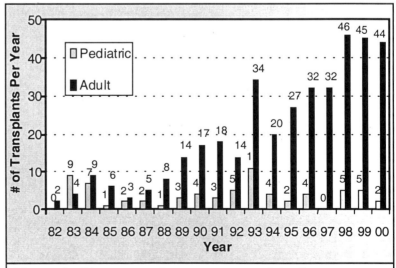

Figure 1. Liver transplant program activity by year.

transplants have been performed in 358 adult patients since the start of the program. This includes 3 split grafts that we have done since 1998 and 16 adult-to-adult live donor transplants since March 1999. Two hundred sixty-two (262) of these 358 adult patients (73%) transplanted at our center are currently alive between 1-17 years after transplantation. Actuarial patient and graft survival rates are shown in Figures 2 and 3 for adult and pediatric recipients, respectively. There were 3 (0.8%) cases of primary non-function in the 380 adult transplants. There were 3 cases (0.8%) of portal vein thrombosis, one of which was diagnosed immediately and successfully treated by surgical thrombectomy. This patient is alive with good liver function and a patent portal vein 8 years later. The second case of portal vein thrombosis required retransplantation and the third patient is living with a thrombosed portal vein with excellent liver function for 7 years and has spontaneously re-opened a pre-existing splenorenal shunt. There were 8 (2.1%) cases of hepatic artery thrombosis, 5 of which occurred early after transplantation and 3 occurred late and were segmental. All 8 patients were retransplanted. Overall, we have retransplanted 22 (5.7%) of our adult patients in 18 years. Other indications for retransplantation included Hepatitis C recurrence (n=4), chronic rejection (n=5), and fulminant liver failure of pregnancy (n=1).

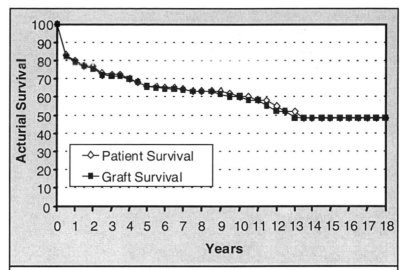

Figure 2. Patient and graft survival in adult liver transplant recipients University of Tennessee.

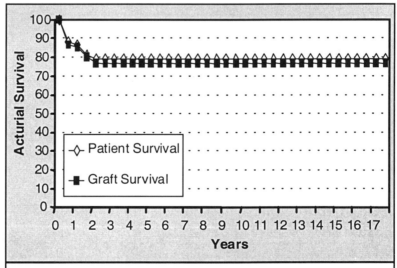

Figure 3. Patient and graft survival in pediatric liver transplant recipients University of Tennessee.

Since Hepatitis B immunoglobulin (HBIG) became available, we have transplanted 27 patients with Hepatitis B liver disease. In each of these patients, we have kept the Hepatitis B antibody titer above 500. By using this regimen, we have had an 86% long-term patient and 79% graft survival in patients receiving HBIG only, compared with 100% long-term patient and graft survival after combining HBIG with lamivudine (2).

Since 1983, 70 liver transplants were performed in 54 pediatric patients at our center. Two patients were retransplanted twice and 12 patients were retransplanted once. We had 2 cases (2.85%) of primary non-function

and 11 cases (15%) of hepatic artery thrombosis in the 70 grafts. Forty-two of 54 pediatric patients (78%) are currently alive between 4 months and 17 years following transplantation. Our retransplant rate in children was 22.8%, with a total retransplant rate of 8.4% for both adult and pediatric patients.

In our pediatric recipients, we have performed 16 reduced-size grafts. In 1997 we started splitting cadaveric livers *in situ* in order to transplant 2 patients with one liver. At this time we are splitting only high quality livers and use the *in-situ* technique because of our belief that *in-situ* splitting reduces cold ischemia time and will result in less bleeding from the cut surface.

Between 1992-1997, we transplanted 12 reduced-size grafts (left lateral segment n=8, left lobe n=2, right lobe n=2) in pediatric patients. Since 1997, 3 split grafts and one living-related liver transplant were performed in pediatric patients; all were left lateral segment transplants.

Three (5.5%) pediatric patients and one adult (0.27%) were diagnosed with posttransplant lymphoproliferative disease. All 4 were managed by reduction in immunosuppression and other non-specific supportive therapy. All 4 patients are alive with good liver function 6-10 years after diagnosis.

Living Donor Results

One of the 16 living related donors in our adult-to-adult series developed a minor bile leak that responded to percutaneous treatment. Only 6 of the donors required blood transfusion, with 4 patients receiving 1-2 units and 2 patients receiving 4-5 units. No patient required either fresh frozen plasma or platelets. Donors stayed in the hospital between 6-9 days (average 8 days). All 16 donors are currently well and have resumed normal employment within 4-8 weeks after donation. All adult living donors continue to do well with a follow up of 4-22 months.

Techniques

The application of technical innovations in our program has for the most part mirrored the steady evolution of the procedures. Between 1982-1985, all liver transplants were performed with cross-clamping of the inferior vena cava without veno-venous bypass. Following the introduction of veno-venous bypass (3), it was selectively utilized in our patients after cross-clamping of the inferior vena cava between 1985-1987. After 1987, all patients who underwent liver transplantation were placed on complete veno-venous bypass. In 1994, we changed our approach to placement of the veno-venous bypass from performing cutdown on the femoral and axillary veins to percutaneous placement of the catheters.

Liver Transplantation without Caval Excision (piggy-back operation)

Encouraged by a limited initial experience and by early reports from other centers, we started to use the piggy-back technique without cross-clamping the inferior vena cava or veno-venous bypass in 1997. At present, nearly 60% of orthotopic liver transplants at our program are being performed with no veno-venous bypass and no cross-clamping of the inferior vena cava. The variant of the piggy-back technique that we use (4) avoids cross-clamping (complete or partial) of the inferior vena cava. In most cases, we repair the right hepatic vein stump and apply a vascular clamp to the confluence of the middle and left hepatic veins as they enter the vena cava. If this orifice is adequate in diameter for the upper cava anastomosis without compromise of outflow, we proceed with a donor cava-to-recipient middle and left hepatic vein anastomosis. In about 15% of cases in which these orifices are deemed inadequate for caval anastomosis, we have performed the conventional cava-to-cava anastomosis with veno-venous bypass. Another important technical feature in the procedure that we practice is maintaining intact portal vein flow to the liver until we are ready to excise the diseased recipient liver, thus minimizing portal vein clamp time. No temporary porto-caval shunts have been performed in our patients.

By following strict rules about the adequacy of the circumference of the middle and left hepatic vein stumps and by not cross-clamping the inferior vena cava in patients undergoing OLT with the piggy-back technique, we were able to demonstrate a decrease in anhepatic time by 50% and a significant decrease in ICU stay, total hospital stay and total hospital charges compared with a concurrent cohort of patients who underwent orthotopic liver transplantation with caval clamping and veno-venous bypass (5). We were also able to show a significant decrease in blood and blood product utilization during surgery in the piggy-back group. In addition, we observed that patients in the piggy-back group required less intra-operative fluid resuscitation to maintain hemodynamic stability and maintained a higher core temperature during surgery. Post-operative complications, both early and late, were similar between both groups, including the development of posttransplant ascites that occurred with a frequency of ≤4% (4% in piggy-back and 3% in conventional technique). All cases of ascites improved with either medical treatment or angioplasty.

We believe that not all patients can undergo liver transplantation with the piggy-back technique, but performing this technique preferentially will result in substantial cost savings while providing a smooth intra-operative and post-operative course without jeopardizing the results. On the other hand, routine use of the piggy-back technique with dissection of the liver from the inferior vena cava has been of great help in teaching our residents and fellows the techniques for liver resection and in the preparation for living related adult-to-adult liver transplantation. Currently we continue to use both piggy-back and veno-venous bypass techniques and believe that by exposing our fellows and trainees to the different approaches to liver transplantation, that they will be ready for starting comprehensive transplantation practices.

Split-Liver Transplantation and In-Situ Splitting of Donor Livers

We begin the operation with an intraoperative cholangiogram. If the number of bile ducts to both segments II, III, and the remainder of the liver prove to be manageable (6), then we proceed with splitting the liver by using the CUSA ultrasonic dissector. Liver splitting is done in the line between segments II and III and the extended right lobe. It usually takes about 1.5-2 hours of extra time to perform the splitting. The intention to split a donor liver *in situ* is announced to the host OPO prior to the procedure and is discussed in advance with the cardiac team. If the donor becomes unstable during splitting, then rapid flush is performed and the splitting is completed at the backtable. As soon as we determine the suitability of the donor liver for splitting, both the adult and pediatric recipient operations are started in order to minimize the cold ischemic time for both recipients. Organizing the logistics in this fashion ensures immediate function of the divided segments and reduces complications associated with the procedure.

Adult-to-Adult Live Donor Transplants

To address the issue of organ shortage further, we started performing adult-to-adult living-related liver transplants in March 1999 (7). In preparation for this technically demanding procedure, our team utilized the surgical research lab and performed extensive preparatory surgical procedures on large animals. This experience was fundamental to a research program that aimed at defining the minimum amount of transplanted liver tissue that would sustain life. Our surgeons also have extensive experience with major hepatic resections and complicated hepato-pancreatico-biliary procedures. Since the inception of the adult-to-adult living-related transplant program, we have elected to use the right lobe of the donor liver for the transplant.

After performing intraoperative cholangiography, the donor operation with right hepatic lobectomy (50%-55% of the total amount of liver) is performed under ultrasonic guidance to stay 1-2 centimeters to the right of the middle hepatic vein. The right hepatic artery and portal vein to the right lobe of the liver are dissected. Parenchymal transection is performed with the help of the ultrasonic CUSA dissector. At no time do we perform any vascular occlusion. Liver dissection from the inferior vena cava is limited to the level of transection of the right lobe of the liver, leaving all small hepatic branches from the caudate lobe to the inferior vena cava intact. Only when the transection is completed and the right lobe is attached by the right portal vein, right hepatic artery and right hepatic vein (the bile duct is divided early in the course of transection of the parenchyma), and the recipient is ready in the other room, do we cross-clamp the right portal vein, right hepatic artery, and right hepatic vein and divide the vessels and bring the right lobe of liver to the backtable for perfusion with University of Wisconsin solution through both the portal vein and hepatic artery. We usually divide the structures in the hilum leaving a 3-4 millimeter stump of the right hepatic bile duct and right portal vein in order to avoid strictures in the donor. The right hepatic artery dissection is limited to the right side of the common hepatic duct and the right hepatic artery is ligated at this level in order not to induce any ischemic stricture in the bile duct of the donor (7). The donor's safety is of prime importance.

We have modified the bile duct anastomosis from hepaticojejunostomy in the recipient of a living-donor liver transplant to duct-to-duct anastomosis (8). In order to do this safely, we adopted the technique of not dissecting the hepatic artery from the bile duct in the hepatoduodenal ligament. We only dissect the artery in the hilum of the liver and intraparenchymally in order to keep the circulation to the recipient's biliary system as intact as possible. The remainder of the implantation of the lobar allograft is performed in a manner identical to our piggy-back technique, including the use of the confluence of the middle and left hepatic veins for the upper hepatic venous anastomosis.

We observed a favorable outcome with transjugular intrahepatic portosystemic shunt (TIPS) in the management of portal hypertension in patients awaiting liver transplantation. The amount of blood and blood products necessary during OLT has been significantly less in the group of patients with TIPS compared to other adult patients who received OLT during the same time period. During surgery, no major technical difficulties were encountered due to the presence of TIPS (9).

Immunosuppression

At the start of our program, cyclosporine was used as maintenance immunosuppression, first as compassionate use until it became available commercially, and then routinely. Double therapy consisting of cyclosporine plus prednisone was used for maintenance treatment and azathioprine was added to the regimen if a patient developed rejection or nephrotoxicity that mandated lowering of the cyclosporine dose. In 1995, FK506 replaced cyclosporine, and in 1996, mycophenolate mofetil replaced azathioprine in our immunosuppressive protocol. During the first 3 months, patients receive low-dose mycophenolate mofetil (500 mg twice a day) plus FK506 and prednisone. Thereafter, FK506 (levels 8-10) plus prednisone are the mainstay of immunosuppression. With this regimen, our rate of biopsy-proven acute rejection at one year has been reduced to 18% (10). Our protocol for treatment of rejection is with steroid pulses, and steroid-resistant rejection is treated with anti-lymphocyte preparations. Recently, IL2-receptor blockers and Rapamycin have been added to our regimen, particularly in patients with pre-existing renal dysfunction. In hepatitis C patients, we attempt to decrease the total steroids and tend to treat lower grade rejections with increasing baseline immunosuppression.

Long-term Immunosuppression and Patient Care

We follow a strict protocol for diligent and personalized posttransplant management based on scheduled evaluations at 3 months, 6 months, one year and yearly thereafter. These evaluations assess hepatic function and anatomy, renal function, immunosuppression, complications, and general laboratory and radiologic examinations. Immunosuppression is adjusted based on histologic findings and clinical course, aiming to achieve the lowest possible doses of immunosuppressants. In addition, all preventive and treatment aspects of patient care are individually evaluated by the transplant team with appropriate consultants. Local and out-of-town referring physicians are kept up-to-date with patient care status and goals with frequent correspondence and personal contact. We do not have any patients lost to follow-up.

Research Activity

The clinical program has supported significant research activity, most recently in relationship to the development of the adult live donor program. Several years of large animal experimentation using dog and pig models for liver transplantation have resulted in our being able to define the appropriate liver volume for transplantation. Segmental liver transplants (segments I, II, and III) were performed in dog model as autografts or allografts to recipients equal in weight to the donor and to recipients 1.5 times larger than their donors. All autografts and donor-recipient weight-matched allografts survived with excellent function in the recipients. Mismatched donor-recipient allografts produced various degrees of hepatic dysfunction in all recipients and were associated with 20% recipient mortality. Donor liver segment weight-to-recipient liver mass demonstrated that allograft survival was possible with a ratio as low as 32% (11). We used this data as the basis for our decision to use right lobe grafts and factors significantly in our clinical decisions during live donor selection.

Further basic research into the regenerative capabilities of the transplanted right lobe, the degree of liver cell apoptosis, and the impact of various clinical parameters on liver regenerative ability is now underway and should provide interesting insight into clinical problems encountered with this procedure.

SUMMARY AND CONCLUSIONS

1. Since its inception, the liver program at UT Memphis has been striving to serve its population by stressing access, technical innovation, and by its focus on quality of life. The results for both adult and pediatric transplants over the past 18 years demonstrate that small and medium-sized programs can function efficiently and are valuable for their local communities.

2. Patient and graft survival rates exceeded 85% in the pediatric population in the first year with the 5-, 10-, and 15-year results above 75%.

3. Patient and graft survival rates in adults were 83% at one year, 68% at 5 years, and 60% at 10 years.

4. Innovative techniques in liver transplantation have had a dramatic impact on accessibility of pediatric recipients to liver transplantation and recently are becoming crucial for select populations of adults requiring expedited transplantation.

REFERENCES

1. Rosendale JD, McBride MA. Organ donation in the United States: 1990-1998. In: Cecka JM, Terasaki PI, Eds. Clinical Transplants 1999. Los Angeles, CA: UCLA Immunogenetics Center, 2000: 83.

2. Nymann T, Shokouh-Amiri MH, Vera SR, Riely CA, Alloway RR, Gaber AO. Prevention of hepatitis B recurrence with indefinite hepatitis B immune globulin (HBIG) prophylaxis after liver transplantation. Clin Transplantation 1996; 10:663.

3. Shaw BW, Martin DJ, Marquez JW, et al. Venous bypass in clinical liver transplantation. Ann Surg 1984; 200:524.

4. Navarro F, Le Moine M-C, Fabre J-M, et al. Specific vascular complications of orthotopic liver transplantation with preservation of the retrohepatic vena cava: review of 1361 cases. Transplantation 1999; 68(5):646.

5. Shokouh-Amiri MH, Gaber AO, Bagous WA, et al. Choice of surgical technique influences perioperative outcomes in liver transplantation. Ann Surg 2000; 6:814.

6. Grewal HP, Shokouh-Amiri MH, Vera SR, et al. In-situ split-liver transplantation. Tennessee Medicine 1999; Nov:411.

7. Grewal HP, Shokouh-Amiri MH, Vera SR, Stratta RJ, Gaber AO. Surgical technique for right lobe adult living donor liver transplantation without veno-venous bypass or portocaval shunting and with duct-to-duct biliary reconstruction. Ann Surg 2001 (In press).

8. Shokouh-Amiri MH, Grewal HP, Vera SR, Stratta RJ, Bagous W, Gaber AO. Duct-to-duct biliary reconstruction in right lobe adult living donor liver transplantation. J Am Coll Surg 2001 (In press).

9. Shokouh-Amiri MH, Gaber AO, Vera SR,et al. The impact of transjugular intrahepatic portosystemic shunt (TIPS) on liver transplantation: a single center experience. (Submitted).

10. Hardinger KL, Shokouh-Amiri MH, Lo A, et al. A comparison of low dose, short course mycophenolate mofetil and tacrolimus versus full dose, long course mycophenolate mofetil and cyclosporine after liver transplantation. Transplantation 2001 (Submitted).

11. Shokouh-Amiri MH, Nymann T, El-Ella K, Adamec T, Helmy A, Britt LG, Gaber AO. Transplantation of liver segments from smaller donors to larger recipients. 1997 Americas Hepato-Pancreato-Biliary Congress Abstract, p. 42.

ACKNOWLEDGEMENT

We thank Jo Lariviere for her excellent help during preparation of the manuscript.

CHAPTER 23

The University of Toronto Liver Transplant Program: Toronto General Hospital, Hospital for Sick Children

Leslie B. Lilly, Mark S. Cattral, Nigel Girgrah, Atul Humar, Paul D. Greig, Annie Fecteau, Gary Levy, and David Grant

The Toronto General Hospital, Toronto, Ontario, CANADA

The University of Toronto Liver Transplant Program was initiated in 1985. Over the past decade it has developed into the largest program in Canada, with almost 1,100 transplants performed (895 adult and 195 pediatric) and more than 100 new liver transplants per year. This chapter serves as an update to our earlier report (1), and describes our program and its results. In addition, it highlights our interest in viral hepatitis, new monitoring techniques for immunosuppression, and describes a new initiative, adult living-related liver transplantation.

Program Structure

The University of Toronto liver transplant program operates jointly out of The Toronto General Hospital and the Hospital for Sick Children. Although these institutions are independent, geographic proximity and a close working relationship have fostered the development of living-related and split liver transplantation. Since its inception, our program has promoted a combined surgical and medical approach to the management of patients with liver disease. Presently, hepatologists and surgeons manage patients on a rotational basis in both the peri-operative and posttransplant period. Both a surgeon and a hepatologist attend daily ward rounds, which provides an optimal environment for teaching fellows and residents. Each week, the adult and pediatric teams meet to discuss new candidates for transplantation, to match potential adult and pediatric recipients for split liver transplantation, and to assess candidates for living related donation. The liver transplant program falls under the umbrella of the multi-organ transplantation program,

which includes transplantation activity in liver, kidney, heart, lung and kidney/pancreas. All transplant patients are managed in a single unit and most members of all transplant disciplines share a common office area.

Patient Selection

Patient selection criteria at the University of Toronto are generally similar to those used by other programs, and have recently been reviewed (2). Patients referred for transplantation are initially assessed by one of the transplant hepatologists. In appropriate candidates, a detailed assessment of medical, surgical and psychosocial issues follows. In addition, arrangements are made to screen family members as potential donors. Once listed, patients are seen frequently in a clinic by Nurse Practitioners and the attending Hepatologist. Patient management and follow-up throughout the transplant process are summarized in Figure 1.

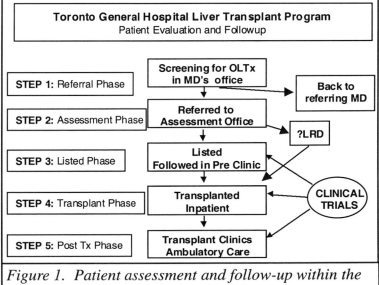

Figure 1. Patient assessment and follow-up within the University of Toronto adult liver transplant program.

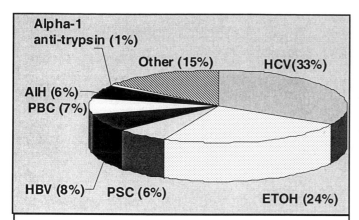

Figure 2. Etiology of end-stage liver disease in adults listed for transplantation (n=140, December 2000).

Patients with end-stage liver disease primarily due to hepatitis C virus (HCV) currently comprise 33% of the waiting list in Toronto (Fig. 2). Alcoholic liver disease (ETOH) is the second major indication, comprising 24% of listed patients. Our program, like most others, requires a minimum of 6 months of abstinence from alcohol and/or drugs before a patient with a history of substance abuse is considered for liver transplantation.

Autoimmune liver diseases, including primary biliary cirrhosis (PBC), primary sclerosing cholangitis (PSC), and autoimmune hepatitis (AIH), are the indication for transplantation in a further 19% of currently listed adult patients. The other important indication in Toronto is hepatitis B (HBV), the etiology of end-stage disease in 8% of listed patients. Fifteen to twenty percent of patients are expected to receive right lobe grafts from living donors.

Hepatocellular carcinoma, almost always on the background of cirrhosis, has been either the primary indication or present incidentally in approximately 10% of patients transplanted at our center. We currently apply the following criteria: a single lesion no larger than 5 cm in diameter, or multiple lesions (no more than 3) none larger than 3 cm in diameter, with no evidence in either case of vascular invasion or extrahepatic spread of disease. Patients are always considered for potential resection prior to referral for transplantation. Appropriate candidates are treated with ablative therapy, either percutaneous ethanol injection or radio frequency ablation, and we are currently reviewing our experience in this regard.

RESULTS

From October 1985 to November 2000, 895 adult liver transplants were performed in 823 patients (Fig. 3). Of these, 72 were retransplants (67 second transplants, 5 third) for a rate of 8.0%. The indications for transplantation since 1995 are shown in Table 1. As predicted from the waiting list, HCV-related end-stage liver disease and cirrhosis due to alcohol were the commonest indications, comprising 30% and 13% of our transplanted patients, respectively.

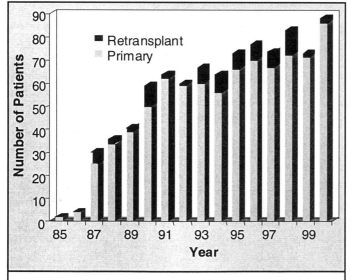

Figure 3. Adult liver transplants performed at the University of Toronto, 1985 – November 2000.

Table 1. Indications for transplantation, adult program (1995-November 2000).	
HCV – hepatitis C virus	30%
ETOH – alcoholic liver disease	13%
PSC – primary sclerosing cholangitis	9%
PBC – primary biliary cirrhosis	9%
RTX - retransplant	8%
HBV – hepatitis B virus	8%
CRYPT – cryptogenic cirrhosis	6%
FHF – fulminant hepatic failure	4%
AAT – alpha 1 anti-trypsin disease	3%
AIH – autoimmune hepatitis	2%
PCLD – polycystic liver disease	1%
FAP – familial amyloidosis	1%
Others	5%

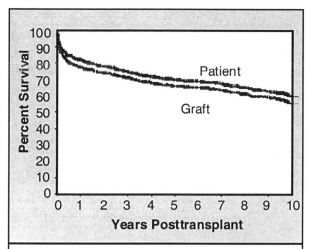

Figure 4. Ten-year graft and patient survival of adults transplanted at the University of Toronto (1985-2000).

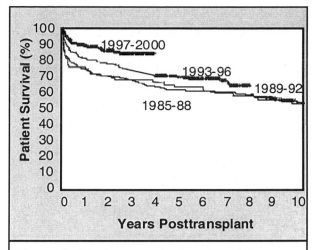

Figure 5. Patient survival grouped by era of transplant.

Ten-year patient and graft survival rates since 1985 (Fig. 4) were 60% and 57%, respectively. However, substantial improvements in patient selection, immunosuppression, surgical methods, and infection management since 1985 have led us to divide this period into 4-year eras (Fig. 5). Forty-eight month patient survival has improved significantly compared with earlier eras, and is currently approximately 85%. Outcomes in patients transplanted for hepatitis B and C will be considered in separate sections to follow.

Immunosuppression

Advances in immunosuppressive therapy have played an important role in the evolution and success of liver transplantation, and our program has been a leader in the evaluation of new agents (3). In the first 10 years of our program, patients were treated with sequential immunosuppression consisting of Minnesota antilymphocyte globulin (MALG) induction in combination with Sandimmune (CsA) and methylprednisolone. More recently, our program has utilized the new microemulsion formulation of CsA, Neoral. The availability of this preparation allowed us to discontinue the routine use of intravenous CsA, which not only resulted in reduced toxicity but also in greater efficacy with rejection rates of 25-30%. Our institution spearheaded a pivotal trial comparing the use of Neoral with tacrolimus and the potential for steroid reduction. In this trial, we demonstrated that both tacrolimus and Neoral are effective agents and steroids can be discontinued in the vast majority of patients using either agent (4).

One of the current challenges in transplant biology is optimizing immunosuppressive protocols to maximize clinical benefits without associated toxicity. Our group, as part of an international team, has examined new markers that provide a better therapeutic index of CsA blood concentrations than can be obtained by the traditional monitoring of trough concentrations and that are closely correlated with positive clinical outcomes (eg., reduction in acute and chronic rejection and reduction of acute CsA nephrotoxicity). A pivotal study completed in liver transplant recipients at our institution clearly identified the value of a simplified single sample point (C_2, 2 hours after dosing) to assess the degree and extent of CsA absorption from Neoral. Based on the findings from studies carried out at our institution, a multicentre, prospective, non-blind, parallel group study was developed to compare C_2 monitoring of Neoral directly with C_0 monitoring in 307 de novo liver transplant recipients. The C_2 group was given Neoral to achieve a mean target of 1 µg/ml and the C_0 target ranged between 0.25-0.4 µg/ml (whole blood mFPIA). At 3 months after transplantation, the overall incidence of acute rejection was 25% lower in the C_2 group versus the C_0 group and the incidence of moderate to severe histologic grading of rejection was significantly lower in the C_2 group versus the C_0 group (47 vs. 73%; p = 0.01). The safety profiles were similar between the 2 groups throughout the 3-month study period, which confirms that the improved clinical benefits seen with C_2 monitoring versus C_0 monitoring are achieved without additional risk of adverse events.

In those patients monitored by C_2, there was a marked effect of time to reach target on incidence of rejection. In those patients who achieved target levels by day 3, the incidence of rejection was 12.5% compared with an incidence of 31% in patients who achieved target by day 7. In contrast, no similar effect was seen in patients monitored by C_0 (5).

We have now examined the impact on renal function and incidence of hypertension of converting maintenance liver transplant recipients to C_2 monitoring. One hundred and ten stable liver transplant patients (with 3-164 months follow-up) on Neoral were converted to C_2 monitoring. At the time of conversion the mean C_0 was 198 µg/ml (range 96-482 µg/ml); the mean C_2 at the time of conversion was 880 µg/ml (range 114-1900 µg/ml) and there was a poor correlation between C_0 and C_2 ($r^2=0.19$). Thirty-three percent of patients at the time of conversion had C_2 levels exceeding recommended targets (0-6 months 1000 µg/ml; 6-12 months 800 µg/ml; > 12 months 600 µg/ml) and 18% had levels below target. There was a poor correlation of C_0 with serum creatinine ($r^2=0.03$), but a better correlation between C2 levels and creatinine ($r^2=0.59$). Within 3 months of conversion to C_2, there was a mean decrease in serum creatinine of 22%: pre-conversion 155 µmol/L (range 76-270 µmol/L); post-conversion mean of 124 µmol/L (range 65-158 µmol/L ($p<0.001$)). Improvement in serum creatinine following conversion and adjustment was seen even 10 years after transplantation. A parallel improvement in blood pressure was seen with C_2 adjustment to target (mean decrease in diastolic blood pressure of 12±3 mmHg ($p<0.03$). For patients exceeding C_2 targets, a mean dose reduction of 12% (range 7-22%) was required. In patients whose C2 levels were below target, adjustments in dose were made to bring patients' target levels in line with recommended C_2 levels with no increase in serum creatinine. No clinical or biochemical evidence of rejection was seen during dose adjustments although protocol biopsies were not performed.

Our Institution has also spearheaded Phase 1 and Phase 2 studies in the development of a rapamycin derivative (RAD) in liver transplant patients. Certican (RAD) is a novel macrolide with potent immunosuppressive and anti-proliferative activities as well as excellent and consistent absorption. A Phase 1 study in de novo liver transplant patients demonstrated that RAD absorption is not influenced by bile diversion or administration site, and that RAD does not affect CsA pharmacokinetics. A Phase 2 study was then undertaken to examine the safety and tolerability of RAD compared to placebo in de novo liver transplant recipients. One hundred and nineteen liver allograft recipients were randomized to one of 4 groups: Group 1 RAD 0.5 mg bid p.o.; group 2 RAD 1 mg bid, p.o.; Group 3 RAD 2 mg bid, p.o. and group 4 placebo. Patients received Neoral to achieve a target trough level of 250-400 µg/ml and prednisone. Overall patient survival (88%) and graft survival (95%) were excellent. The incidence of treated rejection was less in the RAD groups than in the placebo groups: placebo (36.7%); RAD 1 mg/day (28.6%); RAD 2 mg/day (23.3%); 4 mg/day (25.8%). Pharmacokinetic RAD data obtained on day 7, 2 and 3 months after transplantation indicated that RAD steady state is achieved within 7 days of starting RAD, and the PK profiles indicate that there is dose proportionality when looking across the 3 dose groups of RAD. The studies we have performed to date suggest that RAD in combination with Neoral provides effective immunosuppression with excellent patient and graft survival and pave the way for Phase 3 and 4 studies in liver transplant patients.

Our program remains interested in the investigation of new immunosuppressive agents as well as strategies to reduce long-term toxicities in liver transplant recipients. In this regard we are now participating in Phase 3 studies on the effect of a reduced dose regimen of rapamycin/tacrolimus on the incidence of rejection, patient and graft survival, and toxicity as well as a study of C_2 monitoring using Neoral versus Tacrolimus. In addition we continue to examine the effects of conversion of maintenance liver transplant recipients to C_2 Neoral monitoring on renal and non-renal toxicity in an attempt to improve patients' lives.

Liver Transplantation for Viral Hepatitis

Hepatitis B

Due to the demographics of the greater Toronto area, cirrhosis caused by hepatitis B virus has been an important indication for transplantation within our program. Eighty-nine patients who were hepatitis B surface antigen (HBsAg) positive have been transplanted. Severe recurrent disease in the allograft has been observed, particularly in recipients with markers of ongoing viral replication at the time of transplantation. Left untreated, recurrent hepatitis B led uniformly to rapidly progressive liver disease, and viral recurrence was the primary cause of patient death in one-third of transplants. Our group has used prostaglandin E in patients who had recurrent hepatitis B, and a series of 14 patients has been reported (6). During treatment, both serum and liver markers of viral replication decreased or even disappeared, with a concomitant attenuation of biochemical and histological evidence of liver inflammation. The best results were achieved in patients treated early after recurrence, although even patients in early liver failure appeared to receive some benefit from the drug. Initial treatment was with intravenous PGE, and the patients tolerated conversion to the oral preparation well.

Over the years, a number of measures have been instituted in an effort to prevent graft reinfection. Patients who were serum HBV-DNA negative at the time of transplant appeared less likely to develop recurrent disease; thus, only patients with chronic hepatitis B who are serum DNA negative are currently considered for transplantation within our program. A reduction in the recurrence of HBV has been reported with the use of hepatitis B immune globulin (HBIG) administered during both the anhepatic phase and then after transplantation, with dosing titrated to maintain measurable HBsAb levels. In our program, several patients were maintained free of recurrent disease as long as antibody levels greater than 500 U/ml were maintained. This approach, however, only postpones recurrence, and represents a considerable cost, inconvenience and drain on limited supplies, and is no longer being routinely applied in our centre as high-dose monotherapy.

Lamivudine (3TC) has been demonstrated to be effective in lowering HBV-DNA levels in the non-transplant setting. Our program was involved in a multinational trial examining the role of this nucleoside analogue in the prevention and treatment of recurrence in transplant recipients (7). Our experience in the use of lamivudine in these settings has recently been reviewed (8). Thirty-two patients, including 4 with de novo HBV following transplantation for another indication, received lamivudine. Thirteen patients initiated treatment prior to transplantation, and the drug was started only after transplantation for HBV in the remaining 15 patients. Overall patient survival for all treated patients was 81% with a mean follow up of 23 months. Breakthrough infection attributed to the YMDD variant had occurred in 6 patients, for an overall rate of 19%; the majority of these patients have remained clinically stable with no further decline in liver function despite active viral replication.

In view of the experience of treatment failures with HBIG and with lamivudine, we have more recently been managing our HBV patients with combination therapy. Patients who are serum HBV-DNA positive and with active necroinflammatory disease upon referral for transplantation are treated with lamivudine (Heptovir®, 100 mg daily) and transplanted only after serum HBV-DNA levels have fallen below detection. Those who are already serum HBV-DNA negative are started on lamivudine shortly before or on the day of transplantation. Low-dose HBIG treatment is initiated during the anhepatic phase (10 cc, ~2000 units) and continued daily for 7 days, then weekly for 3 weeks and then monthly for a year along with continuation of lamivudine. Patients with fulminant hepatitis B are managed in a similar fashion. At the end of one year, HBIG is discontinued and monotherapy with lamivudine is maintained. In the first 7 patients who have completed combination therapy, there have been no recurrences.

Although many patients who develop breakthrough infection with HBV attributable to the YMDD variant follow a relatively benign course even after transplantation, this is not uniformly the case, and we have had 2 deaths. We are currently managing breakthrough patients who appear to have aggressive disease either with adefovir or with entecavir within the context of clinical trials.

Hepatitis C

Between 1987 and March 1999, 655 patients underwent orthotopic liver transplantation at our centre; of these, 151 patients received 167 transplants for the primary diagnosis of HCV- or non-A non-B hepatitis-related end-stage liver disease. We performed a retrospective analysis of these 151 HCV-positive patients to determine the incidence of recurrent hepatitis and cirrhosis, and the effect of recurrence on graft and patient survival (Malkan, et al. personal communication). The respective one- and 5-year patient survival rates were 90% and 73% after a median follow-up of 1,034 days, and were similar to those of 593 HCV-negative patients who received liver transplantation during the same time period. Among 133 HCV-positive patients followed for longer than 6 months, recurrent hepatitis was diagnosed in 76% at a median of 86 days after liver transplantation as has been reported (9). According to Kaplan-Meier estimates, the probability of developing bridging fibrosis/

(21). We prospectively analyzed the impact of HHV-6 infection in 200 liver transplant recipients using quantitative PCR techniques to measure viral load. Although HHV-6 infection was common, occurring in 28% of patients, we found that disease directly attributable to HHV-6 occurred in only 2/200 (1%) patients (unpublished data). These patients presented with a viral syndrome characterized by fever and bone marrow suppression. Although direct disease due to HHV-6 was uncommon, viral infection may have an immunomodulatory role possibly through cytokine dysregulation or direct interactions with other viruses. We found that HHV-6 infection was significantly associated with the development of CMV disease, other opportunistic infections, and the development of later (after day 30) acute rejection episodes. Therefore, the primary impact of HHV-6 after transplantation appears to be through indirect effects of viral replication.

Other preventative strategies are initiated based on the risk of a particular infectious complication in a given patient. For example, patients at high risk of invasive fungal infections, such as those with biliary tract complications and on broad-spectrum antibiotics, are routinely given fluconazole prophylaxis to prevent infections due to Candida species (22). With the use of these and other strategies, morbidity and mortality due to infectious complications has been minimized in these patients.

Living Donation

The living-donor liver transplantation (LRLD) program began in June 1996 with a transplant between an adult donor and pediatric recipient. With the pressure of an increased number of patients on the waiting list (n=140 as of Dec, 2000), increased time awaiting transplantation (median wait time for patients at home is 16 months for blood type "O", 22 months for "A" and 9 months for "B"), and an increased mortality rate among those awaiting transplantation (15% in 2000), the interest in LRLD has grown enormously. LRLD with right lobe grafts has become our preferred option for adult recipients and is offered during the initial assessment for transplantation.

During 2000, 11 living donor transplants (LDTs) were performed in 2 pediatric and 9 adult recipients. The 2 children were infant recipients of liver segments 2 and 3 from their fathers. The age of the adult recipients (6 male, 3 female) ranged from 31-66 years (mean 50); 4 patients were hospital-bound at the time of transplantation. The adult donors, who were aged 21-56 years (mean 39 years), included one parent, 5 children, 2 siblings and a close friend. All donors underwent a right lobectomy; in all but one case the middle hepatic vein was left intact in the donor. Complications have developed in 4 donors: postoperative bleeding requiring laparotomy (1 patient), right pleural effusion requiring percutaneous drainage (n=1), and wound infection (n=2). All donors are currently alive and well with normal liver tests. In the recipient operation, interposition vein grafts (donor inferior mesenteric vein and recipient left portal vein) were used to drain large venous tributaries draining segment 8 in 2 patients and the middle hepatic vein in one patient. Five adult recipients required separate anastomoses of multiple hepatic ducts (3 ducts in 3 patients and 2 in 2 patients). One late biliary stricture has responded to percutaneous stenting. All recipients are alive and well.

Pediatric Liver Transplantation

The pediatric liver transplant program was developed on a multidisciplinary team model both for the pre- and posttransplant care of patients. The team consists of pediatric transplant surgeons, pediatric hepatologists, transplant nurses, a dedicated anesthesia team, infectious disease specialists, a pharmacist, nutritionist, and a social worker. Hepatologists and surgeons also jointly assume outpatient management. As the pediatric and adult programs are integrated, new or difficult patients are discussed at the weekly conference and pediatric patients are teamed up with the appropriate adult for split-liver transplantation. Each family is assessed and encouraged to proceed with living donation. Joint meetings of the adult and pediatric programs also facilitate the transition of young adults from the pediatric to the adult program.

Pediatric patient selection is similar to that at other centers. From 1986 to November 2000, 195 pediatric liver transplants have been performed. Biliary atresia is the commonest cause of liver disease in our program (41%) followed by fulminant liver failure in 17% of patients. Our program also sees a significant number of patients from the First Nations with cholestatic disease due to our referral area.

Our program has switched to an oral tacrolimus-based dual immunosuppression and we have observed a 28% rate of rejection at one year. All rejection episodes were steroid responsive. Steroids are tapered over 3 months after a 3-month rejection-free period, with a plan to have all patients on monotherapy by the first year after transplantation. All patients receive 3 months of CMV prophylaxis with gancyclovir and CMV immuno-globulins, except for D-/R- patients. No CMV disease has been observed on that regimen. We have achieved both one- and 3-year survival rates of 94% in the last 4-year period. Our graft survival has closely mimicked our patient survival at 92% at one and 3 years.

Posttransplant lymphoproliferative disease (PTLD) has been a challenge for our program. We have been able to decrease our PTLD rate from 16% to 9% in the past 5 years. Patients diagnosed with PTLD are treated with immediate halving of their immunosuppression and reintroduction of gancyclovir and immunoglobulins for a 3-month period. Since the beginning of the program, we have had an overall 33% death rate from PTLD, all patients with high-grade immunoblastic lymphoma. There have been no deaths from PTLD in the last 4 years, as most lymphomas are detected at an early stage. Patients diagnosed with monoclonal monomorphic disease, recurrent or non-responsive PTLD are considered for chemotherapy. Late graft loss due to chronic rejection has been the indication for retransplantation in 11% of the PTLD patients.

SUMMARY

The University of Toronto Liver Transplant Program began in 1985 at a time when the procedure had already evolved from an experimental form of surgery to an accepted treatment for many forms of liver failure. The program was established not only to provide clinical care for patients but also to address academically the barriers that impeded success. The program brought together experts in medicine, surgery, pathology, and the basic sciences of immunology, virology and molecular biology.

Significant advances over the past decade and a half in immunosuppressive drugs and monitoring, patient selection, and infectious management have contributed to markedly improved patient and graft survival rates. Nevertheless, we continue to face 2 major challenges: a growing scarcity of donor organs, a problem partially addressed through development of living-related liver donation, and recurrent viral hepatitis. We expect to remain on the forefront of ongoing research to provide solutions to these and other barriers to the full deployment of liver transplantation in the year 2000.

LIVER — TORONTO, CANADA

REFERENCES

1. Hemming AW, Cattral MS, Greig PD et al. The University of Toronto liver transplant program. In: JM Cecka, PI Terasaki, Eds. Clinical Transplants 1996. UCLA Tissue Typing Laboratory, Los Angeles, 1997:177.

2. Chung SW, Greig, PD, Cattral, MS, et al. Liver transplantation: An evaluation of high risk indications. Brit J Surgery 1997; 84:189.

3. Cattral MS, Lilly LB and Levy GA. Immunosuppression in liver transplantation. In: Seminars in Liver Disease 2001; 20 (in press).

4. Greig PD, Grant DR, Kneteman NM, et al. Early steroid withdrawal following liver transplantation-two year follow up. [abstract] Transplantation 2000; 69:S389.

5. Belitsky P, Dunn, S Johnston, A Levy, G. Impact of absorption profiling on efficacy and safety of cyclosporin therapy in transplant recipients. Clinical Pharmacokinetics 2000; 39:117.

6. Flowers M, Sherker A, Sinclair SB, et al. Prostaglandin E in the treatment of recurrent hepatitis B infection after orthotopic liver transplantation. Transplantation 1994; 58:183.

7. Perrillo R, Rakela J, Dienstag J, et al. Multicenter study of lamivudine therapy for hepatitis B after liver transplantation. Hepatology 1999; 29:1581.

8. Malkan, G, Cattral, MS, Humar, A, et al. Lamivudine for hepatitis B in liver transplantation. Transplantation 2000; 69:1403.

9. Lilly LB, Cattral MS, Levy GA. Hepatitis C and Liver Transplantation. Viral Hepatitis Reviews 2001 (in press).

10. Schalm SW, van Rossum TGJ. Goals of antiviral therapy: viral clearance or ALT normalization. Hepatology 1999; 31:83.

11. Bigam DL, Pennington JJ, Carpentier A, et al. Hepatitis C-related cirrhosis: a predictor of diabetes after liver transplantation. Hepatology 2000; 32:87.

12. Cattral MS, Krajden M, Walness IR, et al. A pilot study of ribavirin therapy for recurrent hepatitis C virus infection after liver transplantation. Transplantation 1996; 61:1483.

13. Cattral MS, Hemming AW, Walness IR, et al. Outcome of long-term Ribavirin therapy for recurrent hepatitis C after liver transplantation. Transplantation 1999; 67:1277.

14. Bizollon T, Palazzo U, Ducerf C, et al. Pilot study of the combination of interferon alpha and ribavirin as therapy of recurrent hepatitis C after liver transplantation. Hepatology 1997; 26:500.

15. Fischer, et al. Treatment of severe recurrent hepatitis C after liver transplantation with ribavirin plus interferon alpha. Transplant Proc 1999; 31:494.

16. El-Amin OA, Poterucha JJ, Zein NN, et al. Interferon/ribavirin therapy for recurrent hepatitis C after liver transplantation [Abstract]. Hepatology 1999; 30:247A.

17. Mazzaferro V, Regalia E, Pulvirenti A, et al. Prophylaxis against HCV recurrence after liver transplantation. Transplant Proc 1997; 29:511.

18. Feray C, Caccamo L, Alexander GJM, et al. European collaborative study on factors influencing outcome after liver transplantation for hepatitis C. Gastroenterology 1999; 117:619.

19. Fiel MI, Schiano TD, Min AD, et al. Histopathologic and clinical features of patients undergoing retransplantation for recurrent hepatitis C viral (HCV) infection [Abstract]. Hepatology 1999; 30:247A.

20. Humar A, Gregson D, McGeer A, et al. Clinical utility of quantitative cytomegalovirus viral load determination for predicting cytomegalovirus disease in liver transplant recipients. Transplantation 1999; 68:1305.

21. Humar A, Malkan G, Moussa G, Greig P, Levy G, Mazzulli T. Human herpesvirus-6 is associated with CMV reactivation in liver transplant recipients. J Infect Dis 2000; 181:1450.

22. Winston DJ, Pakrasi A, Busuttil RW. Prophylactic fluconazole in liver transplant recipients: a randomized, double-blind, placebo-controlled trial. Ann Intern Med 1999; 131:729.

ACKNOWLEDGEMENTS

The authors would like to thank Mr. Robert Smith for assistance in the preparation of survival data and Ms. Charmaine Beal for secretarial support.

CHAPTER 24

Paul Brousse Liver Transplantation: The First 1,500 Cases

Daniel Azoulay, Didier Samuel, René Adam, Eric Savier, Vincent Karam, Valérie Delvard, Faouzi Saliba, Philippe Ichai, Bruno Roche, Cyrille Feray, Jean-Charles Duclos Vallee, Alaova Smail, Denis Castaing, and Henri Bismuth

Centre Hépatobiliaire, UPRES 1596, Assistance Publique-Hôpitaux de Paris, Université Paris Sud, Hôpital Paul Brousse, Villejuif, FRANCE

Between 1984 and November 2000, 1,580 liver transplantations have been performed in 1,370 patients. Data presented in this paper give a comprehensive overview of the status and evolution of liver transplantation in our center.

Indications for Liver Transplantation

The main indications for liver transplantation are summarized in Figure 1. Cirrhosis is by far the most frequent indication (52%). The main causes of cirrhosis were viral infection (56%), alcohol abuse (18%), and primary biliary cirrhosis (14%). Cirrhosis is followed by cancers (18%) related to hepatocellular carcinoma with cirrhosis (76%) or without cirrhosis (29%). Fulminant or subfulminant hepatitis cases represent 17%, mainly related to viral infection (39%) or of unknown cause (41%). Acute hepatic failure is followed by metabolic diseases (6%) with a majority of familial amyloidotic polyneuropathy (69%). Cholestatic disease (5%) is mainly represented by primary sclerosing cholangitis (57%) and biliary atresia (19%). This latter indication is the most frequent (29%) in the pediatric population, followed by metabolic disease (7%).

Patient Survival

Overall patient survival is 83% at one year, 75% at 3 years, 71% at 5 years and, 65% at 10 years. Figure 2 shows the actuarial patient survival following transplantation for cirrhosis, cancer, fulminant hepatitis, and metabolic diseases.

MAIN INDICATIONS FOR LIVER TRANSPLANTATION

Cirrhosis

The most frequent causes of cirrhosis were: Hepatitis C virus (HCV) (13%), alcohol (9%), primary biliary (7%), hepatitis B (HBV) or B-delta (HDV) virus (7%) and HBV, and HDV/HCV co-infection (5%). Patient survival rates in these groups are represented in Figure 3.

Our group did pioneering work on the prevention of

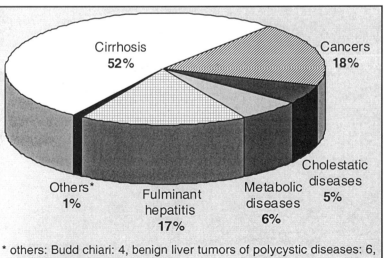

* others: Budd chiari: 4, benign liver tumors of polycystic diseases: 6, parasitic disease: 4, morbus osler: 3

Figure 1. Primary indications for liver transplantation in Paul Brousse Hospital (1,370 patients from 1984-2000).

LIVER – VILLEJUIF, FRANCE

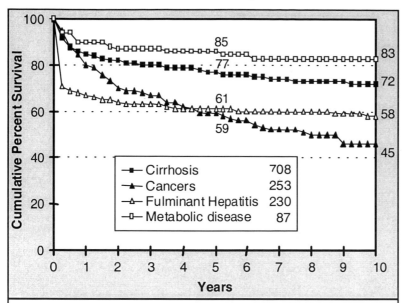

Figure 2. Survival of patients according to the main indication of liver transplantation in Paul Brousse Hospital (1984-2000).

HBV recurrence after liver transplantation with the introduction of anti-HBs (H BIG) long-term passive immunoprophylaxis (1). So far, more than 270 patients have received long-term administration of high-dose H BIG since 1986, with an overall 10-year HBV recurrence rate of 27%. Using this prophylaxis, the 10-year

HBV recurrence rate was 0%, 17%, 52% in fulminant hepatitis B, HDV cirrhotic, and HBV cirrhotic patients, respectively. In the latter group recurrence was higher in those with pretransplant HBV replication as assessed by the presence of HBV DNA in serum. We recently developed a new approach to HBV prevention for this high-risk group by using lamivudine prior to transplantation in association with a posttransplant combination prophylaxis with lamivudine and long-term H BIG administration. This protocol further reduced the rate of HBV reinfection in this high-risk group from 90% to 20%.

HCV reinfection after transplantation of patients suffering from HCV cirrhosis is a major problem for this important group of candidates for transplantation. We showed in a previous study that the 5-year rates of acute and chronic HCV hepatitis, and of cirrhosis were 75%, 60% and 10%, respectively (2). In addition, we expect a 20-25% 10-year rate of HCV cirrhosis of the graft. This outcome seemed to be more severe in our patients infected with genotype 1 (3) and was associated with a high intrahepatic HCV load at the time of acute HCV reinfection. For these reasons, we are developing new strategies to reduce HCV recurrence and its consequences on graft histology. These strategies will include modulation of immunosuppression with reduced steroid doses and treatment of HCV reinfection using an interferon-ribavirin combination, which gave promising results achieving a 20% sustained virologic response.

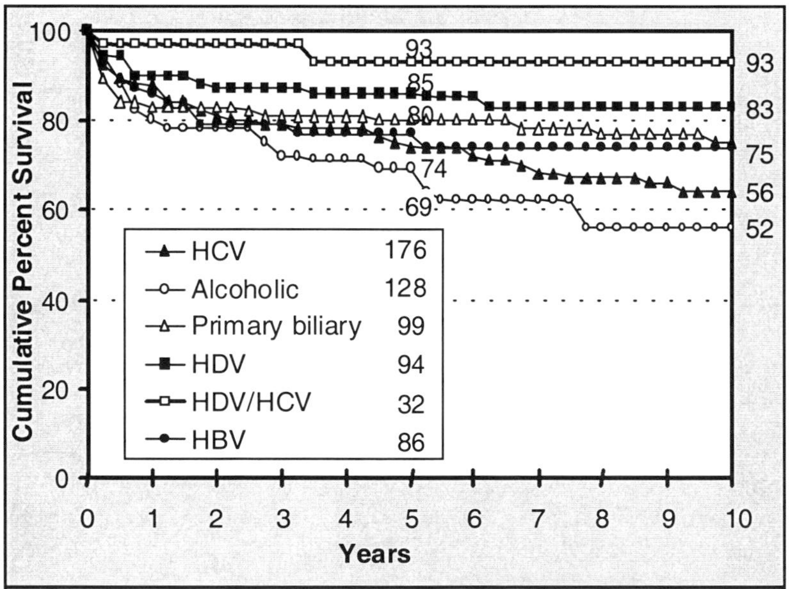

Cancers

Hepatocellular carcinoma (HCC) with cirrhosis is the major cancer indication in our center (14% of overall cases and 76% of cancers). Patient survival is 80% at one year, 65% at 3 years, 59% at 5 years and, 45% at 10 years (Fig. 2). Liver transplantation is the treatment for hepato cellular

Figure 3. Survival of patients with cirrhosis as the main indication of liver transplantation in Paul Brousse Hospital (1984-2000).

carcinoma of the cirrhotic liver. We recognize that this approach may be radical and controversial because it is associated with a high risk of recurrence. Ten years ago, the consensus was to resect the patients with resectable lesions and to transplant those with non-resectable lesions. However, by comparing liver resection with transplantation for hepatocellular carcinoma in the cirrhotic patients of our series (60 patients in each group) we observed that transplantation provided much better results than resection for patients with uni- or binodular HCC (<3 cm) (survival without recurrence was 83% vs. 18% - p<0.001). Conversely, the group of patients classically defined as non-resectable, either because of larger nodules (>3 cm), a diffuse form, or the presence of a portal thrombus, had a high risk of recurrence and a survival rate of only 46% (44% without recurrence). Because of the organ shortage, these latter patients obviously appear to be questionable candidates for liver transplantation since patients with benign disease have much better survival rates. Therefore, our message has been to transplant the patients usually considered as resectable (<3 nodules and <3 cm) and to resect those who presented with a contraindication to liver transplantation (4).

This concept, which initially was controversial, is presently accepted in the transplant community and has recently been confirmed by the results at other centers. In addition, this new policy has been subsequently reinforced by more recent experience using these selection criteria. The overall survival rate of 53% in the period 1985-1991 improved significantly to 76% in the period 1992-1995. The disease-free survival rate increased from 43% to 74%. By appropriately selecting HCC patients for transplantation, it has been possible to obtain results similar to those obtained for benign disease (5,6).

This policy continues to be used by our group. However, HCC still remains a matter of controversy for what we may call "a good indication" because of its increasing frequency. Indeed, while a survival rate of 40-50% at 5 years could appear to be unacceptable when compared with the 70-80% for benign disease in the present era of organ shortage, liver transplantation in patients with more than 3 nodules or tumors more than 3 cm may represent the only chance for long-term survival. The current use of domino liver transplants and living-related transplantation will probably lead to increasing modifications of the very strict selection criteria adopted for cadaver liver transplantation. These alternative techniques have the potential to rescue some "untransplantable" patients and provide a reasonable hope of cure. Our program is open to the more marginal indications of HCC and long-term follow-up will definitely provide the answer as to whether or not we should expand the indications of transplantation for HCC.

Fulminant Hepatitis

Fulminant hepatitis represents 17% of indications related mainly to Hepatitis B infection. Patient survival is 67% at one year, 63% at 3 years, 61% at 5 years and, 58% at 10 years (Fig. 2). Our emergency program for fulminant hepatitis started in 1986 (7) and we have now evaluated more than 200 patients with fulminant hepatitis as candidates for transplantation. We used the French criteria for emergency liver transplantation (7), which includes encephalopathy stage 3 or 4 associated with a factor V level below 20% in a patient less than 30 years old or with a factor V level below 30% in a patient more than 30 years old. We developed an aggressive approach to transplant these patients using poor quality (steatotic) and ABO incompatible grafts (8) in order to increase the feasibility of transplantation in this high-risk group. Recently we tested a bioartificial liver for extracorporeal support (Circe Biomedical®) in 10 patients awaiting emergency transplantation; all were transplanted and 8 have survived long term.

Metabolic Disease

Familial amyloidotic polyneuropathy (FAP) is the main metabolic disease in our center (4% of overall cases). Patient survival is 85% at 5 years and 83% at 10 years. We have one of the largest experiences in liver transplantation for FAP (9), with more than 60 patients transplanted for this indication. FAP is characterized by the occurrence of ascending sensitive and motor polyneuropathy with symptoms starting after age 20 and leading to death after a median of 10 years. This disease affects all organs including the heart, kidneys and involves the autonomic nervous system. This devastating disease is transmitted through an autosomal dominant gene and occurs secondary to a point-mutation in the gene of a protein named transthyretin. The mutated protein deposits an amyloid form on nerves and tissue. Liver transplantation stops the progression of the disease in the majority of cases. Our extensive experience has led us to conclude that transplantation should be performed early in the course of the disease as soon as symptoms appear, and that transplantation improves the patient survival rate and the long-term quality of life of these patients. Particular attention before transplantation should be given to a careful cardiac and renal evaluation. Pacemakers are frequently mandatory before transplantation for those with cardiac amyloidoisis.

THE ROLE OF INNOVATIVE TECHNIQUES IN THE PAUL BROUSSE EXPERIENCE

The "Surgical Answer" to the Organ Shortage

In an effort to overcome the organ shortage, surgeons familiar with "surgical anatomy and anatomical surgery" have developed techniques of graft modification over the past 2 decades. Thus, only 17 years after Starzl performed the first liver transplant (10), our team performed the first transplantation of a reduced-size graft (11).

Orthotopic Transplantation of Reduced-size Grafts

Orthotopic transplantation of a reduced-size graft was first undertaken by our team (11) out of necessity due to a large size discrepancy between the donor (75 kg) and the recipient, who was an 11-year-old child (26 kg) with end-stage liver failure. Following "bench surgery", the left lobe (segments 2 and 3) was implanted. With experience, reduced-size liver transplantation (RSLT) in pediatric patients has yielded results as good as those after whole liver transplantation (12-15). The RSLT procedure has reduced the unacceptable pretransplant mortality (16,17) and the posttransplant morbidity and mortality by shortening the waiting time during which liver disease progresses (18-20) and the waiting time in the particular situations of fulminant hepatitis, primary non-function of a previous graft and hepatic infarction due to hepatic artery thrombosis (13). Furthermore, RSLT has decreased the risk of hepatic artery thrombosis due to the larger vessels of "cut down" livers compared with pediatric cadaveric livers (12,13,21).

Split-Liver Transplantation

There are 2 drawbacks to the use of reduced-size liver allografts: first there is an allocation shift towards pediatric recipients from the cadaver donor pool, bypass-ing adult recipients who might have otherwise been transplanted, and second, there is an inevitable discarding of a large volume of healthy, viable hepatic parenchyma after graft reduction that evokes a sense of waste. To alleviate the organ shortage, one further step was taken by transplanting 2 patients with one liver, the so-called "split-liver" transplant (SLT). Pichlmayr, et al, in Hannover performed the first partition of the liver in 1987 (22) with one adult receiving the right liver lobe and a child receiving the left lobe. One year later, our team (23) divided one liver graft to obtain 2 orthotopic grafts for 2 adult patients with fulminant hepatitis. The left and right livers were transplanted. Although the initial results were good, both patients died at 20 and 45 days after transplantation due to candidiasis and diffuse cytomegalovirus infection, respectively.

After a learning period (24), the results have improved so that morbidity, graft and patient survival are now identical using either a split or whole liver for transplantation (25,26). SLT, which was initially performed "ex-vivo", is also performed "in-situ" as a natural evolution of the techniques developed for living related donors. The in-situ technique for liver transplantation allows better hemostasis, fewer biliary complications (27) and a shorter ischemia time, although the operating time in the donor is prolonged by 2-3 hours. Whether using the ex-vivo or the in-situ techniques, good results that are comparable to those of conventional OLT are obtained when using an optimal technique and making a strict choice of recipients. The number of transplantable grafts has increased up to 28% in the Paul Brousse series (25). During 1995, we split 20 of 83 transplantable livers allocated to our center, generating 40 grafts; 23 were transplanted locally and 17 were given to partner centers. During the same period we accepted 4 split-liver grafts offered to us by other centers. Overall 27 split-liver transplantations were done in our unit, accounting for 30% of the 90 transplants performed in 1995. One-year patient and graft survival rates for split-liver transplantation were 79.4% and 78.5%, respectively. Arterial and biliary complications rates were, respectively, 15% and 22%; none leading to graft loss. Primary non-function occurred in one case (4%). The incidence of complications has declined as we have gained experience with this procedure.

Split-Liver for Two Adults

Whereas the shortage of liver grafts for children has

been solved by the split technique and by living-related liver transplantation, the shortage of cadaver liver grafts for adults keeps worsening. Using livers from donors defined as optimal, we have been developing techniques for split-liver transplantation for 2 adult recipients at our center (28). From July 1993 to December 1999, 34 adults have undergone split-liver transplantation with grafts from optimal donors prepared by ex-situ split (n=30) or by in-situ split (n=4), and 88 adults received optimal whole-liver grafts which were not split. Four split grafts were transplanted at other centers. For whole-liver, right and left split-liver grafts, the one-year and 2-year patient survival rates were 88%, 74%, 88% and 85%, 74%, 64%, respectively, and the one-year and 2-year graft survival rates were 88%, 74%, 75% and 85%, 74%, 43%, respectively. Patient survival was adversely affected by graft steatosis and when recipients were hospitalized or ICU-bound prior to transplantation. Graft survival was adversely affected by steatosis and when the graft-to-recipient body weight ratio was less than 1%. Primary non-function occurred in 3 left split-liver grafts. The rates of arterial (6%) and biliary (22%) complications were similar to published data from conventional split-liver procedures for an adult and a child. Split-liver procedures for 2 adults increased the number of recipients by 62% compared with whole liver transplantation and were logistically possible in 16/104 (15%) of optimal cadaver donors. This preliminary experience shows that split-liver transplantation for 2 adults is technically feasible. Outcomes and complication rates can be improved by rigid selection criteria for donors and recipients, particularly for the smaller left graft, and possibly also by in-situ splitting for cadaver donors. Wider use will require changes in procedures for graft allocation and coordination between centers experienced in the techniques.

Adult-To-Adult Living-Related Liver Transplantation (LRLT)

In 1998, Kawasaki published the first series of LRLT in adults using whole left liver grafts, with no postoperative liver failure reported even though the liver graft was often small for size (29). To increase the volume of the liver graft of the donor, like others (30,31), we have preferred to use right livers. We started our program of LRLT in adults quite late compared with other centers. In fact, we wanted to exhaust all available alternatives first to be certain this program was justified. From January to July 2000, 7 adult-to-adult LRLT were performed.

Donors included 5 females and 2 males aged 20-53 (median=41) years. The recipients were 5 males and 2 females aged 17-58 (median=50) years transplanted for viral cirrhosis (4 cases including 2 with hepatocellular carcinoma), subfulminant hepatitis (1 case), hepatocellular cacinoma in a healthy liver (1 case), and epithelioid hemangiendothelioma (1 case). The right liver was harvested in all cases and a duct-to-duct biliary reconstruction was performed in 6/7 cases (32). The follow-up of the series ranges from 41-157 (median=117) days. One donor had a biliary fistula that healed spontaneously. The 7 donors are alive at home without any late complications. One recipient was retransplanted for hepatic artery thrombosis and 2 recipients had a biliary fistula that healed spontaneously. The 7 recipients are alive at home with normal liver function. For a given patient the possibility of living-related liver donation might expand the indications for transplantation without penalizing the patients waiting for a cadaver liver graft. From January 2000 to December 2000, alternatives to standard whole cadaver liver transplantation - including split, domino (see below) and living donor - represent 29% of our liver transplant activity.

Sequential Liver Transplantation: The "Domino" Liver Transplant

The liver obtained after hepatectomy in an FAP patient, which is anatomically and functionally normal except for the production of prealbumin, may be transplanted to patients (33) with liver malignancies who are not candidates for surgical resection and who cannot benefit from a cadaver liver because of the organ shortage (4,34). Although the long-term outcome among patients receiving FAP livers is still unknown, it is likely to be better than the grim prognosis of the underlying disease. Patients suffering from other metabolic disorders originating from a metabolic or functional deficiency in the liver (oxalosis, ornithine transcarbylamase deficiency, protein C deficiency) have been proposed as potential donors with the same " domino " approach (34).

We reviewed the Paul Brousse experience with a domino liver transplant program for FAP, with a view to extending the approach to other metabolic disorders. Livers from 10 patients transplanted for FAP type 1 were used for domino transplants to patients with unresectable primary or metastatic liver cancers. There was no perioperative mortality. Neuropathy or cardiomyopathy did not increase the morbidity of the domino liver explant or transplant procedures. The morbidity for the domino recipients did not appear to be increased. Variant transthyretin was detected in the sera of FAP liver recipients, with no immediate clinical consequences. The domino approach is feasible, and requires careful planning of the surgical procedures for liver explantation, in particular for the nature and site of vascular anastomoses. Domino transplantation of metabolically dysfunctional livers creates new categories of potential donors and potential recipients. It raises new ethical, technical, and societal issues. The domino approach could be used in several genetic or biochemical disorders now treated by liver transplantation. It has the potential to increase the number of liver grafts available for transplantation. A further step was taken by combining the domino technique with partition of the liver, giving rise to 3 grafts from a single cadaver donor - one liver for 3 patients (35).

Other Technical Aspects

Our group has participated in the development of many innovative techniques including: heterotopic and orthotopic partial auxiliary liver transplantation for chronic liver disease (11), APOLT for fulminant hepatitis (36), combined liver and small bowel transplants in the adult (37), cavoportal hemitransposition and reno-portal anastomosis for diffuse thrombosis of the portal system (38), percutaneous maneuvers in the transplanted patient (39), endovascular maneuvers (40), and TIPS before and after transplant (41).

SUMMARY

During the past 16 years, more than 1,500 liver transplants were performed at Paul Brousse Hospital. The overall patient survival rates were 83% at one year and 65% at 10 years. Our group has pioneered a variety of new approaches to liver transplantation, including:

1. Anti-HBs (HBIG) prophylaxis for the prevention of HBV recurrence. To date more than 270 patients have received long-term treatment and the overall 10-year recurrence rate was 27%.

2. Transplantation for hepatocellular carcinoma of the cirrhotic liver in patients with uni- or binodular HCC (<3cm). Survival for transplanted patients was 83% compared with 18% if the liver was resected.

3. Transplantation for familial amyloidotic polyneuropathy (FAP). More than 60 patients had 5- and 10-year survival rates of 85% and 83%, respectively. Ten livers obtained after hepatectomy from these FAP patients were transplanted as "domino" living donor livers to patients with unresectable liver cancers with satisfactory short-term results.

4. Reduced-size liver grafts have been used successfully to reduce pretransplant mortality and posttransplant morbidity and mortality by shortening the wait for our pediatric patients.

5. Split-liver transplantation has increased the number of transplantable livers by 28%.

6. Split-liver transplantation for 2 adults. Using optimal livers we have transplanted 34 adults with grafts prepared by ex-vivo or in-situ splitting with good survival rates.

7. Adult-to-adult living-related donor liver transplantation. In 2000, 7 adult-to-adult living donor transplants were performed with no complications from the donor surgeries. One recipient was retransplanted for arterial thrombosis, but all 7 recipients are alive at home.

The Paul Brousse Hospital is committed to exploring new technologies to improve the outcome of and expand the indications for liver transplantation. We have taken a surgical approach to the organ shortage, finding new ways to serve the most patients with the limited number of livers available.

REFERENCES

1. Samuel D, Muller R, Alexander A, et al. Liver Transplantation in European patients with the Hepatitis B surface antigen. N Engl J Med 1993; 329:1842.

2. Feray C, Aigou M, Samuel D, et al. The course of hepatitis C virus infection after liver transplantation. Hepatology 1994; 20:1137.

3. Feray C, Caccamo L, Alexander AJM, et al. European collaborative study on factors influencing outcome after liver transplantation for hepatitis C. Gastroenterology 1999; 117:619.

4. Bismuth H, Chiche L, Adam R, et al. Liver Resection Versus Transplantation for Hepatocellular Carcinoma in Cirrhotic Patients, Ann Surg 1993; 218:145.

5. Adam R, Castaing D, Azoulay D et al : Indications et résultats de la transplantation hépatique dans le traitement des carcinomes hépatocellulaires sur cirrhose. Annales de Chirurgie 1998 ; 52:547

6. Bismuth H, Majno P, Adam R, et al. Liver transplantation for hepatocellular carcinoma. In: GN Hortobagyi, D.Kayat, Eds. Progress in Anti-Cancer Chemotherapy. Blackwell Science, London, 1999;161.

7. Bismuth H, Samuel D, Castaing D, et al. Orthotopic Liver transplantation in fulminant and sub fulminant hepatitis. The Paul Brousse experience. Ann Surg 1995; 222:109.

8. Farges O, Kalil A, Samuel D, et al. The use of ABO incompatible grafts in liver transplantation: a life saving procedure in highly selected patients. Transplantation 1995; 59:1124.

9. Adams D, Samuel, D, Goulon-Goueau C, et al. The course and prognostic factors of familial amyloidotic neuropathy after liver transplantation. Brain 2000; 123:1495.

10. Starzl TE, Marchioro TL, Von Kaula KN, et al. Homotransplantation of the liver in human. Surg Gynecol Obstet 1963; 177:659.

11. Bismuth H, Houssin D. Reduced-sized orthotopic liver graft in hepatic transplantation in children. Surgery 1984; 95:367.

12. Otte JB, De Ville De Goyet J, et al. Size reduction of the donor liver is a safe way to alleviate the shortage of size-matched organs in pediatric liver transplantation. Ann Surg 1990; 211:146.

13. Esquivel CO, Nakazato P, Cox K, et al. The impact of liver reductions in pediatric liver transplantation. Arch Surg 1991; 126:1278.

14. Houssin D, Soubrane O, Boillot O, et al. Orthotopic liver transplantation with a reduced-size graft: An ideal compromise in pediatrics ? Surgery 1992; 111:532.

15. Badger IL, Czemiak A, Beath S, et al. Hepatic transplantation in children using reduced-size allografts. Brit J Surg 1992; 79:47.

16. Zitelli BJ, Malatack TJ, Gartner JC et al. Evaluation of the pediatric patient for liver transplantation. Pediatrics 1987; 78:559.

17. Emond JC, Whitington PP, Thistlethwaite JR, et al. Reduced-size orthotopic liver transplantation: use in the management of children with chronic liver disease. Hepatology 1989; 10:867.

18. Esquivel CO, Koneru B, Karrer P, et al. Liver transplantation before I year of age. J Pediatr 1987; 110:545.

19. Malatack JJ, Schaid ill, Urbach AH, et al. Choosing a pediatric recipient for orthotopic liver transplantation. J Pediatr 1987; 111:479.

20. Broelsch CE, Emond JC, Whitington PP, et al. Application of reduced-size liver transplantation as split grafts, auxiliary orthotopic grafts, and living related segmental transplants. Ann Surg 1990; 212:368.

21. De Ville De Goyet J, Hausleithner V, et al. Impact of innovative techniques on the waiting list and results in pediatric liver transplantation. Transplantation 1993; 5:1130.

22. Pichlmayr R, Ringe B, Gubematis G, et al. Transplantation einer Spenderleber auf zwei Empfanger (Split liver transplantation). Eine neue Methode in der Weitzentwicklung der Lebersegment Transplantation. Langenbecks Archiv fur Chirurgie 1988; 373:127.

23. Bismuth H, Morino M, Castaing D, et al. Emergency orthotopic liver transplantation in two patients using one donor liver. Brit J Surg 1989; 76:722.

24. De Ville de Goyet J. Split liver transplantation in Europe - 1988 to1993. Transplantation 1995; 59:1371.

25. Azoulay D, Astarcioglu I, Bismuth H, et al. Split-liver transplantation: The Paul Brousse policy. Ann Surg 1996; 224:737.

26. Busuttil RW, Goss JA. Split liver transplantation. Ann Surg 1999; 229:313.

27. Rogiers X, Malago M, Gawad K, et al. In situ splitting of cadaveric livers: the ultimate expansion of the donor pool. Ann Surg 1996; 224:331.

28. Azoulay D, Castaing D, Adam R, et al. Split liver tranplantation for two adult recipients: feasibility and long term outcomes. Ann Surg 2001 (in press).

29. Kawaski S, Makuuchi M, Matsunami H, et al. Living related liver transplantation in adults. Ann Surg 1998; 227:269.

30. Markos A. Right lobe living donor liver transplantation: A review. Liver Transplantation 2000; 6:3.

31. Azoulay D, Marin-Hargreaves G, Castaing D. Duct to duct biliary anastomosis in living related liver transplantation:The Paul Brousse technique. Arch Surg (in press).

32. Furtado AIL. Domino liver transplantation using livers from patients with familial amyloidotic polyneuropathy. Curr Opin Organ Transplant 2000; 5:69.

33. Azoulay D, Samuel D, Castaing D, et al. Domino liver transplants for metabolic disorders: Experience with familial amyloidotic polyneuropathy. Am Coll Surg 1999; 189:584.

34. Azoulay D, Castaing D, Adam R, et al. Transplantation of three adult patients with one cadaveric graft: wait or innovate; Liver Transpl Surg 2000; 6:239.

35. Bismuth H, Azoulay D, Samuel D, et al. Auxiliary partial orthotopic liver transplantation for fulminant hepatitis. The Paul Brousse Experience. Ann Surg 1996; 224:712.

36. Azoulay D, Savier E, Castaing D, et al. Combined transplantation of liver and small intestine in an adult. First case in France. Surgical aspects. Presse Med 1999; 28:2211 (in French).

37. Azoulay D, Marin Hargreaves G, Castaing D, et al. Caval inflow to the graft: A successful way to overcome diffuse portal system thrombosis in liver transplantation. JAm Coll Surg 2000; (in press).

38. Castaing D, Azoulay D, Bismuth H. Percutaneous catheterization of the intestinal loop of hepatico-jejunostomy: a new possibility in the treatment of complex biliary diseases. Gastroenterol Clin Biol. 1999; 23:882. (in French).

39. Azoulay D, Castaing D, Ahchong K, et al.. A minimally invasive approach to the treatment of stenosis of the portal vein after liver hepatic transplantation. Surg Gynecol Obstet 1993; 176:599.

40. Azoulay D, Castaing D, Majno P, et al. Salvage Transjugular Intrahepatic Portosystemic Shunt (TIPS) for Uncontrolled Variceal Bleeding in Patients with Cirrhosis. J Hepatol (in press).

CHAPTER 25

Adult Liver Transplantation: The Université Catholique de Louvain Experience

J. Lerut [a], O. Ciccarelli [a], F. Roggen [a], P.F. Laterre [b], P. Goffette [c], E. Danse [c], R. Reding [a], A. Geubel [d], M.S. Reynaert [b], and J.B. Otte [a]

[a]Departments of Digestive Surgery, [b]Intensive Care, [c]Radiology, [d]Hepato-gastroenterology
Université Catholique de Louvain, Brussels, BELGIUM

Since its first application in 1963 by Dr T Starzl, liver transplantation (LT) has evolved to a therapeutic standard in the treatment of end-stage acute and chronic liver diseases as well as of selected cases of hepatobiliary malignancy and liver-based metabolic diseases (1). Here we discuss the indications, morbidity and mortality of adult LT and retransplantation (re-LT) based on the results of our single center experience with 430 consecutive adult patients.

PATIENTS AND METHODS

During the period from February 1984-December 1999, 1,066 LT were performed in 953 patients at Cliniques Universitaires St-Luc in Brussels. Among these, 488 LT's were performed in 430 adult patients (aged >15 years). Their mean age was 46.2 years (range 15-73). Four hundred eighty-five livers were implanted orthotopically and 3 heterotopically. Thirty-six patients (7.8%) had a technical variant of LT (24 right split LT; 11 reduced-size LT and 3 living-related donor LT).

Combined liver-kidney transplantation was performed in 5 patients; one patient had a combined liver-pancreas transplant. Three hundred seventy-eight patients were transplanted once (87.1%); 47 patients twice (11.9%); 4 patients (0.8%) 3 times and finally one patient (0.3%) 4 times. Four of them were retransplanted at another institution. The retransplant index in this series was 1.1.

Several patients had more than one diagnosis, however, they were classified in relation to the disease finally leading to the indication for LT (Table 1). Of the major diagnoses, 71.4% (n=307) were transplanted because of chronic liver disease; 13.7% (n=59) because of

hepatobiliary tumors; 9.7% (n=42) because of acute liver failure in a non-cirrhotic liver and 5.1% (n=22) because of a metabolic liver disease.

Fulminant liver failure was defined as the occurrence of severe encephalopathy within 2 weeks after onset of jaundice; subfulminant failure was defined as occurrence of encephalopathy from the third to the eighth week after onset of jaundice (2). Two patients with Wilson's disease, one patient with autoimmune cirrhosis and one patient with acute liver failure after resection of hepatocellular cancer in a cirrhotic liver were classified in the chronic disease group although they were grafted because of acute liver failure (ALF).

Hepatocellular cancers were staged following UICC-classification (3). Stages I and II, correspond to solitary small, unilobar tumors without or with vascular invasion; Stage III to a solitary large (>2 cm) tumor with vascular invasion or multiple unilobar large tumors with or without vascular invasion and Stage IV to multiple bilobar

Table 1. Indications for adult liver transplantation at St-Luc.

	n	%
Chronic liver disease	307	71.4%
hepatocellular	210	51.1%
cholestatic	83	19.3%
toxic	3	0.7%
vascular	1	0.2%
Hepatobiliary tumor	59	13.7%
malignant	54	12.6%
benign	5	1.1%
Acute liver failure	42	9.8%
Metabolic disease	22	5.1%

tumors presenting macrovascular invasion. Seventeen patients were grafted because of prevailing chronic end-stage liver disease whilst having an hepatocellular cancer detected before or after LT. The risk factors of the transplanted population are listed in Table 2.

Due to modifications in operative and perioperative care, the results of these series were analyzed in 2 periods: 1984-1990 (Grp I; n=171) and 1991-1999 (Grp II; n= 259). Early and late events were determined following the practice of the European Liver Transplant Registry, as events occurring within or after the first 3 posttransplant months. Follow-up was complete for all patients with a minimum of 6 months (median 9 years; range 12-200 mo.).

Surgical Technique (Table 3)

During the first study period, liver procurement and transplantation were performed following the methods described by Starzl (1). The recipient's inferior vena cava (R-IVC) was always removed and a veno-venous bypass (VVB) was almost universally used. Afterwards, the great majority of the patients had LT whilst preserving the R-IVC and VVB was only used selectively (4,5). During the past 6 years, cavo-caval LT (CC-LT) was used in all but one primary and one secondary transplantation (2/164 grafts=1.2%) (Fig.1). VVB was used in one primary and in 2 secondary transplants (3/164 grafts=1.8%).

In case of splanchnic vein thrombosis there was a shift from blind thrombectomy during the first period to eversion thrombectomy and superior mesenteric vein implantation during the second period (6) (Fig. 2). Since

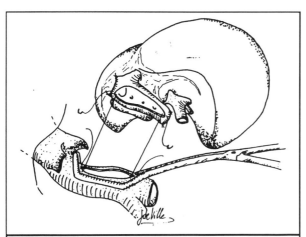

Figure 1. Cavo-caval liver transplantation: partial IVC clamping allows implantation without use of veno-venous bypass.

Table 2. Risk factors in adult LT.

	n	%
- Child-Pugh C classification	193	44.9
- Urgent Transplantation (UNOS 1)	101	23.5
- Previous surgery : upper abdominal	88	20.5
portal hypertension	20	4.7
- Splanchnic vein modification	54	12.6
- Pre-OLT infection	61	14.2
renal failure (organ support)	35	8.1
- Age over 60 years	43	10
- ABO incompatibility	9	2.1
- Previous other transplantation	9	2.1

Table 3. Evolution of surgical technique in adult LT.

Implantation	1984-90	1991-99
Classical	199 (100%)	45 (15.6%)
Piggy-back*		50 (17.3%)
Cavo-caval		194 (67.1%)
VVB-use	181 (94.8%)	69 (23.8%)

* anastomosis between recipient's hepatic vein cuff and donor's suprahepatic inferior vena cava cuff

1994, biliary tract reconstruction was done without stenting. Perioperative cytoprotective therapy, using prostaglandin E1 (Prostin® Upjohn-Pharmacia, S) and ursodesoxycholic acid (Ursofalk® Falk, G) was used since 1993 (7).

Immunosuppression (IS)

Prophylactic

During the period 1984-1990, immunosuppression (IS) was cyclosporine A (CsA) (Sandimmun® Novartis, CH)-based. It consisted of quadruple IS, using methylprednisolone (MP) (Medrol® Upjohn, S), azathioprine (Imuran® Wellcome, UK) and either polyclonal (ALS® or R-ATG® Fresenius, G), monoclonal (OKT3-Orthoclone® Cilag-Jansen, USA) or anti-IL-2-receptor (Lo-Tact-1® Biotransplant, USA) antibodies.

In 1989-1990, a prospective randomized study was done comparing quadruple IS, using OKT3® or Lo-Tact®, and triple IS (8).

Since 1991, IS was reduced substantially and consisted of a CsA-based triple regimen using Sandimmun or Neoral® (Novartis, CH), MP and azathioprine until 1996. Moreover, low-dose steroid therapy (LDSt), representing administration during the first 10 days of 362 mg of MP, as well as systematic steroid withdrawal (STWD) from the third month onwards were applied in the presence of stable graft function (9). In 1997-1998, a prospective randomized study was done comparing triple IS using LDSt, anti-CD-2a antibody (BTI-322 - Biotransplant - USA) and tacrolimus (Tac) (Prograft® Fujisawa) to double IS using Tac and LDSt (10). In 1999 all patients were on double IS using Tac and LDSt.

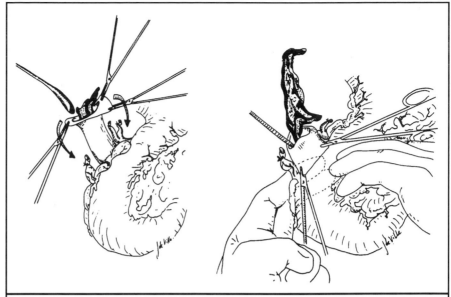

Figure 2. Eversion thrombectomy in a case of extended portal vein thrombosis.

Therapeutic

Treatment of rejection was based on clinical, biochemical and histological findings. In Group I, treatment of rejection consisted of administration of several boli of MP (up to 6.5 g). Corticoresistant rejection was treated with a 10-14 day course of OKT3® or R-ATG®. Since the introduction of our LDSt and STWD protocols (Group II) rejection has been treated with 0.6-1.0 g MP only and corticoresistance has been treated by switching from CsA to Tac. In cases resistant to this switch, a 10-day course of OKT3 was given.

Anti-Infectious Chemotherapy

During the period 1984-1987, antibiotic therapy was not standardized; since 1988, a 4-day course of antibiotic therapy was given according to the status of the patient. In case of elective (low-risk) LT, antibiotic therapy consisted of temocilline (Negaban® Smith-Kline-Beecham, B) and oxacilline (Penstapho® Bristol-Myers Squibb, I); in case of emergency and haemorrhagic (high-risk) LT, ceftazidime (Glazidim® Glaxo-Wellcome, I) and vancomycin (Vancocin® Eli Lilly, USA) were administered.

Since 1990, systemic anti-infectious chemotherapy was completed with selective bowel decontamination consisting of 4 daily intakes of a mixture of polymycine B, netilmicine (Netromycine Shering-Plough, USA) and

amfotericine B (Fungizone® – Bristol-Myers Squibb, F) during the whole posttransplant hospital stay (11). Group II had viral prophylaxis consisting of high-dose acyclovir (Zovirax® Glaxo-Wellcome, UK) or sequential gancyclovir (Cymevene® Roche, CH) and Zovirax® administration for 4-6 months (12). Fungal prophylaxis consisted of a 10-day course of low-dose (10 mg) Fungizone® and protozoal prophylaxis consisted of trimethoprim sulfametoxazole (Bactrim® Roche, CH) 3 times a week until CsA or Tac monotherapy was reached (13).

Since September 1989, hepatitis B viral (HBV) infected recipients were treated, from the anhepatic phase onwards, with high doses of specific anti-HBS immunoglobulins (CAF Red Cross, B) in order to obtain anti-HBS antibody levels above 200 mUI/ml (14). Since 1991, immunoglobulin administration was tailored to the individual clearing of antibodies. There was no prophylactic antiviral treatment in case of LT for hepatitis C viral (HCV) disease.

Cost-Containment Study

Costs of first transplant hospitalization during the years 1990-91, 1992-93, 1994-95 and 1996-97 were analyzed for elective and urgent primary LT and re-LT. The analysis took into account costs related to procurement and transplant procedures, diagnostic procedures, medication, medical care and hospitalization costs. As adaptation of costs to the different time periods was

Table 4. Early mortality (< 3 mo) after adult LT (58/430 patients; 13.5%).

Sepsis +/- multiorgan failure	19
Perioperative haemorrhage	20
Multiorgan failure	7
Recurrent . viral disease	1
. tumor	1
. leukemia	1
Cerebral . haematoma (ICP)[a]	1
. oedema	2
GVHD	1
PTLD	1
Lyell syndrome	2
Iatrogenic pulmonary bleed[b]	1
Myocardial infarction[b]	1
Haemodynamic failure	1

[a] ICP intracranial pressure monitoring
[b] Complication in context of severe early allograft dysfunction

Table 5. Evolution of early mortality after adult LT.

	Deaths	%	Overall
1984-87	11/45	24.4%	
88	10/48	20.1%	
89	10/45[a]	20.0%	20%
90	4/37[a]	10.8%	
1991	5/43[a]	11.6%	
92	2/28	7.1%	
93	3/34	8.8%	
94	3/27[a]	11.1%	
95	3/27[a]	11.1%	8.6%
96	3/25	12.0%	
97	2/24[a]	8.3%	
98	1/25	4.0%	
99	1/35[a]	2.8%	p<0.0006

Overall: 58 (13.5%)

[a] patients transplanted and retransplanted in different years

extremely difficult, the results were displayed in 2-year periods. There were indeed many different price adaptations over the years within cost subgroups such as hospitalization (+41%), medication, and medical interventions (+20%). However, there is no doubt that medical cost expenditure increased markedly over time; during the study period 1990-1997 the index rose by 17%.

RESULTS

One-, 5- and 10-year actuarial survival rates for the total transplant group of 430 patients were 79.6%, 68.0% and 61.2%, respectively. At the end of follow-up, 275 (64%) patients are still alive, 58 patients (13.5%) died during the first 3 months and 97 patients (22.5%) died later.

Posttransplant Mortality

Early mortality was dominated by infectious and bleeding complications (Table 4). This mortality gradually and significantly decreased over the years (Table 5) mainly due to a significantly lower incidence of infections (Table 6) and bleeding complications in Group II (Table 7).

Late mortality was dominated by recurrent allograft disease, infections,

tumors and cardiovascular complications (Table 8). Five (1.1%) patients died of liver failure due to chronic rejection; 4 of them whilst waiting for a retransplant.

Technical Complications

Most complications were related to the biliary tree and to bleeding (Table 9). Ischaemic biliary tract lesions (IBTL) in the absence of angiography-proven hepatic artery occlusion or stenosis accounted for one-third of the biliary complications (Table 10). In contrast to arterial and venous complications, not a single patient died during the early posttransplant period as a consequence

Table 6. Evolution of infectious morbidity and mortality after adult LT.

Infections	1984-90 n=174		1991-99 n=256		P
Bacterial	99	56.9%	104	40.6%	<0.001
Fungal	14	8.0%	11	4.3%	0.1
Viral	87	50.0%	62	24.2%	<0.001
CMV infection	63	36.4%	40	15.6%	<0.001
CMV tissue invasion	47	28.0%	22	8.6%	<0.001
Mortality					
sepsis +/- multiorgan failure	12	6.9%	7	2.7%	0.03
pre-LT infected patient	12/33	39.4%	1/28	3.6%	<0.001

Table 7. Evolution of perioperative bleeding complications of adult LT.

	1984-90	1991-99
Severe perioperative bleeding	92/174 52.9%	1/256 16% p<0.0001
Mortality related to bleeding	18/92 19.6%	2/41 4.9% p<0.02

Table 8. Late mortality (≥3 mo) after adult LT (97/430 patients; 22.5%).

Recurrent Disease	45
Tumor primary/secondary 19/5	
Hepatitis C	11[a]
Hepatitis B	8
Autoimmune	1
Metabolic	1
Infection	14[b]
De novo cancer	6
PostTx lymphoproliferative disease	5
Myocardial infarction	4
Cerebral bleeding	4
Cardiopulmonary failure	2
Chronic rejection	5
De novo Hepatitis C infection	2
Hepatitis B infection	1
Recurrent leukemia	1
Medullary aplasia	1
Suicide	3
Intestinal volvulus	1
Compliance	1
Trauma	1
Unknown	1

[a] tuberculosis (2 patients)
[b] sepsis secondary to hepatic artery thrombosis and intrahepatic biliary tract lesions

Table 9. Technical complications of adult LT (232/430 patients; 66.2%).

	N	Pat.	%	Early mortality
Biliary	93	82	19.1	0
Arterial	28	26	6.0	6 (23.0%)
Venous	21	21	4.9	6 (28.6%)
Haemorrhage	138	133	30.9	20 (14.3%)
VVB-complications	34	34/249	13.7	–

Table 10. Vascular complications of adult LT.

		N	pat. (%)	Early mortality
Arterial	thrombosis	12		2
	stenosis	6	26 pat.	–
	splenic steel	6	(6%)	–
	aneurysm	4		4	23%
Venous				
Portal	thrombosis	10		3
	stenosis	3		–
	torsion	1		1
Hepatic	trombosis	2	21 pat.	2
	torsion	2	(4.9%)	2	28.6%
	stenosis	1		–
IVC	partial thrombosis	1		–
	stenosis	1		–

of biliary complications (Table 11).

Change of technique had a major influence on the incidence of perioperative bleeding and mortality related to bleeding. Intra-operative blood product use (<1 liter) fell significantly (p<0.0001) and the incidence of immediate extubation (p<0.007) increased significantly in Group II recipients (Fig. 3).

Table 11. Biliary complications of adult LT (93/82 patients; 19.1%).

Ischaemic biliary tract lesions		29
Fistula	anastomotic	8
	donor bile duct	6
	section margin	2
Obstruction	anastomotic	19*
	sludge	4
	intrahepatic	3
	ampullary dysfunction	2
	stone	1
	recurrent tumor	1
T-tube	leak	11
	malposition	2
	rupture	4
Cholangitis		1

* Hepatic artery thrombosis complicated with biliary obstruction (4 patients)

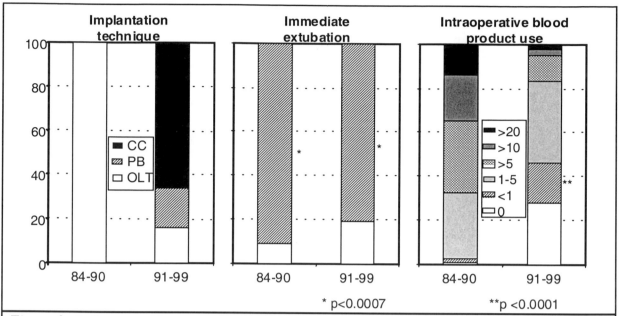

Figure 3. Influence of implantation technique on duration of artificial ventilation and on intraoperative blood product use.

Immunological Complications

With time, the incidence of treated rejections decreased drastically from 96% during the first year of the study towards 8.3% at the end of the study, due to a better integration of biochemical, pathological and clinical data (Fig. 4). The peak (91.7%) of treated rejection in 1994 related to a more rapid withdrawal of steroids often leading to elevated liver tests. Most of these patients were treated with 0.6 g of MP due to inexperience. ABO incompatible grafting led to untreatable rejection in 6 of 8 patients.

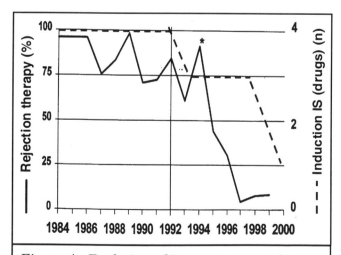

Figure 4. Evolution of immunosuppression strategy in adult LT.

Liver Transplantation for Chronic Benign Liver Diseases

Three hundred seven patients (71.4%) were transplanted because of chronic benign liver diseases. The one, 5- and 10-year actuarial survival rates were 78.5%, 71.0% and 64.0%, respectively. The one-, 5- and 10-year survival rates of patients transplanted because of chronic hepatocellular diseases were 78.5%, 66.7% and 59.5%, respectively. The best results were obtained in the cholestatic patient group with one-, 5- and 10-year survival rates of 82%, 74.1% and 69.7% (Fig. 5).

The majority of LT in chronic benign liver diseases were done for chronic viral diseases (123/220= 55.9%). The one-, 5- and 10-year survival rates among patients transplanted because of postviral HCV liver cirrhosis were 81.7%, 67.4% and 58.8%. A study conducted in 76 HCV long-term (>3 mo) survivors, followed for at least 3 years, showed that 82.9% of patients presented with recurrent viral disease in the allograft; 15.8% died due to recurrent viral allograft disease. Mortality due to recurrent HCV-allograft disease was higher in cases with lower immunosuppression (Table 12).

Patients transplanted for postviral B and B-delta cirrhosis had one-, 5- and 10-year actuarial survival rates of 85.0%, 71.3% and 61.6%, respectively. The prognosis in this group was significantly influenced

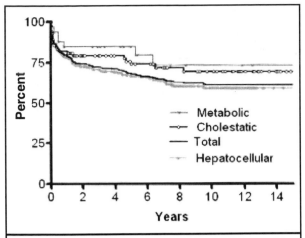

Figure 5. Actuarial survival following LT for benign chronic liver diseases.

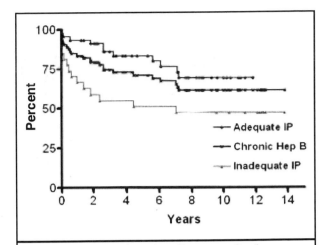

Figure 6. Beneficial influence of adequate immunoprophylaxis on actuarial survival following LT for chronic HBV-disease

by adequate immunoprophylactic therapy (IP) using specific anti-HBs immunoglobulins (93.5% and 83.6% vs. 70.4% and 51.2% one- and 5-year survival in the absence of IP; p<0.01) (Fig. 6) as well by the presence of the co-infection with delta-virus (92.0% and 92.0% vs. 79.2 and 58.5% one- and 5-year survival in the absence of B-delta co-infection; p<0.001). One- and 5-year survival rates among patients with non-replicating and replicating virus were not significantly different (80.5% and 75.4% vs. 84.4% and 64.3%). Individualized monitoring of immunoglobulin clearing reduced the incidence of HBV allograft reinfection to 9.7% (3/31 patients), independent of the patient's pretransplant replicating status.

Table 12. Influence of immunosuppression on HCV recurrent allograft disease and mortality.

	HIS	LDST-IS	MIS	TOTAL
Patients	31	21	24	76
Median follow-up (yrs)	8.2	5.5	3	
Steroid dose	high	low	low	
Antilymphocyte antibody use	90%	57%	8%	
Monotherapy CyA/TAC within 3 yrs post-LT	19%	95%	100%	
Treated rejection	72%	89%	4%	
HCV allograft disease	80%	62%	88%	83%
cirrhosis	10%	10%	17%	12%
HCV-related mortality	10%	14%	29%	16%

HIS: high IS, LDST-IS: low-dose steroid-IS

MIS: minimal immunosuppression: no use of antilymphocyte antibodies and steroid withdrawal within 3 months

Liver Transplantation for Acute Liver Failure

Forty-seven patients (10.9%) underwent LT for acute liver failure (Table 13). Their one-, 5- and 10-year actuarial survival rates were of 76.1%, 66.6% and 58.4%, respectively. The early mortality rate was 19.5%. Group II patients had a significantly reduced mortality (p<0.05) (Table 14). Standardized anti-infectious chemotherapy and perioperative care shifted the causes of death from infectious problems in Group I (6/19=31.6%) towards cerebral failure in Group II (3/28=10.7%). One of the latter patients died because of cerebral bleeding caused by the intracranial pressure-monitoring device.

Liver Transplantation for Hepatobiliary Tumors

The one-, 5- and 10-year actuarial survival rates of 51 patients transplanted because of hepatocellular cancer were 81.1%, 48.7% and 41.2%, respectively. Long-term survival was clearly influenced by the tumor disease stage (Fig. 7). Disease-free survival was significantly better for UICC Stage I, II and III than for Stage IV tumors (26/28= 92% vs. 4/16=25%; p<0.001) (Table 15). The one-, 5- and 10-year survival rates for UICC Stage I, II, III patients were 85%, 62.4 and 62.4%, respectively, compared with survival rates for patients with UICC Stage IV lesions of 79%, 29.5% and 14.7%.

Table 13. *Indications of LT for acute liver failure.*

		Patients	Early mortality
Fulminant hepatic failure (< 2 weeks between jaundice and encephalopathy)			
Hepatitis	A	3	2
	B	14	3
	C	1	
	NANBNC	9	1
	Herpes	1	1
Toxic		3	
Reye's syndrome		1	
Haemorhagic necrosis allograft		1	
Wilson's disease[a]		2	1
Autoimmune cirrhosis[a]		1	
Subfulminant hepatic failure (> 2-8 weeks)			
Hepatitis NANBNC		6	1
Toxic		3	
Autoimmune hepatitis		1	
Post-hepatic resection (HCCA in HCV-cirrhosis)[a]		1	

[a] Acute liver failure in cirrhotic liver

Table 14. *Early mortality after adult LT for acute hepatic failure.*

	1984-90	1991-99	Total series
Fulminant	5/14	3/22	8/36 (22.8%)
Subfulminant	1/5	0/6	1/11 (9.1%)
Total	6/19 (31.6%)	3/28 (10.7%)[a]	9/47 (19.5%)

[a]$p < 0.05$

Table 15. *Hepatocellular cancer in cirrhosis and LT - influence of tumor stratification. (51 patients: 48 long-term (> 3 mo survivors).*

UICC-stage		Disease-free survival	Follow-up
I	14 (12[a])		
II	10 (4[a])	87.1%*	med:60mo.
III	7 (1[a])		(range:5-165)
IV	17	23.5%*	med:60 mo. (range:22-120)
	48	31/48 (64.5%)	*$p < 0.001$

[a] secondary HCCA diagnosis or incidental finding in hepatectomy specimen

Four long-term survivors transplanted because of cholangiocellular carcinoma died of tumor recurrence at 12, 16, 36 and 63 months; one patient transplanted because of bile duct cancer died of tumor recurrence 12 months after LT. Five patients transplanted because of epithelioid haemangioendothelioma were alive at 141, 140, 70, 28 and 12 months; one patient is doing well despite allograft recurrence 10 years after LT. Two patients, transplanted because of colorectal liver metastases, died of recurrent disease at 17 and 65 months; all 3 patients grafted because of neuroendocrine liver metastases died of recurrent disease at 17, 64 and 119 months.

Retransplantation

Fifty-six (13%) patients were retransplanted, 4 of them at another institution. The one-, 5- and 10-year actuarial survival rates of retransplanted patients (75%, 65.7% and 65.7%, respectively) were similar to those of the primary LT patients (80.1%; 68% and 58.8%) (Fig. 8). Early mortality was highest in the patient group retransplanted because of graft dysfunction (5/21=23.8%) or because of acute or chronic graft rejection (7/18=38.9%). Only one (8.3%) of the 12 patients retransplanted because a technical failure died after re-LT (Table 16). Early

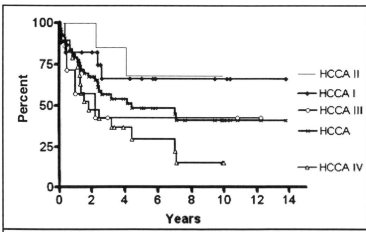

Figure 7. Actuarial survival following LT for hepatocellular cancer and cirrhosis

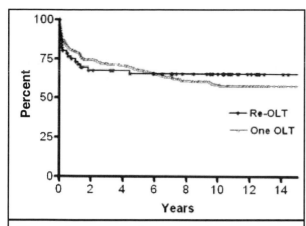

Figure 8. Actuarial survival following primary LT and retransplantation.

mortality after elective re-LT was significantly lower than that after urgent re-LT (2/24= 8.3% vs. 11/32=34.4%; p<0.02).

Early mortality after re-LT in Group II was improved, although not significantly (5/31 Group II patients=16.1% vs. 8/25 Group I patients=32%) (p<0.16).

Liver Transplantation in the Presence of Splanchnic Vein Modifications

Seventy (16.3%) patients were transplanted whilst having major modifications of the splanchnic venous system. Early mortality in this group was 21.4% (15/70 patients). Due to modification of techniques, mortality

Table 17. *Early posttransplant mortality in case of splanchnic venous anomalies*

	1984-90		1991-99	
	26/174	(14.9%)	44/256	(17.1%)
PVT	2/11	(18.2%)	2/30	(6.9%)
PVT-itis	4/4	(100%)	2/8	(25%)
PH Surgery	5/11	(45.5%)	0/6	(0%)
	11/26	(42.3%)	4/44	(9%)*

*p < 0.01
PVT–portal vein thrombosis; PVT-itis–periphlebitis
PH–portal hypertension.

was significantly lower in Group II patients (4/44=9% vs. 11/26 =42.3%; p<0.001) (Table 17). The different technical adjustments necessary in order to perform the transplant procedure are listed in Table 18. Early mortality of eversion and blind venous thrombectomies were 7.1% (2/28) and 33.3% (3/9; p=0.04), respectively.

Cost-containment of LT and re-LT (Table 19)

The cost of elective primary transplants decreased over time. This cannot be said about costs of emergency procedures, which increased especially due to the fact that several of these patients, who had been waiting for a long time, were grafted in extremely advanced stages. The cost of elective re-LT was almost equal to that of elective primary LT. The cost of urgent re-LT was highest, but these figures mostly represented costs related to 2 successive transplant procedures performed during the same hospitalization.

DISCUSSION

After a 20-year period between 1963-1983, when kidneys but few other organs were transplanted, liver transplantation began in earnest with the introduction of cyclosporine. The improvement in results lead to a rapid widening of its indications for different acute and chronic liver diseases (1). A critical review of a large, single centre, adult series is a good means to define progress, possibilities and limitations of the procedure (1, 15, 16).

Table 16. *Indications and outcomes for adult re-LT.*

		Patients	Grafts	Mortality	
				Early	Late
Graft dysfunction	primary	8	8	2	2
	early	13[abc]	14	3	2
Technical failure	art. thrombosis	4[a]	5	1	-
	decapsulation	1	1	-	-
	IBTL	8[b]	9	-	-
Immunological	acute	8[a]	9	5	-
	chronic	10[c]	10	2	1
Recurrent disease	HBV	4	4	-	2
	HCV	2	2	-	
		56 13%	62	13 23.2%	

[a] two re-LT for same indication, [b,c] same patients

Table 18. Splanchnic venous abnormalities and technical adjustments in adult LT.

Venous modification	n	Thrombectomy		SMV implantation	Confluence dissection	Other	Early mortality
PVT	41	blind	6 (1)	7	2 (1)	implantation splenic varix	4
		eversion	25^a (2^b)			1	
PVT-itis	12	blind	1 (1)	3 (1)	4 (3)	implantation ileal varix	6
		eversion	3			1 (1)	
PH-Surgery	17						
portocaval	14	blind	2^c (1)	1^c (1^d)		shunt interruption 14 (2)	4
splenorenal	1				1 and banding		1
mesocaval	2					1	
	70	blind	9 (3)*	11 (2)	7 (5)	15 (3)	15
		eversion	28 (2)*				
		*p=0.04					21.4%

^{a} SPRSh ^{b} PVT ^{c} mortality related to steatosis and procur.trauma ^{d} PVT-itis

Our results reflect the learning curves in relation to indications and perioperative management. Standardization of operative and perioperative care significantly reduced early morbidity and mortality related to bleeding and infectious complications. Modification of recipient hepatectomy, preserving the R-IVC, as well as modification of the allograft implantation technique, using cavo-caval anastomosis contributed to reduced need for blood products (5). Cavo-caval LT allows us to implant the allograft without using VVB, which is responsible for quite a number of specific complications (17). This technique can be done independently of the recipient's status or anatomical condition. Procedures that were adapted in cases with splanchnic vein thrombosis, such as venous eversion thrombectomy and venous iliac graft interposition between the donor portal vein and the recipient's mesenteric vein represent other major technical progress. These technical adaptations must be decided early during intervention in order to minimize hazardous perihilar or retropancreatic dissection; patients having inflammatory changes of splanchnic veins remain the most difficult group to manage (6,18,19).

Arterial and venous technical complications are rather infrequent in adult LT (5%) (19,20). Biliary tract complications, in contrast, are a reason for concern because these occur in about one in 5 patients (1,21). The spectrum of biliary tract lesions has changed since the prolongation of ischaemia times due to introduction in clinical practice of new preservation solutions such as University of Wisconsin solution (21,22). Technical failure of the biliary tract reconstruction, once the Achilles' heel of LT, has been replaced by intra- and extra-hepatic "non-surgical" biliary tract lesions (1,22,23). These modifications are responsible for one third of encountered biliary tract problems. Ischaemic damage of the biliary mucosa, in the absence of a hepatic artery allograft thrombosis, is responsible for diffuse modifications necessitating repetitive interventional

Table 19. Evolution of costs^a of first hospitalization for elective or urgent transplantation and for retransplantation.

Time period	Elective	Urgent LT	Elective	Urgent Re-LT ^{b}
1990-91	1,390,633	2,223,590	1,259,417	2,939,261
	(0.9-4.4)	(1-5.2)	(0.9-1.6)	(1.6-6.2)
1992-93	1,407,898	1,773,558	–	2,284,829
	(0.8-4.2)	(1.4-2.9)		(1.7-5.1)
1994-95	1,228,914	2,009,759	1,257,984	1,970,439
	(0.9-3.9)	(1.2-8.5)	(0.9-1.9)	(1.7-2)
1996-97	1,098,367	2,563,572	–	4,229,477
	(0.8-2.9)	(1.5-8.6)		(3.2-5.2)

^{a} median values in BF (1 USD @ 44 BF)
^{b} includes costs of both transplants if done during same hospitalization

radiological procedures and even re-LT. If biliary infection occurs, re-LT should done in a timely manner. Its incidence can be reduced (but apparently not prevented) by shortening of ischaemia times and by adequate lavage of the biliary system at organ procurement (21,24). Because differential diagnosis between IBTL and rejection can be very difficult, the biliary tree must be aggressively investigated using cholangiography if cholestatic enzymes remain elevated (1,22). Because of its high incidence, we perform percutaneous cholangiography 3-6 months after LT in all recipients.

Improvement in results is also related to standardized systemic and topical, antimicrobial chemoprophylaxis and to less aggressive IS guided by closer correlation between clinical, biochemical and histological findings. Standardized prophylactic systemic and topical antimicrobial, antiviral, antimycotic and antiprotozoal treatments reduce the incidence of infection (11,12,13). Using such prophylactic regimens, successful LT is now possible even in the presence of localized infections.

Late post-LT morbidity and mortality are essentially dominated by viral and tumoral recurrent allograft diseases and by several long-term consequences of IS (1).

Allograft recurrence of hepatitis B viral infection can now be almost completely prevented by a life-long, individualized, adequate use of immunoprophylaxis against the B virus using specific anti-HBs immunoglobulins with or without antiviral nucleoside analogues (14,25). Under these conditions, LT is even successful in the majority of replicating cases (26,27). Selection of HCV patients for LT should be done cautiously as allograft HCV-recurrence is the rule. Recurrence can even have a rapid lethal outcome (28,29). Due to insufficient serological markers and to its aspecific histologic criteria, the "natural" evolution of this viral allograft disease is not yet fully understood. However, there seems to be a tendency towards more severe graft damage in the presence of lower immunosuppression. This explains why HCV-related allograft fibrosis progression has increased in recent years. These findings may indicate that HCV-infection is an immunomediated disease. Inadequate IS may be responsible for an upregulation of the immune response against the HCV infection and for a more aggressive course of the reinfection (30). Effective prophylactic or therapeutic treatments are not yet available (31), but encouraging results have been published recently in relation to the combined pre- and early post-LT use of interferon and ribavirine (32).

Progress in peri-LT care had a major impact on outcome of LT for patients presenting with acute liver failure. The decision for LT should be made before infectious and/or renal complications occur (23). Indications for LT can be made based on the combination of evolution of encephalopathy and of coagulation factors (2). Invasive intra-arterial pressure monitoring should be used selectively as intracerebral bleeding may occur (33). The shift in mortality in our series from infections toward cerebral problems shows that the propensity to infection in acute liver failure can be controlled, but that much research is still needed in relation to pathogenesis and treatment of cerebral oedema. Hepatic (xeno)-assistance may have to play a major role in this context (33,34).

Indications of LT for cholangiocarcinoma and for primary hepatocellular cancer in cirrhotic patients must be strict (3,35,36). Results of LT are excellent if restricted to solitary lesions (up to 3-5 cm diameter) and up to 3 nodules smaller than 3 cm without macrovascular invasion (37). These criteria usually correspond to UICC Stage I, II and III tumors. Results of Stage IV tumors, representing mostly bilobar lesions with macrovascular invasion, are poor; tumor recurrence within 2-3 years after LT is the rule (37,38). Investigations should therefore be done to determine as precisely as possible the extent of the tumor. The final decision for LT must be taken at surgery. The value of pre- and post-LT intra-arterial and/or systemic chemotherapy and of ablative therapies such as alcoolisation and radiofrequency as well as the influence of the different kinds of IS on results of LT for cancer patients needs to be examined by controlled clinical trials (38,39,40).

Negative effects of prolonged and/or inadequate IS are well demonstrated by the development of lymphoproliferative disorders and by the late mortality due to de novo cancers, infectious and cardiovascular complications (1,41). The benefits of the lowest possible IS, of steroid withdrawal and of restrained treatment of rejection have been well demonstrated (42,43,44). Steroid withdrawal, moreover, markedly improves the quality of life by reducing the inherent side effects of IS (44,45,46). More efforts need to be made to avoid acute and chronic nephrotoxicity of the IS schemes. Indeed, there seems to be a slow but sure progression toward functional renal loss despite progressive reduction of nephrotoxic drugs (9) (Table 20).

Re-LT is the only option for severe graft dysfunction, immunological and technical failure as well as for

Table 20. Incidence on side effects of steroid withdrawal and cyclosporine dose reduction in adult LT.

follow-up (mo)	6	12	24	36	48	60
patients at risk	(70)	(69)	(66)	(65)	(63)	(60)
Creatinine (mg/dl)[a]	1.3 ± 0.5	1.3± 0.6	1.4± 0.5	1.4± 0.5	1.6± 1.3	1.56 ± 1[b]
Cholesterol (mg/dl)[a]	211± 65	195± 48.3	194± 48	193± 51.5	193±51	201.4±56.6
Hypertension (%)	37.1	27.1	25.8	36.4	30	26.6
De novo IDD (%)	27.5	10	6	10.6	9.7	13.3
Malignancy (%)	1.4[c]	1.4[d]	–	–	1.6[c]	1.7[d]
Osseous (fracture)	10 (7)	12.8 (7)	5.9	5.9	9.7	14.5[b]
Cataract (%)	2.8	2.8	1.5	1.5	2.1	0
CsA level (ng/ml)[a]	19.22±63.1	180±55.3	160.2±58.6	137.8±51/3	132.9±45.8	113±42
Steroid dose (mg/kg)[a]	0.1±0.1	0.02±0.07	0.2±0.41	0.02±0.07	0.01±0.05	0.01±0.05
Aza dose (mg/kg)[a]	0.5±0.6	0.2±0.4	0.28±1.3	0.1±0.26	0.12±0.27	0.1±0.3

[a] mean ± SD
[b] two patients on haemodialysis, one patient had renal transplantation
[c] PTLD (cumulative incidence of malignancy 5.8% (4/70)), [d] skin cancer

recurrent allograft disease. The incidence of early graft dysfunction has declined due to the introduction of better preservation solutions, to better transplant surgery (5,16,21,41,47), to shortening of ischaemia times and to avoidance of implantation of severely steatotic grafts (1,21). Introduction of protecting prostaglandin E1 during the immediate post-LT period may also have a beneficial effect (7). Re-LT for technical failure has moved from arterial and venous problems towards diffuse biliary tract lesions. Re-LT for graft dysfunction and immunological failure has a high early morbidity and mortality reflecting the urgent degree of the procedure, usually in an overimmunosuppressed patient. ABO incompatible grafts should be avoided as this combination frequently leads to uncontrollable rejection (1). Re-LT, a major rescue operation, can be done with success equal to that for primary LT when aiming at elective surgery; this means early relisting under maximal reduction or even withdrawal of IS (48).

This single-center review of our adult liver transplant series confirms that LT can be performed with success in chronic and acute liver diseases. Major improvements are still necessary in adjuvant treatment of viral diseases (31) and of hepatocellular malignancies (39,40). Our efforts have been focused toward development of a procedure that is medically and economically justified (49). Morbidity and mortality, although still (too) high, have significantly decreased over time due to standardization of surgical, medical and immunological care (1,5,6,14,15,16,47,50,51). Results can be further improved by introducing the concept of operational tolerance making aggressive IS unnecessary (51,52). Better interpretation and correlation of clinical, biochemical and histological criteria of acute cellular rejection makes clear that even severe histological rejection doesn't always deserve aggressive IS treatment (53,54). Immunological attack of the graft may even be beneficial in the long-term; indeed, interplay of donor and recipient immunological systems can lead to a state of tolerance based on the concept of microchimerism (51).

The major problem of the future remains the organ shortage. This must oblige transplant surgeons to develop all available alternative techniques of allograft implantation such as split liver (55,56,57,58), domino (59) and adult living-related LT (60,61).

The lessons learned out of larger experiences must contribute to improve the results of LT thereby consolidating its value in modern hepatology. Indeed, too many patients are still referred to the transplant centre in the final stage of their acute and chronic liver diseases.

SUMMARY

Liver transplantation remains a formidable surgical and medical procedure. The larger single centre experience confirms that standardization of perioperative care and simplification of the surgical procedure markedly improve results. Further efforts must be made in relation to immunosuppressive therapy in order to minimize late morbidity and mortality.

REFERENCES

1. Starzl TE, Demetris AJ. Liver Transplantation Year Book Med Pub, Chicago, 1994.

2. Pauwels A, Mostefa-Kara N, Florent C, Levy VG. Emergency liver transplantation for acute liver failure. Evaluation of London and Clichy criteria. J Hepatol 1993; 17:124.

3. Ringe B, Wittekind C, Bechstein WO, Bunzendahl H, Pichlmayr R. The role of liver transplantation in hepatobiliary malignancy. A retrospective analysis of 95 patients with particular regard to tumor stage and recurrence. Ann Surg 1989; 209:88.

4. Belghiti J, Panis Y, Sauvanet A, Gayet B, Fekete F. A new technique of side-to-side caval anastomosis during orthotopic hepatic transplantation without inferior vena caval occlusion. Surg Gyn Obst 1992; 75:271.

5. Lerut J, Molle G, Donataccio M, et al. Cavocaval liver transplantation without venovenous bypass and without temporary portocaval shunting:the ideal technique for adult liver grafting? Transplant Int 1997; 10:171.

6. Lerut J, Mazza D, Van Leeuw V, et al. Adult liver transplantation and abnormalities of splanchnic veins: experience in 53 patients. Transplant Int 1997; 10:125.

7. Henley KS, Lucey MR, Normolle DP, et al. A double-blind randomized, placebo-controlled trial of Prostaglandin E1 in liver transplantation. Hepatology 1995; 21:366.

8. Reding R, Feyaerts A, Vraux H, et al. Prophylactic immunosuppression with anti-interleukin-2 receptor monoclonal antibody Lo-Tact-1 versus OKT3 in liver allografting. A two-year follow-up study. Transplantation 1996; 61:1406.

9. Lerut JP, Ciccarelli O, Mauel E, et al. Adult liver transplantation and steroid-azathioprine withdrawal in cyclosporine (Sandimmun®) based immunosuppression − 5 year results of a prospective study. Transplant Int 2001(in press).

10. Lerut J, Talpe SF Roggen R, et al. One-year results of Tacrolimus (TAC) and anti-CD antibody (BTI-322) in adult liver transplantation (LT). Abstract Book − XVIII International Congress of the Transplantation Society, 2000:106.

11. Wiesner RH, Hermans PE, Rakela J, Washington JA, Perkins JD, Dicecco S, Krom R. Selective bowel decontamination to decrease gram-negative aerobic bacterial and candida colonization and prevention infection after orthotopic liver transplantation. Transplantation 1988; 45:570.

12. Badley AD, Seaberg EC, Porayko MK, et al. Prophylaxis of cytomegalovirus infection in liver transplantation. Transplantation 1997; 64:66.

13. Castaldo P, Stratta RJ, Wood RP, et al. Clinical spectrum of fungal infections after orthotopic liver transplantation. Arch Surg 1991; 126:149.

14. Samuel D, Muller R, Alexander G, Fassati L, Ducot B, Benhamou JP, Bismuth H, and the Investigators of the European Concerted Action on Viral Hepatitis Study. Liver transplantation in European patients with the hepatitis B surface antigen. N Engl J Med 1993; 329:1842.

15. Bismuth H, Farges O, Castaing D, et al. Evaluation des résultats de la transplantation hépatique:expérience sur une série de 1052 transplantations. Presse Med 1995; 24:1106.

16. Busuttil RW, Shaked A, Millis JM, et al. One thousand liver transplants. The lessons learned. Ann Surg 1994; 219:490.

17. Chari RS, Gan TJ, Robertson KM, Bass K, Camargo CA, Greig PD, Clavien PA. Venovenous bypass in adult orthotopic liver transplantation:routine or selective use ? J Am Coll Surg 1998; 186:683.

18. Seu P, Shackleton CR, Shaked A, et al. Improved results of liver transplantation in patients with portal vein thrombosis. Arch Surg 1996; 131:840.

19. Lerut J, Tzakis A.G, Bron K, et al. Complications of venous reconstruction in human orthotopic liver transplantation. Ann Surg 1987; 205:404.

20. Tzakis A, Gordon RD, Shaw BW, Iwatsuki S, Starzl TE. Clinical presentation of hepatic artery thrombosis after liver transplantation in the cyclosporine era. Transplantation 1985; 40:667-671.

21. Strasberg SM, Howard TK, Molmenti EP, Hertl M. Selecting the donor liver:risk factors for poor function after orthotopic liver transplantation. Hepatology 1994; 20:829.

22. Sanchez-Urdazpal L, Gores GJ, Ward EM, et al. Ischemic-type biliary complications after orthotopic liver transplantation. Hepatology 1992; 16:49.

23. Lerut J, Gordon RD, Iwatsuki S, Esquivel CO, Todo S, Tzakis A, Starzl TE. Biliary tract complications in human orthotopic liver transplantation. Transplantation 1987; 43:47.

24. Lerut J, de Ville de Goyet J. Technique of multiorgan procurement. Curr Opin Organ Transplant 1997; 2:157.

25. Nery JR, Weppler D, Rodriguez M, Ruiz M, Ruiz P, Schiff ER, Tzakis AG. Efficacy of Lamivudine in controlling hepatitis B virus recurrence after liver transplantation. Transplantation 1998; 65:1615.

27. Konig V, Hopf U, Neuhaus P, et al. Long-term follow-up of hepatitis B virus-infected recipients after orthotopic liver transplantation. Transplantation 1994; 58:553.

27. Lerut JP, Donataccio M, Ciccarelli O, et al. Liver transplantation and HBsAG-positive postnecrotic cirrhosis: adequate immunoprophylaxis and delta virus co-infection as the significant determinants of long-term prognosis. J Hepatol 1999; 30:706.

28. Feray C, Caccamo L, Alexander G, et al. European collaborative study on factors influencing outcome of liver transplantation for hepatitis C. Gastroenterology 1999; 117:619.

29. Berenguer M, Prieto M, Rayon J.M, et al. Natural history of clinically compensated hepatitis C virus-related graft cirrhosis after liver transplantation. Hepatology 2000; 32:852.

30. Berenguer M, Ferrell L, Watson J, et al. HCV-related fibrosis progression following liver transplantation: increase in recent years. J Hepatol 2000; 32:673.

31. Araya V, Rakela J, Wright T. Hepatitis C after orthotopic liver transplantation. Gastroenterology 1997; 112:575.

32. Cattral MS, Krajden M, Wanless IR, et al. A pilot study of Ribavirin therapy for recurrent hepatitis C virus infection after liver transplantation. Transplantation 1996; 61:1483.

33. Hoofnagle JH, Carithers RL, Shapiro C, Asher N. Fulminant hepatic failure: summary of a workshop. Hepatology 1995; 21:240.

34. Lerut J, Ciccarelli O, Roggen F, et al. Progress in adult liver transplantation for acute liver failure. Transplant Proc 2001; 32:1.

35. Farmer DG, Rosove MH, Shaked A, Busuttil RW. Current treatment modalities for hepatocellular carcinoma. Ann Surg 1994; 219:236.

36. Madariaga JR, Iwatsuki S, Todo S, Lee RG, Irish W, Starzl TE. Liver resection for hilar and peripheral cholangiocarcinomas: a study of 62 cases. Ann Surg 1998; 227:70.

37. Mazzaferro V, Regalia E, Docl R, et al. Liver transplantation for the treatment of small hepatocellular carcinomas in patients with cirrhosis. N Engl J Med 1996; 334:693.

38. Carr BI, Sally R, Madariaga J, Iwatsuki S, Starzl TE. Prolonged survival after liver transplantation for advanced hepatocellular carcinoma. Transplant Proc 1993; 25:1128.

39. Livraghi T, Giorgio A, Marin G, et al. Hepatocellular carcinoma and cirrhosis in 746 patients: long-term results of percutaneous ethanol injection. Radiology 1995; 197:101.

40. Ryu M, Shimamura Y, Kinoshita T, et al. Therapeutic results of resection, transcatheter arterial embolization and percutaneous transhepatic ethanol injection in 3225 patients with hepatocellular carcinoma:a retrospective multicenter study. Am J Clin Oncol 1995; 27:251.

41. Starzl TE, Porter KA, Iwatsuki S, et al. Reversibility of lymphomas and lymphoproliferative lesions developing under cyclosporin-steroid therapy. Lancet 1984; 17:584.

42. Stegall MD Everson GT, Schroter G, Bilir B, Karrer F, Kam I. Metabolic complications after liver transplantation. Transplantation 1995; 60:1057.

43. Padbury RTA, Gunson BK, Dousset B, et al. Steroid withdrawal from long-term immunosuppression in liver allograft recipients. Transplantation 1993; 55:789.

44. Padbury R, Toogood G, McMaster P. Withdrawal of immunosuppression in liver allograft recipients. Liver Transplant and Surg 1998; 4:242.

45. Stegall MD, Everson G.T, Schroter G, et al. Prednisone withdrawal late after adult liver transplantation reduces diabetes, hypertension and hypercholesterolemia without causing graft loss. Hepatology 1997; 25:173.

46. Belli L, Decarlis L, Rondinara G, et al. Early cyclosporine monotherapy in liver transplantation:a 5 year follow-up of a prospective randomized trial. Hepatology 1998; 27:1524.

47. Deschenes M, Villeneuve JP, Dagenais M, et al. Lack of relationship between preoperative measures of the severity of cirrhosis and short-term survival after liver transplantation. Liver Transplant and Surg 1997; 3:532.

48. Markmann JF, Markowitz JS, Yersiz H, et al. Long-term survival after retransplantation of the liver. Ann Surg, 1997; 226:408.

49. Evans RW, Manninen DL, Dong FB. An economic analysis of liver transplantation. Gastroenterology Clin N Am 1993; 22:451.

50. Cacciarelli TV, Keeffe EB, Moore DH, et al. Primary liver transplantation without transfusion of red blood cells. Surgery 1996; 120:698.

51. Starzl TE, Demetris AJ, Trucco M, et al. Cell migration and chimerism after whole-organ transplantation:the basis of graft acceptance. Hepatology 1993; 17:1127.

52. Mazariegos GV, Reyes J, Marino I, et al. Weaning of immunosuppression in liver transplant recipients. Transplantation 1997; 63:243.

53. McVicar JP, Kowdley KV, Bacchi CE, Barr D, Marsh CL, Perkins JD, Carithers RL. The natural history of untreated focal allograft rejection in liver transplant recipients. Liver Transplant and Surg 1996; 2:154.

54. Neuberger J, Adams DH. What is the significance of acute liver allograft rejection? J Hepatol 1998; 29:143.

55. Pichlmayr R, Ringe B, Gubernatis G, Hauss J, Bunzendahl H. Transplantation einer Spenderleber auf zwei Empfänger (Splitting-Transplantation) – Eine neue Methode in der Weiterentwicklung der Lebersegmenttransplantation. Langenb Arch Chir 1988; 373:127.

56. Broelsch CE, Emond JC, Whitington PF, Thistlethwaite JR, Baker AL, Lichtor JL. Application of reduced-size liver transpantation: split grafts, auxiliary orthotopic grafts and living related segmental transplants. Ann Surg 1990; 212:368.

57. Otte JB, de Ville de Goyet J, Alberti D, Balladur P, de Hemptinne B. The concept and technique of the split liver in clinical transplantation. Surgery 1990; 107:605.

58. Goss JA, Yersiz H, Shackleton CR, et al. In situ splitting of the cadaveric liver for transplantation. Transplantation 1997; 64:871.

59. Furtado A, Tome L, Oliveira FJ, Furtado E, Viana J, Perdigoto R. Sequential liver transplantation. Transplant Proc 1997; 29:467.

60. Tanaka K, Inomata Y. Present status and prospects of living-related liver transplantation. J Hep Bil Pancr Surg 1997; 4:51.

61. Kawasaki S, Makuuchi M, Matsunami H, et al. Living related liver transplantation in adults. Ann Surg 1998; 227:269.

ACKNOWLEDGEMENT

The authors thank Nadine Thiebaut and Killick Paul for their expert help in preparing the manuscript.

ABBREVIATIONS

ALF	acute liver failure
CC-LT	piggyback allograft implantation with cavo-caval anastomosis
Cy	cyclosporine
Gr	group
HCV	hepatitis C viral infection
HBV	hepatitis B viral infection
IBTL	ischaemic biliary tract lesions
IP	immunoprophylaxis
IS	immunosuppression
LDSt	low dose steroid therapy
MP	methylprednisolone
PB	piggyback allograft implantation
PVT	portal vein thrombosis
R-IVC	recipient's inferior vena cava
Re-LT	orthotopic liver (re)transplantation
StWD	steroid withdrawal
Tac	Tacrolimus
VVB	veno-venous bypass

CHAPTER 26

Sixteen-Year Experience with 1,000 Heart Transplants at UCLA

Daniel Marelli, Hillel Laks, Jessica Bresson, Emily Houston, Daniel Fazio, Feng-Chun Tsai, Michele Hamilton, Jaime Moriguchi, Gregg C. Fonarow, Abbas Ardehali, Rocky Camara, Caron Burch, Juan C. Alejos, Barbara George, Nobuyuki Kawata, and Jon Kobashigawa

Department of Cardiothoracic Surgery, UCLA School of Medicine, Los Angeles, California

The decade from 1981-1994 was marked by the popularization of heart transplantation to well over 100 programs in the United States. Essential to this was the development of regional and national organ sharing guidelines, which were facilitated by advances in organ preservation. Waiting lists outgrew the supply of donors (Fig. 1), and the longevity of recipients was limited by graft transplant coronary artery disease (TCAD), requiring retransplantation (1).

The current era may be defined arbitrarily as starting in mid-1994, when pravastatin was introduced and shown to improve survival and decrease the severity of TCAD. In the mid-to-late 1990's, the spotlight shifted from surgical technique and organ preservation to management of congestive heart failure in outpatient settings and refinements in immunosuppression. More recently, the surgical arena has been the focus of intense research to develop alternatives to heart transplantation. Such innovations include the development of the Jarvik 2000 (Jarvik Heart, New York, NY) assist device, the Batista procedure and cell transplantation for myocardial repair, which may help to alleviate the demand for donor hearts (2-5).

The creation of specialized heart failure units with inpatient and outpatient branches, implantable defibrillators and assist devices to bridge patients with cardiogenic shock to heart transplantation (6) came in response to high demand for heart transplantation. These advances in tertiary care lead to the stabilization of the mortality rate on the UNOS waiting list (Fig. 1). Consequently, there has been a trend towards listing more patients as UNOS Status I, and the Status Ia and Ib categories were created (7) to distinguish patients chronically supported by inotropes or assist devices (Fig. 2). The national median waiting time for patients who were listed and transplanted as status II has increased from 235-382 days between 1991-1997.

While patients older than 65 years comprised about 5% of all transplants in 1994, they currently make up about 10% of patients (Fig. 3). We conducted an informal survey of 35 centers performing more than 20 heart transplants per year, which revealed that about half had an upper age limit for recipients set between 60-70 years old. In addition to concerns regarding surgical risk, there has been some concern about diversion of organs away from younger patients, leading UNOS to prioritize

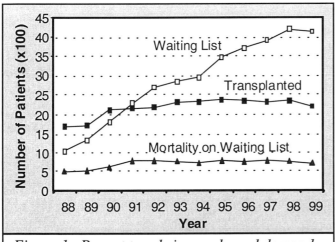

Figure 1. Recent trends in supply and demand for donor hearts (www.unos.org).

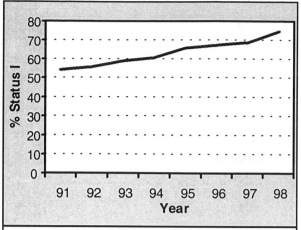

Figure 2. Percentage of recipients transplanted while listed as Status I (UNOS data).

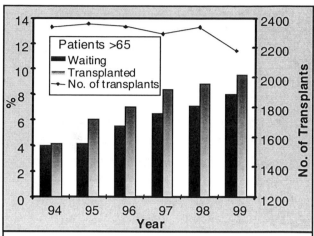

Figure 3. Demand for organs by recipients over age 65 (UNOS data).

hearts from donors under age 18 to similarly aged recipients since 1999.

This review of the UCLA experience with 1,000 consecutive transplants in 943 patients spans the past 16 years. Our experience is divided into 2 eras separated by 1994.

PATIENTS AND METHODS

Fifty-eight recipient and donor risk factors were recorded (Appendix I). The pre- and post-1994 eras are defined by the introduction of pravastatin for all heart transplant recipients (8). This coincided with the

Table 1. Marginal donor criteria.

Risk Factor [a]	Definition
Cardiac	
Coronary artery disease (5%)	Any coronary artery stenosis evident on coronary angiogram or greater than mild calcified plaque possibly requiring coronary revascularization
Age > 45, coronary angiogram not available (2%)	Normal function on echocardiogram
LVH by ECG criteria (2%)	Abnormal function on ECG in V_5 and V_6
LVH by echocardiogram (15%)	Posterior wall thickness $\geq$14mm
Low LVEF (9%)	<50% on echocardiogram
High-dose inotrope requirement (1%)	1 inotrope at maximal dose or 2 inotropes at greater than ½ maximal dose (Dopamine and Dobutamine maximal dose = 20 mcg/kg/min)
Suspected myocardial contusion secondary to chest trauma (21%)	Significant anterior blunt chest injury with RV or septal wall motion abnormality on echo, complemented by elevated CPK-MB
Recent cardiac arrest (15%)	Organ retrieved less than 24 hours after cardiac arrest
Reused Donor Heart (1%)	Perioperative WA in a heart transplant recipient leading to brain death and organ donation
Non-Cardiac	
Older age (17%)	Age greater than 55 years
Hepatitis B positive (1%)	IgG core antibody positive; IgM unknown
Hepatitis C positive (11%)	Positive antibody

[a] Percentages (%) of all marginal donors identified since 1994 are shown.
LVH: left ventricular hypertrophy; LVEF: left ventricular ejection fraction; ECG: electrocardiogram;
RV: right ventricle; CPK-MB: creatinine phosphokinase MB fraction

introduction of the University of Wisconsin (UW) solution for preservation in mid-1994 (9). Excluding retransplants, there were 452 recipients in the pre-1994 era and 491 recipients since then.

Definition of Terms

Marginal Donor: A marginal donor was defined as any donor not meeting standardized criteria (Table 1) (10). In general, such donors were offered to Status I or II patients for whom the potential increased short- or long-term risk was felt to be justified because of the risk of imminent death.

Alternate Recipient: In 1992, our program began to use a second adult recipient list for heart failure patients that we felt were well enough to tolerate surgery but who had an unknown long-term prognosis due to medical risk. This category became increasingly important, since at that time our program had set a recipient age limit of 65 years. An opportunity was created for patients who would typically not be transplanted due to age alone to receive hearts that would otherwise not be used (11).

Marginal hearts were first offered to regularly listed patients (usually Status I). If they remained unused, then they were offered to alternate recipients. For example, from July 1994 to 1998, our institution accepted 149 marginal donor hearts. Of these, 104 went to status I regular patients and 45 were allocated to alternates. The age for listing on the alternate list was set at 65 in 1992. In 1998, as we observed that transplantation in selected elderly recipients was successful, the age limit was raised to 70. We subsequently observed that a higher percentage of standard donor hearts were being allocated to the older recipients. In 1999, the age for listing on the alternate list was changed again to include recipients who were aged 65-70. Since then, candidates between 65-70 years old are simultaneously listed on the alternate and the regular lists while those over age 70 are alternates only. Informed consent is obtained from all patients at the time of listing and organ acceptance.

Mechanical Support: Mechanical support as a bridge to transplant was defined as any ventricular assist device (VAD) used in a Status I patient. External devices were extra-corporeal membrane oxygenation (ECMO) circuits in small children, intra-aortic balloon pumps (IABP), and external VADs. External VADs comprised mostly the pulsatile BVS 5000 (Abiomed, Inc, Danvers, MA) and occasionally the centrifugal Biomedicus pump (Medtronic, Inc., Edenprairie, MN) (Fig. 4). Implantable VADs were the pneumatic and electric Heartmate (ThermoCardiosystems, Inc, Woburn, MA) and the Thoratec pneumatic system (Thoratec, Inc, Berkeley, CA) (Fig. 5).

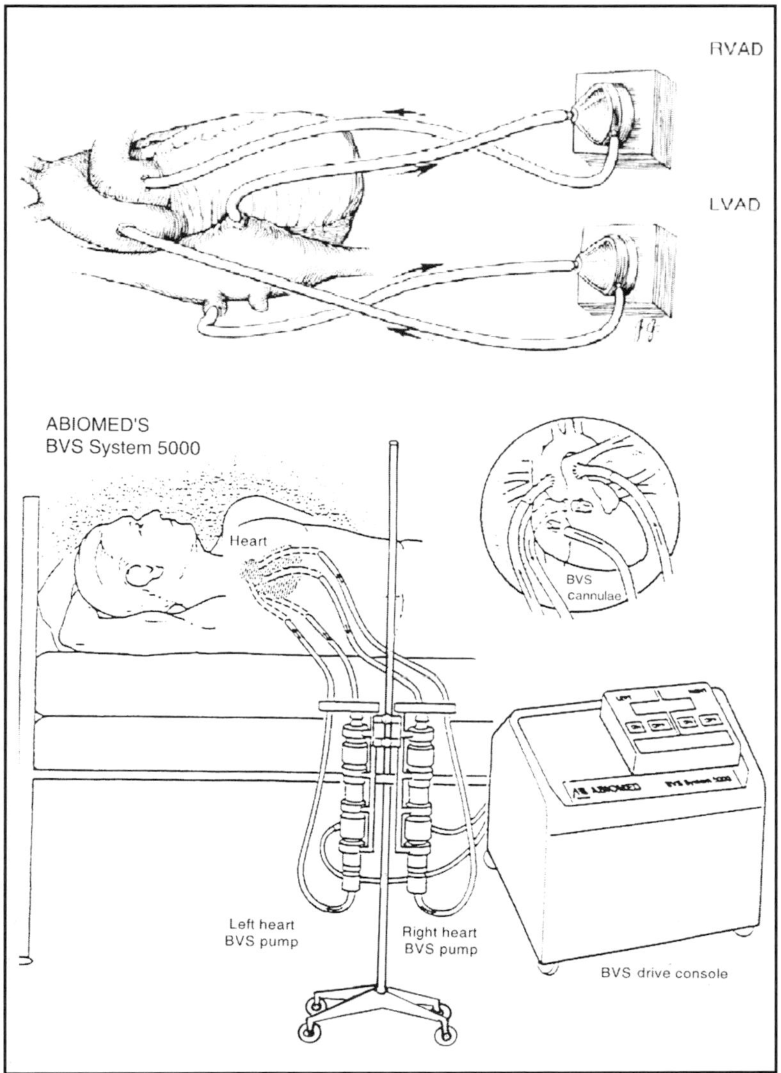

Figure 4. External VADs, Biomedicus (top), and Abiomed BVS 5000 (bottom).

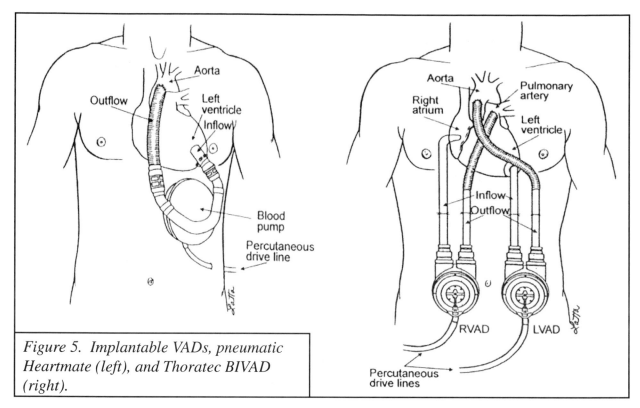

Figure 5. Implantable VADs, pneumatic Heartmate (left), and Thoratec BIVAD (right).

Listing and Donor Allocation

Evaluation for transplantation through our cardiomyopathy center includes cardio-pulmonary exercise testing. Patients whose maximum oxygen consumption is less than 50% of predicted values are listed and tested for panel reactive antibodies (PRA). Patients with greater than 10% PRA undergo prospective crossmatching. Samples of the patient's blood are sent to tissue-typing laboratories both locally and to adjacent regions. If antibodies are broadly reactive, then patients are treated with plasmapheresis and cyclophosphamide to reduce the level of circulating antibody and retested. Hearts are offered according to UNOS geographical allocation guidelines. Since 1999, hearts from donors less than 19 years old have been prioritized to similarly aged recipients.

Organ Preservation

Thyroid hormone infusion is started several hours prior to retrieval. In 1994, our preservation solution was changed from Stanford solution to University of Wisconsin (UW) solution. Hearts are perfused at a constant pressure of 60 mmHg over a 7-minute period, and are transported immersed in hypothermic UW. At the time of implantation, cold Plasmalyte solution is infused into the left ventricle to aid in topical cooling and de-airing. Reperfusion is accomplished via the infusion of leukocyte-depleted, aspartate/glutamate enriched, warm blood cardioplegia (Buckberg Solution) for 3 minutes, followed by leukocyte-depleted blood for 5 minutes. Bicaval anastomosis is used for the right atrium. Postoperatively, patients receive inhaled nitric oxide if mean pulmonary artery pressure is greater than 25 mm Hg (12).

Immunosuppression

Right heart catheterization and myocardial biopsies are performed at regular intervals. Transplant coronary artery disease (TCAD) is monitored with angiography and intra-vascular ultrasound. Our program has not used induction therapy to complement 3-drug regimens. Methylprednisolone (7 mg/kg) is given at the time of reperfusion and upon separation from cardiopulmonary bypass. Cyclosporine (CsA) is administered with the aim of achieving a level of 250 ng/ml. Azathioprine (Aza) is administered at 2 mg/kg/d. Methyl prednisone is given at a dose of 125 mg every 12 hours for 3 doses. Prednisone is initiated at 1mg/kg/d and tapered to 0.1 mg/kg/d over 3 months.

Sample spleen and lymph nodes are obtained from all donors at retrieval and lymphocytes are tested against serum from recipients. Every other day flow cytometry

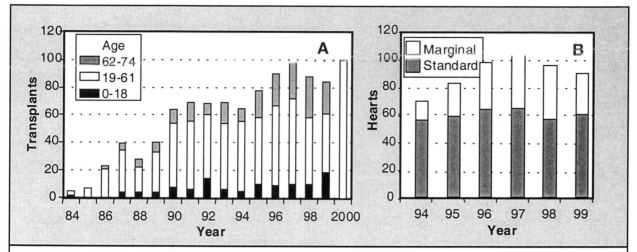

Figure 6. (A) number of transplants per year by recipient age group (Data for 2000 is projected based on 11 months). (B) Marginal and standard donor hearts used at UCLA, showing an increase in the use of marginal hearts

studies are obtained for high-risk patients in the early postoperative period. For those patients with few rejections at 6 months, complete weaning from steroids is attempted and has been achieved in 80% of selected recipients. If patients develop severe, repeated episodes of rejection, then CsA is changed to tacrolimus or Aza to mycophenolate mofetil (MMF). More recently, we have used MMF as a common element of the initial postoperative 3-drug regimen replacing Aza (13). Pediatric patients with congenital heart disease and previous surgery (with blood transfusions) have received tacrolimus and MMF routinely since the mid-1990's. Pravastatin is currently used in all adult and pediatric recipients.

Study Groups

Patients were grouped into 3 age categories according to current national trends; 0-18 years old (group I), 18-61 years old (group II), and greater than 62 years old (group III). An additional group was used for retransplant patients (group IV). Each age group was analyzed in each of the 2 eras for survival,

freedom from TCAD, rejection, and death from TCAD.

Statistical Analysis

Analysis was performed using Excel 97 (Microsoft

Table 2. Clinical data for age groups (1984-1994).

	0-18 n=49 (10.8%)	18-61 n=334 (73.9%)	62-70 n=69 (15.3%)*
Age (median)	10.1 yr	50.8 yr	64.0 yr
% Male	44.9	74.9	75.4
Diagnosis			
ischemic	0	183	53
dilated	15	101	11
congenital	27	7	0
other	7	43	5
Status at OHT			
I	16 (33%)	41 (12%)	9 (13%)
II	33 (67%)	293 (88%)	54 (78%)
Alternate	0	0	6 (9%)
Wait Time (median)	42 days	54 days	63 days
Donor			
Standard	49	334	63 (91%)
Marginal	0	0	6 (9%)
ABO			
match	20	124	22
compatible	6	20	2
Ischemia Time (median)	176.5 min*	155.5 min*	141 min*
Donor Age (median)	11.5 yr	23.0 yr	38.0 yr

*p<0.05 using means or proportions; compared to previous era

Corp, Redmond, WA) and SPSS 8.0 (SPSS Inc, Chicago, IL). Averages were compared using Student's t-test; proportions by Pearson chi-square analysis. Kaplan-Meier analysis with log rank test stratified across time intervals was used for survival and freedom from transplant coronary artery disease. Analysis of the later era was carried out using a Cox logistic regression model. Multivariate hazard ratio was applied if p was less than 0.2. An adjusted selection model was created with significance set at p <0.005. Early mortality was defined as less than 30-day survival.

RESULTS

Trends and Clinical Data

The total number of heart transplants performed per year at UCLA has not increased since 1998 (Fig. 6A). The proportion of elderly recipients has significantly increased in the current era. As expected, there was a significant rise in the number of recipients 0-18 years old with a consequent decrease in those over age 18, secondary to the new UNOS guidelines set in 1999. Figure 6B shows that while the number of standard donors has remained relatively constant since 1994, the use of marginal donor hearts has provided most of the expansion seen in the past 6 years. Figure 7 shows the number of patients who were transplanted from a mechanical bridge or retransplanted for TCAD as a proportion of total yearly transplants. There has been a marked increase in the use of external and implantable devices in the last 2 years. This is highlighted by a shift from external to implantable devices.

Clinical data for each age group and era are shown in Tables 2 and 3. There has been a significant increase in the proportion of patients over age 62 in the later era. Elderly recipients had ischemic cardiomyopathy more frequently. There was a significant increase in

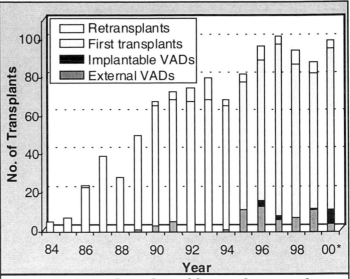

Figure 7. Annual number of first and retransplants at UCLA, including patients with implantable and external ventricular assist devices (VADs).

waiting times and in the percentage of patients receiving a heart transplant while listed as Status I. This was associated with the increased use of VADs shown in Figure 7. The widespread use of marginal donor hearts coincided with the development of our UW preservation

Table3. Clinical data for age groups (1994-1999).			
	0-18 n=62 (12.6%)	18-61 n=292 (59.5%)	62-74 n=137 (27.9%)*
Age (median)	8.4 yr	52.3 yr	65.6 yr
% Male	56.5	71.6	77.4
Diagnosis			
ischemic	0	132	84
dilated	25	114	38
congenital	22	8	0
other	15	38	15
Status at OHT			
I	40 (64%)	174 (60%)*	54 (39%)
II	22 (35%)	118 (40%)	32 (23%)
Alternate	0	0	51 (37%)
Wait Time (median)	13 days	59 days	106 days
Donor			
Standard	56 (90%)	212 (73%)	57 (42%)
Marginal	6 (10%)	80 (27%)*	80 (58%)
Ischemia Time (median)	210 min*	177 min*	185 min*
Donor Age (median)	23.0 yr*	32.0 yr*	35.0 yr
*p<0.05 using means or proportions; compared to previous era			

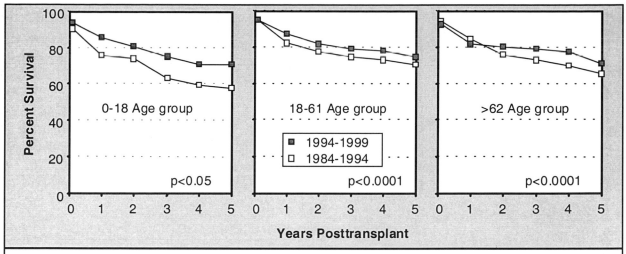

Figure 8. Survival following cardiac transplantation by era for age groups 0-18 years, 18-61 years, and >62 years.

HEART – UCLA

protocol in 1994, which also allowed for significant increases in donor heart ischemia times. There was also a significant increase in donor age from one era to the next for recipients who were less than 62 years old. The cohort of patients receiving retransplants (Table 4) revealed that there were 9 of 943 patients who received a retransplant in the setting of primary graft failure.

Survival

The current 5-year actuarial survival rate for recipients aged 18-61 is 74.5%. This is significantly better

(p<0.0001) than the previous era, when the 5-year actuarial survival rate was 70.4%. Similarly, survival for all age groups improved (Fig. 8). Early graft failure accounted for 1.3% of all deaths in the pre-1994 and 1.8% in the post-1994 era (p=NS).

Rejection and Graft Coronary Artery Disease

Freedom from rejection (ISHLT grade 3A or higher) has improved between the 2 eras, from 14% to 27% (p<0.05). Average number of rejection episodes per patient declined from 2.5 to 1.6. The freedom from TCAD is shown in Figure 9. The results are similar to those observed in our 1994 report which showed 5-year

Table 4. Clinical data for retransplants.

	TCAD n=47	Primary Failure n=9
Age (median)	34.1 yr (4-67)	46.7 yr (0.1-61)
% Male	80.9	66.7
Status at OHT		
I	11	6
II	28	1
Alternate	8	2
Donor		
Standard	33	6
Marginal	14	3
Ischemia Time (median)	180 min	270 min
Donor Age (median)	26 yr	40 yr
Time from previous tx (median)	49.9 mo	1.0 mo
Pre-op Creatinine Level (mean)	2.1 mg/dl	2.0 mg/dl

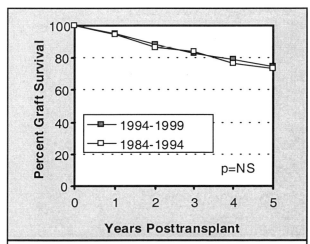

Figure 9. Freedom from TCAD in the pre- and post-1994 eras.

freedom from TCAD of 73%. Further analysis of the current era revealed that there were proportionately fewer deaths attributable to TCAD among all recipients (5% pre-1994 vs. 2.5% post-1994; p<0.0005).

Analysis of Database Variables for the 1994-1999 Era

Recipients were analyzed in 2 groups: those receiving standard donor hearts (n=325) and those receiving marginal donor hearts (n=166). This grouping was used for univariate and unadjusted multivariate analysis after exclusion of patients less than 12 years old. Both groups were compiled to create an adjusted selection model for logistic regression. End points comprised early mortality, late mortality, and TCAD.

Donor Variables

Univariate comparisons revealed that donor non-traumatic intracranial bleed, LVH by ECG, CAD, and history of hypertension were significant risk factors for early mortality for both standard and marginal donor hearts. Donor non-traumatic intracranial bleed as a cause of death persisted as a risk factor for late mortality when using marginal donors.

Significant protective and potentially hazardous donor variables for early and late mortality for both marginal and standard donors are summarized in Tables 5 and 6, respectively.

In the selection model, marginal donors were not found to affect early mortality, late mortality, or TCAD. However, there was a trend for a significant (p<0.09; hazard ratio 1.57) effect on late mortality in the unadjusted model. Factors that approached significance were donor-to-recipient height ratio greater than 0.97 (HR=0.13; p=0.01), donor gram-negative sepsis (HR=2.33; p=0.02), female donor-to-male recipient (HR=3.4; p<0.03), and donor ischemia greater than 4 hours (HR=10.4; p=0.04). Only donor non-traumatic intracranial bleed as a cause of death proved significant as a hazard for early mortality (OR=4.58; p=0.003).

Donor effects on late mortality in the selection model are shown in Table 7. Donor age approached significance as a mild hazard ratio (HR=1.03; p=0.008). Other factors that approached significance were donor-to-recipient height ratio > 0.97 (HR=0.4; p=0.03) and donor hypoxia (pO$_2$ < 60-70 mmHg) crossed with donor hypertension (HR=1.01; p=0.02).

Table 5. Significant results of unadjusted multivariate analysis of donor factors for early mortality.

Donor	Odds Ratio	p value
Standard		
Minimal inotropes	0.08	<0.05
Gram-negative infection	8.90	<0.05
History of hypertension	57.00	<0.01
Marginal		
Local retrieval	0.02	<0.05

Table 6. Significant results of unadjusted multivariate analysis of donor factors for late mortality.

Donor	Odds Ratio	p value
Standard		
Donor-to-recipient weight ratio >1	0.10	<0.05
Blood transfusion	0.20	<0.005
Male	0.40	<0.05
High inotropes [a]	4.60	<0.01
Marginal		
Gunshot wound to the head	0.09	<0.05
Chest trauma	0.09	<0.05
Age >32 yr	1.10	<0.01
Male donor	3.30	<0.05
LVH by EKG	22.90	<0.005

[a] median donor age 28 yr

Table 7. Significant results of selective logistic regression model of donor and recipient variables and their effect on late mortality.

Covariate	Hazard Ratio	p value
Donor blood transfusions	0.34	0.001
Female donor-to-male recipient	2.84	0.003
Retransplant for TCAD	5.74	<0.001

Significant unadjusted model donor variables influencing TCAD are shown in Table 8. Only a donor history of hypertension persisted as a hazard (ratio=3.32; p=0.001) in the adjusted model once pre-existing coronary artery disease was excluded. Set significance was

Table 8. Significant unadjusted model donor variables for TCAD

Donor variable	Odds Ratio	p value
Standard		
History of hypertension	4.1	<0.05
LVH by Echo	4.2	<0.005
Marginal*		
Donor Age (>32 yr)	1.1	<0.005
History of hypertension	2.6	0.1
Male (median age 37 yr)	6.6	<0.01
*includes pre-existing donor CAD		

Table 9. Significant results of unadjusted multivariate analysis of recipient factors for early mortality

Recipient Variable	Odds Ratio	p value
Standard Donor Group		
Dilated Cardiomyopathy	0.006	<0.05
Marginal Donor Group		
Waiting time >7 mo	1.1	<0.05

Table 10. Significant results of unadjusted multivariate analysis of recipient factors for late mortality

Recipient Variable	Odds Ratio	p value
Standard Donor Group		
ABO Match	0.2	<0.005
Dilated Cardiomyopathy	0.2	<0.005
Previous Transplant	8.4	<0.005
Marginal Donor Group		
Previous Cardiotomy	42.0	<0.005
Previous Transplant	10.1	<0.005
Lives Alone	5.5	<0.05

approached for donor blood transfusion (HR=0.44; p<0.01) and donor age (HR=1.03; p=0.02).

Recipient Variables

Factors that were significant on univariate comparisons, but not in the multivariate model were pre-operative intra-aortic balloon pump and mechanical ventilation.

Significant protective and potentially hazardous

recipient risk factors for early and late mortality in association with both marginal and standard donors are summarized in Tables 9 and 10. Recipient retransplantation persisted in the selection model for late mortality (Table 7).

Table 11 summarizes significant recipient variables for TCAD in the unadjusted multivariate model. Recipient variables did not influence TCAD in the adjusted selection model.

Retransplantation

Five-year survival following retransplantation for TCAD (n=47) was 43% (compared with 75% in primary transplantation). Early mortality at 60 days was 19% for patients being retransplanted for TCAD and 67% in the 9 patients receiving retransplants for acute graft failure. Multi-system organ failure (MSOF) was the predominant cause of early and late death. Univariate comparisons revealed age, creatinine, and shorter time from previous

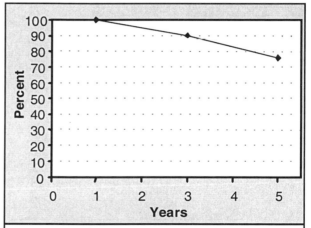

Figure 10. Freedom from TCAD recurrence after retransplantation for TCAD.

Table 11. Significant recipient variables affecting TCAD in the unadjusted multivariate analysis.

Recipient Variable	Odds Ratio	p value
Standard Donor Group		
Male (mean age 49 yr)	0.40	<0.05
Dilated Cardiomyopathy	0.03	<0.005
Non-Ischemic Cardiomyopathy	0.06	<0.05
Marginal Donor Group		
Male (mean age 56 yr)	6.6	<0.01
Previous Transplant	44.7	<0.005

transplant were significant predictors of MSOF for patients undergoing retransplantation for TCAD. Although based on few retransplants, the log rank test revealed that diagnosis (as per Table 4) had an important effect on early survival but little impact on late survival. More than one previous cardiotomy (OR=9.8; p=0.04) and preoperative serum creatinine greater than 1.8 (OR=3.9; p=0.10) were predictors of poor outcome on regression analysis. Freedom from TCAD recurrence after retransplantation for TCAD is shown in Figure 10.

Transplantation in the Elderly and Alternate List Recipients

Since 1992, 102 alternate recipients aged 34-74 were listed (Table 12). Age alone accounted for alternate status in 82 of these patients. Of these, 57

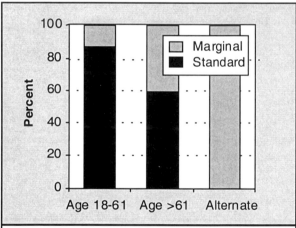

Figure 11. The use of marginal (top) and standard (bottom) donors.

Table 13. Elderly recipient clinical data.

	Age		
	>61, reg n=158	>61, alt n=57	18-61 n=599
Median weight (lb)	155	177	158*
Male (%)	77.0	83.3	81.0
Median age	64.2	68.0	51.5
Ischemic cmp (%)	55.2	68.5	42.6*
Previous heart surgery (%)	46.6	53.7	28*
Pretransplant status (%)			
UNOS I	61.5	0	49.6
UNOS II	38.5	0	48.7
Alternate	0	100	1.7
Donor age (median)	33.4	46.5	27.8*
Ischemic time (median)	174	185	170

* p<0.05 using means or proportions

Table 14. The wait time for recipients according to listing status.

Age	18-61	>61
UNOS I		
Median	27	46
Mean	141±278	177±364
UNOS II		
Median	334	252
Mean	258±325	343±349
Alternate		
Median	203	104
Mean	240±198	159±150*

*p<0.05 compared with UNOS II

Table 12. Characteristics and risk factors for alternate recipients 1992-99.

Characteristic	n=102	Reason for Alternate Status	n=102
Patient demographics		Age alone	82
Mean age (years)	66	Retransplant in combination with:	
Gender (% male)	84%	Renal insufficiency	7
Diagnosis		Age	2
Ischemic cardiomyopathy	66	Peripheral vascular disease	1
Dilated cardiomyopathy	22	Obesity	1
Transplant coronary artery disease	11	Other risk factors:	
Valvular disease	3	Obesity	4
Cardiac profile		Peripheral vascular disease	2
Left ventricular ejection fraction	25%	Renal dysfunction	1
Left ventricle end diastolic dimension	68 mm	Jehovah's witness	1
Maximum O_2 consumption	12.4 l/kg/min	Chagas Disease	1
Best mean pulmonary artery pressure	19 mmHg		

underwent transplantation as alternate elderly recipients and are included in the cohort of patients aged over 62 in the present study. Elderly recipients from both eras were combined for analysis (Table 13). All recipients aged 18-61 spanning both eras (n=626) served as controls for comparisons.

Use of marginal donor hearts versus standard donor hearts is shown in Figure 11. Wait time analysis revealed significantly shorter wait times for alternate recipients (Table 14). Hospital mortality among the elderly recipients was 6.2%, predominantly due to graft failure (1.5%) and MSOF (2.5%). The 5-year actuarial survival rate spanning the 2 eras was 67% (vs. 69% in controls, p<0.05). Rejection greater than ISHLT grade 3A was significantly less frequent during the first year after transplantation for elderly recipients (0.38 per patient vs. 0.77 in controls, p<0.05).

The impact of the alternate list on use of standard donors is shown in Figure 12. In 1997, when all patients over 65 years old were transplanted as alternates, they comprised 10% of total transplants and received 2% of standard donors used. In 1998, when patients between 65-70 years old were taken off the alternate list and placed on the regular list, there was a sharp rise in the distribution (17.8% of total transplants) of standard donors to recipients between 65-70 years old, who made up about 20% of total transplant recipients that year. When patients aged 65-70 were dual listed in 1999, they comprised 20% of total transplants but received only 10% of standard donors. Survival of elderly recipients listed as regular was compared with that of those listed as alternates (Fig. 13). Despite having received marginal donor hearts, alternate elderly recipients had the same 4-year survival rate as the elderly who were transplanted on the regular list.

DISCUSSION

The 2 eras compared in this review demonstrated improved survival for all age groups undergoing heart transplantation in our institution. As seen in our data, this can be linked to improved preservation and surgical technique, better immunosuppression agents, and less severe TCAD, which translated into less mortality attributable to TCAD in the pravastatin era (after 1994). Not shown in our data, but likely to have contributed to improved survival is a better understanding of infection and a greater choice of antibiotic and antiviral agents.

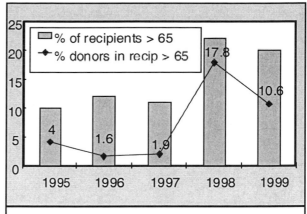

Figure 12. The impact of the alternate list on use of standard donors.

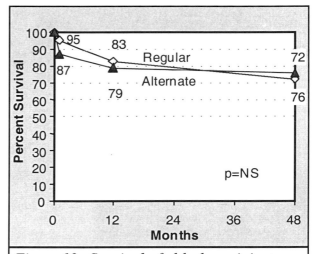

Figure 13. Survival of elderly recipients listed as regular or alternate candidates.

In response to increasing recipient demand and longer wait times, we have expanded our program using marginal donor hearts. The use of marginal donors also has its limits, particularly in the younger age groups who require hearts with greater expected longevity, and who are more likely to tolerate assist device surgery. Such younger adults have dilated cardiomyopathy more often and have had previous surgery less commonly. As seen in our survival analysis of the last 16 years, elderly recipients have a slightly decreased long-term survival rate compared with younger adults. Thus, our use of marginal hearts for Status I patients and alternate elderly recipients matches donor and recipient risks (11).

Our data demonstrated that use of a marginal heart as defined in our institution approached a small incremental hazard, which was not statistically significant. Early graft failure in the post-1994 era was as low as in the previous era despite the increased use of marginal donor hearts and longer ischemla times. This is likely attributable to the improvement of our preservation protocol, the use of bicaval anastomoses and a better immunosuppression strategy including prospective crossmatching in selected cases. Multivariate analysis of the post-1994 (pravastatin/UW) era revealed that a donor history of systemic gram-negative infection, hypertension, and non-traumatic intracranial bleeds were important markers for risk. These do not necessarily contraindicate organ donation but should indicate a specific management. We have found that antibiotics and our preservation protocol can improve the results with donor infection and hypertension, and that long distance, ECG criteria for LVH, and posterior wall thickness >14mm aggravate the risks associated with such intracranial bleed donors (14). We also observed that younger age and shorter ischemia time could compensate for other perceived hazards. As expected, with respect to late mortality, donor blood transfusion was protective and female donor and retransplant were hazards (15). Interestingly, TCAD occurred with equal frequency but was less lethal in recipients of the post-1994 era. This result has a multifactorial basis since these patients received pravastatin and possibly improved immunosuppression. Unexpectedly, the high potassium content of UW did not seem to have a clinically significant effect on TCAD in our series (9). Improved organ preservation with UW decreasing early graft dysfunction has already been described.

Heart transplantation in well-selected elderly recipients yielded clinical results similar to those of younger patients. Because of immune scenesence, elderly recipients also had less rejection, perhaps compensating for the increased surgical risk that they may present. This also justified the use of marginal donors in this age group listed as alternates; both the donor heart and recipient characteristics potentially increased long-term risk, making the use of such marginal donor hearts inappropriate in younger adults who were not at risk of imminent death. The benefit for elderly recipients listed as alternates was a shorter waiting time. Only 4-year survival analysis was feasible since this was a small cohort of patients, most of whom were transplanted in the last few years. Excellent outcome was achieved and we detected no negative trend for the alternate list recipients when compared

with regularly listed elderly patients. Since such patients have fewer rejection episodes and ultimately require less immunosuppression, we cannot estimate their long-term survival, which may be limited either by donor factors or pathology related to aging (eg., malignancies).

The alternate list for elderly recipients proved useful to prevent diversion of standard donors away from younger recipients. Such a 2-list strategy for adult recipients permitted expansion of the donor pool with

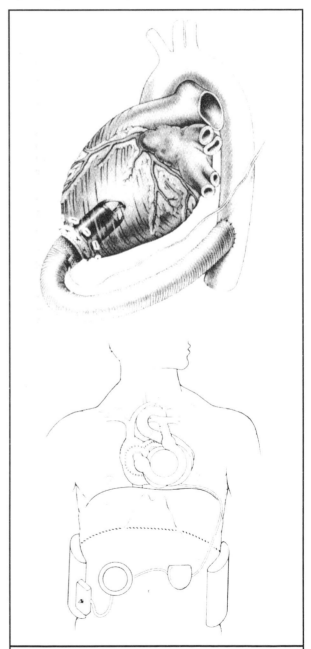

Figure 14. Future mechanical strategies for heart failure, Jarvik 2000 LVAD (top), and Abiomed total artificial heart (bottom).

organs that were not being used, for recipients who would otherwise not be listed. It is important to note that two-thirds of the marginal donor hearts were allocated to younger patients who were Status I. We also demonstrated that the upper age used for alternate listing can be adjusted according to allocation trends and ongoing experience. A formal alternate list facilitates the use of marginal organs in Status II patients since they can be consented ahead of time.

Results of retransplantation were acceptable for TCAD but much less satisfactory for acute graft failure. We observed that mortality within 30-days reflected operative risk and that 60-day survival more accurately reflected recipient risk. Because MSOF remained a cause of late mortality, it is important to have careful selection criteria for retransplantation, particularly for older patients who have renal dysfunction. As a result of this experience, we generally do not offer retransplantation in the first posttransplant year.

By combining short-term external mechanical cardiac assist with an aggressive donor retrieval strategy, our institution has minimized the use of long-term implantable devices (16). Such devices usually require more complex procedures, which require cardiopulmonary bypass possibly resulting in longer hospital stays.

Mean waiting time for Status I patients in our institution has been 22 days. For patients with blood type O or more than 2 m^2 body surface area, this has been 33 days (unpublished data). The trend observed in the last 2 years indicates that despite our strategy, implantable device use will be more common in the future.

On the horizon are smaller implantable left-sided VADs and the possibility of heart replacement therapy with a total artificial heart (Fig. 14). A total artificial heart offers the advantage of functioning as a fully implantable biventricular assist/replacement device. Currently, the only implantable device conceived this way is the Thoratec, with 2 pumps placed immediately outside the abdominal wall. Other implantable devices, such as the Heartmate, require the creation of an intraabdominal pocket and therefore offer only left-sided long-term support. Such devices rely on the fact that in the setting of chronic cardiomyopathy, right-sided failure is usually secondary to left-sided failure. Future studies will identify certain patients for destination therapy with left-sided VADs, while others may require total heart replacement. We anticipate that such therapies will complement heart transplantation, which has achieved excellent and predictable results in the most recent era.

SUMMARY

1. The consecutive pre- and post-1994 eras have demonstrated improved survival for all age groups. This is linked to improved preservation methods, surgical technique and immunosuppression agents.
2. The use of marginal donor hearts for Status I and alternate elderly patients has followed the model of matching donor and recipient risk without affecting patient outcome and minimized the use of implantable assist devices.
3. A donor history of systemic gram-negative infection, hypertension, or traumatic intracranial bleeds was an important marker for risk. Younger age and shorter ischemia time could compensate for other hazards.
4. Heart transplantation in carefully selected elderly recipients yielded clinical results similar to those of younger patients with less rejection.
5. An adult alternate recipient list proved useful to prevent diversion of standard donors away from younger recipients.
6. Retransplantation for TCAD is acceptable but much less satisfactory for acute graft failure.
7. Trends show an increase in the use of implantable devices; refinement in technology for mechanical assist and replacement is forthcoming.

REFERENCES

1. www.unos.org

2. Batista, R, Santos, J, Takeshita, N, Bocchino, L, Lima, P, Cunha, M. Partial left ventriculectomy to improve left ventricular function in end-stage heart disease. J Card Surgery 1996; 11:96.

3. Laks, H, Marelli, D. The current role of left ventricular reduction for treatment of heart failure. Journal of the American College of Cardiology 1998; 32:1809.

4. Marelli, D, Desrosiers, C, El-Alfy, M, Kao, R, Chiu, R. Cell transplantation for myocardial repair: an experimental approach. Cell Transplantation 1992; 1:383.

5. Pouzet, B, Ghostine, S, Vilquin, J, et al. Is skeletal myoblast transplantation clinically relevant to the era of angiotensin-converting enzyme inhibitors? Circulation 2000; 102(18):682.

6. Fonarow, G, Feliciano, Z, Boyle, N, et al. Improved survival in patients with nonischemic advanced heart failure and syncope treated with an implantable cardioverter-defibrillator. Am J Cardiol 2000; 85:981.

7. Renlund, DG, Taylor, DO, Kfoury, AG, Shaddy, RS. New UNOS rules: historical background and implications for transplantation management. J Heart Lung Transplant 1999; 18:1065.

8. Kobashigawa, JA, Katznelson, S, Laks, H, et al. Effect of pravastatin on outcomes after cardiac transplantation. N Engl J Med 1995, 333:621.

9. Drinkwater, DC, Rudis, E, Laks, H, et al. University of Wisconsin solution versus Stanford cardioplegic solution and the development of cardiac allograft vasculopathy. J Heart Lung Transplant 1995; 14:891.

10. Laks, H, Marelli, D, Fazio, D, Kobashigawa, J. Expanding the heart donor base. Curr Opin Organ Transplant 2000; 5:134.

11. Laks, H, Marelli, D. The alternate recipient list for heart transplantation: A model for expansion of the donor pool. Adv Card Surg 1999; 11:233.

12. Ardehali A, Hughes K, Sadeghi A, et al. Inhaled nitric oxide for pulmonary hypertension after heart transplantation. Transplantation 2000 (in press).

13. Kobashigawa JA, Miller I, Renlund D, et al. A randomized active-controlled trial of mcophenolate mofetil in heart transplant recipients. Transplantation 1998; 66:507.

14. Marelli D, Laks H, Fazio D, Moore S, Moriguchi J, Kobashigawa J. The use of donor hearts with left ventricular hypertrophy. J Heart Lung Transplant 2000; 19:496.

15. Young, JB, Naftel, DC, Bourge, RC, et al. Matching the heart donor and heart transplant recipient: clues for successful expansion of the donor pool: a multivariate, multiinstitutional report. J Heart Lung Transplant 1994; 13:353.

16. Marelli D, Laks H, Fazio, D, et al. Mechanical assist strategy using the BVS 5000 for patients with heart failure. Ann Thoracic Surg 2000; 70:59.

Appendix I. Recipient and donor characteristics collected for analysis.

Recipient Information		Donor Information	
Age	Lives alone	Age	Recent alcohol use
Height	Creatinine	Height	Drug use
Weight	Total bilirubin	Weight	Tobacco
Sex	Mechanical ventilator	Sex	A-a gradient
CMV	Previous transplant	ABO	Blood transfusions
Waiting time	Previous cardiotomies	CMV	Echo wall
ABO	Ischemic time (donor)	Brain death interval	Echo LVH
PRA's	CMV	Cause of death	ECG LVH
PVR	Diagnosis	Chest trauma	EF
HLA mismatches	Inotropes	Hepatitis B	MVR >mild
Transplant date	Balloon pump	Hepatitis C	TVR >mild
Assist device	Type of assist device	Thyroxine infusion	CAD
Assist device transfer		CVP (>12)	
Diabetes mellitus (None, NIDDM, IDDM)		Remote alcohol use	
Peripheral artery insufficiency		Local or distant donor hospital	
Rejection episodes (>/= ISHLT 3A)		History of hypertension	
Recipient status (UNOS I, UNOS II, or Alternate)			
Donor status (Normal or Marginal)			

CHAPTER 27

Clinical Cardiac and Pulmonary Transplantation: The Hannover Experience

Stefan Fischer, Martin Strueber, and Axel Haverich

Division of Cardiovascular and Thoracic Surgery, Hannover Medical School
Hannover, GERMANY

Thoracic organ transplantation including heart, lung, and heart-lung transplantation has become a well accepted standard treatment modality for end-stage cardiac and pulmonary diseases, such as ischemic cardiopathy (IC), dilative cardiomyopathy (DCM), congenital anomalies, cystic fibrosis (CF), emphysema, primary pulmonary hypertension (PPH), idiopathic pulmonary fibrosis (IPF) and others (1,2). Since the first report on a successful human lung transplantation procedure in 1986 (3), 13,846 pulmonary transplants, including heart-lung transplants, have been performed worldwide. When compared with cardiac transplantation, approximately one-fourth as many lung transplant procedures have been performed worldwide (4). In their seventeenth official report on the Registry of the International Society for Heart and Lung Transplantation (ISHLT) in 2000, Hosenpud and colleagues demonstrate that during the past 5 years the number of lung transplant procedures has more than doubled with an average of 1,263 lung transplants being performed each year (4). During the same time period, the number of cardiac transplants has increased by 52%. While a remarkable increase in heart and lung donors' ages has occurred during the past 10 years, the average lung recipient's age has decreased due to the increasing number of CF patients being transplanted. In contrast, the mean age of heart transplant recipients slightly increased. The most common indication for bilateral lung transplants is CF, whereas chronic obstructive pulmonary disease dominates the indications for single-lung transplantation (5). Coronary artery disease and myopathy account for approximately 90% of all indications for heart transplantation (6,7).

As with other forms of organ transplantation, there remains a significant shortage of available donor organs. Approximately 22% of patients die while waiting for suitable organs during the first year after being listed (8). After 2 years, the waiting list mortality almost doubles to approximately 42% (8). Human lung transplantation is further limited by the fact that only approximately 20% of lungs from potential donors are suitable for transplantation due to factors such as trauma, pulmonary edema and aspiration (9,10). In a multivariate logistic regression analysis (4) certain risk factors have been identified that affect the one- and 5-year survival after heart and lung transplantation, including mechanical ventilation prior to transplantation, retransplantation, congenital diagnosis, female donor, female recipient, donor age, ischemic time, and others. The actual 5-year survival for the entire lung recipient population (pediatric and adult patients) is about 50% compared with 68% following heart transplantation (4). It appears that double-lung transplants have a survival advantage compared with single-lung transplants (p<0.03). The actual one-year survival for the same patient population is about 75% with no advantages for any type of transplant (single- or double-lung transplant). The major cause of death in lung transplant recipients beyond the first year after transplantation is chronic rejection of the pulmonary graft, which appears histologically as obliterative bronchiolitis. The histological correlate in chronic posttransplant heart dysfunction is transplant vasculopathy. In comparison, the major causes of death in the first year following lung transplantation are infection, rejection and ischemia-reperfusion injury in transplanted pulmonary grafts (11).

METHODS AND RESULTS

The data on all patients in this analysis were collected prospectively. We report on our experience and outcome following clinical heart, lung and heart-lung transplantation at the Hannover Thoracic Organ Transplant Program with a total of 1,033 procedures.

Thoracic transplantation was introduced into our program in 1983, when the first heart transplant procedure was performed. The first pulmonary transplantation in Hannover was performed in 1987. Today heart and lung transplantation have become routine treatment modalities at our institution for patients suffering from end-stage heart and/or lung failure. Table 1 illustrates the distribution of heart, heart-lung and lung transplant procedures. The overall proportion of retransplants is 6.2% (5% for heart transplants only and

Table 1. Number of thoracic transplantation procedures that were performed at our program since 1983 (n=1,033).

	HTx	HLTx	DLTx	SLTx
Primary Tx	632	50	186	101
Re-Tx	35	–	17	12
Total	667	50	203	113

Figure 1 demonstrates the number of different types of thoracic transplantation procedures performed annually in Hannover since 1983. Whereas in the 1980's heart transplantation was the predominant type of transplant, a switch occurred to more lung transplants than hearts each year starting in 1993, 6 years after the introduction of pulmonary transplantation into our program.

Indications for lung and heart-lung transplantation are illustrated in Figure 2. It is noteworthy that the number of retransplantation procedures is high at 9%. In contrast to the ISHLT Registry data, the most frequent indication for pulmonary transplantation is IPF (26%). Emphysema and CF are also very common indications, whereas vascular diseases such as PPH and secondary pulmonary hypertension, as well as rare indications such as sarcoidosis or lymphangioleiomyomatosis, are less common.

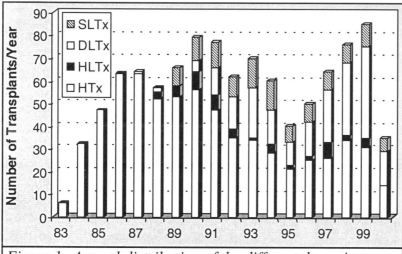

Figure 1. Annual distribution of the different thoracic organ transplantation procedures in our program.

9% for lung and heart-lung transplants only). This is a 1.9-fold higher rate of cardiac and 3.9-fold higher rate of pulmonary retransplantation procedures than that reported in the ISHLT Registry data (4). The number of patients who are waiting for transplantation at our institution varies from 150-200. These patients are considered for elective transplantation and do not include so-called "highly urgent organ requests" in cases of rapid, progressive organ failure with no other treatment option. Of all patients who are listed for thoracic organ transplantation at our program, 70% are listed for lung transplantation, approximately 30% for heart transplantation and only selected patients for heart-lung transplantation.

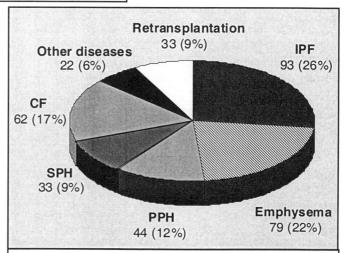

Figure 2. Indications for lung and heart-lung transplantation in the Hannover patient collective.

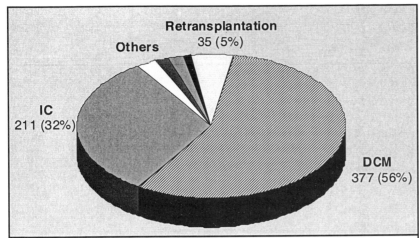

Figure 3. Indications for heart transplantation in the Hannover patient collective.

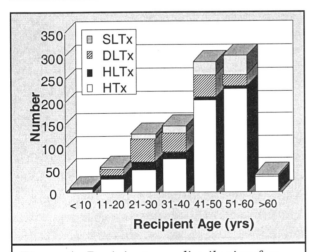

Figure 4. Recipient age distribution for different types of thoracic organ transplantation.

ischemic heart disease and DCM reach the highest incidence. In contrast, heart-lung transplants are most often performed in patients between ages 20-30. This is explained by the fact that congenital cardiac anomalies result in secondary pulmonary failure (secondary pulmonary hypertension and Eisenmenger's syndrome) mainly at this age.

Bilateral lung transplant procedures are performed with about the same frequency in patients in each of the age groups, 20-30, 30-40, and 40-50. This is due to the different indications for bilateral lung transplants such as CF, which occurs in younger patients, and emphysema, which peaks in the older population. IPF seems to occur with no age preference in the age range of 20-50 years. Single-lung transplants are indicated in patients suffering from non-infectious lung diseases such as IPF and emphysema, which explains why most single lungs were transplanted in patients aged 40-50.

The gender distribution in recipients is indicated in Figure 5. While there were no significant differences between the number of male and female recipients in the single-lung, bilateral-lung, and heart-lung transplantation population, the number of male patients in the heart transplant group was 5.9-fold higher compared with the number of female recipients. This is well explained by the fact that diseases such as ischemic heart disease occur with a higher incidence in men than in women.

Figure 3 illustrates the distribution of different indications for heart transplantation in our patient population. The predominant underlying disease is DCM accounting for 56% (n=377) of patients. Another common indication is ischemic heart disease (IC) and coronary vasculopathy patients (n=211, 32%). Again, when compared with the ISHLT Registry data, the number of cardiac retransplants is almost double in our program at 5% (n=35) of cases. Other indications including congenital anomalies, hypertrophic disease, and valvular disease account for 6% (n=38) of all indications for heart transplantation.

The age distribution of our organ recipients is shown in Figure 4. The main peak in heart transplant patients is seen between the fourth and sixth decades, when

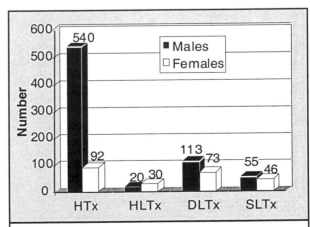

Figure 5. Gender distribution for the different types of transplants.

The current survival rates after heart, lung and heart-lung transplantation at our institution are shown in Figure 6. Although there was no survival advantage between the different types of transplants during the first year after transplantation (ranging from 76-81%), after 9 years we observed a significantly decreased survival in patients that received a single-lung transplant (36±6%) compared with bilateral-lung transplant recipients (56±6%; p<0.05). Interestingly, the heart-lung transplant recipients showed the poorest long-term survival with 18±14% 9 years after transplantation. The one-, 5-, 10-, and 15-year survival rates following heart transplantation in our patients were 81±2%, 70±2%, 52±2%, and 33±3%, respectively. When compared with the ISHLT Registry heart transplant data (4), the survival in our cohort is identical. Regarding the survival after lung transplantation, we see an increased survival following bilateral-lung transplantation compared with the Registry results and an identical outcome after single-lung transplantation.

Some diseases may lead to failure of more than one organ such as CF (lung failure + occlusion of the biliary tract and secondary liver failure) or the development of lung failure after transplantation of other organs. At our program we have performed lung transplant procedures in patients who either received a simultaneous transplantation of another organ or developed secondary lung failure following extrathoracic organ transplantation. The first patient developed ARDS 14 days after liver-kidney transplantation and received a single lung transplant. This patient is alive after 8 years. Another patient received a single lung-liver transplant and died of severe bleeding. A 30-year old CF patient developed acute liver failure following bilateral-lung transplantation and received a liver transplant 5 days after his lungs were transplanted. This patient is alive one year after his liver transplantation. A woman with liver cirrhosis and PPH was treated with a liver and bilateral lung transplant. She died of acute perioperative liver failure with excellent lung function. Another liver and single lung was transplanted into a male patient suffering from cryptic cirrhosis, PPH, and recurrent pulmonary embolism. This patient is alive one year following his transplantation. A 24-year old woman with IPF and autoimmune liver cirrhosis received a liver and bilateral-lung transplant and died perioperatively of multi-organ failure. The seventh patient with α-1-anti-trypsin deficiency emphysema received a bilateral-lung and liver

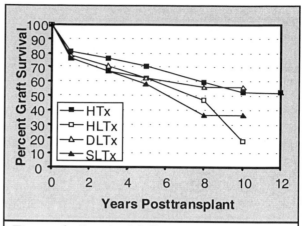

Figure 6. Survival following heart, lung and heart-lung transplantation at the Hannover Thoracic Organ Transplant Program.

transplant and is doing well now one year after transplantation. These data suggest that simultaneous lung-liver transplantation leads to a successful outcome in carefully selected patients.

We recently analyzed the data of all pulmonary retransplant patients at our program retrospectively. The main endpoints were survival and the occurrence of bronchiolitis obliterans syndrome (BOS) in repeat lung grafts. Minor endpoints included age, gender, time between primary transplant and retransplantation, cause of death, reason for retransplantation and the respiratory status prior to the retransplant (O_2-dependant, ECMO, ventilator). The mean age in the group of all retransplanted patients was 35±10 years. Twenty-two recipients were transplanted for chronic (CGF) and 11 for acute graft failure (AGF). The reasons for primary transplantation included cystic fibrosis (n=11), pulmonary fibrosis (n=9), primary pulmonary hypertension (n=8), emphysema (n=3), sarcoidosis (n=1), and a heart-lung transplant in a case of Eisenmenger's syndrome. At the time of retransplantation, 19 patients were O_2-dependant, 11 were mechanically ventilated and 3 were on ECMO. The time between primary and retransplantation was 891±957 days (AGF: 37±31 days; CGF: 1,380±881 days). The mean time in the intensive care unit after retransplantation was 22±18 days (AGF: 23±22 days; CGF: 21±17 days). Eight patients (24%) died within the first 90 days after retransplantation (AGF: 38%; CGF: 29%). The overall survival time was 1,109±1,141 days (AGF: 1,180±1,376 days; CGF 1,045±1,015 days). The one-year survival rate for the entire retransplant population was 70%. Interestingly, the one-year survival in patients who received a retransplant for CGF was 74%. The one-year survival rate for patients after retransplantation for AGF was significantly decreased at only 50%. Among all patients that survived for at least 90 days, BOS in retransplants occurred in 7 cases (21%); in 3 of 4 recipients with AGF after primary transplantation (75%), and in 4 of 15 cases (27%) with CGF.

DISCUSSION

Thoracic transplantation has expanded rapidly in the past 10 years. The shortage of suitable donor organs, however, will soon prohibit further growth. Alternative strategies have been developed experimentally and partially tested clinically in order to identify new sources of transplantable organs such as transplanting organs from non heart-beating donors, the development of artificial organs, xenotransplantation, living-related organ transplantation procedures as well as the improvement of graft preservation techniques, the successful use of so-called "marginal" donor organs and the treatment or prevention of transplantation-related organ dysfunction following transplantation, for instance, due to ischemia-reperfusion injury.

The perioperative and one-year mortality is still high at approximately 25%. This is due to the unfortunate combination of very sick patients with end-stage organ failure on one hand and a high-risk operation on the other hand. The intermediate results are obviously improving. However, when compared with other organ transplants such as the kidney and the liver, the results after thoracic organ transplantation cannot be satisfying. The development of more selective immunosuppressants and a better understanding of the underlying mechanisms of tolerance, acute and chronic rejection and graft injury will ultimately help to improve the outcome following heart and lung transplantation.

Our results reflect the international trend in thoracic organ transplantation towards better outcome. One of our special focuses in lung transplantation is pulmonary retransplantation for patients with acute and chronic organ dysfunction following primary lung transplantation. We have obtained significant experience in the field and conclude that retransplantation for AGF after lung transplantation leads to increased perioperative mortality compared with retransplantation for CGF. The appearance of BOS in lungs appears to be reduced after retransplantation for CGF compared with the primary lung grafts in the same patients. Our data suggest that pulmonary retransplantation leads to acceptable long-term results in patients suffering from CGF after lung transplantation. However, in cases of AGF it should only be performed in carefully selected patients. We suggest considering pulmonary retransplantation as a standard treatment modality for patients with end-stage pulmonary graft dysfunction following lung transplantation.

HEART/LUNG – HANNOVER, GERMANY

SUMMARY

Thoracic organ transplantation has evolved from an experimental to a standard treatment modality for patients suffering from end-stage heart and lung failure. Based on our experience after 1,033 heart, lung, and heart-lung transplantation procedures performed at the Hannover Thoracic Organ Transplant Program, we report:

1. Survival rates following thoracic organ transplants were similar and ranged from 76-81% after one year.
2. The one-, 5-, 10- and 15-year survival rates for heart transplant recipients were 81%, 70%, 52% and 33%, respectively.
3. The 9-year survival rate for bilateral-lung transplant recipients (56%) was significantly better than that for single-lung recipients (36%, p<0.05).
4. Heart-lung recipients had the poorest long-term survival rate in our program – 18% surviving after 9 years.
5. Retransplantation has been an effective treatment for chronic graft dysfunction in lung transplant recipients, but was less successful when used to treat acute graft failure. The one-year regraft survival rate was 74% among 15 patients retransplanted for chronic graft failure compared with only 50% for 4 patients retransplanted for acute failure.

REFERENCES

1. Haverich A, Watanabe G. Heart transplantation, assist devices, and cardiomyoplasty. Curr Opin Cardiol 1992; 7:259.

2. Patterson GA, Cooper JD. Lung Transplantation. In: FG Pearson, J Deslauriers, RJ Ginsberg, CA Hiebert, MF McKneally, HS Urschell, Eds. Thoracic Surgery. New York, Churchill Livingstone, 1995 931.

3. Toronto Lung Transplant Group. Unilateral lung transplantation for pulmonary fibrosis. N Engl J Med 1986; 314:1140.

4. Hosenpud JD, Bennett LE, Keck BM, Boucek MM, Novick RJ. The Registry of the International Society for Heart and Lung Transplantation: Seventeenth Official Report—2000. J Heart Lung Transplant 2000; 19:909.

5. Patterson GA. Indications. Unilateral, bilateral, heart-lung, and lobar transplant procedures. Clin Chest Med 1997; 18:225.

6. Hosenpud JD, Bennet LE, Keck BM, et al. The Registry of the International Society for Heart and Lung Transplantation: Fifteenth Official Report-1998. J Heart Lung Transplant 1998; 17:656.

7. Wagner TO, Haverich A, Fabel H. Lung and heart-lung transplantation: indications, complications and prognosis. Pneumologie 1994; 48:110.

8. Geertsma A, Ten Vergert EM, Bonsel GJ, de Boer WJ, van der Bij W. Does lung transplantation prolong life? A comparison of survival with and without transplantation. J Heart Lung Transplant 1998; 17:511.

9. Egan TM, Boychuk JE, Rosato K, Cooper JD. Whence the lungs? A study to assess suitability of donor lungs for transplantation. Transplantation 1992; 53:420.

10. Sundaresan S, Semenkovich J, Ochoa L, et al. Successful outcome of lung transplantation is not compromised by the use of marginal donor lungs. J Thorac Cardiovasc Surg 1995; 109:1075.

11. Trulock EP. Lung transplantation. Am J Respir Crit Care Med 1997; 155:789.

CHAPTER 28

Hematopoietic Stem Cell Transplantation in the New Millennium: Report from City of Hope National Medical Center

Arturo Molina, Leslie Popplewell, Ashwin Kashyap, and Auayporn Nademanee

Division of Hematology and Bone Marrow Transplantation, City of Hope National Medical Center Duarte, California

The first bone marrow transplant (BMT) performed at City of Hope National Medical Center (COH) was in 1976. Since then more than 3,500 patients with malignant and non-malignant hematological disorders have undergone hematopoietic stem cell transplantation (HSCT) at COH. Over the last 2 decades, there have been significant evolutions in HLA typing techniques, preparative regimens, stem cell sources, graft-versus-host disease (GVHD) prophylaxis and treatment, treatment and prevention of infectious complications and supportive care measures. These developments have led to a substantial reduction in transplant-related morbidity and mortality.

During the first decade of our program, all transplants were from matched sibling donors or from identical twins. The following decade, we initiated our autologous HSCT program in 1986 followed by unrelated donor transplantation in 1989. Bone marrow was the only source of stem cells until 1989, when we started adding peripheral blood progenitor cells (PBPC) to bone marrow to enhance engraftment in patients undergoing autologous transplants. Mobilized PBPC were used instead of autologous bone marrow since 1992 when growth factors such as granulocyte-colony stimulating factor (G-CSF) and granulocyte-macrophage colony stimulating factor (GM-CSF) became commercially available.

The observation that the use of cytokine-mobilized PBPC led to faster hematopoietic reconstitution after autologous transplantation suggested a potential role for this approach in an allogeneic transplant setting. A prospective randomized study conducted at the Fred Hutchinson Cancer Research Center (FHCRC), COH and Stanford University recently showed that mobilized PBPC resulted in faster engraftment, reduced transplant-related morbidity and mortality and improved survival in patients with hematological malignancies undergoing allogeneic HSCT from matched sibling donors (1). Thus, mobilized PBPC are now increasingly being used in both allogeneic matched sibling and unrelated donor transplants.

The combination of total body irradiation (TBI) and high-dose cyclophosphamide (TBI/CY) has been the mainstay regimen for the last 3 decades. A phase I/II study of high-dose etoposide (VP-16) in combination with TBI (TBI/VP-16) conducted at COH showed that this is a very effective regimen for patients with advanced leukemia. Excellent results have been reported with this conditioning regimen when used for acute leukemia in first remission and in chronic myelogenous leukemia. Based on our favorable experience with intensified doses of VP-16, the combination of TBI/VP-16 and cyclophosphamide (TBI/VP-16/CY) was developed at COH for use as a preparative regimen in autologous HSCT for patients with non-Hodgkin's lymphoma (NHL), Hodgkin's disease and acute myelogenous leukemia (AML). Since there is a synergistic effect between busulfan and etoposide, high-dose busulfan has also been added to intensify the combination of TBI/VP16 in an attempt to prevent relapse after HSCT. Currently, we are conducting a phase I/II study to evaluate the toxicity and efficacy of high-dose busulfan, TBI and VP-16 (Bu/TBI/VP-16) in leukemia patients undergoing allogeneic and autologous HSCT.

As we enter the new millennium, we are expanding the disease indications for HSCT to include autoimmune disorders and multiple sclerosis. We are also developing innovative HSCT strategies in an attempt to reduce the toxicities associated with high-dose therapy and extending the application of these techniques to older patients, or to patients with co-existent medical conditions that would ordinarily make them ineligible for transplantation. Herein, we report updated results of HSCT clinical studies performed at COH over the last 2 decades and provide the readers with future directions in the field. Our focus will be primarily in the area of acute leukemia and NHL.

ACUTE LEUKEMIA

Allogeneic Bone Marrow Transplantation for Acute Myelogenous Leukemia

Primary induction therapy for *de-novo* AML leads to complete remission (CR) in 65-80% of patients treated, however, without aggressive post-remission therapy, a high percentage of patients relapse. Post-remission therapy options include repeated courses of intensive consolidation chemotherapy, autologous HSCT, or allogeneic HSCT. Aggressive post-remission therapy administered in first complete remission (CR1) is more likely to result in a durable remission than aggressive therapy given at the time of relapse. Allogeneic transplantation offers the therapeutic potential of a graft-versus-leukemia effect, but also carries with it a higher potential for complications, including increased risk of preparative regimen-related toxicity, infection, and GVHD.

Because of the toxicities peculiar to allogeneic transplantation, much study has focused on determining which patients are most likely to benefit from allogeneic HSCT while in first complete remission. The decision to proceed to allogeneic transplantation thus becomes less controversial as patients move beyond CR1, and towards first relapse, second complete remission (CR2), or in primary refractory disease (induction failure).

Who to transplant? Importance of cytogenetics

Cytogenetic abnormalities are highly predictive of outcome of both standard chemotherapy (2,3) and of allogeneic HSCT in AML (4). A recent SWOG/ECOG Intergroup trial prospectively collected data on disease karyotype prior to intensive post-remission therapy (5). Karyotypes were divided into favorable [inv(16)/t(16;16)/del (16q), t(15;17), or t(8;21) lacking del(9q) or complex karyotypes], versus intermediate [+8, -Y, +6, del(12p), or normal], versus unfavorable [(-5/del(5q), -7/del(7q), ab-

normalities of 3q, 11q, 20q, or 21q, del(9q), t(6;9), t(9;22), abn17p, and complex karyotypes defined as ≥3 unrelated abnormalities] categories. Patients received intensive chemotherapy, autologous HSCT or allogeneic HSCT from an HLA-matched, related donor. In 83 patients treated with autologous HSCT, survival was sharply reduced in the unfavorable karyotype groups compared to the favorable groups, while the differences in relative risk of death were smaller in the allogeneic HSCT arm (5). This observation suggests that allogeneic HSCT is more effective in overcoming poor-risk cytogenetics than autologous HSCT (5) and supports the recommendation that allogeneic HSCT should be offered to all patients with poor-risk cytogenetics and an HLA-matched donor (4).

New Conditioning Regimens

FTBI/VP-16

Five-year disease-free survival (DFS) in patients treated with allogeneic bone marrow transplantation in CR1 varies from 46-62% (6-11). Causes of death following allogeneic HSCT vary from regimen-related toxicity, to infection, to GVHD, to disease relapse. One approach at City of Hope, as at other transplant centers, has been to design alternative conditioning regimens in an attempt to decrease the incidence of death from disease relapse. Replacement of the alkylating agent cyclophosphamide with the epipodophylotoxin etoposide in combination with fractionated TBI (FBTI) represents one attempt to decrease relapse rates following BMT (12). First reported in a phase I/II study from COH in 1987, the combination of FTBI/VP-16 produced DFS of 43% and a relapse rate of 32% in 47 patients with advanced hematologic malignancies (13). A 1993 phase III SWOG study randomized leukemia patients who had failed prior conventional therapy to allogeneic transplantation from a histocompatible donor after conditioning with FTBI/VP16 vs. busulfan/cyclophosphamide (BU/CY) (14). Patients were stratified according to risk criteria. Although neither overall survival nor DFS differed significantly between the 2 treatment groups, a trend toward improved outcomes was seen in patients with good-risk disease treated with the FTBI/VP16 regimen (14).

Encouraged by favorable results in patients with relapsed disease, the same regimen was used by the COH group in patients in first CR (15). Ninety-nine consecutive patients with acute leukemia in first CR under

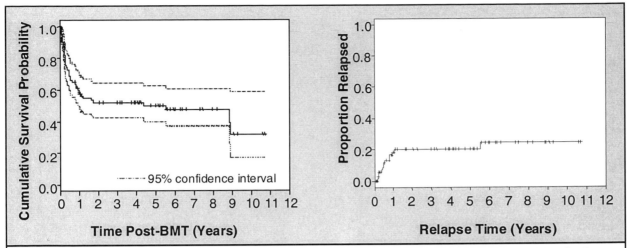

Figure 1. Allogeneic BMT for acute myeloid leukemia in CR1, utilizing FTBI and high-dose etoposide (VP-16) – disease-free survival and relapse rate.

age 50 with a histocompatible sibling donor were treated with FTBI (1320cGy), and high-dose VP-16 (60 mg/kg). Cumulative probabilities of DFS and relapse at 3 years were 61% and 12%, respectively, for the 61 patients with AML and 64% and 12%, respectively, for the 34 patients with ALL. Complications related to acute and chronic transplant-related toxicity rather than relapse of leukemia were the major causes of death (15). An update of these patients was presented by COH in 1999 (16). One hundred forty-seven patients with leukemia (88 with AML, 59 with ALL) were treated with the similar regimen of FTBI to a total dose of1320 cGy, and high-dose VP16 at a dose of 60 mg/kg followed by histocompatible sibling allogeneic BMT. Cumulative probabilities of DFS and relapse rate at 5 years were 54% and 14%, respectively, for the 88 patients with AML (Fig. 1) and 51% and 13% for the patients with ALL with a median follow-up of 5.7 years. This reports demonstrates that patients with AML and ALL in CR1 can achieve durable remission when treated with FTBI/VP16 followed by allogeneic HSCT. A similar observation was made in a larger group of 140 patients with AML in first remission reported by the combined COH/Stanford teams (17). Late complications of allogeneic HSCT were a more common cause of late failure than relapse of disease. Relapses were rare after the first 2 years following allogeneic HSCT (16,17). This conditioning regimen also produces a relatively low relapse rate in patients with Philadelphia chromosome-positive ALL in CR1 as described below (18). However, in the absence of randomized trials, it is unknown whether the FTBI/VP-16 regimen is superior to the FTBI/CY regi-

men when used in the setting of allogeneic HSCT.

BU/VP16/TBI

In a continuing effort to decrease relapse rates following allogeneic HSCT, busulfan (BU) has been added to FTBI and VP16 in a phase I/II clinical trial at COH. Based on in-vitro data suggesting synergy between VP16 and BU, BU was added in escalating doses to a preparative regimen containing a fixed dose of FTBI (1200 cGy), and VP16 (60mg/kg). All patients received marrow from an HLA-identical sibling donor. Forty-six patients with advanced disease (induction failure, overt relapse or blast crisis of CML) were treated. The maximum tolerated dose (MTD) was 12 mg/kg of BU, with one patient developing grade IV pulmonary toxicity. With a median follow-up of 11.5 months, the 2-year DFS was 32%. Patients treated with BU dose >7mg/kg had a significantly decreased risk of relapse and death compared to those with BU dose less than or equal to 7 mg/kg (19) (Fig. 2).

Use of PBPC in Allogeneic Matched Sibling Transplant

Another recent innovation in allogeneic HSCT has been the use of G-CSF primed PBPC in lieu of bone marrow, a development that was previously established in autologous transplantation. Based on the successful treatment of posttransplant disease relapse by infusions of peripheral blood mononuclear cells, a pilot trial was published in 1993 on the use of bone marrow followed by 4 daily transfusions of G-CSF-mobilized blood stem

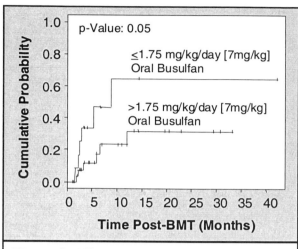

Figure 2. Allogeneic BMT for advanced leukemia – relapse rate by busulfan dose.

cells from HLA-matched sibling donors (20). The transfusions of the blood stem cells were tolerated well. A phase II trial was conducted using blood stem cells alone in 19 patients with hematologic malignancies (21). Recovery of platelet counts was faster than in historical control groups. The actuarial incidence of acute GVHD was 37%, and 13% for grade II - IV GVHD. Chronic GVHD developed in 33% of patients, with actuarial survival of 75% at a median follow-up of 192 days (21). A retrospective comparison of 37 patients treated with allogeneic PBPC transplantation for advanced hematologic malignancies with a historical control group of 37 similar patients treated with allogeneic BM transplantation suggested that the allogeneic PBPC approach was associated with faster engraftment, fewer transfusions, and no greater incidence of acute or chronic GVHD (22). However, after a follow-up of 2 years, the relative risk of developing clinical chronic GVHD among patients receiving PBPC compared with the marrow recipients was 2.22, and for extensive chronic GVHD, it was 2.37. The correlation held up in multivariate analysis (23). Two prospective, randomized clinical trials with relatively small numbers of patients comparing peripheral blood progenitor cells and bone marrow have been reported (24,25). Time to platelet recovery was shorter in the PBPC group in both studies, and neutrophil engraftment was shorter in one study. Acute GVHD incidence, DFS, and LFS did not differ between the groups in either study, but a trend towards a higher incidence of chronic GVHD was seen in both studies, a finding suggested by a large retrospective study reported by the International Bone Marrow Transplant Registry (IBMTR) (26).

A large prospective randomized study of PBPC or BM for patients undergoing allogeneic HSCT was recently reported by Bensinger, et al, on behalf of investigators from the FHCRC, COH and Stanford University (1). PBPC transplantation was associated with faster engraftment without any difference observed in acute or chronic GVHD at a median follow-up of 20 months. Although survival differences were not seen in patients with good-risk disease, PBPC transplantation was associated with lower transplant-related mortality and relapse in patients with advanced disease (1). Preliminary results from 2 additional large studies from Canada and Europe have also been presented (27,28). The current approach at COH is to perform allogeneic HCT from histocompatible siblings with G-CSF primed PBPC in cases of advanced hematologic malignancy (acute leukemia in relapse, CML in accelerated crisis or blast phase). For patients with CML in chronic phase, accrual continues to the Phase III randomized trial comparing BM versus PBPC.

PBPC for Unrelated Donor Transplantation

Reports of PBPC transplants from unrelated donors have recently been published (29-33). Ringden and colleagues reported in 1995 on 2 patients with leukemia receiving PBPC from histocompatible unrelated donors (29). Acute GVHD was minimal in these 2 cases. Additional reports from the same group in 1996 confirmed successful engraftment without significant increase in acute GVHD (30). Faster engraftment of platelets and neutrophils without differences in acute GVHD or survival has been reported in further studies (31,32). A case-control study of 90 patients receiving transplants from unrelated donors was conducted, with 45 patients receiving PBPC and 45 patients receiving BM (33). A short time to platelet count recovery was seen in the PBPC group. Grade II - IV acute GVHD was 20% in the BM controls and 30% in the PBPC group. The probability of chronic GVHD was 85% in the BM groups and 59% in the PBPC group. One-year transplant-related mortality, and overall survival differences were not significant (33). Because the presence of T cells is believed to mediate development of GVHD, as well as to assist in engraftment, methods of T-cell depletion (TCD) in unrelated donor grafts have been explored. A subgroup of patients with grafts depleted of T cells by CD34-positive cell selection was included in the study by Ringden et al, above (33). Graft failure rates were higher in the patients with TCD transplants. The National Marrow Donor Program is currently conducting a prospective multi-institutional study to evaluate the outcome of TCD versus unmanipulated PBPC transplants from unrelated donors.

HSCT for Acute Lymphoblastic Leukemia (ALL) in CR1

ALL accounts for the majority of childhood leukemias in the United States. A second peak occurs around age 50, and incidence increases with increasing age. Predictors for poor outcome include advanced age, high leukocyte count, non-T-cell phenotype, lack of mediastinal adenopathy, poor performance status, Philadelphia chromosome positivity (Ph+), and presence of other chromosomal translocations such as t(4;11), t(1;19) or t(8;14). Patients requiring more than 4 weeks of induction therapy to achieve remission also have a poorer prognosis (34-37).

Cytogenetics can highlight where aggressive treatment should be strongly considered in ALL. Chromosomal changes are found in 60-85% of all cases (38,39). Numerical chromosome abnormalities are also commonly found. The Third International Workshop on Chromosomes in Leukemia identified several significant differences between groups of patients, based on results of cytogenetic studies. Translocations t(8;14), t(4;11), and 14q+ correlate with a higher risk of CNS involve-ment, while t(4;11) , and t(9;22), the Philadelphia chromosome (Ph+), are associated with a higher leukocyte and blast count and risk for relapse.

Treatment of adult patients with ALL has evolved with dramatic increase in intensity of induction therapy, and with the addition of consolidation and maintenance arms of treatment. Overall CR rates have risen to as high as 80-90% of those patients under age 60 (40). Second remissions, when achieved, tend to be short lived. In several Phase II studies, patients with high-risk disease treated with allogeneic transplantation have achieved a DFS longer than would have been otherwise predicted. Allogeneic HSCT offers some groups of patients long-term DFS rates ranging from 40-60% (41). At COH and Stanford University, a series of 53 patients with high-risk features were transplanted in first CR. The majority of these patients underwent allogeneic HSCT in the first 4 months after achieving a CR. HSCT during first remission led to prolonged DFS in this patient population who would otherwise have been expected to fare poorly. At a median follow-up of greater than 5 years, the actual DFS was 61% with a relapse rate of 10% (42). A recent update in 102 patients with high-risk ALL including those with poor- and intermediate-risk cytogenetics, who underwent allogeneic HSCT during first CR showed similar results and suggested that allogeneic HSCT during first CR may overcome the poor prognostic impact of cytogenetics (43). Their disease-free survival and relapse rates are shown in Figure 3.

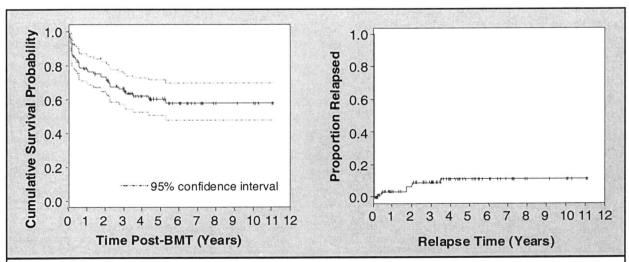

Figure 3. Allogeneic BMT for acute lymphoblastic leukemia in CR1, utilizing FTBI and high-dose etoposide (VP-16) – disease-free survival and relapse rate.

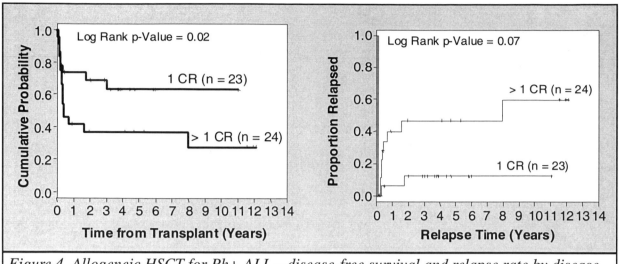

Figure 4. Allogeneic HSCT for Ph+ ALL – disease-free survival and relapse rate by disease status.

In the absence of absolute medical contraindications, allogeneic HSCT during CR1 of Ph+ ALL is recommended. One COH/ Stanford University study reviewed the results of allogeneic transplantation in 38 patients with Ph+ ALL (44). DFS for all patients was 46%, with a relapse rate of 20%, however, patients with more advanced disease at transplant had a DFS of 28% (44). A recent report updated the COH experience on 23 patients with Ph+ ALL transplanted from HLA-identical siblings while in first CR between 1984-1997 (18). All patients but one were conditioned with FTBI (1320 cGy), and high-dose etoposide (60mg/kg). The 3-year probability of DFS and relapse were 65% and 12%, respectively, and is shown in Figure 4. The relatively low relapse rate in this group of patients may reflect the enhanced anti-leukemic activity of etoposide in combination with FTBI. The subset of patients transplanted after 1992 had a DFS of 81% with a relapse rate of 11%, and it is speculated that these patients may have benefited from improvements in supportive care.

Volunteer HLA-matched unrelated donors (URD) are used when no suitable sibling donors can be found. Seattle researchers recently reviewed their URD BMT experience for the 18 patients with Ph+ ALL who underwent transplantation at that center between 1988-1995, and who lacked a suitable family donor (45). The median patient age was 25 years. Seven patients were in first complete remission, one in second remission, 3 in first relapse, and the remaining 7 had more advanced or chemotherapy-refractory leukemia at transplant. All patients were conditioned with cyclophosphamide and to-

tal body irradiation followed by marrow transplants from closely HLA-matched, unrelated volunteers. Graft failure was not observed. Five patients had recurrent ALL after transplantation and another 4 died from causes other than leukemia. Six patients transplanted in first remission, 2 in first relapse, and one in second remission remain alive and leukemia-free at a median follow-up of 17 months (range, 9-73 months). The probability of leukemia-free survival at 2 years was 49% (45). Therefore, URD BMT should be explored in patients with Ph+ ALL who do not have a matched sibling donor.

Autologous HSCT for Acute Myelogenous Leukemia

Adults with de-novo AML will achieve a complete remission (CR) in 60-90% of cases with current induction chemotherapy (46,47). Intensification of post-remission chemotherapy including the use of high-dose cytarabine (HD Ara-C) has led to some improvement in long-term disease-free control, with approximately 20-44% of patients being cured. Results for allogeneic BMT for AML performed in adults in first remission have produced 5-year DFS rates that range from 45-65% and relapse rates between 10-25%. Allogeneic BMT is a treatment option generally limited to patients less than 55 years of age who have a histocompatible sibling, thereby excluding 65-75% of patients who might benefit from high-dose intensive treatment. The treatment-related mortality rate is as high as 30% in many series, and increases with age. The morbidity associated with long-term immunosuppression and with chronic GVHD can compromise quality of life in 15-20% of long-term disease-free survivors.

Since the mid-1970's, interest in autologous HSCT for AML has increased substantially in transplant centers around the world (47-53). Unlike allogeneic BMT for AML in first remission, where the major causes of failure are complications of the therapy, the major causes of failure after autologous transplant using purged or unpurged cryopreserved bone marrow are leukemic relapse and delayed hematopoietic reconstitution, which has been associated with increased morbidity and mortality. Results of syngeneic HSCT and gene marking studies in autologous HSCT demonstrate that the source of relapse after autologous transplant is likely related to the infusion of leukemic cells contained in the stem cell graft and/or the presence of residual leukemic cells after transplantation (54,55). These observations support the concept that an immunotherapeutic effect of the allograft contributes to prevention of relapse after an allogeneic transplant (graft vs. tumor effect).

We have reported previously our results of autologous BMT for AML during first CR using bone marrow as stem cell source (56). The DFS was 49% for all patients enrolled on the study and 61% for those patients who underwent transplantation. In that study, DFS was not correlated with cytogenetic results at diagnosis, however, patients who required 2 courses of induction therapy to achieve a CR had an inferior outcome compared to those requiring only one course of induction therapy. To try to improve the efficacy of the autologous transplant procedure, several modifications were made in the protocol. The first modification was to add Idarubicin to high-dose Ara-C consolidation in an attempt to provide a better in-vivo purge before the collection of PBPC. The second modification was the addition of posttransplant Interleukin-2 (IL-2) to prevent relapse. IL-2 is a cytokine, which has anti-tumor activity in selected tumors (57-59). IL-2 has been administered to patients following recovery from autologous transplants in an effort to reproduce the graft-versus-malignancy effect seen in allogeneic transplants (60-62). This is based on the following observations: 1) human hematological malignant cells can be lysed in vitro by IL-2 activated effector cells; 2) IL-2 responsive cells are present early following transplantation; 3) immunotherapy is likely to be more effective when minimal tumor burden is present; and 4) chemotherapy resistant cells can be lysed by IL-2 activated NK and T

cells. Several centers have explored the use of IL-2 following hematologic recovery with encouraging results (60-65).

Based on laboratory studies which demonstrate that that IL-2 induces effector cells capable of lysing autologous tumor cells and clinical trials which suggest a potential therapeutic effect in patients undergoing autologous transplant for relapsed disease, we have explored the feasibility of administering posttransplant IL-2 in patients undergoing autologous HSCT. The goals of this study were to determine the feasibility, toxicity and therapeutic effect of a treatment program that began with consolidation therapy of AML in first remission. The treatment strategy consists of 1) consolidation post-induction with HD Ara-C and idarubicin followed by G-CSF mobilization and autologous PBPC collection, 2) high-dose therapy using FTBI 12Gy, VP16 60 mg/kg, cyclophosphamide 75 mg/kg followed by autologous PBPC reinfusion and 3) posttransplant IL-2 upon hematological recovery. The IL-2 schedule was 9 x 10^6 IU/m^2/24 hrs on days 1-4 and IL-2 1.6 x 10^6 IU/m^2/24hrs on days 9-18. Patients were eligible if they had de-novo AML (French-American-British [FAB] M0 to M7) in first CR, not receiving any prior consolidation treatment and were between age 16 and physiologic age 60. First remission was defined by standard criteria except patients were required to have normal bone marrow cytogenetics (20 metaphases were analyzed). Patients were excluded if they had acute promyelocytic leukemia (FAB M3), an antecedent myelodysplasia or a myeloproliferative syndrome, previous treatment with chemotherapy or radiation for malignant or non-malignant disorder.

Between August 1994 and November 1999, 56 consecutive patients with AML (non M3) were entered onto this study (65). The median age was 44 years (range, 19-61). FAB classification showed the following: M0 - 4 patients, M1 - 13 patients, M2 - 14 patients, M4 - 8 patients, M4eo - 7 patients, M5 - 6 patients; and M6 – one patient. An FAB type could not be assigned in 3 patients. The WBC count at diagnosis ranged from 1,000-295,000/μL, with a median of 18,200/μL. Cytogenetic studies included: favorable [(t 8;21), inv 16] = 16 (29%), intermediate [normal, +8, -y] = 21 (38%), unfavorable [complex, t(9;11), abn 3q, 11q, -5] = 8 (16%) and missing = 11 (20%). Forty-three percent of patients received standard dose Ara-C and daunorubicin or idarubicin and 57% received HD Ara-C/Idarubicin as induction therapy. The median time from CR to start of consolidation chemotherapy was 34 days (range, 8-98). Two patients (4%) experienced a delay of greater than 3 months. No patients relapsed from the time of CR to the time of starting HD Ara-C/Idarubicin consolidation therapy.

Forty-seven of 56 patients were able to undergo autologous HSCT. The median time from CR to autologous HSCT was 3.7 months (range 2-10). Thirteen percent of patients were transplanted more than 6 months after CR. Delays were attributed to a more protracted hematopoietic recovery post-HD Ara-C/Idarubicin consolidation. The median number of stem cell collections was 5 (range, 1-16) with a median of 3.52 x 10^6 CD34 cells (range 1.1-20.95). Following autologous HSCT, all patients achieved hematopoietic recovery. The median days to achieve an absolute neutrophil count (ANC) of greater than 500/µL and 1000/µL was 10 days (range, 8-22), and 11 days (range, 9-33), respectively. The median days to reach a sustained (untransfused) platelet count of greater than 20,000/µL and 50,000/µL was 22 days (range, 7-183) and 36 days (range 12-320), respectively. The delay in platelet recovery to greater than 50,000 reflects the thrombocytopenic effect of IL-2 given early after engraftment. Thirty-eight patients were treated with IL-2 at a median of 37 days (range, 22-75) from HSCT. Toxicities from IL-2 were mainly thrombocytopenia, leukopenia, fever and fluid retention. No patient required intensive care unit or ventilatory support. There were 2 septic deaths during consolidation (n=1) and during transplant (n=1) for an overall mortality of 4%.

With a median follow-up of 33.3 months (range, 1.2-68.8) for all patients and 44.9 months (range, 3.6-68.8) for surviving patients, the 2-year OS was 66% (95% CI, 55-80%) for all 56 patients entered the study, and 73% (95% CI, 62-88%) for the 47 patients who underwent autologous HSCT (Fig. 5). The probability of relapse was 31% (95% CI, 17-42%) and 25% (95% CI, 11-37%) for the intent-to-treat group and for the autologous HSCT group (Fig. 6), respectively. Univariate analysis revealed that cytogenetics was the only significant prognostic factor that was associated with decreased DFS and increased risk of relapse. However, the impact of cytogenetics became insignificant after HSCT.

This pilot study indicates that it is feasible to use high-dose IL-2 following an FTBI-based high-dose regimen (65). This approach using in-vivo purging with HD Ara-C and Idarubicin consolidation before PBPC collection followed by the TBI/VP16/Cy high-dose regimen and posttransplant IL-2 may improve DFS for patients with AML in first remission. Further studies with larger numbers of patients will be necessary to determine the efficacy of this transplant approach and the role of posttransplant IL-2 in patients with AML.

NON-HODGKIN'S LYMPHOMA

Autologous HSCT for Intermediate-Grade and High-Grade NHL

High-dose therapy and autologous HSCT has been proven to be an effective salvage therapy for patients with relapsed or refractory NHL (66-68). High-dose therapy and autologous HSCT has also been shown to prevent relapse and improve DFS when used as a con-

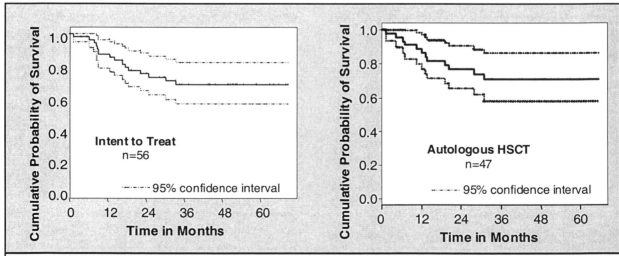

Figure 5. Overall survival from consolidation chemotherapy date for AML patients extend on study (n=56) and for those undergoing autologous HSCT (n=47).

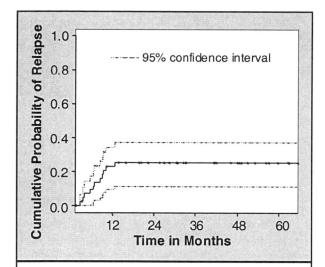

Figure 6. Cumulative probability of relapse after autologous transplant for AML patients (n=47).

solidation therapy during first complete remission in patients with poor-risk NHL (69). Recent randomized studies have confirmed the benefit of high-dose therapy and autologous HSCT both for relapsed NHL as well as for patients with poor-risk NHL in first CR (70-72). Despite the improved outcomes with high-dose therapy and autologous HSCT, relapse remains the most common cause of treatment failure. A number of prognostic factors that predict for relapse and survival after HSCT have been identified in several studies: disease status at HSCT, chemotherapy resistance, bulky mass >10 cm, elevated lactate dehydrogenase (LDH) level, 3 or more prior chemotherapy regimens, time from diagnosis to relapse <12 months, and poor performance status (73-76). These factors can be used to identify patients who are at a higher risk for relapse and who have poor survival after HSCT and therefore may be candidates for alternative novel approaches.

We have previously reported our results of high-dose radiochemotherapy or high-dose chemotherapy during first CR/PR for patients with poor-risk, intermediate- and high-grade NHL (69). Recently, we have updated results of high-dose therapy and autologous HSCT in 264 patients with relapsed, refractory and poor-risk NHL that were performed between February 1987 and August 1998 (77). Patients were eligible for transplant if they had failed to achieve CR after first-line chemotherapy, or if they relapsed after initial chemotherapy induced remission, or during first CR or first PR if they were considered to be at very high risk for relapse. The following

criteria were used to select candidates for transplant during first complete/partial remission: 1) Intermediate-grade and immunoblastic lymphoma patients who were considered to be in the high- or high-intermediate risk groups based on an age-adjusted International Prognostic Index (IPI) (78,79). Autologous HSCT was performed after the patient had achieved a complete or partial remission with conventional chemotherapy. 2) Patients with primary mediastinal large cell lymphoma, who at diagnosis, had elevated LDH level with bulky mediastinal mass >10 cm associated with a pleural effusion on chest radiography or computed tomography (CT) or had persistent mediastinal mass with positive post-treatment gallium 67 (^{67}Ga) scan. 3) Patients with high-grade lymphoma (SNCCL, Burkitt's and non-Burkitt's type) who, at presentation, had all of the following factors: elevated LDH level, unresectable bulky mass >10 cm and Stage IV with bone marrow involvement, or who were in the high- or high-intermediate IPI risk group. 4) Patients with lymphoblastic lymphoma who had bone marrow or central nervous system involvement and/or elevated LDH at diagnosis.

Between February 1987 and August 1998, 264 patients, 169 (64%) Intermediate-grade (Working Formulation D, E, F and G) and 95 (36%) high-grade (Working Formulation H, I, and J) underwent high-dose therapy and ASCT at COH. There were 157 (59%) males and 107 (41%) females with a median age of 44 years (range 5-69). The median number of prior chemotherapy regimens was 2 (range 1-4) and 71 (27%) had received prior radiation as part of induction or as salvage therapy. The median time from diagnosis to ASCT was 10.8 months (range 3-158). Ninety-four patients (36%) were transplanted in first complete/partial remission (1CR/PR), 40 (15%) had induction failure and 130 (49%) were in relapse or subsequent remission. Two preparative regimens were used: total body irradiation (TBI), high-dose etoposide 60 mg/kg and cyclophosphamide 100 mg/kg (TBI/VP/CY) in 208 patients (79%) and carmustine 450 mg/kg (most patients had the dose split over 3 days), etoposide and cyclophosphamide (BCNU/VP/CY) in 56 patients (21%). One hundred and sixty-three patients (62%) received PBPC and 101 (38%) received bone marrow (BM) alone or BM plus PBPC (80,81). Currently, 143 patients (54%) are alive, including 123 (47%) in continuous remission with a median follow-up for the surviving patients of 4.4 years (range 1-12.8). One hundred and twenty-one patients (46%) have died, 94 (35%) due

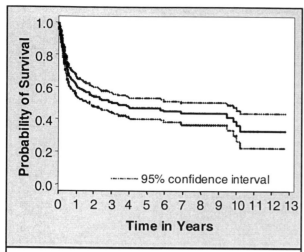

Figure 7. Disease-free survival for intermediate- and high-grade NHL patients receiving an ASCT (n=264).

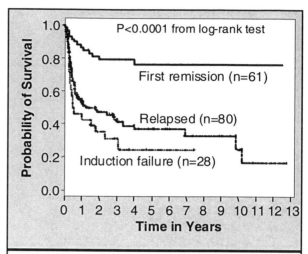

Figure 8. Disease-free survival by status at transplant for intermediate-grade NHL patients receiving ASCT (n=169).

to progressive lymphoma and 27 (10%) due to non-relapse mortality. The 5-year Kaplan-Meier estimates of probability of overall survival (OS), disease-free survival (DFS) and relapse for all patients are 55% (95% confidence interval [CI]: 49-61%), 47% (95% CI: 40-53%), and 47% (95%CI: 40-54%), respectively (Fig. 7). There were 27 deaths (10%) from non-relapse mortality including seven (3%) patients who developed second malignancies (5 with myelodysplasia/acute myelogenous leukemia and 2 solid tumors). By stepwise Cox regression analysis, disease status at ASCT was the only prognostic factor that predicted for both relapse and survival in patients with intermediate grade lymphoma. The 5-year DFS rate for patients transplanted in 1CR/PR was 73% (95%CI: 62-81%) as compared with 30% (95%CI: 16-45%) for induction failure and 34% (95% CI: 26-42%) for relapsed patients and is shown in Figure 8.

Our study represents one of the largest experiences of high-dose therapy and autologous HSCT for intermediate- and high-grade NHL performed at a single large referral-based transplant center. These long-term follow-up results confirm that high-dose therapy and autologous HSCT is an effective salvage therapy for patients with relapsed or refractory NHL. Additionally, these findings confirm our previous experience using high-dose therapy and ASCT as consolidation therapy during first CR in patients with IPI high- and high-intermediate risk aggressive NHL, emphasizing the value of early transplant. Paradoxically, the benefit of early high-dose therapy and ASCT as consolidation therapy in newly di-

agnosed high-risk aggressive NHL has not been confirmed in all the recent phase III randomized studies. In keeping with our observations, 2 phase III randomized studies, the LNH-87 (71,72) trial and the Italian Non-Hodgkin's Lymphoma Study Group (82) in which high-dose therapy was given after a full course of standard induction chemotherapy, support the use of consolidative high-dose therapy. In these 2 studies, patients with age-adjusted IPI high-intermediate and high-risk group were more likely to remain disease-free if they received additional high-dose therapy after achieving a first CR. However, no survival benefits were observed when an abbreviated course of standard induction chemotherapy was given before high-dose therapy in the other 2 randomized studies, the LNH-93 trial (83) and the German High-Grade Lymphoma Study Group trial (84). The difference in results could be due to patient selection, variation in the type and courses of induction regimen and the high-dose regimens utilized. Most patients in our study received a full course of induction chemotherapy before autologous HSCT and TBI-based conditioning high-dose regimen was used preferentially. Given the excellent outcome of autologous HSCT during first CR in our study, this procedure should be considered for patients with IPI high- and high-intermediate risk aggressive NHL. Similarly, high-risk patients with certain subtypes of NHL such as primary mediastinal large-cell lymphoma (85) or peripheral T-cell lymphoma (ie., angioimmunoblastic T-cell lymphoma) may be considered candidates for autologous HSCT in first remission.

Autologous HSCT for Low-Grade NHL

Despite high initial response rates to standard chemotherapy, combined modality regimens and newer agents such as nucleoside analogs and monoclonal antibodies, a continuous pattern of relapse is invariably seen in patients with advanced follicular low-grade lymphoma (FLGL), suggesting that this disorder is incurable with currently available frontline therapies (86-89). The median survival of patients with advanced FLGL ranges from 6-10 years in most single-institution studies and population-based registries.

Autologous bone marrow transplantation (BMT) and peripheral blood stem cell transplantation (PBSCT) have been investigated as a therapeutic modality in follicular lymphoma (90-98). Although prolonged remission can be seen in a subgroup of patients with advanced or relapsed disease, the absence of randomized trials comparing autografting with conventional treatment makes it impossible to demonstrate an improvement in overall survival with the use of transplantation. Equivalent results have been observed in studies utilizing either purged bone marrow or peripheral blood stem cells (PBSC) support (99,100).

We analyzed engraftment, toxicity, treatment outcome and prognostic factors in 58 patients with a history of FLGL who underwent high-dose therapy (HDT) and autologous peripheral blood stem cell transplantation (PBSCT) between 1991-1995 (101). Nineteen (33%) patients were in first complete or partial remission (CR/

PR), 29 (50%) patients were in sensitive relapse (SR), and 10 (17%) patients had evidence of histologic transformation (HT). The median time from diagnosis to HSCT was 31 months. The median number of chemotherapy regimens was 2 (range 1-6). The conditioning regimen consisted of etoposide, cyclophosphamide and FTBI in 43 (74%) patients who had not received radiation or BCNU in 15 (26%) patients who had been previously irradiated. G-CSF-mobilized peripheral blood stem cells and posttransplant G-CSF were used in all patients. All patients engrafted. There was one early treatment-related death from hepatic veno-occlusive disease (VOD) and all other patients recovered from acute regimen-related toxicities. Median follow-up for surviving patients was 62 months (range 17-96). Thirty-nine patients are alive and 23 are free of disease progression. Four (7%) patients developed myelodysplasia and 3 died from this complication. The 5-year Kaplan-Meier estimate probability of overall survival (OS) and progression-free survival (PFS) are 67% (95% CI, 53-78%) and 42% (95% CI, 30-56%), respectively (Fig. 9). Step-wise Cox regression analysis showed that higher age (>50 years) at transplant and no radiation in the conditioning regimen were associated with poor overall survival (p<0.01, p<0.03, respectively) and PFS (p<0.01, p<0.03, respectively (Fig. 10). There were no differences in overall survival and PFS between patients transplanted in first CR/PR, SR or HT. Median survival after relapse was 2.5 years, and the 2-year survival rate after relapse was 65% (95% CI, 45-81%).

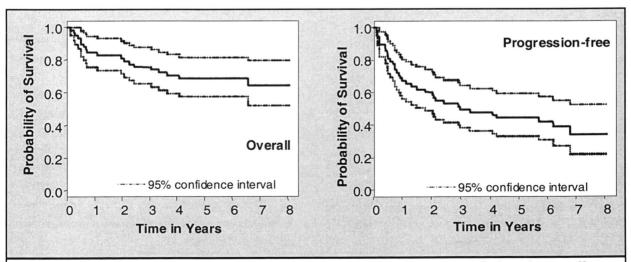

Figure 9. Overall and progression-free survival after ASCT for low-grade lymphoma-all patients (n=58).

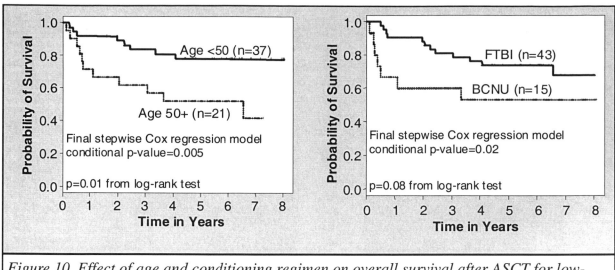

Figure 10. Effect of age and conditioning regimen on overall survival after ASCT for low-grade lymphoma (n=58).

Our results indicate that HDT and PBSCT results in rapid engraftment and low acute treatment-related toxicity in patients with underlying FLGL. Although prolonged PFS can be seen after PBSCT in this patient population, long-term follow-up demonstrates a continuous risk of relapse and an increased risk of secondary myelodysplasia. Additional interventions aimed at decreasing the risk of relapse (ie., rituximab for posttransplant consolidation and/or in-vivo purging) should be investigated in this setting. The higher rate of overall survival and PFS observed in patients receiving an FTBI-containing regimen, which has also been reported in a recent Stanford University study of autologous HSCT for FLGL (102), may reflect the exquisite sensitivity of FLGL to radiation therapy. This observation supports the exploration of using intensified targeted doses of radiation such as radiolabeled antibodies in the conditioning regimen (103-107). Myelodysplasia is a serious posttransplant complication that requires close surveillance, as discussed below.

Efforts to Decrease Relapse

Relapse remains the most common cause of treatment failure after autologous HSCT, especially, in those transplanted in relapse or after induction failure. We evaluated 2 preparative regimens in one of our lymphoma studies and in contrast to reports from others, we found that FTBI/VP/CY regimen was associated with a reduction in relapse rate (41% vs. 67%) and improved survival (52% vs. 31%) when compared to BCNU/VP/CY (77).

However, these findings need to be interpreted with caution because this was not a randomized study. Another approach to prevent relapse is the use of posttransplant immunotherapy. IL-2 has been shown to have anti-lymphoma effects and encouraging results were reported when IL-2 was given after ABMT for resistant NHL patients (64,108). A phase III randomized study comparing posttransplant IL-2 with observation in patients with relapsed or refractory NHL is being conducted by the SWOG using our FTBI/VP/CY conditioning regimen. Another approach under investigation is the use of posttransplant rituximab, a chimeric monoclonal antibody active in the treatment of B-cell malignancies expressing CD20 antigen (89,109).

Since NHL is radiosensitive, and given the availability of monoclonal antibodies for NHL, a novel approach of radioimmunotherapy (RIT) has recently been explored by several groups of investigators both in the low-dose, non-myeloablative setting and in myeloablative doses with autologous stem cell rescue (103-107). This approach may reduce toxicity associated with radiation by directly delivering radiation to tumor sites while sparing the normal tissues. Encouraging results were reported by Press, et al, using escalating doses of [131]Iodine-labeled anti-B1 monoclonal antibody in combination with high-dose etoposide and cyclophosphamide followed by autologous HSCT (106). This study suggests that RIT can be safely given in combination with high-dose chemotherapy in an autologous stem-cell transplant setting. Currently, we are conducting a phase

I/II dose escalating study of Yttrium-90 labeled anti-CD20 monoclonal antibody in combination with high-dose etoposide and cyclophosphamide followed by autologous HSCT for patients with poor-risk and relapsed CD20-positive NHL (107). This approach may not only reduce short-term and long-term toxicity associated with FTBI but may also reduce the relapse rate and improve outcome of autologous HSCT in NHL patients by preferentially targeting higher doses of radiation to tumor sites.

Second Malignancies

Therapy-related myelodysplastic syndrome (t-MDS) and secondary acute myelogenous leukemia (s-AML) have emerged as very serious long-term complications of high-dose therapy and ASCT (110-116). The incidence and risk factors for t-MDS and s-AML vary between studies. At our center, we found that the use of etoposide for stem cell mobilization and pretransplant radiation were the only 2 factors which increased the risk of t-MDS/s-AML in 612 patients with Hodgkin's disease and NHL who underwent autologous HSCT at COH(115). Neither age nor TBI regimen was associated with an increased risk of this complication. A recent study demonstrated that clonality analysis done before transplant using the X-inactivation based HUMARA assay can be predictive of t-MDS and s-AML after autologous HSCT for lymphoma (116). Prospective clonality analyses are being performed at our center to provide more insight into the development of t-MDS and s-AML after autologous HSCT for NHL (117).

The development of solid tumors is another well-known and serious complication of chemotherapy and radiation. The cumulative probability of developing solid malignancies at 2 and 5 years after transplant was 1.6% (0.5%-5.0%), and 3.5%(1.4%-8.6%), respectively, for patients with NHL (77). Similar to t-MDS/s-AML, it is unclear whether second malignancies are related to pretransplant chemotherapy and radiotherapy, or are the result of the conditioning regimen, or a cumulative effect of both. In a retrospective analysis of 2,129 patients who underwent allogeneic and autologous HSCT for hematologic malignancies at COH, the estimated cumulative probability of developing a solid cancer was 6.1±1.6% at 10 years (118). The incidence was significantly higher in younger patients and for those who had received total body irradiation. Furthermore, the risk of radiation-associated second malignancies is likely to in-

crease with longer follow-up. Thus continued surveillance and longer follow-up will be necessary to evaluate the risk of this serious complication.

Autologous and Allogeneic HSCT for Mantle Cell Lymphoma

Mantle cell lymphoma is associated with a poor prognosis and a median overall survival of 3 years when treated with standard chemotherapy. Although not recognized by the Working Formulation, mantle cell is now diagnosed in approximately 6-9% of all new lymphoma diagnoses based on unique clinicopathologic features. Advanced-stage disease, including bone marrow (BM) and peripheral blood/leukemic involvement (PBLI) are commonly seen at diagnosis. Response to conventional treatment approaches such as CHOP chemotherapy tends to be poor and progression of disease is usually seen within 12-18 months (119).

In an attempt to improve treatment outcome in these patients, autologous and allogeneic HSCT has been offered to MCL patients referred to our institution (120,121). Between 8/94 and 12/99, 33 patients (26 male, 7 female) with MCL underwent HSCT (24 autologous and 9 allogeneic). The median time from diagnosis to HSCT was 12 months (range 5-192). The median age was 51 years (range 32-64). Thirty-one patients (94%) had Stage IV disease with BM involvement at diagnosis. PBLI at presentation was seen in 18 patients: (55%) had PB involvement (11 autologous and 7 allogeneic) and 6 had leukemic manifestations (4- autologous and 2 allogeneic) with the white blood cell count ranging from 15,800-138,000/uL. The disease status at HSCT included 11 patients (33%) in CR1 and 22 patients (67%) with refractory or relapse disease. The median number of prior regimens was 2 (range 1-5) and 3 (range 2-5) for autologous and allogeneic patients, respectively. All autologous patients received G-CSF-primed PBSC as a source of stem cells whereas within the allogeneic patients, 8 received BM and one received a PBSC transplant. At apheresis, none of the autologous patients had morphologic PBLI. The conditioning regimen was FTBI-based in 27 patients (82%) and chemotherapy-based in the remaining 6 patients (18%). Twenty-two patients (67%) are alive, and 19 (57%) are in clinical remission. The median follow-up for the surviving patients is 38 months (range 7-68). Causes of death in the 11 patients were as follows: 7 autologous patients died, 6 from relapse/disease pro-

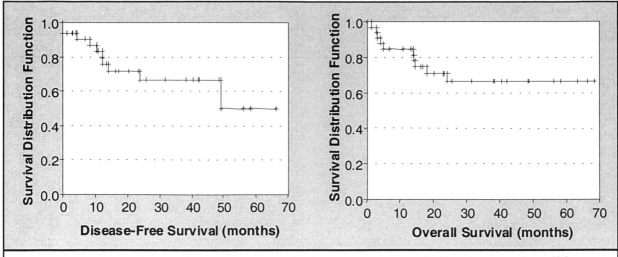

Figure 11. Disease-free and overall survival after SCT (auto and allo) for mantle cell lymphoma (MCL) (n=33).

gression and one from treatment-related mortality; 4 allogeneic patients are dead, one from central nervous system (CNS) relapse and 3 from treatment-related mortality. In this small study, the treatment-related mortality rate was higher for the allogeneic group (p=0.05). The 3-year overall survival and PFS for the entire group are 67% (95% CI, 49-84%) and 58% (95% CI, 40-76%), respectively, with no significant differences between the autologous and allogeneic patients (Fig. 11). Relapse rates for autologous and allogeneic patients were 38% and 17%, respectively, (p=NS). The 3-year overall survival and PFS for patients in CR1 were 91% (95% CI, 74-100%) and 81% (95% CI, 57-100%), respectively,

compared to 55% (95% CI, 32-77%) and 47% (95% CI, 25-69%), respectively, for the other patients (p=0.09 for both overall and PFS) (Fig. 12). No difference in 3-year overall survival and PFS was detected between patients with and without PBLI at diagnosis, even when stratified by autologous and allogeneic groups.

Peripheral blood and leukemic involvement are frequently observed at diagnosis in MCL patients referred to our center for HSCT (121). However, with conventional therapy, most patients clear the peripheral blood and become candidates for an autologous HSCT, if an HLA-matched donor is not available. In MCL, the presence of PBLI at diagnosis is not associated with a worse

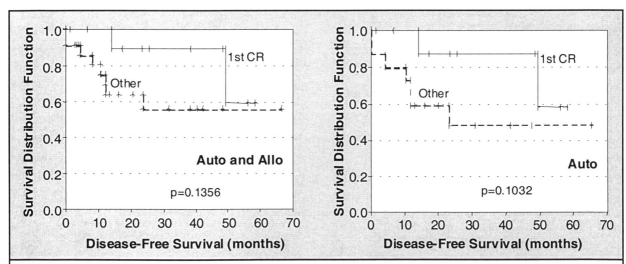

Figure 12. Disease-free survival after SCT (auto and allo, n=33) and auto SCT (n=24) for MCL based on disease status at SCT.

outcome after HSCT. The primary causes of treatment failure are relapse and treatment-related mortality for autologous and allogeneic patients, respectively. There is a trend towards improved overall survival and PFS for patients transplanted in CR1, a finding suggested by other retrospective studies of autologous HSCT for MCL.

We are currently analyzing the combined City of Hope /Stanford University experience with autologous HSCT in 45 patients with MCL: City of Hope (n=24) and Stanford University (n=21) (122). The patients were predominantly male (69%) with a median age of 54 (range, 35-68). The median number of prior chemotherapy regimens was 2, with 12 pts (26%) having 3 or greater prior treatments. Sixteen patients (35%) were in CR1 at the time of HSCT, with an average time from diagnosis to HSCT of 560 days (166-1959). There were no significant differences in sex, age, remission status, number of prior regimens, time to HSCT or preparative regimens between the 2 institutions. Similar conditioning regimens were used at both institutions. FTBI/VP-16/CY (n=34) or BCNU/VP-16/CY (n=11) were administered followed by autografting with antibody-purged (n=21; Stanford University) or unpurged (n=24; City of Hope) stem cell products. The majority of patients received mobilized PBPC products (43 patients) and 2 received purged BM. HSCT was associated with minimal toxicity and low treatment-related mortality (<3%). In this combined study the median follow-up is shorter at 2.6 years (range, 0.6-7.1) in the 35 surviving patients (78%). The overall and event-free survival (EFS) rates at 3 years were 94% and 87% in patients transplanted in CR1 compared to 61% (p=0.09) and 38% (p=0.03), respectively, for patients beyond CR1 (Table 1). The relapse rate was lower (8% vs. 56%, p=0.01) in CR1 patients. Time from diagnosis to HSCT was shorter among CR1 patients (median 228 vs. 441 days, p=0.0001), which showed a trend by univariate analysis towards improved EFS (p=0.09) and lower relapse (p=0.06). The number of prior regimens,

type of preparative regimen and purging were not predictors of overall survival or EFS by univariate analysis. A preliminary analysis of this study suggests that the use of autologous HSCT in MCL patients is able to achieve CR1 results in improved EFS and lower risk of relapse compared to transplantation at a later time in the course of the disease. Other investigators have reported similar findings (123,124). Longer follow-up is needed to determine if this approach improves overall survival. Further studies of more aggressive induction regimens (ie., Hyper-CVAD) followed by autologous HSCT and the use of posttransplant consolidation with IL-2 and/or rituximab are warranted.

Autologous HSCT for HIV-Related NHL

We recently reported long-term follow-up on the use of myeloablative chemotherapy with autologous HSCT in 2 HIV-positive patients with NHL (125). The first patient (patient 1) underwent ASCT in first remission for poor-risk diffuse large-cell NHL as defined by the IPI score and the second patient (patient 2) had multiply-relapsed chemosensitive-Burkitt's lymphoma. Autologous HSCT was performed in both patients using a transplant conditioning regimen of high-dose cyclophosphamide, BCNU and VP-16 (CBV). The target dose of ≥ 5 x 10^6/kg CD34+ peripheral blood stem cells (PBSC) utilized for transplantation was collected using G-CSF following chemotherapy for mobilization while both patients were receiving concomitant highly active anti-retroviral therapy (HAART) for HIV infection. HARRT was continued during CBV conditioning. Prompt hematopoietic recovery was observed and no unexpected toxicites were seen after autologous HSCT. Both patients remain in clinical remission from their lymphoma at 34 and 26 months post-transplant, respectively.

Patient 1 presented with NHL as his AIDS-defining diagnosis and had a viral load of 1,323,013 copies/ml. After initiation of HAART and CHOP chemotherapy, the viral load became undetectable and the CD4 counts improved after transplant (Fig. 13). Patient 2 had multiply-relapsed Burkitt's lymphoma, with none of her initial remissions lasting more than a few months. At present, she remains free of disease more than 26 months after transplant, suggesting that her lymphoma has been cured by the autologous HSCT.

Based on our preliminary results with these 2 patients, we have initiated a prospective trial of autologous HSCT for patients with HIV-associated NHL in first com-

Table 1. City of Hope/Stanford University experience with HSCT in mantle cell lymphoma.

Status	# of pts	OS*	EFS*	REL*
1 CR	16	94%	87%	8%
>1 CR	29	61%	38%	56%
P-value		0.09	0.03	0.01

* estimated @ 3 yrs.

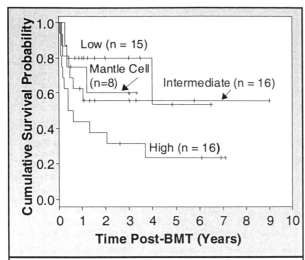

Figure 15. Allo HSCT for poor-risk non-Hodgkin's lymphoma: overall survival by histologic grade.

60%) and 53% (95% CI, 40-66%), respectively (Fig. 14). The 2-year overall survival probability by histologic subtype were: low grade - 80% (95% CI, 53-93%), intermediate grade - 55% (95% CI, 31-77%), high grade - 38% (95% CI, 18-62%) and mantle cell lymphoma - 60% (95% CI, 25-87), with a statistically significant difference seen between low grade and high grade, ($p \leq 0.03$) (Fig. 15).

Our results suggest that allogeneic HSCT is an effective therapeutic strategy in selected patients with poor-risk or refractory lymphoma, particularly low-grade lymphoma patients (138,139). This approach may be considered as an alternative treatment option in select younger patients with a suitable HLA-matched donor who are otherwise ineligible for, or incurable with autologous transplantation. The relatively low risk of relapse observed in this study is in agreement with other observations, which suggest that allogeneic HSCT introduces a GVL or adoptive immunotherapuetic effect. The use of reduced intensity conditioning regimens and allogeneic HSCT as part of a clinical trial may allow for the utilization of this technique in an older, less robust patient population (141-144).

FUTURE DIRECTIONS

HSCT has expanded dramatically in the 3 decades since its first clinical use. As we enter the new millennium reductions in toxicity of this therapy will open new avenues for its application. Herein, we review 2 emerging new facets: treatment of autoimmune diseases and reduced intensity conditioning regimens.

HSCT for the Treatment of Autoimmune Diseases

Autoimmune diseases are a major health problem in terms of mortality and cost of care. Most treatment strategies currently employed are largely palliative with varying degrees of efficacy leaving open the way for novel approaches to treatment such as HSCT. The current conceptual view of autoimmune disease is that it occurs as a consequence of a disturbed and altered immune response leading to an attack of the immune system against host antigens. The reaction is polyclonal and contains B- and T-cell components. The basic mechanisms are still poorly understood, however, once established, the disease process usually continues and leads to tissue destruction and sometimes death (145). All cells of the immune system are derived from hematopoietic stem cells and, as in the case of the monoclonal origin of hematological malignancies, it is unknown whether the true stem cell itself is affected or only its progeny (146).

In genetic (spontaneous) animal models, allogeneic HSCT from healthy, non-affected HLA-compatible donors may not only prevent the development of disease but also reverse associated organ damage (147). In antigen induced (acquired) models, myeloablative conditioning and autologous or syngeneic HSCT can also lead to disease eradication (148). This animal experience is further validated by reports of patients with life-threatening hematological disorders who have been treated by allogeneic or autologous HSCT with control of coincidental autoimmune diseases (149).

Autoimmune diseases have long held a fascination for hematologists. The above observations precipitated suggestions of applying HSCT as a therapy for the treatment of severe autoimmune diseases. These discussions have culminated in a series of consensus conferences and initiation of pilot studies (150). Even though allogeneic transplantation holds more appeal as a potentially curative strategy, the relatively high mortality and morbidity associated with this approach has resulted in the general adoption of autologous transplantation as the preferred therapy to be tested initially. Many aspects of the transplant procedure itself remain highly controversial such as the choice of conditioning regimen and the use of positive or negative graft manipulation. However, a consensus is slowly emerging regarding certain aspects, most notably patient selection.

At City of Hope we have been interested in this subject for a number of years with active protocols open since 1997. We employ intravenous busulfan with cyclophosphamide as conditioning with further immunosuppression using CD34+ graft selection and anti-thymocyte globulin (ATG) as part of an autologous PBPC transplant approach. Our pilot experience has been similar to the worldwide experience as reported to the European Bone Marrow Transplant (EBMT) database (151). The latter identifies multiple sclerosis, systemic sclerosis, rheumatoid arthritis, juvenile chronic arthritis and systemic lupus erythematosus as the leading indication for transplantation – collectively accounting for almost 85% of all patients with autoimmune disorders prospectively treated to date. Preliminary reports of efficacy have been encouraging – particularly in systemic sclerosis and perhaps multiple sclerosis resulting in continued enthusiasm and a growing interest in this treatment strategy for highly selected patients with autoimmune diseases.

Reduced Conditioning Regimen Intensity Allogeneic HSCT

Allogeneic HSCT has emerged as the treatment of choice for a variety of otherwise incurable hematological malignancies. Traditional allogeneic HSCT has been largely limited to younger (age less than 50) and otherwise healthy patients because of unacceptable treatment-related toxicities that have resulted in significant mortality and morbidity. If these toxicities could be overcome or reduced, without compromising efficacy, patients currently excluded from standard allogeneic HSCT may be successfully treated. This would represent a significant advance as: a) the median age of presentation of most hematologic malignancies is over 60 and b) there are few alternative curative strategies for older or otherwise unfit patients.

There are 2 principal forms of allogeneic HSCT toxicity: directly related to the conditioning regimen (regimen-related toxicity [RRT]) and immune mediated – GVHD. The role of the conditioning regimen in allogeneic HSCT is 2-fold. First, to reduce total tumor burden through direct cytotoxic activity and second, to immunosuppress the recipient (in conjunction with drugs such as cyclosporine) in order to facilitate durable engraftment. Two recent advances in transplantation technology have

allowed the latter goal to be achieved without the need for an intensive, toxic conditioning regimen. First, the use of G-CSF mobilized donor PBPC, which can result in more rapid engraftment than the traditionally used marrow derived progenitors and second, the availability of mycophenolate mofetil – a new immunosuppressive agent (152).

The Seattle team was the first to use these in combination in a canine model and show that the need for radiation could be reduced to the point of largely eliminating myeloablation, and thus, a significant degree of RRT (152). The subsequent testing of this strategy in humans led, initially, to an unacceptable degree of graft failure. However, the addition of fludarabine to the original canine regimen overcame this problem without introducing a significant increase in toxicity. This conditioning approach is used to facilitate engraftment and is followed by donor lymphocyte infusion (DLI) – which mediates the bulk of the anti-leukemic effect. The anti-leukemia responses observed after DLI in CML patients who relapsed after an allogeneic HSCT is direct evidence that, in some circumstances, the GVL effect mediated by lymphocytes may be enough to control disease (153-156). This then forms the basis for GVL as the primary therapeutic modality employed in an effort to control hematologic malignancies by reduced intensity transplantation.

Teams from other centers such as Jerusalem and Houston have also developed other "reduced-intensity" conditioning regimens (142,155). However, at City of Hope, we have adopted the Seattle regimen for our phase II trials for a variety of reasons (157). First, it was logically derived by combining 2 technologies that enhance engraftment. Second, the regimen was carefully tested in animals by a team that is very experienced in translating animal results into humans and third, this approach is truly non-myeloablative (as opposed to the "medium-intensity" regimens of other centers).

At the present time the use of this strategy is in its infancy and many questions still remain:

1. Will the reduction in conditioning regimen intensity lead to a loss in efficacy?

   Preliminary data suggests that fast growing hematologic malignancies – such as blast crisis CML – may not respond well to non-myeloablative transplantation implying that the immunologically mediated anti-leukemic effect (GVL) is inadequate in this setting (158).

2. Will the incidence of GVHD be increased?

This treatment approach relies solely on the use of allogeneic PBPC transplantation. Phase II studies of this source of stem cells have suggested that, while engraftment rates may be enhanced, the incidence and severity of chronic GVH may be also markedly increased. Whether this will occur in the setting of reduced intensity conditioning remains to be seen.

CONCLUDING REMARKS

Over the past 2 decades there have been major improvements in the field of HSCT, which have led to a reduction in the morbidity and mortality associated with the procedure. Consequently, the use of HSCT can now be extended to selected older patients without excessive toxicity (159--163). As our knowledge of stem cell engraftment kinetics and graft-versus-tumor reactions has increased, we are now able to devise approaches to further decrease the risks of allogeneic transplantation by utilizing reduced-intensity conditioning regimens that are less toxic but still capable of facilitating allogeneic stem cell engraftment and graft-versus-malignancy reactions. In some settings we are exploring a tandem autologous followed by allogeneic transplant approach. An autologous transplant is performed to reduce the tumor burden in patients with otherwise refractory disease. This is followed by a reduced-intensity allogeneic transplant to facilitate an immune reaction as a form of adoptive immunotherapy against the residual malignant cells, which may persist after the initial autologous procedure (144,159).

HSCT has evolved from being an experimental treatment of last resort to a standard procedure that is often utilized as part of the initial treatment for patients with hematologic malignancies and non-malignant hematologic disorders. As the use of HSCT and success rates of the procedure increase, there will also be an increasing number of survivors who are sometimes faced with delayed or chronic complications such as GVHD and secondary malignancies (115,118). Assessment of quality-of-life issues has shown that psychosocial problems such as unemployment, and financial, and sexual difficulties may also follow HSCT (164). Increased research efforts are needed to reduce long-term complications and to maintain and improve quality of life after HSCT.

SUMMARY

Progress in the in the field of human stem cell transplantation (HSCT) has led to a reduction in transplant-related toxicities and an improvement in survival rates. In the allogeneic setting, conditioning regimens containing FTBI and high dose VP-16 produce high rates of long-term progression-free survival in patients with AML and ALL. Because of more rapid engraftment, peripheral blood stem cells are increasingly being used for allogeneic HSCT, however, longer follow-up will be required to determine whether there are differences in overall survival and long-term complications such as chronic graft-versus host disease (GVHD). Results of autologous transplantation for acute leukemias are improving as new strategies are used to decrease the risk of relapse. For diffuse aggressive NHL, high-dose therapy and autologous HSCT has been established as a potentially curative therapy when performed at the time of relapse or as part of the frontline treatment in selected patients with poor prognostic features at presentation. Patients with HIV-associated NHL may also benefit from autologous HSCT. In other subtypes of NHL such as mantle cell lymphoma and low-grade lymphoma, the curative potential of autologous transplantation is less certain and the graft-versus-lymphoma effect which can be seen in allogeneic HSCT may be required for cure of these histologic subtypes. Our current research efforts focus on reducing the risk of relapse as well as acute and long-term complications.

REFERENCES

1. Bensinger W, Martin P, Clift R, et al. A prospective randomized trial of peripheral blood stem cells (PBSC) or marrow (BM) for patients undergoing allogeneic transplantation for hematologic malignancies. N Engl J Med 2001 (in press).

2. Keating MJ, Smith TL, Kantarjian H, et al. Cytogenetic patterns in acute myelogenous leukemia: A major reproducible determinant of outcome. Leukemia 1988; 2:403.

3. Stein A, O'Donnell MR, Slovak ML, et al. Cytogenetics predict complete remission rate (CR) for adult patients with de novo acute myelogenous leukemia (AML) treated with high dose cytarabine (HD Ara-C). Blood 1997; 90(Suppl 1):64a.

4. Gale RP, Horowitz MM, Weiner RS, et al. Impact of cytogenetic abnormalities on outcome of bone marrow transplants in acute myelogenous leukemia in first remission. Bone Marrow Transplant 1995; 16:203.

5. Slovak ML, Kopecky KJ, Cassileth PA, et al. Karyotypic analysis predicts outcome of preremission and postremission therapy in adult acute myeloid leukemia: a Southwest Oncology Group/Eastern Cooperative Oncology Group study. Blood 2000; 96:4075.

6. Forman SJ, Spruce WE, Farbstein MJ, et al. Bone marrow ablation followed by allogeneic marrow grafting during first complete remission of acute nonlymphocytic leukemia. Blood 1983; 61:439.

7. Bostrom B, Brunning RD, McGlave P, et al. Bone marrow transplantation for acute nonlymphocytic leukemia in first remission: Analysis of prognostic factors. Blood 1985; 65:1191.

8. Clift RA, Buckner CD, Thomas Ed, et al. The treatment of acute nonlymphoblastic leukemia by allogeneic transplantation. Bone Marrow Transplant 1987; 2:243.

9. Helenglass G, Powles RL, McElwain TJ, et al. Melphalan and total body irradiation (TBI) versus cyclophosphamide and TBI as conditioning for allogeneic matched sibling bone marrow transplants for acute myeloblastic leukemia in first remission. Bone Marrow Transplant 1988; 3:21.

10. McGlave PB, Haake RJ, Bostrom BC, et al. Allogeneic bone marrow transplantation for acute nonlymphocytic leukemia in first remission. Blood 1988; 72:1512.

11. Kim TH, McGlave PB, Ramsay N, et al. Comparison of 2 total body irradiation regimens in allogeneic bone marrow transplantation for acute nonlymphoblastic leukemia in first remission. Int J Radiat Oncol Biol Phys 1990; 19:889.

12. Blume KG, Forman SJ. High-dose etoposide (VP-16)-containing preparatory regimens in allogeneic and autologous bone marrow transplantation for hematologic malignancies. Semin Oncol 1992; 19:S63.

13. Blume KG, Forman, SJ, O'Donnell MR, et al. Total body irradiation and high-dose etoposide: A new preparatory regimen for bone marrow transplantation in patients with advanced hematologic malignancies. Blood 1987; 69:1015.

14. Blume KG, Kopecky KJ, Henslee-Downey JP, et al. A prospective randomized comparison of total body irradiation-etoposide versus bulsulfan-cyclophosphamide as preparatory regimens for bone marrow transplantation in patients with recurrent leukemia: A Southwest Oncology Group Study. Blood 1993; 81:2187.

15. Snyder DS, Chao NJ, Amylon MD, et al. Fractionated total body irradiation and high-dose etoposide as a preparatory regimen for bone marrow transplantation for 99 patients with acute leukemia in first complete remission. Blood 1993; 82:2920.

16. Fung HC, Snyder D, Kashyap A, et al. Long term follow-up report of allogeneic bone marrow transplantation for patients with acute leukemia in first complete remission utilizing fractionated total body irradiation (FTBI) and high dose etoposide: late relapse is an uncommon cause of treatment failure. Proc Am Soc Clin Oncol 1999; 18:8a.

17. Fung H, Jamieson C, Snyder D, et al. Allogeneic bone marrow transplantation (BMT) for AML in first remission (1CR) utilizing fractionated total body irradiation (FTBI) and VP-16: analysis of risk factors for relapse and disease-free-survival (abstract 730). Blood 1999; 94(Suppl 1):167a.

18. Snyder DS, Nademanee AP, O'Donnell M, et al. Allogeneic bone marrow transplantation for Philadelphia chromoscome-positive acute lymphoblastic leukemia in first complete remission: long-term follow-up. Leukemia 1999; 13:2053.

19. Stein A, O'Donnell MR, Parker R, et al. Phase I/II Study of escalating doses of Busulfan (BU) in combination with fractionated total body irradiation (FTBI) and etoposide (VP16) as a preparative regimen for allogeneic bone marrow transplant (BMT) for patients with advanced leukemias. Blood 1998; 517a.

20. Nemunaitis J, Rosenfeld C, Collins R, et al. Allogeneic transplantation combining mobilized blood and bone marrow in patients with refractory hematologic malignancies. Transfusion 1995; 35:666.

21. Rosenfeld C, Collins R, Pineiro L, et al. Allogeneic blood cell transplantation without posttransplant colony-stimulating factors in patients with hematopoietic neoplasm: a phase II study. JCO 1996; 14:1314.

22. Bensinger WI, Clift R, Martin P, et al. Allogeneic peripheral blood stem cell transplantation in patients with advanced hematologic malignancies: a retrospective comparison with marrow transplantation. Blood 1996; 88:2794.

23. Storek J, Gooley T, Siadak M, et al. Allogeneic peripheral blood stem cell transplantation may be associated with a high risk of chronic graft versus host disease. Blood 1997; 90:4705.

24. Schmitz N, Bacigalupo A, Hasenclever D, et al. Allogeneic bone marrow transplantation vs. filgrastim-mobilised peripheral blood progenitor cell transplantation in patients with early leukemia: first results of a randomised multicentre trial of the European Group for Blood and Marrow Transplantation. BMT 1998; 21:995.

25. Vigorito AC, Azevedo WM, Marques JF, et al. A randomised, prospective comparison of allogeneic bone marrow and peripheral blood progenitor cell transplantation in the treatment of haematological malignancies. BMT 1998; 22:1145.

26. Champlin RE, Schmitz N, Horowitz MM, et al. Blood stem cells compared with bone marrow as a source of hematopoietic cells for allogeneic transplantation. IBMTR Histocompatibility and Stem Cell Sources Working Committee and the European Group for Blood and Marrow Transplantation (EBMT). Blood 2000; 95:3702.

27. Simpson DR, Couban S, Bredeson C, et al. A Canadian study comparing peripheral blood (PB) and bone marrow (BM) in patients undergoing matched sibling transplants for myeloid malignancies (abstract 2067). Blood 2000; 96:481a.

28. Schmitz N, Beksac M, Hasenclever D, et al. A randomised study from the European Group for Blood and Marrow Transplantation comparing allogeneic transplantation of filgrastim-mobilized peripheral blood progenitor cells with bone marrow transplantation in 350 patients (PTS) with leukemia (abstract 2068). Blood 2000; 96:481a.

29. Ringden O, Lonnqvist B, Hagglund H, Ljungman, et al. Transplantation with peripheral blood stem cells from unrelated donors without serious graft-versus-host disease. Bone Marrow Transplant 1995; 16:856.

30. Ringden O, Potter MN, Oakhill A, Cornish J, et al. Transplantation of peripheral blood progenitor cells from unrelated donors. BMT 1996; 17(Suppl 2):S62.

31. Hagglund H, Ringden O, Remberger M, Lonnqvist B, et al. Faster neutrophil and platelet engraftment, but no difference is acute GVHD or survival, using peripheral blood stem cells from related and unrelated donors, compared to bone marrow. BMT 1998; 22:131.

32. Ringden O, Remberger M, Runde V, Bornhauser M. Faster engraftment of neutrophils and platelets with peripheral blood stem cells from unrelated donors: a comparison with marrow transplantation. BMT 2000; 25(Suppl 2):S6.

33. Ringden O, Remberger M, Runde V, Bornhauser M et al. Peripheral blood stem cell transpalntation from unrelated donors: a comparison with marrow transpalntation. Blood 1999; 94:455.

34. Hoelzer D, Thiel E, Loffler T, et al: Prognostic factors in a multicentric study for treatment of acute lymphoblastic leukemia in adults. Blood 1988; 71:123.

35. Hoelzer D, Ludwig WD, Thiel D, et al: Improved outcome in adult B-cell acute lymphoblastic leukemia. Blood 1996; 87:495.

36. Copelan EA, McGuire EA: The biology and treatment of acute lymphoblastic leukemia in adults. Blood 1995; 85:1151.

37. Laport GF, Larson RA. Treatment of adult acute lymphoblastic leukemia Semin Oncol 1997; 24:70.

38. Third International Workshop on Chromosomes in Leukemia: Chromosomal abnormalities and their clinical significance in acute lymphoblastic leukemia. Cancer Res 1983; 43:868.

39. Faderl S, Kantarjian M, Talpaz M, Estrov Z. Clinical significance of cytogenetic abnormalities in adult acute lymphoblastic leukemia. Blood 1998; 91:3996.

40. Linker CA, Levitt LJ, O'Donnell M, et al. Treatment of adult acute lymphoblastic leukemia with intensive cyclical chemotherapy: A follow-up report. Blood 1991; 78:2814.

41. Forman SJ. The role of allogeneic bone marrow transplantation in the treatment of high-risk acute lymphocytic leukemia in adults. Leukemia 1997;11(Suppl 4):S18.

42. Chao NJ, Forman SJ, Schmidt GM, et al. Allogeneic bone marrow transplantation for high-risk acute lymphoblastic leukemia during first complete remission. Blood 1991; 78:1923.

43. Fung HC, Jamieson C, Snyder D, et al. Allogeneic bone marrow transplantation (BMT) for high-risk ALL in first remission (CR1) (abstract 2709). Blood 1999; 94(Suppl 1):609a.

44. Chao NJ, Blume KG, Forman SJ, Snyder DS. Long-term follow-up of allogeneic bone marrow recipients for Philadelphia chromosome-positive acute lymphoblastic leukemia. Blood 1995; 85: 3353.

45. Sierra J, Radich J, Hansen JA, et al. Marrow transplants from unrelated donors for treatment of Philadelphia chromosome-positive acute lymphoblastic leukemia. Blood 1997; 90:1410.

46. Stein AS, O'Donnell MR, Nademanee A, et al. Idarubicin (IDA) and High-dose cytosine arabinoside (HD ARA-C) for induction therapy for AML and AML arising from myelodysplasia (MDS/AML) (abstract 1531). Blood 1995; 86:386a.

47. Stein AS, Forman SJ. Autologous hematopoietic cell transplantation for acute myeloid leukemia. In: Forman SJ, Blume KG, Thomas ED, Eds. Hematopoietic Cell Transplantation 2nd ed. London: Blackwell Science, Inc. 1998; 963.

48. Ball ED, Mills LE, Cornwell GG 3rd, et al. Autologous bone marrow transplantation for acute myeloid leukemia using monoclonal antibody-purged bone marrow. Blood 1990; 75:1199.

49. Cassileth PA, Andersen J, Lazarus HM, et al. Autologous bone marrow transplant in acute myeloid leukemia in first remission. J Clin Oncol 1993; 11:314.

50. Löwenberg B, Verdonck LJ, Dekker AW, et al. Autologous bone marrow transplantation in acute myeloid leukemia in first remission: Results of Dutch prospective study. J Clin Oncol 1990; 8:287.

51. Burnett AK, Pendry K, Rawlinson PM, et al. Autograft to eliminate minimal residual disease in AML in first remission – update on the Glasgow experience. Bone Marrow Transplant 1990; 6:59.

52. Gorin NC, Aegerter P, Auvert B, et al. Autologous bone marrow transplantation for acute myelocytic leukemia in first remission: A European survey of the role of marrow purging. Blood 1990; 75:1606.

53. Burnett AK, Goldstone AH, Stevens RM, et al. Randomized comparison of addition of autologous bone-marrow transplantation to intensive chemotherapy for acute myeloid leukaemia in first remission: Results of MRC AML 10 trial. Lancet 1998; 351:700.

54. Gale RP, Horowitz MM, Ash RC, et al. Identical-twin bone marrow transplants for leukemia. Ann Intern Med 1994; 120:646.

55. Brenner MK, Rill DR, Moen RC, et al. Gene-marking to trace origin of relapse after autologous bone-marrow transplantation. Lancet 1993; 341:85.

56. Stein AS, O'Donnell MR, Chai A, et al. In vivo purging with high-dose cytarabine followed by high-dose chemoradiotherapy and reinfusion of unpurged bone marrow for adult acute myelogenous leukemia in first complete remission. J Clin Oncol 1996; 14:2206.

57. Foa R. Does Interleukin-2 have a role in the management of acute leukemia? J Clin Oncol 1993; 11:1817.

58. Sznol M, Parkinson DR. Interleukin-2 in therapy of hematologic malignancies. Blood 1994; 83:2020.

59. Fefer A. Graft-versus-tumor responses. In: Forman SJ, Blume KG, Thomas ED, Eds. Hematopoietic Cell Transplantation, 2nd ed. London: Blackwell Science, Inc. 1998; 316.

60. Margolin KA, Wright C, Forman SJ. Autologous bone marrow purging by in situ IL-2 activation of endogenous killer cells. Leukemia 1997; 11:723.

61. Weisdorf DJ, Anderson PM, Kersey JH, Ramsay NKC. Interleukin-2 therapy immediately after autologous marrow transplantation: Toxicity, T cell activation and engraftment (abstract). Blood 1991; 78:226.

62. Klingemann HG, Eaves CJ, Barnett MJ, et al. Transplantation of patients with high risk acute myeloid leukemia in first remission with autologous marrow cultured in interleukin-2 followed by interleukin-2 administration. Bone Marrow Transplant 1994; 14:389.

63. Robinson N, Benyunes MC, Thompson JA, et al. Interleukin-2 after autologous stem cell transplantation for hematologic malignancy: A phase I/II study. Bone Marrow Transplant 1997; 19:435.

64. Margolin K, Forman SJ. Immunotherapy with interleukin-2 after hematopoietic cell transplantation for hematologic malignancies. Cancer J Sci Am 2000; 6(Suppl 1):S33.

65. Stein A, O'Donnell MR, Parker P, et al. Interleukin-2 (IL-2) post high-dose cytarbine mobilized autologous stem cell transplant (ASCT) for adult patients with acute myelogenous leukemia (AML) in first complete remission (CR) (abstract 1196). Blood 1998; 92(Suppl 1):292a.

66. Philip T, Armitage JO, Spitzer G,et al. High-dose therapy and autologous bone marrow transplantation after failure of conventional chemotherapy in adults with intermediate-grade or high-grade non-Hodgkin's lymphoma. N Engl J Med 1987; 316:1493.

67. Vose JM, Anderson JR, Kessinger A, et al. High-dose chemotherapy and autologous hematopoietic stem- cell transplantation for aggressive non-Hodgkin's lymphoma. J Clin Oncol 1993; 11:1846.

68. Stiff PJ, Dahlberg S, Forman SJ, et al. Autologous bone transplantation for patients with relapsed or refractory diffuse aggressive non-Hodgkin's lymphoma: value of augmented preparative regimens- a Southwest Oncology Group Trial. J Clin Oncol 1998; 16:48.

69. Nademanee A, Molina A, O'Donnell MR, et al. Results of High-dose therapy and autologous bone marrow/stem cell transplantation during first remission in poor-risk intermediate- and high-grade lymphoma: International Index high and high-intermediate risk group. Blood 1997; 90:3844.

70. Philip T, Guglielmi C, Hagenbeek A, et al. Autologous bone marrow transplantation as compared with salvage chemotherapy in relapses of chemotherapy-sensitive non-Hodgkin's lymphoma. N Engl J Med 1995; 333:1540.

71. Haioun C, Lepage E, Gisselbrecht C, et al. Benefit of autologous bone marrow transplantation over sequential chemotherapy in poor-risk aggressive non-Hodgkin's lymphoma: Updated results of the prospective study LNH87-2. J Clin Oncol 1997; 15:1131.

72. Haioun C, Lepage E, Gisselbrecht C, et al. Survival benefit of high-dose therapy in poor-risk aggressive lymphoma: Final analysis of the prospective LNH87-2 protocol - a Groupe d'Etude des Lymphomes de l'Adulte study. J Clin Oncol 2000; 18:3025.

73. Mills W, Chopra R, McMilan A, et al. BEAM chemotherapy and autologous bone marrow transplantation for patients with relapsed or refractory non-Hodgkin's lymphoma. J Clin Oncol 1995; 13:588.

74. Weaver CH, Petersen FB, Appelbaum FA, et al. High-dose fractionated total-body irradiation, etoposide, and cyclophosphamide followed by autologous stem-cell support in patients with malignant lymphoma. J Clin Oncol 1994;12:2559.

75. Wheeler C, Strawderman M, Ayash L, et al. Prognostic factors for treatment outcome in autotransplantation of Intermediate-Grade and High-Grade Non-Hodgkin's lymphoma with cyclophosphamide, carmustine, and etoposide. J Clin Oncol 1993; 11:1085.

76. Guglielmi C, Gomez F, Philip T, Hagenbeek A, et al. Time to relapse has prognostic value in patients with aggressive lymphoma enrolled onto the PARMA trial. J Clin Oncol 1998; 16:3264.

77. Nademanee A, Molina A, Dagis A, et al. Autologous stem cell transplantation for poor-risk and relapsed intermediate and high grade non-Hodgkin's lymphoma. Clinical Lymphoma 2000; 1:46.

78. The International Non-Hodgkin's Lymphoma Prognostic Factors Project. A predictive model for aggressive non-Hodgkin's lymphoma. N Engl J Med 1993; 329·987.

79. Shipp MA. Prognostic factors in aggressive non-Hodgkin's lymphoma: Who has "high-Risk" disease? Blood 1994; 83:1165.

80. Kessinger A, Schmit-Pokorny K, Smith D, et al. Cryopreservation and infusion of autologous peripheral blood stem cells. Bone Marrow Transplant 1990; 5:25.

81. Nademanee A, Sniecinski I, Schmidt GM et al. High-dose therapy followed by autologous peripheral blood stem cell transplantation for patients with Hodgkin's disease and non-Hodgkin's lymphoma utilizing unprimed and granulocyte colony-stimulating factor "mobilized" peripheral blood stem cells. J Clin Oncol 1994; 12:2176.

82. Santini G, Salvagno L, Leoni P, et al. VACOP-B versus VACOP-B plus autologous bone marrow transplantation for advanced diffuse non-Hodgkin's lymphoma: Results of a prospective randomized trial by the Non-Hodgkin's Lymphoma Cooperative Study Group. J Clin Oncol 1998; 16:2796.

83. Reyes F, Lepage E, Morel P, et al. Failure of first-line inductive high-dose chemotherapy (HDC) in poor-risk patients with aggressive lymphoma: Updated results of the randomized LNH 93-3 study (Abstract #2640). Blood 1997; 90:594a.

84. Kaiser U, Uebelacker I, Birkmann J, et al. High-dose therapy with autologous stem cell transplantation in aggressive NHL: results of a randomized multicenter study (Abstract # 2716). Blood 1999; 94:611a.

85. Nademanee A, Molina A, Palmer J, et al. High-dose therapy and autologous stem cell transplant (ASCT) for patients with primary mediastinal large cell lymphoma (Abstract#1905). Blood 1998; 92(Suppl 1):462a.

86. Horning SJ. Natural history of and therapy for the indolent non-Hodgkin's lymphomas. Sem Oncol 1994; 20(Suppl 5):75.

87. Dana BW, Dahlberg S, Nathwani BH, et al. Long-term follow-up of patients with low grade malignant lymphomas treated with doxorubicin-based chemotherapy or chemoimmunotherapy. J Clin Oncol 1993; 11:644.

88. Solal-Celigny P, Brice P, Brousse N, et al. Phase II study of fludarabine monophosphate as first-line treatment in patients with advanced follicular lymphoma: a multicenter study by the Groupe d' Etude des Lymphomes de l'Adulte. J Clin Oncol 1996;14:514.

89. McLaughlin P, Grillo-Lopez AJ, Link BK, et al. Rituximab chimeric anti-CD20 monoclonal antibody therapy for relapsed indolent lymphoma: half of patients respond to a four-dose treatment program. J Clin Oncol 1998; 16:2825.

90. Colombat P, Donadio D, Fouillard L, et al. Value of autologous bone marrow transplantation in follicular lymphoma: A france Autogreffe retrospective study of 42 patients. Bone Marrow Transplant 1994; 13:157.

91. Cervantes F, Shu XO, McGlave PB, et al. Autologous bone marrow transplantation for non-transformed low-grade non-Hodgkin's lymphoma. Bone Marrow Transplant 1994; 16:387.

92. Rohatiner AZ, Johnson PW, Price CG, et al. Myeloablative therapy with autologous bone marrow transplantation as consolidation therapy for recurrent follicular lymphoma. J Clin Oncol 1994; 12:1177.

93. Bastion Y, Brice P, Haioun C, et al. Intensive therapy with peripheral blood progenitor cell transplantation in 60 patients with poor-prognosis follicular lymphoma. Blood 1995; 86:3257.

94. Morel P, Laporte JP, Noel MP, et al. Autologous bone marrow transplantation as consolidation therapy may prolong remission in newly diagnosed high-risk follicular lymphoma: a pilot study of 34 cases. Leukemia 1995; 9:976.

95. Haas R, Moos M, Mohle R, et al. High-dose therapy with peripheral blood progenitor cell transplantation in low-grade non-hodgkin's lymphoma. Bone Marrow Transplant 1996; 17:149.

96. Freedman AS, Gribben JG, Neuberg D, et al. High-dose therapy and autologous bone marrow transplantation in patients with follicular lymphoma during first remission. Blood 1996; 88:2524

97. Schouten IC, Raemaekers JJM, Kluin-Nelemans HC, et al. High-dose therapy followed by bone marrow transplantation for relapsed follicular lymphoma. Ann Hematol 1996; 73:273.

98. Bierman PJ, Vose JM, Anderson JR, et al. High-dose therapy with autologous hematopoietic rescue for follicular low-grade non-Hodgkin's lymphoma. J Clin Oncol 1997; 15:445.

99. Armitage JO. Bone marrow transplantation for indolent lymphomas. Sem Oncol 1993; 20(suppl 5):136.

100. Horning SJ. High-dose therapy and transplantation for low-grade lymphoma. Hemat/Oncol Clin North Am 1997; 11:919.

101. Molina A, Nademanee A, O'Donnell MR et al. Long-term follow-up and analysis of prognostic factors after high-dose therapy and peripheral blood stem cell autografting (ASCT) in 58 patients with a history of low-grade follicular lymphoma (FLGL) (Abstract #747). Blood 1999; 94(Suppl 1):171a.

102. Cao T, Negrin RS, Hu W, et al. High-dose therapy and autologous hematopoietic cell transplantation for follicular lymphoma beyond first remission: the Stanford experience (Abstract #2074). Blood 2000; 96:482a.

103. Witzig TE, White CA, Wiseman GA, et al. Phase I/II trial of IDEC-Y2B8 radioimmnotherapy for treatment of relapsed or refractory CD20+ B-cell non-Hodgkin's lymphoma. J Clin Oncol 1999; 17:3793.

104. Press OW, Eary JF, Appelbaum FR, et al. Radiolabeled-antibody therapy of B-cell lymphoma with autologous bone marrow support. N Engl J Med 1993; 329:1219.

105. Liu SY, Eary JF, Petersdorf SH, et al. Follow-up of relapsed B-cell lymphoma patients treated with Iodine-131-labeled anti-CD20 antibody and autologous stem cell rescue. J Clin Oncol 1998; 16:3270.

106. Press O, Eary J, Liu S, Petersdorf S, et al. A phase I/II trial of high-dose Iodine-131-anti-B1 (anti-CD20) monoclonal antibody, etoposide, cyclophosphamide and autologous stem cell transplantation for patients with relapsed B cell lymphomas (Abstract #9). Proc Am Soc Clin Oncol 1998; 17:3a.

107. Raubitschek A, Nademanee A, Molina A, et al. High-dose radioimmunotherapy/ chemotherapy and autologous stem cell transplantation (ASCT) for poor risk and relapsed CD20+ non-Hodgkin's lymphoma (NHL): early feasibility report (Abstract #5372). Blood 2000; 96(Suppl2):374b.

108. Benyunes MC, Fefer A. Interleukin-2 in the treatment of hematologic malignancies. In: Atkins MD, Meier JW, Eds. Therapeutic Application of IL-2. Dekker, New York, 1993; 163.

109. Flinn IW, O'Donnell PV, Goodrich A, et al. Immunotherapy with rituximab during peripheral blood stem cell transplantation for non-Hodgkin's lymphoma. Biol Blood Marrow Transplant 2000; 6:628.

110. Traweek TS, Slovak ML, Nademanee AP, et al. Clonal karyotypic hematopoietic cell abnormalities occurring after autologous bone marrow transplantation for Hodgkin's disease and non-Hodgkin's lymphoma. Blood 1994; 84:957.

111. Stone RM, Neuberg D, Soiffer R, et al. Myelodysplastic syndrome as a late complication following autologous bone marrow transplantation for Non-Hodgkin's lymphoma. J Clin Oncol 1994; 12:2535.

112. Darrington DL, Vose JM, Anderson JR, et al. Incidence and characterization of secondary myelodysplastic syndrome and acute myelogeneous leukemia following high-dose chemoradiotherapy and autologous stem-cell transplantation for lymphoid malignancies. J Clin Oncol 1994; 12:2527.

113. Miller JS, Arthur DC, Litz CE, et al Myelodysplastic syndrome after autologous bone marrow transplantation: An additional late complication of curative cancer therapy. Blood 1994; 83:3780.

114. Micallef INM, Lillington DM, Apostolidis J, et al. Therapy-related myelodysplasia and secondary acute myelogenous leukemia after high-dose therapy with autologous hematopoietic progenitor-cell support for lymphoid malignancies. J Clin Oncol 2000; 18:947.

115. Krishnan A, Bhatia S, Slovak ML, et al. Predictors of therapy-related leukemia and myelodysplasia following autologous transplantation for lymphoma: an assessment of risk factors. Blood 2000; 95:1588.

116. Mach-Pascual S, Legare RD, Lu D, et al. Predictive value of clonality assays in patients with non-Hodgkin's lymphoma undergoing autologous bone marrow transplant: A single Institution Study. Blood 1998; 91:4496.

117. Bhatia R, Miller D, Hyde S, et al. Extensive depletion of primitive hematopoietic progenitors in lymphoma patients following autologous transplantation: implications for the development of therapy-related MDS/AML (t-MDS) (Abstract #1733). Blood 2000; 96(Suppl1):402a.

118. Bhatia S, Louie AD, Bhatia R, et al. Solid cancers after bone marrow transplantation. J Clin Oncol (in press)

119. Molina A, Pezner R. Non-Hodgkin's Lymphoma. In: Pazdur R, Coia L, Wagman L, Hoskins W, Eds. Cancer Management: A Multidisciplinary Approach. (Fourth Edition) PRR, Huntington, NY, 2000; 583.

120. Molina A, Nademanee A, O'Donnell MR, et al. Autologous (AUTO) and allogeneic (ALLO) stem cell transplantation (SCT) for poor-risk mantle cell lymphoma (MCL): the City of Hope (COH) experience (Abstract #1894). Blood 1998; 92(Suppl 1):459a.

121. Molina A, Nademanee A, Carter NH, et al. Mantle cell lymphoma (MCL) with peripheral blood and leukemic involvement (PBLI) at diagnosis: impact of stem cell transplantation (Abstract #3433). Blood 2000; 96(Suppl1):795a.

122. Malone J, Molina A, Stockerl-Goldstein K, et al. Autologous hematopoietic cell transplantation for mantle cell lymphoma: The Stanford/City of Hope experience. (Submitted)

123. Vandenberghe E, Ruiz de Elvira C, issacson P, et al. Does transplantation improve outcome in mantle cell lymphoma (MCL)?: a study from the EBMT (Abstract #2072). Blood 2000; 96(Suppl1):482a.

124. Dreger P, Martin S, Kuse R, et al. The impact of autologous stem cell transplantation on the prognosis of mantle cell lymphoma: a joint analysis of 2 prospective studies with 46 patients. Hematol J 2000; 1:87.

125. Molina A, Krishnan A, Nademanee A, et al. High dose therapy and autologous stem cell transplantation for the treatment of human immunodeficiency virus-associated non-Hodgkin's lymphoma in the era of highly active antiretroviral therapy. Cancer 2000; 89:680.

126. Krishnan A, Molina A, Zaia J et al. HIV infection does not preclude autologous stem cell transplantation (ASCT) for lymphoma (Abstract #1759). Blood 1999; 94(Suppl 1):397a.

127. Zaia JA, Rossi JJ, Krishnan A, et al. Autologous stem cell transplantation using retrovirus-transduced peripheral blood progenitor cells in HIV-infected persons: comparison of gene marking post-engraftment with and without marrow ablation (Abstract #2850). Blood 1999; 94(Suppl 1):642a.

128. Krishnan, AY, Molina A, Zaia J et al. Highly active antiretroviral therapy (HAART) with high-dose therapy (HDC) and autologous stem cell transplantation (ASCT): effects on HIV infection (Abstract #96). Blood 2000; 96(Suppl 1):25a.

129. Ratanatharathorn V, Uberti J, Karanes C, et al. Prospective comparative trial of autologous versus allogeneic bone marrow transplantation in patients with non-hodgkin's lymphoma. Blood 1994; 84:1050.

130. van Biesen K, Mehra RC, Giralt SA, et al. Allogeneic bone marrow transplantation for poor-prognosis lymphoma: response, toxicity and survival depend on disease histology. Am J Med 1996; 100:299.

131. van Biesen K, Thall P, Korbling M, et al. Allogeneic transplantation for recurrent or refractory non-Hodgkin's lymphoma with poor-prognostic features after conditioning with thiotepa, busulfan, and cyclophosphamide: experience with 44 consecutive patients. Bio Blood Marrow Trans 1997; 3:150.

132. Verdonck LF, Dekker AW, Lokhorst HM, et al. Allogeneic versus autologous bone marrow transplantation for refractory and recurrent low-grade non-Hodgkin's lymphoma. Blood 1997; 90:4201.

133. van Besien, Sobocinski KA, Rowlings PA, et al. Allogeneic bone marrow transplantation for low grade lymphoma. Blood 1998; 92:1832.

134. Prezepiorka D, van Besien K, Khouri I, et al. Carmustine, etoposied, cytarabine and melphalan as a preparative regimen for allogeneic transplantation for high-risk malignant lymphoma. Ann Oncol 1999; 10:527.

135. Bierman P, Molina A, Nelson G, et al. Matched unrelated donor (MUD) allogeneic bone marrow transplantation for non-Hodgkin's lymphoma (NHL): results from the National Marrow Donor Program (NMDP) (Abstract #7). ProcAm Soc Clin Oncol 1999;18:3a.

136. Bierman PJ. Allogeneic bone marrow transplantation for lymphoma. Blood Rev 2000; 14:1.

137. Molina A, Nademanee A, Arber D and Forman SJ. Remission of refractory Sezary syndrome after bone marrow transplantation from a matched unrelated donor. Biol Blood Marrow Transpl 1999; 5:400.

138. Molina A, Nademanee A, Parker P, et al. Allogeneic bone marrow transplantation in refractory and recurrent chronic lymphocytic leukemia and leukemic phase of low-grade small lymphocytic lymphoma (Abstract #23). Proc Am Soc Clin Oncol 1998;17:7a.

139. Molina A, Nademanee A, Dagis A, et al. HLA-matched sibling and unrelated allogeneic hematpoietic cell transplantation (ALLO HSCT) for poor-risk non-Hodgkin's lymphoma (NHL): The City of Hope (COH) experience (Abstract #65). Proc Am Soc Clin Oncol 2000; 19:19a.

140. Khouri I, Lee MS, Romaguera J, et al. Allogeneic hematopoietic transplantation for mantle cell lymphoma: molecular remissions and evidence of graft-versus-malignancy. Ann Oncol 1999; 10:1293.

141. Khouri IF, Keating M, Korbling M, et al. Transplant-lite: induction of graft-versus-malignancy using fludarabine-based nonablative chemotherapy and allogeneic blood progenitor-cell transplantation as treatment for lymphoid malignancies. J Clin Oncol 1998; 16:2817.

142. Champlin R, Khouri I, Kornblau S, et al. Allogeneic hematopoietic transplantation as adoptive immunotherapy. Induction of graft-versus-malignancy as primary therapy. Hematol Oncol Clin North Am 1999; 13:1041.

143. Nagler A, Slavin S, Varadi G, et al. Allogeneic peripheral blood stem cell transplantation using a fludarabine-based low intensity conditioning regimen for malignant lymphoma. Bone Marrow Trans 2000; 25:1021.

144. Carella AM, Cavaliere M, Lerma E, et al. Autografting followed by non-myeloablative immunosuppressive chemotherapy and allogeneic peripheral-blood hematoietic stem cell transplantation as treatment of resistant Hodgkin's disease and non-Hodgkin's lymphoma. J Clin Oncol 2000; 18:3918.

145. Theofilopoulos AN. The basis of autoimmunity: Part I. Mechanisms of aberrant self-recognition. Immunology Today 1995; 16:90.

146. Ikehara S, Inaba M, Yasumizu R, et al. Autoimmune diseases as stem cell disorders. Tohoku J Exp Med 1994; 173:141.

147. Good RA, Ikehara S. Preclinical investigations that subserve efforts to employ bone marrow transplantation for rheumatoid or autoimmune diseases. J Rheumatol 1997; 24 (Suppl 48):5.

148. Van Bekkum DW, Kimwell-Bohre EPM, Houben PFJ, Knaan-Shanzer S. Regression of adjuvant-induced arthritis in rats following bone marrow transplantation. Proc Natl Acad Sci USA 1989; 86:1090.

149. Kashyap A, Forman SJ. Autologous bone marrow transplantation (ABMT) for non-Hodgkin's Lymphoma (NHL) resulting in long-term remission of coincidental Crohn's disease. Br J Hematol 1998; Dec 103 (3): 651-2

150. Tyndall A, Gratwohl A, et al. Blood and marrow stem cell transplants in auto-immune disease: a consensus report written on behalf of the European League against Rheumatism (EULAR) and the European Group for Blood and Marrow Transplantation (EBMT). Bone Marrow Transplantation 1997; 19:643.

151. Kashyap A, Passweg JR, Fassas A, et al. for the Autoimmune Disease Working Party of the EBMT. Conditioning regimen intensity and transplant related mortality in patients treated for autoimmune diseases by autologous stem cell transplantation. (Submitted to EBMT 2001).

152. Storb R, Yu C, Wagner JL, et al. Stable mixed hematopoietic chimerism in DLA-identical littermate dogs given sublethal total body irradiation before and pharmacological immunosuppression after marrow transplantation. Blood 1997; 89:3048.

153. Kolb HJ, Schattenberg A, Goldman JM, et al. Graft-versus-leukemia effect of donor lymphocyte transfusions in marrow grafted patients. European Group for Blood and Marrow Transplantation Working Party Chronic Leukemia. Blood 1995; 86:2041.

154. Collins RH Jr, Shpilberg O, Drobyski WR, et al. Donor leukocyte infusions in 140 patient with relapsed malignancy after allogeneic bone marrow transplantation. J Clin Oncol 1997; 15:433.

155. Slavin S. Immunotherapy of cancer with alloreactive lymphocytes. N Engl J Med 2000; 343:802.

156. Brown RA, Adkins D, Khoury H, et al. Long-term follow up of high risk allogeneic peripheral blood stem cell transplant recipients: graft versus host disease and transplant-related mortality. J Clin Oncol 1999; 17:806.

157. Sandmaier BM, Maloney DG, Hegenbart U, et al. Nonmyeloablative conditioning for HLA-identical related allografts for hematologic malignancies (Abstract #2062). Blood 2000; 96:479a.

158. Rezvani K, Lalancette M, Szydlo R, et al. Nonmyeloablative stem cell transplant (NMSCT) in AML, ALL, and MDS: disappointing outcome for patients with advanced phase disease (Abstract #2061). Blood 2000; 96:479a.

159. Molina A, Sahebi F, Maloney DG, et al. Non-myeloablative peripheral blood stem cell (PBSC) allografts following cytoreductive autotransplants for treatment of multiple myeloma (MM). Blood 96(Number 11):480a (abstract 2063), 2000

160. Stockerl-Goldstein KE, Horning SJ, Negrin RS, et al. Influence of preparatory regimen and source of hematopoietic cells on outcome of autotransplantation for non-Hodgkin's lymphoma. Biol Blood Marrow Transplant 1996; 2:76.

161. Kusnierz-Glaz CR, Schlegel PG, Wong RM, et al. Influence of age on the outcome of 500 autologous bone marrow transplant procedures for hematologic malignancies. J Clin.Oncol 1997; 15:18.

162. Spielberger R, Stein A, O'Donnell M, et al. Autologous stem cell transplant (ASCT) as consolidation therapy for patients (PTS) older than 50 years (Y) with acute myelogenous leukemia (AML) in first complete remission (Abstract #1197). Blood 1998; 92(Suppl 1):292a.

163. Fung HC, Nademanee A, Molina A, et al. Very low transplant-related mortality for patients ≤60 years old with poor-prognosis non-Hodgkin's lymphoma treated with autologous stem cell transplantation (ASCT) (Abstract #5016). Blood 1999; 94(Suppl 1):400b.

164. Lee SJ, Fairclough D, Parsons SK, et al. Recovery after stem-cell transplantation for hematologic disease. J Clin Oncol 2001; 19:242.

ACKNOWLEDGEMENTS

AM was supported by an American Cancer Society Clinical Oncology Career Development Award and was a past recipient of a Fellowship from the Lymphoma Research Foundation of America, Inc. LP is a current recipient of a fellowship from the Lymphoma Research Foundation of America, Inc. This work was supported in part by United States Public Service Grants CA30206, CA33572 and AI38592.

CHAPTER 29

Kidney Transplantation Worldwide

International Views of Transplantation at the End of the Twentieth Century

If you only read the English language transplant literature, you are very familiar with renal transplant results from the United States, Canada, and Western Europe. But transplantation is truly a worldwide activity. Based upon reports to the Worldwide Transplant Center Directory, which begins on page 555 of this volume of *Clinical Transplants 2000*, more than 277,000 kidney transplants have been performed outside the United States. For many, access to information about transplants around the world may be limited to presentations at the biannual Congresses of the Transplantation Society or through Transplantation Proceedings. For this millennium edition of Clinical Transplants, we asked leading transplant professionals from more than 50 countries to provide us with the numbers of cadaveric, living-related and living-unrelated donor renal transplants performed in their country each year during the past decade and to provide the one- and 5-year graft survival rates for each donor cohort over that period. In addition we requested a brief summary describing the practice of renal transplantation in their country. The content of each summary was not specified.

The result was a fascinating compilation of results and descriptions, which are reproduced in the following pages. The accounts are informative, often entertaining, and sometimes poignant. In the end, we did not achieve our goal of 50 countries. Some initially responded with enthusiasm, but discovered that collecting data from many transplant centers could not be accomplished within the short interval that was available. Thus, our information about transplantation in China and India will remain limited as neither country could assemble the information we requested. Hungary and Austria provided the data we requested but we never received the narratives. Their data are reproduced below.

A recurring theme in many of the accounts that follow is the frustration with the shortage of organs for transplantation. The approaches to solving the problem are varied and reflect the different cultural, societal, and religious backgrounds unique to each country. The minichapters from 30 countries follow (Italy and North Italy each provided separate accounts). They are arranged alphabetically. We hope you will enjoy reading about Kidney Transplantation Worldwide.

Kidney Transplants in Austria.												Graft Survival (%)	
	1990	1991	1992	1993	1994	1995	1996	1997	1998	1999	Total	1-year	5-year
Rel	14	6	15	7	12	12	14	20	40	24	164	92.0	70.2
Unrel							4	4	9	15	32	95.0	95.0
Cad	410	390	302	377	338	293	347	310	325	382	3,474	86.3	68.4

Kidney Transplants in Hungary.												Graft Survival (%)	
	1990	1991	1992	1993	1994	1995	1996	1997	1998	1999	Total	1-year	5-year
Rel	5	2	1	2	3	3	0	2	8	5	31	96.9	96.9
Unrel										3	3		
Cad	105	136	186	177	241	278	260	307	233	216	2,139	87.2	73.6

Organ Transplantation in Argentina

Félix Cantarovich [a], María del Carmen Bacqué [b] and Domingo Casadei [c]

[a]*Former National Director of the CUCAI, Advisor of the National Under-Secretary of Health,* [b]*President of the INCUCAI,* [c]*Former President of the Argentine Transplantation Society and the Latin-American Transplantation Society, ARGENTINA*

Organ and tissue transplantation began in the middle of the 20th century in Argentina, starting with corneas in 1928, bone in 1948, kidneys in 1957, and hearts in 1968. The use of cadaver donors was unusual until the "Guidelines on organ procurement and sharing" (Transplantation Law N° 21.541) was passed by the National Assembly in 1977. This law created the National Direction of Transplantation (CUCAI), a centralized organization (1). In 1990, law N° 23.885 established the current organ *sharing organization (INCUCAI), an autocratic organization. The current law is N° 24.193 and passed in 1993.

Overview on Organ Transplantation in Argentina (1978-2000)

There are 2 periods in the evolution of transplantation in Argentina. The first, under the CUCAI started in 1978 and the second, under the current INCUCAI organization began in 1991. Here we review aspects of the legal process, the program organization (2-4) and the results of transplantation in Argentina.

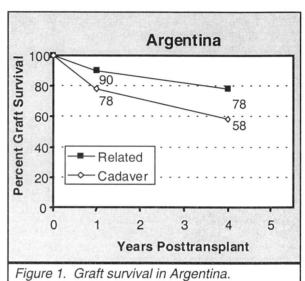

Figure 1. Graft survival in Argentina.

Table 1. Kidney transplants in Argentina.

	1990	1991	1992	1993	1994	1995	1996	1997	1998	1999	Total
Rel	*	*	183	150	162	166	158	137	110	75	2,231
Cad	*	*	108	147	212	416	379	335	330	385	3,026

*714 cadaveric and 1,090 living related grafts between 1984-1991

Legal Processes

Express consent for organ and tissue donation was required initially in Argentina. The donor card was considered a legal document, however, in the absence of a donor card, consent of relatives was mandatory. In practice, consent of relatives was usually requested. The current law N° 24193, established a presumed consent alternative, if a national referendum is positive by 70%. The referendum has not yet been held.

Argentina has a single national list of recipients with established selection criteria (HLA and ABO as first matching criteria).

For cadaver donors, a brain death diagnosis, following the Harvard criteria, is required and it is a mandatory responsibility of any medical doctor to determine brain death. In any case of non-natural death, the re-

sponsible judge must authorize organ retrieval. Organ procurement and sharing are under the exclusive responsibility of the national organization, which today is the INCUCAI. The State is responsible for supporting continuous information campaigns addressed to the public. The State is also obliged to organize procedures for organ donation request and gathering information whenever personal documents are requested by the public (identity cards, driver's licenses, passports, etc). A Presidential decree in 1998 created the National Education Commission. The objective of this commission is to develop educational programs on organ donation. This program is mainly addressed to school-age students.

The law permits authorization for institutions and medical teams by the National Organ Procurement and

Sharing Organization in agreement with the responsible regional program.

The law accepts related living donors, however, spouses, concubines, adoptive parents or offspring are also occasionally accepted.

Program Organization

The purpose of the transplantation organization in Argentina is threefold:
1. To solve social, medical and economic problems of organ transplantation.
2. To guarantee transparency, security and efficacy.
3. To provide equal possibilities to every patient on the waiting list.

Transplant Coordinators Training Program

Since 1981, a national coordinator-training program developed by CUCAI has been in place. Its purpose was to provide collaboration and support concerning procedures of organ procurement and public education. The new approach is to appoint a psychologist to perform this role. The results of this initiative have been fruitful and helpful in developing the program all over the country.

Organ Procurement Organization (INCUCAI)

The model is a non-centralized system of organ procurement. The National Institute (INCUCAI) maintains a continuous relationship with each of the 8 regional procurement organizations. INCUCAI establishes rules and guidelines and also supervises and coordinates all the activity concerning organ sharing in the country. The main goal of the program is to insure a uniform development of organ procurement and sharing all over the country.

Results

During the initial period (1978-1990, CUCAI) 1,989 kidney transplants (969 cadaver and 1,020 living-related donor kidneys) were performed. Multiorgan procurement and heart and liver transplantation started in 1984. In 1988 the first partial liver transplantation from a living hepatic donor was performed.

Since 1993 (INCUCAI), the organ procurement rate has increased from 10.7 per million inhabitants to 21.2 (4). Negative family responses to requests for organ donation decreased from 34.6% in 1996 to 28.8% in 1997.

The graph and table show the graft survival and the yearly number of living-related and cadaver renal grafts since 1992 based on validated current information. Patient survival rates for these were 86% for living-related and 79% for cadaver donor transplantation. Between 1984 and 1991, 714 cadaver and 1,090 living-related donor kidneys were transplanted.

Conclusion

The Argentine transplant program is developing well. Current results are affected by the use of marginal donors (between 15% and 20% of kidneys are discarded) and the still considerable number of grafts with cold ischemia time >24 hours. Two new programs are being instituted, "hospital coordinators", which places a physician in charge of organ procurement in each hospital, and the recent national educational program on organ donation, which is directed towards schools, universities and the general public. These are potential pathways to improve our results in the near future.

References

1. Cantarovich F, Castro LZ, Wilberg R, et al. Argentina Transplant (CUCAI): The first four years' experience of a National Organ Exchange Program. Transplant Proc 1984; 26:193.

2. Cantarovich F, Castro LZ, Dávalos M, et al. Sectarianism, uncertainty and fear: Mechanisms that may reverse attitudes towards organ donation. Transplant Proc 1989; 21:1409.

3. Cantarovich F. Values sacrificed and values gained by the commerce of organs: The Argentine experience. Transplant Proc 1990; 22:925.

4. Instituto Nacional Central Unico de Ablación e Implantes. Memoria 1999. Eds. INCUCAI. Ramsay 2250. Buenos Aires. Argentina.

Acknowledgement

The authors thank Dr. José Luis Araujo for his technical collaboration concerning demographics and results.

Renal Transplantation in Australia and New Zealand 1963 to 1999

Graeme R. Russ

ANZDATA Registry, Queen Elizabeth Hospital, Woodville, South Australia, Australia

The Australia and New Zealand Dialysis and Transplant Registry (ANZDATA) maintains a complete database of all renal transplants performed in Australia since 1963 and in New Zealand since 1965. Eleven thousand eight hundred and forty-three (11,843) transplants have been performed in Australia up to 31 December 1999, of which 5,042 were still functioning. In New Zealand the respective figures were 2,418 and 975. Therefore, the prevalence of patients being maintained with a renal transplant in Australia is 266 per million of population and in New Zealand 256 per million of population.

In Australia the number of functioning grafts at the end of 1999 represents a 4% increase over the previous year, an annual rate of increase which has remained steady. Eighty-seven percent of the functioning grafts were primary and 79% were from cadaveric donors. The modal age group for transplant-dependent patients was 45-54 years and the mean and median ages were 47.8 and 48.8 years, respectively.

Transplants Performed in 1999

In Australia 453 renal transplant operations were performed in 1999. This represents a decrease of 14% compared with 1998 and is consistent with a trend towards a gradual reduction in the absolute number of cadaveric renal transplants being performed since 1992 (Fig. 3). In 1999 the cadaveric donor transplant number was the lowest since 1976. Since 1992 there has been an increasing number of living donor transplants, such that in 1999 the rate was 37% of all renal grafts.

The transplant rate in 1999 as a proportion of patients receiving dialysis was 6.1% in Australia and 7.3% in New Zealand. There was considerable regional variation in the renal transplantation rate in Australia varying from 5.1% of dialysed patients in New South Wales to 11.2% in South Australia (Fig. 4).

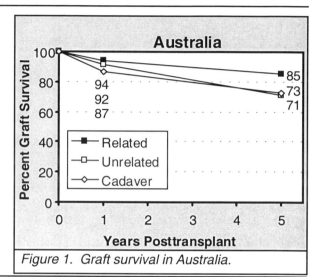

Figure 1. Graft survival in Australia.

Table 1. Kidney transplants in Australia.

	1990	1991	1992	1993	1994	1995	1996	1997	1998	1999	Total
Rel	57	72	68	60	94	87	96	125	126	124	909
Unrel	2	5	1	4	9	6	19	19	35	43	165
Cad	384	392	407	393	337	348	360	358	357	286	3,622

Table 2. Kidney transplants in New Zealand.

	1990	1991	1992	1993	1994	1995	1996	1997	1998	1999	Total
Rel	22	12	17	19	20	23	25	23	19	33	213
Unrel	1	1	0	1	0	1	1	8	12	9	34
Cad	79	64	98	64	63	70	70	81	75	70	734

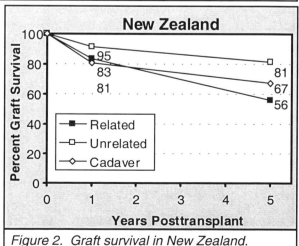

Figure 2. Graft survival in New Zealand.

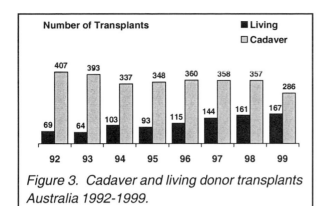

Figure 3. Cadaver and living donor transplants Australia 1992-1999.

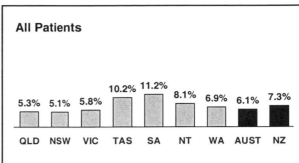

Figure 4. Rate of transplantation 1999 related to patients dialysed.

In New Zealand the transplant rate was 29 per million in 1999 and living donors were used for 38% of all operations.

Outcome of Renal Transplants (Figs. 5, 6)

There has been an improvement in the graft survival of primary cadaver grafts over the past decade. From 1990-1993, the one-year graft survival rate for transplants performed each year was between 84 and 86%. From 1994-1998, the one-year graft survival rate for each year increased to between 89 and 91%. This jump in graft survival is probably related to the more widespread availability of mycophenolate mofetil and tacrolimus as immunosuppresive agents for rescue therapy. In New Zealand, with its smaller transplant numbers, trends in primary cadaver graft survival are more difficult to detect, but for grafts performed in 1998 the one-year survival rate was 87% and this was the highest result recorded in that country.

Living Donor Transplants

In Australia, 1999 saw the largest number and proportion of living donor transplants being performed, representing 37% of all transplant operations. In New Zealand, 38% of all grafts were from a living donor. There has been an increase in the proportion of living donor operations in all recipient age groups but this has been most marked in those recipients over age 45 (Table 3). This has been associated with an increase in the proportion of unrelated donors, which comprised 26% of all living donors in 1999. Most of the unrelated donors were spouses.

Immunosuppressive Therapy for Primary Cadaver Grafts

In 1999, 41% of primary cadaver graft recipients received triple therapy with cyclosporin A, mycophenolate and prednisolone as their initial immunosuppressive regimen. This proportion of patients has

ANZDATA

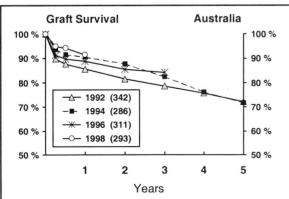

Figure 5. Primary cadaver graft survival 1992-1998 related to year of transplant.

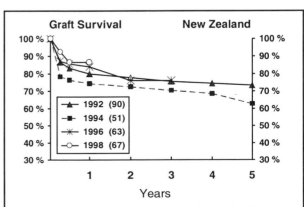

Figure 6. Primary cadaver graft survival 1992-1998 related to year of transplant.

Table 3. Living donor operations as proportion (%) of annual transplantation Australia.

Living Donor Operations as Proportion (%) of Annual Transplantation Australia

Recipient Age Groups	Year of Transplantation							
	1992	**1993**	**1994**	**1995**	**1996**	**1997**	**1998**	**1999**
00-04 years	43%	60%	67%	83%	50%	100%	67%	100%
05-14 years	73%	55%	73%	65%	50%	60%	47%	58%
15-24 years	31%	22%	44%	36%	36%	57%	54%	61%
25-34 years	15%	23%	24%	26%	32%	44%	37%	39%
35-44 years	19%	13%	24%	21%	27%	27%	32%	41%
45-54 years	4%	7%	17%	12%	12%	18%	21%	26%
55-64 years	2%	5%	13%	5%	13%	10%	21%	27%
65-74 years	0%	5%	8%	0%	18%	0%	19%	0%
All Recipients	**14%**	**14%**	**23%**	**21%**	**24%**	**29%**	**31%**	**37%**

been constant since 1997. Prior to that year, approximately 80% of recipients received triple therapy consisting of cyclosporin A, azathioprine and prednisolone. In 1999, 14% of recipients received a regimen including tacrolimus. Prior to this year, very few patients received such a regimen because the listing of tacrolimus for renal transplantation in Australia occurred in September 1998.

Cadaveric Organ Donation

In 1999 the Australian cadaveric organ donation rate was 9 per million and in New Zealand it was 10 per million. These figures have been relatively stable over the past 5 years. The mean donor age was 39 years and 7% of donors were older than age 65. Of the 160 donors for whom consent for renal donation was given in 1999, 20 kidneys were not retrieved and 9 were retrieved but not transplanted because of disease of the organ. In 1999, 2 patients received double adult transplants from donors aged 73 and 77 years, respectively. There were 5 en-bloc kidney transplants from paediatric donors.

Exchange of Kidneys Between Regions

A National Exchange Scheme is currently in place in Australia. This scheme mandates that zero HLA - A,B,DR mismatched kidneys are exchanged. In addition kidneys with one HLA-mismatch are also exchanged for sensitized recipients and to maintain balance between the contributing regions. There is considerable variation in the organ donation rate between the regions. In South Australia in 1999, there was a cadaveric organ donation rate of 20 donors per million of population and in Queensland the rate was 6 donors per million of population.

Summary

The main feature of transplantation in Australia and New Zealand over the last few years has been the increasing proportion of living donor transplants on the background of a cadaveric organ donation rate, which is very low by international standards. The increase in living donor transplants has occurred predominantly as a result of an increase in the number of unrelated grafts. The success rate in transplantation in Australia is excellent with a one-year primary cadaveric graft survival rate of around 90% for each year since 1994 to the present. The accummulated one-year graft survival for unrelated living-donor grafts performed between 1990-1999 was 91.6%, which compares favourably with graft survival for all cadaveric grafts over the same period of 86.5%.

Organ Transplantation in Brazil

Jose O. Medina Pestana

Brazilian Organ Transplant Association (ABTO), Sao Paulo, BRAZIL

Brazil is a country with 160 million inhabitants distributed in an area of 8,200,000 square kilometers and 27 states. The Brazilian economy is the eighth largest in the world with an annual GDP of US$ 635 billion (in 2000) of which only 5%, roughly US$30 billion, are devoted to the public health system.

According to the latest statistics, there are about 45,000 patients registered in the chronic dialysis program, which is fully financed by the public health system. The Health Ministry has recently regulated the creation of organ donation networks in the health departments of each state. Organ procurement organizations are primarily linked to university hospitals. Regional lists of transplant candidates in each state have been established, and organ allocation is centralized and supervised by the attorney general's office.

The law for organ donation (Law #9434 of February 1997) reflects local social values, primarily the need for required consent based on written family authorization. The diagnosis of encephalic death is legally recognized as death and is based on clinical examination and at least one test demonstrating the absence of cerebral blood flow. Transplants between living donors are also state regulated, requiring judicial authorization in cases of donation between non-family members. There is no suspected or confirmed evidence of organ commercialization in the last 4 years.

The numbers of authorized transplant centers and of transplants performed have been steadily increasing in the last few years. The first intestinal transplant was performed in December 2000 in the hospital "Santa Casa" de São Paulo. The number of solid organ transplants performed increased from 2,127 in 1997 to 3,485 in 2000. The majority of the staff transplant physicians received their post-graduate medical training in Europe or in the United States. Their training was financed by Brazilian government agencies. Table 1 shows the number of authorized centers and the number of transplants performed in 2000, as well as the amount in US$ paid by the public health system for each procedure, including hospital expenses and professional fees. Compared with the United States or Europe, the percentage of renal transplants with living donors is considerably higher but transplants from cadaver donors are increasing. The number of living donor transplants appears to have reached a plateau, but cadaver donor transplants are still growing and are projected to increase 4-5-fold in the coming years, as organ procurement network programs grow and become more organized.

The public health system finances more than 95% of the transplants performed in Brazil. Those transplants performed in private institutions usually charge up to 2 times more, either from the health care providers or from the patient. The public health system also provides all registered immunosuppressive drugs to all patients indefinitely, including cyclosporine, tacrolimus, mycophenolate mofetil and anti-lymphocyte receptor antibodies (OKT3, anti-IL-2R). This government-sponsored program of drug supply is similar to that seen with drugs used to treat AIDS disease, which has placed Brazil among those countries with highest efficacy in controlling HIV syndromes as recently published by Rosenberg (Look at Brazil – The AIDS epidemic. The New York Times Magazine, January 28, 2001).

Thanks to this public network, the results achieved by the Brazilian transplant program have surpassed all expectations, considering the resources dedicated to the public health system. Currently, Brazil is second in the world in the absolute number of kidney transplants performed (Table 2). When absolute numbers of transplants are expressed per million inhabitants, Brazil falls to ninth place. Interestingly, when absolute numbers of transplants are corrected to GDP per capita, Brazil becomes the country with the best performance in the world. The world's largest active kidney transplant center is currently located in São Paulo (UNIFESP - Universidade Federal de São Paulo), and performed 427 and 507 kidney transplants in 1999 and 2000, respectively. These high numbers were made possible by the August 1998 opening of a new kidney disease facility dedicated mainly to kidney transplantation and related procedures (Hospital do Rim e Hipertensão).

BRAZIL

The transplant surgeons and physicians are represented by a national organization (ABTO – Associação Brasileira de Transplante de Órgãos), which has recently set up a National Transplant Registry and is working to analyze the effects of many transplant outcome variables.

Brazil, with all its shortcomings, has achieved an outstanding performance in the area of transplantation, similar to what takes place in the area of AIDS control and treatment. The regulation, allocation, financing, and execution of these programs have been possible through the enlightened and active participation of the public health system.

Table 1. Total number of organs transplanted, number of authorized centers and reimbursement for each procedure by the Brazilian Public Health System in year 2000.

Organ	Number of Transplants Living	Cadaver	Authorized Centers	Cost per procedure (US$)
Heart	0	110	36	11,121.24
Liver	43	437	36	25,949.73
Pancreas	0	9	4	4,189.08
Pancreas/Kidney	0	37	10	13,640.35
Lung	0	24	8	18,535.45
Kidney	1,631	1,194	153	9,636.38

Source (ABTO, Decree # 92 2001-Jan-19)

Table 2. Total number of renal transplants performed by country in 1999 (latest data available for all countries).

Country	Population (million)	GDP (US$billion)	Transplants	Transplants per million of pop.	Transplants per $1000 GDP per capita
Brazil	172,86	558.2	2,825	16	605
USA	275,56	9,237	12,162	44	359
Spain	39,99	647	2,006	50	132
Mexico	100,35	483.3	630	6	127
Germany	82,79	2,603	1,895	23	74
France	59,33	1,697	1,760	30	74
UK	59,51	1,254	1,432	24	59
Canada	31,28	663.3	1,025	33	49
Australia	19,16	518	518	28	24
Portugal	10,05	385	385	38	34

Sources (ABTO, U.S. Bureau of the Census, Handbook of International Economic Statistic, International Congress of Transplant Society, Daily Congress News   Letter 30-Ago-2000, " Revista Conjuntura Economica")

Kidney Transplantation in Chile

Alfredo M. Mocárquer and Jacqueline P. Pefaur

Department of Nephrology, Hospital Barros Luco-Trudeau, San Miguel, Santiago, CHILE

Chile is a country located at the most southern part of South America with a population of 15 million habitants. This country has a National Health System that delivers health care to about 75% of the population in state-run clinics and hospitals throughout the country. The other 25% of the population, being more affluent, usually has private insurance and receives medical care in private clinics. Chileans have an average annual income of around US$ 4,700 per capita. As of August 2000, there are more than 7,000 patients on chronic maintenance dialysis (473 patients per million population).

Kidney transplantation was initiated in Chile in the second half of the 1960's in university hospitals, but was later discontinued until 1976 when several hospitals started again with this activity. This form of treatment for end-stage kidney failure has been the main objective of the physicians caring for these patients and also has been encouraged by the state agencies financing medical care. In the 1970's, it was not easy to place a patient on chronic hemodialysis and transplantation by a living related donor was often the only option for survival.

In 1976, the physicians involved with transplantation formed the National Commission on Transplantation based at the National Institute of Public Health (Instituto de Salud Pública) and dependent on The Ministry of Health. At the same time, this Institute initiated the first Laboratory of Histocompatibility, to provide all the transplant centers with the histocompatibility studies that were needed and to maintain all the information on HLA typing, lymphocytotoxic antibodies and sera for the patients on the national waiting list for cadaver kidney transplantation. This information is used for organ sharing and allocation between different centers.

In 1981, the Chilean Transplantation Society was founded. In 1982, the first National Law regulating Organ Donation and Transplantation of Organs was approved. It was amended in 1996. Basically, this law defines brain death and allows for organ procurement after

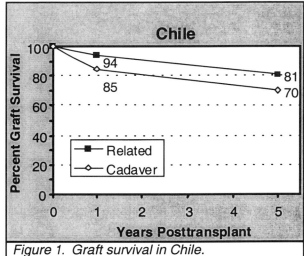

Figure 1. Graft survival in Chile.

Table 1. Kidney transplants in Chile.

	1990	1991	1992	1993	1994	1995	1996	1997	1998	1999	Total
Rel	89	59	46	65	71	47	45	38	43	24	527
Cad	69	71	78	90	122	103	188	167	218	238	1,344

the family gives written consent. It also allows for a living consent given previously by the deceased and registered on the national identity card. The National Corporation for Organ Transplantation, a private entity, was founded with the objective of increasing cadaver organ donation through public awareness and to provide hospitals with the ancillary services they may need in this field.

Cadaver organs are shared among patients on a national waiting list based on HLA matching, but the hospital that procured the donor has the right to use one of the organs for the best HLA-matched patient on their local list. HLA matching, anti-HLA antibody titers and waiting time are all considered in the distribution of organs; but HLA matching is the most important factor both for the national and local list. Any given patient waiting for a kidney is on both the local and national list at the same time.

Since 1976, there have been 3,071 kidney transplants done in Chile (55% from cadaver donors and 45%

from living related donors). At this time, this treatment of end-stage renal failure is performed in 20 hospitals and private clinics with 262 transplants performed in 1999 (90.8% from cadaver donors and 9.2% from living related donors). The rate of kidney transplantation was 17.4 per million population (pmp) for the year 1999 (15.8 pmp received cadaver kidneys and 1.6 pmp received living related kidneys). We do not have living-unrelated kidney transplantation, except for anecdotal cases of organ donation between spouses. Pediatric kidney transplantation is done at 3 centers in Chile. Of the total kidney transplants performed, 8% are in recipients younger than 15 years old. Sixty-nine percent of them received a kidney from a living related donor.

Most of our transplant patients (88%) are treated with cyclosporine, azathioprine and prednisone. Several groups combine this therapy with ketoconazole and others use diltiazem as a cyclosporine-sparing strategy. They all report excellent results with less than a 22% incidence of acute rejection episodes in the first year. Another group of patients receives mycophenolate mofetil together with cyclosporine and prednisone. A minority of patients has been given induction therapy with monoclonal antibodies against IL-2R, or polyclonal anti-lymphocyte antibodies. Acute rejections are usually treated with a bolus of methylprednisolone and rarely with OKT3 in cases of steroid resistance. At the annual meetings of the Chilean Society of Transplantation, there have been reports on a series of simultaneous kidney-pancreas transplantations, reports on a series of non-heart beating donors, transplantation in the elderly and transplantation in diabetics, among others.

The National Health System covers hospital, surgical and basic immunosuppressive treatments for the patients under its care. Patients belonging to the private insurance sector do not have coverage for immunosuppressive drugs once they are ambulatory.

Chile has a well-organized and successful kidney transplant program with more than 25 years of experience with this therapy. Some centers have recently reported over 92% graft survival for cadaver kidney recipients at one year. Although organ donation from cadavers has increased notably in the last few years, we are still behind in the availability of organs needed to keep up with the increasing demand.

Kidney Transplantation at The University Hospital Zagreb, Croatia

A. Kastelan, I. Humar and Z. Marekovic

Univ Clin Hosp-Rebro Zagreb, National Referral Organ Transplant & Tissue Typing Centre, Department of Urology, Zagreb, CROATIA

Twenty-seven years ago, in 1973, the first kidney transplantation was performed in Zagreb. Kidney transplantation has been the treatment of choice for patients with renal failure since the first transplantation was successfully performed. Croatia operates under presumed consent legislation, whereby any individual could make a pledge to donate the organs after death for the purpose of transplantation.

Croatia has 38 dialysis centres, 3 tissue-typing laboratories and 8 transplant centers (2 for kidney, 2 for heart, 2 for liver, 1 cornea center and 1 bone marrow centre). Our country has 4.5 million citizens. Every year there are new cases of end-stage renal disease, yielding an annual increase in the incidence of patients who need a kidney transplant. The majority of patients have access to one of the 38 dialysis centers with 485 dialysis places and during the year 2000, there were 2,692 patients on dialysis. However, fewer than 50 kidney transplantations are performed annually, numbers much lower than the current national demand (Fig. 2).

During its 27-year span, the kidney transplant program has maintained requirements that were considered particularly important. There has been a strong emphasis on HLA matching and a high quality of crossmatch testing. Living-related donor kidney transplantation has been encouraged whenever possible; of the total of 378 transplants, 96 were from familial donors (Fig.1).

Our organ procurement and transplant center has not included non-heart-beating donors in the donor pool. A central feature of the transplant program at our center is continuous follow-up by the dialysis department of our outpatient clinic, with nephrologists and transplant surgeons. Such cooperation plays an important role in follow-up and this has resulted in good graft and patient survival rates as shown in Figure 1.

The 20-year survival results were 71% for patients, 35% for living-related kidney grafts and 27% for cadaver

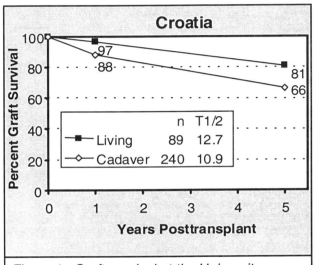

Figure 1. Graft survival at the University Hospital, Zagreb, Croatia (1985-1999).

Table 1. Kidney transplants in Croatia.

	1990	1991	1992	1993	1994	1995	1996	1997	1998	1999	Total
Rel	15	9	6	8	3	4	8	5	4	5	67
Unrel	0	0	0	0	0	0	0	0	0	0	
Cad	27	16	1	14	10	19	14	23	27	33	184

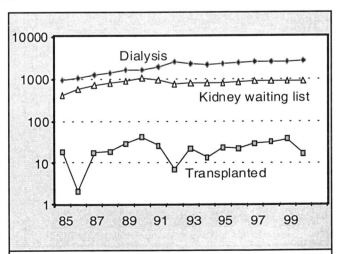

Figure 2. Waiting list compared with patients transplanted.

Organization and Results of Kidney Transplant Activity in Italy During 1995-99

S. Venettoni [a], **G. Scuderi** [b], **D.A. Mattucci** [c], **P. Diciaccio** [a], **F. Quinteri** [b], **O. Pugliese** [b], **P. Chistolini** [c], **G. Frustagli** [c] **V. Macellari** [c], **and A. Nanni Costa** [a]

[a]National Transplant Center, [b]Immunology and [c]Medical Engineering Laboratories, Italian National Institute of Health (ISS), Rome, ITALY

Since January 1995, the Italian National Institute of Health (ISS) through its Immunology and Medical Engineering Laboratories has started to collect and assemble data concerning every transplant performed in Italy using a questionnaire similar to the one used by the Collaborative Transplant Study Registry in Heidelberg (1). Data are recorded when the transplant is performed and the form is sent to ISS within 30 days. This allows us to monitor national transplant activity, including the characteristics of donors and recipients. From 1995-1999, data for 9,777 transplants for all organs have been collected, by the Italian National Transplant Registry.

Based upon the new transplant law (Law 91 of April 1999), the National Transplant Centre (CNT) was created at ISS in March 2000 (2). The collection and communication of transplant data now fall under its jurisdiction. In this report, we describe the characteristics of kidney transplants performed in Italy over the period 1995-1999 at the 38 kidney transplant centres that have been operational in Italy during this period.

Organization of the Italian Transplant Network

In Italy, the network that coordinates organ procurement and transplant activities operates on 4 levels: local, regional, inter-regional and national. The *local coordination level* is made up of local transplant coordinators who are present in each hospital for the identification and maintenance of potential donors. They are in charge of managing all procedures regarding organ and tissue procurement, keeping relations and contacts with the donor's families and communicating donor data to regional and inter-regional centres. They also organize information campaigns in collaboration with the regional centre and inter-regional centres. Organ transplantations have to be authorized by the Ministry of Health, and presently, 172 hospitals are authorized to perform transplants.

The *regional coordination level* is made up of regional reference centres that are responsible for their area. They manage waiting lists, organ donations, organ procurement policy, and relationships with intensive care units, transplants and with transplant centres and relations with the inter-regional centre.

Table 1. Kidney transplants in Italy.

	1995	1996	1997	1998	1999	Total
Rel	42	48	52	25	29	196
Unrel	10	13	12	7	8	50
Cad	911	1,071	1,170	1,081	1,059	5,229

The *inter-regional coordination level* is composed of 3 inter-regional reference centres that cover nearly the whole national territory: AIRT (Inter-regional Transplant Association) includes 6 regions (Piemonte, Valle d'Aosta, Tuscany, Emilia-Romagna and Puglia) and the district of Bolzano; NITp (Nord Italia Transplant Program) includes 6 regions (Friuli, Liguria, Lombardia, Marche and Veneto) and the district of Trento; OCST (South Central Transplant Organization) includes 7 regions (Abruzzo, Basilicata, Calabria, Campania, Lazio, Molise, Sardinia and Umbria).The Sicily region is not yet assimilated. The inter-regional centres manage relationships with regional centres in their area in order to identify donors and to allocate the organs. They manage urgent requests, the national paediatric waiting list, relationships with other inter-regional reference centres and with the CNT. According to law 91/99, regional and inter-regional centres may have different functions depending on different regional policies. The preceding description applies only to to 2 inter-regional organizations (AIRT and OCST). Acitvity performed by the inter-regional centre of the Nord Italy Transplant organization includes additional functions, such as organ allocation.

The *national coordination level* operates through the CNT, which was created on the 26th of February 2000 under the terms of law 91/99 (2). It is composed of a president (the director of ISS), a general director, a representative for each of the inter-regional centres, personnel from ISS and selected experts. The CNT keeps the lists of patients waiting for a transplant on a computer information system, checks criteria and procedures to allocate organs, fixes guidelines for regional and inter-regional centres, identifies indicators and parameters for checking quality and activity of transplant centres; monitors organ procurement and transplant activity over the national territory and maintains relationships with foreign organizations working in this field.

Methods

Within 15 days after a transplant has taken place, the transplant centre sends a completed 3-part questionnaire for data collection. The first part is for the recipient data, the second is for the type and conditions of transplantation and the last is for the donor's characteristics. More than 100 information fields have been introduced and can be linked.

The recipient record includes personal data, time on the waiting list, dialysis duration and kind of treatment, clinical data, HLA typing, serological data, original disease, and therapeutic treatments before transplant and immunosuppressive therapy. The transplant record includes the date, relation to the donor, kind of transplant, transplant number and how many days the previous graft had been working, and the sensitization status for the highest and the most recent serum tested against panels of total lymphocytes, T-cells, B-cells and B-cells at 5°C. The donor record includes personal data, clinical assessment data, HLA typing, serological data, cause of death for cadaveric donors, ischemia time and preservation solution. All data are stored in an electronic file called the Italian National Transplant Register, using a filing and analysis program based on Access software (a dedicated database was created by using Microsoft Access software).

The data format has been adapted to the information requirements of the CTS in Heidelberg.

Results and Conclusions

Table 1 shows the number of kidney transplants carried out in Italy over the period 1995-1999 from both cadaver and living donors. Most transplanted kidneys (95.6%) came from cadaver donors. A smaller percentage (4.3%) came from living donors and 79.6% of these

were family-related living donors. Only 50 transplants were from unrelated living donors. To date, follow-up data on 738 kidney transplants performed during this period have been received and 58 failures within one year of the operation have been reported, but these data are not sufficient to perform statistically significant analyses. It has been possible to evaluate the one-year organ survival rate, which was 89.7%.

The distribution of recipient ages was: 5% over age 60; 40% in the 46- 60 age group; 33% in the 31-45 age group; 17% in the 16-30 age group; 4% in the 0-15 age group (based on 5,270 transplants with data available). Sixty-five percent of recipients were males and 35% were females. Forty-one percent of transplants were for patients with glomerular diseases; 15% were for cystic-congenital diseases; 9% were for systemic diseases (including diabetes); 9% were for pyelonephritis and tubular necrosis diseases and 26% were for other pathologies. The total number of kidney transplants in the paediatric age group (<18 years) performed between 1997-1999 was 147 (4.2%) of the 3,451 transplants in that period. HLA-A,-B,-DR typing data were available for both donor and recipient for 5,030 out of 5,717 (88%) kidney transplants. The number of mismatches (mm) between the corresponding donor-recipient pairs was analysed with the following results: 0.5% 0mm, 5% 1mm, 19% 2mm, 34% 3mm, 27% 4mm, 12% 5mm, 2.5% 6mm. The cause of death was known for 2,790 cadaver kidney donors, and included: vascular diseases (49.2%), cranioencephalic trauma (47.8%), other causes (1.8%). The donor ages were distributed as follows: ages 0-15 (7.0%), 16-60 (80.6%) and over 60 (12.4%). The over-60 age group has grown from 6% in 1995 to 17% in 1999.

Immunosuppressive therapies adopted during the transplant were reported on 80.6% of the forms we received. The most commonly applied therapies were: CsA+steroids (1,771/4,610=38.4%), CsA+steroids +azathioprine (1,569/4,610=34.0%), CsA+steroids+ mycophenolate mofetil (450/4,610=9.7%) and FK506+steroids (73/4,610=1,5%). Other therapies have been added and amount to 6.2% (747/4610) of cases.

Table 2 shows the number of kidney transplants referred to ISS each year during 1995-1999 stratified by type of transplant. Over these 5 years, 5,717 total kidneys were transplanted, of which 5,617 were single kidney transplants, 7 were double kidney transplants and 93 were kidney with other organ transplants.

Table 3 provides the number and rate (pmp) of

ITALY

cadaver donors during the 1995-2000 period. Data regarding 2000 activity were calculated on the basis of 11 months activity. Based on the available data, the number of transplants performed each year in Italy has progressively increased during this period. The 1999 rate of transplantation was 23.5 pmp. The law (578/93) on cerebral death assessment (3) that passed in 1994, the progressive changes in criteria for donor age selection, and a better hospital organization for donation processes have undoubtedly contributed to the increased activity. The number of waiting patients has been stable since 1998 (4). However, the number waiting for a kidney transplant (about 7,000 patients) strongly calls for further increases in transplant activity.

During the 1995-1999 period, the new transplant law 91/99 had not yet been put into effect. The National Transplant Centre, which currently monitors the transplant system, will progressively take on the several functions that the law assigns to it.

Data activity in the year 2000 seems to confirm the positive trends started in 1993, at least regarding cadaver organ donors, with an increase of about 5%. The overall transplant activity in Italy as reported to the ISS before creation of the CNT is presented in Table 4. Altogether 9,777 transplants were performed, including the 5,717 kidney transplants (cadavers and living donors), 2,193 liver transplants, 1,573 heart transplants, 144 double-lung transplants, 136 single-lung transplants, 5 heart-lung transplants and 9 pancreas transplants.

References

1. Opelz G. Transfusion and cadaver kidney transplants. The CTS data. Clin Transplantation 1987; 2:239.
2. ITALIA. Legge 1° aprile 1999, n.91. Disposizioni in materia di prelievi e trapianti di organo. G.U. 15 aprile 1999, n. 87.
3. ITALIA. Legge 29 dicembre 1993, n.578. Norme per l'accertamento e la certificazione di morte. G.U. 8 gennaio 1994, n.5.
4. Benagiano G, Curtoni ES, Sargentini A, Eds. "I Trapianti di Organo e la collaborazione nazionale in Italia". Annali dell'Istituto Superiore di Sanita. 2000.
5. Pugliese O, Scuderi G, Mattucci DA, Chistolini P, Quintieri F. A 5-year analysis of organ donation & recipient in Italy. Prog. in Transplantation (In press).

Table 2. Number of kidney transplants referred to the Italian National Institute of Health during 1995-99.

Type of kidney/Yr	1995	1996	1997	1998	1999	TOTAL
Total Kidney	1,108	1,158	1,234	1,119	1,098	5,717
Single kidney	1,105	1,139	1,205	1,084	1,084	5,617
Double kidney					7	7
Kidney+Pancreas	3	19	26	31		79
Kidney+Liver			3	1	5	9
Kidney+Heart				3	2	5

Table 3. Number of cadaver donors and relative pmp during 1995-2000.

Donors/Year		95	96	97	98	99	2000[ab]	2000[ac]
	North	419	443	459	509	520	569	596
	Middle	80	97	103	103	153	130	152
	South	77	89	105	95	115	126	132
	Italy	576	629	667	707	788	825	880
pmp	North	16.5	17.4	18	19.9	20.3	22.2	23.2
	Middle	7.3	8.8	9.3	9.3	13.8	11.7	13.7
	South	3.7	4.3	5	4.5	5.5	6	6.3
	Italy	10.1	11	11.6	12.3	13.7	14.3	15.2

[a] Data obtained through yearly estimated value of activity performed in the period 1st January - 31st October.
[b] Utilized donors defined as stated by European Organ Exchange Organization.
[c] Effective donors defined as stated by European Organ Exchange Organization.

Table 4. Number of organ transplants referred to the Italian National Institute of Health during 1995-99.

Organ/Year	1995	1996	1997	1998	1999	TOTAL
Kidney	1,108	1,158	1,234	1,119	1,098	5,717
Pancreas only			3	6		9
Heart	363	330	330	266	284	1,573
Single Lung	2	33	32	27	42	136
Double Lung	3	20	43	26	52	144
Heart+Lung			1	1	3	5
Liver	392	420	438	422	521	2193
TOTAL	1,871	1,980	2,113	1,908	2,000	9,777

Kidney Transplantation in the North Italy Transplant Program

M. Cardillo, M. Scalamogna [a], C. Pizzi, F. Poli, P. Rebulla, E. Taioli [b] and G. Sirchia on behalf of the North Italy Transplant program

Centro Trasfusionale e di Immunologia dei Trapianti, [a]Servizio per il Prelievo e la Conservazione di Organi e Tessuti, [b]Laboratorio di Epidemiologia, IRCCS Ospedale Maggior, Milano, ITALY

Renal transplantation in the clinical setting started in Italy in 1966, when Professor Paride Stefanini performed the first successful kidney graft in Rome in a 17-year-old girl from a living donor. Later, the same team performed a xenotransplantation from a chimpanzee to a 19-year-old boy. The kidney had a good function for one month, then the patient died from an infectious complication. In the same period Professor Piero Confortini in Verona was organizing the dialysis program and in 1968, he was the second surgeon to perform a kidney transplant from a cadaver donor in Italy, using an organ harvested soon after cardiac arrest. After more than 30 years the transplanted patient is still in good health, with excellent graft function. A third great surgical school left an unforgettable mark in the Italian history of transplantation: in 1969, Professor Edmondo Malan and his team performed their first cadaver kidney transplant in Milano, the third in Italy.

During that period clinicians became aware of the importance of HLA matching in kidney transplantation (1), thus identifying the need to select the proper recipient for each donor. It soon became clear that kidney allocation could not be performed by the clinicians responsible for the transplants, but it had to be committed to a *super partes* facility with no patients of its own, able to allocate kidneys following defined and accepted criteria. In those years in Italy, Edmondo Malan, Piero Confortini and Girolamo Sirchia developed a reference center for a broad area in Northern Italy, responsible for organ allocation, with competence in immunology and without actually having clinical care of the patients. This center was centered in Milano, where the Blood Transfusion Center of the Maggiore Hospital had already acquired knowledge of leukocyte immunology (2). The first transplant organization in Italy, named the North Italy Transplant program (NITp), began activity on June 18, 1972.

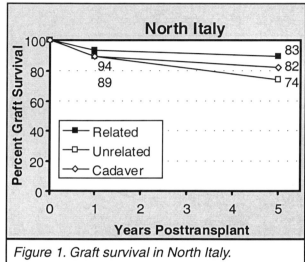

Figure 1. Graft survival in North Italy.

Table 1. Kidney transplants in North Italy.

	1990	1991	1992	1993	1994	1995	1996	1997	1998	1999	Total
Rel	16	22	29	34	37	35	32	47	26	27	305
Unrel*	5	3	3	4	6	7	11	6	6	6	57
Cad	261	299	311	320	416	541	536	559	596	604	4,443

* Spouse

The North Italy Transplant Organizational Model

At present, the NITp includes an area of about 18 million inhabitants in Northern Italy, and is coordinated by a reference center in Milano. It serves 48 procuring hospitals and 40 transplant centers located in 15 hospitals. The tasks of the reference center are management of the waiting list, immunological evaluation of recipients and donors, organ allocation, organization of transportation, data collection, definition of protocols together with the operative units, development of information campaigns, psychological support of donor families and promotion of research and development in the field of organ procurement and transplantation.

New HLA Typing Methods

In the beginning, HLA typing was based on serological methods. Now, HLA specificities are better defined by molecular biology techniques (3). Patient and donor genomic class II HLA typing was introduced as a routine procedure in the NITp 5 years ago. As described below, donor-recipient HLA matching is the basis of the NITp kidney allocation algorithm.

The NITp Working Groups and the Scientific Committee

The NITp Working Groups periodically discuss donor procurement, transplantation safety, education programs, criteria for patient registration and organ allocation, organ retrieval, paediatric transplantation, tissue transplantation, ethics and costs in transplantation. The aim is to establish and update protocols that then must be approved by the NITp Assembly during the annual technical-scientific meeting. The NITp Scientific Committee was created in 1998 with the goal of stimulating the operative units to participate in collaborative studies. Among the projects implemented in the field of kidney transplantation, at least 2 are to be mentioned: 1) the role of Celsior versus UW perfusion solutions on graft functional recovery, and 2) the efficacy of double kidney transplantation from marginal donors.

The NITp Kidney Allocation Algorithm (NITK3)

In the NITp, allocation criteria are discussed and updated during the annual meeting, which involves all NITp unit delegates. Kidney allocation criteria include AB0 identity, HLA compatibility, age matching, time on the waiting list, priority for patients resident in NITp regions, balance between organs procured and transplanted by each center and a negative pretransplant crossmatch. Based on our data, on those of the Collaborative Transplant Study (CTS), and on those of other large international registries, an NITp working group revised the allocation algorithm for adult cadaver donor kidney transplantation in 1997. It was named NITK3, to indicate the third kidney allocation algorithm used in the NITp, and it is extensively discussed elsewhere (4). NITK3 was validated after a 6-month period of use and it is continuously adjusted by the working group on the

basis of data analysis.

The Results of NITK3, 3 Years After Implementation

The main goals of allocation - transplanting patients with better HLA matching and patients with more serious immunological problems - have been achieved. In fact, significantly higher proportions of patients with a waiting time longer than 3 years (34.7% vs. 24.1%, p=0.001), of sensitized recipients (5.1% vs. 2.2%, p=0.001), of patients waiting for a regraft (7.9% vs. 6%, p=0.05) and of patients in the best HLA matching level (20.4% vs. 14.1%, p=0.001) have been transplanted when compared with the 3 previous years. Furthermore, the fraction of kidneys used locally has steadily increased (46.1% vs. 31.7%, p=0.001). These results were obtained without significantly affecting the one-year graft survival rates (91.5% vs. 89.7%) in the same periods.

Transplantation and Donor Procurement Activity

From June 18, 1972 to December 31, 1999, 7,824 kidney transplants were performed in the NITp, more than half of all the renal grafts performed in Italy. A total of 7,353 grafts were from cadaver donors and 471 from living donors, 395 of them related and 76 unrelated. Table 1. shows the data from the past 10 years. In our graft survival analysis, (Fig. 1) only adult recipients (age>15 years) are considered and combined transplants are excluded. Graft failure and patient death (independent of the cause) are both counted as end-points.

In 2000, a total of 341 (18.7 per million population) cadaver donors were procured, with a 1.5% increase as compared to 1999. This value is above the European mean. These results were mostly due to NITp initiatives, including education courses for the ICU personnel on technical aspects of donor procurement and communication with donor families. In the last few years, we observed a significant increase in the number of elderly donors that previously had not been used. In 1999, donors over 60 years of age accounted for 22% of the total, compared with 17% in 1998 (5). Twelve donors were used in the Double Kidney Program, in which donor kidneys are transplanted to a single recipient after histological evaluation. In our series, results obtained in cadaver and living transplantation were not significantly different. When we consider cadaver donor grafts performed from 1990-1999, donor age over 60 years was a major factor impacting on kidney graft survival, determining a 7.7% decrease in the 5-year survival rate compared with younger donors. Nevertheless, older donors may be a precious resource for older recipients. Other factors which influence graft outcome are HLA-A,-B,-DRB1 matching and pretransplant transfusions. The 5-year graft survival rate of 0-1 HLA mismatched (MM) grafts was 89.5%, compared with 86.1% and 77.8% for 2-4 and 5-6 MM grafts, respectively (p=0.02). Grafts performed in non-transfused recipients show better results than those in transfused patients, with 5-year survival rates of 84.2% and 79.8% respectively (p=0.01). Results obtained with double kidney transplants are not significantly different from those of single transplants from standard donors over 50 years of age. From 1996-1999, we observed a 10.3% increase in 5-year graft survival compared with transplants performed from 1990-1995. On December 31, 2000, the NITp kidney waiting list included 2,600 patients, with a 25.3-month median waiting time (range 7-35 in different centers), while 920 patients were newly enrolled in 2000.

Transplantation from Living Donors

Transplantation from living donors bears some ethical problems. Italian law N. 458-67 foresaw the possibility of living-related kidney transplantation and provided the possibility for using living unrelated donors if no related donor was available. However, this possibility may arouse the suspicion of organ trafficking. In fact, rumours of possible economic transactions between the patient and the donor sometimes appeared in the newspapers and resulted in a reduction of cadaver donors. Even in the case of a related donation, psychological pressure on the donor must be avoided. Taking these considerations into account, in 1987 the NITp officially decided to endorse living transplantation only from related donors or spouses, in agreement with the official position expressed by the Council of Europe in the same year. The NITp position was recently reaffirmed, when the Italian Parliament issued a new law on liver transplantation from living donors. The priority is the utilization of cadaver organs, while living donation is a secondary option, which should be considered only after evaluation of donor free choice, information and motivation by an *ad hoc* commission, including a psychiatrist, and after a suitable time on the waiting list for a cadaver organ. Moreover living donation should include careful follow-up of both donor and recipient and the activation of a long-term donor registry.

Conclusions

A number of organizations all over the world have played a major role in developing the social, organizational and technical aspects of transplantation. In Italy, the NITp has acquired a 28-year experience that represents a sound basis for the future. Nevertheless, improvements are possible and desirable, particularly in the field of cadaver donor procurement and organ allocation. From a clinical point of view, we want to improve long-term results and reduce the effects of immunosuppressive therapy; tolerance, perhaps xeno-transplantation or, more likely, tissue repair, are hopes for the future and should be supported by the Health Authority. For the time being, however, more effective measures should be taken to improve cadaver organ procurement, which is insufficient to meet the current patients' needs.

References

1. Bodmer J, Bodmer WF, Payne R, et al. Leucocyte antigens in man: a comparison of lymphocytotoxic and agglutination assays for their detection. Nature 1966; 210:28.

2. Sirchia G, Ferrone S, Mercuriali F, et al. Il candidato al trapianto. Aspetti immunologici. Editrice Ancora, Milano, 1969.

3. Mytilineos J, Sherer S, Dunckley H, et al. DNA HLA-DR typing results of 4000 kidney transplants. Transplantation 1993; 55:778.

4. Sirchia G, Poli F, Cardillo M, et al. Cadaver kidney allocation in the North Italy Transplant program on the eve of the new millennium. In: JM Cecka and PI Terasaki, Eds. Clinical Transplants 1998. Los Angeles, UCLA Tissue Typing Laboratory. 1998:133.

5. North Italy Transplant Program. 1999 Activity Report, Milano, 2000.

Acknowledgements

This study was supported in part by grants of *Progetto a Concorso 2001 "Analisi delle variabili cliniche, strumentali e bio-umorali del donatore cadavere predittive di ripresa funzionale degli organi trapiantati"*, IRCCS Ospedale Maggiore, Milano. We gratefully acknowledge the 101 donor hospitals and 19 transplant centers in the 6 NITp regions and their directors and staffs who participate in NITp and contribute to this work.

Status of Kidney Transplantation in Japan

Kazuo Ota [a], Shiro Hinotsu [b], Miyuki Kawado [b], and Yasuo Ohashi [b]

[a] Ota Medical Research Institute and Biostatistics / Epidemiology and Preventive Health Sciences,
[b] School of Health Sciences and Nursing, University of Tokyo, JAPAN

Amongst the Asian countries, Japan was a leader in the beginnings of organ transplantation. The first kidney and the first liver transplant were done in March 1964, and the first heart transplantation was done in August 1968. The first simultaneous pancreas and kidney transplantation was performed in 1984. The development of transplantation, since its beginnings, has been slow in Japan. This may be due to the fact that there have been difficulties in obtaining donors and obstacles in the acceptance of brain death. The law allowing for the procurement of kidneys and corneas was enacted in March 1980, and the law legalizing organ procurement from brain-dead donors was enacted in October 1997.

In June 1977 distribution of donor cards started in Japan at Jinishoku Fukyukai and the development of a kidney-sharing network was started in 1978 at Sakura National Hospital. At this time, Sakura National Hospital was functioning as one of the main hospitals for kidney transplantation in Japan. This led members of the transplant community to believe that it might be better to have an organization that was not involved in actual transplantation to function as the kidney-sharing center to ensure impartiality. Then the transplant center was switched to the Jinishoku Fukyukai and it was decided to have Sakura Hospital serve as an HLA center for organ sharing.

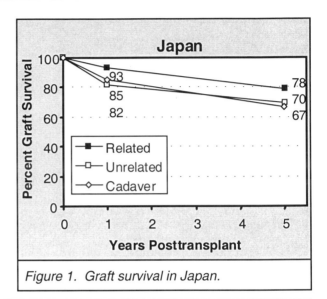

Figure 1. Graft survival in Japan.

Table 1. Kidney transplants in Japan.

	1990	1991	1992	1993	1994	1995	1996	1997	1998	1999	Total
Rel	548	441	414	379	367	404	420	403	507	551	4434
Unrel	36	27	26	38	28	25	35	34	*	*	249
Cad	230	238	228	247	199	168	183	159	149	158	1,959

* unrelated donor transplants are included with related

Number of Kidney Transplants

The annual number of cadaver kidney transplants prior to 1981 was less than 50. In 1981, with the help of Professor Terasaki, who developed a program for sending kidneys from the United States to Japan, the annual number of cadaver kidney transplants reached 160 over the next 2 years. The impact of this program was significant in increasing the total number of kidney transplants in Japan. As a result of the introduction of cyclosporin in the United Stated combined with the growing demand for kidneys domestically, the United States was forced to decrease its export of kidneys to Japan. Since this time the number of cadaver kidney donations in Japan has remained at approximately 160 per year, which is 3 times the number at the start of the project.

The number of kidney transplants in Japan reached a peak in 1989. The total number of kidney transplants that year was 838 including 573 living and 265 cadaver donor transplants. Since then the number of transplants, particularly those from living related donors, decreased drastically and reached its lowest number of 399 in 1994.

This trend was observed during the time when the new law regarding brain death was being discussed. Many family members of kidney transplant candidates postponed their donation in hopes that a cadaver kidney would be available after the legislation passed. The number of kidney transplantations using family donors began to increase again after 1998 because the new law did not result in any increase in the number of cadaver kidney donations. The increasing age of the prospective family donors and their strong desire to donate contributed to the increased activity.

Actually, to our surprise, the cadaver donation rate decreased every year after the enactment of the new law and reached 149 in 1998. There may be several reasons for this, but the most serious one is the confusion regarding the donor card. Many Japanese people are inclined to misunderstand that the donor card is indispensable to provide consent for kidney donation. Moreover, the number of transplant coordinators is small and they are still inexperienced in their work. In the meantime, the number of dialysis patients has increased steadily and reached 197,213 at the end of 1999. Amongst them, 13,422 were on the waiting list for kidney transplantation.

Network and Sharing System

The national network for organ sharing in Japan is called the Japan Organ Transplant Network (JOTN), and was developed at the same time Japan was drafting laws regarding organ transplantation. JOTN divided Japan into 7 blocks excluding Okinawa, which was classified as a sub-block. Prospective recipients are registered with JOTN through the hospital where they want to be transplanted. HLA testing is usually done in the specific hospital or at HLA centers in the block, and the patient is then registered as a candidate on the waiting list. The average waiting time is 5-6 years once a patient is listed for kidney transplantation.

The most important criterion for recipient selection after ABO matching is HLA compatibility. If a 6 HLA antigen-matched recipient is found on the national waiting list, the kidney is sent to the hospital where the prospective recipient is registered. If a 6 HLA antigen-matched patient is not found, then a 5 HLA antigen-matched prospective recipient is selected. If more than one 5 antigen-matched patient is identified in the block waiting list, the one who has the longest waiting time is selected.

Before the JOTN started, a "keep one, share one" rule was used in many regions in Japan. The change to the new sharing system is considered to be one cause of the decrease in cadaveric donation.

Kidney Transplantation in Korea: Past and Present

Kiil Park, Yu Seun Kim, Soon Il Kim, Myoung Soo Kim, Hyun Jeong Kim, and Kyung Ock Jeon

Department of Surgery and The Research Institute for Transplantation, Yonsei University College of Medicine, Seoul, KOREA

The first successful renal transplant in Korea was performed in 1969 and by the end of 1999, more than 10,500 transplants had been undertaken in 44 medical facilities. Both graft and patient survival rates have improved markedly during this time. Reviews on the kidney transplantation activities and survival statistics have been published by the Yonsei University Medical Center and Catholic Medical Center in previous volumes of the *Clinical Transplants* series (1-3). Currently, 5-year graft survival in our center exceeds 82% for more than 1,900 living related and unrelated transplants. These compare well with data reported from the major centers in western countries. A sharp increase in renal transplants over such a short period of time is due to many factors.

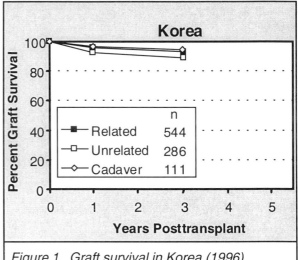

Figure 1. Graft survival in Korea (1996).

Enactment of Government-initiated Health Care System

In 1979, the government initiated the state-run health care system. Although it applied to only a small percentage of the population, kidney transplants were included in the health care benefits, and the financial burden on patients was reduced. However, in the absence of effective immunosuppressive agents, such as cyclosporine A (CsA) or antibodies, the outcome of transplantation was not satisfactory. This meant that only 50-88 transplantations were performed annually. In 1984, CsA was introduced in our practice, and consequently, one-year graft survival rates increased by more than 15%. As the results improved, more transplants were performed and more than 360 were carried out in 1988 alone. In 1989 provision of health care was extended to include most of the population. As the whole nation became beneficiaries of health care, the financial burden on patients was decreased further and the annual number of transplants increased (4).

Table 1. Kidney transplants in Korea.

	1990	1991	1992	1993	1994	1995	1996	1997	1998	1999
Rel	n/a	n/a	n/a	n/a	n/a	n/a	544	459	450	n/a
Unrel	n/a	n/a	n/a	n/a	n/a	n/a	286	327	329	n/a
Cad	n/a	n/a	12	34	63	121	111	176	233	298
Total*	624	680	911	719	686	898	941	962	1,012	1,089

* individual annual breakdown by donor not available

Efforts to Promote Organ Transplantation

As of the end of 1997, approximately 20,000 patients were dependent on various kinds of renal replacement therapy estimated at 431.9 per million population. Of these, only about 30% are enjoying the benefits of transplantation. In 1997, approximately 4,000 new patients (86.8 per million population) requiring renal replacement were reported, but only 962 renal transplants (23%) were performed (5,6). This means that each year there are more than 3,000 patients in need of a kidney. The principal cause for this disparity is the absolute shortage of kidney donors. In Korea, living-related donor transplants have been considerably more common than cadaver transplants for a variety of reasons. In the absence of any legal recognition of brain death, some leading centers, such as our own, initiated living-unrelated donor programs like the family donor exchange (SWAP) program. This was done to alleviate the shortage of donor kidneys. This program, unique to our country, was successful, and we eventually expanded its scope to a multiple donor exchange (SWAP-around) program. We have already presented the indication, the process and outcome for these programs (1,3,7). Currently, the 3-year graft survival rate for 52 swap recipients from our center is 96%.

Recognition of Brain Death

The declaration of brain death as another manifestation of the cessation of life, and its recognition by The Korean Medical Association in 1993, improved the availability of organ donors. This declaration was made at the highest level of the most influential medical association in the country and, while brain death was not accepted legally, the declaration demonstrated its acceptance by the medical fraternity (4). With this approval, medical centers have subsequently been allowed to tacitly use cadaver organs. After the declaration, the number of cadaver kidneys made available increased sharply. In 1999 alone, of the 1,089 renal transplantations reported nationally, cadaver kidney transplants accounted for a recorded high of 298, or 27.3% of the total. As of February 2000, the "Law on The Transplantation of Human Organs" took effect, legally allowing the transplantation of organs from patients who are declared brain dead. The law lays the groundwork for the prevention of the sale of human organs by intermediaries. The decree stipulates that all the information regarding the donor and recipient will be handled by a centralized national organization, with prospective recipients selected fairly in accordance with medical standards in the designated geographic regions.

Korean Network for Organ Sharing (KONOS)

The KONOS, the state-run central agency established by the new law, was launched in February 2000 under the wing of the National Medical Center in Seoul. Its principal responsibility will be to manage all the procedures related to transplants from both brain-dead and live (related or unrelated) donors on a national basis. The major objectives of the KONOS would be to improve the effectiveness of the nation's organ procurement, distribution and transplantation system by increasing the

availability of donor organs, to prevent the illicit handling of human organs, to collect and analyze the data on procurement, preservation, and tissue typing, and to monitor the clinical outcome of transplantation. The KONOS divided the nation into 3 large geographical regions. Basically, organs removed from the deceased in one region must be transplanted to patients in the same region. Hospitals have to obtain licenses from the Ministry of Health and Welfare if they want to perform organ transplants. Those hoping to donate or receive human organs are required to register and get permission from the KONOS. During the 6-month period after the launch of the KONOS, organs from 32 brain-dead donors were made available (58 kidneys, 19 livers, 6 hearts). In addition, 400 kidney, and 156 liver transplants were performed from living related or unrelated donors through the KONOS.

Evolution of Immunosuppression

Immunosuppression protocols have changed over the years as new immunosuppressive agents have emerged. Since the introduction of CsA early in 1984, CsA-based double and triple (including azathioprine [Aza]) therapy constituted the major method by which immunosuppression was maintained. From the late 1980's, cadaver donor kidney recipients frequently received anti-lymphocyte globulin (ATGam or OKT3) for the first 7-10 days according to the functional status of their grafts. After early 1995, microemulsion CsA (Neoral) replaced conventional CsA for a short period. However, mycophenolate mofetil (MMF), introduced early in 1997, has slowly been used in preference to Aza. A clear benefit of MMF in reducing the incidence of acute rejection even after living-donor kidney transplantation was demonstrated by us (8). According to the 1998 Kidney Transplant Registry report, CsA-based triple therapy (including MMF or Aza) was most popular (68.5%), with Neoral and steroids preferred in HLA-identical recipients, and tacrolimus-based double or triple therapy being administered to 9.3% of patients (9).

Nationwide Kidney Transplant Registry

The Kidney Transplant Registry was established within the Korean Society for Transplantation, and annual reports have been published since 1998 (6,9). The total number of kidney transplants since 1996 has increased slowly, with a high of 1,089 recorded in 1999. During these 3 consecutive years, the sharp increase in

KOREA

the number of cadaver kidney transplants is noteworthy. The one- and 2-year actual graft survival rate among 941 transplants performed in 1996 was 94.9% and 93.6%; 96.0% and 95.2% among recipients of living-related, 92.3% and 90.8% among recipients of living-unrelated, and 96.4% and 95.8% among recipients of cadaver donor transplants, respectively, with no significant differences. The high graft survival among the cadaver transplant recipients might be attributed to the short cold preservation time (less than 12 hours in more than 90% of recipients) resulting in injury-free organs. A one-year graft survival rate of 94.8% was reported in 962 recipients transplanted in 1997. Our nationwide Kidney Transplant Registry data show that higher graft survival has been well maintained since the time of its inception. This reflects the proliferation of renal transplantation activities and the maturation of transplantation medicine through the State.

References

1. Park K, Kim YS, Lee EM, Lee HY, Han DS. Single-center experience of unrelated living-donor renal transplantation in the cyclosporine era. In: Terasaki PI, Cecka JM, Eds. Clinical Transplants 1992. Los Angeles, UCLA Tissue Typing Laboratory, 1993; 249

2. Yoon YS, Bang BK, Jin DC, et al. Factors influencing long-term outcome of living donor kidney transplantation in the cyclosporine era. In: Terasaki PI, Cecka JM, Eds. Clinical Transplants 1992. Los Angeles, UCLA Tissue Typing Laboratory, 1993; 257.

3. Park K, Kim SI, Kim YS, et al. Results of kidney transplantation from 1979 to 1997 at Yonsei University. In: Cecka JM, Terasaki PI Eds. Clinical Transplants 1997. Los Angeles, UCLA Tissue Typing Laboratory, 1998; 149.

4. Kim YS. Advances in renal transplantation. JAMA Korea 1997; 12:5.

5. Ahn SJ, Choi EJ. Renal replacement therapy in Korea - Insan Memorial Registry 1997- Korean J Nephrol 1999; 18:1.

6. Organ transplant registry committee, The Korean Society for Transplantation. Solid organ transplantation in Korea – 1997- J Korean Soc Transplant 1998; 12:151.

7. Park K, Moon JI, Kim SI, Kim YS. Exchange donor program in kidney transplantation. Transplantation 1999; 67: 336.

8. Kim YS, Moon JI, Kim SI, Park K. Clear benefit of mycophenolate mofetil-based triple therapy in reducing the incidence of acute rejection after living donor renal transplantations. Transplantation 1999; 68:578.

9. Organ transplant registry committee, The Korean Society for Transplantation. Solid organ transplantation in Korea – 1998- J Korean Soc Transplant 1999; 13:185.

Kidney Transplantation in Mexico

J.L. Melchor [a], C. Gracida [a], A. López [a], M.A. Sanmartin [a], A. Ibarra [a], J. Cancino [a], R. Espinoza [a], L. Terán [b], and H. Aguirre-Gas [a]

[a] Transplant Service Especialidades CMN Siglo XXI, [b] National Transplant Registry
Mexico City, MEXICO

The first kidney transplant in Mexico was performed at Especialidades Hospital CMN Siglo XXI on October 23, 1963. Argentina transplanted its first patient in 1957, and Brazil and Colombia followed in 1965. Between 1963-1968 Especialidades CMN Siglo XXI performed 18 transplants, 13 of them from cadaver donors. Thereafter, activity was scarce until the mid-1970s when the same center transplanted 50 patients in 1975, 18 of them from cadaver donors. In the meantime, 60 kidney transplant centers had been opened around the country. By 1995, a total of 5,965 kidney transplants had been performed in Mexico. New activity began between 1995-1999 when 4,071 patients were transplanted in the country, representing an increase of a 68.2% since 1995. Especialidades CMN Siglo XXI became the first kidney transplant center in Mexico with 1,000 transplants in 1998. In a summary of the past 10 years (1), we reported results from 520 transplants: 367 (70.5%) from living related donors (LRD), 54 (10.3%) from living emotionally-related donors (LERD) and 99 (19%) from cadaver donors (CD). Graft survival at one and 6 years was 99.4% and 85.5% for recipients of LRD kidneys, 98.4% and 75.4% for LERD, and 96.9% and 64.2% for CD transplants, respectively. As of October 2000, we have 118 kidney transplant centers registered and distributed among 29 of 32 federal states in Mexico.

Mexico is one of the most active Latin American countries in transplantation. In Mexico, kidney transplantation is recognized as the best treatment of chronic renal failure and new programs for kidney transplantation are opening. Three kidney transplant centers performed more than 100 transplants annually in 1999: Especialidades No. 71 at Torreon Coahuila (n=126); Especialidades Occidente at Guadalajara (n=125) and Especialidades CMN Siglo XXI at Mexico City (n=107).

There are new attitudes about how to expand the

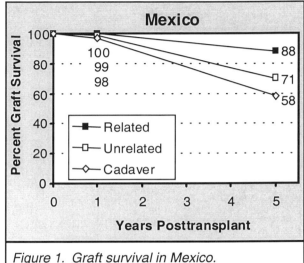

Figure 1. Graft survival in Mexico.

Table 1. Kidney transplants in Mexico.

	1990	1991	1992	1993	1994	1995	1996	1997	1998	1999	Total
Rel	401	456	454	487	495	634	680	776	859	1,016	6,258
Unrel	41	46	54	55	54	67	71	80	89	116	673
Cad	40	45	110	97	104	120	159	170	188	223	1,256

number of kidney transplants. It has been estimated than 60,000 Mexicans have chronic renal failure and 12,000 are in dialysis programs. But just 1,000 kidney transplants are performed annually and we need to perform at least 4,000 to supply the annual demand for transplants. Cadaver organ procurement programs are opening in many federal states. Recently, the National Council of Transplantation (CONATRA) was founded which will organize a National Network for Organ Procurement with advice from the United Network for Organ Sharing (UNOS) in the United States.

Immunosuppression

Immunosuppression is used according to world standards. Initially, we began using azathioprine and when Dr. Starzl reported a better graft survival with prednisone and azathioprine, this combination became the standard Immunosuppression for cadaver and living donor transplants until 1983. Graft irradiation was used for prophylaxis and for treatment of acute rejection and splenectomy was practiced for a short time. Polyclonal antibody was used for induction of transplants. Donor-specific transfusions were used in HLA haplo-identical recipients until the practice was replaced by the introduction of cyclosporine in 1983. Cyclosporine became the baseline immunosuppression with prednisone and azathioprine for the next 15 years for all types of transplants except HLA-identical recipients who were treated with prednisone and azathioprine in some centers. Monoclonal antibody against CD3 (OKT3) was introduced in 1989 and was used as induction and treatment for acute rejection. Induction treatment was used in cadaver or living donor transplant recipients who were at risk because of previous graft loss or high panel antibody reactivity. Since 1990, OKT3 has been used for rescue in cases with steroid-resistant acute rejection. Neoral has been used in Mexico since September 1994, before it was available to transplant centers in the United States and Canada and now we have reported 6 years of experience. Since 1997 we have been involved in many collaborative trials using mycophenolate mofetil, as well as tacrolimus (1998), basiliximab (1999) and sirolimus (2000). In the year 2000, most transplant centers in Mexico are still using the standard immunosuppression based on triple therapy with Neoral, prednisone and azathioprine, but mofetil and tacrolimus have been used as alternatives since 1998.

Kidney Donors

The majority of transplants (73%) are from living related donors; cadaver donors account for 17% and living emotionally related donors for the remaining 10%. Cadaver donors are scarce because of cultural, educational and social factors. On the other hand, transplant coordinators are now recognized as one of the most important professionals in the transplant procurement organizations and many centers have increased their efforts to train them. We think that living related and living emotionally- related donors are important as a source of kidneys for transplantation in Mexico, but centers need to increase cadaver donations to supply the demand for transplants.

Social Issues

A new adjusted general Law of Organ Transplantation was approved by the Mexican Congress in 2000. Improvements were made to the definition of brain death as a loss of life, all deaths are to be considered as potential donors, transplant coordinators are to be the main professionals in procurement programs and more facilities were allocated to deal with legal cases. The governmental National Council of Transplantation (CONATRA) will promote and organize a Network for National Organ Sharing based on a national waiting list and patients will be ranked fairly according to time on the waiting list, histocompatibility, disease status, antibody panel reactivity and previous transplants. Distribution will be local, regional and national. The main obstacle to organized transplantation in Mexico is that there are many levels of governmental and non-governmental health systems performing transplants without a network which have different interests and kinds of patients. Probably the newly elected Government will promote changes and support our efforts to provide the 3,000 transplants that we need, at least in the short term.

References

1. Melchor JL, Gracida C: Kidney transplantation with living donors: Better long-term survival. Transplant Proc 1999; 31:2294.

Kidney Transplantation in Pakistan

S. A. H. Rizvi and S. A. A. Naqvi

Sindh Institute of Urology and Transplantation (SIUT), Dow Medical College, Karachi, PAKISTAN

Pakistan has a population of 133 million people with a per capita income of $500/annum and one third of the people fall below the poverty line. Health expenditures represent about 3% of the GNP. The estimated incidence of end-stage renal disease (ESRD) is 100 per million population. Chronic hemodialysis facilities began to appear in the early 1970's and the first renal transplant was performed in 1979. At that time there were 2 dialysis centers and one transplant center in Pakistan. By 1986 this figure had grown to 5 dialysis centers and 3 transplant centers. In 1999 there were 51 dialysis centers and 9 transplant centers, the majority in the private sector. These facilities are prohibitively expensive increasing the burden on the few government centers with poor resources and a large number of patients. There is a marked urban bias for renal replacement services although two-thirds of the patients reside in the rural areas. In 1999, 1,500 patients were on dialysis and about half of them were waiting for transplants.

Donor Issues

There is a general lack of awareness about transplantation and organ donation and there is no brain death law in Pakistan. Hence, the majority of donors are living. However, 16 non-heart beating cadaveric kidneys have been transplanted at the Sindh Institute of Urology and Transplantation (SIUT) since 1995 with the cooperation of the Eurotransplant Foundation. The first 2 locally procured heart-beating cadaveric kidney transplants were also performed at this center in 1998. Although there are no published figures for the total transplants performed in Pakistan, estimates show that the annual rate is around 6 per million population. The majority of donors are family members although roughly 40% of kidneys are from non-related donors and all of these are performed in private centers.

Studies show that the prospective living donor pool is between 6-10 for every patient. However, poor health, education and cultural constraints reduce this number to one per patient, providing most of them with no more than a once in a lifetime chance of transplantation. In

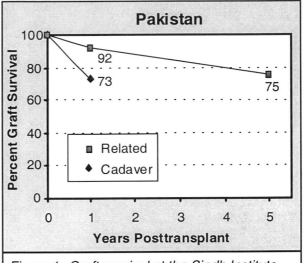

Figure 1. Graft survival at the Sindh Institute, Pakistan.

Table 1. Kidney transplants in Pakistan.

	1990	1991	1992	1993	1994	1995	1996	1997	1998	1999	Total
Rel.	70	80	122	118	147	178	260	360	355	401	2,091
Unrel.	NI	NI	NI	NI	50	80	106	248	267	324	1,075
Cad	0	0	0	0	0	2	3	2	7	4	18

NI: no information

the last decade, SIUT, the largest public sector institution in Karachi has focused on the need for renal replacement services by registering more than 1,000 ESRD patients each year. This activity and the growing number of patients on dialysis all over the country, have alerted the government to the need for state support for dialysis both in public and private sector hospitals. The number of dialysis centers mushroomed from 20 in 1997 to 40 in 1998. Furthermore, in 1998 the state announced financial support for transplantation. Unfortunately, in the absence of cadaver organs this support has provided an impetus for living-unrelated donor renal transplants. These developments are likely to delay the chances for brain-death legislation, which has been pending in the State Senate for the last 5 years and jeopardize the possibility of extra-renal transplants from cadaveric donors.

Tissue Matching

There are 7 tissue-typing centers in Pakistan. Four of the centers perform serological testing for HLA matching. In 1994 SIUT initiated DNA typing methods and by 1999, 3 centers, 2 in the South and one in the North were performing DNA-based HLA typing using PCR with sequence-specific primers. The majority of transplant centers, both public and private, selects donors based on tissue typing criteria.

Immunosuppression

Immunosuppression is based on a triple-drug regimen comprised of steroids, azathioprine and cyclosporine in all centers. Steroid bolus is the mainstay of anti-rejection therapy. Biological agents (ATG or OKT3) are used sparingly for anti-rejection therapy due to their high costs. Two other immunosuppressive drugs, Cellcept and Simulect, have recently become available in Pakistan. Tacrolimus is not available locally but has been used in some centers after direct import. Newer generic cyclosporine formulations have recently been introduced in Pakistan. Drug monitoring facilities for Cyclosporin are available in 3 centers and all use monoclonal antibody assays.

Outcome of Transplants

All of the published literature from Pakistan is based on living-related transplants mostly from one center [1,2]. There is no report on the outcome of living-unrelated transplants nor of their follow-up. Eight hundred and fifty living-related transplants have been performed at SIUT since 1986. The mean age of recipients was 32 years with a male gender bias (M:F ratio of 3:1). SIUT is also the only center that performs pediatric transplants. Of the 850 transplants, 75 (9%) were in pediatric recipients. The mean age of the pediatric recipients was 12 years with a range of 6-17 years and a gender ratio (M:F) of 1.7:1.

The overall mean age of donors was 36 years with a M:F ratio of 1:1. Most of the donors were parents or siblings (84%), but 4% were spouses. Prior to transplant, 92% of the recipients had received blood transfusions because erythropoietin is expensive and sparingly used. Forty percent of the dialysis patients were anti-HCV positive and overall, 15% of the transplanted patients were HCV positive. Pretransplant sensitization was low and 90% of the recipients had a PRA of <10%. Most recipients had 3 HLA antigens matched (69%), 12% had 4-5 antigens matched and 17% were HLA identical. Acute rejections were encountered in 29% of the recipients within the first year. Eighty percent of these were steroid sensitive and the rest required ATG or OKT3 therapy. Overall one- and 5-year graft survival was 92% and 75% and one- and 5-year patient survival was 94% and 81%, respectively. For pediatric patients, the one- and 5-year graft survival was 88% and 65% while patient survival was 90% and 75%, respectively.

Causes of Patient Death and Graft Loss

Posttransplant infections are a major problem in our clinical setting. The incidence of infections requiring hospitalization was 2.1 episodes/patient/year in the first year. After transplantation, 15% of recipients developed TB, 30% had CMV infection and 54% had other bacterial infections. The urinary tract was involved in 60% of the infections. The most common cause of death was infection, which accounted for 74% of deaths with functioning grafts and 23% of deaths with failed grafts. The main causes of graft loss were chronic rejection (58%), infection (23%) and acute rejection (19%). Early detection and control of infection are 2 factors that can improve the outcome of transplants in our setting. Development of newer techniques for TB and CMV diagnosis based on molecular technology at SIUT has contributed to early diagnosis and treatment.

Conclusions

An estimated 6,000-10,000 people require renal transplantation each year in Pakistan, but the overall transplant activity remains around 6 per million population. This maintains a wide gap between the need and number of transplants performed. Government support for dialysis will certainly improve awareness of the ESRD problem in Pakistan. However the absence of a brain-death law and the government's support for transplantation will unfortunately direct transplant activity towards living-unrelated donor transplantation. Any hint of commerce in organs would compromise the ethics and quality of the transplant activity in Pakistan. Keeping in perspective the cultural norms and the lack of public awareness of the benefits of cadaveric donation, there is an urgent need to publicize cadaveric donation. This will help to hold back commercialism in renal transplantation and to promote extra-renal organ transplantations.

References

1. A. Rizvi. Present State of Dialysis and Transplantation in Pakistan. Am. J. Kidney Diseases 1998; 31:xvi-xviii.

2. S. A. Rizvi, S. A. Naqvi, Z. Hussain et al. Factors influencing renal transplantation in a developing country. Transplant Proc 1998; 30:1810.

Organ Transplantation in The Philippines

Enrique T. Ona, Rose Marie Liquete, Benito Purugganan, Antonio Paraiso, and Carlo Ramirez

Departments of Organ Transplantation and Nephrology, National Kidney and Transplant Institute (NKTI), Quezon City, PHILIPPINES

The Philippines is a country of 78 million people with an area the size of New York, New Jersey, Connecticut and Massachusetts combined. It is located just above the equator in Southeast Asia and the people are predominantly of Malay origin. During 350 years of Spanish (1521-1900) and 46 years of American (1900-1946) colonization, both Spanish and American-Filipino intermarriages have produced a sizeable "mestizo" population. Filipino-Chinese interracial mixture has also been going on for several hundred years, so that about 30% of Filipinos have some Chinese blood.

Eighty percent of Filipinos are Catholics, 15% are non-Catholic Christians and 5% are Muslims, the latter found principally in the south, in Mindanao. English is spoken or understood by more than 90% of the population, although Tagalog is the national language with 15 major dialects spoken in the 13 regions of the country. High school and college education, as well as all official documents in courts and in the legislature, use the English language.

Pneumonia and gastroenteritis are still the principal causes of death in children, especially among the poor, but among adults, heart disease, cancer and stroke are now the 3 leading causes of death. End-stage renal disease is the tenth leading cause of death, with an estimated 8,000 Filipinos developing renal failure annually. Hepatoma is the fourth most common cancer and more than 60% of Filipinos have been exposed to Hepatitis B, of whom 12% are carriers. Almost all Filipinos are CMV positive (IgM). Diseases considered to be well under control or non-existent in developed countries, eg. ascariasis, amoebiasis, typhoid fever, malaria and tuberculosis are still common and a source of considerable morbidity and mortality.

The development of organ transplantation in the Philippines followed the advances of transplantation in the United States and Europe. Filipino surgeons and

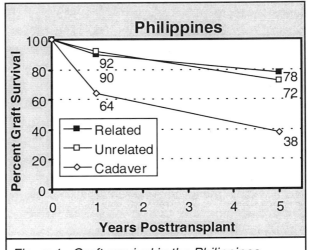

Figure 1. Graft survival in the Philippines.

Table 1. Kidney transplants in the Philippines.

	1990	1991	1992	1993	1994	1995	1996	1997	1998	1999	Total
Rel	77	76	71	99	105	88	101	107	52	81	857
Unrel	3	6	6	6	7	8	11	20	16	37	120
Cad	29	12	23	20	17	17	18	7	7	6	156

nephrologists, most of whom have obtained their postgraduate training abroad, were aware of the epochal works of Medawar, Murray, Hamburger, Starzl, Hume and Calne, but it was the world-wide publicity of the first successful heart transplant performed by Barnard in 1967 that galvanized Filipino surgeons to attempt the first human kidney transplant from a cadaver donor. In December 1968, Dr Enrique Esquivel, a urologist, and Dr Manuel Tayao, a cardiovascular surgeon at the Philippine General Hospital, attempted the first kidney transplantation in the Philippines. The first successful kidney transplant, performed by Dr Antonio Domingo at the UST Hospital in 1969 from a sibling donor, soon followed. The recipient is still alive today with normal creatinine.

In 1970, Drs Picache, who trained under Starzl in Denver, Alano, a nephrologist who trained under Hamburger in Paris, and Ona, after a fellowship with Calne in

Kidney Transplantation in Poland

Piotr Kalicinski, Wojciech Rowinski, Ryszard Grenda, and Janusz Walaszewski

Department of Pediatric Surgery & Organ Transplantation, Children's Memorial Health Institution
Al. Dzieci Polskich, Warsaw, POLAND

The first cadaver kidney transplant in Poland was performed on January 26, 1966, in Warsaw, by Professor Jan Nielubowicz and his team in the first Surgical Department of the Medical University of Warsaw. The operation went well and the patient was discharged home 3 weeks after transplantation. Since then up to December 31, 1999, there have been 6,084 transplants in 5,832 recipients in Poland, including 271 transplants in children. There are 12 kidney transplant centers for adults and one for children (The Children's Memorial Health Institute in Warsaw).

Brain death was not recognized in Poland before 1984, so that harvesting was only possible after the donors' cardiac arrest. The result was a low number of transplants (200-250 in the early 1980's) and a high incidence of ischemic graft dysfunction after transplantation. An announcement of the diagnostic criteria of brain stem death by the Committee nominated by the Ministry of Health in 1984 helped to increase the number of renal transplants to 300-350 per year in the late 1980's as well as to start other organ transplant programs. In the early 1990's, public discussion about organ donation lead to the passage of the Transplant Act by the Polish Parliament in 1996 with the acceptance of presumed consent for organ donation. This Act regulates all legal aspects of the transplantation of cells, tissues and organs from cadaver as well as living donors. The Act introduces the concept of brain stem death and establishes its criteria, regulates the principles of organ allocation, allows for living genetically and emotionally related transplantations and prohibits any attempt at commercial tissue and organ transplantation, specifying severe penalties for such procedures. The Central Registry of Objections to Donation began operating in 1997. Information concerning the right of each citizen to object to donation has been made available in all the media and posted in public places. In 1992, the National Organ Procurement Coordinating Center,

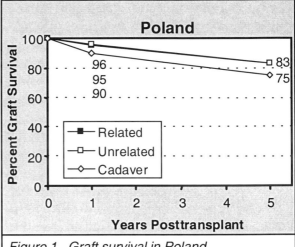

Figure 1. Graft survival in Poland.

Table 1. Kidney transplants in Poland.

	1990	1991	1992	1993	1994	1995	1996	1997	1998	1999	Total
Rel	2	2	3	4	4	2	3	8	8	8	44
Unrel					2	1	3	2	6	8	22
Cad	383	365	309	316	340	350	359	522	541	595	4,080

POLTRANSPLANT, was founded and became an agency of the Ministry of Health in 1996.

Despite the increasing numbers of transplants being performed each year, the application of this treatment still cannot satisfy the need for transplants. Although the number of patients on renal replacement therapy has been rising steadily (in 1999, it reached 200 per million population), still more than 3,000 patients die of chronic renal failure each year (approximately 80-100 per million population).

For a number of reasons, living-related kidney transplantations are performed infrequently in Poland. Only 2.5% of kidney transplants were from living donors in 1999.

The Pediatric Kidney Transplantation Program was started in Poland in 1984 at the Children's Memorial Health Institute in Warsaw and this hospital continues to serve as the only pediatric transplant center in Poland.

Table 2. Pediatric kidney transplants in Poland during last 10 years.

	1990	1991	1992	1993	1994	1995	1996	1997	1998	1999	Total
Rel			1	2	2	2	0	0	2	2	11
Cad	21	18	9	12	11	25	19	22	24	30	191

From 1984 through November 24, 2000, 309 pediatric renal transplants were performed, including 284 cadaver transplants, and 26 living-related donor transplants (8,4% of all pediatric transplants). About 175 children are waiting for a kidney transplant, and the average waiting time is 24-30 months. Two cases of combined liver-kidney transplantations were performed for the first time in Poland in 2000. Since 1996, pediatric patients have been offered all kidneys from donors less than 15 years of age, resulting in a clear increase in the number of children transplanted each year (from 19 in 1996 to 38 in 2000). Overall, the cumulative one- and 5-year patient survival rates are 97% and 96%, respectively. The overall one- and 5-year renal graft survival rates are 90% and 78%, respectively.

Data on kidney transplantations in Poland in the past 10 years are presented in Tables 1 and 2.

Donor-Recipient Immunology

The donor-recipient selection process is decentralized and is done by most centers from their waiting lists. However, all patients awaiting transplantation must be registered on the National Kidney Transplant Waiting List, which also serves as the central tissue typing laboratory for all regional transplant centers. HLA matching between donors and recipients is relatively poor in Poland. In 1999 (595 transplants), 1.2% of recipients were identical at all 4 HLA Class I antigens to their donor, 7.0% had 3 identical antigens, 47.2% had 2 identical antigens, 31.4% had one antigen matched and 9.7% were completely mismatched. For HLA Class II antigens, the respective numbers were: 22.4% (2 matches), 68.5% (1 match), 9.04% (no matches). The average highest panel reactive antibody (PRA) in patients transplanted in 1999 was 8.4% and the average pretransplant PRA was 1.9%.

Immunosuppression

Before 1986, basic immunosuppression after renal transplantation consisted of azathioprine and steroids. Cyclosporine (CsA) was introduced as a third drug in 1986. Mycophenolate mofetil (since 1996) and tacrolimus (since 1999) have been used in selected patients. This year we began a pilot study with sirolimus therapy at the Institute of Transplantology in Warsaw. Inhibitors of interleukin-2 receptor (basiliximab, daclizumab) have been used with increasing frequency during the past few years. The introduction of these new immunosuppressants has significantly improved graft survival.

The history of posttransplant immunosuppression in pediatric recipients includes double- and triple-drug therapy: CsA, azathioprine (AZA) and steroids (P) from 1984, sequential protocols (ATG/OKT3®CsA+AZA+P) from 1988, Neoral® CsA microemulsion formula from 1996, tacrolimus (Prograf®) from 1997, mycophenolate mofetil (MMF, CellCept®) from 1998 and daclizumab (Zenapax®) from 1998. Up to 40% of pediatric renal graft recipients remain on triple therapy, including microemulsion CsA formula (Neoral®) + MMF+P, 10% are on tacrolimus + P and about 20% (high-risk patients) receive quadruple therapy with daclizumab induction.

Future Perspectives of Kidney Transplantation in Poland

An active program of donor identification was initiated 3 years ago within the medical community to increase the number of organs available for transplantation. Improved cooperation between local community hospitals and transplantation centers and the support of society are important factors, which may help to expand cadaver donor organ transplantation. At the same time, more centers are activating living related donor programs to increase number of patients transplanted.

POLAND

Kidney Transplantation in Portugal

Alfredo Mota and Linhares Furtado

University Hospital of Coimbra, Dept of Urology and Transplantation, 3030 Coimbra, PORTUGAL

Renal transplantation in Portugal began in June 1969 at the University of Coimbra with a transplant from a woman to her brother. Later in the same year, 2 additional living-related donor transplants were performed in Lisbon. The first legislation regarding issues of brain death and organ and tissue procurement from brain-dead cadaver donors and from living donors was enacted in 1976. Four years later, in 1980, cadaveric renal transplantation programs were established in Coimbra and Lisbon. These were the only transplant centers in Portugal at that time. By 1999, there were 2 centers in Oporto, one in Coimbra and 4 in Lisbon – 7 centers serving a population of 10 million people. Portugal has a "presumed consent" law for cadaver donations. A National Registry database (RENNDA) was created by the State Department of Health and any citizen may simply declare to opt out and that will be registered. The number of people who register as non-donors has been very low (fewer than 0.5%).

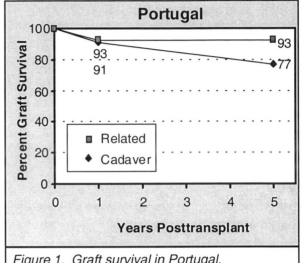

Figure 1. Graft survival in Portugal.

Tissue Typing and Selection of Donor and Recipient Pairs

There are 3 tissue-typing centers in Portugal, one each in Coimbra, Lisbon and Oporto. Their work is coordinated through a national organization called *Luso-Transplante*. These 3 centers provide all histocompatibility testing for transplants performed in Portugal. The waiting list for kidney transplantation in Portugal includes 1,409 patients among the approximately 7,000 patients on dialysis. Of these, 1,242 are awaiting a first transplant, 161 are waiting for a second graft and 6 are waiting for their third transplant. Five coordinating centers, one in Coimbra, 2 in Lisbon and 2 in Oporto, complete the transplantation organization in Portugal.

The selection of recipients when a cadaver donor is available is based on the following criteria:
1. ABO blood group compatibility
2. A negative crossmatch with the donor
3. Clinical urgency
4. Better HLA matching (HLA-DR>HLA-B>HLA-A)
5. The length of time waiting
6. Weight (body mass index<30 kg/m^3) and age (ages 3-70 are accepted) compatibility

We consider 3 grades of clinical urgency: maximum urgency, for patients without vascular access who cannot be placed on peritoneal dialysis; urgency I, for patients with clinical considerations such as diabetes or pediatric patients with 2 HLA antigens matched with the donor (one in HLA-DR); and urgency II for all other patients. Patients with a status of maximum urgency are transplanted with an ABO and crossmatch compatible donor without regard to the other criteria. Kidneys are allocated on a regional basis, except for maximum urgency patients, broadly sensitized patients (>50% PRA) and pediatric patients, who are selected from the national waiting list.

Table 1. Kidney transplants in Portugal.

	1990	1991	1992	1993	1994	1995	1996	1997	1998	1999	Total
Rel	1	0	0	0	2	2	3	6	4	9	28*
Cad	256	304	367	286	341	361	402	385	309	367	3,378

* 2 LRDTx in 1986

The Number of Renal Transplants (1980-1999)

Between June 1980 and December 1999, 4,429 transplants were performed in Portugal. They included 4,213 first grafts, 208 second grafts and 8 patients who received a third transplant. All but 28 transplants (99.4%) were from cadaver donors, 80% of whom died from trauma and 20% of whom had suffered cerebrovascular accidents. The mean waiting time for a kidney transplant was 22 months. Twenty-eight patients received living-related donor transplants. Living donation is permitted between third degree relatives, however, Portuguese law does not permit unrelated living donor transplants.

The mean age of transplant recipients in Portugal is 40.8 years (range of 3-69) and 65% of recipients are male. Nearly all recipients (99.5%) are caucasian with the remainder of African descent. The primary diseases are distributed among glomerular diseases (19.8%), tubulointerstitial diseases (14.7%), cystic/congenital diseases (14.2%) and systemic vascular diseases (16.2%). The disease has not been reported or was unknown for 35.1% of recipients. The mean number of HLA antigen matches is 2.2 and the median cold ischemia time is 21.0 hours.

Immunosuppression consisted of azathioprine and prednisone until 1984. After December 1984, all centers introduced cyclosporine A. In 1998, according to the Portuguese Society of Transplantation, the breakdown of baseline immunosupression for 3,548 transplants was: Pred/Aza/CsA (44.7%), Pre/CsA (22.6%), Pred/CsA/Antithymocyte globulin [ATG] (8.5%), Pred/Aza/CsA/ATG (7.7%), Pred/Aza (5.5%) and Pred/CsA/MMF (5.1%). Graft survival rates over the past 10 years are shown in Figure 1.

Overall, 2.3% of kidneys never functioned, and 23.3% had delayed graft function. During the past 5 years, the acute rejection rate has fallen from 43.7% in 1995 to 34.6% in 1996 (when mycophenolate mofetil was introduced in October) to 33.6% in 1997 and to 23.7% in 1998 and 1999. The major causes of graft loss were death with graft function (40.4%), chronic rejection (29.0%), acute rejection (6.7%), technical or thrombosis (5.8%), noncompliance (3.8%), infection (2.8%, recurrent disease (2.0%) and other deaths (7.4%). Most deaths were cardiovascular (46.4%), followed by infection (25.4%), hepatic failure (6.5%), malignancies (6.5%) and all others (15.2%).

Conclusion

The cadaver renal transplant programs in Portugal have benefitted our end-stage renal disease patients as our actuarial graft survival rates for first cadaveric transplants (91% and 75% one and five years, respectively) attest. The rate of transplantation in Portugal is between 35-40 per million population per year and is the sixth highest in Europe. However, we recognize that the very low rate of living donations must be increased quickly.

Kidney Transplantation in Puerto Rico

E. A. Santiago-Delpín, Z. González-Caraballo, L. Morales-Otero, N. Cruz, C. Guerra, J. O. Pérez, E. Rivé-Mora, and A. Acosta-Otero

The Puerto Rico Transplant Program, Auxilio Mutuo Hospital; and the Departments of Surgery, Pediatrics and Medicine, University of Puerto Rico Medical School, San Juan, PUERTO RICO

The island of Puerto Rico, a United States commonwealth and the smallest of the Caribbean Greater Antilles (3,500 square miles of territory), has a population of 3.8 million inhabitants of mixed European, African, and Native American origin who speak Spanish as native language although the majority can also speak English.

Although the first kidney transplants in Puerto Rico were performed between 1968-1974, it was not until 1977 that a program was inaugurated at the San Juan Veteran's Administration Hospital, and that the first protocol-monitored patients were transplanted within the context of a formal program with trained dedicated personnel. After the first 135 successful transplants, the program was transferred to the Auxilio Mutuo Hosptial because of the non-veteran caseload and personnel constrains, where it has performed the rest of the transplants, which now total more than 800 cases. Auxilio Mutuo Hospital is a 613-bed university-affiliated general hospital with a full complement of tertiary services and consultants.

The program currently consists of 3 transplant surgeons, 4 donor surgeons, 3 additional surgical associates, 2 urologists, 3 adult nephrologists, 3 pediatric nephrologists, an administrator, 2 managers, a medical social worker, a transplant dietitian, 6 transplant coordinators, a data coordinator, 5 secretaries, plus residents, fellows and students. The organ procurement organization, LifeLink of Puerto Rico, includes an executive director, a medical director, 6 organ and tissue coordinators, 3 hospital developers, and 2 secretaries. The histocompatibility laboratory consists of a medical director, a technical supervisor, and 5 tissue typing technicians. A 27-bed transplant ward services all transplant admissions. The program and all its components are accredited by the appropriate local and United States federal agencies.

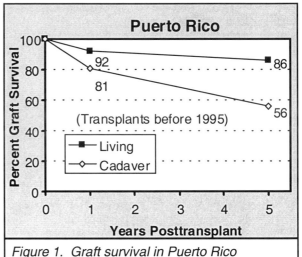

Figure 1. Graft survival in Puerto Rico

Table 1. Kidney transplants in Puerto Rico.

	1990	1991	1992	1993	1994	1995	1996	1997	1998	1999	Total*
Rel	18	20	23	20	19	19	14	20	28	19	427
Unrel	4	7	6	4	0	6	4	6	3	5	54
Cad	13	9	9	13	13	12	7	15	40	32	317

*Total count:1977-2000

Donation and Transplantation

As in most Latin-American countries, cadaver donation in Puerto Rico was meager until recently. A number of local and Latin-American studies demonstrated that the main reasons for low donation were cultural, eg., a particularly severe grief reaction and an ill-defined decision making process by the family were major obstacles. A poor relationship with intensive care units as well as low staffing and mistrust completed the cultural block against donation. Importantly, the Program started living emotionally-related transplantation in 1990 with excellent results. The donation situation changed dramatically when LifeLink of Tampa agreed to develop an organ procurement organization in Puerto Rico. Calls with offers increased 100-fold and organ donation increased 6-fold. With this collaboration, cadaver transplantation not only increased in absolute numbers, but also became more prevalent than living donor transplantation.

Immunosuppression and Survival

Patients in Era-I (1977-1980) received prednisone, azathioprine, and prophylactic Minnesota anti-lymphoblast globulin (MALG), while Era-II (after 1980) patients received low-dose prednisone, azathioprine, and MALG both prophylactical and for rejection. In 1984 we incorporated cyclosporine alone and later as triple therapy, while continuing the use of MALG. In 1990, the monoclonal, OKT3, and anti-thymocyte globulin were used for rejection. We started using tacrolimus as rescue therapy in 1994, and with its use we achieved 86% graft survival for acute intractable rejection and 67% for acute and chronic rejection. Before 1995, the graft survival rate for living donor transplants was 92% and for cadaver donor transplants it was 81% at one year. The corresponding 5-year graft survival rates were 86% and 56%, respectively.

In 1995, we started using mycophenolate mofetil (MMF) and discontinued Aza in new transplants. In January of 1999, basiliximab was started routinely in living and cadaver donor transplants, and in October 1999 rapamycin was started in combination either with Neoral, tacrolimus, or MMF as part of an ongoing center study. Low-dose prednisone (5-7.5 mg per day at 6 months) is our current practice. Basiliximab is used in all cases. The 3-month rejection-free survival rate is 100% and graft survival is 100%. The current one-year patient survival rate is 97.1% and graft survival is 94.2% (data from US Healthcare Financing Administration).

Morbidity

Postoperative bladder leaks and wound infections are seen in only 1.5% and 1.0% of patients, respectively, and lymphoceles in 6%. Common and rare infections occur in our transplant program as they do in the rest of the world. However, we have a very high incidence of cutaneous and nail fungi, especially in our old series based on high-dose prednisone and azathioprine. Gancyclovir is used routinely in high-risk patients. Trimethoprim/sulfamethoxazole is used in all cases, as is oral mycostatin. Varicella is seen frequently, and a prevention protocol has resulted in a very low mortality. Cancer incidence is 2%. Abdominal and gastrointestinal complications are frequent, but early diagnosis and aggressive treatment have resulted in a low mortality, with zero mortality for gastrointestinal bleeding.

Academic, Administrative, and Legal

A brain death law was passed in 1983, and in 1985 – a precedent, we think – a law was approved for the state financing of cyclosporine, which was subsequently extended to other immunosuppressive drugs. The transplant program has participated in the development of administrative, clinical, patient, and research societies locally and internationally including the Latin American Transplant Registry and has actively helped in the development of at least 2 Latin American and one international society. A multi-author, 79-chapter, 915-page, 2-edition textbook on organ transplantation was produced and co-edited in our program, as well as more than 200 research publications.

The transplant program in Puerto Rico has served the Island for 23 years, with more than 800 transplants and thousands of operations on renal patients, and it has made multiple academic, legal, administrative, research, and clinical contributions as well.

PUERTO RICO

Renal Transplants in Russia

L.P. Alexeev [a,] *A.G. Dolbin* [b] *and A.V. Sechkin* [b]

[a] *National Research Center Institute of Immunology,* [b] *Moscow Coordinating Center for Organ Donation, Moscow, RUSSIA*

The first successful related renal transplant was conducted in the USSR in 1965. By 1991, 21 republican and regional renal transplant centers had been established in the territory of the USSR, including 7 centers in Moscow. At that time the Soviet scientists participated in the "Intertransplant" international program, which involved all countries of the former socialist camp. At that stage of the transplant program, donor kidneys were exchanged both within the Soviet Union and among the transplant centers in East Germany (DDR), the Czech Republic (ChSSR), Hungary (PRH), Poland (PRP), and Bulgaria (PRB). The methods to evaluate, monitor, condition and manage donors and to preserve donor organs were standardized. Common approaches for both tissue typing of donors and recipients as well as immunosuppressive therapies were used. By 1990, 7,500 cadaver donor and 225 living related renal transplants had been performed. The actuarial one- and 5-year survival rates (Fig. 1) were 81% and 61%, respectively.

The healthcare system established in the Soviet Union as an integral part of the whole totalitarian society created special terms and difficulties for developing transplantation clinics. It was only in 1985 that an official law was enacted permitting the diagnosis of brain death. The wait resulted in a considerable delay both in time and statistics for heart transplants, heart-lung complex, lung, liver and pancreas transplants.

Because of economic difficulties and the complete absence of a national program, we have not been able to perform the number of vital organ transplants that are needed. At the time of the USSR, no legislative basis for regulating organ transplants was established and financing mechanisms were not sufficiently developed. Society was not well informed about the aims, opportunities, results and problems of transplantation.

However, after the Soviet Union disintegrated at the end of 1992, the law on the transplantation of organs and/or tissues was established. In accordance with the

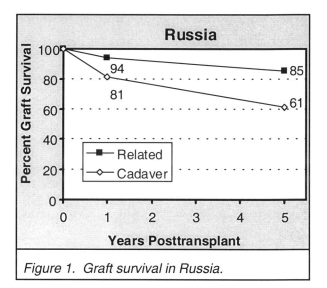

Figure 1. Graft survival in Russia.

Table 1. Kidney transplants in Russia.

	1990	1991	1992	1993	1994	1995	1996	1997	1998	1999	Total
Rel	31	36	39	34	23	20	15	13	10	14	235
Cad	361	355	433	399	352	400	369	405	459	343	3,876

World Healthcare Organization it regulates all legal relationships in the field of transplantation. As far as organ donation is concerned, a judicial model of "presumed consent" is used. According to the law, organ donations from living unrelated donors are prohibited and donor commercialization is prosecuted.

Currently there are 9 cities in the territory of Russia where transplant centres function: Moscow, Saint-Petersbourg, Novosybirsk, Ekaterinbourg, Omsk, Barnaul, Kemerovo and Ufa. The total number of transplantations performed annually is 470-520. About 350-400 of them are performed at 8 transplant centres in the Moscow region. Seven of the Moscow centres perform transplantations on recipients from different areas of Russia. Thus, the 8 Moscow transplant centers perform 90% of the total transplants in our country. In 1995, the Moscow Coordinating Center for Organ Donation was established to coordinate a single waiting list of candidates for each kind of organ transplant. The Coordinating Center provides for the management and preservation of donor kidneys and other organs for transplantation as well as for donor and recipient tissue typing. The Coordinating Center distributes donor organs for transplants and facilitates their exchange among regional centers according to the single waiting list and based on a computerized selection algorithm. Its structure comprises a tissue typing laboratory and surgical team. The tissue typing laboratory provides:

- HLA genotyping and monitoring of the pre-existing antibody level in the waiting patients under treatment in one of the Moscow transplant centers.
- HLA-genotyping and selection of potential donors.

The surgical team is responsible for identification, evaluation and monitoring of potential donors, as well as the management, removal and storage of organs. Independent neurological and forensic medicine teams are an integral part of the surgical team. The neurological team confirms brain death and the forensic medicine team issues permission for organ removal based on qualified forensic expertise.

Moscow has the only established and functioning Coordinating Center for Organ Donation in Russia; however, other regional centers are being organized according to the same scheme in our country. In the near future a similar transplant center will open in Saint Petersbourg.

Since 1995 the waiting list for renal transplants has included 2,380 recipients; 794 donors were used and 1,576 kidney transplants, 36 heart transplants (127 since 1987), and 29 liver transplants were performed. We have selected donor and recipient pairs based on HLA DNA genotyping since 1996 and the graft survival rates for renal transplants have significantly increased during the past 4 years. Our transplantation results over the past 10 years averaged 81% and 61% one- and 5-year graft survival, respectively, but after 1996 the survival rates significantly increased to 86% and 78% at one and 5 years. We should note that in the group where donors and recipients were compatible for 2 HLA-DRB1 specificities, the one-year survival rate was 94% and at 5 years it was 84%. HLA-DRB1-compatible transplants were given to 37% of recipients.

HLA-DRB1 compatibility provided better transplant function. After one year of follow-up, rejection episodes were registered in 32% of these recipients compared with 48% who had rejections among the group of transplants sharing only one HLA-DRB1 specificity. After one year of follow-up, the group of DRB1-compatible patients had no irreversible rejections compared with 7.5 % irreversible rejections in the group with one DRB1 compatible specificity. At the 5-year follow-up, irreversible rejections were observed in 4% and 22%, respectively.

Hence, due to the selection based on HLA-DRB1 genotyping, the efficacy of transplantation was increased. The 5-year graft survival rates were 12% higher (84% vs. 72%) when comparing HLA-DRB1 compatible grafts with those that shared only one HLA-DRB1 specificity with the recipients.

RUSSIA

Renal Transplantation in South Africa

D. Kahn [a], J.R. Botha [b], S. Naicker [c], V.O.L. Karrusseitt [d], A. Haffejee [d] and M.D. Pascoe [a]

Universities of [a] Cape Town, [b] Witwatersand, [c] Natal and [d] Pretoria, SOUTH AFRICA

South Africa has a very rich history of renal transplantation. The first kidney transplant was performed in Johannesburg in 1967 and currently transplants are performed in each of the major centers. Initially, transplantation was limited to the 7 academic teaching institutions. However, in recent years, private institutions in Johannesburg, Cape Town and Durban have established renal transplant programmes.

In this study, we report the results of renal transplantation from the centers in Johannesburg (academic and non-academic), Cape Town, Pretoria and Durban.

Patients and Methods

All patients undergoing renal transplantation in the 4 major centers in South Africa, between January 1990 and December 1999, were included in the study. Standard surgical techniques were used for the procurement of kidneys and the subsequent implantation into the recipients. All kidneys were preserved in Eurocollins solution. The immunosuppression protocol consisted of cyclosporine, steroids and azathioprine. Center A introduced induction therapy with ATG for high-risk patients, including black patients, in October 1988. At Center B, cyclosporine was withdrawn at one year after transplantation and the patients were maintained on steroids and azathioprine.

Cadaver kidneys were allocated according to a negative lymphocytotoxic crossmatch, ABO compatibility and HLA matching. In Center A, kidneys were shared equally between the academic and private institutions. At Center B, kidneys were shared equally between the 2 academic institutions in that region. Centers C and D were the only transplant programmes in those regions.

The patient and graft survival rates were calculated using the Kaplan-Meier method. In the analysis of graft survival, death with a functioning graft was included as a lost graft.

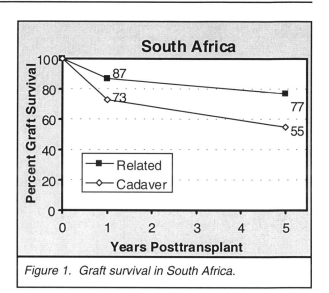

Figure 1. Graft survival in South Africa.

Table 1. Kidney transplants in South Africa.

	1990	1991	1992	1993	1994	1995	1996	1997	1998	1999	Total
Living	9	27	37	42	46	61	58	46	64	56	446
Total	229	186	194	235	256	279	247	219	225	229	2,299

Results

During the 10-year study period, a total of 2,299 cadaver donor renal transplants were undertaken. The number of transplants performed at Centers A, B, C and D were 1,014, 811, 258 and 216, respectively. There were a total of 446 (19.7%) living-related donor transplants included in the study. The proportion of living-related donor transplants increased from below 10% initially to over 20% currently. The proportion of living-related donor transplants at Centers A, B, C and D was 16.3%, 12.3%, 59.7% and 13.9%, respectively.

The total number of transplants performed each year has remained unchanged over the 10-year study period (Table 1). However, there has been a steady increase in the number of living-related donor transplants from 27 in 1991 to 64 in 1998.

The graft survival rates at one and 5 years for cadaver donor transplants were 73% and 55%, respectively (Fig. 1). In contrast, the graft survival rates at one and 5 years for living-related donor transplants were 87% and 77%, respectively. The overall patient survival rates at one and 5 years were 90% and 75%, respectively (Fig. 2). The overall graft survival rates at one and 5 years were 76% and 59%, respectively.

Discussion

Renal transplantation is performed on a routine basis in all the major centers in South Africa. The concept of brain death, the mechanisms for organ donor referral and the network of the transplant co-ordinators are well established. The 5-year graft survival rate with cadaver kidneys was 55%. There are several factors which impact negatively on graft survival. South Africa has a very heterogeneous population and the chances of getting an HLA well-matched cadaver transplant are very low. Many of our patients were from a lower socio-economic background and sometimes have difficulty in follow-up. In addition, many of the transplants were in black patients.

South Africa has a multi-racial, multi-cultural and multi-religious society. All of these factors influence attitudes towards transplantation and organ donation. For example, Muslim families almost never consent to organ donation. Similarly, black families are reluctant to agree to organ donation, although the consent rate has increased in recent years and now exceeds 40%.

Infection with HIV has not been as much of a problem as expected. The non-acceptance rate due to HIV positivity amongst potential cadaver donors has been less than 5%.

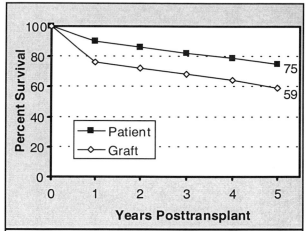

Figure 2. Overall patient and graft survival rates in South Africa.

The majority of transplants in South Africa are from cadaver donors. However, the proportion of living-related donor transplants has increased from less than 10% in the early part of the study, to more than 20% currently. The 5-year graft survival rate was 77% for living-related donor transplants. Very few living-unrelated donor transplants have been performed.

Donor hearts and livers are shared on a national basis for transplantation. In contrast, sharing of kidneys occurs to a limited extent and is on a regional basis. One of the difficulties with sharing is the distance between centers and the problems with transportation.

In conclusion, renal transplant programmes are well established in South Africa. Of concern is the fact that the number of cadaver donor transplants has not changed in the past 10 years.

SOUTH AFRICA

Kidney Transplantation in Spain – 1990-2000

B. Miranda, M.T. Naya, E. Fernández-Zincke, R. Matesanz, and J.J. Amenábar[a]

Organización Nacional de Trasplantes (ONT)[a] the Spanish Group for Dialysis and Kidney Transplant Registry, Madrid, SPAIN

Spain is a European Community country with a population of 39.6 million people. The National Health System is composed of all facilities and public services devoted to health. Today public health assistance is available for 99.4% of the population.

The first kidney transplants were performed in 1965 at the Clinic Hospital in Barcelona. Since then, more than 26,000 kidney transplants have been performed in Spain. Table 1 lists the activity during the past decade and Figure 1 shows survival rates for living and cadaveric kidney transplants for the same time. The living and non-heart beating donor kidney survival rates shown are the results from one different single center in each case (1,2).

Several developments have contributed to the increase in the number of transplants in Spain. Our transplant law was enacted in 1979, and it has been reviewed and updated in 1980, 1986, 1996 and 1999. It provides an adequate legal framework, similar to corresponding laws in other countries. But the law was not the only factor that motivated the change in transplant activity. The need for offering an integrated treatment to patients with end-stage renal disease resulted in the establishment of a real transplant culture, based on the belief that it was necessary to identify donors and to establish a suitable infrastructure to take advantage of donations. In 1989, a unique organization within the Spanish administrative system was born. The Organizacion Nacional de Trasplantes (ONT) began with the charge of coordinating all the activities related to organ donation and the transplantation of organs, tissues and cells within the whole state. However, its work is focused on organ procurement and developing a network of professionals working at all levels - national, regional and hospital. The ONT has a formal but flexible structure that ensures efficacy, guarantees transparency and equity and is accountable for performance (3).

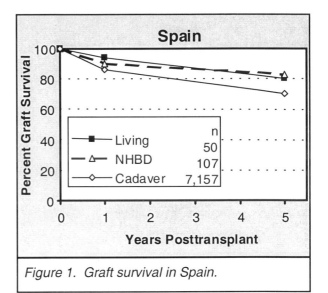

Figure 1. Graft survival in Spain.

Table 1. Kidney transplant activity in Spain.

	1990	1991	1992	1993	1994	1995	1996	1997	1998	1999	2000	Total
Living	16	16	15	20	20	35	22	20	19	17	19	219
Cad	1224	1355	1477	1473	1613	1765	1685	1841	1976	2006	1919	18,334
Non-heart beating donor (NHBD)						41	52	42	43	42		220

Evolution of Organ Donation and Transplantation

The organ donor rate in Spain has increased from 18 to 34 donors per million population (pmp) since 1990. Table 2 shows this remarkable evolution. The rate of family refusal has decreased in the past 10 years from 28% to 21-22% and has remained stable since 1997.

We have noticed important changes in the characteristics of solid organ donors during the past 10 years. The average donor age has increased by more than 10 years from (38 ± 12 to 49 ± 13 yrs) and more than 32% of our current donors are older than age 60. More than 11% of donors are now older than age 70! Traditionally, most potential donors were cranial trauma victims, but we have seen a reversal in the percentage of deaths caused by trauma and stroke. In 1992, 39% of our do-

Table 2. Improving donation rates in Spain.											
	1990	1991	1992	1993	1994	1995	1996	1997	1998	1999	2000
Cadaveric donors	681	778	832	869	960	1037	1032	1155	1250	1334	1345
Organ donors rate pmp	17.1	20.2	21.7	22.6	25.0	27.0	26.8	29.0	31.5	33.6	33.9

nors died from stroke and 43% died in car accidents. In 2000, these percentages were 57% and 21%, respectively. These changes in the donor age and cause of death profiles have also led to an increase in the number of organs discarded once examined. Between 8-10% of our donors, since the mid-1990's, were donors from whom no solid organ could be used after the retrieval, because of a lack of recipients or histological findings in the kidney itself. Age, hypertension or diabetic antecedents are clear determining factors that influence the organ discard rate (4).

References

1. Felipe C, Oppenheimer F, Plaza JJ. Trasplante Renal de vivo: una opción terapéutica real. Nefrología 2000; 20:8.

2. Alvarez J, del Barrio R, Arias J, et al. Non heart-beating donors: Estimated actual potential. Transplant Proc 2001; 33 (In press).

3. Matesanz R, Miranda B, Felipe C. Organ procurement in Spain: The impact of transplant coordination. Clin Transplantation 1994; 8:281.

4. Miranda B, Cañon J, Cuende N. The Spanish organizational structure for organ donation: update. Transplant Rev 2001; 15:1.

Kidney Transplantation in Switzerland

Markus Weber [a], Nicolas Demartines [a], Patrice Ambühl [b], Zakiyah Kadry [a], and Pierre-Alain Clavien [a]

[a]*Clinic of Visceral and Transplantation Surgery,* [b]*Division of Nephrology, University Hospital Zürich, SWITZERLAND*

Solid organ transplantation in Switzerland started 36 years ago with the first kidney transplantation performed at the University Hospital of Zürich in December 1964 (1). During the past 4 decades, almost 5,000 kidneys were grafted at 6 transplantation centers in Switzerland (Basel, Bern, Geneva, Lausanne, St. Gallen and Zürich). Leukocyte antigen matching between donor and recipient was introduced 4 years after the first kidney transplantation and rapidly became a routine procedure in most centers. HLA tissue typing has evolved from a technique using serological methods to one that employs a polymerase chain-reaction procedure and is performed in each transplantation center under the surveillance of the national reference laboratory in Geneva. Since the foundation of SwissTransplant in 1985, transplantation activities have been coordinated by this private organization, including a national exchange program for highly sensitized patients (2). Although, the first kidney transplantation from a living donor was performed very early in 1966 at the University Hospital of Zürich, the living donation program did not become clinically important until the early 1980's. The University Hospital of Basel introduced the first register for living kidney donation. This national register gives us full transparency regarding the origin of all transplanted organs from living donors, and should prohibit any commerce of these organs. The organ shortage has encouraged the development of living donation at most centers in Switzerland, and today approximately 25% of all transplanted kidneys are from living donors (Table 1). Thanks to the introduction of living donation, it has been possible to maintain a stable equilibrium between the demand and supply of renal grafts with a waiting time between 1.5-2.5 years. Recently, a laparoscopic approach to kidney procurement from living donors was introduced at 3 centers (Basel, Lausanne, Zurich) and might facilitate the promotion of living donation.

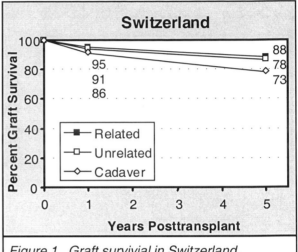

Figure 1. Graft survivial in Switzerland.

Table 1. Kidney transplants in Switzerland.

	1990	1991	1992	1993	1994	1995	1996	1997	1998	1999	Total
Rel	13	11	26	32	30	32	25	36	52	33	290
Unrel	1	2	0	12	7	8	17	17	15	29	108
Cad	207	201	190	208	209	166	157	190	201	198	1,927

The organ shortage problem has also been approached by the use of non heart-beating donors; however, non heart-beating donors are presently accepted at only 2 centers (Zürich and Geneva) in Switzerland. This approach has added approximately 10% more organs to the kidney program at the University Hospital of Zürich since 1985. Moreover, the long-term outcome of these organs at our institution is almost identical to that of kidneys retrieved from heart-beating donors and the results provide a rationale to establish such non-heart-beating programs at other centers.

Combined renal and pancreatic transplantation was also initiated at a very early stage in Switzerland - in 1973. Since then, approximately 180 such procedures have been carried out, beginning with a segmental pancreas graft using the duct occlusion technique, then evolving to bladder drainage. Since 1996, enteric drainage has been performed in most cases. Although, the first clinical islet transplantation was done in 1978 in Zürich, this program was interrupted for several years due to a lack of success. Presently with the introduction of new isolation techniques and new immunosuppressive protocols, combined islet and kidney transplantation has experienced a renaissance in the last few years in Geneva and Zürich.

New immunosuppressive agents such as mycophenolate mofetil, tacrolimus and IL-2-receptor antagonists have advanced kidney transplantation in Switzerland as in other centers around the world. However, cyclosporine and prednisone are still the first choices for primary immunosuppression at most centers. Several national and international studies are currently testing new protocols, including steroid- or calcineurin-free immunosuppression.

One major obstacle in the field of transplantation over the last years in our country has been the lack of a national transplantation law. The Swiss health system is governed by cantonal authorities (there are 24 cantons in Switzerland), and this has led to a variety of different regulations regarding legal aspects of transplantation and organ procurement. Until now, important aspects of transplantation, including brain death diagnosis, have been based on guidelines of the Swiss Academy for Medical Sciences. In February 1997, a nationwide vote changed the federal constitution of Switzerland, which now allows the development of a new law for transplantation. Several important aspects of this new legislation are being thoroughly discussed. One key element of the new law is the regulation of organ allocation and whether organs should be allocated on a center-based list with regional distribution (as is currently done) or on a national waiting list. A second point of discussion will focus on the form of consent (presumed or informed consent) for cadaver donation, which will be applied in Switzerland in the future. Currently the legal situation for this question remains confusing since every canton has its own legislation.

In summary, during the past 4 decades kidney transplantation has became routine in a number of transplantation programs throughout Switzerland. Living donation and the use of non heart-beating donors have helped us to control the organ shortage for kidney transplantation. The new federal transplantation law will soon give us a legal basis with which to face future problems in the fast-moving field of transplantation.

References

1. Candinas D, Schlumpf R, Röthlin R, et al. In: JM Cecka and PI Terasaki, Eds. Clinical Transplants 1996. Los Angeles UCLA Tissue Typing Laboratory, 1997:241.

2. SwissTransplant. Annual review 1999. Geneva, Swisstransplant, 1999.

Transplantation in Taiwan

Chen-Jean Lee

National Taiwan University Hospital, Taipei, TAIWAN

Renal allograft transplantation was not a promising mode of treatment for end-stage renal disease (ESRD) in Asia before 1967. The first successful living-related kidney transplantation was performed by C.J. Lee at the National Taiwan University Hospital (NTUH) on May 27, 1968. Since then, we have been increasingly successful in restoring relatively normal lives to otherwise dying patients with end-stage organ failure by means of solid organ transplantation. In addtion to the kidney, we have also had good fortune with heart, lung, liver, pancreas, and heart-lung transplantation in Taiwan.

Renal Transplantation

Kidney transplantation is already a clinical reality with a very favorable outcome. The one-year graft survival rate after living-related renal transplantation is 91% and at 5 years it is 77%. The one- and 5-year graft survival rates for cadaver renal transplant recipients are 80% and 63%, respectively, in Taiwan.

In this part of the world, most living donors are relatives of the recipient. Some Asian countries are using spouses and unrelated living donors, but as a result, organ purchase, organ snatching and kidnapping are not infrequently reported in those areas. We rarely harvest unrelated living donor kidneys for transplantation since our Transplantation Act legislation, which was passed in 1987, prohibits organ purchase in Taiwan. However, on very few occasions, kidneys from spouses are used. These transplants are indicated in Table 1. as "off-shore". In Taiwan, 89.1% of renal grafts are from cadaver donors pronounced dead either by conventional or brain death criteria.

The hepatitis B virus (HBV) carrier rates are the same in the pre- and posttransplant periods (20.5%), and that is the same incidence as that of the general population. Hepatitis C virus (HCV) antibody prevalences are 32.8% and 46.3% in the pre- and posttransplantation periods, respectively. These rates are significantly higher than

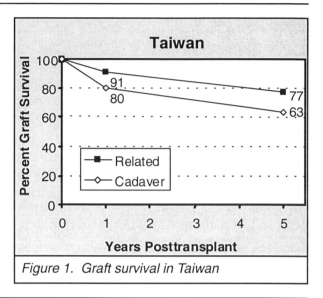

Figure 1. Graft survival in Taiwan

Table 1. Kidney transplants in Taiwan.

	1990	1991	1992	1993	1994	1995	1996	1997	1998	1999	Total
Rel	25	29	10	16	10	8	10	8	11	12	139
Unrel*	5	102	91	37	26	36	34	45	44	62	482
Cad	77	235	229	172	135	116	124	183	177	146	1,594

* off-shore (Mainland China)

the prevalence in the general population (4.2%). Renal transplantation is one of the routes by which HCV is transmitted. The prevalence of chronic liver disease is high in renal transplant recipients, and hepatoma is among the main causes of patient death after renal transplantation.

Among those renal transplant recipients with positive anti-HCV, the hepatitis B surface antigen (HBsAg)-positive group had a significantly higher incidence of chronic hepatitis (50.0% vs. 25.5%, p=0.026) and liver cirrhosis (21.4% vs. 0%, p=0.001), than the HBsAg-negative group. Coinfection with hepatitis HBV and HCV may lead to aggressive liver disease and cirrhosis. The difference in the incidence of chronic hepatitis between azathioprine (Aza)-treated and cyclosporine (CsA)-treated groups was not statistically significant (78.6% in the Aza group vs. 52.4% in the CsA group, p=0.12).

Moreover, HBsAg-positive patients have an increased risk of hepatitis D virus superinfection after renal transplantation, and this may result in rapid progression to liver cirrhosis. Wu, et al. noted that Taiwanese renal transplant recipients have a higher incidence of cancer and that the most frequent type of cancer is hepatocellular cancer, which differs from the cancer reported in transplant recipients in the United States and Europe.

Transplantation of Other Organs

C.L. Chen at Chang Gung Memorial Hospital (CGMH) in Taipei carried out the first whole organ liver transplant in the orthotopic position on March 23, 1984. He had an excellent success in a series of patients with metabolic liver failure (Wilsonian Cirrhosis). The average adult one-year survival rate has been 86.0% and 5-year survival generally has been 42.0%. Children undergoing orthtopic liver transplantation have better results; the one- year survival rate is 80.2% and at 5 years it is 63.0%. Reduced-size liver transplants, either from cadaver or related living donors, have been remarkably successful in 34 cases transplanted between 1994-1999.

The first successful heart transplantation in Taiwan was performed on July 6, 1987 by S.H. Chu at NTUH. As of December 1999, 325 cases of heart whole organ transplantation had been performed with one- and 5-year patient survival rates of 70% and 50%, respectively. These results are comparable with those reported from the International Registry of Heart Transplantation. The perioperative death rate and late deaths have decreased tremendously since 1994 and the patient survival rate has remained at 92% for the past 5 years. The majority of heart transplants in Asia have been preformed in Taiwan (51.2%) followed by Thailand (18.7%), Saudi Arabia (18.7%), Singapore (6.5%), the Peoples' Republic of China (2.5%), Korea (1.6%) and Hong Kong (0.8%). Japan recently passed their Transplantation Act in 1997 recognizing brain death. Japan has performed only a few heart transplants so far.

C.L. Chen of CGMH in Taipei performed the first pancreatic transplant in Taiwan in 1984. The patient died afterward of graft pancreatic vein thrombosis. Eight consecutive pancreatic transplants with primary or secondary renal transplantation were performed successfully by S.H. Chao of NTUH in 1995. The metabolic derrangements caused by pancreatic and renal insufficiency were restored to normal ranges in those patients.

Y. C. Lee of NTUH in Taipei performed the first successful lung transplantation on December 9, 1995. As of December 1999, 32 lung transplantations were undertaken with one- and 4-year survival rates of 50% and 40%, respectively.

Heart-lung transplantation was first performed in Taiwan at NTUH in 1993. Unfortunately, the patient died of septicemia afterwards. We succeeded in heart-lung transplantation in March 1999 and the subsequent 3 patients undergoing heart-lung transplantation are doing fine with a very high degree of rehabilitation.

TAIWAN

Kidney Transplantation in Thailand

Sopon Jirasiritham and Vasant Sumethkul

Ramathibodi Hospital Medical School, Mahidol University, Bangkok, THAILAND

Thailand is a country of 65 million population. The prevalence of ESRD patients is about 11,000 while the yearly incidence of new patients is 3,000 or 46 patients per million population per year. Only half of all ESRD patients can access renal replacement therapies. About 80% of the treated patients receive chronic dialysis (hemodialysis or continuous ambulatory peritoneal dialysis) and 20% treated ESRD patients eventually receive a kidney transplant.

The first kidney transplantation in Thailand was performed in 1972. At that time, progress in organ transplantation was slow due to the poor performance of conventional immunosuppression. Cyclosporine was first introduced into this country in 1986 and since then, transplantation of kidneys and other organs has expanded rapidly. Now, 26 centers provide kidney transplantation; most of these centers are located in Bangkok, the capital city of Thailand. The official criteria of brain death were announced in 1989. Only cadaver donors, living-related donors and spouses are legally allowed for kidney transplantation. At the present time, the Organ Donation Centre of the Thai Red Cross Society acts as the center for organ donation and allocation of cadaver donors. Up to October 2000, 1,824 kidney transplantations had been performed in Thailand.

In Thailand, Ramathibodi Hospital is the largest center for kidney and also liver transplantation. We started our kidney transplantation program in 1986. From 1986-1990, we performed 103 kidney transplantations, and among these, 91% were kidneys from cadaver donors. Table 1 shows the number of kidney transplantations in our hospital from 1991 to October 2000.

Seventy percent of recipients in our institute are given a double-drug maintenance immunosuppressive regimen (Neoral and steroids) and 30% receive a triple regimen (Neoral, steroids and either azathioprine or mycophenolate mofetil). The anti-IL-2 receptor antibody is used as induction therapy for high-risk patients,

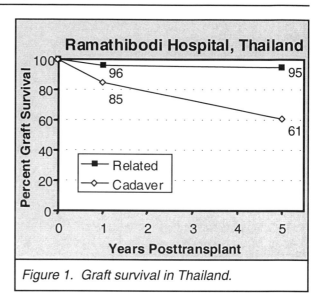

Figure 1. Graft survival in Thailand.

Table 1. Kidney transplants in Ramathibodi Hospital, Thailand.

	1990*	1991	1992	1993	1994	1995	1996	1997	1998	1999	Total**
Rel	13	10	19	12	13	24	44	62	51	45	320
Cad	90	28	15	27	30	22	14	14	29	33	315
Total	103	38	34	39	43	46	58	76	80	78	635

* 1986-1990, ** data up to Oct. 2000

including those with high PRA (>80%), retransplantations, and those with a poorly HLA-matched kidney or with a marginal cadaver donor with prolonged cold ischemia time. Tacrolimus has been used only in a few selected cases. With these protocols, the rate of acute rejection is 20% (21.4% in the cadaveric donor group and 9.1% in the living-related donor group). Most acute rejection episodes (85%) can be reversed by pulse steroid therapy while 15% are steroid resistant and require additional therapies that include OKT3, tacrolimus or mycophenolate mofetil.

At the beginning of the program, our perioperative mortality was 4%, but now the rate has fallen to 1.2%. The one- and 5-year actuarial graft survival rates are 85% and 61%, respectively for cadaver donor transplants and 96% and 95%, respectively for living-related donor transplants (Fig. 1). The one- and 5-year actuarial patient survival rates are 90% and 73% for cadaver and 98% and 95% for living-related donor transplants, respectively.

The prevalence of viral hepatitis infection in our dialysis patients is high (6% for HBV infection and 12-25% for HCV infection). Unexpectedly, the short-term outcome of kidney transplantation for hepatitis patients is acceptable. The one- and 5-year actuarial graft survival rates for HBV patients are 85% and 51%, respectively. The one- and 5-year actuarial graft survival rates for HCV patients are 85% and 60%, respectively. The survival of HCV patients is not lower than that of the non-hepatitis group for up to 7 years of follow-up, but appears to decline thereafter.

Chronic rejection or chronic allograft nephropathy is the major cause (70%) of late allograft dysfunction in Thai patients. The incidence of chronic rejection in kidney transplant recipients is 29% (2). The progression of chronic rejection can be slowed or even stabilized by the addition of mycophenolate mofetil (3). However, 30% of late allograft dysfunction among our patients is attributed to posttransplant recurrent IgA nephropathy (4). The latter is the most common cause of recurrent and de-novo glomerulonephritis in the allograft among Thai recipients. The recurrence of glomerular diseases other than IgA nephropathy is low, but is being closely monitored. The incidence of posttransplant lymphoproliferative disorders is extremely low in our population (0.2%). Instead, our major posttransplant solid organ

malignancies are gastrointestinal in origin like hepato-cellular carcinoma (5).

The future of kidney transplantation in Thailand is challenged by the cadaver organ shortage, which limits the number of kidneys that are available for transplantation. However, the better quality of life and lower cost of treatment experienced by kidney transplant recipients (compared with chronic dialysis) are more and more appreciated by both the patients and the public. The changing attitudes may alleviate the organ shortage in the near future.

References

1. Sumethkul V, Jirasiritham S, Chiewsilp P. Role of HLA matching as a prognostic factor for cadaveric renal transplantation: Analysis of Thai and Thai-Chinese ethnics. Transplant Proc 1994; 26:1897.

2. Jirasiritham S .The kidney transplantation in Thailand : Transplant Proc 1994; 26:2076.

3. Jirasiritham S, Sumethkul V, Mavichak V, Chalermsanyakorn P. The treatment of chronic rejection with Mycophenolate Mofetil (MMF) vs. Azathioprine (Aza) in kidney transplantation. Transplant Proc 2000; 32:2040.

4. Sumethkul V, Jirakranont B, Chalermsanyakorn P, Oralratmanee S. The clinico-pathological correlation of patients with chronic allograft dysfunction. Transplant Proc 2000; 32:1884.

5. Jirasiritham S, Jirasiritham Si, Sumethkul V, Chiewsilp P. Incidence of post transplantation neoplasm in Thailand. Transplant Proc 1996; 28:1586.

THAILAND

Renal Transplantation in Turkey

M. Haberal, R. Emiroglu, G. Arslan, H. Karakayali, G. Moray, and N. Bilgin

Baskent University, Transplantation Center, Ankara, TURKEY

Solid-organ transplantation began in Turkey in 1969, with 2 heart transplantations that, unfortunately, were not successful. By the early 1970s, M. Haberal and his team had initiated experimental studies on renal and liver transplantation (1), and Turkey's first living-related renal transplantation was performed on November 3, 1975 (2). This was followed by the country's first cadaver kidney transplantation on October 10, 1978, with an organ supplied by the Eurotransplant Foundation. After the enactment of a law pertaining to transplantation, the team performed the first local cadaver-donor kidney transplantation in 1979 (3).

The surgical advances of the past 25 years have been exciting, and the new potential for treatment has caused the need for donor organs to swell exponentially. Today, the supply of cadaver kidneys in Turkey lags far behind the demand, and the number of potential transplant recipients has dramatically increased with the rising incidence of end-stage renal disease. These factors have spurred the expansion of living-related renal transplantation in this country. As a consequence, our kidney transplantation program remains largely dependent on first- and second-degree relatives and spouses. This article reviews our 25 years of work in the field of renal transplantation, and presents our results with various recipient subgroups.

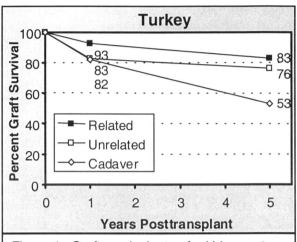

Figure 1. Graft survival rates for kidneys at BUTC, Turkey (1990-1999).

Table 1. Kidney transplants at BUTC, Turkey.

	1990	1991	1992	1993	1994	1995	1996	1997	1998	1999	Total
Rel	44	45	31	37	27	16	25	49	28	42	144
Unrel	1	4	5	6	2	1	1	5	3	5	33
Cad	14	18	15	20	11	10	8	18	15	15	144

Patients and Methods

From 1975-1999, our transplantation team at Hacettepe and Baskent University Transplantation Center (BUTC) performed 1,275 kidney transplantations. Of these, 967 (75.8%) involved living donors and 308 (24.2%) involved cadaver organs. The total number of kidney transplantations done in Turkey during the same period was 4,259, with 3,371 (79.2%) of these transplants coming from living donors and 888 (20.8%) coming from cadavers. In Turkey, any individual who is free of chronic disease and is willing to donate his or her kidney is informed, with no obligation, about the risks, benefits, and

procedures involved in living donor transplantation. At our transplantation center, after obtaining the donor's consent, we undertake a routine examination that includes blood pressure measurement and physical examination; ABO blood-group testing; HLA typing and crossmatching (including both complement-dependent cytotoxicity and flow cytometry methods); routine laboratory testing with complete blood count, blood chemistry, urinalysis, urine culture, and 24-hour creatinine clearance; serology for hepatitis-B and -C viruses, and cytomegalovirus; electrocardiogram; and chest x-ray. If all findings are normal, the candidate then undergoes renal angiography. Although the presence of multiple ureters, multiple veins, renal cysts, and ectopic kidneys are not considered contraindications, we prefer to harvest kidneys that have a single long arterial pedicle.

We have significantly modified our surgical technique since 1975. First, we introduced the 4-quadrant running suture technique for arterial anastomosis; second, we replaced renal artery-internal iliac artery anastomosis with renal artery-external iliac artery anastomosis; and third, we adopted the Lich-Gregoir technique, which involves placing a temporary stent that is removed before ureteral reimplantation is completed (4-6). Recently, with the aim of improving patient compliance and decreasing postoperative discomfort, we have changed our protocol from general anesthesia to epidural anesthesia for recipients, and we have introduced combined spinal-epidural anesthesia for donors.

Regarding immunosuppression, we have used the standard triple-drug low-dose regimen since 1985. Doses of 1 mg/kg prednisolone, 5 mg/kg cyclosporine A, and 2 mg/kg azathioprine are given daily in the postoperative period. In living donor transplantations, azathioprine and prednisolone are started 3 days prior to the surgery. Prednisolone is tapered to the maintenance dose of 10 mg/day at 2 months after transplantation, and is tapered to 5 mg/day if problems such as diabetes, aseptic necrosis, or obesity are present. Cyclosporine doses are adjusted according to target serum levels, and doses of azathioprine are altered according to leukocyte counts and liver function tests. In 1999, we modified our immunosuppression protocol by replacing azathioprine with mycophenolate mofetil and, in select cases, replacing cyclosporine with tacrolimus.

Acute rejection episodes are treated with intravenous bolus doses of methylprednisolone (250-500 mg/day) for 3 consecutive days, and steroid-resistant cases are treated with monoclonal antibody (OKT3) and plasmapheresis.

In addition to the pioneering steps in transplantation mentioned earlier, over the past 25 years our transplant center has also broken new ground in other areas of our field. In May 1992, we were the first to harvest multiple organs (segmental liver and kidney) from one living donor, and performed simultaneous liver and kidney transplantation in 2 patients with these grafts (7). We have also performed retransplantations in 55 patients. Two of these individuals had undergone 3 renal transplantations, and the other 53 patients had received 2 kidney grafts (8).

The severe shortage of kidney transplants in Turkey has forced us to expand our list of criteria for donor eligibility. In 1985, we began to use organs from cadaveric and living donors older than 55 years of age (9). Later, our group also started to do cadaveric kidney transplantations with prolonged cold ischemia times of more than 100 hours (10). Over the 10-year span from 1989-1999, we transplanted 144 cadaveric grafts with a mean cold ischemia time of 32.9±18.7 hours. During this period the mean age of our cadaveric donors was 38.8 ± 21.2 years (range, 2-75 years), while that for living donors was 41.6±11.8 years (range, 18-78 years).

Patient and graft survival rates for the various reported group results were calculated using the log-rank test and the software program SPSS for Windows.

Results

The yearly distribution of living-donor and cadaver-donor renal transplantations done at BUTC from 1990-1999 is listed in Table 1 and similar data compiled from 16 other transplantation centers in Turkey for the same time period are summarized in Table 2. Between 1975-1999, our team performed 30% of all the renal transplantations done in Turkey.

Over the past decade, the one-, 3-, and 5-year patient survival rates for the first-degree living-related kidney transplantation group were 96%, 93%, and 91%, respectively, and the corresponding graft survival rates were 93%, 84%, and 81% (Fig. 1). In the second-degree living-related group, the one-, 3-, and 5-year patient survival rates were 94%, 90%, and 87%, respectively, and the corresponding graft survival rates were 93%, 86%, and 84%. For living-unrelated transplantations, the one-, 3- and 5-year patient survival rates were 93%, 90%, and 83% respectively, and the corresponding graft survival rates were 83%, 78%, and 76%. In the cadaver kidney transplantation group, the one-, 3-, and 5-year patient survival rates were 85%, 78%, and 70%, respectively, and the corresponding graft survival rates were 82%, 64%, and 53%. The one-, 3-, and 5-year graft survival rates related to cadaver and living donors older than 55 years were 80%, 52%, 46% and 88%, 69%, 61%, respectively.

Table 2. Kidney transplants from 16 other transplant centers in Turkey.

	1990	1991	1992	1993	1994	1995	1996	1997	1998	1999	Total
Living	UN*	UN	UN	UN	UN	UN	UN	269	255	273	3,371
Cad	UN	UN	UN	UN	35	24	19	71	129	95	888

*UN=Unknown

Discussion

The total number of renal transplantations fell in 1995 and 1996, but started to rise again in 1997. For the year 1998, the number of procedures done rose by just slightly more than 11%, but the proportion involving cadaver donor organs increased significantly, from 21% to 36.3% as shown in Tables 1 and 2. This rise likely reflects increased collaboration between the transplantation centers, as well as a change in the attitude of Turkish people towards organ donation. The latter has been achieved through the dedicated efforts of staff at transplantation centers and the Ministry of Health, and through persuasive speeches by officials at the Department of Religious Affairs, who have explained that organ donation is not forbidden in Islamic belief.

In Turkey, the leading cause of chronic renal failure (CRF) is chronic glomerulonephritis. The 1998 Turkish Nephrology Society registry had logged 22,766 CRF patients up to that year, and stated that approximately 9,380 new patients were added to the log in 1998. However, of the 1,931 CRF patients who were placed on renal transplant center waiting lists in 1998, only 384 (19.8%) received a kidney graft that year.

In our country, many people with ESRD remain unaware of the possibility of renal transplantation, and the number of patients who receive transplants is far below the number who could benefit from this procedure. There is a great need to inform this group that kidney transplantation is the most effective and rational mode of renal replacement therapy. For those who are aware of the surgery, aside from the general problems of organ supply and demand, there is a specific issue with pediatric transplantation in Turkey. Although pediatric ESRD patients are given priority over adults, only 118 pediatric patients in Turkey had undergone renal transplantation as of 1999, and 42 (35.5%) of these were transplanted at BUTC.

At our center, only first-degree (father, mother, siblings, offspring) and second-degree (aunt, uncle, cousin, nephew, grandmother, grandfather) relatives are considered "related" donors. In order to expand our donor pool, in 1986 we started to use grafts from "unrelated" donors, which include individuals joined by marriage or those who are emotionally close to the recipient (spouses, emotionally attached friends). In the past 10 years, most (93.9%) of the living-unrelated transplantations done at our facility have involved spouses as donors. Interest-

ingly, although these donor-recipient pairings invariably have poorer HLA matches than those typical of living-related pairings, the graft and patient survival rates were comparable (11).

In another move to increase organ availability, we have also expanded the acceptable donor age range. Although we found that patient survival rates are similar in the older and younger donor age groups, survival rates for kidneys from older donors have been slightly lower than the rates for grafts from younger donors. After increasing the acceptable donor age range, we also began to use grafts with longer ischemia time. This innovation has added a new dimension to our field, and soon after our initial work was published, reports of renal transplantations involving cold ischemia times of 48-72 hours started to appear in the literature throughout the world (12).

Conclusion

In the past 25 years, Turkey has seen impressive progress in the field of transplantation. The significant reductions in morbidity and mortality that have been achieved in our kidney transplant patients are the rewards of thorough preoperative evaluation and meticulous surgical technique. Although careful dissection and mastery of the latest surgical methods has led to a steep drop in postoperative complications, infectious complications and graft loss due to chronic rejection continue to be major challenges. In the future, we plan to focus our efforts on solving these problems, and on raising Turkish public awareness about transplantation to a much higher level.

References

1. Haberal M, et al. Köpekte baypas kullanilmadan yapilan ortotopik karaciger homotransplantasyonu. Hacettepe Tip/ Cerrahi Bülteni 1972; 5:462.

2. Haberal M, Bilgin G, Arslan G, Büyükpamukçu N et al. Twenty-two years of experience in transplantation. Transplant Proc 1998; 30:683.

3. Haberal M, Moray G, Karakayali H, et al. Ethical and legal aspects, and history of organ transplantation in Turkey. Transplant Proc 1996; 28:382

4. Haberal M, Karakayali H, Bilgin N, et al. Four-quadrant running-suture arterial anastomosis technique in renal transplantation: A preliminary report. Transplant Proc 1996; 28:2334.

5. Moray G, Bilgin N, Karakayali H, et al. Comparison of outcome in renal transplant recipients with respect to arte-

rial anastomosis: The internal versus the external iliac artery. Transplant Proc 1999; 31:2839.

6. Haberal M. Böbrek Transplantasyonu. In: Haberal M, Eds. Doku ve Organ Transplantasyonlari. Haberal Egitim Vakfi. 1993:159.

7. Haberal M, Moray G, Karakayali H, et al. Transplantation legislation and practice in Turkey: a brief history. Transplant Proc 1998; 30:3644.

8. Karakayali H, Moray G, Demirag A, et al. Long-term retransplantation and graft survival rates at our center. Transplant Proc 1998;30:762.

9. Bilgin G, Karakayali H, Moray G, et al. Outcome of renal transplantation from elderly donors. Transplant Proc 1998; 30:744.

10. Haberal M, et al. Cadaver kidney transplantation with prolonged cold ischemia time. Transplant Proc 1988; 20:932.

11. Haberal M, Gülay H, Tokyay R, et al. Living unrelated donor kidney transplantation between spouses. World J. Surg. 1992; 15:1183.

12. Cicciarelli J, Iwaki Y, Mendez R et al. Effects of cold ischemia time on cadaver renal allografts. Transplant Proc 1993; 25:1543.

Kidney Transplants in Uruguay

I. Alvarez [a,b,c], F. González [b,c], S. Orihuela [c], R. Toledo [a,b,c], M. Bengochea [a,b,c], and L. Curi [c]

[a]*Banco Nacional de Organos y Tejidos - Ministerio de Salud Pública,* [b]*Hospital de Clínicas - Universidad de la República,* [c]*Sociedad Uruguaya de Trasplantes, Montevideo, URUGUAY*

Uruguay is a country located in the southeast part of South America, with 176,215 square kilometers and 3,322,141 people (19/Km^2). The population is 48% male and 52% female and the life expectancy is 74.5 years. Uruguay plays an active role in the Mercosur, and the total gross domestic product (GDP) is 21 billion dollars.

The first kidney transplant was done in 1969 at the University Hospital with a cadaver donor kidney. This activity forced the establishment of a legal framework and in the 1980's, the cadaver renal transplant program started and 571 renal transplants were performed. By 2000, the rate of renal transplantation had risen to 19.1 per million population (pmp). This transplantation activity is governed by transplant law 14.005, the National Bank of Organs and Tissues (BNOT), and has financial support from the Found of National Resources (FNR).

The transplant law of 1971 was the first in Latin America. Based on informed consent, it allows people to register positive or negative willingness to be a donor upon death. The government Institution, the National Bank of Organs and Tissues, opened its doors in 1978. This service operates through the State University Medical School and the Public Health Secretary, sharing academic, normative and administrative responsibilities. BNOT takes care of 1) the National Register of donors through signed informed consent; 2) the procurement of donors; 3) the national histocompatibility laboratory (1-3); 4) the allocation and sharing of organs and tissues; and 5) the tissue bank. Since 1980, national financial support for dialysis and transplantation for all of the Uruguayan population was created using resources from the prepaid health insurance system and the Public Health Secretary. Initially, the same team of nephrologists from 2 transplant institutions (one university and one private) performed 397 renal transplants (4). In 1997-98, 2 other private transplantation institutions began transplanting.

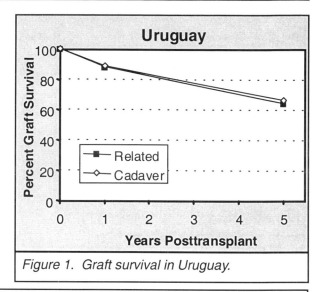

Figure 1. Graft survival in Uruguay.

Table1. Kidney transplants in Uruguay.

	1990	1991	1992	1993	1994	1995	1996	1997	1998	1999	Total
Rel	4	6	13	1	6	4	11	6	12	2	105*
Unrel					1				1	1	4
Cad	20	18	15	21	13	25	40	26	43	41	467*

* including 1980-90 and 2000 data

Patients and Methods

Four hundred fifty-one patients are on the national waiting list. These were selected from the 2,163 ESRD patients (683/pmp) who are on dialysis treatment (5,6), 41.5% of whom are more than 64 years old (7). The patient is placed on the active list after clinical evaluation and a complete study by the histocompatibility laboratory, including PRA status, ABO blood group and Rh typing, and HLA Class I and II, serological typing. Since 1997, "split" resolution of the HLA-A, -B, -DR, and -DQ antigens using monoclonal antibody reagents and fluorescent dye have been reported. The median waiting time after activation on the waiting list until transplant was 45 months (range 1-176 months).

The selection of cadaver donors is made by the donor procurement team. The cause of death was 28%

stroke, 63% brain trauma and 9% others. All donors are routinely screened for infection and disease. The mean donor age was 29 years±14 (range 18 months - 62 years); the upper age limit has been increasing lately. Donors were 71% male and 39% female. Until now, non heart-beating donors have not been used in our program. The donor procurement strategies employed in recent years have provided the Institution with a donation rate of 10 cadaver organ donors pmp.

One hundred eight living donor transplants were performed: 59% from female donors and 41% from males. The donor relationships were: 51% parents, 45% brothers and 4% spouses (all wives).

Organs from donors who test positive for HIV, Hepatitis B antibody or core antigen or Hepatitis C were discarded. Eighty-one percent of donors who were accepted had positive CMV serology and 10% tested positive for Toxoplasma. Two donors with a positive Chagas test were used to transplant negative recipients. The histocompatibility laboratory allocates kidneys based on pre-established algorithms that include: a negative crossmatch on B and T cells, ABO blood group identity, HLA-DR, followed by -B, and -A locus antigen matching, children's age, waiting time and clinical status (3,4).

The immunosuppression protocols have evolved in 3 general eras during our experience with 576 patients who were transplanted since 1980: 1980-1986 - corticosteroids, azathioprine; 1987-1996 - cyclosporine, steroids and azathioprine; and 1997-2000 – cyclosporine, steroids and mycophenolate mofetil. Acute rejection is treated with a methylprednisolone bolus and steroid-resistant rejections are treated with poly- or monoclonal antibody. Patients received induction treatment with lymphoglobulin or OKT3, depending on the era.

Actuarial patient and graft survival rates were calculated by the Kaplan-Meier method and multiple Cox regression. Chi-square and appropriate "t" tests were used for comparing means.

Results

Of the 571 renal transplants, 463 (81%) were from cadaver donors, 104 (18%) were from living-related donors and 4 (1%) from living unrelated donors (spouses). Second transplants were performed in 6.5% of the recipients and 6.5% were diabetic patients. The median follow up was 55.3±52 months (range 1-231 months).

The Figure 1.shows overall similar results at one and 5 years for recipients of cadaver and living related donor transplants and the number of transplants that were performed each year are listed in Table 1.

Table 2. Patient and cadaver kidney survival rate (%).

Survival year	1980-1989 Patient	Graft	1990-1995 Patient	Graft	1996-2000 Patient	Graft
1	92	77	97	87	98	90
5	81	59	88	66	93	77
7	77	50	83	59		
10	71	37	79	52		

Table 2 shows the one-, 5-, 7- and 10-year patient and graft survival rates for the different immunosuppression eras. The one-year graft survival rate was significantly higher in the most recent era (90% vs. 77% in the 1980's). A similar improvement was noted for the 5-year survival rates (77% vs. 59%).

Six variables: age, donor sex, recipient sex, immunosuppression, delayed graft function (>48 hr) and different eras, were analyed for graft survival. Two risk factors had a significant association with graft survival - delayed graft function (p<0.003) and era (p< 0.02).

Comments

Transplant activity and graft survival rates have been increasing, but we need to establish a better donation rate. Our first objective is to increase cadaver donor procurement.

Acknowledgement

We acknowledge the efforts of the clinical teams from the Institute of Nephrology and Urology, Hospital de Clínicas, Hospital Evangélico, Hospital Americano and the BNOT technical and administrative staff.

References

1. Alvarez I, Sans M, Toledo R, Sosa M, Bengochea M, Salzano F. HLA Gene Haplotype Frequencies in Uruguay. Int J Anthro 1993; 8:163.
2. Alvarez I. Nociones Básicas de Histocompatibilidad. In: Departamento de publicaciones de la Facultad de Humanidades y Ciencias de la Educación Eds. In: Bases para el estudio de la población uruguaya. Montevideo, 1994:25.
3. Alvarez I, Toledo R, Bengochea M, González F. In: PI Terasaki, Ed. Visuals of the Clinical Histocompatibility Workshop. Outcome of Renal Transplant in Uruguay 1996.
4. Rodriguez L, González F., Orihuela S, et al. Evolución de Trasplantes Renales en el Uruguay – Nefrología 1993; 8: supp 2.
5. Registro Uruguayo de Diálisis. Unpublished. Date of December, 31,1999.
6. Mazzuchi N, González F, et al. Comparation of survival for hemodialysis patients vs. renal transplant recipients treated in Uruguay. Neprol Dial Transplant 1999; 14:2849.
7. Mazzuchi N, Schwedt E, González C, et al. Archivos de Medicina Interna 2000; 8:1.

CHAPTER 30

Annual Literature Review – Clinical Transplants 2000

James F. Markmann, Luis Campos, Ergun Velidedeoglu, T. Sloan Guy, Sina L. Moainie, Niraj M. Desai, Robert C. Gorman, Kenneth L. Brayman, Ali Naji, and Clyde F. Barker

The Department of Surgery, University of Pennsylvania Health System, Philadelphia, Pennsylvania

As in previous years, the intent of this chapter is to review the major published literature for the year 2000 in the field of transplantation. We have limited the scope of the chapter to solid organ transplantation (kidney, liver, heart and lung) except for the addition of pancreatic islet transplantation for which a major advance has been reported during 2000.

RENAL TRANSPLANTATION

According to UNOS, 12,529 renal transplants were performed in the year 1999. Of those, 8,097 were derived from cadaveric donors and 4,432 were made available through living related and unrelated donation. A total of 47,312 patients were awaiting renal transplantation in 1999, and 3,046 patients died while waiting. In the last 12-years, the number of cadaveric renal transplants increased 13% from 7,062 in 1988 to 8,097 in 1999. Grafts from living donors increased 2.5 fold from 1,800 in 1988 to 4,432 in 1999 (1,2).

Living Donors

Schweitzer, et al (3) analyzed the increase in living renal donation, which has occurred due to laparoscopic donor nephrectomy. They found that the rate of referrals for kidney transplantation doubled following the introduction of laparoscopic donor nephrectomy. This increase was more marked in recipients who were young and Caucasian, than in older patients and Blacks. Donor-recipient relationships also changed, 10% being of only distant family relationship and up to a third being non-family donors. There was no difference in patient or graft survival whether the donor operation was an open or laparoscopic procedure (97.1% and 95% patient survival, and 94.3% and 88.5% graft survival at 1 and 3 years respectively).

The increase in the living donor pool due to utilization of unrelated donors was reviewed by Cecka (4). For several years, the shortage of cadaver kidneys and increasing waiting times have encouraged acceptance of living donors whose relationship to the recipient was emotional rather than genetic. At the University of Wisconsin, 150 living unrelated kidney transplants have been performed since 1981. The 10-year graft survival rate was 65%, compared with 75% for HLA-identical sibling donor kidneys and substantially better than the 44% for cadaveric renal grafts. The excellent survival of unrelated grafts is paradoxical with regard to the importance of HLA antigen matching since over 70% of the living unrelated donors reported to UNOS between 1991-1997 had 4 or more of the 6 HLA antigens mismatched with the recipient. However, the advantages of using living donor transplants include the opportunity for thorough preoperative assessment of the kidney donor, the preemptive initiation of immunosuppression, and the increased compliance with medications and minimizing ischemic damage. Nevertheless, a cautious approach to utilization of living unrelated donors was emphasized since the mortality associated with the procedure was 0.03%, and the morbidity 8-48%.

Matas (5) described "non-directed" donation of living renal allografts as another method for increasing the donor pool. At the University of Minnesota, potential donors are informed of the risks of such donation and questioned regarding reasons for their interest in the procedure. A detailed psychosocial evaluation is performed to assess the donor's competence and understanding, and to rule out psychiatric disorders. To avoid any conflict of interest, the team that accepts an individual for non-directed donation is separate from the team caring for the potential recipient. Recipients are selected

Clinical Transplants 2000, Cecka and Terasaki, Eds. UCLA Immunogenetics Center, Los Angeles, California

from patients on the waiting list for cadaveric transplantation with allocation being based on HLA matching and length of time on the waiting list. Of 98 individuals initially expressing interest on non-directed donation, 38 pursued further evaluation. Eleven potential donors were turned down because of medical or psychosocial factors; 18 were fully evaluated and 6 were finally accepted as donors.

Financial compensation of donors has been proposed by the State of Pennsylvania, and is currently provided by the University of Minnesota in nominal amounts and intended only for food, housing and transportation expenses. However, Levinsky (6) questioned compensation for living unrelated donors, postulating that monetary compensation "might" drive the competition for unrelated living donors to "potentially unethical and dangerous practices", since competing transplant centers might be tempted to use less stringent criteria for donor selection or to offer larger payments.

Spital, et al (7) analyzed the attitude at US transplant centers toward kidney donation from unrelated living donors. In a mail-in survey completed by 62% (129) of the UNOS renal transplant centers, 60% preferred living related donors, 30% had no preference and 5% favored the cadaveric source. Ninety-three percent of the centers would accept a friend of the recipient as a kidney donor (74% had actually performed one such transplant). 38% would consider an altruistic undirected donation, an increase from 8% and 15% in prior surveys 12 and 6 years ago, respectively. Only 18 centers had actually performed an undirected transplant from a living donor.

Halpern, et al (8) compared CT with MR angiography in evaluation of donor kidneys. CT angiography of 26 kidneys demonstrated 33 accessory arteries while MRI of 20 of the same kidneys identified 26 accessory arteries. Since in some cases the identification of accessory arteries of one kidney caused the surgeon to utilize a contra-lateral kidney which had only a single artery, surgical confirmation of pre-operative imaging was possible in only 18 donors. These 18 kidneys had a total of 23 vessels, of which 22 had been identified, both by CT and MR. In one case, a 2-mm upper pole accessory artery was interpreted by CT as a proximal upper pole branch of the main renal artery and was not detected at all by the MR angiogram. In addition, one proximal arterial branch was missed both by CT and MR angiograms. Finally, the presence of 2 small accessory arteries that were suggested by CT was not confirmed at nephrectomy. The authors concluded that the disagreement in CT and MR angiograms is likely only with small diameter vessels of 1-2 mm, which are unlikely to be of clinical relevance.

Kuo, et al (9) reported their experience with a 23-hour hospital stay for laparoscopic donor nephrectomy. Of 41 patients enrolled in this protocol, 36 (88%) were able to leave the hospital after 23 hours of stay. Five patients failed to do so, because of pain in 2 cases and urinary retention in another. Two patients who had expected a longer hospital stay were unwilling to leave the hospital in 23 hours. Open nephrectomy donors had a considerably longer length of stay (5.6 days). Time out of work was also shorter for the 23-hour admit laparoscopic donors than for open donors (2.6 weeks vs. 5.8 weeks). Hospital stays and time out of work were roughly the same for another group of laparoscopic donor patients who were not on the 23-hour protocol. In the 23-hour stay group, one patient required readmission to the hospital for dehydration and nausea, and required an additional 4-day hospitalization. The 23-hour protocol resulted in a savings of almost 100% over the open nephrectomy patients, and about a 65% savings over a group of laparoscopic donors not on the 23-hour protocol. Mosimann, (10) in an editorial comment on this paper viewed the 23-hour stay as an interesting approach, but suggested caution on premature general acceptance of this protocol before long-term outcomes are assessed. In his institution, a 4-7 day hospital stay of a donor requires minimal nursing care and incurs minimal incremental costs over a 25-hour stay, which he regards as negligible in the global context of expenditures for managing end-stage renal failure.

Cadaver Donors

The donor shortage has also encouraged the use of cadaveric kidneys from donors that would have been considered unacceptable in the past. Gridelli and Remuzzi (11) reviewed the outcome of transplantation with kidneys from marginal donors including those whose hearts had stopped beating, were older than 55 or younger than 5 years of age, had hypertension, diabetes mellitus, or hepatitis C infection. In addition, grafts having anatomical abnormalities or prolonged cold ischemia times are also being considered for transplantation. The so-called marginal kidneys derived from donors between the ages of 60-74 have shown actuarial graft survival rates of more than 90%, provided there were fewer than 15% sclerotic glomeruli on a pretransplantation biopsy. However, the transplantation of 2 marginal kidneys with sclerosis of up to 40% of glomeruli transplanted into one recipient showed a similar one-year graft survival to that of transplants from donors who were 50 years of age or older.

Dietl, et al (12), reviewed transplantation of both kidneys from marginal donors into a single aged recipient. The decision to transplant 2 kidneys was evaluated by an algorithm that considered donor age (greater than 65 years), degree of glomerulosclerosis (0-10%, 10-30% and >30%), donor serum creatinine (>1.8), and the combined weight of both kidneys (<300 grams). Grafts that would have otherwise been discarded were transplanted into recipients of a mean age of 59 years. After an average follow up of 18 months, 88% of the recipients were alive. The calculated one- and 2-year graft survival rates were 98.4% and 92%. The rejection rate was only 14%. A similar study evaluating double versus single renal allografts from aged donors was reported by Andres, et al (13). Their recipients were stratified depending on donor characteristics and whether a double or a single transplant was performed: Group I patients received a double cadaveric renal transplant from donors whose mean age was 75 years; Group II received a single cadaveric renal transplant from donors older than 60 years (mean age of 67 years); and Group III patients received a single cadaveric renal transplant from donors younger than 60 years of age (mean age of 37 years). Although group I, those who received the 2 kidneys from elderly donors, consisted of only 21 patients, 76% of them showed immediate renal function compared with only 43% of the recipients who received the single aged cadaveric renal transplant, and 50% of the recipients that received a single graft from an ideal donor. Actuarial one-year patient survival was 100%, 95% and 98% (groups I, II, III, respectively) and overall one-year graft survival was 95%. Interestingly, recipients of the double transplant had a higher rate of thrombosis compared with the other 2 groups.

Carter, et al (14), evaluated the impact of donor hypertension and creatinine clearance on the function and survival of grafts from older cadaveric donors. The actuarial graft survival in recipients transplanted with donors younger than 55 years of age was 88%, 83.4% and 78% at one, 2, and 3 years, respectively. In contrast, patients who received renal allografts of donors age 55 or

older had inferior actuarial graft survival (80.6%, 73.5% and 65.3% at one, 2 and 3 years, respectively). At 6 months, recipients with non-hypertensive donors had lower serum creatinine than those with hypertensive donors. However, after one year, the recipients of kidneys from hypertensive donors had higher creatinine levels than those with non-hypertensive donors only if hypertension had been present for more than 10 years. At 2 years after transplant and beyond, no significant differences in serum creatinine were found between these cohorts. However, recipients of kidneys from donors who had been hypertensive for more than 10 years were at increased risk of delayed graft function and their graft survival was significantly reduced by 8% at 2-3 years compared with recipients of non-hypertensive donor kidneys or those with hypertension of less than 10 years duration. A progressive decline in graft survival was also noted if the donor's creatinine clearance was less than 80 ml/min. Actuarial graft survival at one, 2 and 3 years was 77%, 69% and 62%, respectively, in the recipients of kidneys from donors with a creatinine clearance less than 80 ml/min versus 83%, 76% and 66%, respectively, in the recipients whose donors had a creatinine clearance greater than 80 ml/min. The combination of both donor hypertension and low creatinine clearance resulted in the poorest actuarial graft survival. The recipients of kidneys from donors with hypertension for years and a creatinine clearance less than 80 ml/min had an actuarial graft survival of 77%, 61% and 53.6% at one, 2 and 3 years, respectively.

Randhawa, et al (15) studied the correlation of histologic findings in pretransplant biopsies of marginal donor kidneys with posttransplant renal function. The degree of interstitial fibrosis, tubular atrophy, arteriosclerosis and arteriolar hyalinosis were graded using the Banff schema. The mean donor age was 51 years. The mean recipient age was 47.7±14.5 years. Glomerulosclerosis, tubular atrophy and arteriosclerosis increased positively with donor age. In biopsies with 0% glomerulosclerosis, 1-10% glomerulosclerosis and 11-20% glomerulosclerosis, the incidence of graft dysfunction at 12 months was 25%, 45.9% and 60%, respectively. Graft dysfunction at 12 months after transplantation was 100% when donor biopsies revealed greater than 20% glomerulosclerosis. The authors concluded that donor kidneys that have greater than 20% glomerulosclerosis, more than one grade of arteriosclerosis, or interstitial fibrosis should not be used for transplantation.

Alvarez, et al (16) reported their experience using uncontrolled non-heart beating donors. Patients that arrived in the emergency room with active resuscitation maneuvers in progress but found to have neither spontaneous respiration or a beating heart were declared dead, taken to the operating room and placed on cardio-pulmonary bypass. They were considered acceptable as donors only if it was known that the period of total circulatory arrest was less than 15 minutes. Of 111 evaluated, 62 were found to be acceptable by these criteria and 53 actually became donors. The initial graft function was 16%; with a delayed graft function of 80% and 4% never functioned. Their results corresponded to 67%, 23% and 10% for recipients of heart beating brain dead donors. The 3-year graft survival rate was 78% for non-heart beating donors compared with 83% for brain-dead heart beating donors.

Whiting, et al (17) examined the economic impact of utilizing expanded criteria donors in cadaveric renal transplantation. The Medicare End-Stage Renal Disease Program is the responsible payer for approximately 70% of all kidney transplants making payments of more than $1.2 billion a year for transplantation. According to UNOS, between 1991-1996 there were 25,600 non-high-risk recipient transplants; in 5,718 (22%) of them, expanded criteria donors were utilized. At the same time, there were 8,134 high-risk recipient transplants; in 2,200 (25%) of them, expanded criteria donors were used. Non-high-risk recipients of a non-expanded criteria donor had one- and 5-year graft survival rates of 89% and 70%, respectively. Expanded criteria donor kidneys transplanted into high-risk recipients resulted in 79% and 51% graft survival at one and 5 years. Cost analysis indicated that the 5-year payments for non-expanded criteria donors into non-high-risk patients was $121,698. This compared with $143,329 for expanded criteria donors into non-high-risk patients. Similarly, non-expanded criteria donors into high-risk recipients cost $134,185 versus $165,716 for expanded criteria donors into high-risk recipients. Analysis of "break-even point" for the different donor- recipient pairings (ie., the time at which transplantation becomes less expensive than hemodialysis) showed that non-expanded criteria donors to non-high-risk recipient pairings break even at 4.4 years. However for expanded criteria donors into high-risk recipients, 13 years were required to reach the break-even point.

In "Triumph of Hope over Experience", Tilney (18)

examined the current donation crisis. The "presumed consent" or "opting out" legislation in which the law mandates that organs may be removed after death unless the individual specifically declines to participate has increased donation in countries, like Austria, Spain, and Belgium (19). Gubernatis and Kliemt propose a solidarity plan based on the hypothesis that potential organ recipients who have made clear during their lifetimes that they are willing to donate their own organs at the time of their death will be given priority if they ever need a transplant over those who opt not to donate. Such a plan does not preclude transplantation in any patient, but it does award priority to individuals who themselves expressed willingness to donate. The author suggested that the solidarity scheme could probably work and perhaps should be tried. Daar (20) proposed a similar donation scheme. Cadaveric donation would still be based on altruism and thus people from the general population would not be liable to have a "presumed consent". In this reciprocity proposal, the members of the society who are conscious objectors would compensate by playing a role in public education to raise donor awareness or by raising funds for transplantation or volunteer time in transplant hospitals.

Access to Transplantation

Equitable access to transplantation was a hot topic in the year 2000. Ayanian, et al (21) investigated the influence of patients' preferences and race on access to renal transplantation. The desire for a transplant by renal failure patients was similar for African Americans and Caucasians (76.3% vs. 79.3% respectively for females and 80.1% vs. 85.5% for males). However, larger racial differences were found in the referral of patients for transplantation. Only 50.4% of African-American women were referred to transplant as compared with 70.5% of white women, and only 53.9% of African-American men were referred in contrast to 76.2% of white men.

Gender also appeared to influence access to transplantation. Schaubel (22), using data of the Canadian Transplant Registry, found that the probability of receiving a kidney transplant within 5 years was 47% for men but only 39% for women. In addition, males were more likely to undergo hemodialysis than females, who were treated preferentially with peritoneal dialysis. After adjustments for age, waiting period, race and dialytic modality, males were found to be 20% more likely to receive a kidney transplant than females. This discrepancy increased with age and was greater in Blacks, Asian Indians and American Indians, than in Caucasians.

Racial differences in the access to kidney transplantation were also apparent in an analysis of children and adolescents with end-stage renal disease (23). Data from the USRDS Standard Analysis Files identified 5,448 patients younger than 19 years of age who began dialysis therapy between 1993-1998. Of these, 31.5% were Black and 60.7% were White. Active status on the transplant waiting list was determined prior to the initiation of dialysis, and after 2 and 5 years of therapy. Although only 7.7% of the patients were on a waiting list prior to dialysis, 76% of these patients were White. After 2 years of dialysis, 56% of White and only 50% of Black patients had been activated on the waiting list. After 5 years, 66% of White and 63% of Black patients were on an active wait list. The median time from first dialysis to activation on the waiting list was 215 days for White patients and 275 days for Black patients. Further analysis indicated that only 52% of females were on a waiting list after 2 years of dialysis compared with 64% of males. Socioeconomic analysis suggested that patients who lived in lower income areas had the least access to transplantation. In high-income areas, no racial difference was found.

Racial disparity in simultaneous pancreas and kidney transplantation was analyzed by Isaacs (24) and indicated that Caucasians represented about 65% of all patients with end-stage renal disease and 70% of the patients with end-stage renal disease caused by type I diabetes. Nonetheless, Whites received 72% of all the kidney transplants and 92% of all of the simultaneous pancreas-kidney transplants. Blacks received 21% of the kidney and only 5% of the simultaneous pancreas-kidney transplants, despite representing 29% of patients with end-stage renal disease, and 22% of patients with diabetic nephropathy.

Although males appear to be favored as recipients of renal transplants from living donors, Zimmerman, et al (25) found that females comprise a greater proportion of donors. This study revealed that 54.5% of the acceptable donors were women. This difference began with females being more willing to undergo HLA typing, and culminated in their acceptance as donors. Of the potential donor pool, 28.3% of females became donors compared with 20.3% of males. Thus, 62.5% of living donors were female. The greatest gender difference was

seen in spousal donation in which only 2 out of 20 donors were from men. The authors postulated that women were more likely than men to perceive donation as a family obligation.

The Federal Health Care Financing Administration, (HCFA) has expressed concern over the disparities in access to transplantation and wants to ensure equal opportunity for transplantation, regardless of race or gender. HCFA publications emphasize the need for dialysis centers to provide better patient education and assume responsibility for referring patients to transplant programs for consideration of transplantation (26).

Complications – Infections

CMV infection is the single most frequent infectious complication in renal transplant recipients. Sagedal (27) studied the natural course of the cytomegalovirus (CMV) infection and CMV disease. In this prospective study, the authors evaluated the utility of the CMV PP65 antigenemia assay in monitoring of CMV infections. Data was obtained on 397 first transplants and 80 retransplants. The overall incidence of CMV infection in all patients was 63%. The relative incidence of primary infection and CMV reactivation was the same. However, the rate of CMV disease was nearly 3 times higher in the primary infection group (56% vs. 20%). Quantitative analysis of CMV PP65 antigenemia was done in seronegative recipients of seropositive donors. There was no statistically significant difference in maximum CMV PP65 antigen in-patients with CMV disease and asymptomatic CMV infection. Of patients with reactivated CMV infection, 50% developed disease when the number of CMV PP65 antigen positive leukocytes was between 50-99 per 100,000 cells and greater than 90% developed disease when the number of positive cells was more than 600 per 100,000 cells (sensitivity of 99% and a specificity of 51% with regard to CMV disease). In primary CMV disease, CMV PP65 was always positive. Not all renal transplant recipients at risk develop CMV infection or disease. In this study, 68% of first renal graft recipients in the seronegative, donor-positive group, had an active CMV infection, and of these 82% developed disease. Patient age and rejection were significant risk factors for active infection. For development of CMV disease, rejection and the combination of donor positivity and recipient negativity were significant risk factors. On the basis of this study, patients in the donor-positive, recipient-negative category and patients undergoing anti-rejection therapy (except those who were donor negative and recipient negative) would profit from pre-emptive anti-CMV therapy.

Humar, et al (28) analyzed the association in kidney transplant recipients between CMV disease and cardiac complications. Of 1,859 adults who underwent kidney transplantation, 377 developed cardiac complications after transplantation including myocardial infarction, angina, arrhythmia, congestive heart failure, and coronary artery occlusion. By multivariant analysis, significant risk factors for one of the above cardiac complications were recipient age greater than 50 years, diabetes, a history of cardiac disease, and CMV disease. Of the patients that had no CMV disease, only 19% developed cardiac complications versus 27.5% for the patients with CMV disease. Statistically significant differences were reached when the patients were assessed for arrhythmia (14.1% for patients with CMV disease vs. 5.7% with patients without CMV disease). When the recipient characteristics were analyzed, diabetes, history of smoking, hypertension, cardiac history and age were similar in both groups. The only difference was in the percentage with coronary artery disease prior to transplantation, with the patients with CMV disease having 58.7% versus 48.2% for the patients with no CMV disease. Possible mechanisms for CMV-induced atherosclerosis have been proposed including: direct endothelial injury, smooth muscle proliferation, and inhibition of P53.

Kletzmayr, et al (29) investigated long-term oral ganciclovir prophylaxis for prevention of CMV infection and disease in high-risk renal transplant recipients. In the study group of this prospective open-labeled study, seronegative recipients of CMV-positive grafts were treated prophylactically with IV ganciclovir for 2-3 weeks after transplantation and then switched to oral ganciclovir for 3 months. The control group received IV ganciclovir only during anti-rejection therapy with antilymphocyte antibodies. When assessed serologically at a year after transplantation, 45% of the patients treated prophylactically with ganciclovir tested positive for CMV in comparison to 75% of the controls. In addition, CMV disease occurred in 29% of the study group versus 60% of the controls. Likewise, the severity of the disease was significantly reduced in the ganciclovir treated patients. The onset of CMV disease was significantly delayed in the ganciclovir group at 138 days after transplantation compared with 52 days for the control group. Biopsy-proven rejection was 41.9% for the ganciclovir treated group and

71% for the controls. Steroid-resistant rejection requiring monoclonal or polyclonal antibody treatment was 16% for the group treated prophylactically and 64.2% for the control group. A limitation of the study, as cited by the authors, is that there was a difference in the dose of MMF between the study and the control group due to the higher incidence of rejection. The control group also had more courses of antilymphocytic antibody therapy. Excluding those patients who were treated with antilymphocyte therapy, the study group still showed a reduced incidence of CMV disease.

Limaye, et al (30) report the emergence of ganciclovir-resistant CMV disease among organ transplant recipients. In their study, patients were treated prophylactically for CMV if they were seronegative and their donor was seropositive. Resistance to CMV treatment was defined as no clinical response to 14 days of IV ganciclovir with positive PP65 antigenemia assay or continued symptoms of CMV disease. Infections resistant to ganciclovir were treated with IV foscarnet. Twenty-five of 240 transplant recipients developed CMV disease and only 2.1% were ganciclovir resistant. Only one kidney recipient had ganciclovir-resistant CMV disease. Ganciclovir resistance was more common among pancreas or kidney-pancreas recipients, presumably due to the more intense immunosuppression used in these patients. Two of the 5 patients that developed ganciclovir-resistant CMV responded to higher ganciclovir doses. The authors recommend prophylaxis for up to 12 months in patients who receive antibody induction therapy, such as pancreas recipients.

Bienvenu, et al (31) also reported a ganciclovir patient. A 40-year-old male presented with primary CMV disease with leukopenia and fever and CMV PP65 antigenemia with positivity in 340 cells out of 200,000. The patient initially responded to IV ganciclovir, but by day 100 became positive again for CMV antigen. At this time, he responded to immunoglobulin administration. PCR analysis of the CMV isolate suggested a mutation that was thought to confer resistance to ganciclovir.

Kidd, et al (32) investigated the effect of co-infection of human herpes virus 7 (HHV-7) and human herpes virus 6 (HHV-6) and CMV and the development of acute rejection after renal transplantation. In this prospective study, patients were serologically assessed before transplantation and periodically for as long as 120 days after transplantation. In their series of 52 patients, the pretransplant sero-positivity for CMV, HHV-6 and

HHV-7 was 72.2%, 92.3%, and 94.4%. As assessed by PCR during the surveillance period, CMV viremia occurred in 58% of patients, HHV-6 viremia in 23%, and HHV-7 viremia in 46% of patients. CMV-PCR positive patients had an increased number of rejection episodes compared with CMV-PCR negative patients. CMV-positive patients with HHV-7 co-infection developed CMV disease in 66% of the cases. Neither HHV-7 or HHV-6 viremia appeared to have any obvious clinical importance.

Frances, et al (33) reported the outcome of kidney transplant recipients with previous human herpes virus 8 infection (HHV-8). Eight percent of their renal transplant recipients were positive for HHV-8 prior to transplantation. Twenty-eight percent of the HHV-8 positive patients developed Kaposi's sarcoma (KS), which occurs in only 2.3% of kidney recipients overall. HHV-8 genome was positive in all of the KS tissue samples but negative from all the peripheral blood mononuclear cells. Patient and graft survival rates for anti-HHV-8 antibody positive patients were 90.6% and 84.4% at one year, and 81.2% and 72%, respectively, at 3 years. In comparison, HHV-8 negative transplant recipients had patient and graft survival rates of 96% and 90% at one year, and 90% and 81% at 3 years, respectively. Donor HHV-8 status was not assessed.

Luppi, et al (34) report bone marrow failure associated with HHV-8 infection after transplantation in 3 patients, 2 with renal transplants and one recipient of peripheral blood stem cells. One of the renal transplant recipients developed persistent fever, splenomegaly, and marked cytopenia. He was found to have a high level of HHV-8 viremia and HHV-8 seroconversion. The finding of HHV-8, LANA in this patient within the immature bone marrow cells was found to be indicative of bone marrow failure by primary HHV-8 infection. HHV-8 in the study was transmitted by the donor kidney as ascertained by the K-1 sequence of the HHV-8 DNA, which proved to be the same for the donor and the 2 recipients. The simultaneous occurrence of disseminated Kaposi's sarcoma in one renal transplant recipient and bone marrow failure in the other suggests that the same virus may have distinct pathogenic potential in different human hosts.

Tong, et al (35) investigated the association of the human herpes virus 7 with cytomegalovirus disease in renal transplant recipients. In their study, a cohort of 37 renal transplant recipients were monitored for HHV-6 and HHV-7 using DNA detection as well as serology. The patients were kept on triple immunosuppressive therapy consisting of CsA, azathioprine, and prednisolone. HHV-7 DNA was detectable in 13 patients and 8 of these were among the patients with CMV disease. In 7 of the 8 patients, appearance of the HHV-7 DNA preceded the onset of CMV disease. In the remaining patient, the occurrence coincided with the onset of CMV disease. The authors speculate that HHV-7 may potentiate CMV disease either by direct interaction with CMV or by immunomodulatory effects of the host's system. HHV-7 DNA detection was associated with significantly higher plasma CMV loads. This could be explained by HHV-7 transactivation of CMV.

Pamidi, et al (36) described the persistent anemia seen in a renal transplant recipient secondary to infection with human parvovirus B19 (HPV-B19), a non-enveloped, single-stranded DNA virus which has tropism for human erythroid precursor cells. A 46-year-old white male with end-stage renal disease secondary to Henoch-Schonlein purpura was found to be anemic one year after transplantation. His bone marrow demonstrated hypocellularity with slightly decreased myeloid to erythroid ratio. Intra-nuclear eosinophilic inclusions were found which were confirmed to be of the HPV-B19 by immunoperoxidase staining. A similar case was seen in a 40-year-old white woman with end-stage renal disease secondary to TTP. The authors conclude that HPV infection should be considered in the differential diagnosis of persistent anemia in transplant recipients. Reticulocytopenia and bone marrow erythroid hypoplasia should further raise suspicion of this infection. Treatment with IV IgG should resolve the aplastic anemia.

Randhawa and Demetris (37) reviewed the nephropathy caused by Polyomavirus Type BK, a double-stranded DNA virus, which has a 70% homology with simian virus 40. Sero-prevalence of this virus in adults is estimated between 60-80%. Renal transplant recipients receiving immunosuppressive therapy have reactivation of the polyoma virus in 10-60% of cases. The BK virus has been implicated as a cause of interstitial nephritis in 5% of renal transplant recipients. Graft failure occurs in as many as 45% of affected patients. Afflicted patients can develop high serum creatinine levels mimicking rejection or ATN. The diagnosis is established by recognizing the BK virus inclusions in the renal tubular cells and glomerular epithelial cells of biopsy specimens. Unfortunately, patients with interstitial nephritis due to

BK virus may slip into a cycle alternating between viral interstitial nephritis and rejection precipitated by virus-induced immune activation and reduction of immunosuppression. The detection of virally infected transitional epithelial or "decoy" cells in urine has limited usefulness in diagnosis since BK virus can be detected by this method in only 28% of the cases.

Nickeleit (38) performed PCR assays to detect the BK virus DNA in plasma samples from 9 renal allograft recipients with BK virus nephropathy, 41 renal allograft recipients who did not have signs of nephropathy, and 16 who had "decoy" cells in the urine. As immunocompromised controls, 17 patients who had HIV Type I infection were also studied. The patients with BK virus nephropathy had high serum creatinine concentrations and shedding of "decoy" cells in the urine. The allograft biopsy specimen showed extensive viral infection with necrosis of tubular cells. The BK virus DNA was detected in the plasma samples of all of the patients. In contrast, BK virus was detected in only one of the 16 renal allograft recipients who had "decoy" cells in the urine, but no evidence of BK virus nephropathy. Viral DNA was no longer detectable in the plasma after 5 of the 9 patients had changes in their immunosuppressive therapy, 3 because of loss of the allograft with subsequent nephrectomy and 2 had a change in the doses of immunosuppressive drugs. Repeat biopsies showed endstage allograft nephropathy in one of the patients and acute rejection in another, but no BK virus nephropathy. A clear relationship between plasma viral DNA and BK virus nephropathy could not be established since 50% of the patients had positive serum virus DNA at the time of their nephropathy and 50% had positive virus DNA 16-30 weeks prior to development of BK nephropathy. The author suggests screening for "decoy" cells in the urine by cytologic tests in patients with impaired graft function and if these are present, they recommend PCR analysis of plasma samples for BK virus DNA followed by allograft biopsy.

Vachharajani, et al (39) reviewed the diagnosis and treatment of tuberculosis in hemodialysis and renal transplant patients. In this single-center retrospective study of 177 patients on hemodialysis, 24 (13%) were diagnosed with TB. 109 patients who received a renal transplant had a similar incidence of TB (14.6%). Loss of appetite and nausea was found in 60% of the renal transplant patients with high intermittent fever and persistent low-grade fever seen in up to 75% of the patients. Nearly one-third (31.3%) had diabetes and 12.5% were hepatitis B surface-antigen positive. Patients were treated with a 4-drug regimen. Thirteen of the 16 patients in the transplant group completed one year of therapy with good response. One patient relapsed and required retreatment. Three months after completing the course, 3 patients died, 2 of graft rejection and one of AIDS-related complex. The authors conclude that since resistant strains of *Mycobacterium tuberculosis* have emerged in Western countries, a diagnosis of TB should be considered in transplant patients who develop fevers of unknown origin, pulmonary infiltrates or effusions.

Knirsch, et al (40) described an outbreak of a *Legionella micdadei* pneumonia in a transplant center. In their study, the second most common *Legionella* species, *Legionella micdadei* infected patients that were severely immunosuppressed. The source was found to be the hot water system. Thirty-eight renal or cardiac transplant recipients were tested serologically. At the time of the outbreak, only 12 of these had evidence for *Legionella micdadei* pneumonia. The authors concluded that hospitals with transplant programs must suspect *Legionella* in immunosuppressed patients who have pneumonia of uncertain etiology. They recommend a first-line screen with the *Legionella* urine antigen test followed by specific *Legionella* cultures to identify other *Legionella pneumophila* serogroups and the non-pneumophila *Legionella* species that are not identified by the urine antigen test.

Battaglia, et al (41) report 2 cases of true mycotic arteritis by *Candida albicans*. In this report, 2 recipients of cadaveric renal allografts from the same donor developed complications secondary to *Candida albicans*, presumably transferred from the donor. The first patient developed dehiscence of the arterial anastomosis requiring removal of the renal allograft and ultimately iliac arterial ligation and a fem-to-fem bypass. The explanted renal artery and renal parenchyma were positive for *Candida albicans*. The second case was a patient that developed a high fever and pain in the iliac fossa after transplantation and was diagnosed with an aneurysm of the external iliac artery near the renal arterial anastomosis. This patient also required allograft nephrectomy, aneurysm excision, and arterial repair with a vascular graft. Again the explanted allograft tested positive for *Candida albicans*.

Complications – Tumors

Danpanich, et al (42) analyzed risk factors for the development of potentially life-threatening malignancy in renal transplant recipients. In a group of 1,500 patients, 88 malignancies were found, which - in decreasing order of frequency - included: lymphomas, lung, colorectal, prostate, brain, breast, liver, and other. The incidence of malignancy was 5.9% with a 0.89 per year annual incidence. Recipient age was a major risk factor. Patients 46-59 years of age had a 2.8-fold greater likelihood of developing an invasive malignancy than those younger than 46. Patients 60 years of age or older had a 5-fold greater risk. Pretransplant splenectomy was also strongly associated with cancer in multivariant analysis. Cigarette smoking of more than 25 pack-years had a 2.6-fold risk of cancer compared with those who smoked less or never smoked. Several factors found not to increase the risk of malignancy included: acute rejection episodes and the immunosuppressive regimen utilized either for treatment of acute rejection or maintenance.

Using the Danish registries, Birkeland, et al (43) investigated the risk of cancer in patients on dialysis and renal transplant patients. The dialysis group was comprised of 2,154 men and 1,438 women with mean ages of 50.5 and 49.8 years, respectively. The renal transplant group was comprised of 1,104 men and 717 women with mean ages of 38.7 and 39.2 years. The observation times were 6-6.4 years. There were 130 cancers in the dialysis group (relative risk of 1.35 for men and 1.47 for women). Most cancers in women were of the skin and genitourinary tract. In the transplant group, there were 209 cancers (relative cancer risk of 3.57 in men and 3.61 in women). These included cancer of the lip, skin, and lungs in both sexes, the genitourinary system in women, and non-Hodgkin's lymphomas in men. Posttransplant lymphoproliferative disease (PTLD) was found to be comprised mainly of B-cell lineage tumors. Occasional T-cell lymphoproliferative disorders have also been described. A case of PTLD of natural killer (NK) cell lineage has also been reported (44).

Marshall, et al (45) investigated glutathione S-transferase (GST) polymorphism and skin cancers after renal transplantation. GST is a complex of antioxidant enzymes, which may protect cells from cytotoxic and carcinogenic agents by conjugating reactive chemical species to reduced glutathione. Some isoenzymes have intrinsic organic peroxidase activity. Since many human GSTs have been isolated, the purpose of this study was to investigate whether the presence of any of these isoenzymes correlated with the development of skin cancer in Caucasian transplant recipients. The study was performed on 222 renal transplant recipients, 48 of whom had developed at least one skin tumor. Genotyping was performed by PCR with isoenzyme sequence-specific primers. The duration of immunosuppressive therapy, male sex, and age at the time of the first transplant were all found to be associated with the development of skin cancer, particularly of the squamous cell variety. In addition, the presence of the GST P1 isoenzyme was associated with the occurrence of skin tumors, squamous cell carcinoma in particular. No associations between GST polymorphism and basal cell carcinomas were identified. The authors concluded that GST genes could help identify transplant recipients with increased risk for skin cancer, warranting regular dermatologic review for surgical excision of suspicious lesions and possible aggressive therapy with antioxidant agents such as retinoids.

Post-operative adenotonsillar enlargement is thought to represent early presentation of PTLD in children. In this retrospective study, Huang, et al (46) analyzed children with solid organ transplants who presented with adenotonsillar hypertrophy and underwent removal of lymphoid tissue. The time between transplantation and adenotonsillectomy ranged from 14 months to almost 12 years. The indication for surgery was obstructive sleep disorder or nasal airway obstruction in 13 out of 15 patients. EBV-related lymphoid hyperplasia was demonstrated in 11 patients. This was characterized by lymphoid proliferation with preservation of the lymphoid architecture. *In-situ* hybridization for EBV and colloid RNA in these patients showed strong nuclear staining. The authors conclude that adenotonsillar hypertrophy in a child who has undergone solid organ transplantation may represent PTLD. Factors conferring increased risk for the disease include young age, liver as opposed to kidney allograft, pre-transplant EBV seronegativity, and use of tacrolimus as an immunosuppressive agent.

Herzig, et al (47) described the transmission of B-cell lymphoma by renal transplantation. Two female patients were recipients of kidneys from the same 72-year-old male donor. At the time of transplantation, one of the donor kidneys was biopsied because of donor age. Histological examination revealed a patchy infiltrate of small intermediate size lymphocytes suggestive of lymphoma. Percutaneous biopsy of the other organ after transplantation revealed similar infiltrates. Donor lymphoid tissue samples demonstrated a monoclonal B-cell subpopulation, and CD19- and CD20-positive cells with lambda light chain restriction. Immunosuppression was withdrawn in both recipients and the grafts were allowed to undergo acute rejection, and were removed. Histologic examination showed small B-cell lymphocytic lymphoma, which involved approximately 30% of the cortical and cortical medullary tissue. The presence of donor-derived cells in the peripheral blood of the transplant recipients was determined using a nested PCR approach. This micro-chimerism constituted 0.01-0.1% of the total peripheral blood mononuclear cells of the recipients on both day 6 after transplantation and day one after graft removal. No donor cells could be detected one, 3, and 6 months later.

Results

Wolfe, et al (48) compared mortality of chronic dialysis patients with those on dialysis, who were awaiting transplantation and recipients of a first cadaveric renal transplant. The US Renal Data System was used for this retrospective analysis. From 1991-1996, 228,552 patients under age 70 began treatment for renal failure. The unadjusted annual death rates per 100 patient-years for all patients on dialysis, on the transplant waiting list, and transplant recipients were 16.1, 6.3 and 3.8, respectively. The standardized mortality ratio was 49% lower for the patients on the waiting list and 69% lower among the recipients of a cadaveric renal transplant (compared with all patients on dialysis). When analyzed for each subgroup, the standardized mortality ratio was also lower (whites, blacks, Asians, Native Americans, females, males, diabetics, non-diabetics). The risk of death among transplant recipients during the first 2 weeks after transplantation was 2.8 times higher than for the patients on the waiting list. It remained elevated until 106 days after transplantation, becoming equal to the other groups by day 244. Overall the projected years of life remaining were 10 for the patients on the waiting list and 20 for the patients who received a transplant. The greatest benefit was seen in the age group from 20-39 years, where life expectancy was increased by 17 years with renal transplantation. Nonetheless, 60-74 year-old renal recipients had a projected increase in life-span of 4 years, with a decrease in long-term risk of death of 61%. The survival benefit was observed in all of the subgroups of patients. When analyzed by cause of renal failure, diabetic

patients had the greatest increase in long-term survival (11 years compared with 7 years for glomerulonephritis and 8 years for the other causes of end-stage renal disease). Although much of the mortality risk reduction observed in the renal transplant recipients was actually by being placed on the transplant waiting list (due to probable selection of healthier patients), the authors clearly demonstrated a mortality risk reduction and thus a survival advantage for the patients that were recipients of a renal transplant. With the documented 68% reduction in the long-term risk of death by Wolfe, et al (48), in his editorial review Hunsicker (49) voices the sentiment that renal transplantation should now be considered a lifesaving procedure. He analyzed the potential weaknesses and the possible biases that could have brought the results observed by Wolfe, et al, but ultimately considered them only remotely possible.

Hariharan, et al (50) reviewed the improvement in renal allograft survival in the United States, which took place between 1988-1996 by analysis of 93,934 transplants reported to UNOS by 276 transplant centers. The survival rate at one year for transplants from living donors increased from 88.8% in 1996 to 93.9% in 1998 and for cadaveric grafts from 75.7% to 87.7%. The projected half-life for transplants from living donors rose 70% from 12.7 years in 1988 to 21.6 years in 1995. After censoring data for patients who died with functional grafts, the respective half-life values were 16.9 years in 1988 and 35.9 years in 1995 for live donor transplants. For cadaveric grafts, the projected half-life was 7.9 years in 1988 and 13.8 years in 1995; this represents an increase of 75% in 1995 without censoring, and 11 years and 19.5 years with censoring those who died with functioning grafts. Patients who had an episode of clinical acute rejection during the first year had a reduction in projected half-life of cadaveric transplants (7 years in 1988 and 8.8 years in 1995) compared with patients who did not have an episode of clinical rejection in the first year after transplantation (8.8 years in 1988 and 17.9 years in 1995). The proportion of transplants from cadaveric donors who were more than 50 years old increased from 10.4% in 1988 to 18.2% in 1996 and the projected median half-life of the grafts was 5.5 years in 1988 and 7.5 years in 1995, an increase of 36%. The authors identified acute rejection as the primary obstacle to successful transplantation, and the introduction of CsA in the early 1980's as the most important factor in reducing the incidence of acute rejection and improving early (one-year) graft survival. In the long term, the most important cause of graft loss was chronic rejection with the most important predictor of chronic rejection being prior episodes of acute rejection. The poor outcome found in the black population was attributed to higher incidences of acute and chronic rejection due to differences in immunologic responsiveness, HLA matching, and blood pressure control.

Humar, et al (51) reported the survival of living unrelated kidney transplants. In this single-institution experience, 116 living-unrelated renal transplants were compared with 595 living related allografts. The characteristics of the groups were comparable in respect to donor age, recipient age, recipient gender, incidence of diabetes, and initial graft function, but there was a higher degree of HLA mismatch in the living-unrelated donor group (4.3 mismatches compared 2.6 for related donors). Recipients of living unrelated grafts received induction therapy with an antilymphocyte agent. Recipients of both groups were maintained on CsA, azathioprine, and prednisone. Five years after transplantation, patient survival was greater than 85% in both groups and graft survival was 77% for living-related and 79% for living-unrelated donor transplants. No difference was found in the incidence of acute rejection in the first posttransplant year. 34% of the living unrelated recipients had had an episode of acute rejection versus 33% of living-related donor recipients. The incidence of late acute rejection (greater than 6 months after transplant) was higher for living-related than for living-unrelated donor recipients (8.6 vs. 2.6%). By five years, 10% of the living-unrelated donor recipients had biopsy-proven rejection versus 16.7% of living-related donor recipients. The incidence of CMV disease was slightly higher in the living-unrelated donor recipients (17.2% vs. 13.7%) than in the living-related donor recipients. Despite the negative factors characterizing living-unrelated donor recipients, eg., older age, inferior HLA matching, the incidence of acute rejection and patient and graft survival were essentially the same for both groups.

Tandon, et al (52) analyzed the impact of cold ischemia time on the outcome of cadaveric renal transplants. The kidneys from 31 donors were procured and, due to staff and operating room availability, transplanted after either short or long cold ischemia time. Recipient age, gender, HLA match and PRA percentage was similar in both groups. The only difference between the groups was the cold ischemia time, which was 14.1±5.7

hours for group 1 and 19.2±6.7 hours for group 2. The incidence of ATN was higher for the group with longer cold ischemia (30% vs. 6%). Recipients of grafts that had a longer cold ischemia time also had a longer hospital stay (20.7±10.6 days vs. 16.3±6.2 days).

Healey, et al (53) reported single-institution results of 28 living donor adult kidneys transplanted to infants and small children between 1984-1999. Group 1 included transplants from 1984-1991 and Group 2 from 1992-1999. A major difference between the 2 groups was noted in that Group 1 patients received Minnesota anti-lymphoblast globulin induction therapy, azathioprine, and CsA-based immunosuppression with a tapering dose of CsA during the first 6 months, whereas Group 2 patients were treated with MMF instead of azathioprine and Neoral instead of CsA. Group 2 patients did not receive induction therapy with MALG. In addition, tacrolimus was used for Group 2 as rescue immunosuppression therapy for both chronic rejection and recurrent acute rejection. In Group 1, patient and graft survival rates were 92% and 78% at one year with graft survival rates of 85% at 3 years and 54% at 5 years. Biopsy-proven acute rejection within 6 months after transplantation was similar in the groups (30% for Group 1 and 40% for Group 2). All the recipients in Group 2 were alive with functioning grafts. The authors attributed the excellent results in this group to improved surgical management with aggressive intravascular support and central vascular anastomoses in the infant population, as well as to the advances in immunosuppression and vigilant clinical surveillance.

Nicholson, et al (54) analyzed the impact of allograft size to recipient body weight ratio on the long-term outcome of 104 cadaveric renal transplants. Ultrasonographic index of renal size-to-recipient body weight was determined one week after transplantation. Patients were stratified into 3 groups: transplant-to-body weight ratio; high (0.5); medium (0.3-0.45), or low (<0.3). The patients were then followed with glomerular filtration rates measured by isotope scanning at one, 6, and 12 months after transplantation. The 3 groups were well matched for age, sex, and number of previous transplants, as well as for HLA-DR mismatches, panel-reactive antibody status, donor age, sex, and ischemic times. In the first 5 years after transplantation, the serum creatinine level was significantly lower in patients with a high graft-to-body weight ratio than those with a low or medium transplant-to-weight ratio. Five-year allograft survival rates in the high, medium, and low graft-to-body weight ratio groups were 88%, 71%, and 74%, respectively. This study failed to demonstrate a convincing association between transplant size and graft survival, although the authors suggest that there is a trend toward improved graft survival in recipients with high transplant to weight ratios.

HLA Matching

Takemoto, et al (55) analyzed the outcome of national sharing of 7,614 HLA matched cadaveric kidneys transplanted between 1987-1999 as reported to UNOS. HLA-matched cadaveric renal transplants (defined as identical with the recipient for HLA-A, -B, and -DR antigens) were compared with HLA-mismatched ones. Homozygosity at the same loci by donor and recipient was later added to the definition of an HLA match. Donor grafts that had no HLA mismatches with the recipients HLA were subsequently also included within the definition HLA matched. Microcytotoxicity tests were used for HLA typing. Allocation was performed based on the results of 14 HLA-A loci, 45 HLA-B and 10 HLA-DR loci. Five percent of donor-recipient pairings were 6-HLA-antigen matches. Phenotypic HLA-identical pairing increased this to 7% and the "no-mismatch" criteria to a total of 13%. The estimated half-life of the HLA-matched group was 12.5 years compared with 8.6 years for the HLA-mismatched transplants. The estimated 10-year rate graft survival was 52% for the HLA-matched renal transplants and 37% for the HLA-mismatched transplants. There were no significant differences in the long-term survival of HLA-matched transplants when subdivided into the 6-antigen match, phenotypic match, and no-mismatch subgroups suggesting that these are appropriately grouped together.

The incidence of delayed graft function did not differ significantly between the HLA-matched and HLA-mismatched kidneys (21 vs. 19%). Recipients of HLA-matched renal grafts had higher creatinine levels at the time of discharge, but had a lower incidence of rejection (13 vs. 19%) and fewer days of hospitalization after the initial transplant procedure (10 vs. 11). During the first year after transplantation, 397 HLA-matched transplants failed, 70 due to rejection (18%); 485 HLA-mismatched transplants were lost, 117 due to rejection (24%). Of 141 HLA-matched grafts between 1-3 years after transplantation, 36 failed secondary to rejection (26%) and 62 were lost due to patient death (44%); 239 HLA-mismatched grafts were lost, 85 (36%) due to chronic rejec-

tion and 75 (31%) due to patient death. Despite the national sharing of HLA-matched kidneys, the increase of cold ischemia time was only one hour when compared with HLA-mismatched renal grafts. Thus, it appeared that the benefit of HLA matching was reflected in fewer episodes of rejection during the first 3 years as well as a decrease in both acute and chronic rejection that lead to graft loss.

Saadeh, et al (56) analyzed the impact of HLA-DMA allele polymorphism on kidney allograft outcome. HLA-DMA proteins play a major role in the processing of MHC class II molecules. Thus, different HLA-DMA alleles in kidney allograft recipients may be differentially associated with a more vigorous presentation of foreign donor MHC allopeptides and possibly a state of immune hyperresponsiveness. In this study, 92 renal allograft recipients were typed for the classic HLA class I and II antigens by serology and for the non-classical HLA-DMA alleles by automated DNA sequence analysis. The HLA-DMA allele frequencies were determined for the 0101, 0102, 0103, and 0104 alleles and their distribution was similar to the German and French controls. Patients with different HLA-DMA allele subgroups were compared for graft rejection, with the finding of no increased graft rejection rates attributed to a specific HLA-DMA allele.

Complete HLA-antigen matching is difficult due to the extremely polymorphic nature of the HLA system. One way of increasing the number of patients that can receive a well-matched transplant is by "shared" or "public" cross-reactive group (CREG) antigen matching. CREGs characterize immune reactivity to HLA antigens and can be defined in terms of topological features on the HLA molecule at the molecular level. Mckenna and Takemoto reviewed the benefit of CREG HLA matching (57). Similar or better graft survival has resulted from CREG matching, and been attributed to a decrease in the allogeneic humoral response. In addition, such matching promotes racial equity by considering antigens such as A2 (common in Caucasians) equivalent to A28 (common in minority groups). CREG matching also reduces the chances for a positive crossmatch and thus increases the transplantation rate of highly sensitized recipients (since CREGs are the major target of the anti-HLA antibodies). If the goal of CREG matching is reached (minimal level of matching that still confers histocompatibility); superior graft survival, decrease in PRA status and decrease in ethnic inequality would decrease the need for immunosuppression and shorten the time on the waiting list for minorities and high-PRA recipients.

Hollenbeak, et al (58) analyzed the economic benefit of the allocation of cadaveric renal transplants using CREG matching. The 3-year cost of renal transplantation was compared in the following groups: "0" HLA-mismatched, "0" CREG/DR-mismatched and CREG/DR-mismatched donor-recipient pairings. The best graft survival was seen in "0" HLA-mismatched recipients, 5% higher graft survival than the "0" CREG/DR-mismatched and 7% better than the CREG/DR-mismatched grafts.

Lee, et al (59) analyzed the impact of cold ischemia time (CIT) in "0" HLA mismatched renal transplantation. The average CIT for cadaveric renal allografts according to the UNOS transplant registry was 21.6 hours (62% of the kidneys preserved for less than 24 hours, 30% for 24-36 hours and 8% for longer than 36 hours). Shorter CIT was associated with improved graft and patient survival. Five-year graft and patient survival rates of 68.3% and 85.4%, 63.1% and 82.2%, and 59.9% and 81.3% were found, respectively, for CIT of <24, 24-36 and >36 hours. Recipients of "0" mismatched kidneys with >36 CIT did not have a survival advantage compared with patients with 1+HLA mismatches with a CIT <24 hours.

Acute Rejection

Although the incidence of acute rejection (AR) has decreased in the last decade, it still accounts for increased morbidity, increased cost, and patient re-hospitalization. In addition, AR is thought to be the single most important risk factor for chronic rejection. Multiple episodes of AR have an especially poor prognosis. Humar, et al (60) analyzed the clinical determinants of patients at risk for multiple rejection episodes. In this single-institution study, renal transplant recipients were retrospectively grouped as patients who had a single episode of AR or multiple ARs. Of the 1,793 recipients, 661 (36.9%) were treated for AR. Of the group requiring treatment for AR, 354 (53.6%) had one episode and 307(46.4%) had more than one episode. The 2 groups were similar with regard to donor source (CAD vs. LD), HLA mismatches and recipient PRA level. Patients that had multiple episodes of AR were younger (37.4 years vs. 41.4 years), were re-transplants (25% vs. 18%), had higher rates of delayed graft function requiring dialysis (DGF) and slow graft function (SGF)(24.1% vs. 17.0%). Multivariate analysis with multiple ARs as a dependent variable evidenced DGF and SGF as significant risk fac-

tors (RR=1.71), as well as AR less than 6 months after transplant (RR=1.71), steroid-resistant AR (first episode)(RR=1.61) or presence of vascular rejection (RR=1.34). Patients with multiple AR episodes had a 5-year graft survival rate of 53% compared with 85% in recipients with only one episode of AR.

There was renewed interest in the use of markers for the diagnosis of acute rejection (AR) in biopsy specimens and non-invasive testing. Dugre et al (61) measured cytokine and cytotoxic molecule gene expression in peripheral blood mononuclear cells for the diagnosis of AR. Twenty-one renal transplant recipients were considered for the study, 13 with diagnosed AR. Weekly PBMC samples were collected and analyzed retrospectively for the cytokines IL-2, 4, 5, 6,10 and IFN-g, and the cytotoxic molecules, granzyme (GrB) and Perforin. IL-4, 5 and 6 mRNA of PBMC was significantly higher in patients undergoing an episode of AR. The same applied to GrB and Perforin. IL-2, 10,15 and Fas L mRNA expression did not correlate with AR. When at least 2 of the cytokine markers were elevated, 75% of the rejecting recipients were identified, vs. 15% of the non-rejecting. Two patients with borderline rejection by biopsy had no elevation in cytokine mRNA. This method is suggested as non-invasive test for graft surveillance.

Pascoe, et al (62) performed immuno-cytochemical analysis of fine needle aspiration (FNA) allograft biopsies to investigate the relationship between Perforin, Granzyme B and Fas ligand gene product expression and AR. Fifty-six patients were followed during the first month after renal transplantation who had poor allograft function or a decline in function. Perforin, Granzyme B and Fas ligand positive staining of lymphocytes was present in the specimen of 97%, 88% and 88% respectively of the patients with an AR and in 47%, 23% and 22% of patients with no rejection. In addition, Fas ligand stained positive in renal tubule cells of 40% of the patients who had AR and in none without AR. The sensitivity of FNA immuno-cytochemistry was calculated at 96.5% for one marker positive for the diagnosis of AR, 91.2% for 2 markers positive and 84% when all 3 markers were required to be positive for the diagnosis of AR.

Chareandee, et al (63) measured renal tubule Endothelin-1 (ET-1) in percutaneous renal biopsies as means of diagnosing tubulo-interstitial damage. ET-1 is a mitogenic and pressor peptide that correlates well with chronic rejection when present in the neointima of the renal vessels with transplant vasculitis. The study sought to determine whether renal tubular ET-1 levels were elevated in both acute and chronic rejection. Eighteen patients with acute and 7 with chronic rejection were studied. ET-1 was determined by immuno-histochemistry staining. ET-1 was abundant in the tubular cytoplasm of cortical proximal and distal convoluted tubules and at sites in the interstitium adjacent to the epithelium at localized sites of injury in all of the patients undergoing acute rejection. Similar findings were seen in chronic rejection specimens with tubular ET-1 present in areas of interstitial injury and fibrosis. In contrast to vascular expression of ET-1 in chronic rejection, vascular ET-1 was normal or depressed in specimens of patients undergoing acute rejection.

Teppo, et al (64) studied the changes of urinary β1-microglobulin (β1-M) in the assessment of prognosis in renal transplant recipients. β1-M is a 26-33 kD glycoprotein with a constant serum level, and is both bound to albumin and freely circulating. The free portion is filtered in the glomeruli and is reabsorbed by the proximal tubule cells. β1-microglobinuria correlates with proximal tubule damage/dysfunction. Patients were grouped into cadaveric renal transplant recipients (n=106), cadaveric renal transplant recipients with evidence of AR (n=30) and normal controls. β1-M was measured in daily urine samples. Control individuals had 3.47 mg/24 hr of β1-M in urine with a β1-M /creatinine ratio of 0.27. All of the renal transplant recipients had elevated β1-M in urine after transplant (related to ischemic damage) with a β1-M /creatinine ratio of 19.3. Patients in the AR group had an increase in the β1-M /creatinine ratio to a mean of 22.2 and 26.4, respectively, by the second and third week after transplant. In contrast, uncomplicated transplant recipients had a decrease in their ratios to 10.3 and 8.1 by the second and third weeks. The authors calculated the sensitivity and specificity of decreased urinary β1-M /creatinine ratio to detect patients with an uncomplicated posttransplant course at 88.5% and 85.7%, respectively, with a 95% predictive value.

Bonsib, et al (65) studied the importance of the disruption of tubular basement membranes (TBMs), secondary to acute rejection in the development of chronic allograft nephropathy. Patients were selected based on the presence of acute tubulointerstitial rejection (Banff 97 and NIH/CCTT type 1 rejection). TBM breaks usually consisted of short segments of absent staining associated with foci of acute interstitial rejection and tubulitis. The initial biopsies contained few atrophic tubules, with 7-103 TBM breaks per mm^2. Control biopsies contained only 0-2.91 TBM breaks per mm^2. TBM breaks correlated with development of atrophic tubules from 2.8 to 96.4/mm^2 in the final biopsy. This correlated clinically with increase in Cr level from a mean of 2.2 to a mean of 6.3 mg/dl compared with controls (1.7-1.9).

Chronic Rejection

McLauren, et al (66) performed a multivariate analysis of the risk factors that lead to chronic renal allograft failure. Of the 862 patients transplanted at a single institution, 117 were excluded due to transplant failure within the first 6 months after transplantation. Seventy-seven patients went on to develop biopsy confirmed chronic allograft failure (CAF). Late acute rejection (>6 months posttransplant) was a major risk factor (odds ratio (OR)= 5.91) while acute rejection during the first 3 months was a significant risk (OR 2.31). Patients <50 years old had an increased risk (OR 2.51), but male sex had a protective effect (OR 0.35). The severity of the AR correlated well with a higher incidence of chronic graft failure; patients that developed AR within the first 3 months had a 14.1% incidence of CAF if the serum Cr level returned to within 10% of the baseline level. If the Cr remained elevated, the risk was 26.2% for the development of CAF. In addition, a steroid-resistant AR episode was correlated with a 19.4% incidence of CAF.

Meier-Kriesche, et al (67) studied the impact of AR on the development of chronic renal failure in the recent era. Using data from the US Renal Transplant Scientific Registry, patients from 2 different eras were evaluated for AR and CAF. The incidence of AR in the first 6 months after transplantation decreased from 31.4% in the 1988-89 group, to 14.2% in the 1996-97 group. Since the graft loss due to CAF has remained unchanged, the authors calculate a 5-fold increase in the relative risk for chronic graft failure with an episode of AR. The decrease in the incidence of AR has been attributed to better immunosuppressive regimens.

The relationship between recipient age and chronic renal failure was studied in the Caucasian population (68). Retrospective analysis of the US Renal Transplant Scientific Registry was performed on 3 recipient age groups (18-49 years, 50-64 and >65 years of age). Donors of the >65 years group had a longer cold ischemia time as well as a greater incidence of DGF. The recipients of older donor kidneys also had a higher percentage of cadaveric grafts. Graft survival was decreased in the older age group and markedly decreased in patients older then 65 (death censored). Graft loss due to CAF was likewise increased in the older age groups, with 29% higher relative risk for the age group 50-64 years, and 67% higher for the >65 years group. Hypertension and diabetes also conferred a significant risk increase for the development of CAF. The risk for acute rejection was calculated with a logistic regression model to be decreased in the extreme age group.

Wissing, et al (69) performed a retrospective single institution study, to investigate the relationship between CAF and hypercholesterolemia. Seven hundred seventy-two renal transplantation recipients were grouped according to the presence of acute rejection during the first post-transplant year and cholesterol level. Patients who had had an episode of AR with a cholesterol level >250 mg/dl, had proteinuria, higher creatinine levels and a higher incidence of CAF (50% graft loss at 10 years vs. 24.3% for patients with <250 mg/dl cholesterol level). Furthermore, patients with normal cholesterol levels had similar graft survival whether or not they had had an episode of AR. The association of hypercholesterolemia and AR was more significant in male recipients who had a CAF of 36.3% at 5 years and 61.6% at 10 years. This compared with males with normal cholesterol levels with 11.1% and 28.3%, respectively, at 5 and 10 years. Such an association was not found in female recipients. Risk analysis for CAF found proteinuria, HLA immunization and increased creatinine as risk factors. Hypercholesterolemia was a risk factor only in males.

Jain, et al (70) reviewed the role of transforming growth factor beta (TGF-β) in chronic renal allograft nephropathy. TGF-β is a homodimeric cytokine, of which 3 isoforms are known in humans. It is released as an inactive precursor attached to LAP (latency-associated protein). TGF-β can both stimulate and inhibit cell growth and proliferation. It inhibits adhesion of neutrophils to the endothelium and their membrane transmigration. It also decreases monocyte and lymphocyte proliferation and may induce apoptosis of the latter. Fibroblasts are stimulated by TGF-β to produce collagen and fibronectin. Over-expression of TGF-β is associated with fibrosis. The cytokine may have a protective effect in ischemia-reperfusion injury, but if the injury is extensive, persistence of TGF-β is thought to lead to CAF. Recipient factors like hyperlipidemia and hypertension may induce chronic allograft injury via TGF-β cytokine production. Increased TGF-β mRNA expression has been found in recipients of renal allografts with CAF and CsA nephrotoxicity.

Mas, et al (71) studied the expression of TGF-β with quantitative RT-PCR in renal biopsies of patients with CAF. The TGF-β mRNA expression was found to correlate with proteinuria levels. Patients who had >1000mg of protein in urine/24 hours had 3 to 10- fold greater expression of TGF-β mRNA vs. patients with no proteinuria.

Immunosuppression

Melle and Halloran (72) reviewed the use of Mycophenolate Mofetil (MMF) in transplant recipients. This compound blocks the production of guanosine nucleotides required in de-novo DNA synthesis. T- and B-cell proliferation is inhibited as well as the glycosylation of adhesion molecules.

Three double-blind trials were conducted to test MMF in cadaveric renal recipients. In the US Renal study and the Tricontinental study, MMF (2 mg or 3 mg/day) was compared with Azathioprine (1-2 mg/kg/day)(AZA) in patients who also received CsA and steroids (73,74,75). The incidence of graft loss due to rejection was reduced in the MMF groups versus AZA as were the rates of biopsy-proven rejection and the need for additional anti-rejection therapy (US Renal study). Anemia, hypertension and diarrhea were the most commonly reported side effects of immunosuppressive but only diarrhea was more frequent in the MMF group. Tissue invasive CMV was more frequently seen in patients receiving MMF. In the European study, which compared MMF to placebo, a decrease in biopsy-proven rejection rates and treatment failure was observed in the MMF treated group. Again, GI complaints were higher in the MMF groups as was invasive CMV infection. *Pneumocystis carinii* pneumonia and fungal infections were seen only in the placebo group, a result that was attributed to the antimicrobial effects of MMF. The incidence of PTLD and skin malignancy was similar at one year in all groups. The Tricontinental study indicated that one-year graft survival was improved in recipients treated with 2 or 3 mg of MMF versus AZA, respectively, at 88.3%, 89% and 86%. Graft function as defined by serum creatinine level was similar in the 3 groups. Pooled data from the 3 randomized trials confirmed that MMF reduced the incidence of graft loss due to acute rejection by 50% at 3 years after transplantation. The graft survival was similar for patients receiving either MMF or AZA. In contrast, graft loss due to rejection was decreased for MMF 2mg/day and MMF

3mg/day (5.8% and 3.0%) versus AZA (9.9%). CMV infection, GI toxicity and leukopenia were more common for MMF (3mg/day).

Pascual, et al (76) treated biopsy-proven CAF in 17 patients by discontinuing AZA, reducing the CsA dose by 30% and adding MMF (1 g/day). With a follow up time of 11 months, 88% of patients showed improvement of their renal function as evidenced by a decrease in serum creatinine. Progressive deterioration was seen in patients that had nephrotic range proteinuria. There were no episodes of AR.

Houde, et al (77) substituted MMF for CsA in 17 patients for biopsy proven CsA nephrotoxicity. The patients averaged 57 months after transplantation. MMF was given at 2 g/day except in one patient (1 g/day) and CsA was tapered over a 6-week period. There was a significant decrease in the creatinine level, with maximum effect at 3 months after replacement. There was also improvement of proteinuria, hypertension and hyperlipidemia. In this study, no clinical evidence of AR was found in any of the patients at 20±8 months follow up.

Smak Gregoor, et al (78) weaned 64 stable renal allograft recipients (1 year after transplant) off CsA and randomized them to receive either MMF/Prednisone or AZA/Prednisone. Renal function was improved after discontinuation of CsA in both groups, as evidenced by marked decrease in serum creatinine levels. The AZA/Pred group had a higher incidence of AR (at 18 months follow-up), but only 10% required anti-lymphocyte treatment. The CAF rate was equal in both groups (7%).

Comparison of MMF (2 gm per day) to AZA in patients receiving tacrolimus showed a decrease in AR. One-year AR rates of 8.9% were observed for MMF 2 g/day, 34.9% MMF 1g/day and 35.6% AZA. In a prospective randomized study that compared tacrolimus plus steroids (double therapy) with tacrolimus, MMF and steroids (triple therapy), graft survival of 89% was seen in the triple therapy group vs. 85% for the double therapy group. AR incidence at one year was 44% for double therapy, and 27% for triple therapy. Steroid-resistant rejection rates of 7.5% and 2.9%, respectively, were noted. Furthermore 39% of the patients on triple therapy were subsequently successfully weaned off steroids versus 25% of patients on double therapy (79).

Pascual, et al (80) suggested that the combination of MMF and tacrolimus with steroids was useful for the treatment of steroid-resistant rejection. Despite a limited experience, each of the 14 patients responded to this treatment with improved GFR and a decrease in serum creatinine. When the efficacy of the single drugs (MMF, tacrolimus and IV steroids) were compared in a meta-analysis, tacrolimus treatment resulted in lower rates of recurrent rejection (4-11%) when compared with MMF (25%) and high-dose steroids (36%), and with decreased need for anti-lymphocyte therapy (2%, 10% and 25%, respectively). In addition, serious side effects and CMV disease were seen in 14% and 4% of patients receiving tacrolimus, compared with 56% and 23% for MMF and 44% and 17% for steroids, respectively.

Using the US Renal Transplant Scientific Registry, Ojo, et al (81) compared AZA with MMF in a triple drug regimen including calcineurin inhibitors and steroids. The incidence of AR during the first 6 months after transplantation was 24.7% for the AZA group and 15.5% for the MMF group, with 4-year graft survival rates of 85.6% and 81.9% respectively. The risk for CAF was 27% lower in MMF patients than in AZA patients if there had been a previous episode of AR and 20% lower with MMF in patients who had no previous AR.

Kaplan, et al (82) withdrew MMF from 45 patients on triple immunosuppression one year after renal transplantation. The rationale was that the beneficial effect of MMF in reducing AR episodes is mainly seen in the first posttransplant year. With an average follow up of 12 months after withdrawal, 2 out of 45 patients had an episode of AR compared with one in a control group.

Steroid withdrawal has been a major interest of the transplantation community in recent years. The European steroid withdrawal group studied patients on MMF and CsA. They found an increase in AR in patients who received low-dose steroids followed by withdrawal versus full steroid therapy (19% vs. 5%). The majority of rejection episodes were low-grade and occurred in patients who were on low-dose steroids prior to tapering off of the drug. The patients showed improved lipid profiles at 6 months and there was no difference in patient and graft survival between the groups (83).

The US steroid withdrawal study group reported their results in 133 kidney transplant recipients on CsA and MMF. In the study group, steroids were gradually withdrawn over 8 weeks starting 3 months after transplantation. The control group was kept on maintenance doses of the drug. At one year, the control group had an AR rate of 4.4% (and failure of anti-rejection therapy of 14.9%). In the study group, 21% had AR (and failure of anti-rejection therapy of 39.3%). The study was discontinued due to increased AR in the withdrawal group (84).

In contrast, Matl, et al (85) reported a 6.6% AR rate at one year in patients who were tapered off steroids over a 6-month interval. The baseline triple immunosuppression consisted of AZA and CsA (plus continued steroids in the control group). In a study group of 45 patients, 3 had evidence of AR versus 2 (4.7%) in the steroid control group. They also found lower cholesterol levels in patients who were off steroids.

Steroid withdrawal in a pediatric population on tacrolimus immunosuppression was reported by Chakrabarti, et al (86). In this non-randomized study, steroid withdrawal was attempted in all of the pediatric renal allograft recipients. In 92.5% of the patients it was possible to taper the steroid dose to zero; 70% remained off steroids. Graft loss in the group weaned from steroids was due to rejection in 2 patients, to recurrent disease in 2 and in one to non-compliance. Among patients who initially failed weaning, 39% were eventually successfully weaned off steroids. This group had 3 graft failures due to rejection and one to recurrent disease. Actuarial graft survival for patients off steroids was 97%, 96% and 79% at one, 3 and 5 years, respectively. Graft survival for patients that failed the steroid weaning was 100%, 89% and 83% at one, 3 and 5 years, respectively.

Sandrini, et al (87) compared steroid withdrawal in 116 renal transplant recipients treated with CsA and AZA or CsA alone. Recipient and donor characteristics were similar in the 2 groups. In a 5-year follow-up period, steroids were successfully withdrawn in only 48% of the CsA monotherapy patients, compared with 71% in the CsA/AZA group. AR was responsible for all of the failures. Seventy-four percent of AR episodes occurred during the first 6 months, with 33% of AR episodes in the CsA group occurring after 6 months of steroid weaning compared with 13% for the CsA/AZA group. AR episodes responded to steroid therapy, with two-thirds of the patients returning to pre-rejection renal function. The 5-year graft survival was 88% for the CsA monotherapy and 91% for the CsA/AZA group. Cholesterol levels were improved after steroid withdrawal in both groups.

Hurault de Ligny, et al (88) analyzed factors predicting long-term success of CsA used as monotherapy. Of the 728 recipients, 70% were successfully withdrawn from steroids, and of those 240 were placed on CsA monotherapy. The overall graft survival was 91%, 84%, 77% and 64% at one, 3, 5 and 8 years, respectively;

patient survival was 94% and 92% at 5 and 8 years, respectively. Patients on CsA monotherapy had 3- and 8-year survival rates of 100% and 95%, respectively. Graft survival was 96% and 95% at 5 and 8 years, respectively. Variables significant in univariate analysis for the risk of CsA monotherapy failure were: donor >40 years, recipient age <25 years, cold ischemia time >14 hours, creatinine level at initiation of CsA monotherapy >125 mmol/l and a previous episode of AR. Multivariate analysis excluded recipient age and cold ischemia time from this list.

In order to identify the patients whose immunosuppressive medications can be safely discontinued or reduced, van Besouw, et al (89) tested recipients for their T-cell reactivity with peripheral blood mononuclear cells against donor spleen cells in mixed lymphocyte cultures (MLC). They also determined reactive T-helper lymphocyte precursors (HTLpf) and cytotoxic T-cell precursor (CTLpf) frequencies using limiting dilution analysis (against HLA class I). A decreased rate of AR was seen in recipients that had low donor-specific CTLpf before dose reduction of their immunosuppressive drugs. In addition, none of the patients developed an AR if they had no detectable CTLpf. Thus, the absence of donor CTL was predictive of no subsequent AR in stable patients prior to weaning of immunosuppression.

Higgins, et al (90,91) converted stable renal transplant recipients from tacrolimus to CsA based immunosuppression. The authors are aware of the reported 30% lower incidence of AR in patients treated with tacrolimus than with CsA but rationalize this conversion on the basis of 50% lower costs. The patients were converted at 3-6 months after transplant. The presence of more than one episode of AR disqualified the recipient for the conversion. Patient and graft survival was 100% at 3 months. After a mean of 25 months follow up, 3 of 19 patients were placed back on tacrolimus (because of AR in 2 cases and hirsutism in one). There were no changes in creatinine, BUN, or serum glucose levels but serum levels of magnesium and cholesterol increased significantly. The authors considered the conversion from tacrolimus to CsA a safe strategy with no short- term immunologic consequences and obvious economic advantages.

Breidenbach, et al (92, 93) reported a series of 30 renal transplant recipients whose CsA levels were discovered to drop by a mean of 47% because of non-supervised, intake of St. John's wort (Hypericum perforatum). The herbal extract is used for mild

The proposed system is based in part on the work of Malinchoc, et al (104) who developed the MELD (Mayo End-Stage Liver Disease) scoring system which predicts the expected survival of patients with chronic liver disease who undergo elective TIPS. The authors analyzed the survival of 231 patients from 4 centers who required TIPS for prevention of variceal hemorrhage (n=173) or refractory ascites (n=58). The mean Child's Pugh score for the cohort was 9.8. Using logistic regression analysis, the authors found four variables that had independent prognostic value in predicting survival at 3 months: Total bilirubin, creatinine, INR and the cause of liver disease. Patients with liver disease of cholestatic origin or from alcohol had a better outcome than did those with other diagnoses including Hepatitis C. However the contribution of this variable to the overall model was relatively small and it is unlikely to be included in a UNOS supported system of allocation since it would appear to discriminate against specific groups based on their disease etiology.

By inputting data specific for an individual patient into the MELD regression equation, an estimate of the chance of the patient surviving for 3 months can be calculated and assigned a "risk score". A continuum of risk estimates is possible thus allowing stratification of patients waiting for transplant solely by urgency. This fact makes it feasible to reduce the influence of the amount of time on a wait list in liver allocation.

Although the MELD model appears to have a number of advantages over the current system based on Child's Pugh score, it may also suffer from several deficiencies. For example, patients with tumors are given no priority in the MELD model. Despite the fact that such patients may have less severe liver disease as estimated by the MELD formula, they represent a group in which prolonged waiting may allow extrahepatic spread of tumor and preclude transplantation. Clearly provisions will have to be made for such patients who are not handled well by the MELD model.

Kim, et al (105) examined the applicability of a simplified version the Mayo Primary Biliary Cirrhosis natural history model as a means to select candidates for transplant. The original 5-variable regression model (bilirubin, albumin, prothrombin time, age and edema) was modified to a tabular format similar to the currently utilized Child's-Pugh-Turcotte system. The new model, which assigns 0-3 points depending on the status of each of the same 5 variables, was found to correlate well with the original model in its prognostic capability. A formal comparison of the Mayo PBC and MELD models has not been reported. The inclusion of patient age as a variable in the Mayo PBC may raise questions about equitable selection of recipients.

Shakil, et al (106) reviewed the experience with patients referred to the University of Pittsburgh for acute liver failure (ALF). During a 13-year period, 177 patients were evaluated for ALF. Transplantation was performed in 87 (49%); 25 (14%) recovered with medical therapy alone and 65 patients (37%) died without transplant. Of the patients who died, the vast majority had been listed for transplant at least temporarily, suggesting that many of them may have been saved had a liver become available in a timely fashion. The applicability of the King's College (KC) criteria for poor outcome in acute liver failure was evaluated in the Pittsburgh cohort. In general, the KC criteria demonstrated a high level of specificity but a relatively low sensitivity for both acetaminophen and non-acetaminophen related cases. Thus, given the overall 80% mortality in patients managed medically, the authors concluded that the absence of meeting the KC criteria does not adequately predict survival and should not dissuade consideration of prompt transplantation especially in patients with non-acetaminophen induced liver failure.

Retransplantation of the liver is known to have an outcome inferior to that of primary grafts. Appropriate recipient selection may be a critical determinant. Facciuto, et al (107) reported the results in 48 patients requiring late retransplantation (more than 6 months after a previous graft). Recipient age, elevated preoperative creatinine, and the use of intraoperative blood products were all associated with poor outcome in multivariate analysis. The most common cause of death in this cohort, as in prior series, was sepsis. The authors suggest that careful selection of patients with particular attention to recipient age and renal function may improve results in this difficult transplant group.

Severe pulmonary hypertension mean pulmonary artery pressure (MPAP >50) is known to be associated with poor liver transplant outcomes. Reliable, non-invasive methods to allow preoperative identification of these high-risk patients would be of great value. The accuracy of Doppler echocardio-graphy (DE) to identify liver patients with pulmonary hypertension was studied by Kim, et al (108). Thirty-nine patients with DE estimated right ventricular (RV) systolic pressure of >50 mmHg, and 35 patients with RV systolic pressure of <50 mmHg underwent right heart catheterization. Of the 39 with elevated pressures on DE, 29 (72%) had at least moderate pulmonary hypertension (MPAP >35 mmHg as measured by catheter and 12 (30%) had severe disease (MPAP >50 mmHg). DE failed to identify pulmonary hypertension in only one patient who had only moderate pulmonary hypertension. Overall, DE was found to have a sensitivity of 97% and specificity of 77% indicating that it is a useful screening method for identifying those patients in need of preoperative right heart catheterization.

The utility of Dobutamine stress echocardiography (DSE) to identify liver patients at risk for perioperative morbidity due to coronary artery disease (CAD) was assessed by Williams, et al (109). Patients being evaluated for liver transplantation underwent DSE if they had risk factors for CAD such as atypical chest pain or age >60 years but were without documented CAD or ischemic symptoms (in which case cardiac catheterization was performed). Of 59 transplanted patients with a normal or non-diagnostic DSE, 8 major perioperative cardiac events occurred including 5 arrhythmias. Three cardiac arrests occurred, apparently related in part to intraoperative or postoperative hemorrhage. It was concluded that DSE could be performed safely in patients with ESLD, but in those with low to moderate risk it may be a poor predictor of major postoperative cardiac events.

Compromised nutritional status is common with end-stage liver disease (ESLD) and has been associated with poor outcome. Figueiredo, et al (110) studied 69 patients awaiting OLT to determine which of the commonly measured nutritional parameters provided the best assessment of body cell mass as a surrogate for protein calorie malnutrition. Of multiple parameters examined, the authors found that only mid-arm muscle circumference and hand-grip strength were relevant markers of protein calorie malnutrition.

To determine whether nutritional supplementation could reverse the adverse effects of protein calorie malnutrition, Le Cornu, et al (111) performed a randomized study of nutritional supplementation in pretransplant patients. Half of 82 consecutive patients who were in the 25th percentile or less for mid-arm muscle circumference were treated with calorie-dense enteral feeding until transplantation. Although improvement was seen in the nutritional parameters of supplemented patients, no impact on outcome was observed.

The impact of cross-reactive epitope group (CREG)

matching of liver donor and recipient was investigated by Sawyer, et al (112) who studied the outcome of 288 liver transplants. An unexpectedly high rate of late hepatic artery thrombosis (HAT) was observed in patients with zero CREG mismatches (13%) compared with patients with one or more mismatches (2%). This was associated with a reduced graft survival in the zero CREG mismatch group (56%) compared with controls (68%). The authors suggest an immunological basis for the increased incidence of HAT with better class I HLA matching, however a clear mechanism and convincing support of this hypothesis by histopathological evidence is lacking.

The effect of iron overload on the outcome of liver transplantation was studied by Brandhagen, et al (113), who identified 37 patients in whom hepatic iron overload (hepatic iron index >1.9) was present in the explanted native liver and who were negative for hereditary hemochromatosis by PCR testing for HFE gene mutations (C282Y and H63D). Compared with matched controls (who were similar in age, gender, average CPT score and disease etiology), survival was markedly reduced in patients with iron overload. Kaplan-Meier survival at 5 years for the group with iron excess was 48% compared with 77% for controls. The difference in survival was at least in part attributable to the increased number of fatal infections, especially fungal, seen in patients with iron overload. While this suggests iron excess may be associated with compromised immune function, it is of interest that there was no difference in the rate of acute rejection between the groups.

The development of elevated intracranial pressure (ICP) in patients with acute or fulminant liver failure is known to portend poor survival. Invasive ICP monitoring in the context of liver failure is often problematic due to severe coagulopathy and is itself frequently associated with major complications. Helmke, et al (114) utilized a noninvasive approach to monitor ICP in 22 patients with liver failure and hepatic encephalopathy. This method utilized orbital ultrasound to measure the optic nerve sheath diameter. The authors suggest that dilation of the optic nerve sheath is associated with a shift of the CSF to the orbit due to increased ICP. This can be detected earlier than papilledema. Of 10 patients with abnormal dilation of the optic nerve sheath 8 patients died, most from elevated ICP. Although this approach does not provide continuous measurements, it may provide useful prognostic information in patients who are not candidates for invasive monitoring. Clearly the results need to be confirmed in a larger cohort of patients.

Live-Donor Liver Transplantation

The growing organ shortage may have had its greatest impact in encouraging the use of live liver donors, which would substantially increase the donor pool. Until recently, live donor transplantation has been largely limited to adult-to-child grafts utilizing the left lateral segment of the donor liver. More recently, this procedure has been supplanted by adult-to-child *in-situ* split cadaveric grafts (except in cases of fulminant hepatic failure). The experience at the University of Chicago with adult-to-child live donor transplants was reported by Millis, et al (115). Since the introduction of the technique in 1989, 104 LDLT transplants have been performed using 93 left lateral segments and 11 left lobes. The authors detail the technical modifications they believe are responsible for a marked improvement in survival, specifically, the elimination of arterial and portal venous conduits, and the use of a microsurgical approach to arterial reconstruction.

The need for anastomosing multiple hepatic arteries (HA) from segmental grafts was reported by Kubota, et al (116). These authors utilized back-table infusion of the main artery to determine whether collaterals existed between the main and accessory arteries. The findings were confirmed by back-bleeding after reperfusion via the primary artery and by doppler examination to ensure that all segments of the liver had pulsatile arterial flow. In a series of 64 live donor transplants to children, 25 had an accessory artery. In 22 cases it was deemed expendable and was ligated. There were no obvious deleterious sequelae to this approach, and graft survival in these cases was equivalent to grafts without an accessory artery.

More recently, techniques developed and lessons learned both from adult-to-child live donor grafts and from *in-situ* cadaveric liver splitting have provided the foundation for adult-to-adult live-donor liver transplantation (LDLT). During the past year, many groups have reported their initial experience with this technique and important technical refinements have been described. As a result of the rapid expansion of centers initiating adult-to-adult LDLT, the ASTS Ethics Committee generated a position paper on the procedure (117). This report details reasonable guidelines for donor selection and evaluation, recipient selection, consent, and suggested criteria for centers embarking on such a program.

A comprehensive overview of adult-to-adult LDLT using right lobe (RL) grafts was provided by Marcos, et al (118), who previously reported the first major series of LDLT in the US. All aspects of the procedure are reviewed including donor and recipient selection and work-up (also described in detail by Trotter, et al (119) and by Marcos, et al in a separate publication (120)). An even more complete account of the Medical College of Virginia experience is described by Marcos, et al (121) in other reports including an update of their experience with 40 RL LDLT. On the basis of their extensive experience, they recommend: 1) utilization of donors in whom there is a RL graft-to-recipient body weight ratio of >0.8%, with correction for the extent of steatosis in the donor, 2) angiography to define the donor liver's arterial and portal vascular anatomy of segment IV, 3) preservation of any accessory hepatic veins more than 5 mm in diameter, and 4) external stenting of the main biliary duct. In this experience, complications of both donor and recipient were remarkably infrequent. Overwhelming sepsis was the immediate cause of all recipient deaths, most of which occurred in UNOS Status 2A patients during the first half of the series. In the second half of the series, UNOS Status 2A was considered a contraindication to LDLT. Also of note was the complete absence of acute rejections in the LDLT series compared 48% in cadaveric OLT performed during the same period. Whether this difference resulted from the immunological advantage of using related donors in over 60% of the living donor cases remains to be determined.

The surgical approach to variations in donor vascular and biliary anatomy was detailed separately by Marcos for this series of LDLT (122). An important observation was that no potential donor had to be excluded for anatomical reasons. During arterial and portal dissection in the donor, care in preserving inflow to segment IV is emphasized. Intraoperative ultrasound was useful in defining a transection plane to the right of the middle hepatic vein. Finally, multiple bile ducts requiring anastomosis in the recipient were common and stenting was found to reduce postoperative complications.

Biliary leaks represent the most frequent major complication following LDLT with RL grafts. Testa, et al's (123) report on the experience with 30 LDLTs at the Hospital of Essen on biliary complications noted biliary leaks occurred in 8 cases (26.6%) and were related to the necessity to perform multiple bile duct anastomoses in half of their cases. Biliary leaks occurred in 8 patients, all in the first week. Seven were from grafts with more than one biliary anastomosis. Three of the leaks arose from the cut surface of the liver, 4 were anastomotic and one was combined surface and anastomotic. Of interest is that routine stenting was not utilized for biliary reconstruction in this series.

The Kyoto experience reported by Inomata, et al (124) was similar. A graft-to-recipient weight ratio of >1.0 was found to be ideal. This has become possible by a shift from left lobe grafting to preferential use of right lobe grafts. Blood loss and operative time for the donor procedure were only slightly greater for right lobe procurement (338 ± 175 ml, 6.7 ± 0.9 hours) than for left lobe (247 ± 148 ml, 6.2 ± 1.5 hours).

A potential problem with right lobe grafts is inadequate venous outflow, which can lead to congestion and impaired graft function. This probably results from a combination of reduced outflow from loss of accessory hepatic veins that drain into the vena cava, and the absence of the middle hepatic vein that provides venous drainage from the medial portion of the right lobe (especially from segment V). Kaneko, et al (125) have demonstrated by doppler ultrasound studies that intrahepatic venous collaterals may develop. A more aggressive approach has been taken by Fan, et al (126) who routinely utilize extended right lobe grafts, which include the middle hepatic vein with the graft. This more extensive resection leaves the donor with less liver tissue and might be expected to result in greater morbidity. The most recent results of this series suggest excellent donor outcome, however, the small number of procedures performed to date does not permit definitive conclusions regarding the safety of this approach (127).

Liver regeneration was studied by Marcos, et al (128) following LDLT. In both the donor and recipient, the majority of liver regeneration was complete by one week. Donor liver function tests including prothrombin time and transaminases normalized within the first week. The presence of donor liver steatosis (up to 30%) did not impair the regeneration process.

Although LDLT is currently not recommended for UNOS Status 2A patients, it may have a greater role in Status I patients. Two reports in the last year suggest that the outcome in Status I recipients may be acceptable. Uemoto, et al (129) reported transplantation in 15 adults with fulminant hepatic failure over a 7-year period. In 3 left lobe transplants primary non-function occurred probably because of inadequate liver transplant mass. Marcos, et al (130) reported a single case of LDLT for fulminant hepatic failure with excellent outcome. In this case, the donor work-up was completed in <24 hours, raising a concern whether truly informed consent is possible in such a situation because of the abbreviated time frame.

Hepatitis C

Hepatitis C is the leading cause of liver failure in the US and the most frequent reason for OLT. Transplantation for this disease is especially challenging because of early and frequent recurrence of hepatitis in the transplanted liver and its frequent co-existence with rejection episodes. The scope of the problem is evident from the work of Testa, et al (131) who studied 300 patients who underwent liver transplantation for hepatitis C and found the recurrence rate to be 87% within 2 years. Histological evidence of recurrence was demonstrated in 40.3%, but only 27% of these patients progressed to cirrhosis. Surprisingly, patient survival at 2 and 4 years was not different whether or not there was histological evidence of recurrence and hepatitis C. In contrast, histological recurrence within one year of transplant was associated with decreased survival rates at one and 5 years (65% and 56.4% vs. 80.6% and 78.4%). Patients with histological recurrence had a greater incidence of acute cellular rejection, steroid-resistant rejections and greater cumulative doses of corticosteroids. More patients (37.2%) in the recurrent hepatitis C group had received OKT3 than those who did not have recurrence. A point emphasized by the authors is that distinguishing rejection episodes from recurrent hepatitis C is difficult on the basis of histology. This is problematic since increasing immunosuppression to treat rejection also promotes increased viral proliferation and intensifies graft damage. Conversely, mistaking recurrence for rejection may lead to an inappropriate reduction in immunosuppression.

Belli, et al (132) investigated the influence of immunologic factors on recurrent hepatitis C in 83 transplanted patients. HLA-B14, HLA-DRB1*04 and HLA-DRB1 donor/recipient mismatch, showed a significant relation to the risk of hepatitis disease recurrence. None of the 10 patients with severe recurrence was DRB1*11-positive.

Baron, et al (133) discovered that the ischemic rewarming time during graft implantation influenced the severity of recurrent hepatitis C. The chances of severe recurrent disease within the first year were 19%, 40%

and 60% for ischemic rewarming times of 30, 60 and 90 minutes, respectively. This striking correlation of recurrence with hepatic warm ischemia may provide a novel clue to the cellular events that promote viral replication after transplantation.

Bizollon, et al (134) studied a group of 60 patients with HCV infection after OLT and found that 48% (23 patients) had chronic hepatitis on graft biopsy one year after transplantation. The presence of anti-HCV core IgM one month (p=0.004) and 12 months (p=0.003) after OLT were correlated with recurrence of chronic hepatitis. Specificity and positive predictive values were 0.87 and 0.88.

Gaweco, et al (135) examined 11 liver transplant recipients with hepatitis C. They found that in cases with evidence of necroinflammatory activity, features of portal inflammation/ piecemeal necrosis, lobular inflammation and fibrosis, higher NF-kB staining intensity scores within bile ducts, proliferating ductules, hepatocytes and lymphocytes and increased number of NF-kB-positive cells within bile ducts, proliferating ductules, hepatocytes and lymphocytes were observed. The authors postulated that intragraft NF-kB activation in recurrent HCV disease could be a key mechanism by which the virus both inhibits liver cell apoptosis and leads to continued viral replication and disease progression.

McLaughlin, et al (136) investigated a possible association of HCV with PTLD. They compared 57 transplants in patients with HCV to 127 in patients without HCV. PTLD developed in 4 patients who had HCV (7%) but only in one without HCV (0.8%) (p=0.2). In patients with HCV, PTLD occurred after a median of 7 weeks (range 1-20) compared with 196 weeks in the single control patient. All patients who developed PTLD had been given induction therapy with the antilymphocyte preparation, OKT3, and 60% had experienced 2 or more acute rejection episodes. The authors concluded that PTLD may be more prevalent in patients undergoing liver transplantation for HCV-related liver disease who also receive OKT3, and that HCV infection may be a risk factor for developing PTLD.

Fibrosis of liver allograft was studied by Pelletier, et al (137) in 24 patients transplanted for hepatitis C disease. Despite similar degrees of necroinflammatory activity, transplant recipients with persistently elevated serum transaminase levels, defined as an ALT level 1.5 times the upper limit of normal for more than 3 months, had an increased rate of fibrosis evident which occurred on average within 6 months after transplantation.

Two other reports from the same author examine pretransplant and posttransplant factors influential in outcome. In the first study which was done on 12 recipients (6 with biochemical hepatitis and 6 without), the group of patients with biochemical hepatitis displayed significantly more complex quasispecies variability of the HVR1 region in the pretransplant period than the patients without posttransplant hepatitis (138). Also a significantly increased fibrosis score was noted in recipients without a predominant variant. Although pretransplantation differences in HCV quasispecies did not persist postoperatively, it was concluded that pretransplantation quasispecies might be a predictor of HCV-induced hepatitis and graft fibrosis after liver transplantation. In the second study from the same author (139), pretransplant elevation in the viral replication rate, which was defined as a negative-strand HCV RNA: 18srRNA ratio greater than 2.5, was found to correlate with posttransplantation biochemical hepatitis, an increased rate of allograft fibrosis, and increased mortality rate. The observation of elevated posttransplant serum viral loads despite a stable intrahepatic replication rate after transplant was attributed to decreased viral clearance secondary to immunosuppressive therapy.

Taniguchi, et al (140) made a provocative observation regarding a potential interaction of hepatitis D virus (HDV) with HCV after transplant. Thirteen patients with both HbsAg and HCVab positivity were studied. Eight of them did not have antibodies to hepatitis delta virus (group I) while 5 were positive (group II). After liver transplantation all of the group II patients remained HCV RNA negative while the entire group I patients were HCV RNA positive. Serum ALT levels were elevated in 88% of group I patients but in only 20% of the second group. The authors concluded that among liver transplant recipients with HBV and HCV coinfection, HDV infection is associated with the suppression of HCV replication after OLT.

Hepatitis B

Hepatitis B is one of the leading causes of end stage liver disease, and its recurrence remains a major problem after transplantation. Several recent reports provide hope that it may be possible to prevent recurrence. Marinos, et al (141) considered the immune mechanisms that might be involved in recurrence. They compared 17 liver transplant recipients who had experienced HBV recurrence with 11 who had not. They also compared them to 30 non-transplanted patients who had chronic active hepatitis B and to 45 healthy individuals. Patients with HBV recurrence as well as the non-transplant patients with chronic active hepatitis exhibited significant Hep B core antigen-specific T-cell proliferation. Both hepatic and serum IL-2, IFN-γ and INF-α were enhanced without changes in IL-4 and IL-10 in these groups. They concluded that OLT recipients with HBV recurrence are able to mount a significant HBV-specific, HLA class II-restricted T-cell response despite immunosuppression. This response appeared to play a significant role in the pathogenesis of HBV-induced liver allograft damage.

Sanchez-Fueyo, et al (142) reported on a select group of 17 transplanted Hepatitis B patients who received HBV vaccine starting a few weeks after the last dose of HBIG (0-, 1- and 6-month schedule). Fourteen patients developed protective levels of anti-HBsAg and among these only 2 had HBV recurrence during a 14-month follow up period. The authors suggest that in a select group of transplanted Hepatitis B patients, HBV vaccination alone should provide adequate prophylaxis thereby allowing the discontinuation of HBIG.

Han, et al (143) performed a retrospective analysis of 71 transplanted Hepatitis B patients. Fifty-nine patients had been given a combination of HBIG and lamivudine whereas the remaining 12 received HBIG alone. None of the patients who received both agents developed either serum HbsAg or HBV DNA positivity during a mean follow up of 416 days, whereas in the monotherapy group, 3 patients (25%) had recurrent HBV surface antigenemia during a mean follow up of 663 days. It was concluded that combination therapy was more effective in preventing recurrent Hep B infection than HBIG monotherapy. Combination therapy was more cost-effective as well.

Malkan, et al (144) administered lamivudine to 32 transplanted Hepatitis patients as the only prophylactic treatment. All of the patients lost HBV-DNA at a mean of 2.4±1.6 months. Twenty-six (81%) remain free of viral recurrence. The remaining 6 patients had evidence of breakthrough infection and 2 progressed to graft failure. Four patients in the recurrent infection group had HbsAg expression in the explanted liver although they were HBV-DNA negative at the time. It was concluded that disease-free survival of 81% at 22 months is similar to that achieved by HBIG prophylaxis alone and expression of viral antigens in the liver seemed to identify better the patients at risk of recurrence. A comparison of single-agent versus combination HBIG, lamivudine therapy was not provided by this study.

Dodson, et al (145) conducted a similar study examining 16 transplanted patients positive for HbsAg who were converted to lamivudine after a course of HBIG. After an average follow up of 51 months, all 16 patients remained HbsAg (-).

Mutimer, et al (146) followed the clinical course of 4 liver transplant patients whose recurrent Hepatitis B graft infection was resistant to lamivudine therapy. All of them developed liver failure. In 3, recovery of liver function took place when immunosuppression was stopped and alternative antivirals were given. In one patient, introduction of famciclovir was associated with clinical, virological and histological response.

Surgical Technique

Although the technique of whole organ liver transplantation has become fairly well standardized, the role of venovenous bypass continues to be debated. Shokouh-Amiri, et al (147) compared the perioperative outcomes of orthotopic liver transplantations performed with venovenous bypass with those done without using the "piggyback technique". In the piggyback group, core body temperature was better preserved, fluid requirement was less including blood and blood products, patients spent less time in the ICU and in the hospital which was also reflected in the charges accrued. Although patient selection was not random in this study, recipient characteristics appeared to be comparable.

Soliman, et al (148) conducted a retrospective analysis of 23 cases (of 572 total transplants) in which parenchymal donor liver injury was identified. Injuries to the donor liver occurred either during harvesting, implantation or reperfusion. Techniques to treat the injuries included suturing, fibrin glue, hemostyptics, mesh wrapping and mesh packing. None of the patients died as a result of parenchymal injury. The authors concluded that injuries to the donor liver can often be treated successfully and recommended that they be approached aggressively.

Margarit, et al (149) reported one case of auxiliary heterotopic liver transplantation performed on a 25-year-old patient who had acute fulminant liver failure due to anti-tuberculosis drug toxicity. The donor liver's portal vein was arterialized by means of conduit (donor iliac artery) from the recipient aorta. The heterotopic liver was allowed to remain in place for 2 ½ months.

Meanwhile, the native liver fully recovered allowing removal of the allograft. The authors theorized that the high-pressure inflow accomplished by portal vein arterialization overcame the problem of outflow resistance that they believe has been a major obstacle in other auxiliary liver transplants.

Gundlach, et al (150) described 2 cases of a split-cava technique in which the cadaveric liver graft was split into right and left lobes in order to obtain 2 segmental livers for 2 adult recipients. By leaving a patch of vena cava on each half liver they were able to preserve all retrohepatic veins avoiding unnecessary loss of liver tissue.

Surgical and Related Complications

Davidson, et al (151) reviewed 46 post-OLT patients who had choledochojejunostomies performed to treat a biliary complication. The indications were bile leak (n=23) stricture (n=20) biliary stones (n=2) and sludge (n=1). After choledochojejunostomy there were 3 (6%) perioperative deaths. Twenty-six percent of the patients experienced early complications, (mainly pulmonary infections), and 22% had late complications, mainly strictures; 54% of the patients had undergone previous attempts at radiological or endoscopic corrections of their problem prior to the choledochojejunostomy. There was no statistically significant difference in outcome between the groups who had a prior non-surgical attempt at correction of the problem and the ones who proceeded directly to surgery. Of the 10 patients (22%) who developed late complications, 5 had biliary strictures, which were treated successfully with balloon dilatation. Two had hepatic artery thrombosis requiring retransplantation. The authors concluded that patients undergoing Roux-en-Y choledochojejunostomy in the management of biliary complications after OLT have a high incidence of early and late complications but a low mortality. An initial endoscopic or percutaneous approach to management of a complication that subsequently requires surgical treatment, does not increase, and may reduce the overall complication rate. Strictures are the most common late complication of choledochojejunostomy and can be effectively treated by balloon dilatation.

Saab, et al (152) compared nasobiliary drainage (NBD) versus biliary stenting (BS) by ERCP in the management of biliary leaks after T-tube removal in liver transplant recipients. Of the 69 patients who developed biliary leakage after T-tube removal, ERCP was unsuccessful in 3 cases and these required surgery. NBD was used as the primary therapy in 45 and BS was used as primary therapy in 21. In the NBD group, 9% of the patients required further intervention versus 29% in the BS group. The authors found NBD to be the preferred strategy for endoscopic management of biliary leaks because of fewer complications (mainly recurrent leaks). Moreover NBD allows assessment of bile drainage, provides access for cholangiography and is removed more easily than BS.

Cirera, et al (153) reviewed the problem of posttransplant ascites. Of 378 recipients, only 25 (7%) developed massive ascites. This complication occurred more commonly with the piggy-back technique. That outflow obstruction was responsible for the condition was suggested by the fact that all patients with ascites had a significantly elevated hepatic wedge pressure (>12 mm Hg) and gradient between free hepatic vein pressures and right atrial pressure of >6 mm Hg. These parameters were present in only 18% of patients without ascites. The presence of massive ascites after transplantation was associated with increased morbidity and mortality. The authors recommend measurement of hepatic vein and atrial pressures and correction of outflow problems as a priority in the evaluation and management of these patients.

Marcos, et al (154) reported a case in which a patient transplanted with a right lobe from a living donor presented 11 days post operatively with life-threatening hemorrhage from a large laceration in the liver. An H type portocaval shunt between the portal vein and Vena Cava was performed. This controlled the bleeding and allowed the patient to survive until another graft became available (also donated by a family member). Examination of the explanted liver revealed that the main hepatic vein was thrombosed. Whether this was the cause of the intra graft hematoma could not be determined with certainty but it provides reasonable explanation of the late bleeding event and the relief provided by portosystemic shunting.

Bhattacharjya, et al (155) reported a successful percutaneous portal vein-conduit thrombolysis using tissue plasminogen activator (TPA), angioplasty and endovascular stent placement. The portal vein was patent on ultrasound and liver function tests were normal 8 months after this procedure.

Infectious Complications

Singh, et al (156) examined factors predisposing to bacteremia and related mortality. In 59 liver transplant recipients they observed 111 episodes of fever or infection. 29 patients (49%) had documented bacteremia. Diabetes mellitus and serum albumin level less than 3.0 mg/dL were significant independent predictors of bacteremia compared with nonbacteremic infections. Mortality at 14 days was 28% in those with bacteremia compared with 4% in those with nonbacteremic infections. Lack of febrile response in bacteremic patients was correlated with a poorer outcome.

In an analysis of pulmonary infiltrates in OLT recipients, Torres, et al (157) examined 60 episodes in 50 consecutive liver transplant patients finding that opportunistic infections were the most common etiology followed by bacterial infections (mainly gram-negative species). The majority of bacterial pneumonia occurred during the first 28 posttransplant days while opportunistic infections predominated between 1-6 months.

Lautenschlager, et al (158) diagnosed human herpesvirus-6 (HHV-6) infection in 11 (22%) of 51 liver transplant recipients during the first year after transplantation. Significant graft dysfunction was associated with HHV-6 antigenemia in 8 of 11 patients; viral antigens were detected in the liver biopsy specimen of 3 of these patients. The authors concluded that the HHV-6 antigenemia test and demonstration of HHV-6 antigens in the graft might be informative in the differential diagnosis of graft dysfunction.

Singh, et al (159) studied 72 consecutive liver transplant recipients and detected CMV antigenemia in 22 patients (31%) by performing frequent surveillance cultures (weeks 2, 4, 8, 12, and 16). All 22 patients with asymptomatic antigenemia were randomized into 2 groups. One group received oral ganciclovir (GCV) for 6 weeks and the second group received IV GCV for 7 days. None of the patients in the study developed tissue-invasive CMV disease. CMV disease (viral syndrome) occurred in one patient (9%) in the IV GCV group and in none of the patients in the oral ganciclovir group. Of 50 patients without CMV antigenemia, none developed CMV disease. The authors concluded that the absence of CMV antigenemia had a negative predictive value of 100% and eliminated the need for unnecessary antiviral prophylaxis in the vast majority of liver transplant patients. Antiviral therapy instituted upon detection of antigenemia prevented tissue invasive CMV in both ganciclovir groups. Whether a close monitoring approach had clear advantage over a universal prophylaxis approach in high-risk patients as is commonly employed remains to be determined by randomized trial.

Singhal, et al (160) utilized antifungal prophylaxis with amphotericin B-lipid complex on a subset of liver transplant patients who were at high risk for fungal infection. High risk was defined as a postoperative requirement for prolonged (>5 days) intensive care unit (ICU) treatment. Thirty patients out of 130 fulfilled the criteria and received prophylaxis. Six of 30 patients died, of whom 3 underwent postmortem examinations. None showed evidence of fungal infection. The authors recommend antifungal prophylaxis with lipid-based amphotericin B in post liver transplant patients who require prolonged ICU stay.

Kuse, et al (161) measured the procalcitonin (PCT) levels in 40 patients who had liver transplants during the early postoperative period on a daily basis for 2 weeks. Eleven patients experienced an infectious complication accompanied by an increase in PCT concentrations. Eleven patients had a rejection episode and none of these patients showed a rise in PCT concentrations (p <0.05). The authors suggest PCT as a valuable marker to differentiate infection and rejection and to monitor the course of an infectious illness after therapy is initiated.

Long-term Complications

In 120 consecutive liver transplant recipients, Gayowski, et al (162) studied the development of late onset renal failure (defined as serum creatinine persistently above 2 mg/dl occurring more than 6 months after transplant). Late-onset renal failure occurred in 33 (28%) patients and was associated with posttransplant alcohol use, hepatitis C, and diabetes in univariate statistical analysis. After 5 years of follow up, the mortality in patients with late onset renal failure was significantly higher than those without (43% vs. 2%). Mortality at 5 years was even higher in the sub-group of renal failure patients with hepatitis C (52%). Alcohol recidivism after transplantation was an independent predictor of late-onset renal failure in patients with HCV, and represents a potentially modifiable risk factor in these patients.

Results

Yerdel, et al (163) reviewed 779 cases of liver transplantation and found that 63 (8.1%) had operatively confirmed portal vein thrombosis (PVT). They graded PVT based on the degree of occlusion and extension of the thrombus. In general, thrombectomy was performed for nonocclusive PVT and jump grafts or splanchnic tributaries utilized for inflow for more extensive occlusions. Although the patients with grade 1 PVT had a survival rate similar to the controls, the overall actuarial 5-year patient survival in PVT patients was 65.6% while it was 76.3% in controls. The PVT patients had more postoperative complications, higher in-hospital mortality rates, and reduced 5-year survival rates.

Krowka, et al (164) reviewed 43 patients with portopulmonary hypertension who underwent OLT. Overall mortality was 35%. MPAP of 50 mm Hg or greater was associated with 100% morbidity from cardiac or pulmonary complications. In patients with a MPAP of 35 to less than 50 mm Hg and PVR of 250 dynes.s.cm $^{-5}$ or greater, the mortality rate was 50%. No deaths occurred in patients whose pre-OLT MPAP was less than 35 mm Hg or whose transpulmonary gradient was less than 15 mm Hg. The authors recommended aborting the performance of liver transplant (even intraoperatively) if a MPAP of 50 mm Hg or greater is discovered after induction of anesthesia.

Pilatis, et al (165) attempted to identify predictors of pulmonary hyperperfusion in 55 patients undergoing liver transplant evaluation. Significant predictors included: 1) systemic arterial HTN, 2) loud pulmonary component of the second heart sound, 3) right ventricular heave, 4) right ventricular dilatation by echocardiogram, 5) right ventricular hypertrophy by echocardiogram and 6) echocardiogram estimated systolic PAP greater than 40 mm Hg. In particular, echocardiogram-estimated SPAP greater than 40 mm Hg was strongly associated with pulmonary HTN. None of the predictors alone however demonstrated adequate predictive sensitivity, thus the authors recommended using a combination of parameters to identify patients with pulmonary HTN.

Two studies describing the endotoxin and cytokine response in liver transplant recipients were remarkable. Miki, et al (166) found that serum bilirubin level may be an important preoperative factor influencing perioperative cytokine response in patients undergoing liver transplantation. Maring, et al (167) presented the results of a prospective study on 40 patients and concluded that monitoring endotoxins and cytokines during liver transplantation was of very limited value in predicting outcome.

Chang, et al (168) analyzed 50 consecutive liver transplant recipients and found that the nadir in platelet count was significantly lower in non-survivors compared with survivors (16 vs. 36 x 10³/cmm). Forty-three percent (9 of 21) patients with nadir platelet counts of <30 x 10³ /cmm had a major infection within 30 days of the transplant compared with 17% (5 of 23) with nadir platelet counts >30 x 10³/cmm. Persistent thrombocytopenia was associated with a poor outcome in liver transplant recipients and identified a subgroup of liver transplant patients susceptible to early major infections.

Twenty-four liver transplant recipients with autoimmune hepatitis were followed for 27±14 months by Reich, et al (169). Histologically proven recurrent autoimmune hepatitis occurred in 25%, 15±2 months after transplantation. Half of the patients with recurrence required retransplantation, 11±3 months after diagnosis. After retransplantation 2 of 3 patients had re-recurrence within 3 months and one required a third transplant. Autoimmune hepatitis patients also had a high frequency of rejection and often required OKT3 for treatment.

Ayata, et al (170) reviewed biopsies of the native transplanted liver in 12 patients treated for autoimmune hepatitis. Recurrent disease was seen in 5 patients as manifested by lobular hepatitis with acidophil bodies and lymphoplasmacytic infiltrate. As the disease progressed, portal/interface hepatitis was seen and 2 patients developed cirrhosis. Pretransplant duration of autoimmune hepatitis, donor/recipient gender, HLA and rejection episodes could not be correlated with recurrence. The authors concluded that recurrent autoimmune hepatitis was common (42%) and characterized by a slowly progressive course.

Collins, et al (171) performed a retrospective analysis of long-term results of liver transplantation in patients aged 60 and older. Ninety-one patients over age 60 receiving primary liver transplants during a 13-year period were compared with a group of younger recipients (age 18-53). The only significant difference identified between the groups was long-term survival. Five- and 10-year patient survival rates were 52% and 35% in the older group versus 75% and 60% in the younger group. In the elderly group, the most common cause of late mortality was malignancy (35%), while in younger patients it was infectious complications (24.2%). There were no significant differences with regard to length of hospitalization, the incidence of rejection, infection, repeat operation, and readmission or repeat transplantation between the groups.

A large single center analysis of long-term results of liver transplantation was reported by Jain, et al (172). The actuarial 18-year patient survival of 4,000 consecutive liver transplant recipients was 48%. Survival was significantly better in children, female recipients and in patients who had their transplants after 1990. The rates of retransplantation for acute or chronic rejection were significantly lower with tacrolimus-based immunosuppression. The risk of graft failure and death reached a steady state after the first year. Recurrence of disease, malignancies and age-related complications were the major factors for late graft loss.

Ghobrial, et al (173) assessed the predictors of survival in *in-vivo* split-liver transplants by retrospective analysis of 102 pediatric and adult recipients who received either right lobe (n=55) or left lobe (n=55) split grafts. Recipients of split grafts were compared with a contemporary cohort of 628 adult and pediatric liver recipients who had whole organ transplantation. Overall survival rates of patients who received a split-liver transplant were not significantly different from those who received whole organ transplants (77% vs. 74% at 3 years). By univariate comparison 2 variables, UNOS status and multiple transplants per patient were significantly associated with an increased risk of death.

Studies on quality of life after liver transplantation were reported by Moore, et al (174) and Younossi, et al (175). In both studies, it was concluded that liver transplantation clearly improved patients' quality of life, and cognitive functioning. After successful transplantation, mental health scores were indistinguishable from the general population norms.

Immunology

Hahn, et al (176) performed a study on liver transplant recipients to explore the association of peripheral chimerism with graft-versus-host disease. All patients studied had a low degree of chimerism that was most apparent in the CD8+T-/natural killer-cell population. One patient with persistently high levels of donor cells in the CD8+T-cell population developed severe graft-versus-host disease and died of opportunistic infections. Another patient with biopsy-proven graft-versus-host disease was chimeric in several cell populations. As her symptoms resolved, cells carrying donor alleles were reduced to levels undetectable by the same assay. Based on these findings, the authors thought that persistently elevated levels of donor CD8+T cells in the periphery

may indicate graft-versus-host disease in liver transplant recipients and may aid in its rapid diagnosis.

Evans, et al (177) confirmed the association between chronic rejection and CMV infection. In a study performed on 33 recipients of 57 liver transplants, the combination of donor CMV antibody negativity combined with recipient CMV antibody positivity and duration of CMV infection more than 30 days were associated with an increased relative risk of chronic rejection. CMV infection occurred earlier in those undergoing a second transplant for chronic rejection than for those undergoing a second transplant for other reasons. In addition, an HLA-B antigen mismatch was associated with a prolonged CMV infection.

Milkiewicz, et al (178) performed a study on a total of 77 liver transplant recipients with autoimmune hepatitis as the primary disease found that the incidence of chronic rejection was significantly higher in this group than in subjects transplanted for other indications. Twelve out of 77 recipients (15.6%) developed clinical and histological chronic rejection within a median time of 3.5 months after liver transplantation.

Chang, et al (179) evaluated the effectiveness of sirolimus as a substitute when calcineurin inhibitors had to be discontinued because of nephrotoxicity or neurological side effects. Six patients out of 14 subsequently experienced acute rejection episodes but only one of them required antilymphocyte therapy to reverse rejection. Follow up was 2-7 months. It was concluded that sirolimus therapy is a valid alternative when calcineurin inhibitors are undesirable.

Pediatric Liver Transplantation

Grewal, et al (180) performed a retrospective analysis of 12 pediatric patients who underwent both liver and kidney transplantation between 1984-1997. The results were compared with those in 385 pediatric patients who received only liver grafts during the same period. Actuarial patient survival was 67% versus 69% over 5 years in the 2 groups respectively. All allograft losses in the combined liver and kidney transplant group were the result of patient death and occurred in the early postoperative period.

Reyes, et al (181) reported encouraging results in a group of patients treated by liver transplantation for primary liver tumors. A total of 31 children (12 with hepatoblastoma and 19 with hepatocellular carcinoma [HCC]) underwent liver transplantation for tumors deemed otherwise unresectable. The 5-year survival rates were 83% for hepatoblastoma patients and 63% for HCC patients. In hepatoblastoma patients, intravenous tumor invasion, positive hilar lymph nodes and contiguous spread did not have a significant adverse effect on the outcome. In contrast, these factors along with tumor size, distant metastases and gender were significant risk factors for recurrence in HCC patients. The author's pointed out that unlike HCCs, many hepatoblastomas are amenable to resection or chemotherapy plus resection. Indeed, spontaneous regression of hepatic blastomas has been reported. The results of neoadjuvant chemotherapy and OLT for hepatoblastoma indicate that even extensive disease can sometimes be cured by total resection. In HCC patients, transplantation for TNM stages I-III frequently results in cure whereas stage IV patients fare considerably worse. Thus, living-related donor and split-liver transplantation may be justified in children with end-stage HCC. This approach assumes the absence of tumor involvement of the recipient's vena cava that must be preserved with split-liver cadaver or living-related donor transplants.

In a study by Their, et al (182) from Finland, posttransplant infections were analyzed in 56 children who had liver or kidney transplantations. The greatest number of infections was seen in the smallest children, 3-6 months after transplantation. Viral upper respiratory tract infections were most common.

Two studies from the Thomas E. Starzl Transplantation Institute indicate superiority of tacrolimus over CsA in terms of outcome and side effects. Jain, et al (183) and Reyes, et al (184) described 233 pediatric liver transplant recipients on tacrolimus-based immunosuppressive therapy (Group I) comparing them to 120 pediatric liver transplant recipients on CsA-based regimen (Group II). The 9-year patient survival rates were 85.4% in group I versus 63.8% in Group II (p=0.0001). The 9-year graft survival rates were 78.9% in tacrolimus-treated patients versus 60.8% in CsA patients (p=0.0003). The mean steroid dose was significantly lower in Group I compared with Group II at all time points after transplantation. Although the rate of PTLD was not significantly different (13% in Group I vs. 8.3 % in Group II, p=0.13), the survival after PTLD was significantly better for Group I at 81.2% than for Group II at 50% after 5 years (p=0.034).

Results reported by UCLA Dumont Transplant Center (185) were at odds with the Pittsburgh data regarding the incidence of PTLD and the use of tacrolimus- versus CsA-based regimens. In the UCLA study, there was a 5-fold increase in the incidence of PTLD in the primary tacrolimus group when compared with the primary CsA group (p<0.001). Although the number of patients in each group in the UCLA and Pittsburgh studies was similar, the duration of follow-up times in the Pittsburgh study was longer (91 months for tacrolimus- and 128 months for CsA-based therapy vs. 52 months and 77 months for the UCLA study, respectively).

Krieger, et al (186) evaluated the significance of detecting EBV-specific sequences by PCR in the circulation of asymptomatic pediatric liver transplant recipients. Nine of 13 patients who were initially asymptomatic and EBV PCR positive, ultimately developed symptoms typical of EBV infection (fever, rash, adenopathy, GI dysfunction, hepatitis etc). Five of these 9 went on to develop PTLD. The authors concluded that detection of EBV-specific sequences in the absence of symptoms may herald impending EBV-associated disorders and provide a window for preventive therapy.

Liver Transplantation for Cancer

Iwatsuki, et al (187) reported the Pittsburgh experience with 344 consecutive patients who underwent transplantation for HCC. This series, which is probably the largest in the world, was characterized by a predominance of men (75%), a predominance of cirrhotic patients (92%) and of those with hepatitis C (or non-A, non-B hepatitis) as the primary cause of liver disease (44%). After exclusion of 26 patients who had positive lymph nodes, metastases or positive surgical margins (all of whom had tumor recurrence within 2 years), 3 factors were found by multivariate analysis to independently predict poor outcome: 1) bilobar tumor distribution, 2) tumor size, and 3) vascular invasion. Using relative risk factors derived from the Cox equation for each variable, a risk score grade was developed to categorize patients. Patients received points for: 1) bilobar tumor (3.1 points), 2) a tumor of 2-5cm (4.5 points), 3) a tumor of >5 cm (6.7 points), 4) microvascular invasion (4.4 points), and 5) macrovascular invasion (15 points). Patients with <11.0 total points were considered low risk (grade 1 or 2) and found to have excellent 5-year survival rates (>60%). A total of >15 points (grade 4 or 5) predicted an unacceptable outcome (<10% 5-year tumor-free survival). Grade 3 patients (score 11-14 points) had an intermediate tumor-free survival rate of approximately 40%. This model appeared to discriminate groups of patients better than did the standard TNM system. Based on this large experience, macrovascular invasion (which can usually be detected by preoperative imaging) should be considered an exclusion.

Majno, et al (188) proposed a novel strategy in the management of HCC patients based on a hypothetical mathematical model. They suggested that liver resection be performed as the primary therapy in patients with solitary HCC <5 cm in size and preserved hepatic function. Liver transplantation was reserved as a salvage procedure for tumor recurrence or deteriorating liver function after resection. The estimated life expectancy was 8.8 years for primary transplantation versus 7.8 years for primary resection and salvage transplantation. The benefit of the proposed strategy was evident in a reduced number of transplants required. The calculated use of grafts at 5 years was 52% for primary transplantation versus 23% for salvage transplantation. This difference is relevant in the current setting of increasing donor organ shortage.

Meyer, et al (189) analyzed the Cincinnati Transplant Tumor Registry to obtain data on 207 patients who underwent liver transplantation for otherwise unresectable cholangiocarcinoma or cholangiohepatoma. The 5-year survival estimate was 23%. Survival after recurrence was rarely more than one year. Because of the high rate of recurrent tumor and lack of positive prognostic variables, the authors do not recommend transplantation as a treatment for this disease.

DeVreede, et al (190) studied 11 patients with unresectable cholangiocarcinoma in which the tumor was above the cystic duct and showed no evidence of intra- or extrahepatic metastases. Patients received external beam irradiation plus bolus fluorouracil (5-FU), followed by brachytherapy with iridium and concomitant protracted venous infusion of 5-FU. 5-FU was administered continuously through an ambulatory infusion pump until transplantation could be carried out. Eleven patients completed the protocol with successful OLT. All patients are currently alive but 3 patients have been followed 12 months or less. The remaining 8 patients have a median follow up of 44 months. Only one patient has developed recurrent tumor. The authors concluded that OLT in combination with preoperative irradiation and chemotherapy can be associated with prolonged disease-free and overall survival in highly selected patients with early-stage cholangiocarcinoma.

Donor Selection

Zamir, et al (191) retrospectively studied the fate of liver grafts recovered but declined for use by all local centers of an OPO for either objective reasons (size, malignancy, serologies, etc) or subjective reasons (donor history, graft quality). The outcomes of those organs if accepted for transplantation at distant centers were reported. Thirteen percent of 555 livers procured over a 3-year period were exported under these circumstances. There was a significantly high rate of non-function (17.1%) in the subjectively declined group versus 0% in the objectively declined group. There was also a significant difference in one-year graft survival (79% success in those declined for objective reasons vs. 46% for the declined-for-subjective-reasons group). The authors concluded that livers declined for local use based on a subjective assessment of experienced surgeons have a high non-function rate, high morbidity and low graft survival. They recommended that such grafts be used in recipients of urgent status.

Reich, et al (192) analyzed their experience with controlled non-heart beating donors (NHBD). Eight livers were procured from a total of 16 controlled NHBDs. Patient and graft survival rates were 100% at 18±12 months. There was no intraoperative complication, reperfusion syndrome, poor graft function, primary non-function, arterial thrombosis or any other serious complication. The authors concluded that NHBDs can significantly and safely expand the donor pool.

Bioartificial Livers and Hepatocyte Transplantation

Two potential alternatives to liver transplantation are bioartificial livers and hepatocyte transplantation. Mitzner, et al (193) reported the results of 13 patients treated with a bioartificial liver. Eight out of 13 patients had cirrhosis with hepatorenal syndrome. The average Childs Pugh Turcotte score was 12.4±1. The authors employed a molecular absorbent recirculating system (MARS method) using an albumin-containing dialysate that is re-circulated and perfused on line through charcoal and anion exchanger columns. MARS enables the selective removal of albumin-bound substances. The remaining 5 patients received HDF (hemodiafiltration). Mortality rates were 100% in the control (HDF) group at day 7 and 62.5% in the MARS group at day 7 (75% at day 30) (p<0.01). The authors thought that removal of albumin-bound substances with the MARS method could contribute to the treatment of hepato-renal syndrome.

Levy, et al (194) reported on 2 cases, in which they performed extracorporeal perfusion of blood of patients with fulminant hepatic failure through the liver of a pig transgenic for human complement regulators (CD59 and CD55). The perfusions were carried out for 6.5 and 10 hours, respectively. In both cases there was evidence of function of the *ex-vivo* liver as evidenced by decreases in the patient's prothrombin time and bilirubin. Both patients were subsequently transplanted successfully with liver allografts. The authors conclude that this strategy may provide an approach to bridge patients until a suitable liver becomes available.

In a clinical experiment performed by Bilir, et al (195), 5 patients with severe acute liver failure who were not candidates for liver transplantations underwent intrasplenic and intrahepatic hepatocyte transplantation. The donor liver cells were delivered through a percutaneous catheter in the hepatic artery. Three of the 5 patients lived longer than 48 hours (12, 28 and 52 days) and showed improvement in encephalopathy scores, arterial ammonia levels and prothrombin times. Postmortem examination showed the presence of transplanted hepatocytes in liver and spleen by light microscopy and fluorescent *in situ* hybridization. Function of transplanted hepatocytes was not observed for the first 48-72 hours possibly representing a period necessary for their posttransplant recovery or engraftment. Three of the patients survived long enough so that the procedure could theoretically have been useful as a bridge to OLT, had they been candidates for transplantation.

Miscellaneous

Lowell, et al (196) investigated the demographics and the outcome of the domino organ transplants, which were done between 1987-1996. During this period 16 liver recipients became organ donors. There was no difference in graft survival when comparing kidney or liver recipients (p=0.11) of donors who had been previously transplanted.

Dalmau, et al (197) attempted to address the effect of tranexamic-acid and epsilon-aminocaproic acid on blood transfusion requirements during liver transplantation. One hundred twenty-four liver transplant recipients were randomized into 3 groups: 42 patients were given tranexamic acid at a rate of 40 mg/kg/hr, 42 patients were given epsilon amino caproic acid (EACA) at a rate of 16 mg/kg/hr, and 40 patients in a control group received an equal volume of normal saline 10 ml/kg/hr. At the end of surgery, there was no significant difference in coagulation parameters or hemoglobin values between the groups. Packed red cell transfusion requirements were significantly reduced during OLT in the tranexamic acid group but not in the epsilon-aminocaproic acid group. There were no differences in transfusion requirements after OLT. The incidence of thromboembolic events did not show any statistically significant difference among the groups with four arterial thrombosis events in the tranexamic acid group and 2 arterial thrombosis events in both the EACA and the control groups. The authors concluded that additional patients need to be studied to establish the risks involved in administration of this dose of tranexamic acid, especially in relation to arterial thrombosis.

PANCREAS TRANSPLANTATION

As of August 2000, nearly 14,000 pancreas transplants had been reported to the International Pancreas Transplant Registry, about 75% of them from the United States (198). In 1999 alone, more than 1,300 pancreas transplants were performed by US Centers. The majority of pancreas transplants continue to be performed simultaneously with a kidney transplant (SPK) in uremic patients. Although in recent years the number of pancreas after kidney (PAK) grafts has increased to 12% of US pancreas transplants, pancreas transplants alone (in pre-uremic patients) have remained relatively constant at 4-5% per year. Pancreas graft survival remained best for SPK (84% at 1 year) though graft survival for PAK and PTA has improved over the last few years to 73% and 72%, respectively. These graft survival rates represent improvement during the last decade by almost 10% for SPK and about 20% for PAK and PTA. Several sizable individual center reports suggest that even better graft survival is possible (199-201), and that the risks of the procedure have diminished considerably in recent years (202). One-year patient survival for recipients of pancreas transplants since 1996 was at least 94% in all of the above categories according to the registry report (198).

Technical considerations, which have played a prominent role in the history of pancreas transplantation, continue to evolve. Management of secretions of the exocrine pancreas has been the most controversial issue. Prior to 1994, more than 95% of US transplants were performed with bladder drainage. This method has the advantage of sterility and access to serial urinary amylase determinations as a potentially useful index of rejection, which can be treated more effectively when diagnosed in an early stage prior to the onset of hyperglycemia. However, fluid and bicarbonate losses and other urinary tract complications necessitate eventual conversion to enteric drainage in 10-20% of bladder-drained recipients. This has led to an increasing use of primary enteric drainage, which was employed in 60% of US cases by 1998 (198). Duct management did not influence SPK graft survival but for solitary pancreas grafts (PAK and PTA), one-year survival of bladder-drained grafts was 13-15% superior to that of enteric-drained grafts. This suggests usefulness in monitoring function of the simultaneously transplanted kidney as an index of rejection when urinary amylase cannot be followed. The technical failure rate for enteric-drained pancreas grafts, which was formerly high because of the incidence of infection, has fallen from over 20% in 1992 (twice that of bladder-drained grafts) to about the same level as that of bladder drainage in 1998-99 (10%).

Regardless of the method chosen for draining exocrine secretions, vascular thrombosis of pancreatic grafts remains an unresolved problem and was the cause of about 70% of technical failures. The prevalence of thrombosis is presumed to be related to the relatively sluggish flow of blood through pancreatic grafts. Either arterial or venous thrombosis virtually always results in graft loss, though Ciancio reported 3 cases in which prompt venous thrombectomy via the distal splenic vein followed by systemic anticoagulation salvaged the graft (203).

An additional technical factor of possible importance is whether venous drainage should be systemic (via the iliac vein) or by the portal system. Stratta, et al (204) have championed portal venous drainage since it prevents the hyperinsulinemia resulting from systemic venous drainage. Whether normal serum insulin and the somewhat more physiologic lipoprotein profile seen in patients with portal vein drained grafts will have long-term benefits is debatable, but Stratta, et al in a randomized prospective comparison of systemic bladder (SB) versus portal enteric (PE) drained grafts found that these procedures have comparable results with regard to rate of complications and graft survival (205). In view of the well documented but subtle immunologic advantage of portal vein drainage of allografts in rodent models, it is

intriguing that both Stratta, et al and Bartlett, et al found that portal vein drained pancreas grafts had considerably fewer acute rejection episodes than systemically drained grafts (personal communication).

It seems likely that histocompatibility matching would have some impact on the outcome of pancreas grafts but this is difficult to substantiate. The most recent registry report of results (from 1969-99) indicates no benefit of HLA matching for SPK grafts. However for PAK and PTA transplants, matching for HLA-A and B (but surprisingly not for HLA-DR) was associated with better graft survival (198).

Immunosuppressive regimens used for 1996-1999 US pancreas transplants were analyzed in the August 2000 Registry report. Reddy, et al (206) reported excellent results without anti-lymphoctye antibody induction therapy. However according to the Registry report, two-thirds of the recipients received anti-T-cell antibody therapy as induction (198). In PAK transplants antibody therapy was advantageous but for SPK or PTA transplants it had no impact on graft survival. For maintenance immunosuppression, SPK graft survival at one year was about 10% better in recipients who received regimens including MMF instead of azathioprine, whether in combination with CsA or tacrolimus. Regimens including MMF were also noted to be advantageous for solitary pancreas grafts (PAK and PTA). In addition to the Registry report, individual institution reports called attention to the advantage of MMF (207).

According to the Registry report, almost all pancreas recipients were treated with steroids. To avoid their known diabetogenic action and other drawbacks, several groups have attempted to withdraw steroids. In pancreas recipients on tacrolimus therapy, Jordan, et al (208) successfully withdrew steroids in 58 of 124 patients (47%) 4-40 months after transplantation (mean 15.2 months). Overall one-, 2- and 4-year pancreas graft survival in this series was 98%, 91.5% and 83%, with even better results in those patients in whom steroids were successfully withdrawn. The same group (Corry, et al (209)) reviewed their experience with steroid withdrawal in pancreas recipients who received (3-6x10^8) donor bone marrow cells at the time of transplantation. Twenty-two percent of bone marrow recipients were off steroids at one year, 45% at 2 years and 67% at 3 years. In patients not given bone marrow, withdrawal of steroid was less successful (19%, 38%, 45%) at the same intervals.

Overall pancreas graft survival was excellent in both groups (83% for bone marrow recipients vs. 79% for non-bone marrow recipients).

Autoimmune Recurrence

In addition to rejection, an immunologic threat to pancreas transplants is the autoimmune response, which was responsible for elimination of the native pancreatic beta cells. In rodent models of spontaneous diabetes, it is well known that the autoimmune process is sufficient to destroy transplanted syngeneic islets. Early experience with identical twin donor pancreas transplants at the University of Minnesota indicated that transplanted human islets can also be destroyed by this process. Recipients of pancreas grafts from identical twin donors who were not given immunosuppression suffered recurrent diabetes within 6-12 weeks. Pathologic examination showed insulitis with beta-cell destruction and sparing of alpha cells. Subsequently, the Minnesota group found that immunosuppression could prevent failure of identical twin pancreas transplants.

Recurrence of autoimmune diabetes with selective beta-cell destruction has also been observed in pancreas allografts from living related HLA-identical donors. Until recently, it was thought that this would be unlikely in HLA-mismatched cadaveric transplants, either because the disease was MHC restricted or because the more intensive immunosuppression routinely utilized to prevent rejection of mismatched allografts would easily prevent autoimmune islet damage. Recently, however, in several recipients of cadaveric pancreas transplants it appears that failure was from autoimmunity rather than rejection (210). In these patients, histology of the failed graft exhibited selective destruction of islet beta cells but preservation of alpha and delta cells, a pattern seen in the native pancreas of humans soon after onset in patients with insulin-dependent diabetes. Additional evidence of the impact of autoimmunity was provided by Thivolet (211) who described a group of pancreas transplant recipients in whom late failure of the graft was accompanied by increases in titers of islet autoantibodies (GAD 65 and IA2). The same antibodies are known to appear frequently before the onset of hyperglycemia in type I diabetics. Broghi, et al (212) also reported that rising titers of GAD and 1A2 antibodies was almost invariably followed by functional failure of pancreas allografts.

Course of Microvascular Complications of Diabetes in Pancreas Recipients

Evaluating the impact of successful pancreas transplantation on the secondary complications of diabetes is difficult since randomized control studies are for the most part lacking. Although it appears that there is a benefit to pancreas transplantation in reducing complications, many years of normoglycemia may be necessary before it is detectable.

Neuropathy: In non-uremic diabetic PTA recipients at the University of Minnesota, improvement in nerve conduction velocities was observed after one year. Evoked muscle and nerve action potentials and amplitudes remained stable or improved in patients with long-standing pancreas grafts while amplitudes continued to worsen in recipients whose pancreas transplants failed early (213). In patients studied by the Stockholm group one year after successful SPK transplantation, minimal improvement in neuropathy was noted but after 4 years, nerve conduction had improved significantly (214).

Retinopathy: Several investigators have reported improvement in retinopathy in uremic diabetic patients after successful pancreas transplantation, but most of these studies have been poorly controlled. In non-uremic patients at Minnesota, the retinas of successful pancreas recipients were compared over a 5-year period to those of patients whose grafts failed early. In the first 3 posttransplant years, the incidence of progressive of retinopathy was the same (30%) in both groups. After 3 years, retinopathy appeared to stabilize in patients with successful pancreas transplants while it continued to worsen in those with failed grafts. After 5 years, 55% of patients with failed grafts exhibited progressively severe retinopathy while in successful recipients, progression of retinopathy had occurred in only 30% (215,216). A possibly more sensitive method of evaluating microangiopathy is to study the conjunctival microcirculation. Utilizing this method, Cheung seems to have shown earlier benefit of pancreas transplantation. Computer-assisted intravital microscopy of venules and arteries indicated abnormalities in all of their pretransplant patients and significant improvement in the same studies within 18 months of successful pancreas transplantation (217).

Nephropathy: Microscopic lesions of diabetic nephropathy commonly appear within 1-2 years in kidneys transplanted to diabetic patients who are treated only with insulin. However in recipients of successful SPK transplants at Minnesota, development of diabetic nephropathy in the transplanted kidney was generally prevented. Whether restoration of normoglycemia with a pancreas transplant can influence the course of already established nephropathy in the native kidneys of diabetic patients has been controversial. In a preliminary report by Bilous, et al (218) from the University of Minnesota, native kidneys were biopsied in 7 non-uremic PTA recipients who exhibited early-to-moderate diabetic nephropathy. During the first 2 years after successful pancreas transplantation, the creatinine clearance deteriorated in these patients from 90 ml/min to 60 ml/min. The nephrotoxic effect of CsA may have contributed to this since after this early period of functional deterioration the creatinine clearance stabilized. The microscopic lesions of diabetic nephropathy in the native kidneys did not improve even 5 years after successful pancreas transplantation. However, after 10 years of normoglycemia these recipients exhibited amelioration of the characteristic glomerular and tubular lesions of diabetic nephropathy (219). Thus, there is encouraging histological evidence that restoring euglycemia can prevent or halt progression of diabetic nephropathy. Whether this benefit is sufficient to offset the nephrotoxic effect of immunosuppressive agents such as CsA or tacrolimus is a critical question. Unquestionably, there are patients who benefit greatly from pancreas transplants, some of which have now been functioning for almost 2 decades without deterioration of their renal function (220). Some interesting evidence has been presented by Becker, et al (221) suggesting that simultaneous pancreas-kidney transplantation also reduces mortality (as well as morbidity from the vascular complications) compared with the results of kidney transplantation alone.

TRANSPLANTATION OF ISOLATED PANCREATIC ISLETS

Conceptually, transplantation of isolated pancreatic islets would be the ideal treatment for patients with insulin-dependent diabetes since it has the potential to normalize blood glucose without the operative risks of whole pancreas transplantation. In rodent models, the technical and immunologic barriers to islet isolation and transplantation have been overcome routinely allowing success. In contrast, until very recently human islet allografts have met with consistent failure. Even temporary

correction of hyperglycemia by islet allografts has been unusual in human type I diabetic recipients (222).

Possible explanations for the poor clinical results include the technical difficulty in separating islets from compact fibrous human pancreas often leading to transplantation of inadequate numbers of islets or damaged ones. There is also a suggestion that transplanted isolated islets are more vulnerable than whole pancreas to rejection, autoimmunity or damage from immunosuppressive drugs. This could explain why human islet autotransplants have been so much more successful than allografts.

Autografts

More than 20 institutions have reported a combined series of 170 human islet autotransplants to the International Registry (222). These transplants were done in patients who were undergoing total or near-total pancreatectomy for relief of pain from chronic pancreatitis. Islets isolated from the excised organ were isolated and transplanted to prevent the otherwise inevitable diabetes. Since the islets were autologous, neither rejection nor islet-damaging immunosuppressive drugs were threats. In addition, since the patients were not type I diabetics, there was no concern over recurrent autoimmune damage. About 50% of these patients have remained normoglycemic without the need for insulin.

Allografts

By far the largest numbers of candidates for islet allografts are patients with type I diabetes. Of 29 diabetic patients who were transplanted worldwide from 1985-1989 (222), only in 6 (21%) was any islet function discernible after a month (defined as basal C-peptide levels of at least 1 ng/ml). Only 2 of these patients (7%) ever achieved insulin independence. Between 1974-1996, 305 type I diabetics were transplanted worldwide at 35 institutions. Of these, 215 were transplanted between 1990-1996. In the latter subset, temporary insulin independence was achieved in 30. However, insulin independence at one year was only 6%.

Until recently, the best results so far reported in diabetic recipients were those from the University of Giessen where 27 islet transplants were done between 1992-1996. These patients had a previous or concurrent kidney transplant except for 5 non-uremic type I diabetics, in which the indication was dangerous hypoglycemic unawareness. Three months after transplantation, 64%

of the kidney and islet transplanted patients had discernible function of the transplanted islets. In the non-uremic recipients of islet transplants without kidney transplants, all 5 initially exhibited islet function. However, when immunosuppression was withdrawn, all 5 soon lost all evidence of islet function (222).

Even more encouraging results of clinical islet transplants were reported in 2000 by the Edmonton group who successfully reversed hyperglycemia in 7 consecutive recipients (223). Since these patients were not uremic, none received a kidney transplant. The indications for the islet transplant were a history of severe hypoglycemia with unawareness, coma or metabolic instability. The risk of transplantation and chronic immunosuppression was considered less than that of continued uncontrolled diabetes. These patients received a mean islet mass of $11,547\pm1604$ islet equivalents per kg body weight. Before stable normoglycemia was established, 6 of them required 2 islet transplants and one of them 3 transplants. All of these recipients have maintained excellent glycemic control without insulin therapy for a median duration of 11.9 months. The striking improvement over previous transplants has been attributed to a change in immunosuppression, which was designed to minimize islet damage. The immunosuppressive agents generally used for pancreas or islet transplantation (steroids and CsA or tacrolimus) are known to damage islets. The Edmonton immunosuppression consisted of anti-IL-2 receptor antibody for the first 10 weeks, low-dose tacrolimus and sirolimus. No steroids were administered. Additional features by which the Edmonton series differed from most previous trials were the multiple transplants employed and the choice of non-uremic recipients. The success of the Edmonton experience is likely to encourage many others to conduct similar clinical trials.

CARDIAC TRANSPLANTATION

Recipient Selection

The growing shortage of donor hearts for transplantation has continued to spur the study of optimal patient selection. Emphasis is placed on pursuing alternatives to transplantation such as aggressive medical therapy, revascularization, and weaning patients from ventricular assist device support. Selecting only those patients unlikely to survive without transplantation has become paramount.

Deng, et al (224) from Muenster University studied the severity of heart failure in prospective heart transplant recipients as it related to the eventual outcome of the transplant. Eight hundred eighty-nine patients were grouped into low, medium, and high risk for death based on degree of heart failure at the time they were listed for transplant. No differences in outcome after transplantation were observed between groups. Only in the high-risk group was transplantation associated with a reduction in mortality during the period of observation.

Whellan, et al (225) at Duke University Medical Center examined heart transplant center practice patterns as related to donor access and survival of patients classified by the United Network of Organ sharing as Status 1 patients. A retrospective cohort analysis of Status 1 patients listed by 4 transplant centers within a single regional organ procurement organization was performed. The center at which a patient was listed was an independent predictor of receiving a transplant although only one center had a significantly increased mortality rate.

Tjan, et al (226) from Munster Germany compared the role of coronary artery revascularization versus cardiac transplantation in patients with ejection fractions less than 20%. They found similar survival between the 2 groups and concluded that in view of the donor shortage, patients with viable myocardium and graftable coronary arteries should undergo coronary revascularization rather than heart transplantation.

Hosenpud, et al (227) from Medical College of Wisconsin studied the results of cardiac transplantation in patients who were hepatitis B surface antigen-positive prior to transplantation. The ISHLT/UNOS Thoracic Registry identified 78 such patients and data on 53 of these was made available by the transplant institutions. Of the 53 patients, centers reported that 23 patients had incorrectly been identified as being surface antigen-positive resulting in 30 patients for the cohort analysis. Of the 25 patients receiving follow-up testing, 20 patients continued to be positive for hepatitis B surface antigen. Although 37% of these patients had evidence of active hepatic inflammation and cirrhosis, no survival difference was found between this cohort and a reference cardiac transplant cohort. However, 5 of 9 deaths in the surface antigen-positive patients were attributed to hepatitis. The authors advised continued caution in selecting hepatitis B surface antigen-positive patients for cardiac transplantation.

McCarthy, et al (228) reported on the long-term outcome of fulminant myocarditis as compared with acute non-fulminant myocarditis. Lymphocytic myocarditis may be persistent or reversible. One hundred-forty patients with myocarditis on endomyocardial biopsy were studied. Fulminant myocarditis was defined by clinical criteria including severe hemodynamic compromise requiring either inotropes/vasopressors or ventricular assist devices, rapid onset of symptoms, and fever. These patients (n=15) had symptoms consistent with heart failure (fatigue, dyspnea on exertion or at rest, or edema within a one or 2 day period) and viral illness within 2 weeks. Those patients who were categorized as having acute myocarditis (n=132) had a more insidious onset of symptoms of heart failure.

Of the patients with fulminant myocarditis, 93% were alive without transplant 11 years after biopsy (one died and none were transplanted) compared with 43% of patients not meeting the criteria for fulminant myocarditis (48 died and 7 were transplanted). The authors concluded that recognition of fulminant myocarditis and aggressive hemodynamic support of such patients is important in avoiding unnecessary transplantation.

Donor Selection

The shortage of appropriate donors for cardiac transplantation has led to increased interest in expanding the donor pool by using donors who would ordinarily not be considered in the past. Also, better matching of donors and recipients through improved immunologic testing remains a hotly pursued goal.

Subarachnoid hemorrhage has been associated with abnormal ECG's, echocardiograms, and elevated cardiac enzymes. Deibert, et al (229) from Washington University reported on a donor with a subarachnoid hemorrhage associated left ventricular dysfunction and an elevated troponin I level, who was initially thought to be an unacceptable candidate for cardiac donation. However, after a normal cardiac catheterization, successful transplantation of the donor heart was performed. The authors attributed the cardiac dysfunction to metabolic perturbations. Awareness of this phenomenon in neurologically abnormal donors may prevent discarding usable donor hearts.

An analysis of the influence of conventional and cross-reactive group HLA matching on cardiac transplant patients from the UNOS Scientific Registry by Thompson, et al (230) from the University of Kentucky

suggests that new typing and crossmatching techniques make it possible to add HLA criteria to the allocation protocol for donor hearts. They found that in predicting poor outcome, HLA-DR mismatch ranked behind only pretransplant assist device and race. HLA-A mismatching was also statistically significant as an independent risk factor but HLA-A plus B mismatch was significant only in Caucasian patients. Cross-reactive group mismatching was not found to be a significant independent risk factor. They found that 24-36% of patients in one organ procurement organization could be matched with ABO compatible, non-cross reactive, non-HLA-DR-mismatched donor hearts and concluded that using matching in heart allocation should be considered.

Investigators from the Cleveland Clinic examined the impact of HLA sensitization and donor cause of death in 500 heart transplantations (231). Donors were divided into 2 groups, trauma and non-trauma. Patients with pretransplant panel-reactive antibody levels greater than 10% were included in the HLA sensitized group. As expected, sensitized patients experienced a reduced one-year survival rate (76% versus 89%, respectively, p=0.2). Survival among recipients of hearts from "trauma" donors had better one-year survival (92%) than those receiving "non-trauma" hearts (82%, p=0.02). Interestingly, when "trauma" donor hearts were transplanted into sensitized patients, one-year survival was vastly better (93%) than when "non-trauma" donor hearts were used (52%).

The Cleveland Clinic group also studied flow-cytometry crossmatching (FCXM) in patients with a negative cytotoxic crossmatch (232). They grouped such patients into either negative FCXM, HLA Class I-positive FCXM, and HLA Class II-positive FCXM. Out of a total of 357 patients who had negative cytotoxic crossmatches, 50 were Class I FCXM positive, 144 Class II FCXM positive, and 163 were FCXM negative. Freedom from vascular rejection at one month was 64%, 90%, and 96% respectively. At 3 years, survival of the negative FCXM group was significantly higher (94%) than for the Class I (74%) and Class II (76%) groups. Death related to acute rejection at 3 years was 19% in the Class II group and only 3% and 2% in the negative FCXM and Class I FCXM groups. Thus FCXM results in patients with negative cytotoxic crossmatch were predictive of important clinical events after transplantation.

The use of donor hearts with left ventricular hypertrophy (LVH) was examined by Marelli, et al (233) from the University of California Medical Center in

disorder and lymphomas appearing later in the posttransplant period and having a clinical presentation similar to that seen in immunocompetent individuals. Their analysis of 15 patients with lymphoproliferative disorder following heart transplantation also revealed that only 44% demonstrated the presence of the EBV genome. The absence of demonstrable EBV genes was more common in monoclonal lymphomas.

Swerdlow, et al (251) examined the risk of lymphoid neoplasia following cardiac transplantation. Lymphoproliferative disease occurred in 30 out of 1563 patients. Of these, 6 were non-EBV related (and appeared to result from immunosuppression).

Results from the Italian Study Group of Fungal Infections in Thoracic Organ Transplant Recipients were reported by Grossi, et al (252). One thousand nine hundred and sixty-three patients undergoing thoracic organ transplants were studied (1,852 heart, 35 heart-lung, 30 double lung, 46 single lung). Fifty-one patients (41 heart, 9 heart-lung, one single lung) developed invasive fungal infections at a median of 58 days (range 6-2,479 days). Aspergillosis was the most common organism (64%). Twenty-two percent developed invasive candidiasis. Mortality was 29.4% for invasive aspergillosis and 33.3% for candidiasis. The authors concluded that while invasive fungal infections are rare, mortality is high.

Fortina, et al (253) from Padova, Italy examined risk factors among cardiac (n=252) and renal transplant (n=228) patients for the subsequent development of skin cancer. Skin cancer occurred in 40 heart transplant recipients (16%) and 16 kidney transplant recipients (7%). Using multivariate analysis, age at transplant, skin type, and sun exposure were found to be significant risk factors.

Results of transmyocardial laser revascularization to treat cardiac allograft vasculopathy were reported by Mehra, et al (254) from the Oschner Heart Transplant Center. They found that despite initial enthusiasm for this technique, it provided neither consistent symptomatic improvement, nor improved survival.

Magnani, et al (255) from Bologna, Italy reported results from a randomized control trial in 39 patients, comparing the efficacy and safety of atorvastatin with pravastatin to manage dyslipidemia after cardiac transplantation. They found that atorvastatin was significantly more effective than pravastatin in reducing cholesterol levels. Graft survival was not studied.

Keogh, et al (256) from Sydney, Australia,

prospectively examined the efficacy and safety of pravastatin (n=42) versus simvastatin (n=45) after cardiac transplantation. No differences in lipid profile were seen between the 2 groups. No differences in rejection or infection were seen. However, 6 patients treated with simvastatin experienced rhabdomyolysis or myositis and one-year survival in the pravastatin group (97.6%) was higher than in the simvastatin group (83.7%, p=0.078). The authors concluded that for safety reasons, pravastatin was the preferred drug.

Researchers from The Heart and Lung Institute of The Ohio State University examined plasma atherogenic markers in cardiac transplant patients (257). Cardiac allograft vasculopathy remains a daunting problem among long-term cardiac transplant survivors. This study examined 93 post-cardiac transplant patients compared with a control group of 18 healthy patients and 31 patients with congestive heart failure. Laboratory analysis included lipids, homocysteine, vitamin B12, folate, fibrinogen, von Willebrand factor antigen, and renin. Angiography and intravascular ultrasound was used to evaluate posttransplant coronary artery disease. Levels of atherogenic serum markers were elevated both in the transplant group and in the congestive heart failure group. However, serum marker levels did not correlate with the severity of coronary artery disease in the transplant group. Vasculopathy was associated with prior CMV infection, was increased with time after transplantation, and was decreased by use of 3-hydroxy-methyl-glutaryl-coenzyme A reductase inhibitors.

Labarrere, et al (258) examined serial troponin I levels in 110 patients during the first year after transplantation. All patients had elevated troponin I levels during the first month. During the first year, however, only 56 patients (51%) had persistent elevation. The investigators found that persistent elevation of troponin I was associated with increased risk of subsequent coronary artery disease, increased severity of coronary artery disease and more common graft failure.

Densen, et al (259) from Manchester, UK, found that polymorphism of the transforming growth factor-beta-1 gene correlated with the development of vasculopathy following cardiac transplantation. Genetic polymorphism at position +915 of the TGF-beta1 gene determines the degree of cytokine production in response to injury.

Positivity for circulating intracellular adhesion molecule-1 (ICAM-1) in cardiac allograft recipients has been purported to predict vasculopathy and graft failure.

Campana, et al (260) from Rome, Italy found elevated ICAM-1 levels in 5 of 32 transplant recipients after transplantation. None of the 5 patients demonstrated clinical signs of graft rejection. Fifteen patients had coronary artery disease but their titers of ICAM-1 were not higher than those of patients without coronary artery disease.

Technical Issues

Grande, et al (261) from Pavia, Italy compared orthotopic cardiac transplantation using the standard atrial anastomotic technique with the bicaval technique. Seventy-one patients underwent transplantation using standard technique while 46 patients underwent transplantation with bicaval anastomoses. No significant differences in conduction disturbances were seen. Five patients in the standard group required a permanent pacemaker, whereas no one in the bicaval group required one (P=NS). Atrial fibrillation occurred in 13.1% in the standard group compared with 4.6% in the bicaval group (p=NS). Tricuspid valve regurgitation was higher in the atrial anastomotic group (p=NS). Significantly less blood loss and decreased duration of isoproterenol use was observed in the bicaval group.

Use of Ventricular Assist Devices

DeNofrio, et al (262) from the University of Pennsylvania correlated the detection of anti-HLA antibody in patients with left ventricular assist devices with early rejection in an analysis of 18 patients. They pointed out that while such patients have been shown to have high panel-reactive antibodies (PRA), the significance of anti-HLA antibodies has not been elaborated.

The use of the HeartMate left ventricular assist device to bridge 12 adolescent patients to heart transplantation was reported by Helman, et al (263). All patients were less than 21 years old with a range of 11-20 years (mean 16). Body surface area ranged from 1.4-2.2 m² (mean 1.8 m²). The authors used prosthetic graft abdominal wall closure when necessary in small patients. The duration of VAD support ranged from 0-397 days (mean 123 days). Seven patients were sent home with the VAD in place. Eight patients (62%) were successfully bridged to transplant, 2 patients had their VAD explanted, and 3 patients died with a VAD in place. Complications included 4 patients with systemic infection, 3 with re-operation for hemorrhage, one patient with an embolic event, and one with intra-operative fatal air embolus.

Bank, et al (264) from the University of Minnesota studied the effect of left ventricular assist devices on the outcome of subsequent heart transplantation. A group of Status 1 patients with pretransplant VAD support (n=20) were compared with a group treated with only inotropic therapy. Although survival at 6 months did not differ, event-free survival was lower in the VAD group. Significantly better clinical parameters (hemodynamic stability, renal function) were seen in the VAD group. Costs were significantly higher for the VAD group.

Pediatric Heart Transplantation

Dent, et al (265) from Washington University in St. Louis examined the prevalence of transplant coronary artery disease in 51 pediatric heart transplant recipients. At a median of 3.4 years after transplantation, 74% of patients exhibited intimal thickening on angiography and intracoronary ultrasound. Only time since transplant was a significant predictive factor.

Di Russo, et al (266) from The Children's Hospital of Philadelphia reported the use of prolonged extracorporeal membrane oxygenation as a bridge to transplantation in a child with Epstein's anomaly.

Niles, et al (267) from Loma Linda University studied craniofacial growth in 28 infant heart transplant recipients receiving CsA-based immunosuppression and demonstrated that both craniofacial and axial skeletal growth was unaffected compared with standard growth tables. Previous reports had suggested an adverse effect of CsA on skeletal growth.

Chin, et al (268) from Stanford University examined the safety and utility of routine surveillance biopsy in 56 pediatric heart transplant recipients 2 years after transplantation. Among the 456 biopsies performed for surveillance, 3% were positive for rejection in a symptomatic patients and 20% were positive in the symptomatic patients. However, 75% of positive biopsies were in asymptomatic individuals, leading the authors to recommend continuation of late surveillance biopsies. In contrast, Leonard, et al (269) from Freeman Hospital in the UK studied the role of endomyocardial biopsy in the long-term follow-up of pediatric cardiac transplant recipients treated with a steroid-free immunosuppressive regimen. A review of annual biopsies in 40 asymptomatic pediatric patients revealed no evidence of rejection suggesting that routine endomyocardial biopsies for long-term follow up are not justified.

The pediatric cardiac transplant group from the Children's Hospital of Boston described the use of non-invasive serologic and echocardiographic data to predict biopsy-proven rejection (270). Load independent measures of cardiac function such as shortening fraction and stress velocity index were predictive of rejection (sensitivity 91.8%, specificity 66.7%). They did not find concordance between rejection and elevation of serum markers of myocardial damage (troponin, creatine kinase-MB, C-reactive protein).

Rosenthal, et al (271) from Stanford University reported on the outcome of children awaiting cardiac transplantation with either congenital heart disease or cardiomyopathy. They studied 96 patients listed for heart transplantation between 1977-1996 of whom 67 were successfully transplanted. Survival at 90 days was 81% with no difference between those with congenital heart disease or cardiomyopathy. Those with congenital heart disease experienced less morbidity.

Intermediate-term results of heart transplantation in 20 neonates or children were reported by Azeka, et al (272) from Brazil. Actuarial survival at one and 6 years after transplant was 90% and 78.2% respectively, with a mean follow up of 3.6 years.

Miscellaneous Topics

An excellent review of the status of cardiac xenotransplantation appeared in the Annals of Thoracic Surgery in July 2000 (273). The authors point out that physiological, ethical, and infectious considerations indicate that pigs are likely to be the best source of xenografts. The introduction of results of transplantation of hearts from transgenic pigs expressing human complement regulatory proteins to non-human primates indicates that hyperacute rejection can be avoided.

Until 1997 brain death was not legally recognized in Japan preventing the development of heart transplantation. Thus, Hori, et al (274) from Osaka University was the first from that country to report a successful cardiac transplant under this legislation. The patient transplanted in February 1999 had cardiomyopathy and was supported before transplantation by a ventricular assist device.

An interesting study from the University of Minnesota from Wilson, et al (275) examined sympathetic reinnervation and exercise tolerance among heart transplant recipients. Thirteen early transplant patients, 28 late transplant patients ($\geq$one year), and 20 control subjects were studied. Sinus node sympathetic reinnervation was

confirmed by injecting the artery to the sinus node with tyramine. Heart rate increase of $\geq$15 beats per minute was defined as marked reinnervation. None of the early transplant patients and 12 of the late transplant patients had marked reinnervation. The late transplant patients who did exhibit marked reinnervation demonstrated restoration of normal heart rate response to exercise although exercise duration and maximal oxygen consumption were not related significantly to reinnervation status.

LUNG TRANSPLANTATION

Patient Selection

Vizza, et al (276) from Rome, Italy, reported the outcome of patients with cystic fibrosis awaiting transplantation. The goal of their study was to evaluate factors apparent at the initial evaluation that were predictive of death on the waiting list. One hundred forty-six patients listed for transplantation were studied retrospectively. Patients who died while waiting were compared with those who either received a transplant or were alive at the conclusion of the study. Multivariate statistical analysis identified several risk factors increasing the risk of death on the waiting list including high pulmonary pressures, diabetes mellitus, and short 6-minute walk distance. However, considerable overlap was found in the groups compared. The authors concluded that prediction of death while waiting for a lung transplant based on initial evaluation was unreliable and suggested that further work is needed in this area in order to improve donor lung allocation.

Milstone, et al (277) from Vanderbilt University studied the risks of transplantation in patients with active CMV infection. Patients with preoperative urine cultures positive for CMV (n=5, all idiopathic pulmonary fibrosis patients) were compared with those patients with idiopathic pulmonary fibrosis with urine cultures negative for CMV (n=27). Three of 5 patients (60%) with CMV positive urine cultures subsequently developed CMV disease compared with 3 of 27 (11%) of those with negative CMV urine cultures (p=0.03). They also found that the culture-positive group was more likely to have a CD4/CD8 ratio <1.

Paloyan, et al (278) from Loyola Medical Center in Maywood, Illinois described lung transplantation in 2 patients with bronchioalveolar carcinoma, a condition in which high local recurrence rates after transplantation have been reported. Their patients had advanced disease that was unresectable by usual criteria but limited to the lung parenchyma without nodal involvement. The first patient had recurrence of the tumor in the transplanted lungs 9 months after transplantation but was retransplanted with cardiopulmonary bypass and careful irrigation of the native airway and has subsequently survived 4 years without evidence of disease. The second patient underwent lung transplantation using this modified technique and died 16 months after the transplant of an unrelated cause. An autopsy revealed no recurrent bronchioalveolar carcinoma. The authors believe that the use of cardiopulmonary bypass and careful airway irrigation is important in reducing tumor recurrence.

Results

Investigators from Washington University School of Medicine in St. Louis recently reviewed their 10-year experience with single versus bilateral lung transplantation for idiopathic pulmonary fibrosis (279). Forty-five patients were studied retrospectively including 32 single lung transplants and 13 bilateral sequential lung transplants. Perioperative mortality was 8.9%. One patient underwent retransplantation after primary graft failure and reperfusion injury. Actuarial survival at one and 5 years was 75.5% and 53.5%, respectively. Late deaths were secondary to bronchiolitis obliterans (n=9), malignancy (n=3), and CMV pneumonitis (n=2). Median hospital stay was 22 days. Survival and hospital stay were similar for patients treated by single or double lung transplantation.

Limbos, et al (280) from Toronto compared the psychological function and quality of life of 73 recipients of lung transplants with that of 36 patients awaiting lung transplantation. Multiple well-accepted measures of psychological functioning and quality of life were utilized. They found that although lung transplant recipients have better health (general, physical, and psychologic) compared with their non-transplanted counterparts, that both groups remain significantly impaired.

Wisser, et al (281) from the University of Vienna examined the outcome of lung transplantation in 15 patients who previously had undergone lung volume reduction surgery, a treatment that has been proposed as either an alternative to or as a bridge to lung transplantation. Lung function studies (FEV1) were performed before and after lung volume reduction. Eight patients (53%) experienced no improvement in FEV1 whereas 7 patients (47%) had significantly improved pulmonary

function. Those without improvement were transplanted an average of 10 months earlier than those with improvement. All mortalities (20%) at 3 months belonged to the group not improved by lung volume reduction leading the authors to conclude that if volume reduction improves FEV1 the need for lung transplantation may be substantially delayed.

Rejection

Pham, et al (282) from the University of Pittsburgh studied the effect of donor bone marrow infusion in clinical lung transplantation. Twenty-six patients underwent donor bone marrow infusion with lung transplantation and were found to have a significantly reduced incidence of bronchiolitis obliterans and decreased donor specific reactivity on mixed lymphocyte testing.

Hoffmeyer, et al (283) from Hannover, Germany, reported on the results of a prospective study of azathioprine withdrawal in 7 stable lung and heart/lung transplant recipients who had received a transplant more than 4 years before. These patients had stable graft function, and absence of bronchiolitis obliterans or episodes of rejection for at least 2 years. The study was discontinued at one year after 4 of the 7 patients experienced deteriorating graft function which did not respond to conventional treatment with high-dose corticosteroids and reinstitution of azathioprine therapy. The authors conclude that continuation of potent immunosuppression is necessary for maintenance of stable graft function.

Investigators from Stanford University measured inducible nitric oxide synthase (iNOS) mRNA expression in bronchoalveolar lavage specimen (284). Fifty-one samples were studied from patients with normal transplant function (n=21), acute rejection (n=15), or infection (n=15) based on histologic and bacteriologic examination of the same specimens. INOS mRNA expression was significantly more elevated in the infection group than in either the normal or acute rejection group suggesting possible use of this testing to differentiate infection from rejection.

Hasegawa, et al (285) from the University of Pittsburgh studied the anatomic distribution of acute cellular rejection in allograft lungs. They reviewed transbronchial biopsy specimens in 73 patients in whom biopsies were taken from more than one lobe. Findings included identical rejection grades for each specimen in 45% of patients. Cases with different grades among samples demonstrated a higher grade in 65% of "lower" lobe specimens compared with "upper" lobe specimens suggesting that biopsies of the lower lobes may be more informative.

Investigators from Duke University examined the influence of panel-reactive antibodies (PRA) on posttransplant outcomes in the center's first 200 lung transplant recipients (286). In comparison with non-sensitized patients, those with PRA>10% (sensitized, n=18) were found to have increased median ventilator days (9 ±8 vs. 1±11; p=0.0008), increased incidence of bronchiolitis obliterans (56% vs. 23%, p=0.044), and a trend toward decreased 2-year survival (58% vs. 73%, p=0.31). No difference in incidence of acute rejection was seen. The authors concluded that sensitized lung transplant recipients experience increased complications and may warrant different management strategies.

Quantz, et al (287) from London, Canada, analyzed 3,549 lung transplant patients from the United Network for Organ Sharing/International Society for Heart and Lung Transplantation registry to determine whether HLA antigen matching influences the outcome of lung transplantation. They found that HLA mismatches at the HLA-A and HLA-DR loci predicted 3- and 5-year mortality, as did the total number of HLA mismatches. However, the effect of each covariate was small. The incidence of acute rejection and bronchiolitis obliterans was not affected by HLA matching. The authors concluded that prospective study of HLA matching in lung transplantation was not yet warranted given small numbers of patients with <2 HLA mismatches and the modest effect of HLA matching on outcome as determined retrospectively.

Technical Issues

Garfein, et al (288) from Columbia University reviewed bronchial anastomotic complications in 130 patients and related them to technique. In 41 telescoped bronchial anastomoses, 3 major complications were seen: ischemia (32%), dehiscence (24%), and severe stenosis (32%). In 135 end-to-end anastomoses, these complications were less frequent: ischemia (19%), dehiscence (10%), and severe stenosis (8%). These differences were statistically significant for dehiscence and severe stenosis (p=0.0350 and p=0.0004, respectively). Early post-operative pneumonia was also more common in the telescoped anastomosis group (57%) compared with the end-to-end anastomosis group (35%, p=0.0271). Lick, et al (289) from The University of Texas, Galveston,

used an interesting technique of controlled reperfusion of the transplanted lung in humans. Based on work in a porcine model, they collected 1,500 cc of blood in a cardiotomy reservoir during lung implantation, mixed it to make a 4:1 solution of blood-modified Buckberg perfusate and passed it through a leukocyte filter into the pulmonary artery at 200cc/min immediately prior to removal of the vascular clamp. Five patients underwent this procedure and were extubated on or before the first postoperative day. Although not conclusive, the results of using white-cell filtered, nutrient-enriched blood yielded successful functional results in this small pilot study.

Complications

King, et al (290) from the University of Virginia studied the possible relationship of reperfusion injury after lung transplantation to post-operative pulmonary dysfunction, mortality, and morbidity. They also sought to relate occurrence of reperfusion injury to recipient lung disease and donor organ ischemic time. One hundred patients received 120 organs during the study period with 22% of patients experiencing reperfusion injury. As expected, mortality, morbidity, pulmonary dysfunction, and duration of hospital stay were higher in the reperfusion injury patients. Interestingly, ischemia time was not related to the incidence of reperfusion injury. They also found that the incidence and clinical impact of reperfusion injury was higher in those with preexisting pulmonary hypertension.

Investigators from the University of Kiel, Germany, studied the detection of CMV pneumonitis after lung transplantation using PCR of DNA from bronchioalveolar cells (291). Rapid diagnosis of this infection is important. A total of 28 patients with 105 bronchioalveolar lavage (BAL) specimens, 96 peripheral blood samples, and 14 brushings were studied using PCR detection of viral antigens in the BAL specimens and in the blood samples. These finding were compared with clinical status. A total of 8 episodes of clinical CMV pneumonitis occurred in 6 patients. All episodes of CMV pneumonitis were detected by BAL PCR. In 14 patients, CMV antigen was detected in blood while BAL PCR was negative. However, none of these patients had clinical pneumonitis. The authors concluded that BAL PCR is a sensitive and specific indicator of clinical CMV pneumonitis.

Meyers, et al (292) from Washington University in St. Louis presented evidence that the selective use of extracorporeal membrane oxygenation is warranted after lung transplantation. Out of a total of 444 single or bilateral lung transplants performed during the retrospective study period, 12 (2.7%) experienced graft dysfunction severe enough to warrant extracorporeal membrane oxygenation after conventional therapies failed (sedation, paralysis, nitric oxide). Of the 12 patients, 7 recovered and were ultimately discharged from the hospital. Mean duration of support was 4.2 days. Four patients died during support. Two patients underwent retransplantation while on support and one of these survived to discharge. All 3 patients with more than 4 days of support died. In all of the survivors, extracorporeal membrane oxygenation support was initiated by postoperative day one. There were 3 delayed deaths after discharge (at 12, 13, and 72 months) due to bronchiolitis obliterans. The 4 remaining survivors are alive at 2, 12, 25, and 54 months after transplant.

Kelly, et al (293) from University of Washington in Seattle studied the efficacy and cost of preemptive therapy directed at CMV antigenemia versus prophylaxis with ganciclovir in 19 lung transplant recipients. They found that preemptive therapy is as safe and effective as universal prophylaxis in preventing CMV disease and is less expensive.

Miscellaneous

Gertner, et al (294) from Thomas Jefferson University reported the outcome in 8 lung transplant recipients who became pregnant after transplantation. There were 4 live births, 3 therapeutic abortions, and one spontaneous abortion. Three of the 4 live babies were premature with low birth weights. Rejection occurred during 3 of the pregnancies. All of the transplant patients had at least one complication during pregnancy including either shortness of breath, rejection, or infection. All of the babies subsequently did well without residual problems.

Kulick, et al (295) from the University of Minnesota studied the survival of transgenic pig lungs (with human complement regulatory protein CD59) in a whole human blood perfusion circuit. Survival of the transgenic lungs was 240 ±0 minutes compared with 35±14.5 minutes for the control (non-transgenic) group.

Fischer, et al (296) from Toronto General Hospital examined apoptosis induction in human lungs during ischemia and after lung transplantation. Biopsies were taken after cold preservation, warm ischemic time, and reperfusion. Increased apoptosis was seen after reperfusion and increased with time after reperfusion suggesting that this cell loss may be responsible for organ dysfunction seen after transplantation.

ANNUAL REVIEW

CITED LITERATURE

1. UNOS Critical Data. www.unos.org

2. Cecka JM. The UNOS Scientific Renal Transplant Registry. In: JM Cecka PI Terasaki, Eds. Clinical Transplants 1999, UCLA Immunogenetics Center, Los Angeles, 2000; 1-21.

3. Schweitzer EJ, Wilson J, Jacobs S, Machan C, Philosophe B, Farney A, Colonna J, Jarrell BE, Bartlett SE. Increased rates of donation with laparoscopic donor nephrectomy. Ann Surg 2000; 232(3):392-400.

4. Cecka JM. Kidney transplantation from living unrelated donors. Ann Rev Med 2000, 51:393-406.

5. Matas AJ, Garvey CA, Jacobs CL, Kahn JP. Nondirected donation of kidneys from living donors. N Engl J Med 2000; 343 (6):433-6.

6. Levinsky NG. Organ donation by unrelated donors. N Engl J Med 2000; 343(6):430-2.

7. Spital A. Evolution of attitudes at US transplant centers toward kidney donation by friends and altruistic strangers. Transplantation 2000; 69(8):1728-31.

8. Halpern EJ, Mitchell DG, Wechsler RJ, Outwater EK, Moritz MJ, Wilson GA. Preoperative evaluation of living renal donors: comparison of CT angiography and MR angiography. Radiology 2000; 216(2):434-9.

9. Kuo PC, Johnson LB, Sitzmann JV. Laparoscopic donor nephrectomy with a 23-hour stay: a new standard for transplantation surgery. Ann Surg 2000; 231(5):772-9.

10. Mosimann F, Bettschart V, Schneider R. Laparoscopic live donor nephrectomy: a "23-hour stay" procedure? Transplantation 2000; 70(3):555.

11. Gridelli B, Remuzzi G. Strategies for making more organs available for transplantation. N Engl J Med 2000; 343(6):404-10.

12. Dietl KH, Wolters H, Marschall B, Senninger N, Heidenreich S. Cadaveric "two-in-one" kidney transplantation form marginal donors: experience of 26 cases after 3 years. Transplantation 2000; 70(5):790-4.

13. Andres A, Moralses JM, Herrero JC, Praga M, Morales E, Hernandez E, Ortuno T, Rodicio JL, Martinez MA, Usera G, Diaz R, Polo G, Aguirre F, Leiva O. Double versus single renal allografts from aged donors. Transplantation 2000; 69(10):2060-6.

14. Carter JT, Lee CM, Weinstein RJ, Lu AD, Dafoe DC, Alfrey EJ. Evaluation of the older cadaveric kidney donor: the impact of donor hypertension and creatinine clearance on graft performance and survival. Transplantation 2000; 70(5):765-71.

15. Randhawa PS, Minervini MI, Lombardero M, Duquesnoy R, Fung J, Shapiro R, Jordan M, Vivas C, Scantlebury V, Demetris A. Biopsy of marginal donor kidneys: correlation of histologic findings with graft dysfunction. Transplantation 2000; 69(7):1352-7.

16. Alvarez J, Barrio R, Arias J, Ruiz F, Iglesias J, Elias R, Yebenes C, Matesanz J, Caniego C, Elvira J. Non-heart-beating donors from the streets. Transplantation. 2000:70(2):314-17.

17. Whiting JF, Woodward RS, Zavala EY, Cohen DS, Martin JE, Singer GG, Lowell JA, First MR, Brennan DC, Schnitzler MA. Economic cost of expanded criteria donors in cadaveric renal transplantation: analysis of Medicare payments. Transplantation 2000; 70(5):755-60.

18. Tilney NL. Triumph of hope over experience. Transplantation 2000; 70(4):706-7.

19. Kennedy I, Sells RA, Daar AS. International Forum for Transplant Ethics. The case of "presumed consent" in transplantation. Lancet. 1998; 351:1650.

20. Daar AS. Altruism and reciprocity in organ donation: compatible or not? Transplantation 2000; 70(4):704-5.

21. Ayanian JZ, Clearly Pd, Weissman JS, Epstein AM. The effect of patient's preferences on racial differences in access to renal transplantation. N Engl J Med 1999:341:1661-69.

22. Schaubel DE, Stewart DE, Morrison HI, Zimmerman DL, Cameron JI, Jeffery JJ, Fenton SSA. Sex inequality in kidney transplantation rates. Arch Intern Med 2000; 160:2349-54.

23. Furth SL, Garg PP, Neu AM, Hwang W, Fivush BA, Powe NR. Racial differences in access to the kidney transplant waiting list for children and adolescents with end-stage renal disease. Pediatrics 2000; 106(4):756-61.

24. Isaacs RB, Lobo PI, Nock SI, Hanson JA, Ojo AO, Pruett TL. Racial disparities in access to simultaneous pancreas-kidney transplantation in the United States. Am Kidney Dis 2000; 36(3):526-33.

25. Zimmerman D, Donnelly S, Miller J, Stewart D, Albert SE. Gender disparity in living renal transplant donation. Am J Kidney Dis 2000; 36(3):534-40.

26. SoRelle R. Health Care Financing Administration wants to make kidney transplant availability equal, regardless of race. Circulation. 2000; 101(3):E37.

27. Sagedal S, Nordal KP, Hartmann A, Degre M, Holter E, Foss A, Osnes K, Leivestad T, Fauchald P, Rollag H. A prospective study of the natural course of cytomegalovirus infection and disease in renal allograft recipients. Transplantation 2000; 70(8):1166-74.

28. Humar A, Gillingham K, Payne WD, Sutherland DE, Matas AJ. Increased incidence of cardiac complications in kidney transplant recipients with cytomegalovirus disease. Transplantation 2000; 70(2):310-3.

29. Klctzmayr J, Kreuzwieser C, Watkins-Riedel T, Berlakovich G, Kovarik J, Klauser R. Long-term oral ganciclovir prophylaxis for prevention of cytomegalovirus infection and disease in cytomegalovirus high-risk renal transplant recipients. Transplantation 2000; 70(8):1174-80.

30. Limaye AP, Corey L, Koelle DM, Davis CL, Boeckh M. Emergence of ganciclovir-resistant cytomegalovirus disease among recipients of solid-organ transplants. Lancet 2000; 356(9230):645-9.

31. Bienvenu B, Thervet E, Bedrossian J, Scieux C, Mazeron MC, Thouvenot D, Legendre CH. Development of cytomegalovirus resistance to ganciclovir after oral maintenance treatment in a renal transplant recipient. Transplantation 2000; 69(1):182-84.

32. Kidd IM, Clark DA, Sabin CA, Andrew D, Hassan-Waker AF, Sweny P, Griffiths PD, Emery VC. Prospective study of human beta herpesviruses after renal transplantation: association of human herpesvirus 7 and cytomeglaovirus co-infection with cytomegalovirus disease and increased rejection. Transplantation 2000; 69(11):2400-4.

33. Frances C, Mouquet C, Marcelin AG, Barete S, Agher R, Charron D, Benalia H, Dupin N, Piette JC, Bitker MO, Calvez V. Outcome of kidney transplant recipients with previous human herpesvirus-8 infection. Transplantation 2000; 69(9):1776-9.

34. Luppi M, Barozzi P, Schulz TF, Setti G, Staskus K, Trovato R, Narni F, Donelli A, Maiorana A, Marasca R, Sandrini S, Torelli G. Bone marrow failure associated with human herpesvirus 8 infection after transplantation. N Engl J Med 2000; 343(19):1378-85.

35. Tong CY, Bakran A, Williams H, Cheung CY, Peiris JS. Association of human herpesvirus 7 with cytomegalovirus disease in renal transplant recipients. Transplantation 2000; 70(1):213-6.

36. Pamidi S, Friedman K, Kampalath B, Eshoa C, Harihan S. Human parvovirus B19 infection presenting as persistent anemia in renal transplant recipients. Transplantation 2000; 69(12):2666-69.

37. Randhawa PS, Demetris AJ. Nephropathy due to polyomavirus type BK. N Engl J Med 2000; 342(18):1361-3.

38. Nickeleit V, Klimkait T, Binet I, Dalquen P, Del Zenero V, Thiel G, Mihatsch M, Hirsch H. Testing for polyomavirus type BK DBA in plasma to identify renal-allograft recipients with viral nephropathy. N Engl J Med 2000; 342(18):1309-15.

39. Vachharajani T, Abreo K, Phadke A, Oza U, Kirpalani A. Diagnosis and treatment of tuberculosis in hemodialysis and renal transplant patients. Am J Nephrol 2000; 20:273-77.

40. Knirsch CA, Jakob K, Schoonmaker D, Kiehlbauch JA, Wong SJ, Della-Latta P, Whittier S, Layton M, Scully B. An outbreak of Legionella micdadei pneumonia in transplant patients: evaluation, molecular edpidemiology, and control. Am J Med 2000; 108(4):290-5.

41. Battaglia M, Ditonno P, Fiore T, De Ceglie G, Regina G, Selvaggi FP. True mycotic arteritis by candida albicans in 2 kidney transplant recipients from the same donor. J Urol 2000; 163(4) 1236-8.

42. Danpanich E, Kasiske B. Risk factors for cancer in renal transplant recipients. Transplantation; 68(12):1859-64.

43. Birkeland SA, Lokkegaard H, Storm HH. Cancer risk in patients on dialysis and after renal transplantation. Lancet 2000; 355(9218):1886-7.

44. Kwong YL, Lam CCK, Chan TM. Post-transplantation lymphoproliferative disease of natural killer lineage: a clinicopathological and molecular analysis. Br J Haematol 2000; 110(1):197-202.

45. Marshall SE, Bordea C, Haldar NA, Mullighan CG, Wojnarowska F, Morris PJ, Welsh KI. Glutathione S-transferase polymorphisms and skin cancer after renal transplantation. Kidney Int 2000; 58(5):2186-93.

46. Huang R, Shapiro N. Adenotonsillar enlargement in pediatric patients following solid organ transplantation. Arch Otolaryngol Head Neck Surg 2000; 126(2):159-64.

47. Herzig KA, Falk MC, Jonsson JR, Axelsen RA, Griffin AD, Hawley CM, Rigby RJ, Cobcroft R, Nicol DL, Powell EE, Johnson DW. Novel surveillance and cure of a donor-transmitted lymphoma in a renal allograft recipient. Transplantation 2000; 70(1):149-52.

48. Wolfe RA, Ashby VB, Milford EL, Ojo AO, Ettenger RE, Agodoa LYC, Held PJ, Port KF. Comparison of mortality in all patients on dialysis, patients on dialysis awaiting transplantation, and recipients of a first cadaveric transplant. N Engl J Med. 1999; 341(23):1725-30.

49. Hunsicker LG. A survival advantage for renal transplantation. N Engl J Med. 1999; 341(23) 1762-3.

50. Hariharan S, Johnson C, Bresnahan B, Taranto S, McIntosh M, Stablein D. Improved graft survival after renal transplantation in the United States, 1988 to 1996. N Engl J Med 2000; 342(9):605-12.

51. Humar A, Durand B, Gillingham K, Payne WD, Sutherland DE, Matas AJ. Living unrelated donors in kidney transplants: better long-term results than with non-HLA-identical living related donors? Transplantation 2000; 69(9):1942-5.

52. Tandon V, Botha JF, Banks J, Pontin AR, Pascoe MD,Kahn DA. A tale of two kidneys - how long can a kidney transplant wait? Clin Transplantation 2000; 14:189-92.

53. Healey PJ, McDonald R, Waldhausen JH, Sawin R, Tapper D. Transplantation of adult living donor kidneys into infants and small children. Arch Surg 2000; 135(9):1035-41.

54. Nicholson ML, Windmill DC,Horsburgh T, Harris KPG. Influence of allograft size to recipient body-weight ratio on the long-term outcome of renal transplantation. Br J Surg; 87(3):314-19.

55. Takemoto SK, Terasaki PI, Gjertson DW, Cecka JM. Twelve years' experience with national sharing of HLA-matched cadaveric kidneys for transplantation. N Engl J Med 2000; 343(15):1078-84.

56. Saadeh E, Szatkowski M, Vary CPH, Smith JD, Himmelfarb J, Mahoney RJ.HLA-DMA allele polymorphism: no impact on kidney allograft outcome. Human Immunology 2000; 61:345-47.

57. McKenna RM, Takemoto SK. Improving HLA matching for kidney transplantation by use of CREGs. Lancet 2000; 355:1842-3.

58. Hollenbeak CS, Woodward RS, Cohen DS, Lowell JA, Singer GG, Tesi RJ, Howard TK, Mohanakumar T, Brennan DC, Schnitzler MA. The economic benefit of allocation of kidneys based on cross-reactive group matching. Transplantation 2000; 70(3):537-40.

59. Lee CM, Carter JT, Alfrey EJ, Ascher NL, Roberts JP, Freise CE. Prolonged cold ischemia thime obviates the benefits of O HLA mismatches in renal transplantation. Arch Surg 2000; 135(9):1016-9; discussion 1019-20.

60. Humar A, Payne WD, Sutherland DE, Matas AJ. Clinical determinants of multiple acute rejection episodes in kidney transplant recipients. Transplantation 2000; 69(11):2357-60.

61. Dugre FJ, Gaudreau S, Belles-Isles M, Houde I, Roy R. Cytokine and cytotoxic molecule gene expression deter-mined in peripheral blood mononuclear cells in the diagnosis of acute renal rejection. Transplantation 2000; 70(7):1074-80.

62. Pascoe MD, Marshall SE, Welsch KI, Fulton LM, Hughes DA. Increased accuracy of renal allograft rejection diagnosis using combined perforin, granzyme B, and Fas ligand fine-needle aspiration immunocytology. Transplantation 2000; 69(12):2547-53.

63. Chareandee C, Herman WH, Hricik DE, Simonson MS. Elevated endothelin-1 in tubular epithelium is associated with renal allograft rejection. Am J Kidney Dis 2000; 36(3):541-9.

64. Teppo AM, Honkanen E, Ahonen J, Gronhagen-Riska C. Changes of urinary alpha1-microglobulin in the assessment of prognosis in renal transplant recipients. Transplantation 2000; 70(8):1154-9.

65. Bonsib SM, Abul-Ezz SR, Ahmad I, Young SM, Ellis En, Schneider DL, Walker PD. Acute rejection-associated tubular basement membrane defects and chronic allograft nephropathy. Kidney Int 2000; 58(5):2206-14.

66. McLaren AJ, Fuggle SV, Welsh KI, Gray DW, Morris PJ. Chronic allograft failure in human renal transplantation: a multivariate risk factor analysis. Ann Surg 2000; 232(1):98-103.

67. Meier-Kriesche HU, Ojo AO, Hanson JA, Cibrik DM, Punch JD, Leichtman AB, Kaplan B. Increased impact of acute rejection on chronic allograft failure in recent era. Transplantation 2000; 70(7):1098-100.

68. Meier-Kriesche HU, Ojo AO, Cibrik DM, Hanson JA, Leichtman AB, Magee JC, Port FK, Kaplan B. Relationship of recipient age and development of chronic allograft failure. Transplantation 2000; 70(2):306-10.

69. Wissing KM, Abramowicz D, Broeders N, Vereestraeten P. Hypercholesterolemia is associated with increased kidney graft loss caused by chronic rejection in male patients with previous acute rejection. Transplantation 2000; 70(3):464-72.

70. Jain S, Furness PN, Nicholson ML. The role of transforming growth factor beta in chronic renal allograft nephropathy. Transplantation 2000; 69(9):1759-66.

71. Mas V, Diller A, Albano S, Giraudo C, Alvarellos T, Sena J, Massari P, de Boccardo G. Intragraft expression of transforming growth factor-beta 1 by a novel quantitative reverse transcription polymerase chain reaction ELISA in long lasting kidney recipients. Transplantation 2000; 70(4):612-6.

72. Mele TS, Halloran PF. The use of mycophenolate mofetil in transplant recipients. Immunopharmacology 2000; 47:215-45.

73. European mycophenolate mofetil cooperative study group. Placebo controlled study of mycophenolate mofetil combined with CsA and corticosteroids for prevention of acute rejection. Lancet 1995; 345:1321-25.

74. Tricontinental Mycophenolate mofetil renal transplant study group. A blinded, randomized clinical trial of mycophenolate mofetil for the prevention of acute rejection in cadaveric renal transplantation. Transplantation 1996; 61:1029-37.

75. US renal transplant mycophenolate mofetil study group. Sollinger HW. Mycophenolate mofetil for the prevention of acute rejection in primary cadaveric renal allograft recipients. Transplantation 1995; 60:225-32.

76. Pascual M, Williams WW, Cosimi AB, Delmonico FL, Farrell ML, Tolkoff,-Rubin N. Chronic renal allograft dysfunction: a role for mycophenolate mofetil? Transplantation 2000; 69(8):1749-50.

77. Houde I, Isenring P, Boucher D, Noel R, Lachanche JG. Mycophenolate mofetil, an alternative to CsA A for long-term immunosuppression in kidney transplantation? Transplantation 2000; 70(8):1251-3.

78. Smak Gregoor PJ, van Gelder T, van Besouw NM, van der Mast BJ, Ijzermans JN, Weimar W. Randomized study on the conversion of treatment with CsA to azathioprine or mycophenolate mofetil followed by dose reduction. Transplantation 2000; 70(1):143-8.

79. Miller J, Mendez R, Pirsch JD, Jensik SC. Safety and efficacy of tacrolimus in combination with mycophenolate mofetil (MMF) in cadaveric renal transplant recipients.Transplantation 2000; 69(5):875-80.

80. Pascual M, Williams WW, Cosimi AB, Delmonico FL, Farrell ML, Tolkoff=Rubin N. Chronic renal allograft dysfunction: a role for mycophenolate mofetil? Transplantation 2000; 69(8):1749-50.

81. Ojo AO, Meier-Kriesche HU, Hanson JA, Leichtman AB, Cibrik D, Magee JC, Wolfe RA, Agodoa LY, Kaplan B. Mycophenolate mofetil reduces late renal allograft loss independent of acute rejection. Transplantation 2000; 69(11):2405-9.

82. Kaplan B, Meier-Kriesche HU, Vaghela M, Friedman G, Mulgaonkar S, Jacobs M. Withdrawal of mycophenolate mofetil in stable renal transplant recipients. Transplantation 2000; 69(8):1726-8.

83. Vanrenterghem Y, Lebranchu Y, Hene R, Oppenheimer F, Ekberg H. Double-blind comparison of two corticosteroid regimens plus mycophenolate mofetil and CsA for prevention of acute renal allograft rejection. Transplantation 2000; 70(9):1352-9.

84. Steroid withdrawal study group. Prednisone withdrawal in kidney transplant recipients on CsA and mycophenolate mofetil-a prospective randomized study. Transplantation 2000; 68(12):1865-74.

85. Matl I, Lacha J, Lodererova A, Simova M, Teplan V, Lanska V, Vitko S. Withdrawal of steroids form triple-drug therapy in kidney transplant patients. Nephrol Dial Transplant 2000; 15(7):1041-5.

86. Chakrabarti P, Wong HY, Scantlebury VP, Jordan ML, Vivas C, Ellis D, Lombardozzi-Lane S, Hakala TR, Fung JJ, Simmons RL, Starzl TE, Shapiro R. Outcome after steroid withdrawal in pediatric renal transplant patients receiving tacrolimus-based immunosuppression. Transplantation 2000; 70(5):760-4.

87. Sandrini S, Majorca R, Scolari F, Cancarini G, Setti G, Gaggia P, Cristinelli L, Zubani R, Bonardelli S, Maffeis R, Portolani N, Nodari F, giulini SM. A prospective randomized trial on azathioprine addition to CsA verus CsA monotherapy at steroid withdrawl, 6 months after renal transplantation. Transplantation 2000; 69(9):1861-7.

88. Hurault de Ligny B, Toupance O,Lavaud S, Bauwens M, Peyronnet P, Le Meur Y, Ryckelynck JP, Jolly D, Leroux-Robert C, Touchard G. Factors predicting the long-term success of maintenance CsA monotherapy after kidney transplantation. Transplantation 2000; 69(7):1327-32.

89. Van Besouw NM, van der Mast BJ, de Kuiper P, Smak Gregoor PJ, Vaessen LM, Ijzermans JN, van Gelder T, Weimar W. Donor-specific T-cell reactivity identifies kidney transplant patients in whom immunosuppressive therapy can be safely reduced. Transplantation 2000; 70(1):136-43.

90. Higgins RM, Hart P, Lam FT, Kashi H. Conversion from tacrolimus to CsA in stable renal transplant patients. Transplantation 2000; 69(8)1736-39.

91. Higgins RM, Hart P, Lam FT, Kashi H. Conversion from tacrolimus to CsA in stable renal transplant patients: safety, metabolic changes, and pharmacokinetic comparison. Transplantation 2000; 70(1):199-202.

92. Breidenbach T, Kliem V, Burg M, Radermacher J, Hoffmann MW, Klempnauer J. Profound drop of CsA A whole blood trough levels caused by St. John's wort. Transplantation 2000; 69(10):2229-30.

93. Breidenbach T, Hoffmann MW, Becker T, Schlitt H, Klempnauer J. Drug interaction of St. John's wort with CsA. Lancet 2000; 355:1912.

94. Pham PT, Peng A, Wilkinson AH, Gritsch HA, Lassman C, Pham PC, Danovitch GM. CsA and tacrolimus-associated thrombotic microangiopathy. Am J Kidney Dis 2000; 36(4):844-50.

95. Pham PT, Peng A, Wilkinson AH,m Gritsch HA, Lassman C, Pham PC, Danovitch GM. CsA and tacrolimus-associated thrombotic microangiopathy. Am J Kidney Dis 2000; 36(4):871-4.

96. Kreis H, Cisterne JM, Land W, Wrammer L, Squifflet JP, Abramowicz D, Campistol JM, Morales JM, Grinyo JM, Mourad G, Berthoux FC, Brattstrom C, Lebranchu Y, Vialtel P. Sirolimus in association with mycophenolate mofetil induction for the prevention of acute graft rejection in renal allograft recipients. Transplantation 2000; 69(7):1252-60.

97. Kahan BD. Efficacy of sirolimus compared with azathioprine for reduction of acute renal allograft rejection of acute renal allograft rejection: a randomized multicentre study. The Rapamune US Study Group. Lancet 2000; 356:194-202.

98. Halloran PF. Sirolimus and CsA for renal transplantation. Lancet 2000; 356:179-80.

99. Morelon E, Stern M, Kreis H. Interstitial pneumonitis associated with sirolimus therapy in renal-transplant recipients. N Engl J Med 2000; 343(3):225-6.

100. Thistlethwaite JR Jr, Nashan B, Hall M, Chodoff L, Lin TH. Reduced acute rejection and superior 1-year renal allograft survival with basiliximab in patients with diabetes mellitus. The Global Simulect Study Group. Transplantation 2000; 70(5):765-71.

101. Meier-Kriesche HU, Kaza H, Palekar SS, Friedman GS, Mulgaonkar SP, Ojo AO, Kaplan B. The effect of Daclizumab in a high-risk renal transplant population. Clin Transplantation 2000; 14:509-13.

102. Flechner SM, Goldfarb DA, Fairchild R, Modlin CS, Fisher R, Mastroianni B, Boparai N, O'Malley KJ, Cook DJ, Novick AC. A randomized prospective trial of low-dose OKT3 induction therapy to prevent rejection and minimize side effects in recipients of kidney transplants. Transplantation 2000; 69(11):2374-81.

103. Chisholm MA, Vollenweider LJ, Mulloy LL, Jagadeesan M, Wynn JJ, Rogers HE, Wade WE, DiPiro JT. Renal transplant patient compliance with free immunosuppressive medications. Transplantation 2000; 70(8):1240-4.

104. Malinchoc M, Kamath PS, Gordon FD, Peine CJ, Rank J and TerBorg, PCJ. A Model to Predict Poor Survival in Patients Undergoing Transjugular Intrahepatic Portosystemic Shunts. Hepatology 2000; 31:864-871.

105. Kim WR, Wiesner RH, Poterucha JJ, Therneau TM, Benson JT, Krom RAF, and Dickson ER. Adaption of the Mayo Primary Biliary Cirrhosis Natural History Model for Application in Liver Transplant Candidates. Liver Transplantation 2000; 6:489-494.

106. Shakil AO, Kramer D, Mazariegos GV, Fung JJ and Rakela J. Acute Liver Failure: Clinical Features, Outcome Analysis, and Applicability of Prognostic Criteria. Liver Transplantation 2000; 6:163-169.

107. Facciuto M, Heidt D, Guarrera J, Bodian CA, Miller CM, Emre S, Guy SR, Fishbein TM, Schwartz ME and Sheiner PA. Retransplantation for Late Liver Graft Failure: Predictors of Mortality. Liver Transplantation 2000; 6:174-179.

108. Kim WR, Krowka MJ, Plevak DJ, Lee J, Rettke SR, Frantz RP and Wiesner RH. Accuracy of Doppler Echocardiography in the Assessment of Pulmonary Hypertension in Liver Transplant Candidates. Liver Transplantation 2000; 6:453-458.

109. Williams K, Lewis JF, Davis G and Geiser EA. Dobutamine Stress Echocardiography in Patients Undergoing Liver Transplantation Evaluation. Transplantation 2000; 69:2354-2356.

110. Figueiredo FA, Dickson ER, Pasha TM, Porayko MK, Therneau TM, Malinchoc M, DiCecco SR, Francisco-Ziller NM, Kasparova P and Charlton MR. Utility of Standard Nutritional Parameters in Detecting Body Cell Mass Depletion in Patients with End-Stage Liver Disease. Liver Transplantation 2000; 6:575-581.

111. LeCornu KA, McKiernan J, Kapadia SA and Neuberger JM. A Prospective Randomized Study of Preoperative Nutritional Supplementation in Patients Awaiting Elective Orthotopic Liver Transplantation. Transplantation 2000; 69:1364-1369.

112. Sawyer RG, Pelletier SJ, Spencer CE, Pruett TL and Isaacs RB. Increased Late Hepatic Artery Thrombosis Rate and Deceased Graft Survival After Liver Transplants With Zero Cross-Reactive Group Mismatches. Liver Transplantation 2000; 6:229-236.

113. Brandhagen DJ, Alvarez W, Therneau TM, Kruckeberg KE, Thibodeau SN, Ludwig J and Porayko MK. Iron Overload in Cirrhosis – HFE Genotypes and Outcome After Liver Transplantation. Hepatology 2000; 31:456-460.

114. Helmke K, Burdelski M, and Hansen H-C. Detection and Monitoring of Intracranial Pressure Dysregulation in Liver Failure by Ultrasound. Transplantation 2000; 70:392-395.

115. Millis JM, Cronin DC, Brady LM, Newell KA, Woodle ES, Bruce DS, Thistlehwaite JR and Broelsch CE. Primary Living-Donor Liver Transplantation at the University of Chicago. Ann Surg 2000; 1:104-111.

116. Kubota K, Makuuchi M, Takayama T, Harihara Y, Hasegawa K, Aoki T, Asato H, Kawarasaki H. Simple Test on the Back Table for Justifying Single Hepatic-Arterial Reconstruction in Living Related Liver Transplantation. Transplantation 2000; 70:696-697.

117. Ethics Committee, American Society of Transplant Surgeons. American Society of Transplant Surgeons' Position Paper on Adult-to-Adult Living Donor Liver Transplantation. Liver Transplantation 2000; 6:815-817.

118. Marcos A. Right Lobe Living Donor Liver Transplantation: A Review. Liver Transplantation 2000; 6:3-20.

119. Trotter JF, Wachs M, Trouillot T, Steinberg T, Bak T, Everson GT and Kam I. Evaluation of 100 patients for Living Donor Liver Transplantation. Liver Transplantation 2000; 6:290-295.

120. Marcos A, Fisher RA, Ham JM, Olzinski AT, Shiffman ML, Sanyal AJ, Luketic VAC, Sterling RK, Olbrisch ME and Posner MP. Selection and Outcome of Living Donors for Adult to Adult Right Lobe Transplantation. Transplantation 2000; 69:2410-2415.

121. Marcos A, Ham JM, Fisher RA, Olzinski AT, and Posner MP. Single-Center Analysis of the First 40 Adult-to-Adult Living Donor Liver Transplants Using the Right Lobe. Liver Transplantation 2000; 6:296-301.

122. Marcos A, Ham JM, Fisher RA, Olzinski AT and Posner MP. Surgical Management of Anatomical Variations of the Right Lobe in Living Donor Liver Transplantation. Ann Surg 2000; 231:824-831.

123. Testa G, Malago M, Valentin-Gamazo C, Lindell G and Broelsch CE. Biliary Anastomosis in Living Related Liver Transplantation Using the Right Liver Lobe: Techniques and Complications. Liver Transplantation 2000; 6:710-714.

124. Inomata Y, Uemoto S, Asonuma K, Egawa H, Kiuchi T, Fujita S, Hayashi M, Kawashima M and Tanaka K. Right Lobe Graft in Living Donor Liver Transplantation. Transplantation 2000; 69:258-264.

125. Kaneko T, Kaneko K, Sugimoto H, Inoue S, Hatsuno T, Sawada K, Ando H and Nakao A. Intrahepatic Anastomosis Formation Between the Hepatic Veins in the Graft Liver of the Living Related Liver Transplantation: Observation by Doppler Ultrasonography. Transplantation 2000; 70:982-984.

126. Fan S-T, Lo C-M, Liu C-L, Yong B-H, Chan JK-F, and Ng I O-L Safety of Donors in Live Donor Liver Transplantation Using Right Lobe Grafts. Arch Surg 2000; 135:336-340.

127. Fan ST, Lo C-M and Liu C-L. Technical Refinement in Adult-to-Adult Living Donor Liver Transplantation Using Right Lobe Graft. Ann Surg 2000; 231:126-131.

128. Marcos A, Fisher RA, Ham JM, Shiffman ML, Sanyal AJ, Luketic VAC, Sterling RK, Fulcher AS and Posner MP. Liver Regeneration and Function in Donor and Recipient after Right Lobe Adult to Adult Living Donor Liver Transplantation. Transplantation 2000; 69:1375-1379.

129. Uemoto S, Inomata Y, Sakurai T, Egawa H, Fujita S, Kiuchi T, Hayashi M, Yasutomi M, Yamabe H and Tanaka K. Living Donor Liver Transplantation for Fulminant Hepatic Failure. Transplantation 2000; 70:152-157.

130. Marcos A, Ham JM, Fisher RA, Olzinski AT, Shiffman ML, Sanyal AJ, Luketic VAC, Sterling RK and Posner MP. Emergency Adult to Adult Living Donor Liver Transplantation for Fulminant Hepatic Failure. Transplantation 2000; 69:2202-2205.

131. Testa G, Crippin JS, Netto GJ, Goldstein RM, Jennings LW, Brkic BS, Brooks BK, Levy MF, Gonwa TA and Klintmalm GB. Liver Transplantation for Hepatitis C: Recurrence and Disease Progression in 300 Patients. Liver Transplantation 2000; 6:553-561.

132. Belli LS, Zavaglia C, Alberti AB, Poli F, Rondinara G, Silini E, Taioli E, DeCarlis L, Scalamogna M, Forti D, Pinzello G, and Ideo G. Influence of Immunogenetic Background on the Outcome of Recurrent Hepatitis C After Liver Transplantation. Hepatology 2000; 31:1345-1350.

133. Baron PW, Sindram D, Higdon D, Howell DN, Gottfried MR, Tuttle-Newhall JE, Clavien P-A. Prolonged Rewarming Time During Allograft Implantation Predisposes to Recurrent Hepatitis C Infection After Liver Transplantation. Liver Transplantation 2000; 6:407-412.

134. Bizollon T, Ahmed SNS, Guichard S, Chevallier P, Adham M, Durerf C, Baulieux J and Trepo C. Anti-hepatitis C virus core IgM antibodies correlate with hepatitis C recurrence and its severity in liver transplant patients. Gut 2000; 47:698-702.

135. Gaweco AS, Wiesner RH, Porayko M, Rustgi VK, Yong S, Hamdani R, Harig J, Chejfec G, McClatchey KD, and VanThiel DH. Intragraft Localization of Activated Nuclear Factor kB in Recurrent Hepatitis C Virus Disease Following Liver Transplantation. Hepatology 2000; 31:1183-1191.

136. McLaughlin K, Wajstaub S, Marotta P, Adams P, Grant DR, Wall WJ, Jevnikar AM and Rizkalla KS. Increased Risk for Posttransplant Lymphoproliferative Disease in Recipients of Liver Transplants with Hepatitis C. Liver Transplantation 2000; 6:570-574.

137. Pelletier SJ, Iezzoni JC, Crabtree TD, Hahn YS, Sawyer RG and Pruett TL. Prediction of Liver Allograft Fibrosis After Transplantation for Hepatitis C Virus: Persistent Elevation of Serum Transaminase Levels Versus Necroinflammatory Activity. Liver Transplantation 2000; 6:44-53.

138. Pelletier SJ, Raymond DP, Crabtree TD, Iezzoni JC, Sawyer RG, Hahn YS and Pruett TL. Pretransplantation Hepatitis C Virus Quasispecies May be Predictive of Outcome After Liver Transplantation. Hepatology 2000; 32:375-381.

139. Pelletier SJ, Raymond DP, Crabtree TD, Berg CL, Iezzoni JC, Hahn YS, Sawyer RG and Pruett TL. Hepatitis C-Induced Hepatic Allograft Injury is Associated with a Pretransplantation Elevated Viral Replication Rate. Hepatology 2000; 32:418-426.

140. Taniguchi M, Shakil AO, Vargas HE, Laskus T, Demetris AJ, Gayowski T, Dodson SF, Fung JJ and Rakela J. Clinical and Virologic Outcomes of Hepatitis B and C Viral Coinfection After Liver Transplantation: Effect of Viral Hepatitis D. Liver Transplantation 2000; 6:92-96.

141. Marinos G, Rossol S, Carucci P, Wong PYN, Donaldson P, Hussain MJ, Vergani D, Portmann BC, Williams R, and Naoumov NV. Immunopathogenesis of Hepatitis B Virus Recurrence After Liver Transplantation. Transplantation 2000; 69:559-568.

142. Sanchez-Fueyo A, Rimola A, Grande L, Costa J, Mas A, Navasa M, Cirera I, Sanchez-Tapias JM and Rodes J. Hepatitis B Immunoglobulin Discontinuation Followed by Hepatitis B Virus Vaccination: A New Strategy in the Prophylaxis of Hepatitis B Virus Recurrence After Liver Transplantation. Hepatology 2000; 31:496-501.

143. Han S-HB, Ofman J, Holt C, King K, Kunder G, Chen P, Dawson S, Goldstein L, Yersiz H, Farmer DG, Ghobrial RM, Busuttil RW and Martin P. An Efficacy and Cost-Effectiveness Analysis of Combination Hepatitis B Immune Globulin and Lamivudine to Prevent Recurrent Hepatitis B After Orthotopic Liver Transplantation Compared With Hepatitis B Immune Globulin Monotherapy. Liver Transplantation 2000; 6:741-748.

144. Malkan G, Cattral MS, Humar A, Asghar HA, Greig PD, Hemming AW, Levy GA and Lilly LB. Lamivudine for Hepatitis B in Liver Transplantation. Transplantation 2000; 69:1403-1407.

145. Dodson SF, deVera ME, Bonham CA, Geller DA, Rakela J, and Fung JJ. Lamivudine After Hepatitis B Immune Globulin Is Effective in Preventing Hepatitis B Recurrence After Liver Transplantation. Liver Transplantation 2000; 6:434-439.

146. Mutimer D, Pillay D, Shields P, Cane P, Ratcliffe D, Martin B, Buchan S, Boxall L, O'Donnell K, Shaw J, Hubscher S, and Elias E. Outcome of lamivudine resistant hepatitis B virus infection in the liver transplant recipient. Gut 2000; 46:107-113.

147. Shokouh-Amiri MH, Gaber AO, Bagous WA, Grewal HP, Hathaway DK, Vera SR, Stratta RJ, Bagous TN and Kizilisik T. Choice of Surgical Technique Influences Perioperative Outcomes in Liver Transplantation. Ann Surg 2000; 231:814-823.

148. Soliman T, Langer F, Puhalla H, Pokorny H, Grunberger T, Berlakovich GA, Langle F, Muhlbacher F, and Steininger R. Parencyhmal Liver Injury in Orthotopic Liver Transplantation. Transplantation 2000; 69:2079-2084.

149. Margarit C, Bilbao I, Charco R, Lazaro JL, Hidalgo E, Allende E, and Murio E. Auxiliary Heterotopic Liver Transplantation With Portal Vein Arterialization for Fulminant Hepatic Failure. Liver Transplantation 2000; 6:805-809

150. Gundlach M, Broering D, Topp S, Sterneck M and Rogiers X. Split-Cava Technique: Liver Splitting for Two Adult Recipients. Liver Transplantation 2000; 6:703-706.

151. Davidson BR, Rai R, Nandy A, Doctor N, Burroughs A and Rolles K. Results of Choledochojejunostomy in the Treatment of Biliary Complications After Liver Transplantation in the Era of Nonsurgical Therapies. Liver Transplantation 2000; 6:201-206.

152. Saab S, Martin P, Soliman GY, Machicago GA, Roth BE, Kunder G, Han S-HB, Farmer DG, Ghobrial RM, Busuttil RW and Bedford RA. Endoscopic Management of Biliary Leaks After T-Tube Removal in Liver Transplant Recipients: Nasobiliary Drainage Versus Biliary Stenting. Liver Transplantation 2000; 6:627-632.

153. Cirera I, Navasa M, Rimola A, Garcia-Pagan JC, Grande L, Garcia-Valdecasas JC, Fuster J, Bosch J and Rodes J. Ascites After Liver Transplantation. Liver Transplantation 2000; 6:157-162.

154. Marcos A, Fisher RA, Ham JM, Olzinski AT, Shiffman ML, Sanyal AJ, Luketic VAC, Sterling RK and Posner MP. Emergency Portacaval Shunt for Control of Hemorrhage from a Parenchymal Fracture After Adult-to-Adult Living Donor Liver Transplantation. Transplantation 2000; 69:2218-2221.

155. Bhattacharjya T, Olliff SP, Bhattacharjya S, Mirza DF and McMaster P. Percutaneous Portal Vein Thrombolysis and Endovascular Stent for Management of Posttransplant Portal Venous Conduit Thrombosis. Transplantation 2000; 69:2195-2198.

156. Singh N, Paterson DL, Gayowski T, Wagener MM, and Marino IR. Predicting Bacteremia and Bacteremic Mortality in Liver Transplant Recipients. Liver Transplantation 2000; 6:54-61.

157. Torres A, Santiago E, Insausti J, Guergue JM, Xaubet A, Mas A, and Salmeron JM. Etiology and Microbial Patterns of Pulmonary Infiltrates in Patients with Orthotopic Liver Transplantation. Chest 2000; 117:494-502.

158. Lautenschlager I, Linnavuori K and Hockerstedt K. Human Herpesvirus-6 Antigenemia After Liver Transplantation. Transplantation 2000; 69:2561-2566.

159. Singh N, Paterson DL, Gayowski T, Wagener MM and Marino IR. Cytomegalovirus Antiogenemia Directed Pre-Emptive Prophylaxis with Oral Versus I.V. Ganciclovir for the Prevention of Cytomegalovirus Disease in Liver Transplant Recipients. Transplantation 2000; 70:717-722.

160. Singhal S, Ellis RW, Jones SG, Miller SJ, Fisher NC, Hastings JGM and Mutimer D. Targeted Prophylaxis with Amphotericin B Lipid Complex in Liver Transplantation. Liver Transplantation 2000; 6:588-595.

161. Kuse E-R, Langefeld I, Jaeger K, and Kulpmann W-R. Procalcitonin in fever of unknown origin after liver transplantation: A variable to differentiate acute rejection from infection. Critical Care Medicine 2000; 28:555-559.

162. Gayowski T, Singh N, Keyes L, Wannstedt CF, Wagener MM, Vargas H, Laskus T, Rakela J, Fung JJ and Marino IR. Late-Onset Renal Failure After Liver Transplantation: Role of Posttransplant Alcohol Use. Transplantation 2000; 69 383-388.

163. Yerdel MA, Gunson B, Mirza D, Karayalcin K, Olliff S, Buckels J, Mayerj D, McMaster P and Pirenne J. Portal Vein Thrombosis in Adults Undergoing Liver Transplantation. Transplantation 2000; 69:1873-1881.

164. Krowka MJ, Plevak DJ, Findlay JY, Rosen CB, Wiesner RH and Krom RAF. Pulmonary Hemodynamics and Perioperative Cardiopulmonary-Related Mortality in Patients With Portopulmonary Hypertension Undergoing Liver Transplantation. Liver Transplantation 2000; 6:443-450.

165. Pilatis ND, Jacobs LE, Rerkpattanapipat P, Kotler MN, Owen A, Manzarbeitia C, Reich D, Rothstein K, and Munoz SJ. Clinical Predictors of Pulmonary Hypertension in Patients Undergoing Liver Transplant Evaluation. Liver Transplantation 2000; 6:85-91.

166. Miki C, McMaster P, Mayer AD, Kriyama K, Suzuki H, and Buckels JAC. Factors predicting perioperative cytokine response in patients undergoing liver transplantation. Critical Care Medicine 2000; 28(2):351-354.

167. Maring JK, Klompmaker IJ, Zwaveling JH, van derMeer J, Limburg PC and Slooff MJH. Endotoxins and Cytokines During Liver Transplantation: Changes in Plasma Levels and Effects on Clinical Outcome. Liver Transplantation 2000; 6:480-488.

168. Chang FY, Singh N, Gayowski T, Wagener MM, Mietzner SM, Stout JE and Marino IR. Thrombocytopenia in Liver Transplant Recipients. Transplantation 2000; 69:70-75.

169. Reich DJ, Fiel I, Guarrera JV, Emre S, Guy SR, Schwartz ME, Miller CM and Sheiner PA. Liver Transplantation for Autoimmune Hepatitis. Hepatology 2000; 32:693-700.

170. Ayata G, Gordon FD, Lewis WD, Pomfret E, Pomposelli JJ, Jenkins RL and Khettry U. Liver Transplantation for Autoimmune Hepatitis: A Long-Term Pathologic Study. Hepatology 2000; 32:185-192.

171. Collins BH, Pirsch JD, Becker YT, Hanaway MJ, Van der Werf WJ, D'Alessandro AM, Knechtle SJ, Odorico JS, Leverson G, Musat A, Armbrust M, Becker BN, Sollinger HW and Kalayoglu M. Long-Term Results of Liver Transplantation in Patients 60 years of Age and Older. Transplantation 2000; 70:780-783.

172. Jain A, Reyes J, Kashyap R, Dodson SF, Demetris AJ, Ruppert K, Abu-Elmagd K, Marsh W, Madariaga J, Mazariegos G, Geller D, Bonham A, Gayowski T, Cacciarelli T, Fontes P, Starzl TE and Fung JJ. Long-Term Survival After Liver Transplantation in 4,000 Consecutive Patients at a Single Center. Ann Surg 2000; 232:490-500.

173. Ghobrial RM, Yersiz H, Farmer DG, Amersi F, Goss J, Chen P, Dawson S,. Lerner S, Nissen N, Imagawa D, Colquhoun S, Arnout W, McDiarmid SV, and Busuttil RW. Predictors of Survival After In Vivo Split Liver Transplantation. Analysis of 110 Consecutive Patients. Ann Surg 2000; 232:312-323.

174. Moore KA, Jones RMcL and Burrows GD. Quality of Life and Cognitive Function of Liver Transplant Patients: A Prospective Study. Liver Transplantation 2000; 6:633-642.

175. Younossi ZM, McCormick M, Price LL, Boparai N, Farquhar L, Henderson JM and Guyatt G. Impact of Liver Transplantation on Health-Related Quality of Live. Liver Transplantation 2000; 6:779-783.

176. Hahn AB and Baliga P. Rapid Method for the Analysis of Peripheral Chimerism in Suspect Graft-Versus-Host Disease After Liver Transplantation. Liver Transplantation 2000; 6:10-14.

177. Evans PC, Soin A, Wreghitt TG, Taylor CJ, Wight DGD and Alexander GJM. An Association Between Cytomegalovirus Infection and Chronic Rejection After Liver Transplantation. Transplantation 2000; 69:30-35.

178. Milkiewicz P, Gunson B, Saksena S, Hathaway M, Hubscher SG and Elias E. Increased Incidence of Chronic Rejection in Adult Patients Transplanted for Autoimmune Hepatitis: Assessment of Risk Factors. Transplantation 2000; 70:477-40.

179. Chang GJ, Mahanty HD, Quan D, Freise CE, Ascher NL, Roberts JP, Stock PG and Hirose R. Experience with the Use of Sirolimus in Liver Transplantation-Use in Patients for Whom Calcineurin Inhibitors are Contraindicated. Liver Transplantation 2000; 6:734-740.

180. Grewal HP, Brady L, Cronin DC, Loss GE, Siegel CT, Oswald K, Fisher JS, Bruce DS, Aronson AJ, Woodle ES, Millis JM, Thistlethwaite JR and Newell KA. Combined Liver and Kidney Transplantation in Children. Transplantation 2000; 70:100-105.

181. Reyes J, Carr B, Dvorchik I, Kocoshis S, Jaffe R, Gerber D, Mazariegos GV, Bueno J and Selby R. Liver transplantation and chemotherapy for hepatoblastoma and hepatocellular cancer in childhood adolescence. Journal of Pediatrics 2000; 136:795-804.

182. Their M, Holmberg C, Lautenschlager I, Hockerstedt K and Jalanko H. Infections in Pediatric Kidney and Liver Transplant Patients after Perioperative Hospitalization. Transplantation 2000; 69:1617-1623.

183. Jain A, Mazariegos G, Kashyap R, Green M, Gronsky C, Starzl TE, Fung J, and Reyes J. Comparative Long-term Evaluation of Tacrolimus and CsA in Pediatric Liver Transplantation. Transplantation 2000; 70:617-625.

184. Reyes J, Jain A, Mazariegos G, Kashyap R, Green M, Iurlano K and Fung J. Long-term Results after Conversion from CsA to Tacrolimus in Pediatric Liver Transplantation for Acute and Chronic Rejection. Transplantation 2000; 69:2573-2580.

185. Younes BS, McDiarmid SV, Martin MG, Vargas JH, Goss JA, Busuttil RW and Ament ME. Transplantation 2000; 70:94-99.

186. Krieger NR, Martinez OM, Krams SM, Cox K, So S and Esquivel CO. Significance of Detecting Epstein-Barr-Specific Sequences in the Peripheral Blood of Asymptomatic Pediatric Liver Transplant Recipients. Liver Transplantation 2000; 6:62-66.

187. Iwatsuki S, Dvorchik I, Marsh JW, Madariaga JR, Carr B, Fung JJ and Starzl TE. Liver Transplantation for Hepatocellular Carcinoma: A Proposal of a Prognostic Scoring System. J Am Coll Surg 2000; 191:389-394.

188. Majno PE, Sarasin FP, Mentha G and Hadengue A. Primary Liver Resection and Salvage Transplantation or Primary Liver Transplantation in Patients with Single, Small Hepatocellular Carcinoma and Preserved Liver Function: An Outcome-Oriented Decision Analysis. Hepatology 2000; 31:899-906.

189. Meyer CG, Penn I and James L. Liver Transplantation for Cholangiocarcinoma: Results in 207 Patients. Transplantation 2000; 69:1633-1637.

190. DeVreede I, Steers JL, Burch PA, Rosen CB, Gunderson LL, Haddock MG, Burgart L and Gores GJ. Prolonged Disease-Free Survival After Orthotopic Liver Transplantation Plus Adjuvant Chemoirradiation for Cholangiocarcinoma. Liver Transplantation 2000; 6:309-316.

191. Zamir GA, Markmann JF, Abrams J, Macatee MR, Nunes FA, Shaked A and Olthoff KM. The Fate of Liver Grafts Declined for Subjective Reasons and Transplanted Out of a Local Organ Procurement Organization. Transplantation 2000; 70:1149-1154.

192. Reich DJ, Munoz SJ, Rothstein KD, Nathan HM, Edwards JM, Hasz RD and Manzarbeitia CY. Controlled Non-Heart-Beating Donor Liver Transplantation. Transplantation 2000; 70:1159-1166.

193. Mitzner SR, Stange J, Klammt S, Risler T, Erley CM, Bader BD, Berger ED, Lauchart W, Peszynski P, Freytag J, Hickstein H, Loock J, Lohr J-M, Liebe S, Emmrich J, Korten G and Schmidt R. Improvement of Hepatorenal Syndrome With Extracorporeal Albumin Dialysis MARS: Results of a Prospective, Randomized, Controlled Clinical Trial. Liver Transplantation 2000; 6:277-286.

194. Levy MF, Crippin J, Sutton S, Netto G, McCormack J, Curiel T, Goldstein RM, Newman JT, Gonwa TA, Banchereau J, Diamond LE, Bryne G, Logan J and Klintmalm GB. Liver Allotransplantation After Extracorporeal Hepatic Support with Transgenic (hCD55/hCD59) Porcine Livers. Transplantation 2000; 69:272-280.

195. Bilir BM, Guinette D, Karrer F, Kumpe DA, Krysl J, Stephens J, McGavran L, Ostrowska A, and Durham J. Hepatocyte Transplantation in Acute Liver Failure. Liver Transplantation 2000; 6:32-40.

196. Lowell JA, Smith CR, Brennan DC, Singer GG, Miller S, Shenoy S, Ramanchandran V, Dolan S. Miller B, Peters M and Howard TK. The Domino Transplant: Transplant Recipients as Organ Donors. Transplantation 2000; 69:372-376.

197. Dalmau A, Sabate A, Acosta F, Garcia-Huete L, Koo M, Sansano T, Rafecas A, Figueras J, Jaurrieta E, and Parrilla P. Tranexamic Acid Reduces Red Cell Transfusion Better than [epsilon]-Aminocaproic Acid or Placebo in Liver Transplantation. Anesthesia & Analgesia 2000; 91:29-34.

198. Newsletter International Pancreas Transplant Registry (IPTR) Pancreas Transplants Worldwide 2000; 12:4-23.

199. Sudan D, Sudan R and Stratta R. Long-Term Outcome of Simultaneous Kidney-Pancreas Transplantation. Transplantation 2000; 69:550-555.

200. Becker BN, Brazy PC, Becker YT, Odorico JS, Pintar TJ, Collins BH, Pirsch JD, Leverson GE, Heisey DM and Sollinger HW. Simultaneous pancreas-kidney transplantation reduces excess mortality in type 1 diabetic patients with end-stage renal disease. Kidney Int 2000; 57:2129-2135.

201. Jordan ML, Shapiro R, Gritsch HA, Egidi F, Khanna A, Vivas CA, Scantlebury VP, Fung JJ, Starzl TE and Corry RH. Long-Term Results of Pancreas Transplantation Under Tacrolimus Immunosuppression. Transplantation 1999; 67:266-272.

202. Humar A, Kandaswamy R, Granger D, Gruessner RW, Gruessner AC, and Sutherland DER. Decreased Surgical Risks of Pancreas Transplantation in the Modern Era. Ann Surg 2000; 231:269-275.

203. Ciancio G, Julian JF, Fernandez L, Miller J and Burke GW. Successful Surgical Salvage of Pancreas Allografts After Complete Venous Thrombosis. Transplantation 2000; 70:126-131.

204. Stratta RJ, Gaber O, Shokouh-Amiri MH, Reddy KS, Alloway RR, Egidi MF, Grewal HP, Gaber LW and Hathaway D. Evolution in Pancreas Transplantation Techniques: Simultaneous Kidney-Pancreas Transplantation Using Portal Enteric Drainage Without Antilymphocyte Induction. Ann Surg 1999; 229:701-712.

205. Stratta RJ, Gaber O, Shokouk-Amiri H, Reddy KS, Egidi MF, Grewal HP, and Gaber LW. A prospective comparison of systemic-bladder versus portal-enteric drainage in vascularized pancreas transplantation. Surgery 2000; 127:217-26.

206. Reddy KS, Stratta RJ, Shokouh-Amiri H, Alloway R, Somerville T, Egidi MF, Gaber LW and Gaber AO. Simultaneous Kidney-Pancreas Transplantation Without Antilymphocyte Induction. Transplantation 2000; 69:49-54.

207. Merion RM, Henry ML, Melzer JS, Sollinger HW, Sutherland DER and Taylor RJ. Randomized, Prospective Trial of Mycophenolate Mofetil Versus Azathioprine for Prevention of Acute Renal Allograft Rejection After Simultaneous Kidney-Pancreas Transplantation. Transplantation 2000; 70:105-111.

208. Jordan ML, Chakrabarti P, Luke P, Shapiro R, Vivas CA, Scantlebury VP, Fung JJ, Starzl TE and Corry RJ. Results of Pancreas Transplantation After Steroid Withdrawal Under Tacrolimus Immunosuppression. Transplantation 2000; 69:265-271.

209. Corry RJ, Chakrabarti PK, Shapiro R, Rao AS, Dvorchik I, Jordan ML, Scantlebury VP, Vivas CA, Fung JJ, and Starzl TE. Simultaneous Administration of Adjuvant Donor Bone Marrow in Pancreas Transplant Recipients. Ann Surg 1999; 230:372-381.

210. Petruzzo P, Andreelli F, McGregor B, Lefrancois N, Dawahra M, Feitosa LC, Dubernard JM, Thivolet C and Martin X. Evidence of Recurrent Type 1 Diabetes Following HLA-Mismatched Pancreas Transplantation. Diabetes & Metabolism (Paris) 2000; 26:215-218.

211. Thivolet C, Abou-Amara S, Martin X, Lefrancois N, Petruzzo P, McGregor B, Bosshard S and Dubernard JM. Serological Markers of Recurrent Beta Cell Destruction in Diabetic Patients Undergoing Pancreatic Transplantation. Transplantation 2000; 69:99-103.

212. Braghi S, Bonifacio E, Secchi A, DiCarlo V, Pozza G and Bosi E. Modulation of Humoral Islet Autoimmunity by Pancreas Allotransplantation Influences Allograft Outcome in Patients with Type 1 Diabetes. Diabetes 2000; 49:218-224.

213. Kennedy WR, Navarro X, and Goetz FC, et al. The effects of pancreas transplantation on diabetic neuropathy. N Engl J Med 1990; 15:1031-1037.

214. Solders G, Tyden G, and Tibell A., et al Improvement in nerve conduction 8 years after combined pancreatic and renal transplantation. Transplant Proc 1995; 27:2091.

215. Ulbig M, Kampick A, and Thurau S., et al Long term follow up of diabetic retinopathy for up to 71 months after combined renal and pancreatic transplantation. Graefes Arch Clin Exp Ophthalmol 1991; 229:242-245.

216. Wang Q, Klein R, and Moss SE, et al The influence of combined kidney-pancreas transplantation on the progression of diabetic retinopathy. Ophthalmology 1994; 101:1071-1976.

217. Cheung ATW, Perez RV and Chen PCY. Improvements in Diabetic Microangiopathy After Successful Simultaneous Pancreas-Kidney Transplantation: A Computer-Assisted Intravital Microscopy Study on the Conjunctival Microcirculation. Transplantation 1999; 68:927-932.

218. Bilous RW, Mauer SM, and Sutherland DER, et al Glomerular Structure and Function Following Successful Pancreas Transplantation for insulin-dependent diabetes mellitus. Diabetes 1987; 36:43A.

219. Fioretto P, Steffes MW, Sutherland DER, Goetz FC, and Mauer M. Reversal of Lesions of Diabetic Nephropathy after Pancreas Transplantation. N Engl J Med 1998; 339:69-75.

220. Robertson EP, Sutherland DER and Lanz KJ. Normoglycemia and Preserved Insulin Secretory Reserve in Diabetic Patients 10-18 Years After Pancreas Transplantation. Diabetes 1999; 48:1737-1740.

221. Becker BN, Brazy PC, Becker YT, Odorico JS, Pintar TJ, Collins BH, Pirsch JD, Leverson GE, Heisey DM and Sollinger HW. Simultaneous pancreas-kidney transplantation reduces excess mortality in type 1 diabetic patients with end-stage renal disease. Kidney Int 2000; 57:2129-2135.

222. Hering BJ and Ricordi C. Islet Transplantation for Patients with Type 1 Diabetes. Graft 1999; 2:12-27.

223. Shapiro AMJ, Lakey JRT, Ryan EA, Korbutt GS, Toth E, Warnock GL, Kneteman NM and Rajotte RV. Islet Transplantation in Seven Patients with Type 1 Diabetes Mellitus Using a Glucocorticoid-free Immunosuppressive Regimen. N Engl J Med 2000; July 27.

224. Deng MC, De Meester JM, Smits JM, Heinecke J, Scheld HH. Effect of receiving a heart transplant: analysis of a national cohort entered on to a waiting list, stratified by heart failure severity. Comparative Outcome and Clinical Profiles in Transplantation (COCPIT) Study Group [see comments]. BMJ 2000; 321:540-5.

225. Whellan DJ, Tudor G, Denofrio D, Abrams JD, Loh E. Heart transplant center practice patterns affect access to donors and survival of patients classified as status 1 by the United Network of Organ Sharing. American Heart Journal 2000; 140:443-50.

226. Tjan TD, Kondruweit M, Scheld HH, Roeder N, Borggrefe M, Schmidt C, Schober O, Deng MC. The bad ventricle—revascularization versus transplantation. Thoracic & Cardiovascular Surgeon 2000; 48:9-14.

227. Hosenpud JD, Pamidi SR, Fiol BS, Cinquegrani MP, Keck BM. Outcomes in patients who are hepatitis B surface antigen-positive before transplantation: an analysis and study using the joint ISHLT/UNOS thoracic registry. J Heart Lung Transplant 2000; 19:781-5.

228. McCarthy RE, 3rd, Boehmer JP, Hruban RH, Hutchins GM, Kasper EK, Hare JM, Baughman KL. Long-term outcome of fulminant myocarditis as compared with acute (nonfulminant) myocarditis [see comments]. N Engl J Med 2000; 342:690-5.

229. Deibert E, Aiyagari V, Diringer MN. Reversible left ventricular dysfunction associated with raised troponin I after subarachnoid haemorrhage does not preclude successful heart transplantation. Heart 2000; 84:205-7.

230. Thompson JS, Thacker LR, 2nd, Takemoto S. The influence of conventional and cross-reactive group HLA matching on cardiac transplant outcome: an analysis from the United Network of Organ Sharing Scientific Registry. Transplantation 2000; 69:2178-86.

231. Bishay ES, Cook DJ, El Fettouh H, Starling RC, Young JB, Smedira NG, McCarthy PM. The impact of HLA sensitization and donor cause of death in heart transplantation. Transplantation 2000; 70:220-2.

232. Bishay ES, Cook DJ, Starling RC, Ratliff NB, Jr., White J, Blackstone EH, Smedira NG, McCarthy PM. The clinical significance of flow cytometry crossmatching in heart transplantation. Eur J Cardio-Thoracic Surg 2000; 17:362-9.

233. Marelli D, Laks H, Fazio D, Moore S, Moriguchi J, Kobashigawa J. The use of donor hearts with left ventricular hypertrophy. J Heart Lung Transplant 2000; 19:496-503.

234. Pfau PR, Rho R, DeNofrio D, Loh E, Blumberg EA, Acker MA, Lucey MR. Hepatitis C transmission and infection by orthotopic heart transplantation. J Heart Lung Transplant 2000; 19:350-4.

235. John R, Rajasinghe H, Chen JM, Weinberg AD, Sinha P, Itescu S, Lietz K, Mancini D, Oz MC, Smith CR, Rose EA, Edwards NM. Impact of current management practices on early and late death in more than 500 consecutive cardiac transplant recipients. Ann Surg 2000; 232:302-11.

236. Srivastava R, Keck BM, Bennett LE, Hosenpud JD. The results of cardiac retransplantation: an analysis of the Joint International Society for Heart and Lung Transplantation/ United Network for Organ Sharing Thoracic Registry. Transplantation 2000; 70:606-12.

237. Aziz T, Burgess M, Rahman A, Campbell C, Deiraniya A, Yonan N. Early and long-term results of heart transplantation after previous cardiac surgery. Eur J Cardio-Thoracic Surg 2000; 17:349-54.

238. Tenderich G, Koerner MM, Stuettgen B, Mirow N, Arusoglu L, Morshuis M, Bairaktaris A, Minami K, Koerfer R. Pre-existing elevated pulmonary vascular resistance: long-term hemodynamic follow-up and outcome of recipients after orthotopic heart transplantation. J Cardiovasc Surg 2000; 41:215-9.

239. Carrier M, White M, Pelletier G, Perrault LP, Pellerin M, Pelletier LC. Ten-year follow-up of critically ill patients undergoing heart transplantation. J Heart Lung Transplant 2000; 19:439-43.

240. Klauss V, Konig A, Spes C, Meiser B, Rieber J, Siebert U, Regar E, Pfeiffer M, Reichart B, Theisen K, Mudra H. CsA versus tacrolimus (FK 506) for prevention of cardiac allograft vasculopathy. Am J Cardiol 2000; 85:266-9.

241. Straatman LP, Coles JG. Pediatric utilization of rapamycin for severe cardiac allograft rejection. Transplantation 2000; 70:541-3.

242. Haddad H, MacNeil DM, Howlett J, O'Neill B. Sirolimus, a new potent immunosuppressant agent for refractory cardiac transplantation rejection: two case reports. Canadian J Cardiol 2000; 16:221-4.

243. Pham SM, Rao AS, Zeevi A, Kormos RL, McCurry KR, Hattler BG, Fung JJ, Starzl TE, Griffith BP. A clinical trial combining donor bone marrow infusion and heart transplantation: intermediate-term results. J Thoracic Cardiovasc Surg 2000; 119:673-81.

244. Beniaminovitz A, Itescu S, Lietz K, Donovan M, Burke EM, Groff BD, Edwards N, Mancini DM. Prevention of rejection in cardiac transplantation by blockade of the interleukin-2 receptor with a monoclonal antibody [see comments]. N Engl J Med 2000; 342:613-9.

245. Baan CC, van Gelder T, Balk AH, Knoop CJ, Holweg CT, Maat LP, Weimar W. Functional responses of T cells blocked by anti-CD25 antibody therapy during cardiac rejection [see comments]. Transplantation 2000; 69:331-6.

246. Dempsey SJ, D'Amico C, Weintraub WS, Lutz J, Smith AL, Ghazzal ZM, Book WM. Angiographic and clinical follow-up of percutaneous revascularization for transplant coronary artery disease [see comments]. J Invasive Cardiol 2000; 12:311-5.

247. Yamani MH, Starling RC, Goormastic M, Van Lente F, Smedira N, McCarthy P, Young JB. The impact of routine mycophenolate mofetil drug monitoring on the treatment of cardiac allograft rejection. Transplantation 2000; 69:2326-30.

248. Birks EJ, Owen VJ, Burton PB, Bishop AE, Banner NR, Khaghani A, Polak JM, Yacoub MH. Tumor necrosis factor-alpha is expressed in donor heart and predicts right ventricular failure after human heart transplantation. Circulation 2000; 102:326-31.

249. Lindelow B, Bergh CH, Herlitz H, Waagstein F. Predictors and evolution of renal function during 9 years following heart transplantation. J Am Soc Nephrol 2000; 11:951-7.

250. Dotti G, Fiocchi R, Motta T, Gamba A, Gotti E, Gridelli B, Borleri G, Manzoni C, Viero P, Remuzzi G, Barbui T, Rambaldi A. Epstein-Barr virus-negative lymphoproliferate disorders in long-term survivors after heart, kidney, and liver transplant [see comments]. Transplantation 2000; 69:827-33.

251. Swerdlow AJ, Higgins CD, Hunt BJ, Thomas JA, Burke MM, Crawford DH, Yacoub MH. Risk of lymphoid neoplasia after cardiothoracic transplantation. a cohort study of the relation to Epstein-Barr virus [see comments]. Transplantation 2000; 69:897-904.

252. Grossi P, Farina C, Fiocchi R, Dalla Gasperina D. Prevalence and outcome of invasive fungal infections in 1,963 thoracic organ transplant recipients: a multicenter retrospective study. Italian Study Group of Fungal Infections in Thoracic Organ Transplant Recipients. Transplantation 2000; 70:112-6.

253. Fortina AB, Caforio AL, Piaserico S, Alaibac M, Tona F, Feltrin G, Livi U, Peserico A. Skin cancer in heart transplant recipients: frequency and risk factor analysis. J Heart Lung Transplant 2000; 19:249-55.

254. Mehra MR, Uber PA, Prasad AK, Park MH, Scott RL, McFadden PM, Van Meter CH. Long-term outcome of cardiac allograft vasculopathy treated by transmyocardial laser revascularization: early rewards, late losses. J Heart Lung Transplant 2000; 19:801-4.

255. Magnani G, Carinci V, Magelli C, Potena L, Reggiani LB, Branzi A. Role of statins in the management of dyslipidemia after cardiac transplant: randomized controlled trial comparing the efficacy and the safety of atorvastatin with pravastatin. J Heart Lung Transplant 2000; 19:710-5.

256. Keogh A, Macdonald P, Kaan A, Aboyoun C, Spratt P, Mundy J. Efficacy and safety of pravastatin vs. simvastatin after cardiac transplantation. J Heart Lung Transplant 2000; 19:529-37.

257. Cooke GE, Eaton GM, Whitby G, Kennedy RA, Binkley PF, Moeschberger ML, Leier CV. Plasma atherogenic markers in congestive heart failure and posttransplant (heart) patients. J Am Coll Cardiol 2000; 36:509-16.

258. Labarrere CA, Nelson DR, Cox CJ, Pitts D, Kirlin P, Halbrook H. Cardiac-specific troponin I levels and risk of coronary artery disease and graft failure following heart transplantation. JAMA 2000; 284:457-64.

259. Densem CG, Hutchinson IV, Cooper A, Yonan N, Brooks NH. Polymorphism of the transforming growth factor-beta 1 gene correlates with the development of coronary vasculopathy following cardiac transplantation. J Heart Lung Transplant 2000; 19:551-6.

260. Campana E, Parlapiano C, Borgia MC, Papalia U, Laurenti A, Pantone P, Giovanniello T, Marangi M, Sanguigni S. Are elevated levels of soluble ICAM-1 a marker of chronic graft disease in heart transplant recipients? Atherosclerosis 2000; 148:293-5.

261. Grande AM, Rinaldi M, D'Armini AM, Campana C, Traversi E, Pederzolli C, Abbiate N, Klersy C, Vigano M. Orthotopic heart transplantation: standard versus bicaval technique. Am J Cardiol 2000; 85:1329-33.

262. DeNofrio D, Rho R, Morales FJ, Kamoun M, Kearns J, Dorozinsky C, Rosengard BR, Acker MA, Loh E. Detection of anti-HLA antibody by flow cytometry in patients with a left ventricular assist device is associated with early rejection following heart transplantation. Transplantation 2000; 69:814-8.

263. Helman DN, Addonizio LJ, Morales DL, Catanese KA, Flannery MA, Quagebeur JM, Edwards NM, Galantowicz ME, Oz MC. Implantable left ventricular assist devices can successfully bridge adolescent patients to transplant. J Heart Lung Transplant 2000; 19:121-6.

264. Bank AJ, Mir SH, Nguyen DQ, Bolman RM, 3rd, Shumway SJ, Miller LW, Kaiser DR, Ormaza SM, Park SJ. Effects of left ventricular assist devices on outcomes in patients undergoing heart transplantation. Ann Thoracic Surg 2000; 69:1369-74; discussion 1375.

265. Dent CL, Canter CE, Hirsch R, Balzer DT. Transplant coronary artery disease in pediatric heart transplant recipients. J Heart Lung Transplant 2000; 19:240-8.

266. Di Russo GB, Clark BJ, Bridges ND, Godinez RI, Paridon SM, Spray TL, Gaynor JW. Prolonged extracorporeal membrane oxygenation as a bridge to cardiac transplantation. Ann Thoracic Surg 2000; 69:925-7.

267. Niles DG, Rynearson RD, Baum M, Neufeld RD, Caruso JM. A study of craniofacial growth in infant heart transplant recipients receiving CsA. J Heart Lung Transplant 2000; 19:231-9.

268. Chin C, Akhtar MJ, Rosenthal DN, Bernstein D. Safety and utility of the routine surveillance biopsy in pediatric patients 2 years after heart transplantation. J Pediatrics 2000; 136:238-42.

269. Leonard HC, O'Sullivan JJ, Dark JH. Long-term follow-up of pediatric cardiac transplant recipients on a steroid-free regime: the role of endomyocardial biopsy. J Heart Lung Transplant 2000; 19:469-72.

270. Moran AM, Lipshultz SE, Rifai N, O'Brien P, Mooney H, Perry S, Perez-Atayde A, Lipsitz SR, Colan SD. Non-invasive assessment of rejection in pediatric transplant patients: serologic and echocardiographic prediction of biopsy-proven myocardial rejection. J Heart Lung Transplant 2000; 19:756-64.

271. Rosenthal DN, Dubin AM, Chin C, Falco D, Gamberg P, Bernstein D. Outcome while awaiting heart transplantation in children: a comparison of congenital heart disease and cardiomyopathy. J Heart Lung Transplant 2000; 19:751-5.

272. Azeka E, Barbero-Marcial M, Jatene M, Camargo PR, Auler JO, Atik E, Ramires JA, Ebaid M. Heart transplantation in neonates and children. Intermediate-term results. Arquivos Brasileiros de Cardiologia 2000; 74:197-208.

273. Adams DH, Chen RH, Kadner A. Cardiac xenotransplantation: clinical experience and future direction. Ann Thoracic Surg 2000; 70:320-6.

274. Hori M, Yamamoto K, Kodama K, Takashima S, Sato H, Koretsune Y, Kuzuya T, Yutani C, Fukushima N, Ohtake S, Shirakura R, Matsuda H. Successful launch of cardiac transplantation in Japan. Osaka University Cardiac Transplant Program. Japanese Circulation Journal 2000; 64:326-32.

275. Wilson RF, Johnson TH, Haidet GC, Kubo SH, Mianuelli M. Sympathetic reinnervation of the sinus node and exercise hemodynamics after cardiac transplantation. Circulation 2000; 101:2727-33.

276. Vizza CD, Yusen RD, Lynch JP, Fedele F, Alexander Patterson G, Trulock EP. Outcome of patients with cystic fibrosis awaiting lung transplantation. American J Resp Crit Care Med 2000; 162:819-25.

277. Milstone AP, Brumble LM, Loyd JE, Ely EW, Roberts JR, Pierson RN, 3rd, Dummer JS. Active CMV infection before lung transplantation: risk factors and clinical implications. J Heart Lung Transplant 2000; 19:744-50.

278. Paloyan EB, Swinnen LJ, Montoya A, Lonchyna V, Sullivan HJ, Garrity E. Lung transplantation for advanced bronchioloalveolar carcinoma confined to the lungs. Transplantation 2000; 69:2446-8.

279. Meyers BF, Lynch JP, Trulock EP, Guthrie T, Cooper JD, Patterson GA. Single versus bilateral lung transplantation for idiopathic pulmonary fibrosis: a ten-year institutional experience. J Thoracic Cardiovasc Surg 2000; 120:99-107.

280. Limbos MM, Joyce DP, Chan CK, Kesten S. Psychological functioning and quality of life in lung transplant candidates and recipients. Chest 2000; 118:408-16.

281. Wisser W, Deviatko E, Simon-Kupilik N, Senbaklavaci O, Huber ER, Wolner E, Klepetko W. Lung transplantation following lung volume reduction surgery. J Heart Lung Transplant 2000; 19:480-7.

282. Pham SM, Rao AS, Zeevi A, McCurry KR, Keenan RJ, Vega JD, Kormos RL, Hattler BG, Fung JJ, Starzl TE, Griffith BP. Effects of donor bone marrow infusion in clinical lung transplantation. Ann Thoracic Surg 2000; 69:345-50.

283. Hoffmeyer F, Hoeper MM, Spiekerkotter E, Harringer W, Haverich A, Fabel H, Niedermeyer J. Azathioprine withdrawal in stable lung and heart/lung recipients receiving CsA-based immunosuppression. Transplantation 2000; 70:522-5.

284. Soccal PM, Jani A, Chang S, Leonard CT, Pavlakis M, Doyle RL. Inducible nitric oxide synthase transcription in human lung transplantation. Transplantation 2000; 70:384-5.

285. Hasegawa T, Iacono AT, Yousem SA. The anatomic distribution of acute cellular rejection in the allograft lung. Ann Thoracic Surg 2000; 69:1529-31.

286. Lau CL, Palmer SM, Posther KE, Howell DN, Reinsmoen NL, Massey HT, Tapson VF, Jaggers JJ, D'Amico TA, Davis RD, Jr. Influence of panel-reactive antibodies on posttransplant outcomes in lung transplant recipients. Ann Thoracic Surg 2000; 69:1520-4.

287. Quantz MA, Bennett LE, Meyer DM, Novick RJ. Does human leukocyte antigen matching influence the outcome of lung transplantation? An analysis of 3,549 lung transplantations. J Heart Lung Transplant 2000; 19:473-9.

288. Garfein ES, McGregor CC, Galantowicz ME, Schulman LL. Deleterious effects of telescoped bronchial anastomosis in single and bilateral lung transplantation. Ann Transplantation 2000; 5:5-11.

289. Lick SD, Brown PS, Jr., Kurusz M, Vertrees RA, McQuitty CK, Johnston WE. Technique of controlled reperfusion of the transplanted lung in humans. Annals of Thoracic Surgery 2000; 69:910-2.

290. King RC, Binns OA, Rodriguez F, Kanithanon RC, Daniel TM, Spotnitz WD, Tribble CG, Kron IL. Reperfusion injury significantly impacts clinical outcome after pulmonary transplantation. Ann Thoracic Surg 2000; 69:1681-5.

291. Bewig B, Haacke TC, Tiroke A, Bastian A, Bottcher H, Hirt SW, Rautenberg P, Haverich A. Detection of CMV pneumonitis after lung transplantation using PCR of NA from bronchoalveolar lavage cells. Respiration 2000; 67:166-72.

292. Meyers BF, Sundt TM, 3rd, Henry S, Trulock EP, Guthrie T, Cooper JD, Patterson GA. Selective use of extracorporeal membrane oxygenation is warranted after lung transplantation. J Thoracic Cardiovasc Surg 2000; 120:20-6.

293. Kelly J, Hurley D, Raghu G. Comparison of the efficacy and cost effectiveness of pre-emptive therapy as directed by CMV antigenemia and prophylaxis with ganciclovir in lung transplant recipients. J Heart Lung Transplant 2000; 19:355-9.

294. Gertner G, Coscia L, McGrory C, Moritz M, Armenti V. Pregnancy in lung transplant recipients. Progress in Transplantation 2000; 10:109-12.

295. Kulick DM, Salerno CT, Dalmasso AP, Park SJ, Paz MG, Fodor WL, Bolman RM, 3rd. Transgenic swine lungs expressing human CD59 are protected from injury in a pig-to-human model of xenotransplantation. J Thoracic Cardiovasc Surg 2000; 119:690-9.

296. Fischer S, Cassivi SD, Xavier AM, Cardella JA, Cutz E, Edwards V, Liu M, Keshavjee S. Cell death in human lung transplantation: apoptosis induction in human lungs during ischemia and after transplantation. Ann Surg 2000; 231:424-31.

CHAPTER 31

Impact of Delayed Graft Function and Acute Rejection on Kidney Graft Survival

David W. Gjertson

The consequences of delayed graft function (DGF) on long-term graft survival (GS) following renal transplantation remain controversial. Some report that DGF is detrimental regarding long-term GS (1-8). Other centers report that DGF affects only acute rejection (AR) and early renal function, but not long-term GS (9-11). For example, Boom et al (11) found that DGF, defined as the absence of a decline in serum creatinine of 10% or more in 3 consecutive days for more than one week after transplantation, effected graft function at one year as well as the incidence of acute rejection episodes, but it did not seem to influence late graft loss since there was no difference in GS after 6 months posttransplant. On the other hand, Shoskes and Cecka (6) demonstrated that DGF reduced graft half-life by ~60% starting one year after transplantation.

Here, we will examine outcomes following renal transplantation using a stratified model that permits direct comparison of the long-term (i.e., 5-yr) GS effects of DGF, early AR (EAR = AR <6 months) and late AR (LAR = AR from 6 months to 1 year). Further, we estimated the effects of 15 pretransplant covariates on early adverse events. After limiting the data to only those recipients whose grafts survived beyond one year, we estimated the effect of the 15 covariates on long-term GS within 4 recipient risk groups: 1) those recipients without DGF or LAR; 2) those with DGF but without LAR; 3) those without DGF but with LAR; and 4) those with both DGF and LAR. Finally, we discussed the impact of these risk factors with respect to immunogenicity and nephrotoxic responses.

MATERIALS AND METHODS

As of April 2000, 86,682 renal transplants grafted between 1991-1998 were reported to the United Network for Organ Sharing (UNOS). All patients were included

for study, and patients who died were considered to have had graft failure. DGF was defined by first-day anuria or the requirement for dialysis during the first week after transplantation. EAR episodes were those reported during hospitalization for transplantation or those reported within 6 months following transplantation. LAR episodes were those reported from 6 months through one full year after transplantation. Indicators for hospital discharge, 6-month, one-year and 5-year graft function, as well as 15 pretransplant variables [1) recipient age, race, sex, original disease, PRA and pretransplant dialysis and medical condition; 2) donor age, race, relationship, cause of death, cold ischemia and CMV status; and 3) transplant year and number of HLA mismatches] were selected for analysis.

The last reported serum creatinine value was used to impute graft function for censored patients (12,13). Based on the imputed failures, overall graft survival was 90.0%, 87.5% and 68.8% at 6 months, 1 and 5 years posttransplant, respectively. These rates nearly equal the corresponding Kaplan-Meier estimates of $90.0\pm0.1\%$, $87.6\pm0.1\%$ and $67.5\pm0.2\%$, indicating a general lack of bias in the imputation scheme. To distinguish short- from long-term effects, it was necessary to partition posttransplant time into 4 consecutive intervals and analyze subsets of patients entering each interval. The initial subset included all 86,682 transplants and was used to assess factors affecting DGF. The second subset consisted of 83,210 grafts that were hospital discharged and was used to assess EAR. The third subset consisted of 78,036 grafts that survived beyond 6 months after transplantation and was used to assess LAR. The fourth subset consisted of 75,812 grafts that functioned beyond one year and was used to assess long-term GS.

The joint effects of pretransplant factors were estimated via logistic regression models with stratified outcomes reiterated on each period posttransplant. For example, 2 separate models assessing the effects of the 15 pretransplant factors on EAR were fitted after grouping the discharged patients according to whether or not they experienced DGF. Again, 4 separate models assessed the effects of the factors on LAR after grouping the patients whose grafts survived beyond 6 months according to whether or not they experienced EAR with and without DGF. For all models, Hosmer-Lemeshow goodness-of-fit tests were not significant, suggesting models were appropriate when comparing factors. The variance associated with a given factor was computed as a pseudo R^2 defined by $1-L_1/L_{[x]}$ where L_1 was the log likelihood of the full model and $L_{[x]}$ was the log likelihood of the model with factor x removed (14). Tests of significance were done using the chi-square method, and all reported P values were two-sided tests.

RESULTS

Results are presented in Figures 1-8 and Tables 1-4. The annual incidences of DGF, EAR and LAR from 1991-1998 are shown in Figure 1. The percent of cases with DGF remained near 21% throughout the period (P = 0.20). In contradistinction, both incidences of EAR and LAR declined significantly (P <0.0001) during the period. In 1991, 37% and 11% of grafts experienced episodes of EAR and LAR, respectively, but, by 1998, just 18% and 5% of grafts experienced episodes of EAR and LAR, respectively. The steepest decline in EAR and LAR occurred after 1993.

The path diagram shown in Figure 2 traces the interrelationships among the rates of DGF, EAR, LAR and GS during the first year of the transplant for the 86,682 renal graft recipients reported to UNOS between 1991-1998. Prior to hospital discharge, 17,893 (21%) recipients experienced DGF, and, among these recipients, 15,364 (86%) were discharged with a functioning kidney graft. Among the 68,789 recipients without DGF, 67,846 (99%) were discharged with a functioning graft. Thus, DGF was associated with lower rates of hospital discharge (P<0.0001).

Before 6 months, 17,635 of 67,846 (26%) discharged recipients without DGF experienced at least one episode of EAR. Whereas, 5,820 of 15,364 (38%) dis-

charged recipients with DGF experienced at least one episode of EAR. DGF was associated with EAR (P<0.0001). If a discharged patient experienced no DGF and no EAR, then they had a 97% change of surviving beyond 6 months after transplantation. Rates of 6-month survival were 90% for patients without DGF but with EAR, 91% with DGF but without EAR, and 82% with DGF and EAR (P< 0.0001). Clearly, DGF and EAR influence early transplant outcomes.

After 6 months, 78,036 grafts remained functioning. Among 6-month surviving patients without DGF and EAR, 4% experienced LAR. 19% of patients without DGF but with EAR experienced LAR, 6% of patients with DGF but without EAR experienced LAR, and 18% of patients with both adverse events experienced LAR. Note that LAR was primarily influenced by the presence/absence of EAR (odds ratio = 4.7, P<0.001) and, to a much lesser extent, by DGF (odds ratio = 1.1, P = 0.002). By one year, 75,812 transplants were still functioning.

Table 1 lists the results of stratified logistic regression analysis using the 15 pretransplant factors to estimate odds ratios for 1) developing DGF before hospital discharge, 2) episodes of EAR with and without DGF before 6 months, and 3) episodes of LAR with and without DGF and/or EAR before one year. Starting from the left column, non-sensitized (PRA <11%), female and non-Black recipients with inherited disease and shorter pretransplant dialysis durations who received a living,

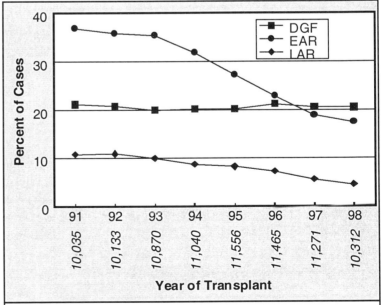

Figure 1. Annual incidences of DGF, EAR and LAR in kidney transplants reported to UNOS from 1991-1998.

young (< 45 years of age), well-HLA-matched, trauma donor's kidney with less than 24 hours of cold ischemia enjoyed the lowest risks of DGF. Continuing to the right across Table 1, prognostic factors for EAR (regardless of DGF status) included younger recipients, transplantation before 1993 and increasing numbers of HLA mismatches. Note that the effects of PRA, donor relationship, pretransplant dialysis and cold ischemia times abated.

The last 4 columns of Table 1 list odds ratios for prognostic factors of LAR stratified by DGF and EAR effects. Black and teenage recipients transplanted with older donors were at the greatest risk of LAR regardless of DGF and EAR events. If DGF and EAR were absent, then year of transplant and number of HLA mismatches were also significant prognostic factors for LAR.

Table 2 ranks as percentages the extent of assignable variation in short-term outcomes of DGF, EAR and LAR attributable to the various factors. Percentages depended on both size and diversity of factor effects. The top 4 factors impacting DGF were cold

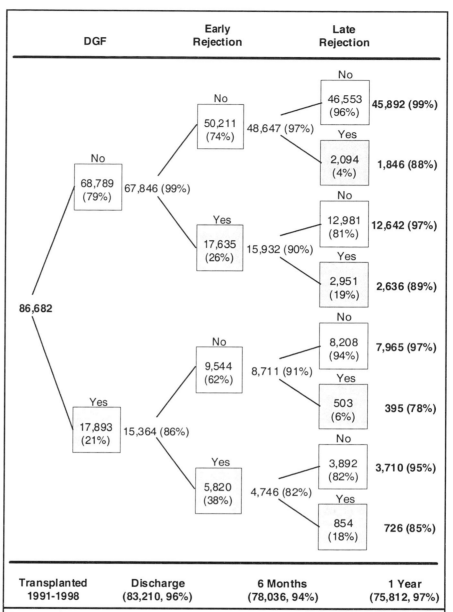

Figure 2. Path diagram showing the relationships among DGF, EAR, LAR and GS during the first year after renal transplantation.

ischemia time (accounting for 28% of explainable variation), duration of pretransplant dialysis (21%), donor age (18%) and PRA (12%). They combined to account for nearly 80% of the assignable variation in DGF. The 4 primary factors for EAR variation were year of transplant, HLA mismatches, recipient age, and recipient race, which accounted for 89% and 77% of assignable variation in EAR when DGF was absent and present, respectively. The dominant factors influencing LAR were recipient age and race, and donor age.

Among the long-term surviving transplants, 45,892 (61%) recipients did not experience any adverse effects during their first GS year; their subsequent 5-year GS was 82.0% and half-life (HL) was 14.1±0.2 years (Figure 3). Further, 7,965 (11%) recipients experienced only DGF (5-yr GS = 71.4%, HL = 8.6±0.2 yrs), 12,642 (17%) experienced only EAR (5-yr GS = 77.0%, HL = 10.5±0.2 yrs), and 1,846 (2%) experienced only LAR (5-yr GS = 54.1%, HL = 4.6±0.2 yrs). Those experiencing 2 events included 3,710 (5%) with DGF and EAR but without LAR

Table 1. Odds ratios for prognostic factors of DGF, EAR and LAR[1].

Factor	DGF (86,682)	EAR Given Discharge		LAR DGF / EAR			
		-DGF (67,846)	+DGF (15,364)	-/- (48,647)	+/- (8,711)	-/+ (15,932)	+/+ (4,746)
Recipient							
Sex: Female	**0.82(.02)**	**0.91(.02)**	1.00(.04)	0.94(.04)	1.05(.10)	0.96(.04)	0.92(.08)
Race: Caucasian (baseline)							
Black	**1.38(.03)**	0.93(.02)	0.96(.04)	**1.72(.10)**	**1.60(.18)**	**1.39(.08)**	**1.35(.12)**
Hispanic	1.03(.03)	**0.69(.02)**	**0.56(.04)**	0.86(.07)	1.02(.17)	0.95(.08)	0.93(.16)
Other	0.98(.04)	**0.70(.03)**	0.92(.08)	0.76(.10)	1.02(.24)	0.79(.10)	0.76(.16)
Age: 46-60 yr (baseline)							
0-12 yr	0.94(.07)	**1.66(.09)**	**1.87(.29)**	**2.17(.28)**	1.26(.68)	1.08(.13)	1.99(.57)
13-25 yr	0.98(.04)	**1.59(.05)**	**1.47(.10)**	**2.50(.29)**	**2.12(.38)**	**1.52(.11)**	**1.61(.23)**
26-45 yr	**0.91(.02)**	**1.31(.03)**	**1.23(.05)**	**1.28(.07)**	**1.57(.17)**	1.07(.05)	1.26(.11)
>60 yr	0.94(.03)	**0.82(.03)**	0.89(.05)	**0.63(.06)**	1.00(.16)	**0.72(.07)**	0.99(.14)
Original disease: other (baseline)							
Systemic	0.94(.02)	1.00(.02)	0.90(.03)	1.01(.05)	1.21(.12)	0.96(.04)	0.87(.07)
Inherited	**0.90(.03)**	0.93(.03)	0.88(.05)	1.03(.08)	0.98(.17)	0.93(.06)	0.94(.12)
Pre-tx medical status: no impairment (baseline)							
Impairment	**1.18(.02)**	1.02(.02)	1.04(.04)	1.05(.05)	1.07(.11)	1.05(.04)	1.03(.08)
PRA: 0% (baseline)							
1-10%	1.06(.02)	1.03(.02)	1.12(.05)	1.10(.06)	1.07(.12)	1.05(.05)	1.31(.12)
11-50%	**1.26(.03)**	1.07(.03)	1.26(.06)	1.19(.08)	0.95(.13)	1.01(.06)	0.99(.11)
51-80%	**1.53(.06)**	**1.24(.06)**	1.18(.09)	1.22(.14)	1.01(.21)	0.94(.11)	1.29(.22)
81-100%	**1.99(.08)**	**1.35(.06)**	**1.46(.10)**	1.30(.15)	1.02(.20)	0.95(.10)	1.10(.17)
Duration pre-transplant dialysis: ≤12 mo (baseline)							
13-24 mo	1.02(.03)	1.00(.02)	0.99(.05)	1.00(.06)	0.93(.13)	1.05(.06)	0.73(.08)
25-36 mo	**1.43(.04)**	0.96(.03)	1.10(.06)	1.00(.08)	0.77(.13)	1.04(.07)	0.77(.10)
>36 mo	**1.80(.05)**	0.95(.03)	1.08(.06)	0.97(.07)	0.96(.14)	0.84(.06)	**0.67(.08)**
Donor							
Relationship: cadaver (baseline)							
Parent	**0.52(.05)**	0.99(.07)	1.21(.24)	0.91(.16)	0.52(.30)	0.96(.15)	0.86(.40)
Living related	**0.48(.04)**	0.86(.05)	1.34(.22)	0.85(.14)	0.63(.30)	0.92(.13)	1.08(.43)
Living unrelated	**0.54(.06)**	1.10(.08)	1.69(.37)	0.86(.18)	0.62(.44)	0.99(.17)	0.60(.32)
Race: Caucasian (baseline)							
Black	0.97(.03)	**1.29(.04)**	**1.23(.07)**	1.11(.08)	1.02(.16)	0.99(.07)	1.11(.13)
Hispanic	1.07(.04)	0.94(.03)	0.99(.06)	1.11(.10)	0.94(.16)	1.14(.09)	0.80(.12)
Other	1.00(.06)	0.95(.06)	1.08(.12)	1.01(.15)	1.14(.33)	1.03(.15)	1.12(.27)
Age: 16-30 yr (baseline)							
1-3 yr	1.17(.08)	0.95(.08)	1.04(.16)	0.98(.21)	1.24(.51)	1.14(.22)	1.08(.43)
4-15 yr	**0.88(.03)**	1.10(.04)	1.24(.09)	1.07(.10)	0.92(.21)	1.12(.09)	0.89(.16)
31-50 yr	**1.39(.03)**	1.06(.02)	1.11(.05)	**1.21(.07)**	1.24(.16)	1.08(.06)	**1.42(.16)**
> 50 yr	**1.90(.06)**	**1.31(.04)**	**1.25(.07)**	**1.60(.12)**	**1.63(.25)**	**1.32(.09)**	**1.52(.19)**
Death: trauma (baseline)							
Non-trauma	**1.25(.03)**	**1.14(.03)**	1.10(.04)	1.12(.07)	1.17(.13)	1.11(.06)	0.99(.09)

Factor	DGF	EAR Given Discharge		LAR DGF / EAR			
		-DGF	+DGF	-/-	+/-	-/+	+/+
Cold ischemia time: 4-12 hr (baseline)							
0-3 hr	0.87(.07)	0.99(.06)	1.17(.19)	0.87(.13)	1.32(.57)	1.05(.14)	0.72(.28)
13-24 hr	**1.42(.03)**	0.99(.02)	1.05(.05)	0.91(.06)	0.91(.12)	1.06(.06)	1.00(.11)
> 24 hr	**2.05(.05)**	0.96(.02)	1.01(.04)	0.87(.06)	0.96(.12)	1.04(.06)	1.21(.12)
CMV status: negative (baseline)							
Positive	1.04(.02)	1.00(.02)	1.06(.04)	1.00(.05)	1.30(.13)	1.03(.04)	1.03(.08)
Transplant							
Year of transplant: 1994-8 (baseline)							
< 1994	0.94(.02)	**1.87(.03)**	**1.50(.05)**	**1.56(.07)**	**1.70(.16)**	1.11(.05)	1.18(.09)
HLA-ABDR mismatches: 0 (baseline)							
1-2	**1.15(.05)**	**1.85(.08)**	**1.41(.12)**	**1.54(.16)**	1.49(.36)	1.29(.14)	1.22(.27)
3-4	**1.30(.05)**	**2.35(.09)**	**1.74(.14)**	**1.73(.17)**	1.32(.30)	1.31(.14)	1.49(.31)
5-6	**1.31(.05)**	**2.80(.12)**	**1.80(.15)**	**1.87(.20)**	1.59(.37)	1.30(.14)	1.54(.33)

[1] Significant (P≤0.001, allowing for multiple comparisons) values are listed in **bold**.

Table 2. Extent of assignable variation in one-year renal graft outcomes of DGF, early and late rejection attributable to various factors stratified by prior events (i.e., DGF and early rejection).

Factor	DGF (86,682)	Early Rejection Given Discharge		Late Rejection (6m-1y) DGF / Early Rej.			
		-DGF (67,846)	+DGF (15,364)	-/- (48,647)	+/- (8,711)	-/+ (15,932)	+/+ (4,746)
Recipient							
Sex	3.3	1.0	0.0	0.3	0.2	0.4	0.9
Race	6.3	5.7	17.8	21.1	17.0	27.4	16.2
Age	0.7	15.0	15.8	39.9	24.5	36.9	16.8
Medical status	2.2	0.0	0.3	0.2	0.4	1.0	0.2
Original disease	0.5	0.2	2.2	0.0	3.5	1.0	2.5
PRA	11.8	1.9	8.6	2.2	0.8	1.1	10.8
Duration pre-transplant dialysis	21.4	0.2	1.3	0.1	2.7	8.1	12.4
Donor							
Relationship	2.6	1.1	1.4	0.3	1.2	0.4	2.1
Race	0.2	3.0	3.0	0.6	0.3	1.6	3.5
Age	17.6	3.0	4.5	7.2	10.7	10.4	17.1
Death	3.0	1.1	1.2	0.7	1.8	2.2	0.0
Cold ischemia time	28.0	0.1	0.5	1.1	1.0	0.8	6.1
CMV status positive	0.2	0.0	0.7	0.0	5.8	0.2	0.2
Transplant							
Year of transplant	0.3	40.8	27.5	17.6	24.9	4.0	4.1
HLA-ABDR mismatches	2.0	27.0	15.2	8.6	5.2	4.4	7.2
Total assignable variation as fraction of variance in outcome	10.6	4.2	2.7	3.7	3.6	1.2	2.6

Table 3. Odds ratios for prognostic factors of long-term survival given the kidney graft survived beyond one year after transplantation.[1]

Factor	All Cases (75,812)	DGF / LAR -/- (58,534)	+/- (11,675)	-/+ (4,482)	+/+ (1,121)
Recipient					
Sex: Female	**0.68(.01)**	**0.67(.02)**	**0.64(.03)**	0.89(.06)	0.72(.10)
Race: Caucasian (baseline)					
Black	**1.80(.04)**	**1.67(.05)**	**1.77(.09)**	**2.14(.18)**	**2.11(.32)**
Hispanic	0.90(.03)	0.89(.04)	0.89(.07)	1.35(.18)	0.83(.21)
Other	**0.79(.04)**	**0.81(.05)**	0.72(.08)	1.20(.22)	0.81(.28)
Age: 46-60 yr (baseline)					
0-12 yr	**0.58(.05)**	**0.55(.05)**	0.43(.12)	0.55(.11)	0.60(.32)
13-25 yr	**1.59(.06)**	**1.49(.06)**	**1.37(.12)**	**1.70(.18)**	1.16(.27)
26-45 yr	**1.08(.02)**	1.07(.03)	1.05(.05)	1.05(.08)	1.12(.17)
>60 yr	1.03(.03)	1.10(.04)	1.01(.07)	0.79(.12)	0.87(.20)
Original disease: other (baseline)					
Systemic	**1.08(.02)**	**1.10(.03)**	1.03(.05)	1.07(.08)	1.25(.17)
Inherited	**0.80(.02)**	**0.77(.03)**	0.85(.06)	0.99(.10)	1.03(.23)
Pre-tx medical status: no impairment (baseline)					
Impairment	**1.15(.02)**	**1.13(.03)**	1.15(.05)	1.22(.08)	0.95(.13)
PRA: 0% (baseline)					
1-10%	0.99(.02)	0.95(.02)	1.14(.06)	1.00(.07)	0.89(.14)
11-50%	1.07(.03)	1.00(.03)	1.18(.07)	1.07(.10)	1.13(.22)
51-80%	1.14(.05)	1.02(.06)	1.29(.12)	1.41(.24)	1.14(.34)
81-100%	1.14(.05)	1.12(.07)	1.03(.09)	1.16(.20)	1.33(.36)
Duration pre-transplant dialysis: ≤12 mo (baseline)					
13-24 mo	1.07(.03)	**1.12(.03)**	0.92(.06)	1.00(.08)	0.86(.15)
25-36 mo	**1.13(.04)**	**1.13(.04)**	1.06(.08)	1.00(.11)	0.92(.20)
>36 mo	**1.18(.03)**	**1.17(.04)**	1.08(.07)	1.20(.12)	1.01(.19)
Donor					
Relationship: cadaver (baseline)					
Parent	0.98(.08)	1.06(.10)	1.45(.38)	0.52(.13)	0.49(.37)
Living related	0.88(.06)	0.92(.07)	1.49(.32)	0.54(.13)	1.71(1.01)
Living unrelated	1.04(.09)	1.10(.11)	1.31(.38)	0.64(.18)	2.78(2.40)
Race: Caucasian (baseline)					
Black	**1.26(.04)**	**1.27(.05)**	**1.36(.09)**	1.04(.10)	1.21(.25)
Hispanic	0.98(.04)	0.95(.04)	1.07(.08)	0.92(.12)	1.02(.26)
Other	1.11(.06)	1.12(.08)	1.13(.16)	1.09(.23)	0.73(.73)
Age: 16-30 yr (baseline)					
1-3 yr	0.89(.08)	0.92(.10)	0.90(.20)	0.79(.25)	2.44(1.73)
4-15 yr	0.98(.04)	1.01(.05)	1.05(.10)	0.82(.10)	0.67(.21)
31-50 yr	**1.39(.03)**	**1.32(.04)**	**1.43(.08)**	**1.42(.12)**	1.41(.25)
> 50 yr	**2.46(.08)**	**2.33(.09)**	**2.70(.18)**	**1.87(.21)**	**2.04(.44)**
Death: trauma (baseline)					
Non-trauma	**1.32(.03)**	**1.31(.04)**	**1.35(.07)**	1.01(.09)	1.18(.18)

Factor	All Cases	DGF / LAR -/-	+/-	-/+	+/+
Cold ischemia time: 4-12 hr (baseline)					
0-3 hr	0.84(.06)	0.83(.03)	0.71(.15)	1.22(.26)	0.83(.47)
13-24 hr	1.03(.03)	0.98(.03)	1.06(.07)	0.94(.08)	1.01(.18)
> 24 hr	**1.11(.03)**	1.06(.02)	1.08(.06)	1.00(.09)	1.25(.21)
CMV status: negative (baseline)					
Positive	**1.12(.02)**	**1.13(.03)**	1.05(.05)	1.15(.08)	0.97(.13)
Transplant					
Year of transplant: 1994-8 (baseline)					
< 1994	**1.20(.02)**	**1.22(.03)**	1.06(.05)	1.05(.07)	0.85(.11)
HLA-ABDR mismatches: 0 (baseline)					
1-2	**1.35(.05)**	**1.37(.06)**	1.14(.11)	1.14(.18)	0.99(.35)
3-4	**1.39(.05)**	**1.39(.06)**	1.07(.10)	1.34(.20)	0.97(.32)
5-6	**1.41(.06)**	**1.38(.07)**	1.11(.10)	1.41(.22)	0.98(.33)

[1] Significant (P≤0.001, allowing for multiple comparisons) values are listed in **bold**.

Table 4. Extent of assignable variation in long-term renal graft outcomes (i.e., 5-yr graft survival given one-year graft survival) attributable to various factors stratified by first-year events DGF and late rejection.

Factor	All Cases (75,812)	DGF / Late Rejection -/- (58,534)	+/- (11,675)	-/+ (4,482)	+/+ (1,121)
Recipient					
Sex	13.6	16.2	14.6	1.4	7.8
Race	24.1	19.1	25.9	36.2	39.2
Age	9.3	9.2	4.2	23.6	3.9
Medical status	1.7	1.6	1.4	4.2	0.2
Original disease	2.9	4.6	1.0	0.4	3.4
PRA	0.6	0.6	2.1	2.2	4.1
Duration pre-transplant dialysis	1.3	1.4	1.4	1.9	1.5
Donor					
Relationship	0.4	0.6	0.5	3.4	8.0
Race	2.1	2.6	3.1	0.4	1.9
Age	31.9	30.1	37.9	20.2	22.9
Death	4.4	4.6	5.3	0.0	1.5
Cold ischemia time	0.9	0.6	1.7	0.6	3.5
CMV status positive	1.1	1.6	0.2	1.9	0.1
Transplant					
Year of transplant	2.9	3.9	0.3	0.2	2.0
HLA-ABDR mismatches	2.9	3.4	0.4	3.4	0.0
Total assignable variation as fraction of variance in outcome	6.4	5.3	6.5	5.5	6.3

(5-yr GS = 68.2%, HL = 7.1±0.2 yrs); 395 (1%) with DGF and LAR but without EAR (5-yr GS = 49.8%, HL = 3.5±0.3 yrs); and 2,636 (3%) with EAR and LAR but without DGF (5-yr GS = 61.3%, HL = 5.6±0.2 yrs). Finally, 726 (1%) recipients experienced all 3 adverse effects (5-yr GS = 51.5%, HL = 4.3±0.2 yrs). Based on actual and imputed 5-year outcomes, effects of DGF, EAR and LAR were adjusted via logistic regression for the 15 cofactors (data not shown). Following adjustment, the main effects of DGF, EAR and LAR on long-term survival remained significant, with relative risks equal to 1.4, 1.4 and 2.6, respectively (P<0.0001).

In Figure 3, subgroups with and without EAR did not significantly differ with respect to their long-term survival rates except for comparing "event-free" recipients to those with just EAR. On average, HL's were reduced ~30% by the presence of DGF, ~3% by EAR, and ~50% by LAR (non-cumulative). In the subsequent multi-factor analysis, the 8 groups were condensed into 4 groups based solely on DGF and LAR categories. The results of regrouping are shown in Figure 4. Both DGF and LAR independently affect long-term graft as well as patient and functional survival rates.

Table 3 lists the relative risks for prognostic factors on long-term survival given the kidney graft survived beyond one year. The values in the first column are estimated overall categories of DGF and LAR. Subsequent columns list long-term risks for factors depending on whether or not DGF and LAR occurred. When DGF and LAR were absent, most factors had one or more levels significantly affecting long-term graft survival. The exceptions included cold ischemia time, PRA and donor relationship.

As adverse early events mounted, the effects of pretransplant factors generally diminished. Specifically, Black recipients and older donors were the only additional risk factors affecting long-term survival when DGF and LAR were both present. Female and teenage recipients, and Black and older donors, demonstrated larger odds ratios when LAR was absent regardless of DGF. Whereas, the risk of long-term failure was greatest for Black recipients when DGF was absent regardless of LAR.

Percentages of accountable variation in outcomes beyond one year are shown in Table 4. Ranking long-

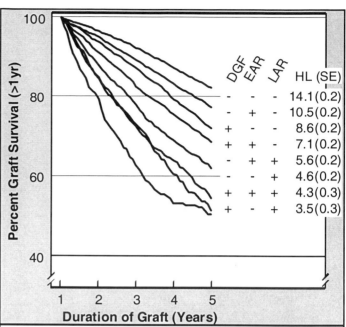

Figure 3. Kaplan-Meier survival curves for kidney grafts with good function starting one year after transplantation based on the absence (-) or presence (+) of DGF, EAR or LAR.

term outcomes from all studies demonstrated that recipient race and donor age accounted for the majority of changes in long-term kidney graft survival. Recipient sex, cause of donor death and donor age exhibited stronger impacts when LAR was absent; recipient age and number of HLA mismatches exhibited stronger influences when DGF was absent.

Interactions of 4 factors (recipient race, recipient age, donor age and number of HLA mismatches) with DGF/LAR categories are explored further in Figures 5-8. Each figure displays 4 panels corresponding to the four categories: -DGF/-LAR (top left panel); +DGF/-LAR (top right panel); -DGF/+LAR (bottom left panel); and +DGF/+LAR (bottom right panel). Within each panel, the GS beyond one year is plotted at various levels of the 4 factors.

In Figure 5, the inferior long-term GS for Black recipients compared to non-Blacks is shown. Without DGF or LAR, Blacks demonstrated a half-life of 8 years compared to 15 years for non-Black counterparts. Differences between Blacks and non-Blacks were more pronounced when LAR had occurred. With an incidence of LAR, the half-life was 3 years for Blacks compared to 6 years for non-Blacks.

The long-term effects of recipient age are shown in Figure 6. Based on previous results, recipients were

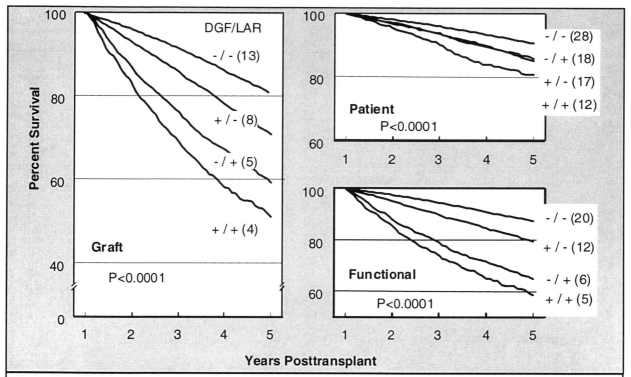

Figure 4. Long-term graft, functional and patient survival based on the absence (-) or presence (+) of DGF and LAR.

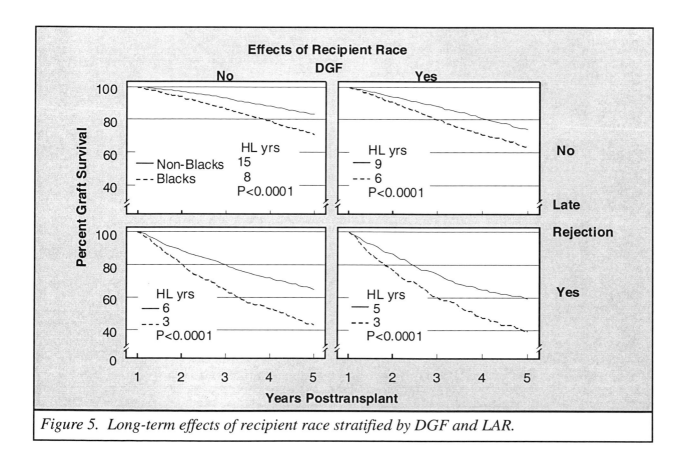

Figure 5. Long-term effects of recipient race stratified by DGF and LAR.

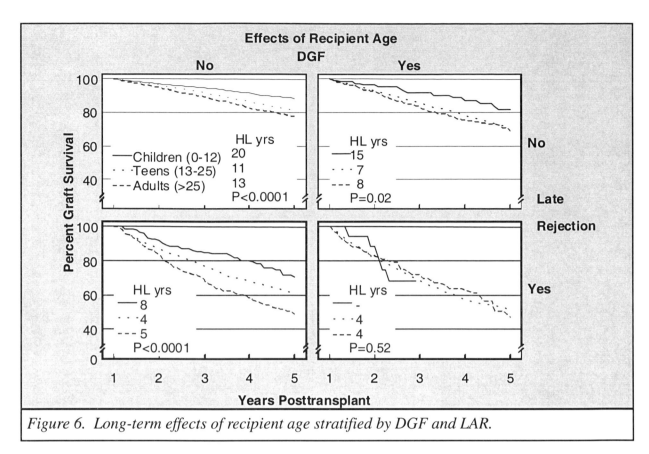

Figure 6. Long-term effects of recipient age stratified by DGF and LAR.

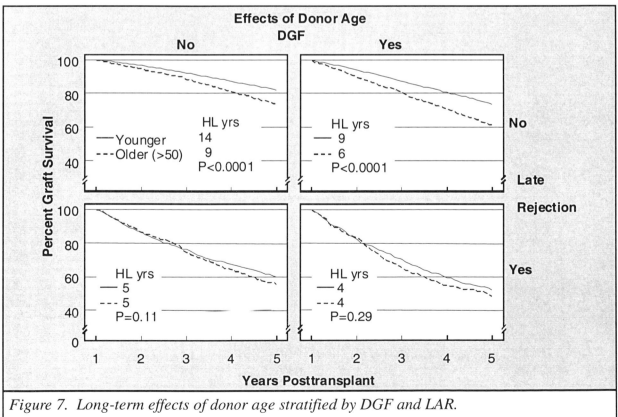

Figure 7. Long-term effects of donor age stratified by DGF and LAR.

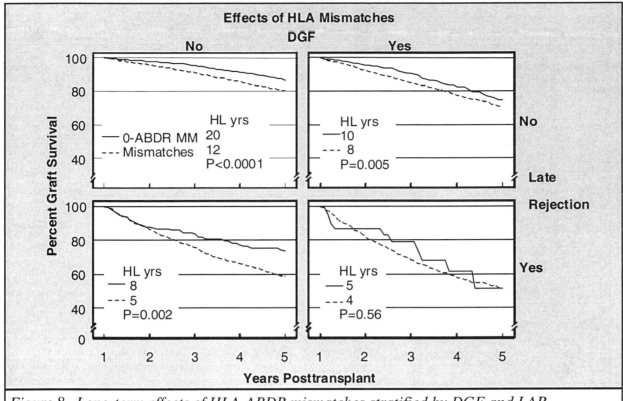

Figure 8. Long-term effects of HLA-ABDR mismatches stratified by DGF and LAR.

grouped into 3 age cohorts: children (0-12 yrs), teens (13-25 yrs) and adults (>25 yrs). Although children tended to have the best long-term survival and teenagers the worst, the differences were significant only when DGF was absent. Without DGF and LAR, the half-life for children receiving a kidney graft was 20 years compared to 11 years for teens and 13 years for adults. Similarly, for grafts without DGF but with LAR, the half-lives for children, teens and adults were 8, 4 and 5 years, respectively. When both DGF and LAR occurred, varying the recipient's age did not alter long-term GS.

When donor kidneys are grouped into younger ($\leq$50 yrs) and older (>50) age groups based on the age of the donor at the time of transplantation, donor age was a long-term factor when LAR was absent (Fig. 7). Without LAR, half-lives for transplants using kidneys from older donors were reduced by ~33% compared to transplants using younger kidneys. As shown in the bottom 2 panels of Figure 7, LAR uniformly lowered kidney graft half-lives such that the age of the donor was no longer a factor.

In Figure 8, the effects of HLA-ABDR mismatches on long-term GS are shown. Here, the zero-mismatched kidney transplants enjoyed significantly better long-term

outcomes provided that DGF was absent. When LAR was concurrently absent, the half-life for the 0-MM group was 20 years compared to 12 years for the mismatched group. With LAR, half-lives were reduced but 0-MM grafts still demonstrated a significantly higher value of 8 years compared to 5 years for mismatched grafts. Zero-MM grafts with DGF and LAR had equal long-term GS rates as mismatched ones with DGF and LAR.

DISCUSSION

In this study of the UNOS Renal Scientific Registry, we examined the effects of pretransplant risk factors, DGF, EAR and LAR on one another and on short- and long-term kidney GS provided an effect was antecedent to an outcome. Starting with pretransplant risk factors for DGF, we found that PRA over 80%, pretransplant dialysis durations over 3 years, kidneys from donors over 50 years of age, and cold ischemia times over 24 hours each increased the risk of DGF by a factor of ~2 (Table 1). These increases are associated with mechanisms of decreased glomerular filtration rate in DGF. High PRA might result in very early and subclinical AR, which could necessitate dialysis (11). Also, total metabolism, renal function and renal blood flow decrease with time on dialysis and age (15), and tubular damage can result from ischemia injury (16). These damages are associated with a decrease in the nephron mass, a decrease in the glomerular volume and interstitial fibrosis (17).

Next, we found that DGF significantly increases the chance of EAR but not LAR (Fig. 2). This supports the hypothesis that DGF may increase the immunogenicity of the graft (18). Twenty-six percent of patients discharged without DGF experienced EAR, but 38% of patients with DGF experienced EAR. Concerning LAR, 6% and 4% of patients without EAR and with and without DGF, respectively, experienced LAR. Further, 18% and 19% of patients with EAR and with and without DGF, respectively, experienced LAR. Notice that, while DGF did not greatly impact LAR, EAR increased the incidence of LAR by 13-15 percentage points.

While non-immune pretransplant factors tended to influence DGF, immune factors explained most of the variation in EAR (Table 2). Black and younger recipients, increasing numbers of HLA-ABDR mismatches, and transplantation before 1993 contributed to higher risks for EAR and combined to explain over 75% of the total variation in EAR outcomes. The increased immunogenicity of the first 3 factors is well documented (19), and year of transplant could be a surrogate marker for changing immunosuppressive regimens, where newer drugs (e.g. MMF) have been shown to significantly lower AR.

The same factors that impacted EAR impacted LAR, and, additionally, donor age emerged as a strong factor. Kidneys procured from donors over 50 demonstrated relative risks of LAR from 1.3 to 1.6 compared to baseline donors who were 16-30 years old. Donor age accounted for 3-5% of variation in EAR, but accounted for 7 to 17% of the variation in LAR (Table 2).

Long-term GS results from this study confirmed that DGF was an independent and deleterious long-term risk factor (Figs 3 & 4). By stratifying recipients who survived beyond one year after transplantation into 8 groups according to their histories of DGF (-/+), EAR (-/+) and LAR (-/+), we were able to demonstrate that half-lives for groups with DGF were always less than half-lives for corresponding groups without DGF. On par, DGF lowered half-lives by 30%. EAR demonstrated a lesser role by reducing long-term GS only when no other adverse effects were present. LAR reduced half-lives by 50% across the spectrum of DGF and EAR strata.

Lastly, we showed that the long-term effects of some pretransplant risk factors are confounded by DGF and LAR (Tables 3 & 4). Some risk factors, like recipient race, had strong effects regardless of DGF and LAR (i.e., Black recipients exhibited poor long-term GS in all strata, Fig. 5). Other factors, like recipient sex, exhibited varying effects depending on DGF and LAR. Although female recipients generally do better long-term than male recipients, the effects of recipient sex were much stronger among patients without LAR but nearly the same among patients with and without DGF. Other examples of interrelationships among DGF, LAR and 3 risk factors (recipient age, donor age and HLA) on long-term GS were shown in Figures 6-8. Provocatively, the effects of the 2 immune factors (i.e., recipient age and HLA) were strongest when DGF was absent, and the effect of the non-immune factor (donor age) was strongest when LAR was absent. Other factors that exhibited heightened effects when DGF was absent included recipient medical status pretransplant and donor CMV status; other factors that exhibited heightened effects when LAR was absent included donor race and cause of donor death (Table 4). Further study is needed to firmly establish whether DGF principally mitigates the long-term effects of immune factors and whether LAR chiefly mitigates the effects of non-immune factors.

The findings in this study support the theory that DGF and AR, in and of themselves, can both influence long-term graft survival. Thus, immune and non-immune mechanisms are acting to cause the chronic long-term loss of kidney grafts. Clearly, in order to improve the short- and long-term outcome of renal transplants, strategies aimed at reducing both DGF and AR must be developed.

SUMMARY

1. From 1991 to 1998, the incidence of DGF remained at 21% of all kidney grafts (n = 86,682) reported to the UNOS Scientific Transplant Registry. In contrast, percentages of early acute rejection (EAR) and late acute rejection (LAR) have dropped precipitously to half their starting values. (EAR started at 37% and dropped to 18%, and LAR started at 11% and dropped to 5%.)

2. Among discharged recipients, DGF was associated with increased EAR (odds ratio = 1.7) within 6 months of transplant; whereas, EAR (odds ratio = 4.7) but not DGF (odds ratio = 1.1) was associated with increased LAR for recipients from 6 months to one year after transplantation.

3. Non-immune factors (e.g., duration of pretransplant dialysis, donor age, and cold ischemia time) primarily influenced the risk of DGF, and immune factors (e.g., recipient race, recipient age, HLA) mainly determined the risk of EAR and LAR.

4. DGF, EAR and LAR were independent risk factors for long-term graft loss. DGF and LAR exhibited the strongest influences, reducing half-lives by 30% and 50%, respectively.

5. Some long-term risk factors demonstrated consistent effects regardless of DGF and/or LAR. For example, Black recipients always had poor long-term GS. On the other hand, some risk factors, mostly immune-type factors, exhibited effects only in the absence of DGF (e.g., recipient sex, age and HLA matching). Many non-immune factors exhibited long-term effects only in the absence of LAR (e.g., donor age, cause of donor death).

6. Strategies aimed at reducing both DGF and AR are necessary to improve the long-term outcome of kidney transplants.

REFERENCES

1. Sanfilippo F, Vaughn WK, Spees EK, Lucas BA. The detrimental effects of delayed graft function in cadaver donor renal transplantation. Transplantation 1984; 38:643.

2. Kahan BD, Mickey R, Flechner SM, et al. Multivariate analysis of risk factors impacting on immediate and eventual cadaver allograft survival in cyclosporine-treated recipients. Transplantation 1987; 43:65.

3. Halloran PF, Aprile MA, Farewell V, et al. Early function as the principal correlate of graft survival. A multivariate analysis of 200 cadaveric renal transplants treated with a protocol incorporating antilymphocyte globulin and cyclosporine. Transplantation 1988; 46:223.

4. Rosenthal JT, Danovitch GM, Wilkinson A, Ettenger RB. The high cost of delayed graft function in cadaveric renal transplantation. Transplantation 1991; 51:1115.

5. Ojo AO, Wolfe RA, Held PHJ, Port FK, Schmouder RL. Delayed graft function: Risk factors and implication for renal allograft survival. Transplantation 1997; 63:968.

6. Shoskes DA, Cecka JM. Deleterious effects of delayed graft function in cadaveric renal transplant recipients independent of acute rejection. Transplantation 1998; 66:1697.

7. Tejani AH, Sullivan EK, Alexander SR, et al. Predictive factors for delayed graft function (DGF) and its impact on renal graft survival in children: A report of the North American Pediatric Renal Transplant Cooperative Study (NAPRTCS). Pediatr Transplant 1999; 3:293.

8. Kyllonen LEJ, Salmela KT, Eklund BH, et al. Long-term results of 1047 cadaveric kidney transplantations with special emphasis on initial graft function and rejection. Transpl Int 2000; 13:122.

9. Troppmann C, Gillingham KJ, Gruessner RWG, et al. Delayed graft function in the absence of rejection has no long-term impact. A study of cadaver kidney recipients with good graft function at 1 year after transplantation. Transplantation 1996; 61:1331.

10. Lehtonen SRK, Isoniemi HM, Salmela KT, et al. Long-term graft outcome is not necessarily affected by delayed onset of graft function and early acute rejection. Transplantation 1997; 64:103.

11. Boom H, Mallat MJK, de Fijter JW, Zwinderman AH, Paul LC. Delayed graft function influences renal function, but not survival. Kidney Int 2000; 58:859.

12. Mitch WE, Buffington GA, Lemann J, Walser M. A simple method of estimating progression of chronic renal failure. Lancet 1976; 2:1326.

13. Walser M. Progression of chronic renal failure in man. Kidney Int 1990; 37:1195.

14. Judge GG, Griffiths WE, Hill RC, Lutkepohl H, Lee TC. The Theory and Practice of Econometrics. 2nd ed. New York, John Wiley & Sons, 1985.

15. Nyengaard JR, Bendtsen TF. Glomerular number and size in relation to age, kidney weight, and body surface in normal man. Anat Rec 1992; 232:194.

16. Marcussen N, Lai R, Olsen S, Solez K. Morphometric and immunohistochemical investigation of renal biopsies from patients with transplant ATN, native ATN or acute graft rejection. Transplant Proc 1996; 28:470.

17. Seron D, Carrera M, Grino JM, Castelao AM, Lopez-Costea MA, Riera L, Alsina J. Relationship between donor renal interstitial surface and post-transplant function. Nephrol Dial Transplant 1993; 8:539.

18. Shoskes DA, Parfrey NA, Halloran PF. Increased major histocompatibility complex antigen expression in unilateral ischemic acute tubular necrosis in the mouse. Transplantation 1997; 63:519.

19. Kerman RH, Kimball PM, Van Buren CT, Lewis RM, Kahan BD. Possible contribution of pretransplant immune responder status to renal allograft survival differences of black versus white recipients. Transplantation 1991; 51:338.

CHAPTER 32

Maintenance Immunosuppression

Steven K. Takemoto

To understand why certain drugs are combined in current practice to protect transplants from rejection, it is helpful to follow the development of treatment protocols(1). In the 1960s treatment consisted of azathioprine and solumedrol with rejections treated with prednisone or anti-lymphocyte antibody. Success rate was 50% at one year. With the introduction of cyclosporin in the 1980s, one-year survival rates improved above 80%. Cyclosporin is nephrotoxic, so standard treatment modulates its use in "triple therapy" using cyclosporin as the primary agent in conjunction with steroids, and azathioprine as an adjunctive agent. Anti-lymphocyte antibody or the monoclonal anti-T-cell antibody, OKT3, are sometimes given as induction agents at the time of transplantation to bolster immunosuppression in recipients with increased risk for rejection or to provide cover allowing delay in administration of cyclosporin in patients with delayed function or lower doses in patients who may be experiencing cyclosporin nephrotoxicity.

Tacrolimus was approved by the FDA for use as a primary immunosuppressant for kidney transplants in 1997 (2). The mechanism of action is similar to that of cyclosporin in that it selectively inhibits the action of calcineurin, an enzyme necessary for T-cell activation that promotes expression of cytokine genes such as IL-2, TNF-alpha and IFN-gamma (1).

Neoral, a new formulation of cyclosporin that increases absorption and bioavailability of the active compound was introduced at about the same time as Tacrolimus. Some studies have shown significantly lower rejection rates for patients receiving Neoral compared with those receiving cyclosporin. Therefore, this analysis compares usage and outcome between Tacrolimus and Neoral as primary immunosuppression agents.

Mycophenolate mofetil was approved for clinical transplantation after 3 large clinical trials demonstrated its effectiveness as an adjunctive agent in reducing the incidence of rejection compared with azathioprine (1). Mycophenolate prevents synthesis of purines that are necessary for lymphocyte proliferation.

In this chapter, the introduction and impact of Tacrolimus and Neoral as primary agents of maintenance immunosuppression, and the change from azathioprine to mycophenolate as adjunctive agents are chronicled with registry data.

PATIENTS AND METHODS

A total of 101,913 recipients of cadaveric renal allografts, transplanted between 1991-1999 with outcome reported to the UNOS Renal Transplant Registry were included in this analysis. Four classes of immunosuppressive agents were compared: Primary agents included Neoral and Tacrolimus (Tac); adjunctive agents included Azathioprine (Aza) and Mycophenolate Mofetil (MMF); steriods were Prednisone and Solumedrol (methylprednisolone); and induction antibodies included ATG (atgam, anti-thymocyte globulin) and OKT3. First use of each agent was noted by examining the induction and maintenance medication fields on the transplant registration record. Follow-up records through 3 years were used to supplement data for primary, adjunctive or steroid agents for patients lacking this information on the discharge form.

The significance of difference was determined using chi-square analysis. Logistic regression analyses were used to determine the relative effect of various cofactors on the risk of rejection, graft loss and patient death. In the logistic regression analyses, the parameter for each covariate with the lowest level of rejection, graft or patient loss was taken as the baseline. The relative contribution of the remaining cofactors was reported as an odds ratio with values greater than 1 representing the increased percentage of risk of rejection, graft or patient loss compared with baseline values. STATA statistical software (College Station, TX) was used for all statistical analysis.

RESULTS

The results are shown in the following figures and tables:

Clinical Transplants 2000, Cecka and Terasaki, Eds. UCLA Immunogenetics Center, Los Angeles, California

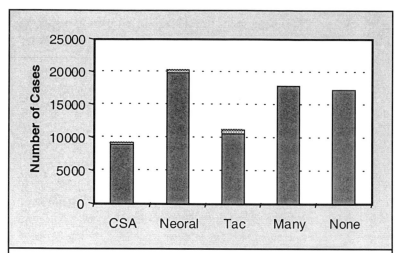

Figure 1. Completeness of primary agent reporting in the UNOS Registry.

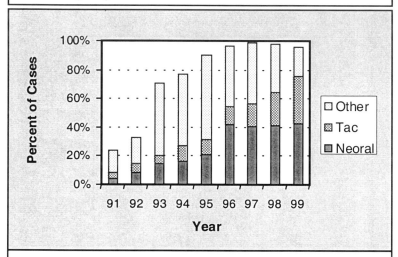

Figure 2. Use of primary agent by year of transplant.

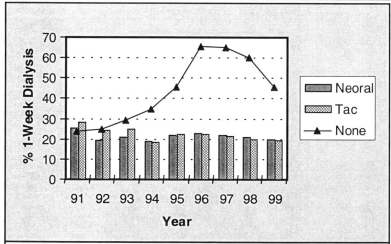

Figure 3. Need for early dialysis by year of transplant for patients receiving calcineurin inhibitors.

Cyclosporin was listed as a maintenance or induction drug for only 12% of cases, compared with 26% for Neoral and 14% for Tacrolimus. There was a small percentage of patients with a different calcineurin inhibitor listed as a maintenance drug on a subsequent followup (indicated by the cross-hatched area above the respective bars). More than one initial calcineurin inhibitor was indicated for 24% of transplants and 23% of recipients did not have a calcineurin inhibitor agent listed.

In 1991, 4% of cadaveric renal transplant recipients received Neoral and 4% received Tacrolimus. In 1995, the percentage of recipients receiving Neoral increased to 21% and 10% received Tacrolimus. From 1996-1999, the percentage of recipients receiving Neoral remained at about 40% while the percentage receiving Tacrolimus increased from 13-33%. Prior to 1995, reporting of calcineurin inhibitor usage is likely incomplete. After 1995, a calcineurin inhibitor was reported for 96-98% of transplants.

Since calcineurin inhibitors can damage transplanted kidneys, their use is often delayed until the transplanted kidney begins functioning. Analysis of graft outcome according to calcineurin inhibitors administered as maintenance immunosuppressants, therefore, is biased because kidneys with poor initial function are not included. After 1994, approximately 20% of patients receiving Neoral or Tacrolimus required dialysis during the first posttransplant week. Up to two-thirds of the patients that never received Neoral or Tacrolimus required dialysis.

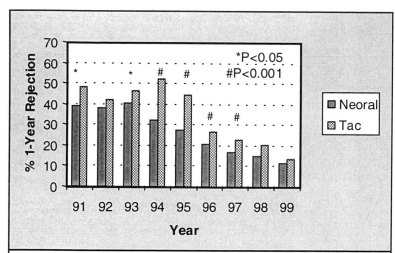

Figure 4. Incidence of first year rejection by year of transplant for patients receiving calcineurin inhibitors.

In 1994, 52% of renal transplant recipients receiving Tacrolimus maintenance therapy had rejections reported in the first post transplant year compared with 32% for those receiving Neoral. This difference remained significant through 1999, but the incidence of rejection for recipients treated with either agent, has decreased in a step-wise manner. In 1999, 14% of patients receiving Tacrolimus had a reported rejection compared with 11% for those receiving Neoral.

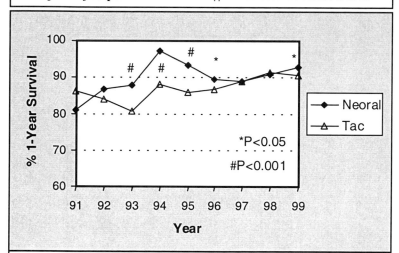

Figure 5. Graft survival at one year by year of transplant for patients receiving calcineurin inhibitors.

In 1994, the one-year graft survival rate for renal transplant recipients receiving Neoral was 97% compared with 88% for those receiving Tacrolimus. As usage became more widespread in 1995 and 1996, one-year graft survival decreased for patients receiving Neoral and increased for those receiving Tacrolimus. One-year graft survival was significantly higher for recipients receiving Neoral transplanted between 1993-1996.

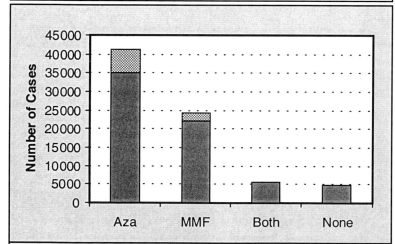

Figure 6. Completeness of adjunctive agent reporting in the UNOS Registry.

The report of adjunctive agent use was more complete than calcineurin inhibitors. Use of azathioprine or mycophenolate as an induction or maintenance agent was missing for only 6% of renal transplant recipients. Over 50% of recipients received azathioprine, 30% received mycophenolate, and 7% had both agents listed in the initial report. The crosshatched area indicates the percentage of patients with the other agent listed in a subsequent report.

IMMUNOSUPPRESSION

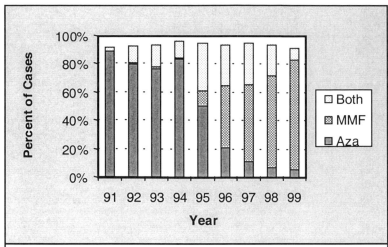

Figure 7. Usage of adjunctive agents by year of transplant.

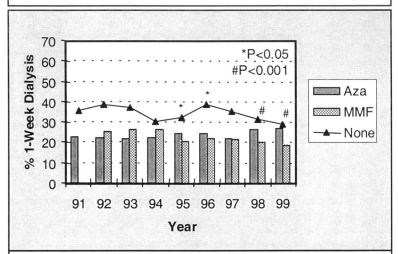

Figure 8. Need for early dialysis by year of transplant for patients receiving adjunctive agents.

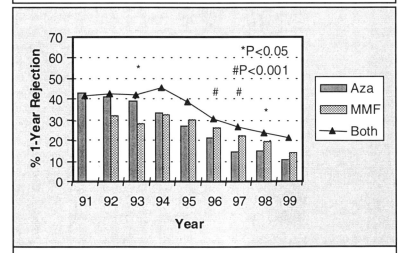

Figure 9. Incidence of first-year rejection by year of transplant for patients receiving adjunctive agents.

Between 1991-1994, 90% of renal transplant recipients received azathioprine and fewer than 200 received mycophenolate. In 1995, 85% of the recipients received azathioprine compared with 11% who received mycophenolate. In 1996, use of mycophenolate increased four-fold to 44%. The percentage of patients receiving mycophenolate has increased by 10% every year between 1997-1999 to 77%. Only 6% of renal transplant recipients in 1999 received only azathioprine, 9% received both azathioprine and mycophenolate, and 8% received neither.

Analysis of graft outcome for adjunctive agents is also biased because a certain percentage of patients with poor initial function never received these agents. Between 20-30% of patients receiving azathioprine or mycophenolate required dialysis compared with 30-40% of patients who did not receive these agents. In 1998 and 1999, 27% of patients receiving azathioprine required dialysis compared with 20% for those receiving mycophenolate.

Another complication in this analysis is the handling of patients switching regimens. From 1996-1999, the incidence of rejection was actually higher in patients receiving mycophenolate than those receiving azathioprine. However, those patients receiving azathioprine who were later switched to mycophenolate had a significantly higher incidence of rejection, suggesting that rejection may have prompted the change in drugs.

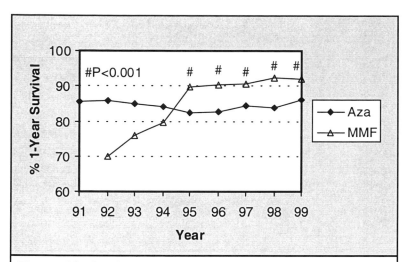

Figure 10. Graft survival at one year by year of transplant for patients receiving adjunctive agents.

One-year graft survival remained at about 85% for patients receiving azathioprine between 1991-1999. Graft survival for patients receiving mycophenolate was actually lower than azathioprine during the first 3 years with at least 50 cases. With more widespread use after approval in 1995, kidney transplant recipients receiving mycophenolate had a significantly higher one-year graft survival rate of 90%. This rate increased to 92% in 1998.

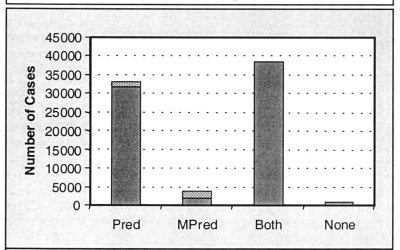

Figure 11. Completeness of steroid reporting in the UNOS Registry.

Unlike calcineurin inhibitors or adjunctive agents where a single agent predominated for each class, both prednisone and solumedrol were administered for over half of the transplant recipients. Prednisone was given alone to 42% of recipients, while 2% received only solumedrol. Neither steroid was listed for only 1% of transplants.

In 1991, prednisone was the only steroid administered to 72% of recipients, while 24% received both solumedrol and prednisone. These percentages reversed in 1994 with 33% receiving prednisone and 65% both solumedrol and prednisone. The distribution for steroids was similar in 1999, except the use of solumedrol without prednisone increased to 3% of recipients.

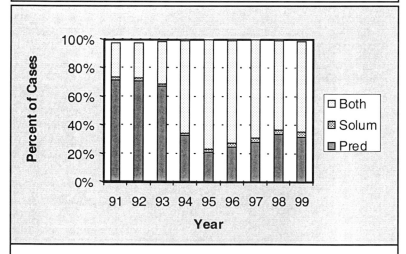

Figure 12. Usage of steroids by year of transplant.

IMMUNOSUPPRESSION

Table 3. Logistic regression adjusting risk of covariates on incidence of rejection, graft loss and death for calcineurin inhibitor vs. adjunctive agent analysis.

	Rejection in 1 year				Failure at 3 years				Death at 3 years			
	RR	95% CI		P	RR	95% CI		P	RR	95% CI		P
Tacrolimus vs Neoral	1.34	1.22	1.47	<0.001	1.12	1.00	1.25	0.046	0.99	0.85	1.16	0.918
MMF vs Aza	1.10	0.98	1.22	0.104	1.61	1.42	1.81	<0.001	1.51	1.28	1.78	<0.001
Both vs Pred	1.10	1.00	1.21	0.045	1.09	0.98	1.22	0.122	1.08	0.92	1.26	0.336
Sol vs Pred	0.73	0.55	0.95	0.02	2.04	1.58	2.63	<0.001	2.18	1.55	3.05	<0.001
ALG vs no Ind Ab	0.84	0.74	0.96	0.009	1.31	1.14	1.51	<0.001	1.20	0.99	1.47	0.069
OKT3 vs no Ind Ab	0.87	0.78	0.97	0.014	1.14	1.01	1.29	0.034	1.12	0.95	1.33	0.179
TX Yr '95-96	1.70	1.55	1.87	<0.001	1.67	1.49	1.86	<0.001	1.76	1.52	2.05	<0.001
White Recip	1.34	1.08	1.66	0.007	1.17	0.92	1.50	0.199	1.28	0.90	1.82	0.162
Black Recip	1.91	1.54	2.39	<0.001	1.70	1.32	2.19	<0.001	1.37	0.95	1.98	0.09
Recip Age (linear)	0.89	0.85	0.93	<0.001	1.16	1.11	1.23	<0.001	1.72	1.57	1.87	<0.001
Recip Age (quadratic)	1.02	0.98	1.05	0.374	1.10	1.06	1.14	<0.001	1.04	0.97	1.11	0.263
Diabetic									1.50	1.30	1.73	<0.001
Multi-organ Transplant	1.41	1.22	1.62	<0.001								
Previous lost Transplant	1.32	1.16	1.50	<0.001	1.38	1.19	1.61	<0.001				
PRA 10-50%					1.10	0.96	1.26	0.191				
PRA >50%					1.40	1.19	1.64	<0.001				
Donor Age (linear)	1.16	1.11	1.21	<0.001	1.19	1.13	1.25	<0.001	1.14	1.06	1.24	<0.001
Donor Age (quadratic)	1.06	1.02	1.10	0.003	1.14	1.09	1.19	<0.001	1.04	0.98	1.11	0.196
Non-trauma donor	1.18	1.07	1.29	0.001	1.18	1.06	1.32	0.003	1.13	0.97	1.32	0.12
Ischemia (linear)	1.02	0.97	1.07	0.352	1.11	1.04	1.17	0.001	1.03	0.96	1.12	0.407
Ischemia (quadratic)	1.00	0.98	1.02	0.958	0.99	0.96	1.01	0.287	1.02	0.99	1.05	0.294
Medium 140 center	1.31	1.10	1.57	0.003	1.37	1.11	1.71	0.004	1.77	1.26	2.47	0.001
Lowest 20 centers	1.44	1.17	1.79	0.001	1.46	1.13	1.89	0.004	1.69	1.14	2.50	0.008
Fewer than 100 tx center	1.35	1.06	1.73	0.016	1.80	1.35	2.40	<0.001	2.27	1.49	3.48	<0.001
1-2 ABDR MM	1.57	1.32	1.87	<0.001	1.15	0.95	1.40	0.161	0.92	0.70	1.20	0.541
3-4 ABDR MM	1.71	1.47	1.99	<0.001	1.28	1.09	1.51	0.003	1.06	0.85	1.32	0.611
5-6 ABDR MM	1.90	1.61	2.23	<0.001	1.53	1.28	1.83	<0.001	1.29	1.02	1.64	0.034
Unknown HLA	1.29	0.98	1.69	0.065	1.27	0.94	1.71	0.113	1.36	0.92	1.99	0.12

ther none or more than one calcineurin inhibitor and also excluded those who received none or more than one adjunctive agent. Almost one-third of patients transplanted between 1995-1999 received both Neoral and Tacrolimus during the induction or initial hospitalization period (Table 4). Another 10% switched from azathioprine to mycophenolate and 5% from mycophenolate to azathioprine after the initial period. Because of this difficulty to categorize patients, the analyses in Tables 1-3 included only one-third of the total kidney recipients transplanted between 1995-1999.

Recipients who continued their initial protocol tended to have better outcome than those who switched during the initial hospitalization or later periods. The rate of re-jection for transplants treated consistently with Neoral, Tacrolimus or mycophenolate was 20%. Only 10% of the grafts for these recipients were lost in 3 years and the rate of patient death was 5%. Rejection rates were higher for patients with multiple protocols. The incidence of rejection for patients receiving more than one calcineurin inhibitor in the initial report was 28%, and was even higher for those recipients who were switched to a different agent in a later report. The modest rates of failure and death for patients switching protocols results from sampling bias since extended kidney function was necessary for this change to be recorded on a subsequent follow-up report.

Table 4. Incidence of rejection, graft loss and death for calcineurin inhibitor categories.

	Cases	%	%1-Yr Rej	%3-Yr Fail	%3-Yr Death
Calcineurin Inhibitors					
CsA	2,985	5.0	23.6	23.4	11.1
Neoral	23,346	38.8	17.1	10.8	5.1
Tacrolimus	10,710	17.8	21.3	11.6	4.8
CsA->Other	498	0.8	45.6	9.2	2.8
Neoral-> Other	544	1.0	37.1	10.5	2.9
Tac->Other	575	1.0	32.0	10.6	4.4
Many	19,314	32.1	28.0	9.5	3.5
None	2,244	3.7	19.8	74.0	29.1
Adjunctive Agents					
Aza	11,880	19.7	21.7	20.6	9.2
MMF	29,956	49.7	19.9	9.6	4.1
Aza->MMF	6,124	10.2	35.7	9.0	2.9
MMF->Aza	2,822	4.7	23.0	8.2	3.3
Both	5,825	6.0	25.3	14.7	6.1
None	3,609	6.0	16.2	32.0	13.1

Between 4-6% of patients never began standard protocol treatment. Graft loss within 3 years (including death) was reported for 74% of recipients with no indicated calcineurin inhibitor, and the rate of patient death was 29%.

DISCUSSION

Reports of clinical trials testing the efficacy of emerging immunosuppressive agents to promote transplant graft acceptance dominate transplant literature, but it is often difficult to translate the impact of these protocols to clinical practice because of the multitude of patient factors and treatment options. Our first attempt to use registry data to provide guidance for administering treatment options was in the form of look up tables to compare outcome after treatment with Tacrolimus or cyclosporin in various patient cohorts (3). This is the first analysis in this series to focus on the impact on graft outcome resulting from the emergence of Tacrolimus, Neoral and mycophenolate.

The rate of rejection during the first year dramatically decreased from over 40% in 1991 to 12% in 1999. This decrease corresponded with notable changes in maintenance immunosuppression protocols. Use of Neoral increased from 4-40% and Tacrolimus from 4-33% of transplants. Use of azathioprine decreased from over 90% to 6% while use of mycophenolate increased from less than 1% to 77% of transplants. Usage of prednisone as the sole corticosteroid decreased from over 70% to about 30% while administration of both solumedrol and prednisone increased from less than 25% to over 60% of transplants. Use of induction antibody increased from 10% to a peak of over 40% in 1996, but again declined to 10% in 1999.

There were significant differences in the usage in maintenance and induction agents depending on risks posed to the transplant. Neoral was more often administered to older recipients, those with multiple pregnancies or those receiving kidneys from older donors while patients receiving Tacrolimus more often were diabetic, received multi-organ transplants (most often a pancreas in conjunction with their kidney), received a regraft (had a previously failed transplant), had broadly reacting HLA antibody (PRA >50%), or a transplant with 5-6 HLA mismatches. Patients given azathioprine more likely were given a kidney from a donor having a non-trauma cause of death, while those given mycophenolate more likely were Black, received a multi-organ or regraft transplant, or had broadly reacting HLA antibody. Patients given induction antibody more likely required dialysis in their first posttransplant week or had broadly reacting HLA antibody.

Another complication was the difficulty categorizing patients into treatment protocols. Only one-third of the cadaveric renal recipients transplanted between 1995-1999 had a clearly defined primary and adjunctive therapy protocol. Patients switching protocols or never enrolled in a protocol because of poor initial function all had poorer outcome than those placed in a protocol for the multivariate analysis. It is also difficult using registry data to determine intent. The higher rate of rejection observed for recipients given mycophenolate mofetil before its licensing may reflect its use in trials for patients with rejection.

This analysis attempts to determine whether a specific new agent was responsible for the declining rates of rejection and improvements in graft survival observed in the 1990s. Mycophenolate was compared with azathioprine in an earlier registry analysis, but this study did not control for year of transplant (4). The comparison of Neoral and Tacrolimus as primary agents and mycophenolate with azathioprine as adjunctive agents may have given an advantage to mycophenolate because it was compared with an agent that was widely used in the 1980s, while both of the calcineurin inhibitors, as well as mycophenolate were introduced in the latter half of the 1990s. If a specific agent were responsible for decreasing the rejection rate, we would expect a dramatic decrease in rejection rates corresponding with its introduction. The yearly declines in rejection rates continued in recipients given the newer calcineurin inhibitors, suggesting that another agent may be responsible. The dramatic increase in survival in 1995 for patients given mycophenolate suggest that this agent has had a greater impact on graft outcome. The multivariate analysis also supports this conclusion.

Earlier analysis suggested induction antibody therapy reduced the rate of rejection in sensitized recipients (5). Induction antibody is also given to patients with delayed function to provide cover so that potentially damaging calcineurin inhibitor treatment can be delayed or given at a lower dosage (1). Here induction antibody reduced the incidence of rejection and improved graft survival in patients with delayed graft function overall, but did not influence rejections when analyzed each year.

Shipping kidneys to HLA-matched recipients improves graft survival despite a marginal increase in ischemia time (6). Since this analysis included only patients able to tolerate standard treatment protocols, it minimized the effect of HLA matching. Patients not receiving standard treatment, or switching treatment protocols had higher rates of rejection and lower rates of survival. Even with the stringent patient selection in this analysis, poorly HLA-matched recipients had 90% increased risk of rejection, and 50% increased risk of graft loss compared with those receiving HLA-matched kidneys.

In 1999, the rejection rate was 12% and only 7% of renal transplants were lost in the first posttransplant year. Newly approved agents such as Rapamycin and monoclonal antibodies specific to T-cell co-stimulatory molecules will likely lead to further improvements in graft outcome. Many other agents will likely prove beneficial in promoting transplant tolerance (1,2). The problem facing the transplant community and the pharmaceutical industry is demonstrating the efficacy of new agents. Chronic rejection continues to be a major cause of long-term graft loss (5). The challenge in facilitating these trials will be to find ways to identify the patients at risk for chronic rejection.

SUMMARY

1. The increased utilization of Neoral, Tacrolimus and mycophenolate mofetil correlated with the dramatic decrease in rejection rates in the 1990s.

2. The 4% difference in the incidence of rejection noted for recipients treated with Tacrolimus (20%) compared with Neoral (16%) corresponded to a 34% increased odds ratio in the multivariate analysis. The risk of graft loss and patient death were similar for the 2 calcineurin inhibitors.

3. Almost every renal transplant recipient received mycophenolate mofetil in 1999. This agent reduced the risk of 3-year graft loss by 60% and halved the risk of death compared with azathioprine.

4. Use of solumedrol as a corticosteriod increased from 26-67% in the 1990s, but this change in practice did not significantly impact outcome.

5. Although recipients given induction ATG or OKT3 had increased risk of graft failure, these recipients more likely were sensitized or required early dialysis.

6. The risk of rejection was 90% higher for recipients with 5-6 HLA mismatches than those with 0 A,B,DR mismatches. Recipients with a poorly HLA-matched kidney had 50% increased risk of graft loss within 3 years compared with HLA-matched transplants.

REFERENCES

1. Danovitch GM: Immunosuppressive medications and protocols for kidney transplantation. In: Danovitch GM Ed. Handbook of Kidney Transplantation. Lippincott, Williams and Wilkens, Philadelphia, 2001; 62.

2. Ciancio G, Burke GW, Roth D, Tzakis AQ, Miller J: Update in transplantation-1997. In: Terasaki PI, Cecka JM Eds. Clinical Transplants 1997. UCLA Tissue Typing Laboratory, Los Angeles, 1998; 241.

3. Gjertson DW: Look-up survival tables for renal transplantation. In: Cecka JM, Terasaki PI Eds. Clinical Transplants 1997. UCLA Tissue Typing Laboratory, Los Angeles, 1998; 337.

4. Ojo AO, Meier-Kriesche HU, Hanson JA, Leichtman AB, Cibrik D, Magee JC, Wolfe RA, Agodoa LY, Kaplan B. Mycophenolate mofetil reduces late renal allograft loss independent of acute rejection. Transplantation 2000; 69:2405.

5. Takemoto S, Cho YW, Gjertson DW: Transplant risks. In: Terasaki PI, Cecka JM Eds. Clinical Transplants 1999. UCLA Tissue Typing Laboratory, Los Angeles, 2000; 325.

6. Takemoto SK, Terasaki PI, Gjertson DW, Cecka JM. Twelve years' experience with national sharing of HLA-matched cadaveric kidneys for transplantation. N Engl J Med 2000; 343:1078.

CHAPTER 33

The HLA-Matching Effect in Different Cohorts of Kidney Transplant Recipients

Paul I. Terasaki

The role of HLA matching for renal transplants has been a controversial issue for many years. Immunosuppression has improved over the years, insuring better control of the immune response. The recipient population has aged and with aging comes diminished immune responsiveness. An increasing proportion of transplants involve marginal donor kidneys that often fail for reasons that are non-immune in nature. As a result of these changes and others, the role of HLA matching has been frequently challenged and re-examined. This chapter focuses on the HLA-matching effect in a variety of different patient groups.

The large volume of data accrued by the UNOS Kidney Transplant Registry since 1987 permits us to group the recipient population according to several different recipient demographic and disease categories and to re-examine the effect of HLA-matching with particular emphasis on 10-year graft survival rates. Because we considered 4 HLA-mismatch categories, the number of patients available was insufficient for analysis for many of the more rare disease categories.

With recently improved immunosuppressive agents and higher graft survival rates, we also examined the HLA-matching effect on transplants performed since 1994 and projected new expected 10-year survival rates based on the graft half-lives computed for kidneys that survived at least one year.

METHODS

The UNOS Kidney Registry data from October 1987–April 2000 was utilized for analysis. It contained 127,769 transplant records. Kaplan-Meier survival statistics and half-life were calculated using Stata software. Graft survival was computed counting graft removal and patient death as graft losses. Functional survival rates counted patient deaths as lost to follow-up.

RESULTS

The following figures show the results of these analyses. In order to have a sufficient number of cases per determination, the HLA-match categories were compressed into 0, 1+2, 3+4 and 5+6 antigen-mismatch groups. Line thickness represents different levels of mismatching.

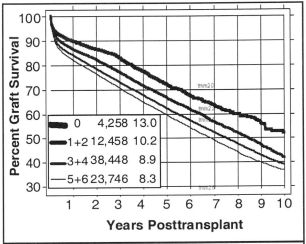

Figure 1. First cadaver donor kidney transplants.

Zero-ABDR-mismatched first cadaver donor transplants (as shown by the thickest line) had the highest survival rate. Increasing levels of mismatches yielded correspondingly lower graft survival rates indicated by the decreasing thickness of the lines representing 1+2, 3+4, and 5+6 ABDR mismatches, respectively. Transplants were performed since October 1987 and the number of cases is given in the second column. Half-life appears in the third column. The HLA-matching effect is apparent.

Clinical Transplants 2000, Cecka and Terasaki, Eds. UCLA Immunogenetics Center, Los Angeles, California

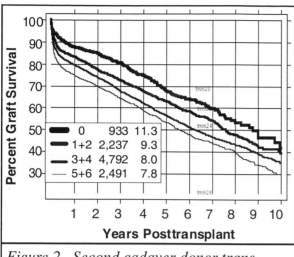

Figure 2. Second cadaver donor transplants.

Second cadaver donor transplants also showed a strong HLA-matching effect, although overall graft survival was about 8% lower at 10 years than for first cadaver donor grafts. Note that most of the difference between first and second cadaver donor grafts occurs in the early posttransplant months.

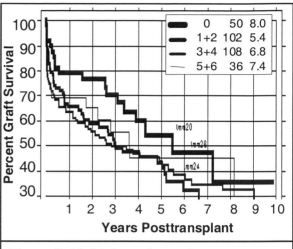

Figure 3. Multiple cadaver donor transplants (third or more).

Multiple cadaver donor grafts (more than 2) resulted in graft survival rates that were substantially lower than second grafts. Note that again, the main survival difference from first grafts occurred very early after transplantation, and the effect of immunization produced by rejection of a prior graft had a relatively small effect on the rate of long-term loss, as shown by the half-lives.

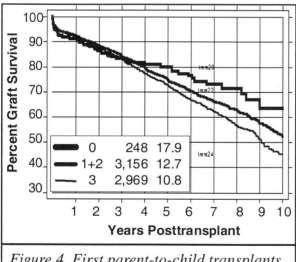

Figure 4. First parent-to-child transplants.

First transplants from parent to child are mismatched for one HLA haplotype. Some exceptional HLA-matched transplants occur as a result of sharing HLA phenotypes by both parents. The survival rate of these HLA-matched grafts was similar to 2 haplotype-matched sibling donor transplants. Note that fewer mismatched antigens produce some long-term benefits.

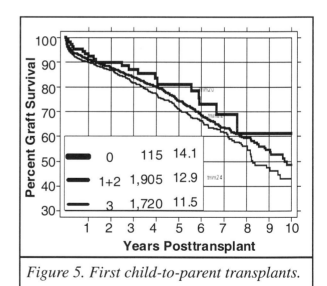

Figure 5. First child-to-parent transplants.

Child-to-parent transplants, which by definition are also one haplotype-matched, produced results similar to those of parent- to-child grafts. Apparently the donor age and recipient age differences in child-to-parent and parent-to-child transplants did not influence graft survival as much as the fact that one HLA haplotype was mismatched. Better survival rates were noted when by chance, all 6 HLA-ABDR antigens were matched.

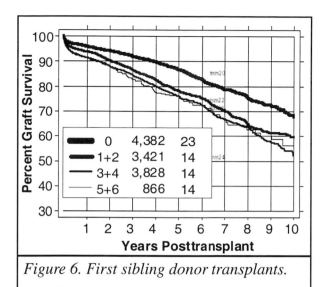

Figure 6. First sibling donor transplants.

First transplants from sibling donors reaffirmed the long-standing finding that HLA-identical sibling donors provided the highest graft survival rates (69% at 10 years). The most striking result shown here is that 2 haplotype-mismatched sibling donors (5+6 ABDR-mismatched transplants) produced graft survival rates similar to those of one haplotype-mismatched sibling donors.

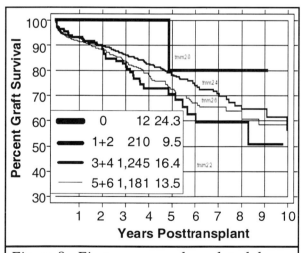

Figure 8. First spouse and unrelated donor transplants.

When spousal and other unrelated-living donor transplants were analyzed together, they had essentially the same graft survival rate as spousal donor transplants alone. Even when combined, few living-unrelated donor transplants were well matched (12 with 0 mismatches and 210 with 1-2 mismatches).

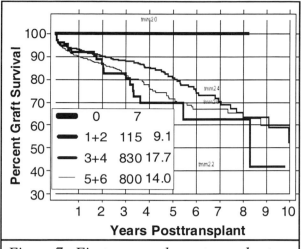

Figure 7. First spouse donor transplants.

Spousal donor transplants produced similar overall graft survival rates when compared with parental and offspring donor transplants (Figs. 4, 5). Only 7 spousal donor grafts were 0 ABDR-mismatched, and all have survived. Most of the transplants had approximately 60% 10-year graft survival, which was higher than the 40% graft survival of cadaver donor transplants and similar to the 2 haplotype-mismatched sibling donor transplants. 10-year graft survival of spousal grafts is based on a relatively small number of transplants when compared with related donor transplants.

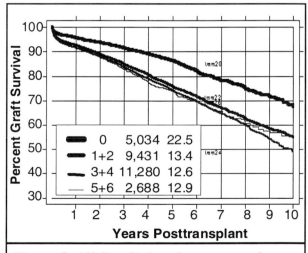

Figure 9. All first living donor transplants.

When all living donor transplants were combined the results showed again that 0 ABDR-mismatched transplants had superior 68% 10-year survival and all other mismatch categories had a similar graft survival rate of 50-56% at 10 years.

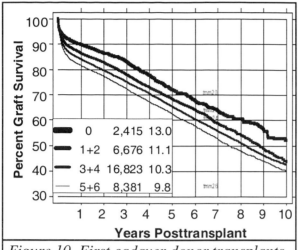

Figure 10. First cadaver donor transplants in Caucasian patients.

The effect of HLA matching among Caucasian recipients of first cadaver donor transplants differed from the overall results shown in Figure 1 in that the worst mismatches had a higher 10-year graft survival rate of 40% rather than 37%. Since the best matches had 52% 10-year graft survival, the difference in 10-year graft survival rates attributable to HLA matching was 12%.

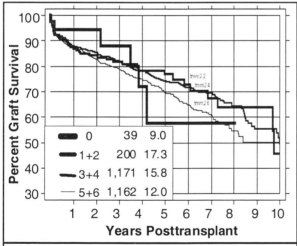

Figure 12. First cadaver donor transplants in Asian patients.

Asian cadaver donor transplant recipients had generally higher graft survival rates than Caucasian recipients. The overall 10-year graft survival was approximately 50% for Asian recipients compared with 42% for HLA-mismatched Caucasian recipients (Fig. 10). Only 39 Asians (1.5%) received 0 ABDR-mismatched kidneys.

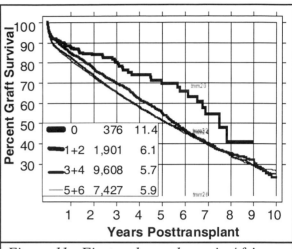

Figure 11. First cadaver donor in African American patients.

African-Americans (AA) received one-tenth as many 0 ABDR-mismatched grafts as Caucasian recipients, and correspondingly had a less stable survival curve. Zero ABDR-mismatched grafts had the highest survival rate, whereas the HLA-mismatched grafts had a 27% 10-year survival rate. Because of this lower long-term graft survival rate and the marked difference in half-life compared with Caucasians, subsequent survival rates were examined in non-African American recipients.

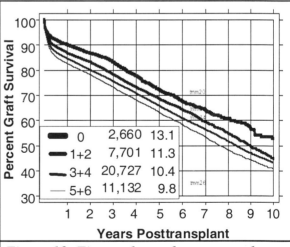

Figure 13. First cadaver donor transplants in non-African American patients.

The survival curves in Caucasian (Fig.10) and non-African American first cadaver donor transplant recipients were almost identical. The main difference was that more patients were in each category. This increased number of patients was useful in that it allowed the total to be grouped into disease categories, as shown below.

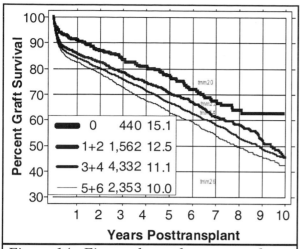

Figure 14. First cadaver donor transplants in non-AA patients with glomerulonephritis.

Glomerulonephritis patients showed an HLA-matching effect similar to the overall patient population shown in Figure 13, although the range of half-lives was larger. The result was a broader difference in long-term survival rates.

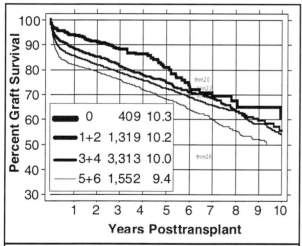

Figure 16. First cadaver donor transplants in non-AA patients with polycystic kidney disease.

Polycystic kidney disease patients showed an HLA-matching effect but differed from the previously noted diseases in that, overall, about 10% higher survival was noted in all mismatch categories. Subsequently we will show this higher graft survival rate can be attributed to a lower frequency of deaths among polycystic kidney disease patients. Presumably, systemic effects of the disease are minimal.

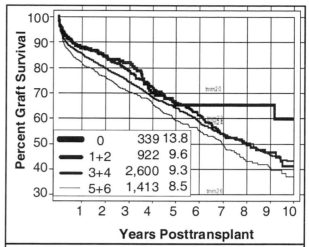

Figure 15. First cadaver donor transplants in non-AA patients with hypertensive nephritis.

Patients with hypertension showed the effect of HLA matching to a lesser degree than those recipients with glomerulonephritis, and had lower overall graft survival rates. In other words, most of the mismatch categories had similar, slightly lower graft survival rates.

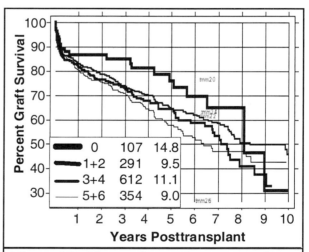

Figure 17. First cadaver donor transplants in non-AA patients with systemic lupus erythematosus.

Systemic lupus erythematosus patients showed no HLA-matching effect for the first 4 posttransplant years, except for the high graft survival rate of 0 ABDR-mismatched transplants.

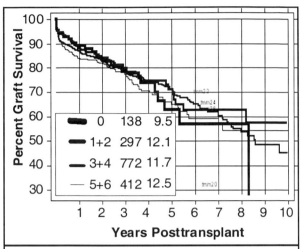

Figure 18. First cadaver donor transplants in non-AA patients with focal glomerulonephritis.

Focal glomerulonephritis patients showed only a small HLA-matching effect for 5 years. Subsequently, the small number of cases did not allow for conclusions.

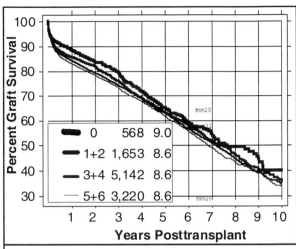

Figure 19. First cadaver donor transplants in non-AA patients with Type I diabetes.

Juvenile-onset diabetic patients had a relatively small HLA-matching effect. There was a uniformly lower overall survival rate of about 36% at 10 years compared with 40% for the worst mismatches in the combined diseases. These findings are examined more closely in Figures 42-48.

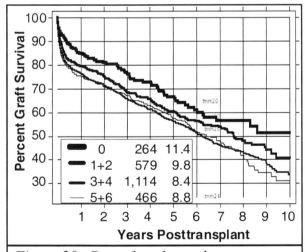

Figure 20. Regraft cadaver donor transplants in non-AA patients with glomerulonephritis.

Retransplanted glomerulonephritis patients manifested an HLA-matching effect. However, the overall graft survival rate was about 10% lower than for first grafts (Fig. 14). Note that most of this difference was evident even 6 months after transplantation.

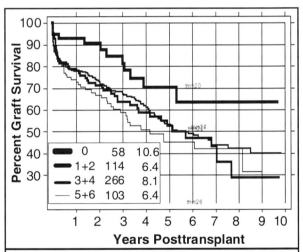

Figure 21. Regraft cadaver donor transplants in non-AA patients with hypertensive nephritis.

Regrafted patients with hypertension showed a high survival rate when given a 0 ABDR-mismatched kidney. An HLA-matching effect for the remaining patients was unclear since the number of patients available for analysis was small.

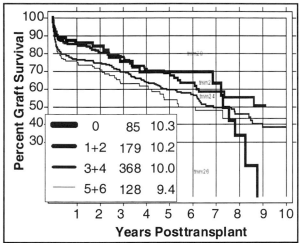

Figure 22. Regraft cadaver donor transplants in non-AA patients with polycystic kidney disease.

Retransplanted polycystic kidney disease patients showed an HLA-matching effect out to 6 years, at which time the number of transplants was too small to evaluate. Again, when compared with first grafts, the lower survival rate was apparent after 6 months.

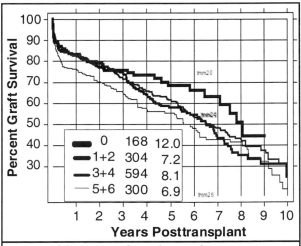

Figure 23. Regraft cadaver donor transplants in non-AA patients with Type I diabetes.

Retransplanted diabetic patients had a strong long-term HLA-matching effect, for the best and worst matches had a very wide spread of difference to 7 years. This contrasts with the smaller role of HLA matching in first grafts (Fig.19).

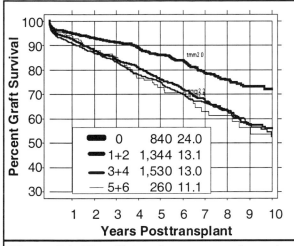

Figure 24. First living donor transplants in glomerulonephritis patients.

Glomerulonephritis patients receiving living donor transplants showed the clear superiority of 0 ABDR-mismatched transplants and almost equivalent survival rates for all other mismatch categories. There was an approximate 17% difference in graft survival at 10 years between the 0 ABDR-mismatch grafts and other mismatched groups.

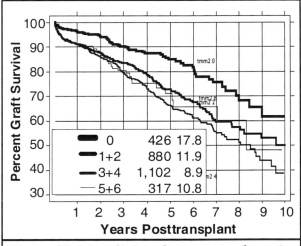

Figure 25. First living donor transplants in hypertensive nephritis patients.

Among hypertensive nephritis patients receiving living donor transplants, graft survival was clearly best for those with 0 ABDR mismatches. For the remainder, graft survival was only slightly better than for cadaver donor transplant recipients (Fig. 15).

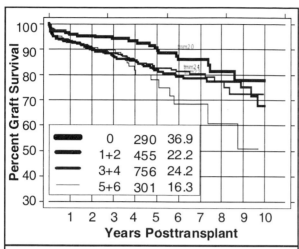

Figure 26. First living donor transplants in polycystic kidney disease.

Polycystic kidney disease patients receiving living donor transplants had an overall 20% higher 10-year survival rate than cadaver donor recipients. Zero ABDR-mismatched patients had a high 77% 10-year survival rate. The worst 5+6 mismatched patients had survival rates similar to those of the worst matched cadaver donor transplants (Fig. 16).

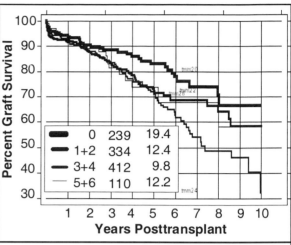

Figure 27. First living donor transplants in systemic lupus erythematosus patients.

Living donor transplants into systemic lupus erythematosus patients also showed an HLA-matching effect, but in contrast to polycystic kidney disease patients, 10-year graft survival was about 15% less in all mismatch categories. This difference probably is due to higher death rates in SLE patients shown in Figures 50 and 57.

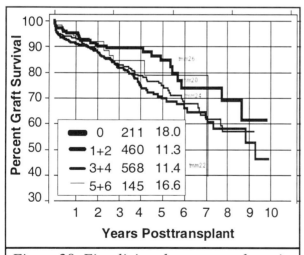

Figure 28. First living donor transplants in focal glomerulonephritis patients.

Focal glomerulonephritis patients receiving living donor transplants showed an approximate 10% superiority overall to grafts from cadaver donors (Fig. 18).

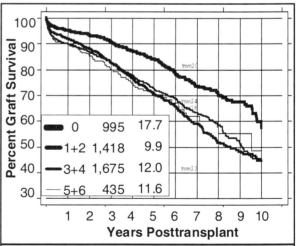

Figure 29. First living donor transplants in Type I diabetes patients.

Type I diabetes patients who received living donor transplants had about a 10% overall survival advantage over recipients of cadaver donor grafts (Fig. 19). HLA-identical donor transplants had the highest survival rate, although the 10-year survival was 60% compared with 77% survival in polycystic kidney disease patients transplanted from HLA-identical donors.

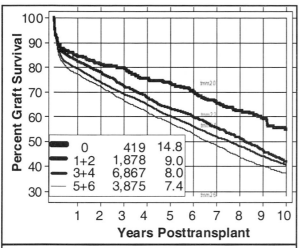

Figure 30. First cadaver donor transplants performed in 1987-1990.

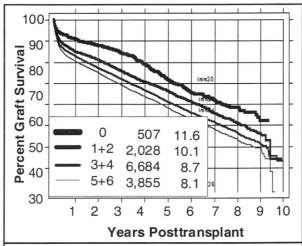

Figure 31. First cadaver donor transplants performed in 1991-1992.

There was a 17% difference in 10-year graft survival rates between the best and worst mismatches in first cadaver donor transplants performed between 1987-1990.

Transplants performed between 1990-1992 had an approximate 16% difference in 8-year graft survival. There was roughly a 10% improvement in survival in all categories over the 1987-1990 period (Fig. 30).

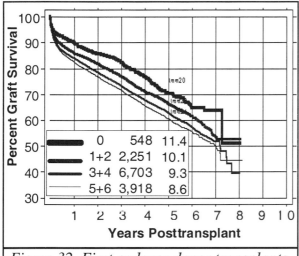

Figure 32. First cadaver donor transplants performed in 1993-1994.

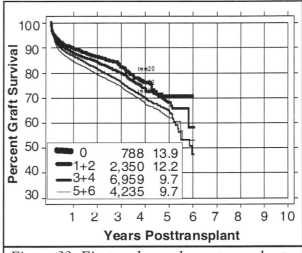

Figure 33. First cadaver donor transplants performed in 1995-1996.

The effect of HLA matching on transplants performed between 1992-1994 produced similar survival rates as were noted in the previous period. At 5 years, the difference between the best and worst mismatches was 10%.

Transplants performed between 1994-1996 had about an 8% difference in graft survival at 5 years comparing the best and worst mismatches.

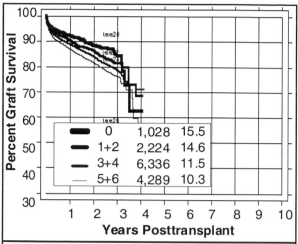

Figure 34. First cadaver donor transplants performed in 1997-1998.

Transplants that were done between 1996-1998 continued to show a matching effect with about a 10% spread in graft survival rates between best and worst mismatches at 3 years.

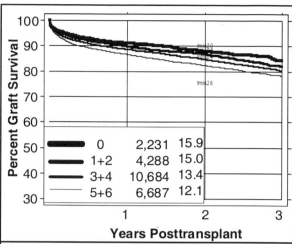

Figure 35. First cadaver donor transplants performed in non-AA after 1994.

First cadaver donor transplants performed after 1994 were pooled to examine the effect of matching in recent years. At 3 years after transplantation, they showed a 7% difference between the best and worst mismatches.

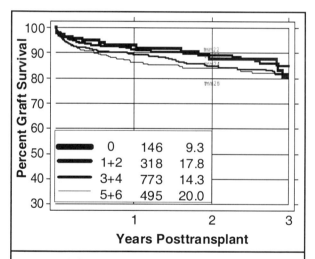

Figure 36. First cadaver donor transplants performed in non-AA after 1994 in patients with glomerulonephritis.

A reduced effect of HLA matching was noted among glomerulonephritis patients, primarily because of improved survival rates in all mismatched categories. When compared with the overall results for glomerulonephritis patients (Fig. 14), at 3 years all the mismatched categories had higher graft survival rates, whereas the survival of 0 ABDR-mismatched patients remained the same.

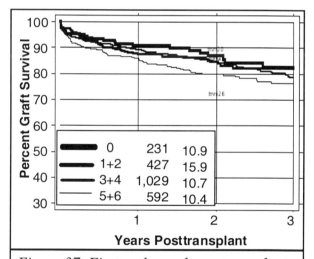

Figure 37. First cadaver donor transplants performed in non-AA after 1994 in patients with hypertensive nephritis.

Patients with hypertensive nephritis had improved 3-year survival since 1994, reaching levels of 80% at 3 years that correspondingly reduced the effect of HLA matching. Survival of 0 ABDR-mismatched patients remained the same as for those in the overall analysis (Fig. 15).

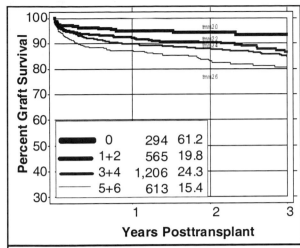

Figure 38. First cadaver donor transplants performed in non-AA after 1994 in patients with polycystic kidney disease.

Polycystic kidney disease patients with 0 ABDR mismatches showed a remarkable 93% 3-year graft survival rate with a 13% differential between the best and worst mismatches at 3 years. Thus, the effect of HLA matching remained the same as in the total file (Fig. 16).

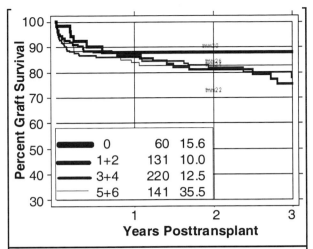

Figure 39. First cadaver donor transplants performed in non-AA after 1994 in patients with systemic lupus erythematosus.

Systemic lupus erythematosus patients showed an approximate 10% improvement in the survival rate for mismatched patients at 3 years when compared with the total file (Fig. 17).

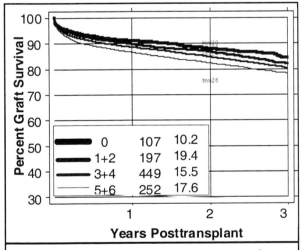

Figure 40. First cadaver donor transplants performed in non-AA after 1994 in patients with focal glomerulonephritis.

Focal glomerulonephritis patients had a 6% matching effect at 3 years. In this disease, the matching effect was more pronounced in recent transplants than in the overall analysis (Fig. 18).

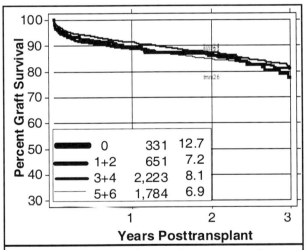

Figure 41. First cadaver donor transplants performed in non-AA after 1994 in patients with Type I diabetes.

In the recent transplants, juvenile-onset diabetic patients did not benefit from HLA matching out to 3 years. In the overall data, there was about a 7% difference between the best and the worst mismatched transplants (Fig. 19).

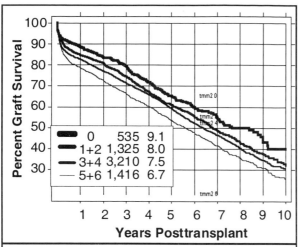

Figure 42. First cadaver donor transplants performed in non-AA after 1994 in patients with Type I diabetes who received a kidney only.

In Type 1 diabetic patients who had received only a kidney transplant, there was a clear HLA-matching effect in contrast to results in all diabetic patients (Fig. 19). The explanation for this difference is seen in the next figure.

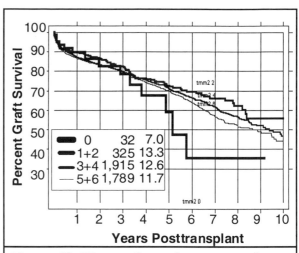

Figure 43. First cadaver donor transplants performed in non-AA after 1994 in patients with Type I diabetes with a kidney and pancreas.

Type 1 diabetic patients who were grafted with a pancreas in addition to the kidney, showed no HLA-matching effect up to 4 years. After that, some degree of matching effect was noted (except for the 7 zero ABDR mismatches). Most strikingly, 10- year graft survival was 50% compared with 30% for patients receiving only a kidney.

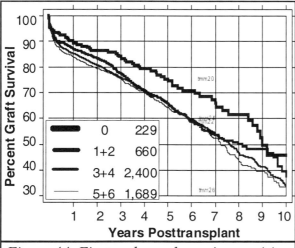

Figure 44. First cadaver donor in non-AA from donors 20-35 years of age in Type I diabetes.

Zero ABDR-mismatched donor transplants showed superior graft survival in diabetic patients out to 8 years when the cadaver donor has between the ages of 20-35. When the donor was older, this effect of zero mismatching was lost (as shown in the next figure).

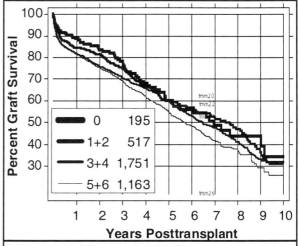

Figure 45. First cadaver donor in non-AA from donors 35-50 years of age in Type I diabetes.

When the cadaver donor was 35-50 years of age, the 0 ABDR-mismatched donor transplants had low graft survival rates. A similar result was obtained when donors were older than age 50 (data not shown).

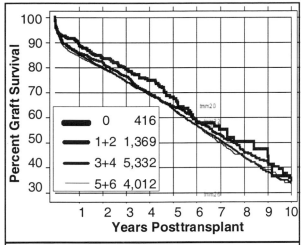

Figure 46. First cadaver donor transplants in non-AA with cold ischemia time <24 hours, in Type I diabetes.

Even when cold ischemia time was less than 24 hours, kidneys from 0 ABDR-mismatched donors did not have clearly superior graft survival rates.

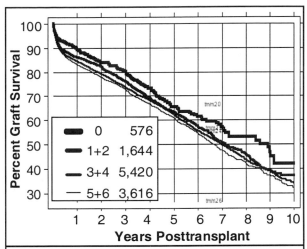

Figure 47. First cadaver donor transplants in non-AA in Type I diabetic patients with <10% PRA.

Non-sensitized diabetic patients (with PRA <10%) showed a small HLA-matching effect.

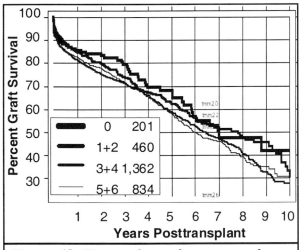

Figure 48. First cadaver donor transplants in non-AA in Type I diabetic patients with >10% PRA.

Diabetic patients who were sensitized (with PRA >10%) had a slightly lower initial graft survival than non-sensitized patients (Fig. 47), and had a small HLA-matching effect.

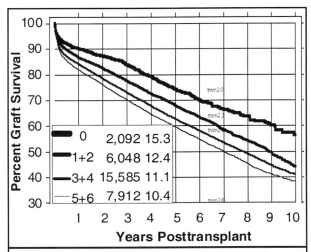

Figure 49. First cadaver donor transplants in non-AA in patients without Type I diabetes.

When diabetic patients were excluded, the overall HLA-matching effect was increased. The survival rate of the zero mismatched transplants was 57% compared with 53% in the total file (Fig. 13). The difference between the 10-year graft survival rates of the best and worst matched grafts was almost 20%.

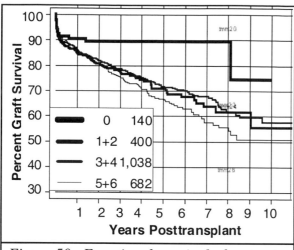

Figure 50. Functional survival of systemic lupus erythematosus patients.

When patient deaths were censored, the functional graft survival rate among non-AA first cadaver transplant recipients with systemic lupus erythematosus was about 10% higher than graft survival rates including deaths as a graft loss (Fig. 17). Zero mismatched transplants had decidedly higher graft survival rates.

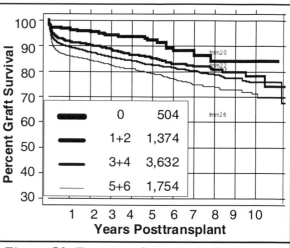

Figure 51. Functional survival of polycystic kidney disease patients.

Functional graft survival rates in non-AA first cadaver transplants with polycystic kidney disease were about 10% higher than the graft survival rates counting death as a graft loss (Fig. 16). The HLA-matching effect was maintained when analyzing functional survival.

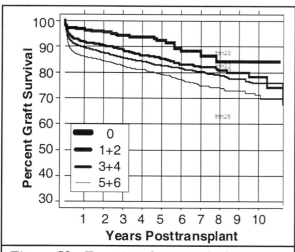

Figure 52. Functional survival of Type I diabetes patients.

The functional graft survival rate was much higher for diabetics than conventional graft survival when deaths were censored. The HLA-matching effect on functional survival was pronounced. Zero mismatched transplants had an 84% 10-year functional graft survival rate compared with 40% when deaths were included. Even the worst mismatches resulted in a 70% functional survival rate compared with 35% graft survival at 10 years.

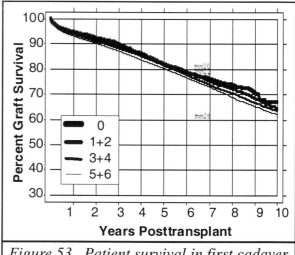

Figure 53. Patient survival in first cadaver donor transplants.

At 10 years, there was a 5% difference in patient survival rates between the best and worst mismatched first cadaver donor transplant recipients. Overall, about 65% of the patients survived to 10 years.

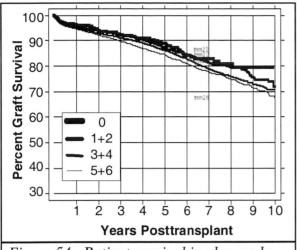

Figure 54. Patient survival in glomerulo-nephritis patients receiving a first cadaver donor transplant.

Patient survival for glomerulonephritis patients was higher than the overall patient survival rate (Fig. 53). The matching effect appears to increase with time.

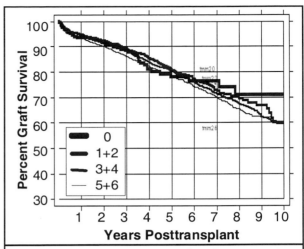

Figure 55. Patient survival in hypertensive nephritis patients receiving a first cadaver donor transplant.

Long-term patient survival in recipients with hypertensive nephritis was influenced by HLA matching.

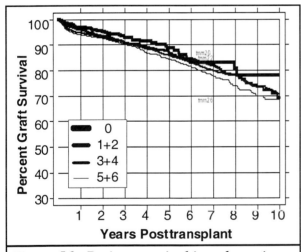

Figure 56. Patient survival in polycystic kidney disease patients receiving a first cadaver donor transplant.

Patient survival in polycystic kidney disease patients was also affected by HLA matching in the long term.

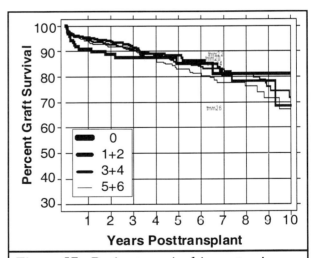

Figure 57. Patient survival in systemic lupus erythematosus patients receiving a first cadaver donor transplant.

Patient survival in recipients with systemic lupus erythematosus was higher than the overall patient survival rate. Zero-ABDR mismatched grafts did not improve patient survival.

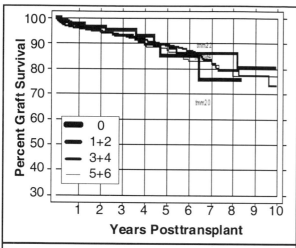

Figure 58. Patient survival in focal glomerulonephritis patients receiving a first cadaver donor transplant.

Patient survival in recipients with focal glomerulonephritis was about 80% at 10 years. It should be noted that patient survival includes survival after returning to dialysis as well as survival following transplantation.

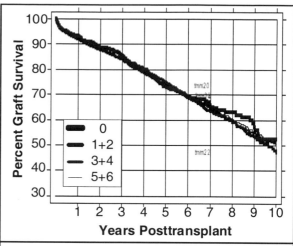

Figure 59. Patient survival in Type I diabetes patients receiving a first cadaver donor transplant.

Patient survival in Type 1 diabetics was the lowest among all the major diseases. Overall, only 50% of diabetics survived 10 years. The higher death rate is responsible for the lower graft survival rate among diabetics (Fig. 52).

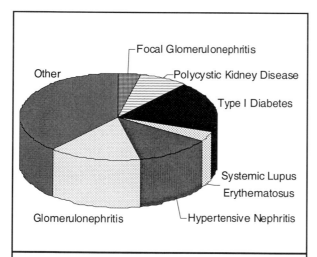

Figure 60. Distribution of disease classifications.

Percentage of transplanted patients classified according to their diseases. The 3 major disease categories are: glomerulonephritis, Type 1 diabetes, and hypertensive nephritis.

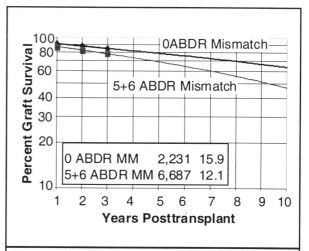

Figure 61. Projected HLA matching effect in non-AA patients based on transplants performed since 1994.

For 0 ABDR-mismatched transplants, the projected 10-year graft survival rate is 64% and for the 5+6 ABDR mismatched transplants it is 47%, a 17% differential. Despite the high initial survival rate in the first few years, the HLA-matching effect has a slightly greater effect than in the data based on transplants since 1987, when the zero mismatched graft had a 53% 10-year graft survival rate and the worst mismatches had a 37% graft survival rate, a difference of 16% (Fig. 1).

DISCUSSION

Recipients of HLA-matched first cadaver donor transplants between 1987-1990 had an overall 10-year graft survival rate of 53%, compared with 37% for recipients of 5-6 HLA-ABDR-mismatched transplants – a 16% survival difference between the best and worst HLA-mismatched patients (Fig. 1). Among patients transplanted since 1994 (Fig. 35), the difference was 7% at 3 years. When these recent transplant survival rates are projected out to 10 years, the HLA-matched transplants had an improved 64% survival rate compared with 47% survival for the 5-6 antigen mismatched transplants – a 17% difference (Fig. 61) which was not different from the experience during 1987-1990. Thus, despite overall higher graft survival, the long-term HLA-matching effect has not changed in recent years.

Considering living donor transplants, HLA-matched grafts showed a 68% 10-year graft survival rate whereas the worst mismatches resulted in a 50% 10-year survival rate. Thus, the worst matched living donor grafts provided survival rates similar to the best matched cadaver donor grafts.

Because the worst matched African-American (AA) cadaver donor transplants had a 10-year survival rate of approximately 26% (Fig. 11) compared with 40% for poorly matched Caucasian patients (Fig. 10), the bulk of the analyses reported in this chapter were performed on non-AA patients.

To our knowledge, there are no published studies on the effect of HLA matching with respect to the original diseases. Most impressive was the finding that first cadaver donor transplant recipients with juvenile onset diabetes had only a small 5% survival difference between the best-to-worst mismatched grafts (Fig. 19). Moreover, in transplants performed since 1994 (Fig. 41), there was no HLA-matching effect. Overall, at 10 years, Type I diabetics had about a 10% lower graft survival rate than recipients with other diseases. When graft survival of kidney-only transplants (excluding simultaneous pancreas-kidney transplants) was examined, however, a strong matching effect was noted (Fig. 42). Transplants with both a kidney and pancreas resulted in a high graft survival, with no effect of HLA matching, at least for the first 4 years (Fig. 43). Thus, the overall combination of diabetic patients with and without a pancreas results in an overall survival with no HLA-matching effect as shown in Figure 19.

Simultaneous pancreas-kidney transplants had a very strong effect in improving overall survival, for at 3 years there was an 80% graft survival rate compared with 66-70% survival for the poorly matched kidneys transplanted without a pancreas. It remains to be seen whether simultaneous pancreas transplants require no HLA matching. The long-term matching effect after 4 years could be the result of either the matching effect becoming apparent later, or transplants performed more than 4 years ago showing the effect.

The effectiveness of HLA matching among Type I diabetics is apparent when we plot the functional survival, which excludes deaths as "lost-to-follow-up" (Fig. 52). There was a 15% difference between survival of the best and worst mismatched patients at 10 years. Higher mortality among Type 1 diabetics is reflected in their lowest patient survival rate compared with other diseases studied here (Fig. 59). Retransplanted Type 1 diabetic patients also showed some effect of HLA matching.

Among Type I diabetics, although 0 ABDR-mismatched transplants had a higher graft survival rate when the cadaver donor was aged 25-35 (Fig. 44), the advantage of good matching was lost when the donor was older than 35. Even the use of kidneys with less than 24 hours of cold ischemia time did not improve graft survival in Type 1 diabetics.

The highest 10-year graft survival in Type 1 diabetics (60%) was obtained with HLA-identical living donor grafts.

First cadaver donor graft recipients with focal glomerulonephritis did not show any HLA-matching effect in the overall data. However, there was a small 6% difference in transplants performed since 1994 (Fig. 40). Focal glomerulonephritis patients who received living donor grafts also showed some HLA-matching effect.

Among patients with other diseases, the matching effect was apparent in first cadaver grafts, regrafts, and living donor grafts. Polycystic kidney disease patients were remarkable in that their survival rates were about 10% higher at 10 years than recipients with other diseases.

SUMMARY

1. The HLA-matching effect in Type I diabetic patients applied only to those receiving a kidney alone. Those receiving simultaneous pancreas transplants did not benefit significantly from HLA-matching, although graft survival was high. Nevertheless, an HLA-matching effect could be shown for grafts from cadaver donors who were 25-35 years of age. Grafts from older donors apparently were more vulnerable to diabetic complications. The highest graft survival in diabetic patients was obtained with HLA-identical living donor grafts - 60% at 10 years, which was in marked contrast to the 35% survival rate of HLA-mismatched cadaver donor grafts.

2. Functional graft survival analysis (censoring deaths) of Type 1 diabetics showed that graft survival was low because of deaths, presumably resulting from diabetic complications.

3. The HLA-matching effect was modest for focal glomerulonephritis patients. However, a small HLA-matching effect was noted in retransplants from cadaver donors and grafts from living donors.

4. Patients with polycystic kidney disease had the highest overall graft survival rates in all HLA-mismatch categories. Zero-ABDR-mismatched first cadaver transplants had a 60% ten-year survival rate and a 78% survival rate from HLA-identical living donors.

5. Patient survival in all the disease groups was not affected by HLA matching. Graft failure and return to dialysis apparently did not affect survival of patients.

6. Overall graft survival rates have improved markedly with newer immunosuppressants and improved patient care. The 3-year graft survival rate for the worst mismatches improved from 67% in 1987-90 to 73% for 1990-92 transplants to 73% for 1992-94, 78% for 1994-96, and 80% for transplants performed in 1996-98.

7. Projected 10-year graft survival for patients transplanted since 1994 was 64% for 0-HLA-mismatched grafts and 47% for 5-6 antigen-mismatched transplants – a 17% differential. Thus, despite newer immunosuppression, HLA matching continues to be an important factor.

WORLD TRANSPLANT RECORDS - 2000

Patients Who Currently Have Functioning Transplants

KIDNEY (LIVING-RELATED)

	TX DATE	NAME	TX AGE	CURR AGE	YEARS CONT'D FUNCTION	CURRENT FUNCTION (SCr)	CENTER

Longest Surviving First Living-Related Renal Allograft:

	TX DATE	NAME	TX AGE	CURR AGE	YEARS CONT'D FUNCTION	CURRENT FUNCTION (SCr)	CENTER
1	10/9/59	C.H.	12	53	41yrs, 2mos	0.9	Oregon Health Sci Univ
2	1/31/63	R.P.	38	75	37yrs,11mos	1.3	Univ Colorado-Denver
3	7/19/63	D.H.	15	52	37yrs, 5mos	0.9	Univ Colorado-Denver
4	10/7/63	N.W.	18	55	37yrs, 2mos	1.0	Univ Colorado-Denver
5	11/13/63	R.R	17	54	37yrs, 1mo	1.2	Univ Colorado-Denver
6	12/27/63	R.J.	8	75	37yrs, -	functng	Univ Minnesota-Mnpls
7	2/10/64	J.W.	18	54	36yrs,10mos	1.6	Univ Colorado-Denver
7	2/17/64	S.H.	15	51	36yrs,10mos	0.9	Univ Colorado-Denver
7	2/22/64	D.M.	15	51	36yrs,10mos	1.7	Univ Colorado-Denver
8	3/3/64	J.N.	32	68	36yrs, 9mos	functng	Univ Colorado-Denver
9	7/8/64	K.S	20	56	36yrs, 5mos	functng	Univ Minnesota-Mnpls
10	10/12/64	M.M.	34	70	36yrs, 2mos	1.0	Univ Colorado-Denver
11	1/26/65	D.S.	24	58	35yrs,11mos	1.6	Univ Minnesota-Mnpls
12	5/25/65	V.B.	33	68	35yrs, 7mos	1.1	Clinic St Luc-Brussels
13	6/15/65	K.A.	28	60	35yrs, 6mos	functng	Univ Minnesota-Mnpls
14	9/7/65	J.M.	—	—	35yrs, 3mos	functng	Univ Colorado-Denver
15	2/15/66	H.M.	22	57	34yrs,10mos	1	U Pennsylvania-Phila
16	3/2/66	C.M.	24	58	34yrs, 9mos	functng	Mayo Clinic-Rochester
16	3/18/66	L.S.	—	—	34yrs, 9mos	functng	Univ Colorado-Denver
17	4/27/66	K.E.	—	—	34yrs, 8mos	functng	Univ Colorado-Denver
18	6/21/66	C.C	—	—	34yrs, 6mos	functng	Univ Colorado-Denver
19	7/1/66	R.H.	31	65	34yrs, 5mos	1.0	Univ Colorado-Denver
19	7/29/66	L.N.	24	58	34yrs, 5mos	1.1	Univ Colorado-Denver
20	9/13/66	M.B.	—	—	34yrs, 3mos	functng	Univ Colorado-Denver
20	9/13/66	E.L.	44	78	34yrs, 3mos	func/alive	Sahlgrenska U-Goteborg
21	10/19/66	J.N.	—	—	34yrs, 2mos	functng	Univ Colorado-Denver
22	11/11/66	R.B.	—	—	34yrs, 1mo	functng	Univ Colorado-Denver
22	11/15/66	M.S.	26	60	34yrs, 1mo	0.9	Univ Wisconsin-Madison
23	12/12/66	C.S.	—	—	34yrs, -	functng	Univ Colorado-Denver
23	12/16/66	I.T.	—	—	34yrs, -	functng	Univ Colorado-Denver
24	1/3/67	R.D.	68	101	33yrs,11mos	1.0	Univ Wisconsin-Madison
24	1/4/67	T.T	26	59	33yrs,11mos	functng	Univ Minnesota-Mnpls
25	2/21/67	L.O.	14	47	33yrs,10mos	1.3	Univ Wisconsin-Madison
25	2/3/67	M.S.	11	45	33yrs,10mos	1.5	Helsinki Univ-Finland
26	6/1/67	J.G.	55	88	33yrs, 6mos	1.0	Univ Wisconsin-Madison
27	7/14/67	R.P.	24	57	33yrs, 5mos	functng	Univ Minnesota-Mnpls
28	9/13/67	C.H.	21	54	33yrs, 3mos	1.6	Cleveland Clinic
29	10/16/67	K.H.	10	43	33yrs, 2mos	1.0	Children's-Cincinnati
30	11/1/67	D.L.	28	61	33yrs, 1mo	functng	Univ Minnesota-Mnpls

	TX DATE	NAME	TX AGE	CURR AGE	YEARS CONT'D FUNCTION	CURRENT FUNCTION (SCr)	CENTER
30	11/17/67	C.O.	22	55	33yrs, 1mo	functng	Univ Minnesota-Mnpls
31	3/7/68	T.R.	24	55	32yrs, 9mos	1.1	Helsinki Univ-Finland
32	4/1/68	M.G.	33	64	32yrs, 8mos	0.8	FMUSP-Sao Paulo
33	5/15/68	P.K.	20	52	32yrs, 7mos	1.0	Cleveland Clinic
34	6/4/68	J.T.	40	72	32yrs, 6mos	0.9	Oregon Health Sci Univ
35	7/18/68	K.K.	22	53	32yrs, 5mos	functng	Univ Minnesota-Mnpls
36	9/19/68	G.M.	19	51	32yrs, 3mos	1.8	Montefiore Med Ctr-Bronx
36	9/24/68	P.Q.	25	57	32yrs, 3mos	1.7	Univ Wisconsin-Madison
37	10/22/68	N.O.	33	65	32yrs, 2mos	2.1	Univ Wisconsin-Madison
38	11/14/68	G.S.	32	64	32yrs, 1mo	functng	Univ Minnesota-Mnpls
39	1/20/69	J.P.	20	52	31yrs,11mos	functng	Univ Minnesota-Mnpls
40	2/6/69	P.K.	25	56	31yrs,10mos	0.7	Helsinki Univ-Finland
41	4/17/69	E.E.	17	48	31yrs, 8mos	1.4	Cleveland Clinic
42	10/16/69	W.G.	26	56	31yrs, 2mos	1.0	Montefiore Med Ctr-Bronx
42	10/28/69	J.A.	25	57	31yrs, 2mos	1.7	Univ Florida-Gainesville
43	12/11/69	D.S.	29	60	31yrs, -	1.2	Univ Hosp-Cincinnati
43	12/22/69	C.L.	17	48	31yrs, -	functng	Univ Minnesota-Mnpls
44	2/10/70	J.P.	37	63	30yrs,10mos	3.1	Cleveland Clinic
44	2/11/70	T.P.	30	60	30yrs,10mos	functng	Univ Minnesota-Mnpls
45	4/2/70	K.A.	43	73	30yrs, 8mos	1.4	Helsinki Univ-Finland
45	4/10/70	S.J.	4	34	30yrs, 8mos	functng	Univ Minnesota-Mnpls
45	4/14/70	D.M.	25	55	30yrs, 8mos	1.7	Cleveland Clinic
45	4/23/70	A.T.	22	52	30yrs, 8mos	0.8	Helsinki Univ-Finland
46	7/3/70	J.O	18	48	30yrs, 5mos	1.0	Univ Wisconsin-Madison
46	7/6/70	K.O.	26	56	30yrs, 5mos	1.2	Nat'l Defense Hosp-Japan
46	7/14/70	J.R.	22	52	30yrs, 5mos	1.5	Cleveland Clinic
47	9/8/70	D.H.	36	66	30yrs, 3mos	0.9	Oregon Health Sci Univ
47	9/17/70	J.P.	29	59	30yrs, 3mos	0.9	Hennepin Cnty M C-Mnpls
47	9/17/70	R.L.	31	63	30yrs, 3mos	functng	Univ Minnesota-Mnpls
48	10/8/70	J.H	33	63	30yrs, 2mos	functng	Univ Minnesota-Mnpls
49	11/10/70	E.E.	14	44	30yrs, 1mo	1.0	Cleveland Clinic
49	11/17/70	W.M.	51	81	30yrs, 1mo	1.4	Cleveland Clinic
50	12/4/70	C.B.	39	58	30yrs, -	1.7	Hennepin Cnty M C-Mnpls
51	1/6/71	W.F.	27	56	29yrs,11mos	1.2	Univ Florida-Gainesville
52	2/23/71	H.H.	48	78	29yrs,10mos	1.9	Yale University-Conn
53	3/30/71	L.B.	15	44	29yrs, 9mos	1.2	Univ Florida-Gainesville
53	3/18/71	A.H.	12	41	29yrs, 9mos	func/alive	Sahlgrenska U-Goteborg
54	4/20/71	D.M.	18	47	29yrs, 8mos	1.0	Univ Florida-Gainesville
55	10/28/71	J.O.	56	85	29yrs, 2mos	func/alive	Sahlgrenska U-Goteborg
56	4/28/72	T.Z.	8	36	28yrs, 8mos	0.8	Health Sci Ctr, Winnipeg-Canada
57	5/12/72	L.P.	21	49	28yrs, 7mos	0.9	Health Sci Ctr, Winnipeg-Canada
57	5/15/72	A.S.	21	49	28yrs, 7mos	1.5	Oregon Health Sci Univ
57	5/31/72	L.L.	25	52	28yrs, 7mos	0.9	Vanderbilt U-Nashville
58	8/7/72	P.S.	38	66	28yrs, 4mos	0.9	Oregon Health Sci Univ
58	8/18/72	C.R.	23	51	28yrs, 4mos	0.9	Health Sci Ctr, Winnipeg-Canada
58	8/21/72	J.W.	24	52	28yrs, 4mos	1.1	Oregon Health Sci Univ

	TX DATE	NAME	TX AGE	CURR AGE	YEARS CONT'D FUNCTION	CURRENT FUNCTION (SCr)	CENTER
59	9/7/72	P.H.	21	49	28yrs, 3mos	0.8	Vanderbilt U-Nashville
60	11/7/72	J.B.	40	68	28yrs, 1mo	1.2	Univ Florida-Gainesville
60	11/14/72	C.M.	21	49	28yrs, 1mo	2.5	Univ Florida-Gainesville
61	?/?/72	E.B.	38	67	28yrs, -	2.6	Fundacion Jimendez Diaz
62	1/22/73	D.E.	10	37	27yrs,11mos	1.3	Oregon Health Sci Univ
63	2/15/73	G.M.	54	81	27yrs,10mos	0.5	Univ Hosp-Cincinnati
64	6/6/73	B.P.	24	51	27yrs, 6mos	1.8	Laikon Gen Hosp-Greece
65	6/19/73	S.E.	35	63	27yrs, 6mos	1.2	CEMIC-Buenos Aires
65	7/5/73	F.G.	24	51	27yrs, 5mos	1.9	Univ Hosp-Cincinnati
65	7/23/73	N.B.	34	61	27yrs, 5mos	1.3	Oregon Health Sci Univ
66	8/1/73	W.T.	21	49	27yrs, 4mos	1.2	So ILL Univ-Springfield
67	9/25/73	A.B.	25	52	27yrs, 3mos	1.2	Univ Florida-Gainesville
68	10/29/73	P.C.	22	49	27yrs, 2mos	2.0	Oregon Health Sci Univ
69	11/20/73	L.C.	43	70	27yrs, 1mo	0.8	Univ Florida-Gainesville
70	12/4/73	C.H.	41	68	27yrs, -	1.0	Univ Florida-Gainesville
70	12/11/73	W.B.	38	45	27yrs, -	2.2	Univ Florida-Gainesville
71	1/15/74	D.D.	38	65	26yrs,11mos	1	Florida Hosp Med Ctr
72	3/20/74	F.P.	32	58	26yrs, 9mos	1.5	Policlinico Univ-Milan
73	7/5/74	M.G.	25	51	26yrs, 5mos	2.5	Oregon Health Sci Univ
74	1/11/77	I.S.	39	58	23yrs,11mos	1.1	Auxilio Mutuo Hosp-PR
75	3/3/77	D.G.	39	62	23yrs, 9mos	2.4	Univ Hosp-Cincinnati
76	12/15/77	R.S.	26	48	23yrs, -	1.3	Univ Hosp-Cincinnati
77	3/22/79	M.B.	36	58	21yrs, 9mos	1.1	Univ Hosp-Cincinnati
78	9/4/79	L.L.	9	30	21yrs, 3mos	1.7	Hosp Infantil La Fe-Valencia

Youngest Recipient With Surviving Living-Related Renal Allograft:

	TX DATE	NAME	TX AGE	CURR AGE	YEARS CONT'D FUNCTION	CURRENT FUNCTION (SCr)	CENTER
1	6/10/82	A.H.	6mos	18	18yrs, 6mos	functng	Univ Minnesota-Mnpls
1	12/21/82	T.G.	6mos	18	18yrs, -	functng	Univ Minnesota-Mnpls
1	12/3/86	J.D,	6mos	13	14yrs, -	functng	Univ Minnesota-Mnpls
1	1/14/93	M.L.	6mos	8	7yrs,11mos	1.1	Univ Pittsburgh
2	12/13/88	B.C.	7mos	12	12yrs, -	1.1	Univ Pittsburgh
2	4/18/95	J.V.	7mos	6	5yrs, 8mos	0.8	Univ Pittsburgh
0	3/20/99	M.D.	9mos	2	1yr, 3mos	0.3	St Francis Med Ctr-ILL
4	10/31/88	E.L.	12mos	13	12yrs, 1mo	1.2	Montefiore Med Ctr-Bronx
5	6/4/84	J.S.	16mos	16	16yrs, 6mos	1.9	Montefiore Med Ctr-Bronx
5	9/21/94	C.S.	16mos	7	6yrs, 3mos	func/alive	Sahlgrenska U-Goteborg
6	10/17/95	T.A.	18mos	6	5yrs, 2mos	0.7	Univ Florida-Gainesville
6	2/13/96	R.D.	18mos	6	4yrs,10mos	0.6	Univ Pittsburgh
6	12/29/97	E.F.	18mos	4	3yrs, -	0.5	St Francis Med Ctr-ILL
7	11/29/85	T.G.	22mos	16	15yrs, 1mo	1.0	Univ Wisconsin-Madison
8	7/27/91	J.R.	2yrs	11	9yrs, 5mos	0.7	Auxilio Mutuo Hosp-PR
8	11/5/84	L.M.	2yrs	17	16yrs, 1mo	1.7	Montefiore Med Ctr-Bronx
8	10/21/86	A.D.	2yrs	16	14yrs, -	3.0	Montefiore Med Ctr-Bronx
8	11/9/93	W.R.	2yrs	8	7yrs, 1mo	1.3	Montefiore Med Ctr-Bronx
8	8/1/94	K.H.	2yrs	7	6yrs, 4mos	1.4	Montefiore Med Ctr-Bronx
9	7/31/96	J.S.	3yrs	6	4yrs, 5mos	1.9	Montefiore Med Ctr-Bronx

TX DATE	NAME	TX AGE	CURR AGE	YEARS CONT'D FUNCTION	CURRENT FUNCTION (SCr)	CENTER

Oldest Living Related-Renal Allograft Donor:

	TX DATE	NAME	TX AGE	CURR AGE	YEARS CONT'D FUNCTION	CURRENT FUNCTION (SCr)	CENTER
1	5/11/98	F.B.	52	81yr mother	2yrs, 7mos	0.9	Sao Paulo Hosp
2	9/29/99	A.D.	53	78yrs donor	1yr, 3mos	2.5	Med Univ Luebeck-Germany
2	12/5/99	W.	77	78yrs donor	1yr, -	good	Univ of San Francisco
2	2/9/00	E.	74	78yrs donor	-,10mos	good	Univ of San Francisco
3	12/20/96	B.R.		74yr mother	4yrs, -	functng	Univ Minnesota-Mnpls
4	12/3/91	S.S.		72yr father	9yrs, -	functng	Univ Minnesota-Mnpls
5	11/17/93	A.I.	38	71yr parent	7yrs, 1mo	2.7	Kakegawa City GH-Japan
5	3/28/90	E.M.		71yr father	10yrs, 9mos	functng	Univ Minnesota-Mnpls
5	4/25/84	S.E.	41	71yr donor	16yrs, 8mos	2.4	Med College of Georgia
5	10/24/94	T.Y.	50	71yr donor	6yrs, 2mos	4.4	Nagasaki Univ Sch of Med
6	5/24/93	M.Y.	41	70yr mother	7yrs, 7mos	1.2	Hamamatsu Univ-Japan
6	5/23/95	R.B.		70yr mother	5yrs, 7mos	functng	Univ Minnesota-Mnpls
6	10/1/92	D.J.		70yr father	8yrs, 2mos	functng	Univ Minnesota-Mnpls
7	11/7/91	M.B.	44	69yr parent	9yrs, 1mo	alive/well	Montefiore Med Ctr-Bronx
7	1/23/95	H.G	37	69yr father	5yrs,11mos	0.5	Ege Univ Med Sch-Turkey
8	10/5/93	T.A.	41	68yr parent	7yrs, 2mos	3.8	Kakegawa City GH-Japan
8	1/25/89	D.P.		68yr mother	11yrs,11mos	functng	Univ Minnesota-Mnpls
8	5/7/97	K.I.		68yr HLA-ID sib	3yrs, 7mos	functng	Univ Minnesota-Mnpls
8	1/18/93	S.M.	38	68yr father	7yrs,11mos	1.0	Hamamatsu Univ-Japan
9	8/24/92	K.F.	40	65yr father	8yrs, 4mos	1.5	Hamamatsu Univ-Japan

Longest Surviving Second Living-Related Renal Allograft:

	TX DATE	NAME	TX AGE	CURR AGE	YEARS CONT'D FUNCTION	CURRENT FUNCTION (SCr)	CENTER
1	3/3/64	J.N.	32	68	36yrs, 9mos	functng	Univ Colorado-Denver
2	8/12/70	W.J.	20	50	30yrs, 4mos	functng	Univ Minnesota-Mnpls
3	6/28/77	B.L.	36	59	23yrs, 6mos	1.3	Univ Florida-Gainesville

Longest Surviving Third Living-Related Renal Allograft:

	TX DATE	NAME	TX AGE	CURR AGE	YEARS CONT'D FUNCTION	CURRENT FUNCTION (SCr)	CENTER
1	9/20/83	L.U.	22	39	17yrs, 3mos	0.9	Univ Florida-Gainesville
2	11/9/83	D.L.	30		17yrs, 1mo	functng	Univ Minnesota-Mnpls
3	7/29/87	J.F.	36	49	13yrs, 5mos	3.3	Univ Florida-Gainesville

Smallest Recipient to Receive Living-Related Renal Allograft:

	TX DATE	NAME	TX AGE	CURR AGE	YEARS CONT'D FUNCTION	CURRENT FUNCTION (SCr)	CENTER
1	6/10/82	A.H.	6mos	18	5.5kg (11.1lbs)	functng	Univ Minnesota-Mnpls
2	12/3/86	J.D.	6mos	14	6.2kg (13.6lbs)	functng	Univ Minnesota-Mnpls
3	12/21/82	T.G.	6mos	18	7.1kg (15.7lbs)	functng	Univ Minnesota-Mnpls

Smallest Recipient to Receive Living-Related Second Renal Allograft:

	TX DATE	NAME	TX AGE	CURR AGE	YEARS CONT'D FUNCTION	CURRENT FUNCTION (SCr)	CENTER
1	12/13/94	S.B.	2	8	6yrs, -	0.9	Univ Pittsburgh
2	2/23/87	C.R.	4yrs, 10kg(22lbs)	18	13yrs,10mos	1.3	Montefiore Med Ctr-Bronx

Oldest Surviving Living-Related Kidney:

	TX DATE	NAME	YEARS CONT'D FUNCTION	CURRENT FUNCTION (SCr)	CENTER
1	9/18/68	G.M. father (donor) 65yrs at Tx.			
		Kidney is now 97yrs old.	32yrs, 3mos	1.8	Montefiore Med Ctr-Bronx
2	4/11/69	V.B. mother(donor) 63yrs at Tx.			
		Kidney is now 94yrs old.	31yrs, 8mos	functng	Mayo Clinic-Rochester
3	2/10/64	J.W. aunt(donor) 58yrs at Tx.			
		Kidney is now 94yrs old.	36yrs,10mos	functng	Univ Colorado-Denver

	TX DATE	NAME	TX AGE	CURR AGE	YEARS CONT'D FUNCTION	CURRENT FUNCTION (SCr)	CENTER
4	11/17/67	C.O. father (donor) 58yrs at Tx.					
		Kidney is now 91yrs old.			33yrs, 1mo	funcntg	Univ Minnesota-Mnpls
5	5/30/72	M.H. donor 60yr old at Tx.					
		Kidney is now 88yrs old.			28yrs, 7mos	1.5	Civile Maggiore-Verona
6	1/26/65	D.S. mother (donor) 52yrs old at Tx.					
		Kidney is now 87yrs old.			35yrs,11mos	functng	Univ Minnesota-Mnpls
7	10/28/71	J.O. donor 54yrs at Tx.					
		Kidney is now 83yrs old.			29yrs, 2mos	func/alive	Sahlgrenska U-Goteborg
8	9/6/89	L.L. mother (donor) 69yrs at Tx.					
		Kidney is now 80yrs old.			11yrs, 3mos	2.3	Auxilio Mutuo Hosp-PR
9	7/16/76	A.V. donor 56yrs at Tx.					
		Kidney is now 80yrs old.			24yrs, -	1.1	Policlinico Univ-Milan
10	11/14/72	C.M. donor 50yr old at Tx.					
		Kidney is now 78yrs old.			28yrs, 1mo	2.5	Univ Florida-Gainesville
10	5/21/92	N.T. donor 70yr old at Tx.					
		Kidney is now 78yrs old.			8yrs, 7mos	4.5	Oyokyo Kidney Rsch Inst
10	11/7/91	M.B. mother (donor) 69yrs old at Tx.					
		Kidney is now 78yrs old.			9yrs, 1mo	1.7	Montefiore Med Ctr-Bronx
11	4/20/71	D.M. donor 48yr old at Tx.					
		Kidney is now 77yrs old.			29yrs, 8mos	1.0	Univ Florida-Gainesville
12	8/22/95	T.P. mother (donor) 71yrs old at Tx.					
		Kidney is now 76yrs old.			5yrs, 4mos	1.6	Oregon Health Sci Univ
13	3/22/94	B.S. mother (donor) 69yrs old at Tx.					
		Kidney is now 75yrs old.			6yrs, 9mos	1.8	Policlinico Univ-Milan

Longest Surviving Living-Related ABO Incompatible Renal Transplant Recipient:

1	11/11/82	D.S. rcv'd an ABO incompatible kidney from her mother.					
			13		18yrs, 1mo	1.0	Clinic St Luc-Brussels

Longest Surviving Living-Related Renal Allograft Without Immunosuppression:

1	1/31/63	R.P.	38	75	37yrs,11mos	functng	Univ Colorado-Denver
2	7/19/63	D.S.	16	53	37yrs, 5mos	functng	Univ Colorado-Denver
3	2/10/64	J.W.	15	52	36yrs,10mos	functng	Univ Colorado-Denver
4	3/3/64	J.N.	32	68	36yrs, 9mos	functng	Univ Colorado-Denver
5	1/17/72	F.A.	29	57	28yrs,11mos	0.8	Civile Maggiore-Verona
6	8/28/72	M.M.	18	46	28yrs, 4mos	0.7	Inst Nacional de Ciencias Medicas
7	5/22/74	M.N.	30	56	26yrs, 7mos	1.3	Civile Maggiore-Verona

Longest Uninterrupted Wait For First Living-Related Renal Allograft

1	2/27/87	M.V. 15yrs, 8mos wait for a suitable donor (father)					
			32	46	13yrs,10mos	1.2	Policlinico Univ-Milan

Longest Surviving Living-Related Transplant Recipients with an Original Systemic Disease that may reoccur
Systemic Lupus Erythematosus

1	6/24/76	J.G.	42	66	24yrs, 6mos	0.8	Univ Hosp-Cincinnati

Diabetes Mellitus

1	3/18/75	C.W.	31	56	25yrs, 9mos	1.1	Univ Florida-Gainesville

TX DATE	NAME	TX AGE	CURR AGE	YEARS CONT'D FUNCTION	CURRENT FUNCTION (SCr)	CENTER

Longest Surviving Cadaver Renal Allograft Recipients with Original Systemic Disease That May Reoccur:

Diabetes Mellitus

	TX DATE	NAME	TX AGE	CURR AGE	YEARS CONT'D FUNCTION	CURRENT FUNCTION (SCr)	CENTER
1	3/9/72	M.L.	30	58	28yrs, 9mos	functng	Univ Colorado-Denver
2	4/16/77	W.B.	31	54	23yrs, 8mos	0.8	Univ Hosp-Cincinnati
3	7/17/78	V.M.	27	49	22yrs, 5mos	1.1	Clinic St Luc-Brussels
4	8/15/78	A.C.	35	57	22yrs, 4mos	1.3	U Saskatchewan-Canada
5	9/24/79	D.M.	33	54	21yrs, 3mos	1.5	Cleveland Clinic
6	6/13/80	P.T.	28	49	20yrs, 6mos	1.4	Cleveland Clinic
7	12/14/87	T.H.	41	54	13yrs, -	3.5	Montefiore Med Ctr-Bronx

Systemic Lupus Erythematosus

	TX DATE	NAME	TX AGE	CURR AGE	YEARS CONT'D FUNCTION	CURRENT FUNCTION (SCr)	CENTER
1	5/15/68	P.K.	20	52	32yrs, 7mos	1.0	Cleveland Clinic
2	6/29/71	K.K.	19	48	29yrs, 6mos	1.1	Cleveland Clinic
3	10/26/71	D.W.	18	46	29yrs, 2mos	1.2	Cleveland Clinic
4	12/12/75	M.C.	25	50	25yrs, -	1.0	Univ Hosp-Cincinnati
5	9/24/80	J.S.	29	49	20yrs, 3mos	1.2	So ILL Univ-Springfield
6	11/19/82	J.J.	40	58	18yrs, 1mo	1.6	Univ Pittsburgh
7	1/24/83	J.M.	35	52	17yrs,11mos	0.6	Montefiore Med Ctr-Bronx

Focal seg GS

	TX DATE	NAME	TX AGE	CURR AGE	YEARS CONT'D FUNCTION	CURRENT FUNCTION (SCr)	CENTER
1	7/8/78	H.J.	19	41	22yrs, 5mos	1.5	Univ Florida-Gainesville
2	7/20/83	P.P.	13	30	17yrs, 5mos	1	Policlinico Univ-Milan
3	3/16/84	J.M.	30	46	16yrs, 9mos	1.6	Montefiore Med Ctr-Bronx

Longest Surviving Cadaver Transplant Recipient with Renal Malignancy as Original Disease

	TX DATE	NAME	TX AGE	CURR AGE	YEARS CONT'D FUNCTION	CURRENT FUNCTION (SCr)	CENTER
1	7/11/86	M.M.	7	21	14yrs, 5mos	1	Policlinico Univ-Milan

PANCREAS

TX DATE	NAME	TX AGE	CURR AGE	YEARS CONT'D FUNCTION	CURRENT FUNCTION (SCr)	CENTER

SIMULTANEOUS PANCREAS-KIDNEY TRANSPLANT (CADAVER)

Longest Functioning Pancreas-Kidney Transplant:

#	TX DATE	NAME	TX AGE	CURR AGE	YEARS CONT'D FUNCTION	CURRENT FUNCTION (SCr)	CENTER
1	4/10/81	A.M.	31	50	19yrs, 8mos	well/func	Univ Hosp-Zurich
2	12/10/81	L.B.	33	52	19yrs, -	gluc 88/0.9	Univ Hosp-Cincinnati
3	6/4/84	J.P.	35	51	16yrs, 6mos	insulin-indep	Huddinge Hosp-Sweden
4	3/15/85	C.E.	37	52	15yrs, 9mos	insulin-indep	Huddinge Hosp-Sweden
5	5/28/85	H.F.	40	55	15yrs, 7mos	insulin-Indep	Huddinge Hosp-Sweden
6	9/2/85	A.A.	35	50	15yrs, 3mos	insulin-indep	Huddinge Hosp-Sweden
6	9/4/85	E.O.	30	45	15yrs, 3mos	insulin-indep	Huddinge Hosp-Sweden
7	12/18/85	J.C.	36	51	15yrs, -	insulin-indep	Univ Wisconsin-Madison
8	1/14/86	F.M.	29	43	14yrs,11mos	insulin/indep	Clinic St Luc-Brussels
8	1/27/86	P.C.	34	48	14yrs,11mos	insulin-indep	Huddinge Hosp-Sweden
9	2/27/86	J.O.	44	58	14yrs,10mos	insulin-indep	Huddinge Hosp-Sweden
10	3/28/86	B.A.	33	47	14yrs, 9mos	insulin-indep	Univ Wisconsin-Madison
11	4/16/86	D.I.	34	48	14yrs, 8mos	well/func	Univ Hosp-Zurich
11	4/21/86	J.N	32	46	14yrs, 8mos	func/alive	Sahlgrenska U-Gotesborg
12	5/4/86	R.K.	37	51	14yrs, 7mos	insulin-indep	Univ Wisconsin-Madison
12	5/9/86	U.R.	32	46	14yrs, 7mos	well/func	Univ Hosp-Zurich
13	6/4/86	S.L.	36	50	14yrs, 6mos	insulin-indep	Huddinge Hosp-Sweden
14	7/9/86	J.W.	40	54	14yrs, 5mos	insulin-indep	Univ Minnesota-Mnpls
14	7/21/86	S.A.	29	43	14yrs, 5mos	insulin-indep	Univ Wisconsin-Madison
15	10/10/86	M.H.	37	51	14yrs, 2mos	insulin-indep	Univ Minnesota-Mnpls
15	10/28/86	V.W.	35	49	14yrs, 2mos	insulin-indep	Univ Minnesota-Mnpls
15	10/30/86	J.J.	43	57	14yrs, 2mos	insulin-indep	Univ Wisconsin-Madison
16	12/28/86	M.P.	33	47	14yrs, -	insulin-indep	Huddinge Hosp-Sweden
17	1/22/87	B.B.	34	47	13yrs,11mos	insulin-indep	Huddinge Hosp-Sweden
17	1/29/87	P.J.	27	42	13yrs,11mos	insulin-indep	Huddinge Hosp-Sweden
17	1/10/87	M.H.	36	48	13yrs,11mos	well/func	Univ Hosp-Zurich
18	2/23/87	T.K.	36	49	13yrs,10mos	insulin-Indep	Univ Minnesota-Mnpls
19	5/10/87	C.S.	43	56	13yrs, 7mos	insulin-indep	Univ Minnesota-Mnpls
19	5/31/87	C.M.	23	36	13yrs, 7mos	insulin-indep	Univ Minnesota-Mnpls
20	7/21/87	J.W.	38	51	13yrs, 5mos	insulin-indep	Univ Wisconsin-Madison
21	10/19/87	D.R.	35	48	13yrs, 2mos	insulin-indep	Univ Wisconsin-Madison
22	1/19/88	A.C.	27	39	12yrs,11mos	insulin-indep	Policlinico Univ-Milan
23	4/15/88	G.O.	38	50	12yrs, 8mos	insulin-indep	Huddinge Hosp-Sweden
24	3/21/91	M.S.	47	56	9yrs, 9mos	0.9	Univ Illinois Hosp
25	8/27/91	K.Z.	32	41	9yrs, 4mos	2.4	Univ Illinois Hosp

Longest Functioning Bladder-Drained Pancreas-Kidney Transplant:

#	TX DATE	NAME	TX AGE	CURR AGE	YEARS CONT'D FUNCTION	CURRENT FUNCTION (SCr)	CENTER
1	12/18/85	J.C.	36	51	15yrs, -	insulin-indep	Univ Wisconsin-Madison
2	3/28/86	B.A.	33	47	14yrs, 9mos	insulin-indep	Univ Wisconsin-Madison
3	5/4/86	R.K.	37	51	14yrs, 7mos	insulin-Indep	Univ Wisconsin-Madison
4	7/9/86	J.W.	40	54	14yrs, 5mos	insulin-indep	Univ Minnesota-Mnpls

TX DATE	NAME	TX AGE	CURR AGE	YEARS CONT'D FUNCTION	CURRENT FUNCTION (SCr)	CENTER

Longest Functioning Third Pancreas-Kidney Transplant:

1	11/19/94	R.S.	58	64	6yrs, 1mo	gd functn	Clarkson Hosp-Omaha

2nd Kidney Regraft Simultaneous With Pancreas After Failure of 1st Kidney:

1 M.F. 29yrs old, rcv'd first kidney 11/15/80 which rejected
08/01/84. 2yrs later, 01/14/86 rcv'd simultaneous
kidney-pancreas TX. 14yrs,11mos ins-ind/1.5 Clinic St Luc-Brussels

2nd Kidney Regraft After Kidney Transplanted Simultaneous With Pancreas Failed:

1 J.O. 31yrs old, rcv'd SPK Tx 07/30/87.
Kidney failed 10/10/88. Regrafted 12/12/89.
Pancreas functioning 13yrs - kidney 11yrs both functng Univ Wisconsin-Madison

2 S.L. 40yrs old, rcv'd SPK Tx 10/28/87. Kidney failed 06/07/96.
Regafted 07/10/96.
Pancreas functioning 13yrs - kidney 4yrs both functng Univ Wisconsin-Madison

3 D.M. 37yrs old, rcv'd SPK Tx 11/01/88 Kidney failed 12/22/94.
Regrafted 12/22/94.
Pancreas functioning 12yrs - kidney 6yrs both functng Univ Wisconsin-Madison

4 M.H. 32yrs old, rcv'd SPK Tx 06/09/92.
Kidney failed 08/09/95. Regrafted.
pancreas functioning 8yrs - kidney 5yr functng Univ Wisconsin-Madison

5 K.M. 31yrs old, rcvd SPK TX 6/16/89.
Second TX 6/3/96 3yrs, 6mos gd functn Clarkson Hosp-Omaha

6 G.W. 42 yrs old, rcv'd SPK Tx 10/25/97 3yrs, 2mos 1.5 Charleston Area-W Va

SIMULTANEOUS PANCREAS-KIDNEY TRANSPLANT (LIVING-RELATED)

Simultaneous Segmental Pancreas (duct-injected), and Kidney Transplant from Living-Related Donor:

1	3/10/94	D.E.	28	34	6yrs, 9mos	ins/dial free	Univ Minnesota-Mnpls

Living-Related Pancreas-Kidney Transplant from Identical Twin

1	6/13/97	K.W.	39	42	3yrs, 6mos	1.0/xclnt func	Univ Illinois Hosp

PANCREAS AFTER KIDNEY TRANSPLANT (CADAVER)

Longest Functioning Pancreas After Kidney Transplant:

1	8/24/84	E.C.	30	46	16yrs, 4mos	insulin-indep	Univ Pittsburgh
2	4/28/85	C.D.	27	43	15yrs, 8mos	insulin-indep	Univ Wisconsin-Madison
3	7/10/85	W.F.	42	57	15yrs, 5mos	insulin-indep	Univ Wisconsin-Madison
4	6/5/86	S.K.	33	47	14yrs, 6mos	insulin-indep	Univ Wisconsin-Madison

PANCREAS AFTER KIDNEY TRANSPLANT (LIVING-RELATED)

Longest Functioning Duct-Drained Pancreas After Kidney Transplant:

1	12/03/80	K.D.	25	45	20yrs, -	insulin-indep	Univ Minnesota-Mnpls

Longest Functioning Enteric-Drained Pancreas After Kidney Transplant:

1	2/18/84	K.H.	31	48	16yrs,10mos	insulin-indep	Univ Minnesota-Mnpls

TX DATE	NAME	TX AGE	CURR AGE	YEARS CONT'D FUNCTION	CURRENT FUNCTION (SCr)	CENTER

Longest Functioning Bladder-Drained Pancreas After Kidney Transplant:

1	4/28/85	C.D.	27	42	15yrs, 8mos	insulin-indep	Univ Wisconsin-Madison
2	7/10/85	W.F.	42	57	15yrs, 5mos	insulin-indep	Univ Wisconsin-Madison

Longest Functioning Second Pancreas After Kidney Transplant:

1	2/18/84	K.H.	30	46	16yrs,10mos	insulin-indep	Univ Minnesota-Mnpls

Longest Surviving Pancreas Transplant Preserved With UW Solution:

1	5/4/86	R.K.	37	51	14yrs, 7mos	insulin-indep	Univ Wisconsin-Madison

PANCREAS AFTER KIDNEY TRANSPLANT (LIVING-UNRELATED)

Longest Surviving Pancreas Graft After Receiving Living Unrelated Kidney Transplant:

1	9/21/95	D.L.	51	52	5yrs, 3mos	insulin-indep	Univ Minnesota-Mnpls

PANCREAS ONLY TRANSPLANT (LIVING-RELATED)

Longest Functioning Enteric-Drained Related Pancreas Transplant:

1	11/4/82	W.L.	30	48	18yrs, 1mo	insulin-indep	Univ Minnesota-Mnpls
2	7/21/83	J.H.	42	58	16yrs, 5mos	insulin-indep	Univ Minnesota-Mnpls

PANCREAS ONLY TRANSPLANT (CADAVER)

Longest Functioning Pancreas Only Transplant:

1	5/21/83	N.H.	33	50	17yrs, 7mos	insulin-indep	Univ Minnesota-Mnpls
2	12/13/85	B.S.	32	47	15yrs, -	insulin-indep	Univ Minnesota-Mnpls
3	3/27/86	S.Y.	33	47	14yrs, 9mos	insulin-indep	Univ Minnesota-Mnpls
4	11/10/86	F.S.	29	43	14yrs, 1mo	insulin-indep	Huddinge Hosp-Sweden
5	10/31/94	R.K.	31	37	6yrs, 2mos	functng	Univ Illinois Hosp

Longest Functioning Enteric-Drained Pancreas Only:

1	11/10/86	F.S.	29	43	14yrs, 1mo	insulin-indep	Huddinge Hosp-Sweden

Longest Functioning Duct-Injected Pancreas Only:

1	5/21/83	N.H.	33	50	17yrs, 7mos	insulin-indep	Univ Minnesota-Mnpls

Longest Functioning Bladder-Drained Pancreas Only:

1	3/27/86	S.Y.	33	49	14yrs, 9mos	insulin-indep	Univ Minnesota-Mnpls

Longest Functioning Third Pancreas Only Tx:

1	6/9/87	K.W.	40	53	13yrs, 6mos	insulin-indep	Univ Minnesota-Mnpls

TX DATE	NAME	TX AGE	CURR AGE	YEARS CONT'D FUNCTION	CURRENT FUNCTION (SCr)	CENTER

Longest Successful Preservation of a Pancreas:

1	3/21/92	O.H. 29hrs-pancreas preserved in UW solution.				
				8yrs, 9mos	xclnt functn	Univ Wisconsin-Madison
2	6/27/92	M.S. 28hrs-pancreas preserved in UW solution.				
				8yrs, 6mos	xclnt functn	Univ Wisconsin-Madison
3	5/29/91	N.L. 27hrs-pancreas preserved in UW solution.				
				9yrs, 7mos	xclnt functn	Univ Wisconsin-Madison
4	6/11/93	C.H. 26.6hrs-pancreas preserved in UW solution				
				7yrs, 6mos	xclnt functn	Univ Wisconsin-Madison

Oldest Recipient With Pancreas Only Transplant:

1	4/6/93	K.L.	62	69	7yrs, 8mos	gd functn	Clarkson Hosp-Omaha

Stapled Vascular Anastomoses in Pancreas Transplant:

1	7/23/97	G.R.	32	35	3yrs, 5mos	gd functng	St Mary's-London

LIVER (CADAVER)

	TX DATE	NAME	TX AGE	CURR AGE	YEARS CONT'D FUNCTION	CURRENT FUNCTION (SCr)	CENTER
Longest Surviving Liver Transplant:							
1	1/22/70	K.H.	3	33	30yrs,11mos	functng	Univ Colorado-Denver
2	7/31/71	S.K.	3	32	29yrs, 5mos	functng	Univ Colorado-Denver
3	2/18/73	K.K.	3	30	27yrs,10mos	functng	Univ Colorado-Denver
4	10/8/73	J.W.	4	31	27yrs, 2mos	functng	Univ Colorado-Denver
5	4/9/74	J.H.	37	63	26yrs, 8mos	functng	Univ Colorado-Denver
6	10/16/74	G.K.	3	29	26yrs, 2mos	functng	Univ Colorado-Denver
8	11/28/74	N.M.	22	48	26yrs, 1mo	functng	Univ Colorado-Denver
7	11/19/75	I.D.	41	66	25yrs, 1mo	gd functn	Med Hochschule Hannover
9	12/30/75	G.B.	31	57	25yrs, -	alive/well	Addenbrookes-Cambridge
10	1/22/76	S.M.	30	54	24yrs,11mos	functng	Univ Colorado-Denver
11	11/27/76	T.L.	15	39	24yrs, 1mo	functng	Univ Colorado-Denver
12	1/8/77	E.T.	33	56	23yrs,11mos	functng	Univ Colorado-Denver
13	1/4/78	H.S.	20mos	24	22yrs,11mos	functng	Univ Colorado-Denver
14	2/26/78	J.F.	5	27	22yrs, 9mos	functng	Univ Colorado-Denver
15	4/17/78	M.S.	39	61	22yrs, 8mos	functng	Univ Colorado-Denver
16	7/15/78	T.C.	15	37	22yrs, 5mos	functng	Univ Colorado-Denver
17	4/16/79	T.C.	45	66	21yrs, 8mos	alive/well	Groningen-Netherlands
18	9/9/79	N.L.	35	56	21yrs, 3mos	functng	Univ Colorado-Denver
19	12/3/79	B.B.	21	42	21yrs, -	functng	Univ Colorado-Denver
20	2/3/80	L.R.	9	30	20yrs,10mos	functng	Univ Colorado-Denver
21	3/5/80	D.V.	53	73	20yrs, 9mos	alive/well	Groningen-Netherlands
22	4/13/80	M.H.	41	61	20yrs, 8mos	functng	Univ Colorado-Denver
23	5/17/80	R.C.	26	46	20yrs, 7mos	functng	Univ Colorado-Denver
24	6/5/80	R.D.	23	41	20yrs, 6mos	functng	Univ Colorado-Denver
25	11/4/83	B.B.	20	37	17yrs, 1mo	norm functn	Yale University-Conn
26	11/3/85	C.K.	25	40	15yrs, 1mo	gd functn	Kaohsiung Chang Gung-Taiwan
27	9/26/86	E.T.	46	61	14yrs, 3mos	func/alive	Sahlgrenska U-Goteborg
28	12/2/88	M.M.	55	67	12yrs, -	gd functn	Hosp Italiano-BsAs-Argentina
Oldest Liver Recipient At Time Of Transplant:							
1	3/31/96	F.A.	76	82	4yrs, 9mo	alive/well	NYU Med Ctr
2	2/28/92	W.M.	74	81	8yrs,10mos	norm functn	Univ Pittsburgh
3	4/10/99	R.M.	73	75	1yr, 8mos	normal	Univ Iowa Hosp
4	6/24/91	M.L.	72	81	9yrs, 6mos	functng	Med Univ So Carolina
5	4/14/91	H.M	71	80	9yrs, 8mos	good	Clinic St Luc-Brussels
5	9/9/91	G.M.	71	80	9yrs, 3mos	good functn	Baylor Univ-Dallas
5	11/22/94	I.L.	71	77	6yrs, 1mo	xclnt/alive	Clinica Univ Navarra-Spain
Youngest Liver Transplant Recipient:							
1	6/12/92	D.E.	12dys	8	8yrs, 6mos	alive/well	Univ Chicago
2	9/27/92	N.L.	13dys	8	8yrs, 3mos	doing great	Children's Hosp-Phila
3	6/2/88	R.G.	14dys	12	12yrs, 7mos	doing well	Univ Pittsburgh
4	5/2/00	J.C.	19dys	8mos	-, 8mos	alive/well	Childrens's-Cincinnati
5	5/25/95	G.S.	28dys	5	5yrs, 7mos	doing well	Cardinal Glennon-St Louis

TX DATE	NAME	TX AGE	CURR AGE	YEARS CONT'D FUNCTION	CURRENT FUNCTION (SCr)	CENTER

Oldest Liver Donor:

	TX DATE	NAME	TX AGE	CURR AGE	YEARS CONT'D FUNCTION	CURRENT FUNCTION (SCr)	CENTER
1	8/11/93	A.T.	61	92yr dnr	7yrs, 4mos	functng	London Hlth Sci Ctr, Canada
2	2/2/99	M.A.	58	86yr dnr	1yr,10mos	functng	Univ Pittsburgh
3	9/7/98	M.M.	63	85yr dnr	2yrs, 3mos	functng	Univ Pittsburgh
4	12/18/97	C.B.	27	79yr dnr	3yrs, -	Excellent	Univ Iowa Hosp
5	2/12/99	R.T.	51	78yr dnr	1yr,10mos	good	Univ of San Francisco
6	11/12/94	T.P.	40	76yr dnr	6yrs, 1mo	norm functn	St Louis Univ Hosp

Longest Surviving Cadaver Liver Retransplant:

1	C.L. rcv'd 1st Cadaveric liver Tx 06/03/81, 21 days later,06/24/81,						
	rcv'd 2nd liver Tx.				19yrs, 6mos	functng	Univ Pittsburgh

Smallest Surviving Liver Transplant Recipient:

1	6/2/88	R.G. 14dy old, weighed					
		2.8kg (6.2lbs) at Tx			12yrs, 6mos	functng	Univ Pittsburgh
2	6/7/92	D.E. 12dy old, weighed					
		2.9kg (6.4lbs) at Tx			8yrs, 6mos	alive/well	Univ Chicago
3	12/5/86	E.H. 3mos old, weighed					
		3.5kg (7.7lbs) at Tx			14yrs, -	xclnt funct	Univ Wisconsin, Madison
4	9/14/91	J.J. 6mos old, weighed					
		5.3kg (11.6lbs) at Tx			9yrs, 3mos	xclnt funct	Univ Wisconsin, Madison

Largest Surviving Liver Transplant Recipient:

1	8/12/93	D.M. 42yrs old, weighed 376lbs at time of Tx.					
				47	7yrs, 4mos	alive/well	Univ Chicago

Longest Surviving Liver Transplant For Histiocytosis X With Cirrhosis Without Recurrence:

	TX DATE	NAME	TX AGE	CURR AGE	YEARS CONT'D FUNCTION	CURRENT FUNCTION	CENTER
1	11/29/85	N.E.	51	66	15yrs, 1mo	alive/well	Osp Maggiore-Milan
2	4/15/90	B.M.	43	53	10yrs, 8mos	alive/well	Osp Maggiore-Milan

Longest Surviving Pediatric Recipient With ABO Incompatible Cadaver Liver Transplant:

1	11/3/81	B.R. <1yr old, ABO - A to O		19yrs, 1mo	functng	Univ Pittsburgh

Longest Surviving Liver Transplant Without Immunosuppression:

1	7/15/78	T.C.20yrs off immunosuppression		functng	Univ Colorado-Denver
2	12/3/79	B.B.17yrs off immunosuppression		functng	Univ Colorado-Denver
3	10/8/73	J.W.14yrs off immunosuppression		functng	Univ Colorado-Denver

Longest Survival of Recipient with a Thrombosed Portal Vein to Receive a Liver Transplant:

	TX DATE	NAME	TX AGE	CURR AGE	YEARS CONT'D FUNCTION	CURRENT FUNCTION	CENTER
1	2/28/84	J.P.	57	73	16yrs,10mos	functng	Univ Pittsburgh
2	8/1/86	R.S.	17	31	14yrs, 4mos	func/alive	Royal Prince Alfred-Sydney

Longest Surviving Child Transplanted With A Cut-Down Adult Liver:

	TX DATE	NAME	TX AGE	CURR AGE	YEARS CONT'D FUNCTION	CURRENT FUNCTION	CENTER
1	8/27/84	E.F.	16	32	16yrs, 4mos	functng	Clinic Univ St Luc-Bruxelles
2	11/4/86	S.P.	2	16	14yrs, 1mo	func/alive	Royal Prince Alfred-Sydney

Successful Liver Transplant for Two Siblings with Crigler Najjar's Disease:

	TX DATE	NAME	TX AGE	CURR AGE	YEARS CONT'D FUNCTION	CURRENT FUNCTION	CENTER
1	7/24/91	F.A.	4	13	9yrs, 5mos	alive/well	Osp Maggiore-Milan
2	7/10/92	F.R.	7	15	8yrs, 5mos	alive/well	Osp Maggiore-Milan

TX DATE	NAME	TX AGE	CURR AGE	YEARS CONT'D FUNCTION	CURRENT FUNCTION (SCr)	CENTER

Reduced Size Heterotopic Auxilary Liver Transplant for Crigler-Najjar Syndrome Type 1:

1	7/14/94	L.D.	9mos	6	6yrs, 5mos	well	Univ Michigan-Ann Arbor

Longest Surviving Split Liver Transplant:

1	11/23/88	C.S.	15	27	12yrs, 1mo	functng	Clinic Univ St Luc-Bruxelles
2	1/24/89	K.K.	20mos	12	11yrs,11mos	alive/well	Univ Chicago (left lobe)
		P.V.	36	42	11yrs,11mos	alive/well	Univ Chicago (right lobe)
3	11/30/89	R.L.	49	58	11yrs, 1mo	alive/well	Univ Pittsburgh
4	9/7/94	I.S.			6yrs, 3mos	gd functn	Rabin Med Ctr-Petach-Tikva
5	5/30/95	H.S.			5yrs, 7mos	gd functn	Rabin Med Ctr-Petach-Tikva

Longest Surviving Recipient With Auxiliary Partial Orthotopic Liver Transplant:

1	11/25/89	G.Z.			3343 with recovered functn of own liver		
					11yrs, 1mo	gd functn	Med Hochschule-Hannover

LIVER (LIVING-RELATED)

Longest Surviving Living-Related Liver Transplant:

1	11/27/89	A.S	1	12	11yrs, 1mo	alive/well	Univ Chicago
2	12/8/89	S.J.	1	12	11yrs, -	alive/well	Univ Chicago
3	2/13/90	K.B.	9mos	11	10yrs,10mos	alive/well	Univ Chicago
4	4/10/90	A.S.	1	11	10yrs, 8mos	alive/well	Univ Chicago
5	6/26/90	P.G.	9mos	11	10yrs, 6mos	alive/well	Univ Chicago
5	6/29/90	H.M.	3	14	10yrs, 6mos	good	Kyoto Univ Hosp
6	10/26/90	Y.K.	3	13	10yrs, 2mos	alive/well	Kyoto Univ Hosp

Youngest Surviving Living-Related Liver Transplant Recipient:

1	8/9/96	R.K.	43dys	4	4yrs, 4mos	good	Kyoto Univ Hosp
2	9/20/91	J.Y.	45dys	11	9yrs, 3mos	alive/well	Univ Chicago
3	5/2/94	S.K.	2mos	6	6yrs,10mos	alive/well	Univ Chicago
4	11/10/94	D.P.	2mos	6	6yrs, 1mo	alive/well	Univ Chicago

Living-Related Liver Transplant without Transfusion of Blood or Blood Products

1	6/15/99	W.J.	44	46	1yr, 6mos	xclnt functn	USC University Hosp

Longest Surviving Liver Transplant without Immunosuppression:

1	9/2/92	H.E.5yrs,10mos off immunosuppression					
		(ABO incompatible)				good	Kyoto Univ Hosp
2	8/5/94	K.T.5yrs, - off immunosuppression				good	Kyoto Univ Hosp
3	8/6/93	E.K.4yrs, 7mos off immunosuppression				good	Kyoto Univ Hosp
4	11/30/90	Y.A.4yrs, 4mos off immunosuppression				good	Kyoto Univ Hosp

HEART

	TX DATE	NAME	TX AGE	CURR AGE	YEARS CONT'D FUNCTION	CURRENT FUNCTION	CENTER
Longest Surviving Heart Transplant Recipient:							
1	1/25/77	R.D.	14	37	23yrs,11mos	alive/well	Stanford Univ
2	8/30/78	R.H.	20	42	22yrs, 4mos	alive/well	Stanford Univ
3	3/30/79	D.O.	36	57	21yrs, 9mos	alive/well	Stanford Univ
4	10/19/79	B.E.	20	41	21yrs, 2mos	alive/well	Stanford Univ
5	11/18/79	D.M.	26	47	21yrs, 1mo	alive/well	Stanford Univ
6	12/17/79	B.D.	16	37	21yrs, -	alive/well	Stanford Univ
6	12/21/79	J.L.	28	49	21yrs, -	alive/well	Stanford Univ
7	1/5/80	P.T.	14	35	20yrs,11mos	NYHA I	Groote Schuur-Cape Tn
8	4/16/82	J.W.	26	44	18yrs, 8mo	alive/well	Univ Pittsburgh
9	10/23/84	R.S.	48	64	16yrs, 2mos	gd functn	Inst of Clin & Exp Med-Prague
10	7/30/85	W.C.	42	57	15yrs, 5mos	alive/well	Northern Indiana Heart Inst
11	2/23/86	G.G.	40	56	14yrs,10mos	alive	Univ Calif-Los Angeles
12	3/29/86	J.N	51	65	14yrs, 9mos	alive/well	Northern Indiana Heart Inst
13	4/8/86	T.M.	57	71	14yrs, 8mos	xclnt functn	Temple U-Philadelphia
14	5/22/86	R.T.	54	68	14yrs, 7mos	alive/well	Northern Indiana Heart Inst
15	6/30/86	L.W.	62	76	14yrs, 6mos	alive/well	Northern Indiana Heart Inst
16	8/24/86	F.G.	52	66	14yrs, 4mos	alive/well	Northern Indiana Heart Inst
17	9/21/86	A.S.	66	80	14yrs, 3mos	alive/well	Univ Calif-Los Angeles
18	11/21/86	C.N.	58	72	14yrs, 1mo	alive/well	Northern Indiana Heart Inst
19	4/12/87	E.B.	59	72	13yrs, 8mos	alive/well	Northern Indiana Heart Inst
20	6/11/87	H.B.	60	73	13yrs, 6mos	alive/well	Northern Indiana Heart Inst
20	6/15/87	R.C.	43	56	13yrs, 6mos	alive/well	Northern Indiana Heart Inst
21	8/16/87	C.H.	61	74	13yrs, 4mos	alive/well	Northern Indiana Heart Inst
22	10/31/87	B.S.	58	71	13yrs, 2mos	alive/well	Northern Indiana Heart Inst
23	1/13/88	C.W.	47	60	12yrs,11mos	alive/well	Univ Mississippi
Longest Surviving Infant Heart Transplant Recipient:							
1	11/20/85	B.M.	4dys	15	15yrs, 1mo	doing well	Loma Linda Univ
2	12/23/86	A.D.	5mos	14	14yrs, -	doing well	Stanford Univ
3	2/7/87	J.D.	3mos	13	13yrs,10mos	doing well	Loma Linda Univ
4	10/16/87	P.H.	3hrs	13	13yrs, 2mos	doing well	Loma Linda Univ
4	10/26/87	M.B.	11dys	13	13yrs, 2mos	doing well	Loma Linda Univ
5	11/20/87	G.B.	3mos	13	13yrs, 1mo	doing well	Loma Linda Univ
6	1/30/88	R.L.	18dys	12	12yrs,11mos	doing well	Loma Linda Univ
7	2/14/88	C.E.	8dys	12	12yrs,10mos	doing well	Loma Linda Univ
8	4/7/88	T.K.	21dys	12	12yrs, 8mos	doing well	Loma Linda Univ
8	4/19/88	A.L.	6mos	12	12yrs, 8mos	doing well	Loma Linda Univ
9	8/6/88	N.K.	16dys	12	12yrs, 4mos	doing well	Loma Linda Univ
10	9/3/88	J.G.	21dys	12	12yrs, 3mos	doing well	Loma Linda Univ
11	10/22/88	D.J.	1mo	12	12yrs, 2mos	doing well	Loma Linda Univ
12	11/12/88	W.P.	17dys	12	12yrs, 1mo	doing well	Loma Linda Univ
12	11/20/88	J.R.	1mo	12	12yrs, 1mo	doing well	Loma Linda Univ
13	12/22/88	K.M.	4mos	12	12yrs, -	alive/well	Stanford Univ
13	12/29/88	K.F.	20dys	12	12yrs, -	doing well	Loma Linda Univ

TX DATE	NAME	TX AGE	CURR AGE	YEARS CONT'D FUNCTION	CURRENT FUNCTION	CENTER

Youngest Heart Transplant Recipient:

	TX DATE	NAME	TX AGE	CURR AGE	YEARS CONT'D FUNCTION	CURRENT FUNCTION	CENTER
1	10/16/87	P.H.	3hrs	13	13yrs, 2mos	doing well	Loma Linda Univ
2	8/1/90	C.Y.	3dys	10	10yrs, 4mos	doing well	Loma Linda Univ
3	11/20/85	N.A.	4dys	15	15yrs, 1mo	doing well	Loma Linda Univ
3	12/30/90	L.S.	4dys	10	10yrs, -	doing well	Loma Linda Univ
3	11/21/94	V.A.	4dys	6	6yrs, 1mo	doing well	Loma Linda Univ
4	10/11/93	D.M.	6dys	8	7yrs, 2mos	alive/well	Univ Texas-San Antonio
5	9/28/89	M.K.	7dys	11	11yrs, 3mos	doing well	Loma Linda Univ
5	2/6/91	S.H.	7dys	10	9yrs,10mos	alive/well	Children's-U Pittsburgh
6	2/14/88	C.E.	8dys	13	12yrs,10mos	doing well	Loma Linda Univ
7	7/26/89	B.W.	9dys	11	11yrs, 5mos	doing well	Loma Linda Univ
7	3/11/90	C.W.	9dys	10	10yrs, 9mos	doing well	Loma Linda Univ
7	4/11/92	J.O.	9dys	9	8yrs, 8mos	doing well	Loma Linda Univ
7	12/2/94	E.C.	9dys	6	6yrs, -	doing well	Loma Linda Univ
7	1/6/95	R.T.	9dys	6	5yrs,11mos	doing well	Loma Linda Univ
7	3/4/95	K.A.	9dys	5	5yrs, 9mos	doing well	Loma Linda Univ
7	1/24/97	R.G.	9dys	4	3yrs,11mos	doing well	Loma Linda Univ
7	4/24/98	D.N.	9dys	2	2yrs, 8mos	doing well	Loma Linda Univ
8	10/4/89	J.N.	10dys	11	11yrs, 2mos	doing well	Loma Linda Univ
8	12/21/89	N.D.	10dys	11	11yrs, -	doing well	Loma Linda Univ
9	10/26/87	M.B.	11dys	13	13yrs, 2mos	doing well	Loma Linda Univ

Oldest Heart Transplant Recipient:

	TX DATE	NAME	TX AGE	CURR AGE	YEARS CONT'D FUNCTION	CURRENT FUNCTION	CENTER
1	12/27/99	R.N.	79	80	1yr, -	xclnt functn	Univ of Alberta Hosp-Canada
2	10/17/95	A.Z.	74	79	5yrs, 2mos	xclnt functn	Hrt Ctr N Rhine-Westfalia
2	11/27/95	G.M.	74	79	5yrs, 1mo	alive/good	Favaloro Foundation
2	11/27/95	G.M.	74	79	5yrs, 1mo	gd functn	ICYCC Favaloro-Argentina
3	11/20/90	W.H.	73	83	10yrs, 1mo	alive/good	Hrt Ctr N Rhine-Westfalia
4	9/5/91	G.D.	71	80	9yrs, 3mos	xclnt functn	Hrt Ctr N Rhine-Westfalia
4	12/29/94	J.W.	71	77	6yrs, -	alive/good	St Vincent Med Ctr-LA
4	12/28/96	E.D.	71	75	4yrs	gd functn	Groote Schuur Hosp.
5	8/24/92	S.T.	70	78	8yrs, 4mos	alive/good	Hrt Ctr N Rhine-Westfalia
5	4/7/93	K.S.	70	77	7yrs, 8mos	xclnt functn	Hrt Ctr N Rhine-Westfalia
5	1/19/95	E.N.	70	75	5yrs,11mos	xclnt functn	Hrt Ctr N Rhine-Westfalia
5	11/6/99	J.J.	70	71	1yr, 1mo	xlnt functn	Vanderbilt U-Nashville
6	3/24/92	J.T.	69	78	8yrs, 9mos	alive/well	Univ Calif-Los Angeles
6	3/18/92	H.P.	69	77	8yrs, 9mos	alive/good	Hrt Ctr N Rhine-Westfalia
6	9/2/92	K.C.	69	77	8yrs, 3mos	alive/well	Hrt Ctr N Rhine-Westfalia
6	5/19/95	H.R.	69	74	5yrs, 7mos	alive/well	Hrt Ctr N Rhine-Westfalia
6	6/6/95	H.H.	69	83	5yrs, 6mos	xclnt functn	Hrt Ctr N Rhine-Westfalia
6	7/7/97	S.H.	69	72	3yrs, 5mos	alive/well	Stanford Univ
6	2/26/98	G.S	69	71	2yrs,10mos	alive/well	Univ Pittsburgh
7	5/4/92	F.R.	68	76	8yrs, 7mos	xclnt functn	Hrt Ctr N Rhine-Westfalia
7	6/17/93	F.N.	68	75	7yrs, 6mos	xclnt functn	Hrt Ctr N Rhine-Westfalia
7	9/12/95	W.V.	68	73	5yrs, 3mos	xclnt functn	Hrt Ctr N Rhine-Westfalia
8	10/16/88	C.Y.	67	79	12yrs, 2mos	alive/well	Univ Calif-Irvine

	TX DATE	NAME	TX AGE	CURR AGE	YEARS CONT'D FUNCTION	CURRENT FUNCTION	CENTER
8	1/20/90	H.H.	67	77	10yrs,11mos	xclnt functn	Hrt Ctr N Rhine-Westfalia
8	9/17/91	H.W.	67	76	9yrs, 3mos	xclnt functn	Hrt Ctr N Rhine-Westfalia
8	11/23/91	H.J.	67	76	9yrs, 1mo	alive/good	Hrt Ctr N Rhine-Westfalia
8	1/23/92	S.G.	67	75	8yrs,11mos	xclnt functn	Hrt Ctr N Rhine-Westfalia
8	4/26/93	S.A.	67	74	7yrs, 8mos	alive/good	Hrt Ctr N Rhine-Westfalia
8	8/26/93	M.B.	67	74	7yrs, 4mos	alive/well	Northern Indiana Heart Inst
8	11/8/95	S.W.	67	72	5yrs, 1mo	xclnt functn	Hrt Ctr N Rhine-Westfalia
8	11/16/95	H.S.	67	72	5yrs, 1mo	alive/well	Hrt Ctr N Rhine-Westfalia
9	9/21/86	A.S.	66	80	14yrs, 3mos	alive/well	Univ Calif-Los Angeles
9	9/3/90	R.G.	66	76	10yrs, 3mos	alive/well	Northern Indiana Heart Inst
9	10/19/91	R.T.	66	75	9yrs, 2mos	alive/well	Northern Indiana Heart Inst
9	9/22/94	L.B.	66	72	6yrs, 3mos	alive/well	Univ Calif-Los Angeles
9	5/24/96	R.W.	66	70	4yrs, 7mos	alive/well	Stanford Univ
9	11/12/96	H.M.	66	71	4yrs, 1mo	alive/well	Northern Indiana Heart Inst
9	2/23/97	E.P.	66	70	3yrs,10mos	alive/well	Stanford Univ

Youngest Heart Donor:

	TX DATE	NAME	TX AGE	CURR AGE	YEARS CONT'D FUNCTION	CURRENT FUNCTION	CENTER
1	4/3/91	R.C.	14dys	1dy dnr	9yrs, 8mos	norm funct	Loma Linda Univ
1	5/6/91	T.U.	2mos	1dy dnr	9yrs, 7mos	doing well	Loma Linda Univ
1	6/29/91	C.A.	2mos	1dy dnr	9yrs, 6mos	doing well	Loma Linda Univ
1	7/3/94	A.J.	36dys	1dy dnr	6yrs, 5mos	doing well	Loma Linda Univ
2	4/24/98	D.N.	9dys	2dy dnr	2yrs, 8mos	doing well	Loma Linda Univ
2	9/22/89	A.Z.	24dys	2dy dnr	11yrs, 3mos	doing well	Loma Linda Univ
2	1/23/91	S.C.	40dys	2dy dnr	9yrs,11mos	doing well	Loma Linda Univ
2	2/7/87	J.D.	3mos	2dy dnr	13yrs,10mos	doing well	Loma Linda Univ
2	10/16/87	P.H.	3hrs	2dy dnr	13yrs, 2mos	doing well	Loma Linda Univ
2	7/23/93	A.L.	50dys	2dy dnr	7yrs, 5mos	doing well	Loma Linda Univ
2	12/2/93	A.M.	2mos	2dy dnr	7yrs, -	doing well	Loma Linda Univ
3	2/14/96	L.T.	84dys	3dy dnr	4yrs,10mos	doing well	Loma Linda Univ
3	4/17/98	H.G.	11dys	3dy dnr	2yrs, 8mos	doing well	Loma Linda Univ
3	11/21/90	T.R.	38dys	3dy dnr	10yrs, 1mo	doing well	Loma Linda Univ
3	5/25/89	D.A.	13dys	3dy dnr	11yrs, 7mos	doing well	Loma Linda Univ
3	1/2/90	A.B.	19dys	3dy dnr	10yrs,11mos	doing well	Loma Linda Univ
3	10/29/94	A.H.	13dys	3dy dnr	6yrs, 2mos	doing well	Loma Linda Univ
4	11/20/85	N.A.	4dys	4dy dnr	15yrs, 1mo	doing well	Loma Linda Univ
4	2/14/88	C.E.	8dys	4dy dnr	12yrs,10mos	doing well	Loma Linda Univ
4	8/17/90	D.O.	17mos	4dy dnr	10yrs, 4mos	doing well	Loma Linda Univ
4	10/12/94	C.B.	17dys	4dy dnr	6yrs, 2mos	doing well	Loma Linda Univ
5	11/12/88	W.P.	17dys	5dy dnr	12yrs, 1mo	doing well	Loma Linda Univ
5	7/10/90	B.S.	14dys	5dy dnr	10yrs, 5mos	doing well	Loma Linda Univ
5	6/8/93	B.M.	3mos	5dy dnr	7yrs, 6mos	excellent	Stanford Univ
6	12/24/97	J.P.	31dys	6dy dnr	3yrs, -	doing well	Loma Linda Univ
7	3/29/92	J.G.	17dys	7dy dnr	8yrs, 9mos	doing well	Loma Linda Univ
8	5/11/92	J.H.	11dys	8dy dnr	8yrs, 8mos	alive/well	Stanford Univ
8	9/21/92	B.M.	2mos	8dy dnr	8yrs, 3mos	doing well	Loma Linda Univ
8	11/28/98	J.P.	49dys	8dy dnr	2yrs, 1mo	doing well	Loma Linda Univ

TX DATE	NAME	TX AGE	CURR AGE	YEARS CONT'D FUNCTION	CURRENT FUNCTION	CENTER

Oldest Heart Donor:

1	4/24/92	I.H.	57	65yr dnr	8yrs, 8mos	xclnt functn	Hrt Ctr N Rhine-Westfalia
1	3/25/94	K.R.	63	65yr dnr	6yrs, 9mos	xclnt functn	Hrt Ctr N Rhine-Westfalia
2	5/19/95	R.H.	69	64yr dnr	5yrs, 7mos	alive/well	Hrt Ctr N Rhine-Westfalia
3	11/18/98	D.G.	71	63yr dnr	2yrs, 1mo	alive/good	Hrt Ctr N Rhine-Westfalia
4	8/26/94	P.R	63	62yr dnr	6yrs, 4mos	xclnt functn	Hrt Ctr N Rhine-Westfalia
5	9/27/93	T.K.	63	61yr dnr	7yrs, 3mos	alive/good	Hrt Ctr N Rhine-Westfalia
5	9/10/94	P.C.	42	61yr dnr	6yrs, 3mos	alive/well	Univ Calif-Los Angeles
6	2/28/91	R.B.	59	58yr dnr	9yrs,10mos	alive/well	Northern Indiana Heart Inst
7	1/16/97	F.M.	59	57yr dnr	3yrs,11mos	alive/well	Univ Pittsburgh
7	6/6/97	M.L.	60	57yr dnr	3yrs, 6mos	alive/well	Northern Indiana Heart Inst
8	7/14/92	H.T.	53	55yr dnr	8yrs, 5mos	alive/well	Univ Pittsburgh
9	4/6/92	J.E.	59	53yr dnr	8yrs, 8mos	NYHA I	Stanford Univ
10	4/1/92	R.C.	62	52yr dnr	8yrs, 8mos	alive/well	Northern Indiana Heart Inst
11	11/16/91	L.T.	52	51yr dnr	9yrs, 1mo	alive/well	Northern Indiana Heart Inst

Longest Survival of Coronary Artery Bypass Graft (CABG) of Donor Heart, (Using vessel of recipient to repair donor heart prior to transplant):

1	3/24/92	J.T.	68	76	8yrs, 9mos	alive/well	Univ Calif-Los Angeles
2	2/9/93	R.R.	64	71	7yrs,10mos	alive/well	Univ Calif-Los Angeles

Longest Surviving Heart Recipient Who Received a Ventricular Device Pretransplant:

1	9/13/84	R.L.	51	67	16yrs, 3mos	alive/well	Stanford Univ
2	6/7/88	R.M.	55	67	12yrs, 6mos	alive/well	Univ Pittsburgh
3	10/2/88	J.L.	43	55	12yrs, 2mos	alive/well	Univ Pittsburgh
4	12/14/88	T.S.	22	34	12yrs, -	alive/well	Univ Pittsburgh
5	1/5/89	J.W.	20	32	11yrs,11mos	alive/well	Univ Pittsburgh
6	7/5/89	J.B.	24	36	11yrs, 5mos	alive/well	Northern Indiana Heart Inst
7	2/9/90	W.B.	48	58	10yrs,10mos	alive/well	Univ Pittsburgh

Youngest Heart Recipient Who Received a Ventricular Assist Device Pre-Transplant:

1	8/28/90	J.W.	15	25	10yrs, 4mos	alive/xclnt	Univ Pittsburgh

Oldest Heart Recipient Who Received A Ventricular Assist Device Pre-Transplant:

1	10/14/94	G.N.	61	67	6yrs, 2mos	alive/well	Univ Pittsburgh
2	4/26/95	L.G.	60	65	5yrs, 8mos	alive/w/ell	Univ Pittsburgh
3	6/7/88	R.M.	55	68	12yrs, 6mos	alive/well	Univ Pittsburgh
4	10/15/88	R.L.	51	63	12yrs, 2mos	alive/well	Northern Indiana Heart Inst

Longest Surviving Recipient Who Received an Artificial Heart Pre-Transplant:

1	4/28/87	N.M.	39	52	13yrs, 8mos	alive/well	Univ Pittsburgh
2	5/3/87	C.L.	15	28	13yrs, 7mos	alive/well	Abbott Northwestern-Mnpls
3	10/15/88	R.L.	51	63	12yrs, 2mos	alive/well	Northern Indiana Heart Inst

Youngest Heart Recipient Who Received an Artificial Heart Pre-Transplant:

1	5/3/87	C.L.15yrs old was implanted with a Jarvik 7-70, 04/08/87-bridge to heart transplant on 05/03/87 one month later.					
				13yrs, 7mos	NYHA I	Abbott Northwestern-Mnpls

TX DATE	NAME	TX AGE	CURR AGE	YEARS CONT'D FUNCTION	CURRENT FUNCTION	CENTER

Longest Surviving Heterotopic Heart Transplant:

#	TX DATE	NAME	TX AGE	CURR AGE	YEARS CONT'D FUNCTION	CURRENT FUNCTION	CENTER
1	1/5/80	P.T.	14	35	20yrs,11mos	NYHA I	Groote Schuur-Cape Tn
2	12/29/84	A.C.	44	60	16yrs, -	alive/well	Univ Pittsburgh

Oldest Heterotopic Heart Donor with Batiste of Native Heart

#	TX DATE	NAME	TX AGE	CURR AGE	YEARS CONT'D FUNCTION	CURRENT FUNCTION	CENTER
1	2/27/97	D.B. 21yr dnr		34	3yrs,10mos	very good	Harefield-UK

Youngest Heterotopic Heart Donor with Batiste of Native Heart

#	TX DATE	NAME	TX AGE	CURR AGE	YEARS CONT'D FUNCTION	CURRENT FUNCTION	CENTER
1	11/23/97	J.M.dnr-newborn anencephalic			3yrs, 1mo	good	Harefield-UK

First Child born to Parents Who Both Had Heart Transplants

#	TX DATE	NAME	TX AGE	CURR AGE	YEARS CONT'D FUNCTION	CURRENT FUNCTION	CENTER
1	9/10/90	C.L.	24	34	died(accident)	gd functn	Wythenshaw-Manchester
2	1/14/94	R.L.	22	28	6yrs,11mos	alive/well	Wythenshaw-Manchester

Longest Surviving Recipient With Both Heterotopic and Orthotopic Heart Transplant:

#	TX DATE	Description	YEARS CONT'D FUNCTION	CURRENT FUNCTION	CENTER
1	1/5/80	P.T. rcv'd an heterotopic heart. Almost 4yrs later rcv'd orthotopic heart-Tx 12/28/83. Alive and well, with both hearts functioning.	20yrs,11mos	NYHA I	Groote Schuur-Cape Tn

Smallest Heart Donor:

#	TX DATE	Description	YEARS CONT'D FUNCTION	CURRENT FUNCTION	CENTER
1	7/10/90	B.S. 14dys old rcv'd the heart of a donor weighing 2.2kg (4.8lbs).	10yrs, 5mos	alive/very well	Loma Linda Univ
2	5/25/89	D.A. 26dys rcv'd the heart of a donor weighing 2.4kg (5.3lbs)	11yrs, 7mos	doing well	Loma Linda Univ

Most Undersized Donor Heart:

#	TX DATE	Description	YEARS CONT'D FUNCTION	CURRENT FUNCTION	CENTER
1	11/13/92	T.L.46 donor/recip ratio .42	8yrs, 1mo	xclnt functn	Temple U-Philadelphia

Weight Mismatch of Recipient-Donor Heart:

#	TX DATE	NAME	Difference	YEARS CONT'D FUNCTION	CURRENT FUNCTION	CENTER
1	9/27/87	E.T.	86lbs difference	13yrs, 3mos	doing well	Loma Linda Univ
2	2/8/97	B.R.	57lbs difference	3yrs,10mos	doing well	Loma Linda Univ
3	1/6/94	J.M.	48lbs difference	6yrs,11mos	doing well	Loma Linda Univ
4	11/15/90	H.B.	32lbs difference	10yrs, 1mo	doing well	Loma Linda Univ
5	1/30/93	A.Y.	31lbs difference	7yrs,11mos	doing well	Loma Linda Univ

Longest Cold Ischemic Time:

#	TX DATE	NAME	TX AGE	Time	YEARS CONT'D FUNCTION	CURRENT FUNCTION	CENTER
1	3/28/93	L.S.	6	9hrs,12mn	7yrs, 9mos	doing well	Loma Linda Univ
2	12/2/86	A.D.	5mos	8hrs,15mn	14yrs, -	alive/well	Stanford Univ
3	11/25/91	A.W.	5	8hrs,10mn	9yrs, 1mo	doing well	Loma Linda Univ
4	6/8/93	B.M	3mos	8hrs, 8mn	7yrs, 6mos	alive/well	Stanford Univ
5	3/27/95	J.S.	14dys	8hrs, 5mn	5yrs, 9mos	doing well	Loma Linda Univ
6	2/20/91	J.A.	34dys	8hrs, 2mn	9yrs,10mos	doing well	Loma Linda Univ
7	1/6/95	R.T.	9dys	8hrs, 1mn	5yrs,11mos	doing well	Loma Linda Univ
8	7/30/93	C.F.	3mos	7hrs,59mn	7yrs, 5mos	doing well	Loma Linda Univ
9	9/20/97	W.H.	11mos	7hrs,53mn	3yrs, 3mos	doing well	Loma Linda Univ
10	7/28/92	J.P.	52dys	7hrs,52mn	8yrs, 5mos	xclnt functn	Temple U-Philadelphia
11	11/6/98	B.M.	153dys	7hrs,49mn	2yrs, 1mo	doing well	Loma Linda Univ
12	3/7/94	M.C.	2	7hrs,40mn	6yrs, 9mos	doing well	Loma Linda Univ
12	11/27/98	J.V.	109dys	7hrs,40mn	2yrs, 1mo	doing well	Loma Linda Univ

	TX DATE	NAME	TX AGE	CURR AGE	YEARS CONT'D FUNCTION	CURRENT FUNCTION	CENTER
13	1/11/97	R.A.	3	7hrs,36mn	3yrs,11mos	doing well	Loma Linda Univ
14	2/14/96	L.T.	84dys	7hrs,30mn	4yrs,10mos	doing well	Loma Linda Univ
15	9/5/93	S.E.	4	7hrs,24mn	7yrs, 3mos	doing well	Loma Linda Univ
16	12/24/97	J.P.	31dys	7hrs,20mn	3yrs, -	doing well	Loma Linda Univ
17	2/15/90	B.M.	4mos	7hrs,19mn	10yrs,10mos	doing well	Loma Linda Univ
17	3/11/90	C.W.	9dys	7hrs,19mn	10yrs, 9mos	doing well	Loma Linda Univ
18	1/23/91	S.C.	40dys	7hrs,17mn	9yrs,11mos	doing well	Loma Linda Univ
19	7/20/93	M.H.	29dys	7hrs,13mn	7yrs, 5mos	doing well	Loma Linda Univ
20	4/24/98	D.N.	9dys	7hrs, 8mn	2yrs, 8mos	doing well	Loma Linda Univ
21	1/26/91	A.R.	3mos	7hrs, 7mn	9yrs,11mos	doing well	Loma Linda Univ
21	4/17/95	E.D.	38dys	7hrs, 7mn	5yrs, 8mos	doing well	Loma Linda Univ
22	4/24/93	Z.A.	50dys	7hrs, 6mn	7yrs, 8mos	doing well	Loma Linda Univ
23	11/1/91	A.G.	2mos	7hrs, 2mn	9yrs, 1mos	doing well	Loma Linda Univ
24	5/28/94	J.R.	5	7hrs,-	6yrs, 7mos	doing well	Loma Linda Univ
25	8/5/93	K.J.	61	5hrs,16mn	7yrs, 4mos	alive/good	Hrt Ctr N Rhine-Westfalia

Rare Indications for Heart Transplant:

Acute VSD-

1	4/8/86	T.M.	57	71	14yrs, 8mos	xclnt functn	Temple U-Philadelphia

B-Thalassemia Major-

1	11/15/89	P.P.	15	26	11yrs, 1mo	xclnt functn	Hrt Ctr N Rhine-Westfalia

Longest Survival Following Heart Transplant In A Patient With A Pre-Existing Malignancy:

1	4/12/87	E.B. breast cancer-8yrs disease free pre-Tx.					
					13yrs, 8mos	alive/well	Northern Indiana Heart Inst
2	2/28/90	M.W. Leukemia-9yrs disease free pre-Tx.					
					10yrs,10mos	alive/well	Northern Indiana Heart Inst
3	6/21/96	E.O. breast cancer-1yr disease free pre-Tx.					
					4yrs, 6mos	alive/well	Northern Indiana Heart Inst

First Child-to-Parent Heart Transplant:

1   C.S. 58yrs rcv'd his 22yr old daughter's heart after she was found brain dead following an auto accident 08/22/94

					6yrs, 4mos	functng	Wm Beaumont-Michigan

Youngest Heart Retransplant:

1   J.M. born 06/14/89 was 20 days old when rcv'd first heart Tx 07/04/89. rcv'd 2nd heart 08/05/89, 51dys old.

			10		11yrs, 6mos	doing well	Loma Linda Univ

Oldest Heart Retransplant Recipient:

1   N.F 67yrs old rcv'd' 1st heart Tx 06/17/93, rcv'd 2nd heart TX 06/21/93.

					7yrs, 6mos	xclnt functn	Hrt Ctr N Rhine-Westfalia

Longest Surviving Recipient To Receive A Liver Transplant After Receiving A Heart Transplant:

1   T.D. 12 yrs old rcv'd a heart transplant 04/01/86. 17 days later, 04/21/86, due to Hypercholesterolemia, Familial Type II A, T.D.rcv'd' a liver.

	Both organs				11yrs	gd functn	Puerta de Hierro-Madrid

HEART-LUNG

TX DATE	NAME	TX AGE	CURR AGE	YEARS CONT'D FUNCTION	CURRENT FUNCTION	CENTER
Longest Survival of Heart-Lung Transplant:						
1	11/21/83	C.J.	26	43	17yrs, 1mo	alive/well	Univ Pittsburgh
2	7/25/84	J.H.	39	55	16yrs, 5mos	alive/well	Stanford Univ
3	1/21/89	L.W.	29	41	11yrs,11mos	alive/well	Univ of Maryland Med. Ctr.
4	7/3/90	R.M.	29	39	10yrs, 5mos	alive/well	Stanford Univ
Youngest Heart-Lung Recipient:						
1	6/14/89	M.M.	4mos	11	11yrs, 6mos	alive/well	Stanford Univ
2	6/2/92	S.K.	1yr	9	8yrs, 6mos	alive/well	Children's-U Pittsburgh
3	1/1/93	J.W.	3yrs	9	7yrs,11mos	alive/well	U No Carolina-Chapel Hill
Oldest Heart-Lung Recipient:						
1	10/21/88	B.R.	52	64	12yrs, 2mos	alive/well	Univ Pittsburgh
2	3/14/95	R.B.	50	55	5yrs, 9mos	alive/well	Univ Pittsburgh
Youngest Heart-Lung Donor:						
1	6/14/89	M.M.	4mos	6dy dnr	11yrs, 6mos	alive/well	Stanford Univ
2	1/1/93	J.W.	3yrs	18mos dnr	7yrs,11mos	alive/well	U No Carolina-Chapel Hill
Oldest Heart-Lung Donor:						
1	7/15/92	A.W.	22	55yr dnr	8yrs, 5mos	allive/w/ell	Univ Pittsburgh

LUNG (SINGLE)

TX DATE	NAME	TX AGE	CURR AGE	YEARS CONT'D FUNCTION	CURRENT FUNCTION	CENTER
Longest Surviving Single-Lung Recipient:						
1	9/15/87	W.M.	46	59	13yrs, 3mos	alive/well	The Toronto Hosp
2	9/27/88	W.C.	42	54	12yrs, 3mos	alive/well	The Toronto Hosp
3	8/2/89	D.F.	35	46	11yrs, 4mos	alive/well	Stanford Univ
4	4/17/90	R.D.	27	37	10yrs, 8mos	alive/well	U No Carolina-Chapel Hill
5	8/5/90	J.C.	48	58	10yrs, 4mos	alive/well	London Health Sci Ctr-
		Ontario					
6	11/27/90	H.B.	48	58	10yrs, 1mo	alive/well	Univ Pittsburgh
7	5/1/91	J.S.	44	53	9yrs, 7mos	alive/well	Univ Pittsburgh
7	5/6/91	M.H.	36	45	9yrs, 7mos	alive/well	Univ Pittsburgh
7	5/14/91	D.W.	43	52	9yrs, 7mos	alive/well	Stanford Univ
8	8/28/91	J.K.	62	71	9yrs, 4mos	alive/well	Northern Indiana Heart Inst
9	3/26/92	R.A.	60	68	8yrs, 9mos	excellent	Univ Calif-San Francisco
10	10/26/93	E.M.	50	57	7yrs, 2mos	alive/well	Univ Geneva Hosp
11	1/27/94	C.J.	47	53	6yrs,11mos	alive/well	Univ Geneva Hosp
12	2/28/94	A.M.	49	55	6yrs,10mos	alive/well	Univ Geneva Hosp
13	6/6/94	P.H.	53	59	6yrs, 6mos	gd functn	Univ Pittsburgh
13	6/6/94	B.M.	51	57	6yrs, 6mos	gd functn	Univ Pittsburgh
14	7/7/94	J.P.	57	63	6yrs, 5mos	alive/well	Univ Geneva Hosp
15	10/10/94	A.R.	43	49	6yrs, 2mos	alive/well	Univ Geneva Hosp
16	3/2/95	H.C.	46	51	5yrs, 9mos	alive/well	Univ Geneva Hosp

TX DATE	NAME	TX AGE	CURR AGE	YEARS CONT'D FUNCTION	CURRENT FUNCTION	CENTER

Oldest Single-Lung Recipient:

	TX DATE	NAME	TX AGE	CURR AGE	YEARS CONT'D FUNCTION	CURRENT FUNCTION	CENTER
1	3/10/00	H.W.	70	70	-, 9mos	alive/well	Univ Pittsburgh
2	5/25/97	P.K.	68	71	3yrs, 7mos	alive/well	Univ Pittsburgh
3	8/28/91	J.K.	62	71	9yrs, 4mos	alive/well	Northern Indiana Heart Inst
3	12/7/98	W.W.	62	64	2yrs, -	alive/well	Stanford Univ
4	12/19/96	D.K.	61	65	4yrs, -	alive/well	Stanford Univ
4	3/11/98	S.W.	61	63	2yrs, 9mos	alive/well	Stanford Univ
5	11/7/93	D.A.	60	67	7yrs, 1mo	alive/well	Stanford Univ
6	12/9/99	V.C.	51	60yr dnr	1yr, -	alive/well	Univ Pittsburgh

LUNG (DOUBLE)

Longest Surviving Double-Lung Transplant:

	TX DATE	NAME	TX AGE	CURR AGE	YEARS CONT'D FUNCTION	CURRENT FUNCTION	CENTER
1	11/26/86	A.H.	42	56	14yrs, 1mo	ad functn	The Toronto Hosp
2	1/9/87	D.M.	32	45	13yrs, 11mos	alive/well	The Toronto Hosp
3	2/27/87	C.U.	36	49	13yrs, 10mos	fair functn	The Toronto Hosp
4	7/23/87	P.R.	43	56	13yrs, 5mos	alive/well	The Toronto Hosp
5	3/26/88	L.W.	29	41	12yrs, 9mos	alive/well	The Toronto Hosp
6	5/6/88	F.S.	60	72	12yrs, 7mos	alive/well	Univ Mississippi
7	10/19/88	P.M	37	50	12yrs, 2mos	alive/well	Univ Pittsburgh
8	1/10/89	S.S.	12	15	11yrs, 11mos	alive/well	Children's-U Pittsburgh
9	10/8/90	D.S.	39	49	10yrs, 2mos	alive/well	Stanford Univ
9	10/8/90	H.G.	28	38	10yrs, 2mos	alive/well	U No Carolina-Chapel Hill
10	10/9/91	D.G.	32	41	9yrs, 2mos	alive/well	U No Carolina-Chapel Hill
11	1/9/92	L.D.	41	49	8yrs, 11mos	alive/well	Stanford Univ
12	9/8/92	N.M.	10	18	8yrs, 3mos	alive/well	Children's-U Pittsburgh
13	1/18/93	B.S.	29	37	7yrs, 11mos	alive/well	Stanford Univ
14	4/18/93	K.L.	29	36	7yrs, 8mos	alive/well	Stanford Univ
15	5/19/93	J.G.	9	16	7yrs, 7mos	alive/well	U No Carolina-Chapel Hill
16	10/21/93	M.O.	9	16	7yrs, 2mos	gd functn	Washington Univ-St Louis
17	12/13/93	A.K.	15	22	7yrs, -	gd functn	Washington Univ-St Louis
17	12/15/93	M.M.	17	24	7yrs, -	gd functn	Washington Univ-St Louis
18	1/2/94	G.L.	29	35	6yrs, 11mos	alive/well	Stanford Univ
18	1/16/94	P.L.	42	49	6yrs, 11mos	alive/well	Univ Geneva Hosp
19	2/21/94	C.F.	32	39	6yrs, 10mos	alive/well	Univ Geneva Hosp
20	7/18/94	M.D.	42	48	6yrs, 5mos	excellent	Univ Calif-San Francisco

Youngest Double-Lung Recipient:

	TX DATE	NAME	TX AGE	CURR AGE	YEARS CONT'D FUNCTION	CURRENT FUNCTION	CENTER
1	3/11/94	A.W.	2mos	5	6yrs, 9mos	good functn	Washington Univ-St Louis
1	6/14/94	M.C.	2mos	5	6yrs, 6mos	good functn	Washington Univ-St Louis
1	5/25/95	G.P.	2mos	7	5yrs, 7mos	good functn	Washington Univ-St Louis
2	7/26/94	S.M.	3mos	5	6yrs, 5mos	good functn	Washington Univ-St Louis
3	4/9/94	M.W.	19mos	5	6yrs, 8mos	good functn	Washington Univ-St Louis

TX DATE	NAME	TX AGE	CURR AGE	YEARS CONT'D FUNCTION	CURRENT FUNCTION	CENTER

Oldest Double-Lung Recipient:

	TX DATE	NAME	TX AGE	CURR AGE	YEARS CONT'D FUNCTION	CURRENT FUNCTION	CENTER
1	6/13/96	D.W.	67	71	4yrs, 6mos	alive/well	The Toronto Hosp
1	7/21/97	M.J.	67	70	3yrs, 5mos	alive/well	The Toronto Hosp
2	3/27/94	R.P.	66	72	6yrs, 9mos	xclnt functn	The Toronto Hosp
3	11/9/92	L.G.	64	72	8yrs, 1mo	xclnt functn	The Toronto Hosp
4	8/26/93	K.M	62	69	7yrs, 4mos	alive/well	Univ Pittsburgh
5	7/23/94	D.K.	54	60	6yrs, 5mos	alive/well	Stanford Univ

Youngest Double-Lung Donor:

	TX DATE	NAME	TX AGE	CURR AGE	YEARS CONT'D FUNCTION	CURRENT FUNCTION	CENTER
1	6/14/94	M.C.	2mos	2mos dnr	6yrs, 6mos	good functn	Washington Univ-St Louis
2	3/11/94	A.W.	2mos	4mos dnr	6yrs, 9mos	good functn	Washington Univ-St Louis
3	7/26/94	S.M.	3mos	14mos dnr	6yrs, 5mos	good functn	Washington Univ-St Louis
3	4/9/94	M.W.	19mos	14mos dnr	6yrs, 8mos	good functn	Washington Univ-St Louis

Oldest Double-Lung Donor:

	TX DATE	NAME	TX AGE	CURR AGE	YEARS CONT'D FUNCTION	CURRENT FUNCTION	CENTER
1	9/3/97	D.M.	27	54yr dnr	3yrs, 3mos	alive/well	Univ Pittsburgh

Youngest Recipient To Survive Two Cadaver Double Lung Transplants:

1 M.C. rcv'd 1st cadaver double Tx 02/21/94 at 2 months of age.

Four months later, lungs failed due to severe infection.

M.C., six months old, rcv'd 2nd cadaver double lung Tx, 06/14/94.

					YEARS CONT'D FUNCTION	CURRENT FUNCTION	CENTER
					6yrs, 6mos	good functn	Washington Univ-St Louis

Youngest Recipient To Receive Double Lung Transplant From Two Living-Related Donors Simultaneously:

1 7/7/94 J.B. 13yrs old rcv'd one lung lobe from his mother, and one lung lobe from his father.

					YEARS CONT'D FUNCTION	CURRENT FUNCTION	CENTER
					6yrs, 5mos	good functn	Washington Univ-St Louis

INTESTINE

TX DATE	NAME	TX AGE	CURR AGE	YEARS CONT'D FUNCTION	CURRENT FUNCTION (SCr)	CENTER

INTESTINE (CADAVER)

Longest Surviving Intestine Tx:

#	TX DATE	NAME	TX AGE	CURR AGE	YEARS CONT'D FUNCTION	CURRENT FUNCTION (SCr)	CENTER
1	3/18/89	V.R.	5mos	12	11yrs, 9mos	xclnt functn	Necker Enfants-Paris
2	7/1/90	T.G.	3	13	10yrs, 1mo	gd functn	Univ Pittsburgh
2	8/3/90	M.C.	27	37	10yrs, 1mo	gd functn	Univ Pittsburgh
3	11/2/91	A.A.	2	11	9yrs, 1mos	gd functn	Univ Pittsburgh

Youngest Recipient to Receive an Intestine Transplant:

#	TX DATE	NAME	TX AGE	CURR AGE	YEARS CONT'D FUNCTION	CURRENT FUNCTION (SCr)	CENTER
1	3/18/89	V.R.	5mos	12	11yrs, 9mos	xclnt functn	Necker Enfants-Paris
2	7/27/92	J.H.	6mos	7	8yrs, 1mo	functng well	Univ Pittsburgh
3	5/10/99	T.R.	7mos	1	1yr, 7mos	functng well	Univ Pittsburgh

INTESTINE (RELATED)

Longest Surviving Intestine Transplant From A Living-Related Donor:

#	TX DATE	NAME/DETAIL	YEARS CONT'D FUNCTION	CURRENT FUNCTION (SCr)	CENTER
1	9/26/96	P.J. 40 yrs old rcv'd intestine from one identical triplet brothers, caval drainage of intestine-no immunosuppression	4yrs, 3mos	xclnt funct	Addenbrookes-Cambridge
2	4/30/98	C.H. 13yrs old rcv'd intestine from his brother	2yrs, 8mos	excellent	HUG-Hosp Cantonal-Switzerland

MULTI-ORGAN GRAFTS

KIDNEY/BONE MARROW:

#	TX DATE	NAME	TX AGE	CURR AGE	YEARS CONT'D FUNCTION	CURRENT FUNCTION (SCr)	CENTER
1	12/14/92	S.M.	50	58	8yrs, -	doing well	Univ Pittsburgh

HEART/BONE MARROW:

#	TX DATE	NAME	TX AGE	CURR AGE	YEARS CONT'D FUNCTION	CURRENT FUNCTION (SCr)	CENTER
1	3/22/94	J.T.	50	56	6yrs, 9mos	doing fine	Univ Pittsburgh
1	3/22/94	D.C.	41	47	6yrs, 9mos	doing fine	Univ Pittsburgh

HEART/KIDNEY:

#	TX DATE	NAME	TX AGE	CURR AGE	YEARS CONT'D FUNCTION	CURRENT FUNCTION (SCr)	CENTER
1	7/18/90	D.C.	51	61	10yrs, 5mos	1.0	Clinic Ct Luc Brussels
2	7/23/90	R.B.	43	53	10yrs, 5mos	xclnt functn	Temple U-Philadelphia
3	5/29/91	J.H.	53	62	9yrs, 7mos	1.2	Univ Calif-San Francisco
4	10/9/94	H.P.	38	43	6yrs, 2mos	alive/well	Univ Pittsburgh
5	1/21/95	P.C.	61	66	5yrs,11mos	alive/well	Methodist M C-Dallas
6	2/11/95	R.J.	46	51	5yrs,10mos	xclnt functn	Temple U-Philadelphia
7	2/14/96	N.M.	43	47	4yrs,10mos	xclnt functn	Temple U-Philadelphia
8	6/3/96	S.P.	59	63	4yrs, 6mos	alive/well	Policlinico Univ-Milan

HEART/KIDNEY/PANCREAS:

#	TX DATE	NAME	TX AGE	CURR AGE	YEARS CONT'D FUNCTION	CURRENT FUNCTION (SCr)	CENTER
1	2/12/92	L.S.	40	48	8yrs,10mos	1.6	Methodist M C-Dallas
2	2/25/95	R.B.	47	52	5yrs,10mos	alive/well	Methodist M C-Dallas

HEART/LIVER/KIDNEY

#	TX DATE	NAME	TX AGE	CURR AGE	YEARS CONT'D FUNCTION	CURRENT FUNCTION (SCr)	CENTER
1	5/1/99	K.S.		60	1yr, 7mos	alive/well	Univ Chicago

	TX DATE	NAME	TX AGE	CURR AGE	YEARS CONT'D FUNCTION	CURRENT FUNCTION (SCr)	CENTER
HEART/LUNG/LIVER:							
1	8/21/98	B.E.	2	4	2yrs, 4mos	well	Children's-U Pittsburgh
HEART/PANCREAS:							
1	11/9/93	G.C.	42	49	7yrs, 1mo	alive/well	Methodist M C-Dallas
2	3/30/95	R.C.	50	55	5yrs, 9mos	alive/well	Methodist M C-Dallas
LIVER/KIDNEY:							
1	12/28/83	J.M.	27	44	17yrs, -	alive/well	Univ Hosp-Innsbruck
2	7/22/84	G.H.	42	58	16yrs, 5mos	norml liver/2.1	Univ Pittsburgh
3	11/24/84	G.F.	15	31	16yrs, 1mo	doing fine	Univ Pittsburgh
4	2/12/85	M.R.	43	58	15yrs,10mos	doing fine	Univ Pittsburgh
5	12/26/85	J.S.	60	75	15yrs, -	alive/well	Univ Hosp-Innsbruck
6	1/28/86	J.L.	34	48	14yrs,11mos	doing fine	Univ Pittsburgh
7	3/6/86	L.F.	55	69	14yrs, 8mos	alive/well	Univ Hosp-Innsbruck
8	2/20/87	P.S.	41	54	13yrs,10mos	alive/well	Univ Hosp-Innsbruck
9	5/6/87	L.C.	11	24	13yrs, 7mos	0.7	Clinic St Luc-Brussels
10	10/18/87	W.L.	48	61	13yrs, 2mos	norm functn	Univ Pittsburgh
Youngest Liver-Kidney Recipient:							
1	7/28/99	A.D.	3mos	1	5mos	good	St. Christopher's Hosp Childrn
LIVER/BONE MARROW:							
1	6/7/92	J.S.	31	39	8yrs, 6mos	doing fine	Univ Pittsburgh
LIVER/HEART:							
1	7/7/92	R.F.	47	55	8yrs, 5mos	alive/well	Mayo Clinic-Rochester
2	6/14/93	R.C.	61	68	7yrs, 6mos	doing fine	Univ Pittsburgh
3	12/2/95	W.R.	47	52	5yrs, -	alive/well	Univ Chicago
4	4/1/96	D.C.	39	43	4yrs, 8mos	alive/well	Univ Chicago
5	3/2/98	S.T.	45	47	2yrs, 9mos	alive/well	Univ Chicago
LIVER/HEART/LUNG:							
1	8/22/98	B.E.	2	4	2yrs, 4mos	functng	Univ Pittsburgh
LIVER/ISLETS:							
1	11/26/92	C.V.	47	55	8yrs, 1mo	gd functn	Nat'l Tumor Inst-Milan
2	7/25/98	P.E.	64	66	2yrs, 5mos	alive/well	Univ Chicago
LIVER/PANCREAS:							
1	7/1/88	A.B.	39	51	12yrs, 5mos		
					adequate liver functn. insulin-indep		Univ Pittsburgh
LIVER/INTESTINE:							
1	7/24/90	T.G.	3	13	10yrs, 5mos	alive/well	Univ Pittsburgh
2	8/3/90	M.C.	26	36	10yrs, 4mos	alive/well	Univ Pittsburgh
3	11/25/90	J.P.	4	14	10yrs, 1mo	alive/well	Univ Pittsburgh
4	3/29/92	G.B.	24	32	8yrs, 9mos	alive/well	Univ Pittsburgh
5	7/21/92	B.V.	9mos	8	8yrs, 5mos	alive/well	Univ Pittsburgh

	TX DATE	NAME	TX AGE	CURR AGE	YEARS CONT'D FUNCTION	CURRENT FUNCTION (SCr)	CENTER
5	7/27/92	J.H.	6mos	8	8yrs, 5mos	alive/well	Univ Pittsburgh
6	8/14/92	B.S.	19	27	8yrs, 4mos	alive/well	Univ Pittsburgh

Longest Surviving Multivisceral Transplant Recipient:

	TX DATE	NAME	TX AGE	CURR AGE	YEARS CONT'D FUNCTION	CURRENT FUNCTION (SCr)	CENTER
1	7/24/90	T.G.	3	13	10yrs, 7mos	functng	Univ Pittsburgh
2	8/3/90	M.C.	27	37	10yrs, 4mos	functng	Univ Pittsburgh

Longest Surviving Upper Abdominal Extraction and Cluster Transplant (liver, pancreas duodenum, and partial stomach):

	TX DATE	NAME	TX AGE	CURR AGE	YEARS CONT'D FUNCTION	CURRENT FUNCTION (SCr)	CENTER
1	10/27/88	D.C.	36	48	12yrs, 2mos	alive/well	Univ Pittsburgh
2	1/12/89	D.H.	40	51	11yrs,11mos	alive/well	Univ Pittsburgh
3	5/19/89	F.G.	38	49	11yrs, 7mos	alive/well	Univ Pittsburgh
4	6/12/89	J.K.	35	46	11yrs, 6mos	alive/well	Univ Pittsburgh
5	8/7/89	J.R.	40	51	11yrs, 4mos	alive/well	Univ Pittsburgh
6	3/16/90	F.S.	52	62	10yrs, 9mos	alive/well	Univ Pittsburgh
7	4/28/90	M.E.	43	53	10yrs, 8mos	alive/well	Univ Wisconsin-Madison

BONE MARROW

TX DATE	NAME	TX AGE	CURR AGE	YEARS CONT'D FUNCTION	CURRENT KARNOFSKY	CENTER

BONE MARROW (SYNGENEIC)

Longest Surviving Syngeneic BMT-(CML)

	TX DATE	NAME	TX AGE	CURR AGE	YEARS CONT'D FUNCTION	CURRENT KARNOFSKY	CENTER
1	5/17/76	B.H.	22	47	24yrs, 7mos	in CR	FHCRC-Seattle
2	10/29/76	D.S.	41	66	24yrs, 1mo	in CR	FHCRC-Seattle
3	1/21/77	A.W.	13	37	23yrs,11mos	in CR	FHCRC-Seattle
4	2/9/79	J.M.	25	47	21yrs,10mos	in CR	FHCRC-Seattle

BONE MARROW (ALLOGENEIC RELATED)

Longest Surviving Allo Related BMT-
Acute Lymphocytic Leukemia (ALL):

	TX DATE	NAME	TX AGE	CURR AGE	YEARS CONT'D FUNCTION	CURRENT KARNOFSKY	CENTER
1	2/21/74	R.L.			26yrs,10mos	80%	FHCRC-Seattle
2	11/4/74	D.D.			26yrs, 1mo	100%	FHCRC-Seattle
3	5/25/76	D.N.			24yrs, 7mos	100%	FHCRC-Seattle
4	6/25/76	T.R.			24yrs, 6mos	100%	FHCRC-Seattle
5	10/8/75	E.F.			24yrs, 2mos	100%	FHCRC-Seattle
6	2/1/77	D.P.			23yrs,10mos	100%	FHCRC-Seattle
6	2/23/77	D.C.			23yrs,10mos	100%	FHCRC-Seattle
7	4/8/77	T.W.			23yrs, 8mos	50%	FHCRC-Seattle
8	8/9/77	J.M.			23yrs, 4mos	100%	FHCRC-Seattle
9	3/29/78	L.B.			22yrs, 9mos	90%	FHCRC-Seattle
10	4/24/78	M.C.			22yrs, 8mos	50%	FHCRC-Seattle
11	9/28/78	C.K.			22yrs, 3mos	100%	FHCRC-Seattle
12	11/10/78	E.B.			22yrs, 1mo	100%	FHCRC-Seattle
13	4/23/79	T.H.			21yrs, 8mos	100%	FHCRC-Seattle
13	4/25/79	N.C.			21yrs, 8mos	100%	FHCRC-Seattle
13	4/30/79	M.S.			21yrs, 8mos	100%	FHCRC-Seattle
14	7/30/79	J.H.			21yrs, 5mos	alive/well	U Minnesota-Mnpls
15	8/13/79	D.L.			21yrs, 4mos	100%	FHCRC-Seattle
16	11/21/78	B.W.			21yrs, 1mo	100%	FHCRC-Seattle
16	11/20/79	D.D.			21yrs, 1mo	100%	FHCRC-Seattle
17	12/26/79	M.F.			21yrs, -	100%	FHCRC-Seattle

Acute Myelogenous Leukemia (AML):

	TX DATE	NAME	TX AGE	CURR AGE	YEARS CONT'D FUNCTION	CURRENT KARNOFSKY	CENTER
1	1/6/72	C.L.			28yrs,11mos	100%	FHCRC-Seattle
2	4/18/72	T.S.			28yrs, 8mos	100%	FHCRC-Seattle
3	5/11/73	L.E.			27yrs, 7mos	100%	FHCRC-Seattle
4	3/25/74	C.V.			26yrs, 9mos	100%	FHCRC-Seattle
5	8/2/74	M.W.			26yrs, 4mos	90%	FHCRC-Seattle
6	3/10/76	S.M.			24yrs, 9mos	70%	FHCRC-Seattle
7	12/11/76	N.V.			24yrs, -	90%	FHCRC-Seattle
7	12/28/76	M.J.	28	51	24yrs, -	alive/well	City of Hope-Duarte
8	2/4/77	T.G.			23yrs,10mos	100%	FHCRC-Seattle

	TX DATE	NAME	TX AGE	CURR AGE	YEARS CONT'D FUNCTION	CURRENT KARNOFSKY	CENTER
9	4/1/77	R.M.			23yrs, 8mos	90%	FHCRC-Seattle
10	6/25/77	L.B.			23yrs, 6mos	100%	FHCRC-Seattle
11	8/11/77	A.S.			23yrs, 4mos	100%	FHCRC-Seattle
11	8/24/77	K.P.			23yrs, 4mos	100%	FHCRC-Seattle
12	11/23/77	J.C.			23yrs, 1mo	70%	FHCRC-Seattle
13	12/2/77	B.D.			23yrs, -	100%	FHCRC-Seattle
14	1/16/78	M.S.			22yrs,11mos	100%	FHCRC-Seattle
15	3/14/78	L.E.			22yrs, 9mos	90%	FHCRC-Seattle
16	6/14/78	D.K.			22yrs, 6mos	100%	FHCRC-Seattle
17	7/7/78	J.C.			22yrs, 5mos	100%	FHCRC-Seattle
18	10/10/78	D.S.			22yrs, 2mos	100%	FHCRC-Seattle
19	11/1/78	J.K.			22yrs, 1mo	disease free	St Francis Hosp-Hawaii
19	11/6/78	J.O.			22yrs, 1mo	100%	FHCRC-Seattle
20	12/15/78	R.Y.			22yrs, -	60%	FHCRC-Seattle
20	12/26/78	V.R.			22yrs, -	100%	FHCRC-Seattle
21	3/7/79	N.F.			21yrs, 9mos	90%	FHCRC-Seattle
21	3/21/79	G.K.			21yrs, 9mos	95%	FHCRC-Seattle
22	4/6/79	M.J.			21yrs, 8mos	90%	FHCRC-Seattle
23	5/7/79	L.H.			21yrs, 7mos	95%	FHCRC-Seattle
24	7/5/79	L.N.			21yrs, 5mos	100%	FHCRC-Seattle
25	9/17/79	D.T.			21yrs, 3mos	100%	FHCRC-Seattle
25	9/21/79	M.C.			21yrs, 3mos	100%	FHCRC-Seattle
26	10/24/79	D.D.			21yrs, 2mos	100%	FHCRC-Seattle
27	11/13/79	W.T.			21yrs, 1mo	100%	FHCRC-Seattle
27	11/28/79	D.B.			21yrs, 1mo	100%	FHCRC-Seattle
28	12/5/79	M.D.			21yrs, -	80%	FHCRC-Seattle
28	12/28/79	S.K.			21yrs, -	100%	FHCRC-Seattle

Bruton's Disease:

	TX DATE	NAME	TX AGE	CURR AGE	YEARS CONT'D FUNCTION	CURRENT KARNOFSKY	CENTER
1	3/27/88	J.G.			12yrs, 9mos	alive/well	Peking U People's Hosp

Chronic Myelogenous Leukemia (CML):

	TX DATE	NAME	TX AGE	CURR AGE	YEARS CONT'D FUNCTION	CURRENT KARNOFSKY	CENTER
1	5/17/76	B.H.	22	47	24yrs, 7mos	0.9	FHCRC-Seattle
2	2/23/79	R.S.			21yrs,10mos	100%	FHCRC-Seattle
3	5/15/79	P.F.			21yrs, 7mos	90%	FHCRC-Seattle
4	8/10/79	L.F.			21yrs, 4mos	alive/well	Hammersmith-London
5	10/12/79	S.H.			21yrs, 2mos	100%	FHCRC-Seattle
6	7/18/80	R.L.			20yrs, 5mos	100%	FHCRC-Seattle
7	9/16/80	C.H.	36	56	20yrs, 3mos	func/alive	U Basel-Switzerland
7	9/16/80	A.W.	36	56	20yrs, 3mos	func/alive	U Basel-Switzerland
8	3/5/81	C.C.			19yrs, 9mos	100%	FHCRC-Seattle
9	4/28/81	R.J.			19yrs, 8mos	100%	FHCRC-Seattle
9	4/30/81	H.D.			19yrs, 8mos	100%	FHCRC-Seattle
10	8/5/81	J.A.			19yrs, 4mos	100%	FHCRC-Seattle
11	11/2/81	E.F.			19yrs, 1mo	100%	FHCRC-Seattle
11	10/29/81	C.M.			19yrs, 1mo	100%	FHCRC-Seattle

	TX DATE	NAME	TX AGE	CURR AGE	YEARS CONT'D FUNCTION	CURRENT KARNOFSKY	CENTER
12	12/30/81	J.L.			19yrs, -	80%	FHCRC-Seattle
13	2/19/82	S.P.			18yrs,10mos	100%	FHCRC-Seattle
14	4/2/82	J.E.			18yrs, 8mos	100%	FHCRC-Seattle
14	4/16/82	W.M.			18yrs, 8mos	100%	FHCRC-Seattle
15	7/30/82	J.R.			18yrs, 5mos	100%	FHCRC-Seattle
16	8/23/82	A.T.			18yrs, 4mos	100%	FHCRC-Seattle
17	9/16/82	J.S.			18yrs, 3mos	100%	FHCRC-Seattle
17	9/17/82	A.C.			18yrs, 3mos	100%	FHCRC-Seattle
18	10/14/82	A.A.			18yrs, 2mos	100%	FHCRC-Seattle
19	11/24/82	S.W.			18yrs, 1mo	100%	FHCRC-Seattle
20	12/7/82	S.K.			18yrs, -	90%	FHCRC-Seattle
21	3/11/83	F.D.			17yrs, 9mos	100%	FHCRC-Seattle
21	3/18/83	W.B.			17yrs, 9mos	70%	FHCRC-Seattle
21	3/24/83	G.A.			17yrs, 9mos	100%	FHCRC-Seattle
21	3/25/83	D.A.			17yrs, 9mos	90%	FHCRC-Seattle
21	3/25/83	J.A.			17yrs, 9mos	100%	FHCRC-Seattle
22	4/25/83	M.R.			17yrs, 8mos	100%	FHCRC-Seattle
23	5/9/83	B.H.			17yrs, 7mos	100%	FHCRC-Seattle
24	7/1/83	M.S.			17yrs, 5mos	100%	FHCRC-Seattle
24	7/22/83	R.F.			17yrs, 5mos	100%	FHCRC-Seattle
25	8/4/83	L.M.			17yrs, 4mos	100%	FHCRC-Seattle
25	8/11/83	G.R.			17yrs, 4mos	100%	FHCRC-Seattle
26	9/20/83	G.E.			17yrs, 3mos	100%	FHCRC-Seattle
27	10/6/83	J.F.			17yrs, 2mos	100%	FHCRC-Seattle
27	10/26/83	M.N.			17yrs, 2mos	100%	FHCRC-Seattle
28	4/24/85	T.B.	32	47	15yrs, 8mos	good	Clin Hosp N.6-Russia
29	5/10/85	J.H.			15yrs, 7mos	90%	FHCRC-Seattle

Diamond/Blackfan Syndrome:

1	6/2/82	R.G.			18yrs, 6mos	100%	FHCRC-Seattle
2	8/12/85	R.S.			15yrs, 4mos	100%	FHCRC-Seattle
3	10/9/92	A.V.			8yrs, 2mos	100%	FHCRC-Seattle

Evans Syndrome:

1	2/10/92	N.T.			8yrs,10mos	100%	FHCRC-Seattle

Fanconi Anemia:

1	3/7/73	L.R.			27yrs, 9mos	90%	FHCRC-Seattle
2	10/24/80	P.A.			20yrs, 2mos	90%	FHCRC-Seattle

Hodgkins Disease (HD):

1	4/27/82	M.H.			18yrs, 8mos	100%	FHCRC-Seattle
2	4/4/86	J.B.			14yrs, 8mos	100%	FHCRC-Seattle
3	5/12/86	K.D.			14yrs, 7mos	100%	FHCRC-Seattle
4	5/27/88	S.V.			12yrs, 7mos	100%	FHCRC-Seattle

	TX DATE	NAME	TX AGE	CURR AGE	YEARS CONT'D FUNCTION	CURRENT KARNOFSKY	CENTER
Malignant Lymphoma (ML):							
1	7/24/70	C.B.			30yrs, 5mos	100%	FHCRC-Seattle
2	10/7/75	D.S.			25yrs, 2mos	alive/well	U Minnesota-Mnpls
3	4/18/80	anon			20yrs, 8mos	alive/well	U Minnesota-Mnpls
Neuroblastoma:							
1	11/25/86	S.H.			14yrs, 1mo	100%	FHCRC-Seattle
2	11/25/87	M.F.			13yrs, 1mo	100%	FHCRC-Seattle
3	6/19/89	C.P.			11yrs, 6mos	100%	FHCRC-Seattle
Paroxysmal Nocturnal Hemoglobinuria (PNH):							
1	11/15/71	C.L.			29yrs, 1mo	90%	FHCRC-Seattle
Severe Aplastic Anemia (SAA):							
1	8/2/71	S.M.			29yrs, 4mos	100%	FHCRC-Seattle
2	5/2/72	G.M			28yrs, 7mos	100%	FHCRC-Seattle
3	12/5/72	C.K.			28yrs, -	100%	FHCRC-Seattle
4	2/9/73	L.L.			27yrs,10mos	100%	FHCRC-Seattle
4	2/21/73	D.T.			27yrs,10mos	100%	FHCRC-Seattle
5	3/29/73	J.B.			27yrs, 9mos	100%	FHCRC-Seattle
6	6/20/73	A.B.			27yrs, 6mos	90%	FHCRC-Seattle
7	10/16/73	P.D.			27yrs, 2mos	alive/well	Leiden U-Netherlands
8	1/14/74	D.K.			26yrs,11mos	100%	FHCRC-Seattle
9	2/25/74	S.S.			26yrs,10mos	100%	FHCRC-Seattle
10	3/27/74	L.C.			26yrs, 9mos	100%	FHCRC-Seattle
11	7/16/74	B.S.			26yrs, 5mos	100%	FHCRC-Seattle
12	9/11/74	N.R.			26yrs, 3mos	100%	FHCRC-Seattle
13	1/28/75	A.V.			25yrs,11mos	100%	FHCRC-Seattle
14	2/21/75	D.B.			25yrs,10mos	100%	FHCRC-Seattle
15	3/11/75	J.G.			25yrs, 9mos	100%	FHCRC-Seattle
15	3/18/75	C.M.			25yrs, 9mos	alive/well	Univ Munich-Germany
16	6/2/75	G.R.			25yrs, 6mos	100%	FHCRC-Seattle
17	8/7/75	R.L.			25yrs, 4mos	100%	FHCRC-Seattle
17	8/26/75	K.K.			25yrs, 4mos	100%	FHCRC-Seattle
18	11/19/75	A.B.			25yrs, 1mo	100%	FHCRC-Seattle
19	1/21/76	T.S.	5	29	24yrs,11mos	func/alive	U Basel-Switzerland
20	2/12/76	A.P.	30	54	24yrs,10mos	func/alive	U Basel-Switzerland
Severe Combined Immunological Deficiency (SCID):							
1	12/19/68	J.M.			32yrs, -	alive/well	Leiden U-Netherlands
Sickle Cell Anemia:							
1	9/19/91	O.O.			9yrs, 3mos	100%	FHCRC-Seattle
Systemic Sclerosis							
1	3/22/99	S.S.			1yrs, 9mos	100%	FHCRC-Seattle

TX DATE	NAME	TX AGE	CURR AGE	YEARS CONT'D FUNCTION	CURRENT KARNOFSKY	CENTER

Thalassemia:

	TX DATE	NAME	TX AGE	CURR AGE	YEARS CONT'D FUNCTION	CURRENT KARNOFSKY	CENTER
1	7/1/82	F.G.			18yrs, 5mos	100%	FHCRC-Seattle
2	2/18/83	C.R.			17yrs,10mos	100%	FHCRC-Seattle

Wiskott-Aldrich Syndrome:

	TX DATE	NAME	TX AGE	CURR AGE	YEARS CONT'D FUNCTION	CURRENT KARNOFSKY	CENTER
1	3/24/80	K.K.			20yrs, 9mos	100%	FHCRC-Seattle
2	10/12/82	C.P.			18yrs, 2mos	100%	FHCRC-Seattle

Oldest BMT Recipient:

	TX DATE	NAME	TX AGE	CURR AGE	YEARS CONT'D FUNCTION	CURRENT KARNOFSKY	CENTER
1	8/4/99	P.S.	72	73	1yr, 4mos	80%	FHCRC-Seattle
2	6/28/00	anon	70	70	-, 6mos	alive/well	Universitatsklinikum Freiburg
3	4/17/97	H.G.	68	68	3yrs, 8mos	alive/well	Ontario Cancer Inst
4	8/22/95	L.M.	67	67	5yrs, 4mos	alive/well	Ontario Cancer Inst
5	8/22/96	A.Mc.	66	66	4yrs, 4mos	alive/well	Ontario Cancer Inst
6	2/23/95	M.T.	65	70	5yrs,10mos	80%	Emory Univ-Atlanta

Youngest BMT Recipient:

	TX DATE	NAME	TX AGE	CURR AGE	YEARS CONT'D FUNCTION	CURRENT KARNOFSKY	CENTER
1	11/26/80	T.W.	20dys	20	20yrs, 1mo	100%	Grt Ormond St Hosp-London
2	11/23/84	H.E.	21dys	16	16yrs, 1mo	alive/well	Children's Hosp-LA
3	1/30/95	Y.H.	22dys	5	5yrs,11mos	alive	Med Ctr Israel-Petach Tikva
4	9/6/90	L.S.	30dys	10	10yrs, 3mos	alive/well	Univ Gothenburg-Sweden
5	2/26/91	R.G.	3mos	9	9yrs,10mos	100%	FHCRC-Seattle
6	7/10/92	Y.Y.	4mos	8	8yrs, 5mos	alive/well	Nagoya Univ Hosp-Japan

Oldest BMT Donor:

	TX DATE	NAME	TX AGE	CURR AGE	YEARS CONT'D FUNCTION	CURRENT KARNOFSKY	CENTER
1	7/9/97	L.T.	76yr dnr		3yrs, 5mos	alive/well	FHCRC-Seattle
2	3/29/88	J.F.	69yr dnr		12yrs, 9mos	alive/well	Virchow Klinikum-Berlin

Youngest BMT Donor:

	TX DATE	NAME	TX AGE	CURR AGE	YEARS CONT'D FUNCTION	CURRENT KARNOFSKY	CENTER
1	9/9/80	A.A.	3mos dnr		20yrs, 3mos	alive/well	FHCRC-Seattle

Longest Surviving After Second Allogeneic BMT:

		YEARS CONT'D FUNCTION	CURRENT KARNOFSKY	CENTER
1	J.L..-1st BMT 1/19/78 from sister for aplastic anemia 2nd BMT 1/25/79 from brother	21yrs,11mos	100%	FHCRC-Seattle
2	D.G. -2nd BMT 2/21/85, after 1st BMT 7/10/84 from same sibling failed.	5yrs,10mos	alive/well	Univ Leuven-Belgium
3	J.G. -2nd BMT 3/27/88 from another sibling, after 1st BMT 11/87 rejected	12yrs, 9mos	alive/well	Peking Univ People's Hosp
4	S.S. -2nd BMT 2/14/89, after failure of 1st BMT 1988.	11yrs,10mos	alive/well	St Francis Hosp-Hawaii
5	D.N. -2nd BMT 7/11/90, after 1st BMT failed 4/18/90.	10yrs, 5mos	100%	Hosp Clin-Sao Paulo

Longest Surviving After Three Allogeneic BMT:

		YEARS CONT'D FUNCTION	CURRENT KARNOFSKY	CENTER
1	A.S. 1st BMT from sibling for Aplastic Anemia 5/27/84, 2nd BMT on 1/3/86, 3rd BMT on 3/10/87 all from same donor.	13yrs, 9mos	100%	FHCRC-Seattle

TX DATE	NAME	TX AGE	CURR AGE	YEARS CONT'D FUNCTION	CURRENT KARNOFSKY	CENTER

2   M.P. 4yrs old rcv'd first BMT on 12/15/89 for Ph-ve CML from 11mos old sister (d.o.b. 01/25/88). 2nd allograft from same donor 08/07/92. 3rd BMT on 07/29/94 also from the same donor.

| | | | | 6yrs, 5mos | alive/well | Hammersmith-London |

Smallest Recipient to Receive a Bone Marrow Transplant:

1   Y.H. born premature on 01/08/95 with SCID. Patient was 22dys old weighing 1570 grams (3lbs,7 ounces), when BMT was rcv'd from 4yr old sibling 01/30/95.

| | | | | 5yrs,11mos | alive/well | Med Ctr Israel-Petach Tikva |

Youngest Double BMT Donor:

1   4/28/92   R.F. 1st BMT(4/28/92) from 14mo old sister, rcv'd 2nd BMT(9/1/92) from same donor. Patient had rcv'd a liver Tx prior to the 2 BMTs

| | | | | 8yrs, 8mos | exclnt hlth | Univ Munich-Germany |
| 2   5/6/86 | S.W. | 2 | 16 | 14yrs, 7mos | | FHCRC-Seattle |

Youngest Triple BMT Donor:

1   M.P. 4yrs old, rcv'd 3 BMTs from 11 month old sibling, 12/15/89; (2) 08/07/92; (3) 07/29/94.

| | | | | 11yrs, - | alive/well | Hammersmith-London |

Longest Surviving BMT Recipient with Heart Transplant:

1   02/15/91 K.B. rcv'd BMT 8yrs 100% 04/01/92 K.B. rcv'd heart

| | | | | 9yrs,10mos | alive/well | Hammersmith-London |

Longest Surviving Recipient to Receive BMT After Liver Transplant:

1   7/24/87 S.E. rcv'd a BMT Tx (13 yrs) 2/20/97 rcv'd liver tx (3yrs)

| | | | | 13yrs, 5mos | alive/well | FHCRC-Seattle |

2   03/—/87 D.S. rcv'd a liver Tx 12yrs,9mos alive/well 04/18/89 D.S. rcv'd a BMT

| | | | | 11yrs, 9mos | alive/well | FHCRC-Seattle |

3   R.F. Rcv'd a liver Tx (11/9/91) prior to rcv'ng two BMTs, 04/28/92 and 09/01/92 from infant sister.

| | | | | 8yrs, 1mo | xclnt/100% | Univ Munich-Germany |

Longest Surviving Recipient to Receive A Liver Transplant After BMT:

1   5/10/91 I.P. 22yrs old with CML recv'd a BMT from his sister. 8/20/91 patient recv'd a liver Tx as a result of severe acute liver GVHD.

| | | | | 9yrs, 7mos | alive/well | Hammersmith-London |

BONE MARROW (ALLOGENEIC UNRELATED)

Longest Surviving Allo Unrelated BMT-
Acute Lymphocytic Leukemia (ALL):

#	TX DATE	NAME			YEARS CONT'D FUNCTION	CURRENT KARNOFSKY	CENTER
1	8/11/87	B.C.			13yrs, 4mos	100%	FHCRC-Seattle
2	12/13/88	A.A.			12yrs, -	100%	FHCRC-Seattle
3	2/24/89	L.H.			11yrs,10mos	100%	FHCRC-Seattle
4	10/24/89	R.C.			11yrs, 2mos	95%	FHCRC-Seattle

Metachromatic Leukodystrophy:

#	TX DATE	NAME			YEARS CONT'D FUNCTION	CURRENT KARNOFSKY	CENTER
1	8/15/91	B.W.			9yrs, 4mos	100%	FHCRC-Seattle

TX DATE	NAME	TX AGE	CURR AGE	YEARS CONT'D FUNCTION	CURRENT KARNOFSKY	CENTER

Hurler's Syndrome (MPS I)

	TX DATE	NAME	TX AGE	CURR AGE	YEARS CONT'D FUNCTION	CURRENT KARNOFSKY	CENTER
1	11/28/88	M.L.			12yrs, 1mo	100%	FHCRC-Seattle
2	6/28/90	E.B.			10yrs, 6mos	80%	FHCRC-Seattle
3	11/14/91	A.U.			9yrs, 1mo	60%	FHCRC-Seattle

Acute Lymphocytic Leukemia (ALL):

	TX DATE	NAME	TX AGE	CURR AGE	YEARS CONT'D FUNCTION	CURRENT KARNOFSKY	CENTER
1	1/27/95	L.D.			5yrs,11mos	100%	FHCRC-Seattle

Chronic Lymphocytic Leukemia (CLL):

	TX DATE	NAME	TX AGE	CURR AGE	YEARS CONT'D FUNCTION	CURRENT KARNOFSKY	CENTER
1	5/11/92	T.F.			8yrs, 7mos	100%	FHCRC-Seattle
2	12/7/92	B.R.			8yrs, -	100%	FHCRC-Seattle

Multiple Myeloma (MM)

	TX DATE	NAME	TX AGE	CURR AGE	YEARS CONT'D FUNCTION	CURRENT KARNOFSKY	CENTER
1	3/11/88	L.C.			12yrs, 9mos	100%	FHCRC-Seattle
2	11/23/88	R.R.			12yrs, 1mo	70%	FHCRC-Seattle
3	7/20/89	A.B.			11yrs, 5mos	90%	FHCRC-Seattle
4	3/15/96	J.W.			4yrs, 9mos	95%	FHCRC-Seattle

Myelodysplastic Syndrome (MDS)

	TX DATE	NAME	TX AGE	CURR AGE	YEARS CONT'D FUNCTION	CURRENT KARNOFSKY	CENTER
1	8/19/82	L.T.			18yrs, 4mos	100%	FHCRC-Seattle
2	9/13/82	V.S.			18yrs, 3mos	90%	FHCRC-Seattle
3	7/12/84	A.M.			16yrs, 5mos	100%	FHCRC-Seattle
4	5/17/85	E.P.			15yrs, 7mos	90%	FHCRC-Seattle

Oldest Stem Cell Transplant

	TX DATE	NAME	TX AGE	CURR AGE	YEARS CONT'D FUNCTION	CURRENT KARNOFSKY	CENTER
1	11/26/98	M.M.	83yr donor		2yrs, 1mo	func/alive	Univ Med Ctr-Ljubljana

WORLDWIDE TRANSPLANT CENTER DIRECTORY
KIDNEY TRANSPLANTS

1)=Director, 2)=Tx Surgeons, 3)=Physicians, 4)=Tissue Typers, 5)=TxCoords	1998	1999	2000	Total

UNITED STATES

ALABAMA

Univ of Alabama at Birmingham, Dept of Surg, 701 S 19th St, Birmingham, AL 35294 Ph: (205) 934-2131 Fax: (205) 975-7549 1,2) M.H. Deierhoi, 2) J.S. Bynon, D. Eckhoff, C.A. Young, M. Sellers, M.H. Gallichio, 3) J. Curtis, B. Julian, R. Gaston, C. Kew, 4) J. Thomas, 5) Hardin, Huey, Mayes, Brasfield	288	282	361	5397
Univ of South Alabama Med Ctr, Transp Surg, 2451 Fillingim St 10F, Mobile, AL 36617 Ph: (334) 471-7391 Fax: (334) 471-7417 Email: bbrowne@jaguar1.usouthal.edu 1,2) B.J. Browne, 3) O. Emovon, M. Culpepper, W. Kirkpatrick, 4) UAB Tissue Typing Lab, 5) C. Holt, L. Oyler	1	19	31*	44

ARIZONA

Good Samaritan Reg Med Ctr, Samaritan Transp Serv, 1410 N 3rd St, Phoenix, AZ 85004-1608 Ph: (602) 251-2700 Fax: (602) 251-2750 1,2) A.J. Fabrega, 1,3) E. Polito, 2) L.J. Koep, A.I. Serota, 3) Yee, Haws, Chang, Schon, Guerra, Hyde, 4) T. Vyvial, DNA HLA, 5) J. Bell, A. Moore, M. Ruocco, K. Helzer, K. Fitzpatrick	95	101	87*	1859
Mayo Clinic Hosp, Div of Transpl Med, 5777 East Mayo Blvd, Phoenix, AZ 85054 Ph: (480) 342-0514 Fax: (480) 342-2324 Email: heilman.ray@mayo.edu/moss.adyr@mayo.edu 1) R.L. Heilman, 1) A.A. Moss, 2) D.C. Mulligan, 3) I.M. Cohen, R.L. Heilman, D.N. Wochos, 4) Donor Network of AZ, 5) T.A. Kriesand, J.S. Mitoff		9	7	16
Univ of Arizona Med Ctr, Dept of Transp Serv, 1501 N Campbell Ave, P.O.Box 245145, Tucson, AZ 85724 Ph: (520) 694-4984 Fax: (520) 694-4983 1,2) J.U. Zamora, 1) II, 2) P. Nakazato, J. Hughes, 3) H. Lein, S. James, 4) C. Spier, 5) L. Maselli, N. Stubbs, S. Anderson, C. Gebremariam	40	51	33	270

ARKANSAS

Arkansas Children's Hosp, Dept of Neph/Renal Transp, 800 Marshall, Little Rock, AR 72202- 3591 Ph: (501) 320-1847 Fax: (501) 320-3551 1,3) E.N. Ellis, 2) C. Wagner, B. Ketel, 3) T. Wells, R. Blaszak, 4) V. Smith, T. Harville, 5) K. Pennington	6	6	7	104
Baptist Med Ctr, Kidney Transplant Program, 9601 Interstate 630 Exit 7, Medical Tower II,Suite 800, Little Rock, AR 72205 Ph: (501) 202-1500 Fax: (501) 202-1357 1,3) S. Young, 2) R. Casali, W.E. Tucker, D. Dean, 4) V. Smith, 5) K. Clingan, J. Mott	35	40	45	416
The Univ Hosp of Arkansas, Dept of Surg, 4301 W Markham, Box 520, Little Rock, AR 72205 Ph: (501) 686-6644 Fax: (501) 686-5725 1,2) B.L. Ketel, 2) G. Barone, 3) M. Bunke, S. Abdul-Ezz, 4) V. Smith, P. Treadway, 5) S. Turton-Weeks, L. Lingo, K. Conery-Reed	36	52	36*	971

CALIFORNIA

Arrowhead Regional Med Ctr, Dept of Transp, 400 North Pepper Ave, Colton, CA 92324 Ph: (909) 580-6103 Fax: (909) 580-2234 Email: tolefree@armc.co.san-bernardino.ca.us 1,2) W. Concepcion, 2) E. Dainko, R. Hadley, O. Ojogho, 3) A. Kavalich, H. Phan, 4) Metic Lab, LLUMC Histo Lab, 5) L. Tolefree	5	8	6	506
Scripps Green Hosp, Ctr for Organ & Cell Transp, 10666 N Torrey Pines Rd, 200-N, La Jolla, CA 92037 Ph: (858) 554-4310 Fax: (858) 554-4311 Email: ahassoun@scrippsclinic.com 1,2) M. Brunson, 2) A. Hassoun, 3) D. Salomon, S. Bhaduri, A. King, 4) UCSD HLA Lab, 5) J. Henry, K. Bounds, K. Thorson, L. Biermann	6	16	19	63
Loma Linda Univ Med Ctr, Transp Inst, 11234 Anderson, Loma Linda, CA 92354 Ph: (909) 558-4252 Fax: (909) 558-0112 1,2) W. Concepcion, 2) O. Ojogho, P. Baron, 3) S. Teichman, S. Sahney, 4) S. Nehlsen-Cannarella, L. Buckert, 5) R. Custodio, C. Maas, J. Vickers, D. Peterson	78	62	94	996

KIDNEY

*Preliminary UNOS data

1)=Director, 2)=Tx Surgeons, 3)=Physicians, 4)=Tissue Typers, 5)=TxCoords	1998	1999	2000	Total
St Mary's Med Ctr, Transp Ctr, 1050 Linden Ave, Long Beach, CA 90813 Ph: (562) 491-9300 Fax: (562) 491-9238 1,3) L.M. Barba, 2) J. Rajfer, M. Sender, P. Werthman, 4) UCLA Immunogenetics Center, 5) N. Scott	17	11	10*	173
Cedars-Sinai Med Ctr, Ctr for Liver & Kidney Transp, 8635 W 3rd St, Ste 590W, Los Angeles, CA 90048 Ph: (310) 423-2641 Fax: (310) 423-0234 1,2) C. Shackleton, 2) S. Colquhoun, W. Arnaout, L. Cohen, 3) S. Jordan, F. Strauss, M. Bunnapradist, 4) S. Jordan, D. Tyan, 5) Jagolino, Oldham, Pacino, Meadows	59	59	68	961
Childrens Hosp Los Angeles, Dept of Neph/Dial/Transp #40, 4650 Sunset Blvd, Los Angeles, CA 90027 Ph: (323) 669-2102 Fax: (323) 668-1829 1,3) C. Grushkin, 2) B. Hardy, N. Sherman, 3) C. Grushkin, G. Lerner, M. Mentser, 4) A. Jenkins, 5) K. VanWert	13	17	7*	727
St Vincent Med Ctr, Dept of Transp, 2100 W 3rd St #500, Los Angeles, CA 90057 Ph: (213) 484-6307 Fax: (213) 413-0190 1,2) R. Mendez, 2) R.G. Mendez, T. Bogaard, U. Khetan, P. Asai, H. Shidban, 3) M. Spira, E. Feinstein, R. Minasian, 4) Y. Iwaki, J. Cicciarelli, 5) Felty, Lozado, Norfles, Park, Uleman, Webb	207	203	162*	3998
Univ Calif-Los Angeles Med Ctr, Renal Transp Serv Dept of Neph, 10833 LeConte Ave, Rm BH-427 CHS, Los Angeles, CA 90095-1796 Ph: (310) 825-6836 Fax: (310) 206-0564 1,3) G.M. Danovitch, 1,2) J.T. Rosenthal, 2) H.A. Gritsch, J. Raifer, 3) R.B. Ettenger, E. Kendrick, A.H. Wilkinson, 4) UCLA Immunogenetics Center, 5) Kaufman, Henderson, Dutton, Butenschoen, Foley, Sanford, Hands, Agra, Needham, Park, Ricci	217	258	194*	2647
Univ Calif-Los Angeles Med Ctr, Dept of Peds Neph, 10833 Le Conte Ave, Rm A2-383 MDCC, Los Angeles, CA 90024 Ph: (310) 206-6987 Fax: (310) 206-0564 1,3,) R. Ettenger, 2) H.A. Gritsch, J.T. Rosenthal, 3) I. Salusky, O. Yadin, S. Al Akash, B. Kuizon, 4) UCLA Immunogenetics Center, 5) J. Marik, R. Lenner	22	23	29	495
Univ Southern Calif Univ Hosp, Dept of Transp, 1500 San Pablo St, Los Angeles, CA 90033 Ph: (323) 442-8419 Fax: (213) 442-6201 1) R.R. Selby, 2) N. Jabbour, Y. Genyk, R. Mateo, 3) M. El-Shahawy, 4) UCLA Immunogenetics Ctr, 5) M. Abe, C. Rooney	22	24	15	237
St Joseph Hosp, Renal Transp Ctr, 1100 W Stewart Dr, PO Box 5600, Orange, CA 92863-5600 Ph: (714) 771-8033 Fax: (714) 744-8803 Email: eruzics@sjo.stjor.org 1,2) E. Ruzics, 2) G. Terzakian, 3) A.E. Jabara, J.F. Sigala, 4) UCLA Immunogenetics Center, 5) M. Weil, P. Gull	41	23	38	606
Univ of Calif-Irvine Med Ctr, Div of Transplantation, 101 The City Dr, Bldg. 26, Room 1001, Orange, CA 92868 Ph: (714) 456-8441 Fax: (714) 456-8796 1,2) D.K. Imagawa, 2) S. Colquhoun, R.M. Ghobrial, D. Farmer, S. Cao, 3) C. Barton, M. Pahl, 4) Metic Lab, 5) J.B. Mize, D. Huddleston, L. Gibson, G. Ginther, R. Heyn-Lamb	14	13	15	587
Stanford Univ Med Ctr, Kidney Pancreas Program, 750 Welch Rd, Suite 200, Palo Alto, CA 94304-1509 Ph: (650) 725-9891 Fax: (650) 723-3997 1,2) C. Esquivel, 2) O. Salvatierra, M. Millan, 3) J.D. Scandling, 4) C. Grumet, 5) Waskerwitz, Knoppel, Salvatierra, Law, Wong	124	97	29*	669
Sutter Mem Hosp, Sutter Transp Serv, 5151 F St, Sacramento, CA 95819-3295 Ph: (916) 733-8133 Fax: (916) 733-1967 1,2) R.E. Ward, 2) C. Brownridge, 3) J. O'Green-Koenig, P. Lim, M.S. Mezger, 4) Sacramento Med Foundation Bld Ctr, 5) K. Guerrero, R. Vrchoticky, M. Basten	26	20	25	375
Univ Calif-Davis Med Ctr, Transplant Program, Housestaff Facility, Room 1018, 2315 Stockton Blvd, Sacramento, CA 95817 Ph: (916) 734-2111 Fax: (916) 734-0432 1,2) R.V. Perez, 2) J. McVicar, 3) S. Gandhi, 4) P. Holland, 5) M. Friend, D. Higgs, M. Sturges, D. Lehe	57	38	58*	585
St Bernardine Med Ctr, Kidney Transp Ctr, 2101 N Waterman Ave, San Bernardino, CA 92404 Ph: (909) 881-4429 Fax: (909) 881-7174 1,2) E. Dainko, 3) H. Le, E. Serros, H. Phan, J. Robertson, C. Sun, G. Grames, S. Shankel, 4) UCLA Immunogenetics Center, 5) L. DeSoucy	12	19	15*	322
Sharp Mem Hosp, Transp Office, 7901 Frost St, San Diego, CA 92123 Ph: (858) 541-3831 Fax: (858) 541-4547 1,2) R. Mendez, 2) P. Asai, T. Boggard, U. Khetan, A. Martinez, R. Mendez, 3) S. Steinberg, I. Cohen, C. Mosley, 4) J. Cicciarelli, L. Lebeck, 5) E. Catlon, T. Kress, N. Valentine	76	69	51*	659

1)=Director, 2)=Tx Surgeons, 3)=Physicians, 4)=Tissue Typers, 5)=TxCoords	1998	1999	2000	Total
Univ Calif-San Diego Med Ctr, Renal Transp Prog, 200 W Arbor Dr, San Diego, CA 92103-8745 Ph: (619) 294-6257 Fax: (619) 296-1852 1,3,5) J. Dunn, 2) M.E. Hart, A. Khanna, 3) R. Steiner, 4) L. Lebeck, 5) M. Masteller, L. Conly, S. Heisterkamp	75	79	78*	1609
Calif Pacific Med Ctr, Dept of Transp, 2340 Clay St, San Francisco, CA 94115 Ph: (415) 923-3450 Fax: (415) 923-3836 1,3) B. Levin, 2) W. Bry, R. Osorio, 3) V. Warvariv, S. Inokuchi, L. Bohannan, S. Katznelson, 5) Healy, Mitnick, Becker, Borgonov, Marcos, DeGraaf-Olson	116	110	120*	2925
Univ of Calif-San Francisco, Transp Serv, Moffitt Hosp, Rm 884, San Francisco, CA 94143-0116 Ph: (415) 353-1551 Fax: (415) 353-8708 1,2) J.P. Roberts, 2) N.L. Ascher, P. Stock, C. Freise, R. Hirose, S. Feng, 3) F. Vincenti, W. Amend, S. Tomlanovich, D. Aden, 4) L.A. Baxter-Lowe, 5) Sabatte-Caspillo, Torres, Moczkowski, Devney, DelGrosso, Driscoll	236	202	296*	5949
Western Med Ctr, Renal Transp Serv, 1001 N Tustin Ave, Santa Ana, CA 92705 Ph: (714) 953-3653 Fax: (714) 953-3547 1,2) G. Tertzakian, 3) R. Ness, R. Nathan, 4) UCLA Immunogenetics Center, 5) V. Koogler, K. Grotewold	31	23	24*	333
Santa Rosa Mem Hosp, Kidney Transp Ctr, 1165 Montgomery Dr,#3D01, PO Box 522, Santa Rosa, CA 95402 Ph: (707) 525-5297 Fax: (707) 525-5298 Email: ktts@6.stjoe.org 1,2) T. Duckett, 2) J. Palleschi, W. Tom, R. James, P. Bretan, 3) P. Ruiz-Ramon, D. Shapiro, J. Robertson, J. Edison, 4) P. Holland, 5) N. Swick, L. Miranda	12	26	25	284
Harbor-UCLA Med Ctr, Dept of Transp, Box 5, 1000 W Carson St, Torrance, CA 90509 Ph: (310) 222-2728 Fax: (310) 222-2856 1,3) L.M. Barba, 2) J. Rajfer, M. Sender, D.A. Shoskes, 3) J.D. Kopple, 4) UCLA Immunogenetics Center, 5) L. Avelino, K. Lomeli	21	22	14*	673

COLORADO

	1998	1999	2000	Total
Centura Porter Adventist Hosp, Transp Serv, 2535 S Downing St, #380, Denver, CO 80210 Ph: (303) 778-5797 Fax: (303) 778-5205 1,2) W.B. Vernon, 2) W. Kortz, E. Kortz, 3) C. Kuruvila, M. Dillingham, M. Yanover, D. Gillum, J. Scott, 4) Laboratories at Bonfils, 5) D. Long, M. Luedtke, G. Lewis, K. Bramley, T. Sandoval	49	37	64	427
Presbyterian/St Luke's Med Ctr, Transp Prog, 1719 E 19th Ave, 1C, Denver, CO 80218 Ph: (303) 869-2155 Fax: (303) 869-2106 1,3) K. Fitting, 1,3) A. Cooper, 2) I. Kam, M. Wachs, T. Bak, 4) IAD, 5) B. Guyon, C. Aberle, K. Jantz, K. O'Dea, R. Otto, I. Sansoucy	32	42	36	812
The Children's Hosp-Denver, Dept of Transp Surg, 1056 E 19th Ave, Box B-323, Denver, CO 80218 Ph: (303) 861-6571 Fax: (303) 764-8077 1,2) F. Karrer, 2) I. Kam, M. Koyle, M. Wachs, T. Bak, 3) G. Lum, D. Ford, 4) Immun Assoc of Denver, UCHSC, 5) K. Orban-Eller, D. Dovel, M. Christopher	8	9	5	70
Univ of Colorado Hosp, Dept of Transp Surg, 4200 E Ninth Ave, Box C-318, Denver, CO 80262 Ph: (303) 372-8750 Fax: (303) 372-8737 1,2) I. Kam, 2) F. Karrer, M. Wachs, T. Bak, 3) L. Chan, A. Wiseman, A. Jani, 4) UCHSC Clinical Immunology & Histocompatibility, 5) J. Millspaugh, R. Williams, N. Dabrowski, B. Britz	71	79	95	797

CONNECTICUT

	1998	1999	2000	Total
Hartford Hosp, Transp Prog, Suite 321, 85 Seymour St, Hartford, CT 06106 Ph: (860) 545-4132 Fax: (860) 545-4208 1,2) D. Hull, 2) S. Bartus, M. Brown, 3) J. D'Avella, M. Lazor, D. Rotenberg, J. Laut, M. Carle, J. Post, M. Izard, 4) L. Bow, T. Alberghini, 5) D. Palmeri, A. White, C. Drouin	59	56	64	1373
Yale New Haven Hospital, Department of Surgery, Div of Organ Transp, P.O.Box 208062, New Haven, CT 06520-8062 Ph: (203) 785-2565 Fax: (203) 785-7162 Email: athy.lorber@yale.edu 1,2,4) M.I. Lorber, 2) G.P. Basadonna, A.L. Friedman, 3) M. Bia, A. Kliger, N. Siegel, 4) L.A. Geiselhart, 5) M. Corrigan, J. Albert, N. Sowers, J. Bates	74	72	74	1135

KIDNEY

1)=Director, 2)=Tx Surgeons, 3)=Physicians, 4)=Tissue Typers, 5)=TxCoords	1998	1999	2000	Total
DELAWARE				
Alfred I DuPont Institute, Dept of Neph/Transp, PO Box 269, 1600 Rockland Rd, Wilmington, DE 19899 Ph: (302) 651-5999 Fax: (302) 651-5990 1,2) M.Z. Schwartz, 2) V.T. Armenti, M.J. Moritz, 3) L. Hopp, C. Mckay, 4) Jefferson Univ Tissue Typ Ctr, 5) M.E. Schofield	1	0	5	17
DISTRICT OF COLUMBIA				
Children's National Med Ctr, Dept of Ped Surg, 111 Michigan Ave NW, Washington, DC 20010 Ph: (202) 884-2151 Fax: (202) 884-4174 1,2) J.C. Gilbert, 2) J.C. Gilbert, T. Sasaki, J.A. Light, 3) K. Kher, A. Moudgil, 4) N. Melhorn, A. Johnson, 5) L. Midgley	11	7	9*	195
Georgetown Hosp, Dept of Surg, 4 PHC, 3800 Reservoir Rd NW, Washington, DC 20007 Ph: (202) 784-3700 Fax: (202) 687-3004 1,2) L.B. Johnson, 2) P.C. Kuo, A. Lu, 3) J. Winchester, 4) S. Rosen-Bronson, 5) A. Cribbs, C. Story, W. Sachau, N. Lawson	52	64	48	939
Howard Univ Hosp, Transp Ctr, 2041 Georgia Ave NW, Tower II-Ste 4200, Washington, DC 20060 Ph: (202) 865-1443 Fax: (202) 865-4462 1,2) M.S. West, 2) J. Stevens, C.O. Callender, 3) I. Cruz, 4) J. Delatorre, N. Kramer, B. Baumgardner, 5) C. Yeager, T. Hoilett, T. Cropper	9	10	6	366
Walter Reed Army Med Ctr, Organ Transp Serv, WD 48, WRAMC, 6900 Georgia Ave,NW, Washington, DC 20307 Ph: (202) 782-6462 Fax: (202) 782-0185 1,2) J. Swanson III, 2) D.S. Batty, A. Kirk, 3) S. Polly, 4) W. Nelson, H. Dinh, J. Gaffney, J. Carr, 5) J. Burke, B. Reinmuth, S. Carson, M. Gooden, B. Barros	49	33	33	834
Washington Hosp Ctr, Transp Serv, 110 Irving St NW, Rm 3B1, Washington, DC 20010 Ph: (202) 877-6029 Fax: (202) 877-6581 1,2) J. Light, 2) C. Currier, Gonzalez, T. Sasaki, Aquino, Haaki, 3) J. Moore, J. Veis, 4) W. Ward, 5) J. FLores, J. Trollinger, D. Lepley, J. Stein, W. Cascon	94	109	99	2117
FLORIDA				
Southwest Florida Regional Med Ctr, Renal Transplant, 2727 Winkler Ave, Fort Myers, FL 33901 Ph: (941) 939-8442 Fax: (941) 939-8298 1,3) J. Van Sickler, 2) G. Burtch, 4) W. LeFor, D. Becker, 5) K. Malavsky, C. McBride, J. Levine	22	42	27*	301
Shands at the Univ of Florida, Transplant Center, Box 100251, 1600 SW Archer Road, Gainesville, FL 32610-0251 Ph: (352) 265-0130 Fax: (352) 265-0108 1,2) R.J. Howard, 1,3) R.S.Fennel, 2) A. Reed, W.J. Van der Werf, A. Hemming, 3) R.E. Neiberger, T.R. Srinivaz, 4) J. Scornik, 5) J. Renderer, S. Morgan, A. Hastings, B. Cicale, J. Lloyd-Turner	114	130	121	2677
Mayo Clinic Jacksonville/St. Luke's, Renal & Pancreatic Transp, 4203 Belfort Rd, Suite 204, Jacksonville, FL 32216 Ph: (904) 296-9075 Fax: (904) 296-5874 1,2) J.L. Steers, 2) J. Nguyen, C. Hughes, V. Gopalan, 3) J.R. Spivey, R.C. Dickson, D.M. Harnois, 4) P. Genco, 5) D. Boyum	0	0	11	11
Shands Jacksonville, Jacksonville Transp Ctr, 580 W 8th St, Jacksonville, FL 32209 Ph: 904 244-9800 Fax: 904 244-9842 1,2) T.G. Peters, 2) K.W. Jones, J.L. Steers, J. Nguyen, C. McCullougn, 3) Harmon, Torres, Vaz, Kawwaff, Baker, Gadallah, Cu, Smart, 4) R.K. Charlton, 5) S. Repper, M. Vincent, B. Black, I. Cruz	52	58	56	452
Univ of Miami Sch of Med, Div of Transp, Dept of Surg, R 440, PO Box 012440, Miami, FL 33101 Ph: (305) 355-5100 Fax: (305) 355-5134 1,2) J. Miller, 1,2) A. Tzakis, 2) G.W. Burke III, G. Ciancio, 3) D. Roth, 4) V. Esquenazi, 5) J. Colona, D. Balboa-Jorge, G. Jefferson	168	168	121	2030
Florida Hosp Med Ctr, TransLife, 2501 N Orange Ave, Ste 137, Orlando, FL 32804 Ph: (407) 303-2474 Fax: (407) 303-2478 1) T. Jankiewicz, 2) Jablonski, Vaughn, Klaiman, Gundian, Thill, 3) Metzger, Warren, Pins, Sackel, Ranjit, Prince, Youell, Kusnir, 4) M. Marschner, M. Soeharsono, K. Woodie, A. Nadeau, 5) Blanton, Conforti, Northcutt, Sooklall, Ruping, Lazarus, Priddle	113	125	123	1541
All Children's Hosp, Dept of Transp, 801 6th St So, Box 795, St Petersburg, FL 33701 Ph: (727) 892-8984 Fax: (727) 897-4803 1,3) S. Perlman, 2) V. Bowers, 3) S. Schurman, 4) W. LeFor, 5) S. DiSano	2	2	3*	34

KIDNEY

1)=Director, 2)=Tx Surgeons, 3)=Physicians, 4)=Tissue Typers, 5)=TxCoords	1998	1999	2000	Total
LifeLink Transplant Inst, Tampa Gen Hosp, LifeLink Transp Immun Lab, 409 S. Bayshore Blvd, Tampa, FL 33606 Ph: (813) 253-2640 Fax: (813) 251-1819 Email: lifelinkfound.org 1,2) V.D. Bowers, 1,3) C.E. Wright, 2) A. Alsina, 3) D. Alveranga, S. Weinstein, C. Sanders, L. Kahana, N. Allison, 4) W. LeFor, D. Becker, M. Lopez, 5) Murphy, Heinrichs, Wahler, Anderson, DelFavero, Brown, Seaman	180	186	165*	2543

GEORGIA

	1998	1999	2000	Total
Egleston Children's Hosp-Emory Univ, Dept of Ped Neph, 2040 Ridgewood Dr NE, Atlanta, GA 30322 Ph: (404) 727-5750 Fax: (404) 727-8213 1,3) B.L. Warshaw, 2) C. Larsen, T. Pearson, 3) L. Hymes, 4) R. Bray, 5) M. Shaw	10	15	12	246
Emory Univ Hosp, Dept of Surg, Room H-124, 1364 Clifton Rd NE, Atlanta, GA 30322 Ph: (404) 727-0717 Fax: (404) 727-8972 1,2) T.C. Pearson, 1,2) C.P.Larsen, 2) P. Tso, 3) C. Zayas, 4) R. Bray, 5) G. McGrath, C. Johnson, M. Jeffrey, T. Ofenloch, B. Begley, W. Wilson	202	144	143	3055
Piedmont Hosp, Dept of Surg, 1968 Peachtree Rd, NW, Atlanta, GA 30309 Ph: (404) 605-3530 Fax: (404) 605-2900 1,2) J.D. Whelchel, 2) D.P. O'Brien, 3) E.L. Hochgelerent, D.C. Lowance, 5) L.A. Bernsteil, J. Donnelly, C. Manley	0	72	104*	835
Med College of Georgia, Dept of Surg, 1120 15th St, Augusta, GA 30912-7700 Ph: (706) 721-2874 Fax: (706) 721-6271 1,2) J. Wynn, 3) L. Mulloy, M. Jagadeesen, 4) S. Helman, 5) J. Barnett, B. Wolff, J. Bowley, J. Maxwell	61	48	56*	1267

HAWAII

	1998	1999	2000	Total
St Francis Med Ctr, Dept of Transp, 2230 Liliha St, Honolulu, HI 96817 Ph: (808) 547-6228 Fax: (808) 547-6750 1,2) W. Limm, 2) F.L. Fan, A. Cheung, L.L. Wong, H. Noguchi, 3) J. Sugihara, 4) Y.K. Paik, 5) P. Bouhan, J. Nekoba, C. Bailey	35	49	42	861

ILLINOIS

	1998	1999	2000	Total
Children's Mem Hosp, Siragusa Transplant Center, 2300 Children's Plaza, PO Box 57, Chicago, IL 60614 Ph: (773) 880-3711 Fax: (773) 880-3339 Email: siragusatx@childrensmemoial.org 1,2) C. Firlit, 2) R. Superina, S. Almond, 3) R.C. Cohn, C. Langman, J. Melnick, 5) T. Zielinski	10	19	17	377
Northwestern Mem Hosp, Div of Organ Transp, 675 North St Clair St, Galter 17-200, Chicago, IL 60611 Ph: (312) 695-8900 Fax: (312) 695-9194 1,2) F. Stuart, 2) M. Abecassis, D. Kaufman, J. Fryer, J. Leventhal, 3) W. Schlueter, L. Gallon, 4) M. Buckingham, 5) P. Gierut, L. Rockley, E. DeMayo	116	142	148	2244
Rush Presbyterian/St Lukes Med Ctr, Organ & Tissue Transp Serv, 1653 W Congress Prkwy, 201 Jones, Chicago, IL 60612 Ph: (312) 942-6242 Fax: (312) 563-1529 1,2) J.W. Williams, 1,2) S. Jensik, 2) H. Sankary,P. Foster, F. Merkel, L. McChesney, D. Mital, 3) E. Lewis, S. Hou, S.M. Korbet, R. Rodby, J.Orlowski, S. Saltzberg, 4) H. Gebel, M. Prod, 5) N. Ebert, L. Moore, L. Mauro, T. Partida, A.Harmon	138	112	152*	1537
Univ of Chicago Med Ctr, Dept of Transp Surg, 5841 S Maryland Ave, m/c 5026, Chicago, IL 60637 Ph: (773) 702-6104 Fax: (773) 702-2126 1,2) J.R. Thistlethwaite, 2) D.S. Bruce, K.A. Newell, J.M. Millis, D.C. Cronin, 3) M. Josephson, 4) V. Lazda, 5) R. Sweda, S. Pellar, L. Gardner, C. Robinson, K. Davis	106	106	36*	1805
Univ of Illinois Hosp & Clins, Dept of Surg, Div of Transp, 840 S.Wood St., Room 402,M/C 958, Chicago, IL 60612-7322 Ph: (312) 996-6771 Fax: (312) 413-3483 1,2) E. Benedetti, 2) A. Bartholmew, L. Cicalese, 3) J. Arruda, 4) V.A. Lazda, 5) F. Pascual, O. Woghiren, X. Lopez	43	60	90	1583
Loyola Univ Med Ctr, Dept of Renal Transp, Bldg 54, Room 037, 2160 S 1st Ave, Maywood, IL 60153 Ph: (708) 216-3454 Fax: (708) 216-6003 1,2) P. Minlch, 2) J. Brems, R. Flanigan, D. Hatch, D. Holt, 4) B. Susskind, 5) B. Kostro, D. Calvert, A. Pakrasi, A. Bordi	49	64	63	1209
OSF St Francis Med Ctr, Transp Serv-Kidney, 420 NE Glen Oak Ave, Ste 102, Peoria, IL 61603 Ph: (309) 655 4101 Fax: (309) 655 2597 1,3) T. Pflederer, 2) F.S. Darras, R. Pollak, 3) Olson, Sparrow, Bryan, Horvath, B. Pflederer, Rosborugh, Dreyer, 4) ROBI, 5) N. Howard, C. Wyzlic, D. Himmel, K. Smith	53	40	65	518

1)=Director, 2)=Tx Surgeons, 3)=Physicians, 4)=Tissue Typers, 5)=TxCoords	1998	1999	2000	Total
So Univ Illinois Sch of Med, Mem Med Ctr, Transp Serv, 701 N 1st, Springfield, IL 62781-0001 Ph: (217) 788-3441 Fax: (217) 788-4610 Email: toconnor@siumed.edu 1,2) T.P. O'Connor, 3) Mitra, Mehta, Smith, Weaver, Tamizuddin, Krall, 4) P. McConnachie, 5) T. Beauchamp, D. Daily, B. Grantham	23	22	42	469
INDIANA				
Indiana Univ Med Ctr, Dept of Surg/Organ Transp, 550 N University Blvd, Rm UH4258, Indianapolis, IN 46202 Ph: (317) 274 4370 Fax: (317) 274 3084 1,2) R.S. Filo, 2) S.B. Leapman, M.D. Pescovitz, M.L. Milgrom, 3) M. Govani, T. Batiuk, M. Kraus, 4) Z. Brahmi, 5) M.L. Sabnin, P. Martin, A.S. Holmes	133	109	106*	2187
Methodist Hosp, Transp Ctr, I-65 at 21st St, PO Box 1367, Indianapolis, IN 46206-1367 Ph: (317) 929-8677 Fax: (317) 929-5768 1,2) B. Haag, 2) L. Stevens, D. Rouch, 3) C. Carter, 4) J. McIntyre, N. Higgins, 5) N. Duncan, C. Brents, C. Newbold-Thompson	53	54	56	1135
IOWA				
Iowa Methodist Med Ctr, Transp Dept, 1221 Pleasant St, Ste 500, Des Moines, IA 50309 Ph: (515) 241-4044 Fax: (515) 241-4100 1,2) C. Franklin, 3) C. Shadur, P. Chandran, M. Flood, 4) S. Dhanwada, G. Dreyfeurst, J. Malatesta, J. Siewert, 5) S. Kauzlarich	14	31	19*	199
Mercy Hosp Med Ctr, Transp Serv, 1111 6th Ave, Des Moines, IA 50314 Ph: (515) 247-4261 Fax: (515) 643-8770 1,2) C. Franklin, 2) A. Isenberg, 3) S. Jagarlapudi, B. Buchsbaum, 4) S. Dhannavada, 5) K. Carlberg, P. Freeman, L. Frost	8	17	13*	148
Univ of Iowa Hosp & Clin, Dept Surg, Transp Serv, University Hospitals, Iowa City, IA 52242 Ph: (319) 356-3585 Fax: (319) 356-1556 1,2) S.C. Rayhill, 2) A. Bozorgzadeh, Y. Wu, 3) Hunsicker, Flanigan, Bertalotus, Thomas, Porter, Weisman, Golconda, 4) N.E. Goeken, E. Fields, 5) Schanbacher, Goddard, Reynolds, Satterly, Cox, Zehr, Schulz	100	90	104*	2212
KANSAS				
Univ of Kansas Med Ctr, Div of Neph, 3901 Rainbow Blvd, Kansas City, KS 66160-7382 Ph: (913) 588-6074 Fax: (913) 588-3867 1,2) G. Pierce, 2) A.S. Hermreck, J.H. Thomas, 3) A. Chonko, B. Cowley, J. Grantham, F. Winklhofer, 4) Midwest Organ Bank, 5) J. Greathouse, D. Todd, P. Hunt	37	48	50*	857
Via Christi Regional Med Ctr-St Fran, Dept of Renal Transp, 929 N St Francis, Wichita, KS 67214 Ph: (316) 268-5890 Fax: (316) 291-7727 1,2) C.F. Shield III, 2) J.L. Smith, 4) E. Thien, T. Hughes, 5) M. Blackmore, J. Lemon, K. Zecha, J. Wenz	42	39	30	745
KENTUCKY				
Univ of Kentucky Med Ctr, Dept of Surg/Uro, 800 Rose St,Rm C416, Lexington, KY 40536-0293 Ph: (859) 323-4661 Fax: (859) 323-1700 1,2) T. Johnston, 2) D. Ranjan, S. Reddy, B. Lucas, 3) T. Waid, W. McKeown, E. Jackson, 4) T. Eichorn, J. Byrne, J.S. Thompson, D. Jennings, F. Lower, 5) N. Dawson, B. Adkins, T. Carter, B. Barnett	62	52	52	1450
Jewish Hosp, Transp Serv, 217 E Chestnut St, Louisville, KY 40202 Ph: (502) 587-4358 Fax: (502) 587-4879 1,2) F.R. Bentley, 2) D. Granger, F. Bentley, H. Randall, 3) R. Ouseph, D. Woo, 4) P. Landrum, J. Ogle, R. Pound, J. Cassin, M. Steele, 5) C. Mattingly, P. Kaiser, N. Bellis, C. Schuhmann, L. Carpenter	89	71	79	1610
Kosair Children's Hosp, Dept of Ped Neph, PO Box 35070, Louisville, KY 40232 Ph: (502) 852-3875 Fax: (502) 852-4201 1,3) H.L. Harrison, 2) F. Bentley, D. Granger, 3) L.R. Shoemaker, 4) Univ of Louisville, 5) K. Lincoln	2	0	3	55

1)=Director, 2)=Tx Surgeons, 3)=Physicians, 4)=Tissue Typers, 5)=TxCoords	1998	1999	2000	Total
LOUISIANA				
Children's Hosp, New Orleans, Dept of Ped Neph, Div of Transp at LSUMC, 200 Henry Clay Ave, New Orleans, LA 70118 Ph: (504) 896-9202 Fax: (504) 896-9240 1,2) J.P. Boudreaux, 2) D. Frey, J. Jerius, 3) M. Vehaskari, D. Aviles, A. Robson, D. Silverstein, 4) P.N. Rao, P. Kumar, 5) L. Dublin	5	3	5	24
Memorial Med Ctr (LSUNO), Transplant Institute, 3535 Bienville St, Ste 225 East, New Orleans, LA 70119 Ph: (504) 488-8121 Fax: (504) 488-9672 1,2) D.J. Frey, 2) J.P. Boudreaux, J. Jerius, 3) F. Gonzales, 4) P. Kumar, 5) P. Ryan, C. Stechman, C.SchraderD. Radcliff	31	37	51	241
Ochsner Foundation Hospital, Multi-Organ Transp Program, 1514 Jefferson Hwy, BH309, New Orleans, LA 70121 Ph: (504) 842-3925 Fax: (504) 842-5746 1,2) J. Eason, 2) G. Loss, 3) J.B. Copley, C.G. Staffeld, 4) G. Stewart, S. Herbert, E.S. Cooper, 5) Bailey, Bouvette, Guillera, Stevenson, McNeil, White	50	50	50	710
Tulane Univ Med Ctr, Dept of Surg, SL 22, 1415 Tulane Ave, New Orleans, LA 70112 Ph: (504) 588-5344 Fax: (504) 584-3563 1,2) D. Slakey, 2) S. Cheng, 3) N.K. Krane, J. Puschett, F. Boineau, L. Hamm, J. Lewy, T. Hammond, 4) K.A. Sullivan, 5) A. Zarifian, M. Sander III, M. White, L. Larmeu, J. Hahn	66	69	82*	1064
LSU-Willis Knighton Med Ctr, Dept of Surg, 2600 Greenwood Rd, Shreveport, LA 71130 Ph: (318) 632-4676 Fax: (318) 632-2425 1,2) J.C. McDonald, 2) R. McMillan, G. Zibari, D. Altman, 3) Work, Abreo, Paulson, Pervez, Gadallah, White, Lynn, 4) T. Roggero, D. Michell, K. Horton, W. Blackburn, R. Jones, 5) N. Noles, E. Kilpatrick	25	20	34*	409
MAINE				
Maine Med Ctr, Dept of Neph, 22 Bramhall St, Portland, ME 04102 Ph: (207) 871-2417 Fax: (207) 871-6306 1,3) J. Himmelfarb, 2) J. Jorgensen, W. Herbert, S. Broaddus, J. Whiting, 3) J. Vella, 4) R. Mahoney, 5) B. White, R. Taylor, C. Cutting, G. Clark	50	53	57	845
MARYLAND				
The Johns Hopkins Hosp, Dept of Surg, Harvey 611, 600 N Wolfe St, Baltimore, MD 21287-4606 Ph: (410) 955-6875 Fax: (410) 614-2079 1,2) L.E. Ratner, 2) Klcin, Colombani, Maley, Lau, Montomery, Markowltz, Burdick, 3) L. Gimenez, P. Scheel, M. Choi, W. Briggs, Watnick, Kraus, Sameniengo, 4) J. Hart, 5) Barshick, Burrell, Refugia, Kusel, Kahan, Dane, Wise, Case, Humphries	128	170	161*	1818
Univ of Maryland Med Sys, Dept of Surg, Organ Transp, 29 S Greene St, Ste 200, Baltimore, MD 21201 Ph: (410) 328-5408 Fax: (410) 328-3837 1) S.T. Bartlett, 2) E. Schweitzer, A. Farney, B. Philosophe, J. Colonna, B. Jarrell, 3) D. Klassen, M. Weir, P. Light, E. Ramos, L. Cango, J. Fink, R. Wali, 4) American Red Cross National Histocompatibility, 5) Evans, Stern, Wilson, Young, Ford, Roberts, Aiken, Lee, Hopkins, Mann	285	348	437	2459
MASSACHUSETTS				
Beth Israel/Deaconess Med Center, Transp Div, 1 Deaconess Rd, Boston, MA 02215 Ph: (617) 632-9700 Fax: (617) 632-9775 1,2) A.P. Monaco, 2) D. Shaffer, 3) Strom, Brown, Steinman, Kuhlik, Cautley, Derman, Solomon, Williams, 4) NEOB, 5) M. Hoar, B. Chizan	53	50	13*	615
Boston Univ Hosp, Dept of Surg/Transp Serv, D-511, 88 E Newton St, Boston, MA 02118 Ph: (617) 638-8430 Fax: (617) 638-8427 1,2) S.I. Cho, 2) G. Carptrito, 3) D. Mesler, 4) NEOB, 5) C. McGandy, L. Stattord	24	41	49	899
Boston VA Med Ctr, Dept of Surg, 150 S Huntington Ave, Transp Office-112, Boston, MA 02130 Ph: (617) 278-4571 Fax: (617) 278-4435 1,2) S.I. Cho, 2) A.G. Hakaim, 3) G. Schmitt, 4) New England Organ Bank, 5) N. Sato	5	10	9	404
Brigham & Womens Hosp, Renal Transp Office, 75 Francis St, Boston, MA 02115 Ph: (617) 732-6446 Fax: (617) 732-7832 1,2) H. Auchincloss, 1,3) Jr, C.B. Carpenter, 2) A.B. Cosimi, S. Feng, D. Ko, J.A. Powelson, 3) D. McKay, M. Sayegh, 5) A. Gramajo, L. Imbaro	42	41	41*	1877

1)=Director, 2)=Tx Surgeons, 3)=Physicians, 4)=Tissue Typers, 5)=TxCoords	1998	1999	2000	Total
Children's Hosp Boston, Renal Transp Prog, 300 Longwood Ave, Boston, MA 02115 Ph: (617) 355-7636 Fax: (617) 232-3739 1) W. Harmon, 2) C. Lillehei, J. Wilson, 3) J. Herrin, D. Briscoe, M. Somers, M. Baum, A. Schachter, 4) NEOB, 5) P. Glidden, E. Hughson	14	15	14	471
Massachusetts Gen Hosp, Dept of Surg, 32 Fruit St, Boston, MA 02114 Ph: (617) 726-2825 Fax: (617) 726-9229 Email: delmonico.francis@mgh.harvard.edu 1,2) F.L. Delmonico, 2) A.B. Cosimi, D. Ko, W. Goggins, J. Powelson, 3) N. Tolkoff-Rubin, W. Williams, L. Fang, H. Bazari, J. Niles, 4) D. Fitzpatrick, S. Saidman, 5) S. Noska, K. Grant	67	65	61	1627
New England Med Ctr, Div of Transp Surg, Box 40, 750 Washington St, Boston, MA 02111 Ph: (617) 636-5592 Fax: (617) 636-8228 1,2) R.J. Rohrer, 2) R.B. Freeman, M. Angelis, 3) R.D. Perrone, 4) A. Rabson, 5) S. Fitzmaurice	36	42	51*	710
Lahey Clinic Med Ctr, Dept of Renal Transp-Dial Unit, 41 Mall Rd, Burlington, MA 01805 Ph: (781)744-8023 Fax: (781)744-5379 1,2) M. Malone, 2) J. Libertino, L. Zinman, W. Bihrle, 3) C. Ying, S. Kassissieh, M. Parker, B. Bouthot, 5) J.E. Kobrenski	8	4	6*	125
Baystate Med Ctr, Dept of Renal Transp, 759 Chestnut St, Springfield, MA 01199 Ph: (413) 750-3440 Fax: (413) 750-3432 1,2) G.S. Lipkowitz, 2) R.L. Madden, 3) M.J. Germain, 4) NorthEast Organ Proc Org, 5) J. O'Shaughnessy	38	35	44*	452
Univ of Massachusetts Med Ctr, Transplantation, 55 Lake Ave N, S3-709, Worcester, MA 01655 Ph: (508) 856-6202 Fax: (508) 856-3920 1) R.C. Harland, 2) P. Ayvazian, 3) J. Stoff, A. Cohen, G. Kershaw, D. Clive, P.Y. Fan, M. Hawley, 4) New England Organ Bank, 5) T. Lovewell, P. Bigwood, J. Lane	32	14	36	408

MICHIGAN

	1998	1999	2000	Total
Univ of Michigan Med Ctr, Dept Gen Surg, Div of Transp, 2926 Taubman Ctr-Box 0331, 1500 E Medical Ctr Dr, Ann Arbor, MI 48109-0331 Ph: (734) 936-5816 Fax: (734) 763-3187 Email: janco@umich.edu 1,2) J.C. Magee, 2) D.A. Campbell, Jr, R. Merion, J.D. Punch, S.M. Rudich, J. Arenas, 3) A. Leichtman, A. Ojo, B. Kaplan, D. Cibrik, H. Meier-Kriesche, 4) J. Baker, 5) M. Fox, S. Hutmacher, A. Moloney, J. Novak	197	187	203	2892
Children's Hosp of Michigan, Dept of Ped Neph, 3901 Beaubien, Detroit, MI 48201 Ph: (313) 745-5604 Fax: (313) 966-0039 1) S. Dabbagh, 2) M. Kaplan, 3) L.E. Fleischman, A. Gruskin, T. Mattoo, R. Valentini, 4) D. Kukuruga, 5) D. McWilliams	11	7	6	291
Harper Hosp, Dept of Transp Surg, 3990 John Rd, Detroit, MI 48201 Ph: (313) 745-7318 Fax: (313) 993-0595 1,2) E.R. Reinitz, 2) M.P. Kaplan, 3) D. Sillix, P. Kissner, J. Sondheimer, 4) D. Kukuruga, 5) S. Callaway, C. Graham, K. Morawski	31	24	22*	865
Henry Ford Hosp, Dept of Surg/Med, 2799 W Grand Blvd, Detroit, MI 48202 Ph: (313) 916-7178 Fax: (313) 916-9147 1,2) V. Douzdjian, 2) M. Abouljoud, 3) K.K. Venkat, M. Goggins, R. Parasuraman, 4) D. Kukuruga, 5) M. Uniewski, G. Banfield, M. Jensen, S. Reese	61	81	58*	1528
St John Hosp and Med Ctr, Transp Surg, Prof Bldg II, Ste 174, 22101 Moross, Detroit, MI 48236 Ph: (313) 343-3048 Fax: (313) 343-7349 1,2) H.K. Oh, 3) R. Provenzano, 4) D. Levin, 5) N. Satmary, K. Heckman, C. McQuerry	42	46	54	466
Hurley Med Ctr, Kidney Transplant Unit, 1 Hurley Plaza, Flint, MI 48503 Ph: (810) 257-9572 Fax: (810) 760-9950 1,3) E. Singson, 2) M. Beer, 3) P. Schroeder, E. Alumit, S. Ponze, 4) R. Bull, (E. Lansing Histo Lab), 5) M. Moore	10	15	20*	785
St Mary's Health Serv, Dept of Neph, 200 Jefferson SE, Grand Rapids, MI 49503 Ph: (616) 752-6235 Fax: (616) 752-6324 1,3) W. Bouman, 2) Alix, Borreson, Robson, Novak, Thompson, Sherman, Kuntzman, Avalloni, 3) M. Boelkins, J. Dean, D. Legault, 4) R. Bull, 5) R. Dressler, T. Winglow, M. Page	53	53	60	1003
William Beaumont Hosp, Nephrology/Transplant, 3535 West Thirteen Mile Rd, Suite 644, Royal Oak, MI 48073 Ph: (248) 551-1033 Fax: (248) 551-2125 1) L. Rocher, 2) M. Frikker, J. Hollander, W. Spencer, S. Cohn, 3) L. Greenberg, F. Dumler, K. Bodziak, 4) T. Fosdick, 5) Harris-Burns, Martens, Ward, Garland, Kulikowski, Wojtylo, Hendrix	59	55	59	1006

1)=Director, 2)=Tx Surgeons, 3)=Physicians, 4)=Tissue Typers, 5)=TxCoords	1998	1999	2000	Total
MINNESOTA				
Abbott Northwestern Hosp, 800 E 28th St, Minneapolis, MN 55407 Ph: (612) 863-5638 Fax: (612) 863-3646 1,2) M.D. Odland, 2) D. Jacobs, A. Ney, 3) T. Davin, M. Johnson, R. Sweet, 5) J. Berken, F. Hoffman, L. Larson, N. Siemers			35*	35
Fairview Univ Med Ctr, The Transplant Center, Box 482, 516 Delware St SE, Minneapolis, MN 55455 Ph: (612) 625-5115 Fax: (612) 625-2190 1,2) A.J. Matas, 2) Dunn, Sutherland, Payne, Najarian, Humar, Kandaswamy, Gruessner, 3) Mauer, Chavers, Nevins, Kashtan, Hostetter, Daniels, Manske, 4) H. Noreen, D. McKinley, N. Henrickson, 5) Rolf, Cook, Garvey, Leister, Gibson, Mova, Halverson, Thomas	228	224	239	5526
Hennepin Cnty Med Ctr, Dept of Surg, 701 Park Ave, Minneapolis, MN 55415 Ph: (612) 347-5931 Fax: (612) 347-8755 1) M.D. Odland, 2) A. Ney, D. Jacobs, A. Mandal, 3) V. Rao, D. Dahl, B. Kasiske, H. Rabb, J. Silkensen, 4) H. Noreen, 5) B. Danielson	73	76	76	1765
Mayo Clinic-Rochester Methodist Hosp, Transplant Center, 200 1st St. SW, Rochester, MN 55905 Ph: (507) 266-8731 Fax: (507) 266-2810 1,2) M.D. Stegall, 2) S. Sterioff, S. Nyberg, M. Prieto, M. Ishitani, 3) Gloor, Larson, Schwab, Velosa, Griffin, 4) S.B. Moore, S. DeGoey, 5) D. Dicke-Henslin, L. Fix, M. Kreps, C. Bauer, M. Murphy	105	142	135	2227
MISSISSIPPI				
Univ of Mississippi Med Ctr, Mississippi Renal Transp Prog, Dept of Neph, 2500 N State St, Jackson, MS 39216-4505 Ph: (601) 984-5065 Fax: (601) 984-5075 1,3) D. Butkus, 1,2) W.H. Barber, 3) S. Schlessinger, 4) J. Cruse, R. Lewis, 5) B. Robinson, D. Munson, K. Temple, A. Peters, G. Tornes	48	31	24*	735
MISSOURI				
Univ of Missouri Hosp and Clin, Transp Dept, One Hosp Dr, Columbia, MO 65212 Ph: (573) 882-8763 Fax: (573) 884-4237 1,2) N. Muruve, 2) S. Weinstein, L. Teague, G. Ross, 3) R. Khanna, V. Venkataraman, M. Misra, 4) A.M. Luger, 5) C. Messina, M. Misplay, C. Russell	39	44	44	731
St John's Mercy Med Ctr, Dept of Renal Transp, 621 So.New Ballas Rd Ste 228A, Creve Coeur, MO 63141 Ph: (314) 569-6225 Fax: (314) 569-6093 1,2) M.D. Jendrisak, 3) M. Ravenscraft, B. Lippnann, 4) Barnes HLA Lab, 5) D. Straatman, J. Olesky	27	17	18*	185
Research Med Ctr, Transp Inst, 6400 Prospect, Ste 328, Kansas City, MO 64132 Ph: (816) 822-8257 Fax: (816) 822-8259 1,2) M. Aeder, 3) A.R. Mir, R. Muther, 4) C. Bryan, 5) J. Giessel, M. White	34	50	45	710
St Luke's Hosp, Renal Transplant Dept, PO Box 11900, 4401 Wornall Rd, Kansas City, MO 64111 Ph: (816) 932-3550 Fax: (816) 932-3973 1) T.T. Crouch, 2) T. Helling, P. Nelson, 3) J.I. Mertz, J.N. Sharma, B. Wood, A. Awad, 4) C. Bryan, 5) B. Brewer, L. Harte, S. Bogner	48	45	45	893
Barnes-Jewish Hosp, Washington Univ Med Ctr, Transp Serv, Lower Level, One Barnes Hosp Plaza, St Louis, MO 63110 Ph: (314) 362-5365 Fax: (314) 362-5470 1,2) J. Lowell, 2) S. Shenoy, V. Ramachandran, 3) D. Brennan, B. Miller, C. Wang, 4) D. Phelan, 5) Jones, Martin, Bowe, Mahon, Anstey, Coletta, Howard, Sizemore	125	122	113	2135
Cardinal Glennon Hosp for Children, Dept of Ped Neph, 1465 S Grand, St Louis, MO 63104 Ph: (314) 577-5662 Fax: (314) 268 6449 1,3) E.G. Wood, 2) P. Garvin, H. Solomon, 3) C. Belsha, M. Loghman-Adham, 4) K. Riordan, 5) A. Sinclair	9	6	4	91
DePaul Health Ctr, Dept of Renal Transp, 12303 DePaul Dr, St Louis, MO 63044 Ph: (314) 344-7009 Fax: (314) 344-6976 1,2) M.A. Castaneda, 1,3) D. Polack, 4) Barnes Hosp, 5) A. Hood, G. Goeltz, J. Spinks, J. Hart-Nitz, D. Dunn	17	17	13*	177
St Louis Children's Hosp, Dept of Dial/Transp, One Children's Pl, St Louis, MO 63110 Ph: (314) 454-6065 Fax: (314) 454-2762 1,2) J. Lowell, 3) B. Cole, P. Hmiel, 4) D. Phelan, 5) M. Nadler, L. Bianchi, S. Stuebgen	10	2	7*	163

KIDNEY

1)=Director, 2)=Tx Surgeons, 3)=Physicians, 4)=Tissue Typers, 5)=TxCoords	1998	1999	2000	Total
St Louis Univ Hosp, Abdom Organ Transp, 3635 Vista Ave at Grand, PO Box 15250, St Louis, MO 63110-0250 Ph: (314) 577-8867 Fax: (314) 268-5133 1,2) P.J. Garvin, 2) H. Solomon, P. Garvin, C. Varma, 3) B. Bastani, 4) K. Riordan, 5) Hoff, Aridge, Lindsey, Carter, Kirkpatrick, Johns, Maxfield, Nagel	34	36	40	1131
NEBRASKA				
Nebraska Health Systems, Clarkson Hosp-Univ Hosp, Kidney/Pancreas Transpl Office, 987555 Nebraska Medical Center, Omaha, NE 68198-7555 Ph: (402) 552-2440 Fax: (402) 552-3052 2) R. Taylor, A. Langnas, B. Shaw, D.SudanK. Iyer, 3) Hammeke, Groggel, Ranga, Guirguis, 4) J. Wisecarver, R. Rubocki, S. Shepherd, 5) S. Miller, T. Baker, M. Krobot, C. Lykke, K. Frisbie, K. McAnally, Livers	72	79	85	1347
St Joseph Hosp, Dept of Surg, 601 N 30th St, Omaha, NE 68131 Ph: (402) 449-4251 Fax: (402) 449-4337 1,2) C.M. Zielinski, 3) M.H. Bierman, 4) Univ of Nebraska Med Ctr, 5) P. Nielsen	5	0	1*	132
NEVADA				
NVUM-Univ Med Ctr, Transp Serv, 1800 W Charleston Blvd, Las Vegas, NV 89102 Ph: (702) 383-2224 Fax: (702) 383-3035 1,2) G. Shen, 3) J. Snyder, 4) C. Lively, 5) L. Scott, P. Hess	26	2	12	192
Sunrise Hosp & Med Ctr, Renal Transp Ctr, 3101 Maryland Pkway #211, Las Vegas, NV 89109 Ph: (702) 731-8659 Fax: (702) 731-5209 1,2) S.A. Slavis, 2) N. Feduska, 3) M. Gross, G. Kantor, D. Makil, M. Takiyyuddin, S. Norris, W. King, 4) Donor Network of Arizona, 5) C. Swift	32	51	50	308
NEW HAMPSHIRE				
Mary Hitchcock Memorial Hosp, Dept Renal Dialysis, One Medical Center Dr, Lebanon, NH 03756 Ph: (603) 650-5102 Fax: (603) 650-5530 1,3) M.C. Chobanian, 2) H.F. Henriques III, 3) B. Remillard, 5) C. Pratt	17	17	20*	128
NEW JERSEY				
Our Lady of Lourdes Med Ctr, Dept of Surg, Ambulatory Care Center, 1601 Haddon Ave, Camden, NJ 08103-3117 Ph: (856) 757-3840 Fax: (856) 757-3519 1,3) J. Capelli, 2) N. Youssef, R. Santos, M. Khan, 3) S.M. Chen, M.A. Torres, P.S. Panebianco, B.E. Michel, 4) G. Kirshnan, S. Borrero, A. Biehl, 5) J.F. Dennis, S. Lay-Martino, M. Naurath	33	58	63	689
St Barnabas Med Ctr, Renal Transp Dept, E Wing-Ste 303, Old Short Hills Rd, Livingston, NJ 07039 Ph: (973) 322-5938 Fax: (973) 322-8465 1,3) S. Mulgaonkar, 2) S. Geffner, S. Fletcher, M. Whang, 3) G. Friedman, P. DeFranco, L. Bonomin, N. Lyman, M.G. Jacobs, N. Shah, 4) C. Pancoska, 5) P. Lipere, R. Dowell, E. Simchera, L. Bogert, C. Lascori, D. Girone	167	181	171	1845
Newark Beth Israel Med Ctr, Div of Organ Transp-Kidney, 201 Lyons Ave; F-4, Newark, NJ 07112 Ph: (973) 926-7555 Fax: (973) 923-0646 1,3) M. Goldblat, 2) S. Geffner, 3) S. Palekar, 4) C. Pancoska (NJOTSN), 5) C. Flores, J. Hinkis, T. Alvarez	43	50	47	1235
UMDNJ Univ Hosp, Dept of Surg-Liver Transp Serv, 150 Bergen St, Rm E-244, Newark, NJ 07103 Ph: (201) 982-7218 Fax: (201) 982-6227 1,2) B. Koneru, 2) A. Fisher, 3) C.M. Leevy, 4) C. Pancoska, 5) B. Smith, D. Nolan	3	2	0	14
Robert Wood Johnson Univ Hosp, One Robert Wood Johnson Pl, New Brunswick, NJ 08901 Ph: (732) 235-8695 Fax: (832) 235-8696 1,2) D.A. Laskow, 3) A. Constantinescu, T. Kapoian, R. Mann, 5) K. Cahill, D. James, D. Max, K. O'Connor			57*	57
NEW MEXICO				
Presbyterian Hosp, Transp Serv, PO Box 26666, 1100 Central SE, Albuquerque, NM 87125 Ph: (505) 841-1434 Fax: (505) 222-2149 1) K. Gabrys, 2) R. Lowe, J. Lopez, R. Lovato, T. Scarborough, 3) L. Fox, R. Goldman, R. Cronin, S. Kanig, K. Gabrys, 5) C. Moore, K. McEvoy	28	31	36*	353

1)=Director, 2)=Tx Surgeons, 3)=Physicians, 4)=Tissue Typers, 5)=TxCoords	1998	1999	2000	Total
Univ Hosp-UNMHSC, Dept of Surg, Transp Serv, 2211 Lomas Blvd NE, Albuquerque, NM 87106 Ph: (505)272-3100 Fax: (505)272-3105 1,3) A. Harford, 2) L. Gibel, A. Smith, B. Eghtesad, W.H. Ecker, 3) J. Brandt, 4) New Mexico Immuno Lab, 5) P.J. Demarest, S. Powell, K. Burrell, J. Dax	32	27	29*	898

NEW YORK

1)=Director, 2)=Tx Surgeons, 3)=Physicians, 4)=Tissue Typers, 5)=TxCoords	1998	1999	2000	Total
Albany Med College, Dept of Transp, A-61-GE, 47 New Scotland Ave, Albany, NY 12208 Ph: (518) 262-5614 Fax: (518) 262-5571 1,2) D. Conti, 2) T.P. Singh, G. Shen, 3) D. McGoldrick, 4) D. Constantino, A. Hahn, 5) F. Taft	78	88	63*	1552
Montefiore Med Cent, Albert Einstein Coll of Med, Dept of Surg-Transplantation, 111 E 210th St, Bronx, NY 10467-2490 Ph: (718) 920-4459 Fax: (718) 547-4773 Email: vtellis@montefiore.org 1,2) V.A. Tellis, 2) S.M. Greenstein, R.S. Schechner, 3) D. Glicklich, I. Greifer, F. Kaskel, 4) C. Sigona, L. Bow, 5) Mallis, Clemetson, Figueroa, Feuerstein, McDonough	73	101	87	2039
SUNY HSC at Brooklyn, Dept of Surg, Div Transp, 450 Clarkson Ave, Box 40, Brooklyn, NY 11203-2098 Ph: (718) 270-1898 Fax: (718) 270-3762 1) B.G. Sommer, 2) J.H. Hong, N. Sumrani, D.A. Distant, 3) E. Friedman, M. Markell, 4) A.J. Norin, 5) A. DiBenedetto, V. Maursky, R. Clayton, L. Neve	75	72	48	2520
Buffalo Gen Hosp, Renal Transp Dept, 100 High St, Buffalo, NY 14203 Ph: (716) 859-1345 Fax: (716) 859-4631 1) J.R. Gerbasi, 2) R.N. Stephan, 3) R. Kohli, Shirdhar, 4) T. Shanahan, 5) K. Paolini, H. Guzowski	21	6	28*	712
Children's Hosp of Buffalo, Ped Kidney Ctr, 219 Bryant St, Buffalo, NY 14222 Ph: (716) 878-7275 Fax: (716) 888-3801 Email: jspringate@upa.chob.edu 1,3) J.E. Springate, 2) M. Caty, R. Stephan, 3) W.R. Waz, 4) T. Shanahan, 5) C. Drabelo	4	5	2	85
Erie County Med Ctr, Dept of Med, Neph Div, 462 Grider St, Buffalo, NY 14215 Ph: (716) 898-4803 Fax: (716) 898-4493 1) R.C. Venuto, 2) J.R. Gerbasi, D. Leary, T. Rasmussen, M. Pell, 3) E. Cunningham, B.M. Murray, J. Hom, J. Tienzo, 4) T. Shanahan, 5) K. Reed	24	64	44	416
Columbia Presbyterian Hosp New York, Dept of Surg, 622 W 168th St, New York, NY 10032 Ph: (212) 305-6469 Fax: (212) 305-9642 1,2) M.A. Hardy, 2) A. Benvenisty, R. Nowygrod, J. Chabot, 3) Cohen, Appel, Stern, Kunis, Williams, Valeri, Radhakrishnan, 4) N. Suciu-Foca, 5) J. Cianci, M.J. Samuels, J. Kelly, R. Rodriguez	73	76	61*	1304
Mt Sinai Med Ctr, Recanati/Miller Transp Insti, Box 1104, One Gustave Levy Pl, New York, NY 10029 Ph: (212) 241-8086 Fax: (212) 426-2015 1,2) J.S. Bromberg, 2) L. Burrows, R. Sung, S. Ames, 3) B. Murphy, E. Akalin, V. Sehgal, 4) M. Fotino, 5) L. Daly, K. McKeough, C. Derrien, R. Ifrah, M. Gonzalez	101	73	96	1157
New York Hosp, Cornell Med Ctr, Depts of Med Surg, 525 E 68th Street, New York, NY 10021 Ph: (212) 517-3099 Fax: (212) 517-4762 1,2) W.T. Stubenbord, 2) M. Kinkhabwala, S. Kapur, 3) J.S. Cheigh, R. Riggio, J. Wang, S. Saal, K. Stenzel, D. Serur, R. Bologa, 4) M. Fotino, 5) R. Billman, E. Carey, J. Hambleton, M. Corpron	106	89	95	2135
NYU Medical Center, Dept of Surg, 403 E 34th St, Third floor, New York, NY 10016 Ph: (212) 263-8134 Fax: (212) 263-8157 Email: thomas.diflo@med.nyu.edu 1) T. Diflo, 2) L. Teperman, G. Morgan, D. John, 3) J. Weistuch, J. Benstein, B. Soberman, 4) Rogosin Inst, 5) L. Irwin, D. Campbell, L. Johnson	28	32	30	200
St Luke's-Roosevelt Hosp Ctr, Dept of Surg/Transp, 1090 Amsterdam Ave at 12th Fl, New York, NY 10025 Ph: (212) 523-4700 Fax: (212) 523-4720 Email: jtomasula@slrhc.org 1,2) J.R. Tomasula, 3) V. Sehgal, 4) M. Fotino, M. Suthantihran, 5) B. Lindower, J. Matson	0	7	11*	441
Strong Mem Hosp, Univ of Rochester, Dept of Transp Surg, 601 Elmwood Ave, Rochester, NY 14642 Ph: (716) 275-5875 Fax: (716) 271-7929 1,2) L. Mieles, 2) O. Bronsther, M. Orloff, 3) M. Zand, D. Ornt, 4) M. Coppage, 5) B. Byer, M. Kramer, J. Moraghan, K. Stewart	65	63	37*	1138
Univ Hosp, SUNY at Stony Brook, Dept of Surg-Transp, Health Science Center T-19, Rm 040, Stony Brook, NY 11794-8192 Ph: (631) 444-2209 Fax: (631) 444-3831 1,2) W.C. Waltzer, 2) Z. Frischer, J. Rilotta, 3) L. Arbeit, R. Barnett, R. Fine, G. Kaloyanides, H. Suh, 4) K. Malinowski, 5) L. Etter	56	54	59*	613

KIDNEY

1)=Director, 2)=Tx Surgeons, 3)=Physicians, 4)=Tissue Typers, 5)=TxCoords	1998	1999	2000	Total
SUNY Upstate Med Univ, Dept of Surg, 750 E Adams St, Syracuse, NY 13210 Ph: (315) 464-4550 Fax: (315) 464-6288 1) D.S. Kittur, 2) F.S. Szmalc, 3) E.T. Schroeder, S. Scheinman, S. Narsipur, R. Giamarco, J. Legger, 4) C. Hubbell, J.B. Henry Sr, 5) M. Leaf, A. Koman, J.B. Henry Jr	39	36	39*	857
Westchester Med Ctr, Transp Serv, Macy East, Rm 1048, Valhalla, NY 10595 Ph: (914) 493-1990 Fax: (914) 493-1983 1,2) K. Butt, 3) V. Delaney, 4) Westchester Med Ctr, I. Argani, 5) M. Collins, K. Farkas, D. Surrusco	108	113	113	1066

NORTH CAROLINA

	1998	1999	2000	Total
Univ of North Carolina Hosp, Comprehensive Transplant Ctr, 3306 West Wing, 101 Manning Drive, Chapel Hill, NC 27514 Ph: (888) 253-5293 Fax: (919) 966-5697 Email: transplant@unch.unc.edu 1,2) M. Johnson, 2) D. Gerber, K. Andreoni, J. Fair, 3) W. Finn, 4) J. Crawford, J. Schmitz, 5) L. McCoy, L. Friedman, B. Rodegast, L. Scott	53	47	57	884
Carolinas Med Ctr, Transpl Center, PO Box 32861, Charlotte, NC 28232 Ph: (800) 562-5752 Fax: (704) 355-7616 Email: bthrasher@carolinas.org 1,3) G. Hart, 2) D. Hayes, P. Gores, L. Eskind, J. Jones, 3) P. Walker, C. Fotiadis, J. Chandler, K. Doman, H. Cremisi, J. Bruce, 4) S. Bruner, S. Mallory, B. Ranson, J. Mattachini, L. Murphy, 5) Thrasher, Floyd-Gimon, Zebedis, Feemster, Derkowsk, Ligon	103	80	90	1399
Duke Univ Med Ctr, Dept of Surg, Box 3522, Erwin Rd, Durham, NC 27710 Ph: (919) 668-1856 Fax: (919) 681-7508 Email: kuo00004@mc.duke.edu 1,2) P.C. Kuo, 2) R. McCann, J. Tuttle-Newhall, J. Weinerth, R. Bollinger, B. Collins, 3) S. Smith, P. Conlon, D. Butterly, R. Mannon, 4) F. Ward, 5) L. Hicks, J. Thompson, C. Boone	74	69	89*	1749
East Carolina Univ Sch of Med, Pitt County Mem Hosp, Div of Immun Transp, Dept of Surg, 4S-10 Brody Bldg, Greenville, NC 27858 Ph: (919) 816-2620 Fax: (919) 816-3021 Email: haisch@mail.ecu.edu 1,2) C.E. Haisch, 2) P. Cunningham, 3) G. Byrum, P. Bolin, R. Detwiler, J. Hoggard, J. Reed, M.J. Barchman, 4) L. Rebellato, 5) K. Parker, K. Bozik, K. Vershave	46	51	56	575
North Carolina Baptist Hosp, Dept of Surg, Bowman Gray Sch of Med, Medical Center Blvd, Winston-Salem, NC 27157 Ph: (336) 716-4541 Fax: (336) 716-5414 1,2) M.S. Rohr, 3) P. Adams, 4) C. Manning, 5) S. Haney	67	64	56	950

NORTH DAKOTA

	1998	1999	2000	Total
North Dakota Transp Ctr, Dept of Surg, Medcenter One Health Systems, 300 N 7th St, Bismarck, ND 58501 Ph: (701) 323-6218 Fax: (701) 323-6267 1,2) N. Koleilat, 3) E. Dunnigan, A. Tells, F. Hassan, 4) T. Chase, D. Reinke, 5) I. Eckroth, L. Ulmer, R. Ward	12	21	18	164
Meritcare Hospital, Transplantation Services, 737 Broadway, Fargo, ND 58123 Ph: (701) 234-6715 Fax: (701) 234-2452 1,2) B. Mistry, 3) T. Ahlin, R. Knutson, 4) T. Sell, 5) M. Miller, P. Olinger, B. McKeeven, M. Johnson	27	9	8*	192

OHIO

	1998	1999	2000	Total
Akron City Hosp, Renal Tx, 525 E. Market St, Akron, OH 44304 Ph: (330) 375-3041 Fax: (330) 375-7569 Email: transplant@summa-health.org 1,2) S. Flechner, 2) C. Modlin, 3) C. Boshkos, J. Jacobs, 4) D. Cook, 5) L. Bridle, S. Hodge, C. Keating, P. Fisher	27	17	23	630
Children's Hosp Med Ctr, Div of Ped Neph, 3333 Burnet Av, CHRF-5, Cincinnati, OH 45529-3039 Ph: (513) 636-4531 Fax: (513) 636-7407 1,3) P.T. McEnery, 2) F. Ryckman, C. Sheldon, M. Alonso, 3) F. Strife, T. Welch, J. Bissler, L. Patterson, 4) Hoxworth Bld Ctr, 5) D. Schoborg, J. Ross	16	11	15	357
The Christ Hosp, Dept of Med, 2139 Auburn Ave, Cincinnati, OH 45219 Ph: (513) 241-5630 Fax: (513) 585-3167 Email: woodlees@uc.edu 1,3) M.A. Cardi, 1,2) E.S. Woodle, 2) J.W. Alexander, R. Munda, J.P. Fidler, J. Buell, M. Hanaway, 3) Mendoza, Clyne, Stephens, Giese, Austin, Shaugnessy, Cohen, Anderson, 4) L. Whitacre, D. Eckels, 5) E. Berilla	68	74	61	996
Childrens Hosp, 700 Childrens Dr, Columbus, OH 43205 Ph: (614) 722-4360 Fax: (614) 722-6482 1, 3) M. A. Turman, 2) R. Ferguson, M. Henry, 3) J. Mahan, Jr, 5) C. Campbell, M. Sprague			2*	2

1)=Director, 2)=Tx Surgeons, 3)=Physicians, 4)=Tissue Typers, 5)=TxCoords	1998	1999	2000	Total
Univ of Cincinnati Coll of Med, Dept of Medicine, Sec of Transp, 231 Bethesda Ave, Cincinnati, OH 45267-0585 Ph: (513) 584-7001 Fax: (513) 584-5571 Email: zavalaey@healthall.com 1,2) E.S. Woodle, 1,3) M.R. First, 2) R. Munda, J.W. Alexander, J. Buell, M. Hanaway, 3) R. Peddi, P. Roy-Chaudhary, 4) L. Whitacre, D. Eckels, 5) P. Weiskittel, M. Bryant	40	37	41	1245
Cleveland Clin Fnd, A110 Transplant Center, 9500 Euclid Ave, Cleveland, OH 44195 Ph: (216) 444-6996 Fax: (216) 445-8141 1,3) A. Novick, 2) D. Goldfarb, S. Flechner, C. Modlin, S. Streem, I. Gill, Krishnamurthi, 3) W. Braun, R. Cunningham, J. Nally, V. Dennis, S. Nurko, R. Fatica, 4) D. Cook, 5) Milner, Mastroianni, Savas, Protiva, Corder, Castle, Pearl, Poling	80	89	110	2345
Univ Hosps of Cleveland, Dept of Surg, Transp Ctr, 11100 Euclid Ave, Cleveland, OH 44106 Ph: (216) 844-3689 Fax: (216) 844-7764 1,2) J.A. Schulak, 2) D.S. Seaman, C.T. Siegel, 3) D.E. Hricik, I. Davis, T. Knauss, B. Vogt, 4) N. Greenspan, 5) M. Bartucci, J. Arnovitz, H. Dorsey	112	90	109	1461
Ohio State Univ Hosp, Dept of Surg, Div of Transp, 363 Means Hall, 1654 Upham Dr, Columbus, OH 43210 Ph: (614) 293-8545 Fax: (614) 293-4541 1,2) R.M. Ferguson, 2) E. Elkhammas, M. Henry, E. Davies, G. Bumgardner, R. Pelletier, 3) Bay, Hebert, Cosio, Middendorf, Nahman, Falkenhain, Pesevento, 4) P. Adams, 5) B. Miller, L. McDonnell	145	143	203*	2779
Miami Valley Hosp, AKU-Div of Transp, One Wyoming St, Dayton, OH 45409 Ph: (937) 208-8000 Fax: (937) 208-2966 Email: actaylor@mvh.org 1,2) H.A. Feller, 2) K. Rundell, 3) N. Christoff, A. Eduafo, 4) K. Balakrishnan, T. Ritz, 5) A. Taylor, P. Finke	29	29	19	607
Medical College of Ohio Hospitals, Transplant Services, 3065 Arlington Avenue, Toledo, OH 43614-5807 Ph: (419) 383-5390 Fax: (419) 383-5728 1,2) S.H. Selman, 2) K.A. Kropp, J.S. Jhunjhunwala, M. Rees, 3) J. Shapiro, D. Malhotra, P. Rao, K. Modi, 4) A. Blair, 5) T. Fite, L. Ferguson	39	46	64*	1013
St Elizabeth Health Center, Transp Ofc, 1044 Belmont Ave, Youngstown, OH 44501 Ph: (330) 480-3642 Fax: (330) 480-2768 Email: kathy-pieton@hmis.org 1,2) C. Modlin, 2) V. Krishnamurthi, D. Goldfarb, S. Flechner, I. Gill, 3) E. Sarac, L. Vassilaros, 4) D. Cook (Cleveland Clin), 5) A. Benedetto, A. Ottney, M. Begala	23	16	14*	255

OKLAHOMA

	1998	1999	2000	Total
Baptist Med Ctr of Oklahoma, Renal Transp Sec, 3300 NW Expressway, Oklahoma City, OK 73112 Ph: (405) 949-3816 Fax: (405) 945-5173 1,2) E.N.S. Samara, 2) B. Voss, W. Miller, 3) Matter, Sholer, Southmayd, Khanna, Aly, Rankin, Bond, Redding, Wilson, 4) Y. Choo, 5) P. Sumpter, D. Johnson, L. Larsen, M. Brumbaugh	33	38	30	444
Childrens Hosp of Oklahoma, Dept of Ped Neph, 940 NE 13th St, Oklahoma City, OK 73104 Ph: (405) 271-4409 Fax: (405) 271-3967 1,3) J.E. Wenzl, 2) E.N. Scott-Samara, 4) S. Oleinick, D.M. Smith, 5) C. Winters	5	6	2*	235
St Anthony Hosp, Dept of Dial/Transp, 1000 N Lee St, PO Box 205, Oklahoma City, OK 73101 Ph: (405) 272-7164 Fax: (405) 272-6203 1,2) E.N.S. Samara, 2) W. Miller, L. Pennington, R. Squires, J. Donavon, 3) O. Llan de Rosos, T.V. Raman, G. Toma, G. Dubois, 4) T. Violett, S. Calhoun, 5) M. Mayandie	4	15	10*	477
Univ Hosp, Transp Serv, Rm 5E190, 800 NE 13th St, Oklahoma City, OK 73104 Ph: (405) 271-7498 Fax: (405) 271-1772 1,2) L.R. Pennington, 2) R. Squires, R. Postier, A. Jacocks, S. Samara, 3) J. Pederson, 4) J. Baker, 5) E. Grubbs	19	29	25*	383
Hillcrest Med Ctr, Kidney Transp Prog, 1124 S St Louis, Tulsa, OK 74120 Ph: (918) 579-7994 Fax: (918) 579-7667 1) T. Kenkel, 2) R. Haglund, V. Robards, S. Miller, 3) A. Paton, J. Keveney, B. von Hartitzsch, R. Gold, R. Kaul, T. Thu, 4) S. Ward, R. Zarrabi, 5) B. Harwell, T. Farmer	24	24	32*	613
St John Med Ctr, Inc, Dept of Renal Transp, 1923 S Utica Ave, Tulsa, OK 74104 Ph: (918) 744-3542 Fax: (918) 744-3341 1,3) T.R. Medlock, 2) V.L. Robards, J.S. Miller, R.U. Haglund, 3) J.J. McCauley, D.D. Schram, 4) Dawn Office, 5) D. Saab	10	8	15*	65

KIDNEY

1)=Director, 2)=Tx Surgeons, 3)=Physicians, 4)=Tissue Typers, 5)=TxCoords	1998	1999	2000	Total
OREGON				
Legacy Good Samaritan Hosp & Med Ctr, 1015 NW 22nd Ave, Portland, OR 97210 Ph: (503) 413-6555 Fax: (503) 413-6563 1,2) J.F. Valente, 2) T. Hatch, K. McEvoy, J. Valente, 3) W. Bennett, K. Douek, 5) D. Dreyer			17*	17
Oregon Hlth Sci Univ, Transp Prog, 3181 SW Sam Jackson Park Rd, Portland, OR 97201 Ph: (503) 494-8470 Fax: (503) 494-8671 Email: barryj@ohsu.edu 1,2) J.M. Barry, 1,3,4) D.J. Norman, 2) M. Lemmers, M. Conlin, E. Fuchs, 3) A.M. Demattos, R. Mak, 4) P. Wetzsteon, 5) Allee, Cannard, Klein, Krause, St. Clair, Hickes, Brice, Sebers	147	161	173	3006
PENNSYLVANIA				
Lehigh Valley Hosp, Dept of Transp, Cedar Crest & I-78, PO Box 689, Allentown, PA 18105 Ph: (610) 402-8506 Fax: (610) 402-1682 1,2) C.R. Reckard, 3) D.E. Johnson, 4) M. Williams, P. Kimble, M. Hoffman, D. Hartzel, M. Wetmore, N. Nolihan, 5) P. Boyer, L. McGovern	36	24	29	239
Geisinger Med Ctr, Dept of Surg, Transp Sec 01-14, 100 N Academy Ave, Danville, PA 17822-0114 Ph: (570) 271-8888 Fax: (570) 271-5126 1,2) J.C. West, 2) S. Chao, 3) Bisordi, Largent, Hartle, Landwehr, Yahya, 4) Hershey Med Ctr, 5) S. Kelley, R. Latsha, N. Fetterolf, G. Maloney-Saxon, B. Shepulski	42	40	23	662
Pinnacle Health System at Harrisburg Hosp, 111 S Front St, PO Box 8700, Harrisburg, PA 1710-8099 Ph: (717) 231-8700 Fax: (717) 231-8753 1,2) H.C. Yang, 2) M. Holman, 3) N. Ahsan, 5) K. Barnett, P. Kratzer, M. Scouten			40*	40
Univ Hosp Penn State Coll of Med, Dept of Surg, Sec of Transp, PO Box 850, 500 University Dr, Hershey, PA 17033 Ph: (717) 531-5852 Fax: (717) 531-6579 1,2) H.C. Yang, 2) M. Holman, J.O. Arenas, M. Jarowenko, 3) J. Cheung, J. Diamond, N. Ahsan, M. Waybill, I. Groff, 4) P.J. Romano, 5) Scouten, Norton, Ulsh, fareell, Kratzer, Bollinger	81	92	115*	1213
Albert Einstein Med Ctr, Sec of Kidney/Pancreas Transpl, 5401 Old York Road, Klein 505, Philadelphia, PA 19141 Ph: (215) 456-6933 Fax: (215) 456-6716 1) F. Badosa, 2) S.L. Yang, 3) R. Raja, 4) R. McAlack, 5) L.F. Lerner, K. Austin, C. Morrison	48	45	35	1060
Children's Hosp of Philadelphia, Dept of Surg, 34th St and Civic Ctr Blvd, Philadelphia, PA 19104 Ph: (215) 590-2449 Fax: (215) 590-3705 Email: petro@email.chop.edu 1,2) K. Brayman, 3) H.J. Baluarte, 4) M. Kamoun, 5) J. Petro, J. Palmer	15	31	16	102
Hahnemann Univ Hosp, Dept of Surg, Div of Transp, Broad & Vine Sts, MS 417, Philadelphia, PA 19102 Ph: (215) 762-1857 Fax: (215) 762-1621 Email: jaya@access1 1,2) M.S.A. Kumar, 2) M.R. Laftavi, 3) J. Brezin, P. Lyons, O. Pankewycz, 4) E. Tecza, N. Burvainis, R. Prophet, R. Devine, 5) K. Phillips, A.M. Damask, M.B. Tomeny	75	89	99	1490
St Christopher's Hosp for Children, Dept of Ped Neph, Erie Ave at Front St, Philadelphia, PA 19134 Ph: (215) 427-5190 Fax: (215) 427-5351 1,2) S.P. Dunn, 2) A.T. Casas, 3) H.J. Baluarte, S.B. Conley, 4) S. Bulova (Hahnemann Univ), 5) C. Braas, J. Palmer	9	13	10*	402
Temple Univ Hosp, Transplant Surg, 3401 N Broad St, PP1, Philadelphia, PA 19140 Ph: (215) 707-8889 Fax: (215) 707-8894 1,2) C. Foster, 2) S. Guy, 3) C. Bastl, P. Silva, 4) S. Leech, 5) G. Libetti, P. Sellers, M. McSorley, K. Wuest	29	33	19	222
Thomas Jefferson Univ Hosp, Transplant Program, 111 S 11th St, Ste 1950G, Philadelphia, PA 19107-4801 Ph: (215) 955-7625 Fax: (215) 923-1848 1,2) M. Moritz, 2) J. Radomski, V. Armenti, D. Dafoe, 3) J.F. Burke, G. Francos, 4) B. Colombe, D. Lacava, C. Lynch, R. VanderHeide, D. Nguyen, M. Bruneau, 5) E. Stefanosky, K. O'Neill, K. Corte, R. Cameron	93	71	85	1444
Univ of Pennsylvania Hosp, The Penn Transplant Center, 3400 Spruce St, Philadephia, PA 19104 Ph: (215) 662-6200 Fax: (215) 349-5096 Email: diane.jakobowski@uphs.upenn.edu 1,2) C. Barker, 2) A. Naji, K. Brayman, J. Markmann, 3) R.A. Grossman, R. Bloom, K. Mange, 4) M. Kamoun, J. Kearns, 5) M. Palanjian, C. Hooper, J. Eyer, T. Holland, K. Kilgarriff, C. Naus	133	154	162	2838
Allegheny Gen Hosp, Dept of Surg, Transp Serv, 320 E North Ave, Pittsburgh, PA 15212 Ph: (412) 359-6800 Fax: (412) 359-4721 1,2) D.D. Nghiem, 2) M.R. Gignac, 3) B.J. Carpenter, R. Marcus, 4) S. Hsia, 5) B.A. Kijanka, M.A. Breckenridge, K. Kinter	100	86	88*	1103

1)=Director, 2)=Tx Surgeons, 3)=Physicians, 4)=Tissue Typers, 5)=TxCoords	1998	1999	2000	Total
Children's Hosp of Pittsburgh, Dept of Renal Transp, One Children's Pl, 3705 Fifth Ave, Pittsburgh, PA 15213-2582 Ph: (412) 648-3200 Fax: (412) 648-3085 1,2) R. Shapiro, 2) V.D. Scantlebury, M.L. Jordan, C. Vivas, A. Jan, 3) D. Ellis, A. Vats, M. Moritz, 4) A. Zeevi, R. Duquesnoy, 5) James, Good, Woods, Flohr, Bauder, Orlofske, Paynter, Barber	6	9	12	285
UPMC-Presbyterian, Starzl Transplantation Inst, 4 Falk Clinic, 3601 Fifth Ave, Pittsburgh, PA 15213 Ph: (412) 648-3200 Fax: (412) 648-3085 1,2) T.E. Starzl, 1,2) J.J. Fung, 2) Hakala, Jordan, Shapiro, Scantlebury, Vivas, 3) S. Kusne, J. McCauley, M. Green, J. Johnston, 4) R. Duquesnoy, A. Zeevi, 5) Good, Woods, Bauder, Flohr, Orlofske, Paynter, James, Barber	147	197	140	3307
Lankenau Hosp, Dept of Renal Transp, 100 Lancaster Ave, West City Line, Wynnewood, PA 19096-3426 Ph: (610) 645-8485 Fax: (610) 645-8509 1,2) J.D. Angstadt, 3) K. Superdock, 5) S. Cole	6	14	18*	104
RHODE ISLAND				
Rhode Island Hospital, Transplant Services, APC Building, Suite 921, 593 Eddy Street, Providence, RI 02903 Ph: (401) 444-8562 Fax: (401) 444-3283 Email: RGohh@Lifespan.org 1,2) A.P. Monaco, 2) P.E. Morrissey, 3) R.Y. Gohh, 4) NEOB, 5) B. Hopkins-Garcia	52	53	60	200
SOUTH CAROLINA				
Med Univ of South Carolina, Dept of Surg, 171 Ashley Ave, R 404 CSB, Charleston, SC 29425 Ph: (803) 792-3553 Fax: (803) 792-8596 1,2) P.R. Rajagopalan, 2) P. Baliga, K. Chavin, J. Roger, 3) M. Budisavljevic, 4) J. Jakubek, 5) T. Sill, G. Magwood, L. Hildebrand, E. Thurman, J. Dauson, R. Hogarth	112	129	156*	1922
Richland Memorial Hosp, 5 Richland Medical Park, Columbia, SC 29203 Ph: (803) 434-3766 Fax: (803) 434-3765 1,2) R.R.M. Gifford, 3) Allen Bowen II, J. Brannigan, Jr, M. Cook, 5) M. Sobral, S. Thomas			6*	6
SOUTH DAKOTA				
McKennan Hosp, Dept of Renal Transp, PO Box 5045, 800 E 21st St, Sioux Falls, SD 57117 Ph: (605) 322-8030 Fax: (605) 322-7501 1,2) D. McQuitty, 3) Jensen, Lankhorst, Santella, Zawada, Kellerman, Nemeh, Burris, 4) Univ Minnesota, 5) E. Bonnema, H. Mitzel	29	34	26	158
TENNESSEE				
Erlanger Med Ctr, Erlanger Regnl Kidney Transp, 975 E.3rd St, Suite 1108, Chattanooga, TN 37403 Ph: (423) 778-8067 Fax: (423) 778-6674 1,2) D.F. Fisher, 1,3) J. Yium, 2) J. Cofer, 3) D. Franklin, 4) L. Allen, 5) T.W. Belknap, J.D. Davis	29	24	30	309
Johnson City Medical Center, Dept of Surg-Transplant, 408 State of Franklin Rd, Transp Ofc, Ste 46, Johnson City, TN 37604 Ph: (423) 431-6164 Fax: (423) 928-6795 1,2) P.N. Joshi, 2) R. Weingart, 3) C.F. Wiegand, L. Panus, 4) Univ of Tenn-Knoxville, 5) L. Walker, K. Kelley, J. Hawkins	27	19	16	234
Univ of Tennessee Med Ctr-Knoxville, Dept of Surg, 1924 Alcoa Hwy, Knoxville, TN 37920 Ph: (865) 544-9236 Fax: (865) 544-9128 1) M.H. Goldman, 2) M. Freeman, S. Stevens, 3) R. Regester, M. Malagon, 4) J.D. Tyler, S. Looney, 5) K. Collins, K. Howard	28	41	44*	513
Le Bonheur Children's Med Ctr, Dept of Ped Transp, 50 N Dunlap, Memphis, TN 38103 Ph: (901) 572-5438/5434 Fax: (901) 572-5052 1,2) A.O. Gaber, 2) H.P. Grewal, H. Shokouh-Amiri, S. Vera, R.J. Stratta, 3) R. Wyatt, D. Jones, B. Ault, 4) C. Miller, B. Loehman, T. Northroi, L. Marek, Y. Cao, 5) S. Powell	4	3	8	159
William F Bowld Hosp, Univ of Tenn, Dept of Surg, 956 Court Ave, Rm A202, Memphis, TN 38163 Ph: (901) 448-5924 Fax: (901) 448-7208 1,2) A.O. Gaber, 2) S. Vera, H. Shokouh-Amiri, R.J. Stratta, H.P. Grewal, 3) M.F. Egidi, S. Acchiardo, F. Kraus, R. Bastnagel, R. Wyatt, 4) B. Loehman, L. Marek, 5) N. O'Keefe, B. Culbreath, R. Vincent	123	94	110*	1779
Centennial Med Ctr, Dept of Organ Transp, 2400 Parman Pl, Ste 8, Nashville, TN 37203 Ph: (615) 342-5626 Fax: (615) 342-5635 1) P. Minich, 2) L. Rehman, 3) R. Atkinson, M. Kaplan, 4) DCI Lab, 5) C. Jackson, T. Poston, R. Waddell	24	49	44	346

KIDNEY

1)=Director, 2)=Tx Surgeons, 3)=Physicians, 4)=Tissue Typers, 5)=TxCoords	1998	1999	2000	Total
St Thomas Hosp, Kidney Transp Dept, 4220 Harding Rd, Nashville, TN 37205 Ph: (615) 222-6618 Fax: (615) 222-6074 1,2) R.E. Richie, 2) D. VanBuren, W. Nylander, 3) M.A. Wigger, 4) DCI Lab/REN Histo Lab, 5) M. Dubuque, K. Gilmartin	13	16	14*	115
Vanderbilt Univ Med Ctr/VA Hosp, Dept of Surg, 912 Oxford House, Nashville, TN 37232-4750 Ph: (615) 936-0404 Fax: (615) 936-0409 1,2) R.E. Richie, 2) W. Nylander, D. VanBuren, 3) J.H. Helderman, S. Goral, 4) D. Crowe, 5) J. Hopkins, G. Kelly, K. Brisendine	81	83	59*	2532

TEXAS

	1998	1999	2000	Total
Brackenridge Hosp, Dept of Transp, 601 E 15th St, Austin, TX 78705 Ph: (512) 323-1374 Fax: (512) 323-1300 1,2) M.T. Stewart, 2) R. Tate, R. Bridges, P. Church, S. Settle, 3) Moore, Simpson, Salmond, Lindley, Moncrief, Nader, Maidment, Decherd, 4) G.A. Beathard, 5) A. Shipe, M. White	6	13	8*	552
Baylor Univ Med Ctr, Transp Serv, Dept of Surg, 3500 Gaston Ave, Dallas, TX 75246 Ph: (214) 820-2050 Fax: (214) 820-4527 1,2) G. Klintmalm, 2) R. Goldstein, M. Levy, E. Molmenti, C. Fasola, 3) T.A. Gonwa, L. Melton, M. Mai, 4) D. Smith, 5) K. Manley, S. Hashim, H. Roman, C. Johnson, P. Fertig	76	135	73*	915
Children's Med Ctr of Dallas, Dept of Neph/Renal Transp, 1935 Motor St, Dallas, TX 75235 Ph: (214) 456-2781 Fax: (214) 640-8042 1,2) P.C. Guzzetta Jr, 2) C.D. Coln, A. Sagalowsky, J. Roden, 3) M. Baum, M. Seikaly Jr, R. Quigley, A. Quan, 4) P. Stastny, 5) D. Haas, T. Romano	8	9	2*	230
Medical City Dallas Hosp, Transplant Center, 7777 Forest Lane, A-14th Floor, Dallas, TX 75230 Ph: (800)348-4318 Fax: (972)566-4872 1,2) S. Seitz, 2) D. Ogden, M. Mack, T. Dewey, M. McGee, R. Bowman, I. Davidsons, S. Reeder, 3) J.E. Rosenthal, M. Lerman, J. Hunt, A. Shulkin, K. Hoang, A. Anderson, 4) A. Nikaein, 5) M. Covin, T. McMellon, D. Stevenson, C. Cava-Bartsch, A. Kuhnel	0	4	13	17
Methodist Med Ctr, Transp Serv, PO Box 655999, 1441 N.Beckley, Dallas, TX 75265-5999 Ph: (214) 947-1800 Fax: (214) 941-8061 1,3) P. Vergne-Marini, 2) G. Trevino, R.M. Dickerman, 3) K. Brinker, L. Melton, D. Nesser, R. Velez, 4) G. Land, 5) A. Louzau, R. Bunton, J. McDonald, C. Cannon	56	47	62	1734
Parkland Mem Hosp, Transp Clin, 5201 Harry Hines Blvd, Dallas, TX 75235-7747 Ph: (214) 590-5656 Fax: (214) 590-6929 1,3) C. Lu, 2) A. Sagalowsky, S. Li, B. Nibhanupudy, 3) M. Vasquez, M. Kielar, 4) P. Stastny, 5) J. Grammer, R. Mangus, M. Qviste, V. Sangworn, D. Sweatt	36	36	22	1632
Sierra Med Ctr, Dept of Transp, 1625 Medical Center Dr, El Paso, TX 79902 Ph: (915) 747-2747 Fax: (915) 544-9264 1,2) H.J. Diaz-Luna, 2) J. Lozano, 3) F. Raudales, 4) K. Patel, 5) I. Kernan, D. Simon, M. Horsch, E. Vuyosevich	26	29	24	246
Cook Childrens Med Ctr, Dept of Renal Transp, 901 Seventh Ave, Suite 410, Fort Worth, TX 76104 Ph: (817) 870-7960 Fax: (817) 885-3943 1,3) W.C. Arnold, 2) R. Sloane, J. Miller, 3) D. Pena, 4) Methodist Hospital of Dallas, 5) P. Brigance	3	7	3	34
Harris Methodist-Fort Worth, Renal Transplant Program, 1301 Pennsylvania Ave, Ste 811, Fort Worth, TX 76104 Ph: (817) 882-2443 Fax: (817) 878-5136 Email: nancypytes@texashealth.org 1,3) C. Andrews, 2) S. Worsham, R. Sloane, 3) R. Mauk, L. Anderson, R. Davda, C. Andrews, 4) G. Land, 5) S. Nicholas, A. Brown	64	41	31	537
Univ of Texas Med Branch-Galveston, Dept of Surg, Old JSH, Rm 6.206, 301 University Blvd, Galveston, TX 77555-0536 Ph: (409) 772-2412 Fax: (409) 772-6368 1,2) K.K. Gugliuzza, 2) J. Daller, L. Echeverri, A. Sankar, 3) J. Rice, TJ. Ahuja, R. Remmers, 4) S. Vaidya, 5) M. Byrd, J. Boughton, D. Devine, M. Armendariz, B. Medina, J. Upchurch	63	72	71*	1825
St Luke's Episcopal Hosp, Texas Heart Inst, Dept of Transp 2-114, 6720 Bertner, PO Box 20269, Houston, TX 77225 Ph: (713) 791-3128 Fax: (713) 794-6696 Email: dhosey@sleh.com 1) O.H. Frazier, 2) C.T. VanBuren, B. Kahan, S. Katz, R. Knight, 3) C. Barcenas, J. Robeson, M. Rubin, R. Esquenaz, 4) R. Kerman, 5) D. Hosey, S. Fife, K. Sanne, M. Zeledon, S. Crockett, M. Turner	87	64	90	757

1)=Director, 2)=Tx Surgeons, 3)=Physicians, 4)=Tissue Typers, 5)=TxCoords	1998	1999	2000	Total
Texas Children's Hosp, Transp Serv, MC 1-2720, 6621 Fannin St, Houston, TX 77030 Ph: (713) 770-2575 Fax: (713) 770-2570 1,3) E. Brewer, 2) G. Noon, W. Rosenberg, J. Cafutrite, E. Gonzales, D. Roth, R. Sutherland, 3) A. Kale, D. Powell, I. Boydstun, S. Goldstein, R. Sleth, 4) R. Kerman, 5) T. Stephens	2	20	11*	119
The Methodist Hosp, Multi-Organ Transp Ctr, 6565 Fannin-SM 447, Houston, TX 77030 Ph: (713) 790-2501 Fax: (713) 793-1335 1,2) W.G. Guerriero, 2) G.P. Noon, W. Rosenberg, 3) R. Johnson, M. Assouad, 4) G. Rodey, 5) L. Coomes-Hill, M.C. Matula	22	35	41*	1028
Univ of Texas-Medical School, Dept of Surg-Organ Transp, 6431 Fannin(MSB6.240), Houston, TX 77030 Ph: (713) 500-7400 Fax: (713) 500-0785 1,2) B.D. Kahan, 2) C.T. VanBuren, S. Katz, 3) T. DuBose, 4) R.H. Kerman, 5) L. Schoenberg	115	116	113	2284
Covenant Med Ctr, Dept of Organ Transp, PO Box 1201, 3615 19th St, Lubbock, TX 79408 Ph: (806) 725-0590 Fax: (806) 723-7103 1,2) G.B. Helfrich, 4) D.M. Dunn, 5) M. Bentley, D. Knox	32	14	28*	239
Univ Med Ctr, Dept of Surg, PO Box 5980, Lubbock, TX 79417 Ph: (806) 743-2308 Fax: (806) 743-2421 1) A. Willingham, 2) G.B. Helfrich, 3) D. Wesson, M. Laski, 4) M. Thurman, L. Spence, C. Sypert, K. Moscola, 5) A. Willingham, A. Mackety	12	15	16*	278
Methodist Specialty & Transplant Hosp, 8026 Floyd Curl Dr, San Antonio, TX 78229 Ph: (210) 692-8250 Fax: (210) 692-8154 1,2) F.H. Wright, Jr, 2) C. Samacki, S. Vick, 3) S. Diamond, C. Hura, K. Irwin, M. Isbell, H. Reineck,S. Rosenblatt,4) J. Morrisey, 5) Farias, Galliardt, Hudson, Leonhardt, Martinez, McNeil, Pineda, Rhoden, Richardson			122*	122
Christus Santa Rosa Med Ctr, 2827 Babcock Rd, San Antonio, TX 78229 Ph: (210) 705-6700 Fax: (210) 705-6094 1,2) G. A. Halff, 2) J. Calhoon, F. Cigarroa, R. Esterl, Jr, W. K. Washburn, 3) M. Isbell, P. Mulgrew, K. Speeg, Jr, H. Villarreal, Jr, 5) C. Kennedy, K. Stutes			44*	44
Univ of Texas HSC, Med Ctr Hosp, Organ Transp Prog, 7703 Floyd Curl Dr, San Antonio, TX 78284-7842 Ph: (210) 567-5777 Fax: (210) 567-4458 1,2) G.A. Halff, 2) R. Esterl Jr, 3) D. Riley, 4) Blackwell, Rocha, Hoog, Magneish, Amont, Vargas, Radnik, 5) A. Lopez, L. Nichols, M. Buecher, C. Castillo, N. Herrera	46	47	70	422
Scott & White Memorial Hosp, 2401 S 31st St, Temple, TX 76508 Ph: (254) 724-8912 Fax: (254) 724-8772 1,2) G. J. Jaffers, 3) C. Foulks, M. Narayanan, 5) R. Sanchez			27*	27
East Texas Med Ctr, Dept of Renal Transp, 1000 S Beckhan, P.O. Box 6400, Tyler, TX 75711 Ph: (903) 531-8126 Fax: (903) 535-6843 1,3) T.A. Lowery, 2) D.N. Andrews, H.D. Short, 3) Gerard, Cotton, Woodard, Bankhead, Dobrowolski, Ahmed, Martin-Diaz, 4) C. Jordan, 5) B. Oden	27	21	19	276

UTAH

	1998	1999	2000	Total
LDS Hosp, Dept of Transp, 8th Ave & C St, Salt Lake City, UT 84143 Ph: (801) 408-3090 Fax: (801) 408-3098 1,2) J. Sorensen, 2) L.P. Belnap, M.H. Stevens, 3) R.C. Lambert, J.B. Stinson, E. Thor, R. Cline, M. McAnult, G. Rabetoyy, 4) T. Fuller, 5) J. Arata, G. Martin, K. Baker, R. Lowrie	74	66	75	1146
Univ of Utah Med Ctr, Renal Transp Office, 85 N Medical Dr, East Rm 201, Salt Lake City, UT 84132 Ph: (801) 581-6403 Fax: (801) 581-5727 1,2) J.H. Holman Jr, 2) E.W. Nelson, 3) F. Shihab, 4) T. Fuller, 5) A. Hansen, M. Ellison, C. Aguayo	72	83	64	1491

VERMONT

	1998	1999	2000	Total
Fletcher Allen Health Care, Dept of Surg/Med/Pathology, 111 Colchester Ave, Burlington, VT 05401 Ph: (802) 847-3572 Fax: (802) 847-3607 Email: jeffrey.reese@vtmednet.org 1,2) J. Reese, 3) V. Hood, J. Rimmer, F.J. Gennar, W. Weise, A. Seagel, M. Weidner, 4) B. MacPherson, 5) M. Taylor	22	19	21*	479

KIDNEY

1)=Director, 2)=Tx Surgeons, 3)=Physicians, 4)=Tissue Typers, 5)=TxCoords	1998	1999	2000	Total
VIRGINIA				
Univ of Virginia HSC, Transp Ctr, Box 265-Univ Station, Charlottesville, VA 22908 Ph: (804) 924-8604 Fax: (804) 982-0099 1,2) T. Pruett, 2) R.G. Sawyer, H. Sanfey, 3) P.L. Lobo, R. Isaacs, 4) C. Spencer, J. Guan, C. Davis, 5) B. Shephard, W. Simmons, C .Lawson	69	63	55	1010
Inova Fairfax Hosp, Dept of Surg, 3300 Gallows Rd, Falls Church, VA 22042 Ph: (703) 698-2986 Fax: (703) 698-2797 Email: johann.jonsson@inova.com 1,2) J. Jonsson, 2) T. Shaver, D. Kelly, 3) R. Mackow, 4) W. Ward, 5) P. Disanto, Hicks, B. Erickson, E. Skipper, V. Charity	60	86	76*	409
Sentara Norfolk General Hosp, Renal Transp Prog, 600 Gresham Dr, Norfolk, VA 23507 Ph: (757) 668-3906 Fax: (757) 668-2814 1,2) R.L. Hurwitz, 2) M. Glickman, M. Fogle, S. McEnroe, G. Stokes, R. Demasi, R. Gayle, 3) Wombolt, McCune, Whelan, Yeh, Chidester, Bundy, Gelpi, 4) A. Arnold, 5) L. Yell, R. French, K. Goad	57	45	37*	1174
Henrico Doctors' Hosp, Virginia Transp Ctr, 1602 Skipwith Rd, Richmond, VA 23229 Ph: (804) 289-4941 Fax: (804) 287-4359 1,2) G. Mendez-Picon, 2) K.B. Brown, 3) J.A. Thompson, 4) C. Duvall, C. Squire, 5) G. Spicer, L. Emery, L. Warden, L. Mathias, C. Rice, L. Pavlat	49	48	61*	430
Med Coll of Virginia, Dept of Surg, Div of Vasc/Transp Surg, 1200 E Broad St, Box 980057, Richmond, VA 23298 Ph: (804) 828-4104 Fax: (804) 828-4858 1,2) M.P. Posner, 2) R.A. Fisher, J. Ham, A. Cotterell, S. Dawson, 3) A. King, 4) P. Kimball, 5) S. Carter, C. Canody	53	59	67*	1412
WASHINGTON				
Children's Hosp & Med Ctr, Dept of Surg-CH-78, 4800 Sand Point Way NE, PO Box C-5371, Seattle, WA 98105 Ph: (206) 526-2039 Fax: (206) 527-3925 1,2) P. Healey, 2) D. Tapper, R. Sawin, J. Waldhausen, J.D. Perkins, 3) R. McDonald, 4) K. Nelson, 5) E. Juel-Medina	14	17	12	145
Univ of Washington Med Ctr, Transplant Services, 1959 N.E. Pacific St, Box 356174, Seattle, WA 98195 Ph: (206) 598-6700 Fax: (206) 598-6706 Email: cmarsh@u.washington.edu 1,2) C.L. Marsh, 2) J.D. Perkins, L. Wrenshall, B. Stevens, P. Healey, A. Levy, C. Kuhr, 3) Davis, Couser, Bomsztyk, Ahmad, Muczynski, Shankland, 4) K. Nelson (Puget Sound Bld Ctr), 5) P. Forg, C. Arp, C. Conover, D. Mullenix	69	69	95	619
Virginia Mason Med Ctr, Div of Renal Transp, 1100 9th Ave, C7-N, Seattle, WA 98111 Ph: (206) 341-0925 Fax: (206) 341-0886 1,3) R.L. Wilburn, 1,2) T.R. Hefty, 2) T.R. Hefty, R. Gibbons, F. Govier, R. McClure, T. Pritchett, R. Weissman, 3) C. Thompson, C. Cryst, M. Cooper, R. Wilburn, 4) K. Nelson, 5) M. Cressman, W. Ryan, J. Buck	100	101	114*	1540
Sacred Heart Med Ctr, Kidney Transp Prog, PO Box 2555, W 101 8th Ave, Spokane, WA 99220 Ph: (509) 474-4500 Fax: (509) 474-4487 Email: kidneytrans@shmc.org 1,2) R.J. Golden, 2) R. Golden, T. Fairchild, 3) Carson, Wickre, Benedetti, Sundberg, Obermiller, Mroch, Wiederkehr, 4) E. Klohe (Inland Northwest Blood Ctr), 5) A. Joyce, C. Nichols, T. Stevens	34	37	56	553
Swedish Medical Center, Organ Transplant Program, 1120 Cherry St, Ste 400, Seattle, WA 98104 Ph: (206) 386-3660 Fax: (206) 386-3644 1,2) W.H. Marks, 2) L.S. Florence, P.H. Chapman, 3) D. Perkinson, J. Eschbach, B. O'Neill, M. Kelly, R. Ochi, 4) Puget Sound Blood Center, K.K. Nelson, 5) S. Canniff, D. Gould, K. Ross, A. Alering, M. Kurtz	67	62	6	1428
WEST VIRGINIA				
Charleston Area Med Ctr, Dept of Renal Transp, 501 Morris St, Charleston, WV 25301 Ph: (304) 348-7823 Fax: (304) 348-7820 1,2) B. Sankari, 2) L. Wyner, 3) Lewis, Rahman, Lamb, Espiritu, Chiang, Szego, 4) D. Cook (Cleveland Clin), 5) D. Claridades, S. Huffman, L. Lipscomb, N. Morganroth	52	65	44	461
West Virginia Univ Hosp, Dept of Uro, Div of Transp, P O Box 9251, Morgantown, WV 26506 Ph: (304) 293-3342 Fax: (304) 293-2807 1,2) W. Tarry, 2) D.L. Lamm, 3) K. MacKay, 4) A. August, 5) J. Guess	22	14	15*	212

1)=Director, 2)=Tx Surgeons, 3)=Physicians, 4)=Tissue Typers, 5)=TxCoords	1998	1999	2000	Total
WISCONSIN				
Univ of Wisconsin-Madison, Transp Ofc H4/785, Clin Sci Ctr, 600 Highland Ave, Madison, WI 53792 Ph: (608) 263-1385 Fax: (608) 262-5624 1,2) H. Sollinger, 2) A. D'Alessandro, S. Knechtle, M. Kalayoglu, J. Odorico, Y. Becker, 3) J. Pirsch, B. Becker, S. Bartosh, A. Freeman, C.Sanchez, 4) D. Lorentzen, 5) Groshek, Armbrust, Spaith, Douglas, Nelson, Jaeger, Breslow, Shanaha	267	303	278	4887
Children's Hosp of Wisconsin, Abdominal Organ Transp, 9000 W Wisconsin Ave, PO Box 1997,MS653, Milwaukee, WI 53201 Ph: (414) 266-2000 Fax: (414) 266-2765 1,3) C.G. Pan, 2) M. Adams, C. Johnson, A. Roza, 3) L. Greenbaum, S. Van Why, C. Pan, 4) Bld Ctr of SE Wisconsin, 5) C. Werner	10	3	9	87
Froedtert Mem Lutheran Hosp, Med Coll of Wisconsin, Dept of Transp Surg, 9200 W Wisconsin Ave, Milwaukee, WI 53226 Ph: (414) 456-6920 Fax: (414) 456-6222 1,2) M.B. Adams, 2) C. Johnson, A. Roza, 3) S. Hariharan, 4) Bld Ctr of SE Wisconsin, D. Eckels, 5) P. Walczak, L. Venturi, C. Weickardt, S. Klenner, D. Pierce	131	86	97*	2462
St. Luke's Med Ctr, 2900 W Oklahoma Ave, Milwaukee, WI 53215 Ph: (414) 649-7222 Fax: (414) 649-5452 1,2) W. C. Stevenson, 2) F. Downey III, A. Tector, 3) C. Fritsche, A. Vidyaranya, 5) N. Contreras, K. Goelz, T. Graham, C. Gumm, N. Kloth, N. Niebauer, P. Schauer			12*	12
ARGENTINA				
Ctr of Med Ed & Clin Investigation, CEMIC - Dept of Med, Sanchez de Bustamente 2560, 1425 Buenos Aires Ph: (54)14 808-8199 Fax: (54)14 808-8115 Email: nefrologia@cemic.edu.ar 1,2) L.J. Jost, 1,2) R. Brunet, 2) A. Bracco, P. Zaefferer, H. Fernandez, A. Rovegno, F. Aulet, M. Pattin, 3) A. Vilches, M. Davalos, M. Turin, A. Cusumano, C. Diaz, 4) J. Egozcue, 5) V. labichella	30	33	19	650
Hosp Italiano de Buenos Aires, Dept of Surg, Gascon 450, Buenos Aires, 1181 Ph: (54)1 981-5010 Fax: (54)1 981-3881 1) S. Algranati, 2) C. Giudice, A. Domenech, 3) R. Groppa, 4) N. Prigoshine	9	18	22	205
Hosp Privado, Ctr Med de Cordoba, Prog de Transp Renales, Naciones Unidas 346, 5016 Cordoba Ph: (54)51 688232 Fax: (54)51 688271 1,3) G. Boccardo, 2) H. Paladini, 3) P. Massari, 4) C. Giraudo	64	52		610
AUSTRALIA				
St Vincent's Hosp, Dept of Nephrology, 376 Victoria St, Darlinghurst, NSW, 2010 Ph: (61)2 361-2362 Fax: (61)2 361-2032 Email: lstrauss@stvincents.com.au 1) J.M. Hayes, 2) R.S.A. Lord, A.R. Graham, A. Grabs, 3) E. Savdie, 4) Red Cross Bld Transf Ctr, 5) C. Windle	8			297
John Hunter Hosp, Newcastle Transp, Dept of Surg, Locked Bag No 1, Hunter Reg Mail Ctr, Newcastle, NSW, 2305 Ph: (61)49 21 4326 Fax: (61)49 21 4339 1,2) A.D. Hibberd, 2) P.W. Robinson, 3) P.R. Trevillian, 4) Bld Transf Serv, Sydney, 5) J. Crooks, A. Stein	17	18	17	276
Royal Prince Alfred Hosp, Univ of Sydney, Kidney Transp Unit, Missenden Rd, Camperdown, Sydney, NSW, 2050 Ph: (61)2 95158647 Fax: (61)2 93513361 1,2) A.G.R. Sheil, 2) D. Verran, G. Stewart, 3) J. Eris, 4) Sydney Red Cross Bld Transf Serv, 5) C. deLeon	59	51	62	1497
Westmead Hosp, Transp Unit, Westmead, NSW, 2145 Ph: (61)29 845 6962 Fax: (61)29 633 9351 Email: paul-robertson@wsahs.nsw.gov.au 1,2) R.D.M. Allen, 2) A.J. Richardson, H.M.H. Lau, 3) J.R. Chapman, P. O'Connell, B. Nankivell, 4) NSW Red Cross Tissue Typ Serv, 5) P. Robertson	39	33	33	464
Royal Perth Hosp, Dept of Clin Immunology, 2nd Flr, N Block, Wellington St, Perth, W. Australia, 6000 Ph: (61)8 92242899 Fax: (61)8 92242920 Email: ftchrist@cyllene.uwa.edu.au 1) F.T. Christiansen, 2) Thompson, House, Mitchell, Heath, Sieunarine, Rao, Mander, Crompton, 3) Irish, Thomas, Saker, Warr, Luxton, Moody, Hutchison, Hewitt, Rhodes, 4) D. Sayer, C. Witt, 5) J. Cusack, S. Foot, M. Smith	36	45	54	546
Princess Alexandra Hosp, Dept of Surg, Ipswich Rd, Woolloongabba, Brisbane, 4102 Ph: (61)7 3240 5716 Fax: (61)7 3240 2560 Email: d.nicol@uq.edu.au 1,2) D. Nicol, 2) D. Wall, P. Woodruff, J. Quinn, A. Griffin, J. Preston, 3) C. Hawley, J. Burke, D. Johnson, S. Campbell, N. Isbel, 4) S. Lee, 5) G. Frohloff	93	64	105	2058

1)=Director, 2)=Tx Surgeons, 3)=Physicians, 4)=Tissue Typers, 5)=TxCoords	1998	1999	2000	Total
Royal North Shore Hospital, Renal Medicine, Pacific Hwy, St. Leonards, Sydney, N.S.W., 2065 Ph: (612) 9926-8255 Fax: (612) 9906-3123 1) J. Mahony, 2) J. Payne, A. Sheil, A. Graham, G. White, 3) R.J. Caterson, D.A. Waugh, S. Roger, L.S. Ibels, C.A. Pollock, 4) N.S.W. Red Cross, T. Doran, 5) D. Morgan	15	12	10	810
Monash Med Ctr, Dept of Neph, 246 Clayton Rd, Clayton, Victoria, 3168 Ph: (61)3 9594-3529 Fax: (61)3 9594-3530 1) R.C. Atkins, 2) D. Scott, A. Saunder, R. Bell, 3) S. Chaoban, 4) B. Tait, 5) G. Scully, O. Maney	31	20	41	789
Austin Repatriation Med Ctr, Renal Transp Office, Heidelberg, Melbourne, Victoria, 3084 Ph: (61)3 9496-5685 Fax: (61)3 9496-5123 1) D. Power, 2) A. Roberts, G. Fell, M. Hoare, 3) Lerino, Francesco, 4) B. Tait, 5) A. Kakris	7	20	9	447
Royal Melbourne Hosp, Dept of Neph, Melbourne, Victoria, 3050 Ph: (61)3 9342-7143 Fax: (61)3 9347-1420 1,2) G. Becker, 1,3) R.Walker, 2) D. Francis, R. Millar, A. Robertson, 3) K. Nicholls, I. Fraser, S. Cohney, 4) B. Tait, 5) D. Yip	57	51	49	1410
Alfred Hosp, Renal Unit, Commercial Rd, Prahran, Victoria, 3181 Ph: (61)3 276 2585 Fax: (61)3 276 3494 1,3) J. Sabto, 2) C. Miles, M. Grigg, R. Snow, D. Westmore, 4) Royal Melbourne Hosp, 5) G. Scully	10			129

AUSTRIA

	1998	1999	2000	Total
Univ Klin for Chir, Dept of Transp Surg, Auenbruggerplatz 29, A-8036 Graz Ph: (43)316 385-2707 Fax: (43)316 385-4446 1,2) K.H. Tscheliessnigg, 3) Holzer, 4) G. Lanzer, 5) F. Iberer, T.H. Auer, A. Wasler, B. Petutuschnigg	38	48		436
Univ Hosp, Dept of Transp Surg, Anichstrasse 35, Innsbruck, 6020 Ph: (43)512 504-2603 Fax: (43)512 504-2605 1,2) R. Margreiter, 2) A. Koenigsrainer, B. Spechtenhauser, W. Steurer, 3) C. Bosriuller, 4) D. Schoenitzer, 5) H. Fetz, P. Schobel	93	88	106	1784
Gen Hosp Linz, II Dept of Intern Med, Krankenhaus Str 9, Linz 4020 Ph: (43)732 7806 Fax: (43)732 3300 Email: georp.biesenbach@akh.linz.at 1) G. Syre, 2) P. Brucke, Mair, Gruss, 3) G. Biesenbach, O. Janko, 4) Gabriel	11	24	12	359
KH d. Elisabethinen, Dept of Neph, Fadingerstr 1, Linz, A-4020 Ph: (43)732 76764305 Fax: (43)732 76764306 Email: stummvo@austglobal.net 1) H.K. Stummvoll, 2) A. Fugger, J. Behrenberg, 3) Leitner, Robl, 4) Artmann (KH Wels), 5) Leitner	27	33	30	587
Allgemeines Hosp, Univ of Vienna, Dept of Surg, Transp Ctr, Wahringer Gurtel 18-20, Vienna, A-1090 Ph: (43)1 40400 4000 Fax: (43)1 40400 6872 1,2) F. Muhlbacher, 2) R. Steininger, G. Berlakovich, 3) J. Kovarik, W. Horl, 4) W. Mayr, 5) M. Bodingbauel, R. Asari	163	202	177	3749

BELGIUM

	1998	1999	2000	Total
Univ Hosp Antwerpen, Dept of Neph/Hyper, Wilrijkstr 10, Edegem, Antwerp, B-2650 Ph: (32)3 821-3000 Fax: (32)3 829-0100 1) M.E. DeBroe, 2) D. Ysebaert, T. Chapelle, G. Roeyen, 3) G.A. Verpooten, M.M. Couttenye, J.L. Bosmans, K. van Hoeck, 4) L. Muylle, G. Mertens, 5) G. van Beeumen, W. van Donink	25	38	37	477
AZVUB, Univ of Brussels Med Ctr, Dept of Med, Laarbeeklaan 101, 1090 Brussels Ph: (32)2 477 6056 Fax: (32)2 477 6053 1) D. Verbeelen, 2) J. Lamote, 3) J. Sennesael, 4) C. Demanet, 5) B. Amerijckx	12	13	12	129
Clin Univ St Luc, Dept of Transp, 10 Ave Hippocrate, 1200 Brussels Ph: (32)2 7642207 Fax: (32)2 7707858 Email: squifflet@chir.ucl.ac.be 1,2) J.P. Squifflet, 2) M. Mourad, J. Malaise, 3) Y. Pirson, 4) D. Latinne, 5) C. Lecomte, V. Dumont, P. van Ormelingen	101	100	118	3003
Erasme-Clin Univ de Bruxelles, Dept Neph, Dial/Transp, 808 Route De Lennik, B-1070 Brussels Ph: (32)2 555-3334 Fax: (32)2 555-6499 1,3) D. Abramowicz, 2) L. DePauw, L. Hooghe, 3) M. Wissing, 4) E. Dupont, M. Andrien, 5) B. van Haelewyck, E, Angenon, V. Duthie	57	75		1561
Univ Hosp Ghent, Dept of Neph, DePintelaan 185, B-9000 Ghent Ph: (32)9 240-4509 Fax: (32)9 240-4599 1,3) N. Lameire, 1,2) B.de Hemptinne, 2) J. DeRoose, F. Vermassen, U. Hesse, 3) R. van Holder, 4) B. van dekerckhove, 5) M. van der Vennet, L. Colenbie	41	62	79	698

1)=Director, 2)=Tx Surgeons, 3)=Physicians, 4)=Tissue Typers, 5)=TxCoords	1998	1999	2000	Total
Univ Leuven, Hosp Gasthuisberg, Dept of Neph, Herestraat 49, Leuven, B3000 Ph: (32)16 344580 Fax: (32)16 344599 1,3) Y. Vanrenterghem, 2) W. Coosemans, J. Pirenne, 3) D. Kuypers, B. Maes, T. Messiaen, P. Evenepoel, 4) M.P. Emonds, J. Dendievel, 5) F. Van Gelder, D. Van Hees, S. Kimpen	115	142	135	2413
Ctr Hosp Univ-Liege, Dept of Surg/Transp, Domaine Univ du Sart-Tilman-B35, Liege, 4000 Ph: (32)43 667206 Fax: (32)43 667517 1,2) M. Meurisse, 2) O. Detry, A. DeRoover, 3) P. Mahieu, M. Beaujean, 4) C. Bouillenne, 5) M.H. Delbouille, M.F. Hans	31	24	25	547

BRAZIL

	1998	1999	2000	Total
FHDF-Hosp de Base do Distrito Fed, Clin Uro/Renal Transp, SMHS 101 B1 "A"-HBDF, Brazilia, DF Ph: (55)61 325-4479/4725 Fax: (55)61 322-6479 Email: urologia.hbdf@ambr.com.br 1) A.T. Franca, 2) DC. Teles, ERR.Faria.L.G. Carvalho, PJA. Moura, 3) VO. Bello, MCSG. Lobo, 4) JAF. Villaca, 5) PJA. Moura	36	43		502
Casa de Saude Santa Maria S/A, Dept of Neph-Renal Transp, Rua Dr Joaquim Ribeiro Filho, 209 Colatina, Colatina, ES 29702-130 Ph: (55)27 722 0777 Fax: (55)27 722 0777 1,5) M.X. Carrera, 2) N. Souza Cardoso, 3) A. Soares	6			20
Hosp Felicio Rocho, Dept of Neph, Rua Odilon Braga 1254, Belo Horizonte, MG 30.310-340 Ph: (55)31 339-7351 Fax: (55)31 227-7297 1) E. Lasmar, 2) A. Bamberg, 3) S. Vilaca, 4) M. Lima, 5) E. Tavora	31	27	20	736
CAJURU, Unidade Transp Renal, Av Sao Jose 300, Curitiba, PR 80050 350 Ph: (55)41 360-3051 Fax: (55)41 336-4141 Email: mcriella@cwb.pam.corn.br 1) M.C. Riella, 2) L.S. Santos, F.M. Martina, 3) R.M. de Carvalho, L.S. Emed, 4) C. von Ghlen, 5) R.M. de Carvalho	22	23		266
Hosp Evangelico de Curitiba, Dept of Neph/Uro, Rua Augusto Stellfeld-1908-8 Andar, Curitiba, PR 80.730-150 Ph: (55)41 224-0906 Fax: (55)41 224-0906 Email: mcriella@cwb.pam.com.br 1) M.C. Riella, 2) S.C. Ziesemer, J.P. Pagani, M. Serpe, H. Contieri, 3) F.C. Contieri, R. Benvenutti, 4) C. von Glehn, M.G. Bicalho, 5) F.C. Contieri	36	45	40	678
Santa Casa de Curitiba, Dept of Neph, Praca Rui Barbosa, 694, Curitiba, PR Ph: (55)41 322-6967 Fax: (55)41 322-6967 1) M. Scaramuzza, 1) S.G. Marks, 2) R. Tambara, L.C. Rocha, 3) J.R.M.M. deCarvalho, H.V. Cassi, 4) N.F. Pereira, A.C. Senegaglia	18	24	24	347
Policlinica Pato Branco S/A, Unidade de Terapia-Dept Neph, Rua Pedro Ramires de Mello, 361, Av Brasil, 530, Pato Branco, PR 85501-250 Ph: (55)46 224-5367 Fax: (55)46 225-5959 Email: utr@qualinet.com.br 1,3,5) J.L.Z. Ramos, 2) A. Freire, E. Guerios, A. Motizuki, S. Janczeski, R. Yamada, 3) M. Engel, 4) N.F. Pereira, C. von Glehn, A.C. Senegaglta, 5) M. Engel	19	19	22	264
Hosp de Clinicas de Porto Alegre, Dept of Neph, Rua Ramiro Barcelos 2350, Sala 2030, Porto Alegre, RS 90035-003 Ph: (55)51 311 6699 Fax: (55)51 331 6598 1,2) W.J. Koff, 2) N.T. Denicol, M. Berger, 3) R.C. Manfro, D. Saitovith, F.J. Veronese, L.F. Goncalves, 4) L.F. Jobim, 5) L.F. Goncalves	34	36	48	460
Santa Casa De Porto Alegre, Serv De Transp (Enf 2), Praca Dom Feliciano S/N, Porto Alegre, RS 90020160 Ph: (55)51 226-0848 Fax: (55)51 228-0496 1,2) V.D. Garcia, 2) G. Cantisani, P. Vitola, 3) J.J. Bianchini, J.C. Goldani, A.E. Bittar, E. Keitel, 4) J. Neumann, 5) N. Hoefelmann	82	80	113	1150
Hosp Clin Med-Ribeirao Preto, Dept of Surg/Intern Med, Campus Da Univ Sau Paula, Ribeirao Preto, SP 14048-900 Ph: (55)16 633 0907 Fax: (55)16 633 5074 1) A. Spallini Ferraz, 2) A.C.P. Martins, H.J. Suaid, A. Cologna, 3) J.A. Cardeal da Costa, T.M. Pisi Garcia, L.T. Santamaria, 4) C, M.P. Santos, 5) N.L. de Almeida	43	56		821
Hosp Dom Silverio Gomes Pimenta, Dept of Neph, Rua Voluntarios da Patria, 3693, Sao Paulo, SP Ph: (55)11 959 2266 Fax: (55)11 959 2388 1,5) J.O. Medina Pestana, 2) J.C.B. Silva, 3) C. Melaragno, 4) M. Gerbase De Lima	3	0	0	535
Instituto de Urologia E Nephrologia, Urol & Nephrol, Rua Voluntarios de Sao Paulo, 3826, 15015 Sao Jose do Rio Preto, Sao Paulo, SP Ph: (55)172 32 2322 Fax: (55)172 32 2230 1,3) M. Abbud-Filho, 2) C. Verona, M. Zerati-Filho, C. D'Avila, S. Zerati, R. Martucci, 3) J.B. Barberato, H.J. Ramalho, 4) E. Gaio	42	50	71	611

KIDNEY

1)=Director, 2)=Tx Surgeons, 3)=Physicians, 4)=Tissue Typers, 5)=TxCoords	1998	1999	2000	Total
Sao Paulo Hosp, Dept of Neph, Rua Pedro de Toledo, 715, Sao Paulo, SP Ph: (55)11 571 6376 Fax: (55)11 571 5197 1,5) J.O. Medina Pestana, 2) C. Almeida, 3) A.P.S. Filho, 4) M. Gerbase de Lima	171	428	507	2108
Univ de Sao Paulo, Hosp das Clin, Kidney Transp Unit, Renal Transp-70 andar-Sala 706-F, Av Dr Eneas de Carvalho Aguiar, 255, Sao Paulo, SP 05403-900 Ph: (55)11 3062-9006 Fax: (55)11 3064-7013 1) L.E. Ianhez, 2) W.C. Nahas, E. Mazzuchi, I.M. Antonopoulos, 3) Chocair, Fonseca, Galvao, Castro, David-Neto, Azevedo, Saldanha, 4) J.K. Filho, 5) F. Jota de Paula, F.C.B. Cavalcanti	99	100	132	2723

CANADA

1)=Director, 2)=Tx Surgeons, 3)=Physicians, 4)=Tissue Typers, 5)=TxCoords	1998	1999	2000	Total
Univ of Alberta Hosp, Dept of Med, Div Neph/Immun, Renal Transplant Office CSB 11-102, 8440 112th St, Edmonton, AB T6G 2B7 Ph: (780) 407-8099 Fax: (780) 407-6389 1) P.F. Halloran, 2) G. Warnock, G. Todd, R. Moore, N. Kneteman, 3) S. Cockfield, P. Campbell, A. Murray, F. Harley, V. Yiu, 4) A. Halpin, 5) T. Voyer, L. McKinstry, S. Comeau, C. Sholter	72	68	79	1413
British Columbia Children's Hosp, c/o British Columbia Transp Sc, 3th Flr W Tower, 555 W 12th Ave, Vancouver, BC V5Z 3X7 Ph: (604) 875-2240 Fax: (604) 877-2111 1) Mr B. Barrable, 2) H.W. Johnson, J. LeBlanc, G.U. Coleman, 3) D. Lirenman, J. Carter, M. Hurley, 4) B. Draney, 5) S. Duncan, J. Waines	8	10	4	97
St Paul's Hosp, Renal Transp Dept, 1081 Burrard St, Vancouver, BC V6Z 1Y6 Ph: (604) 806-8970 Fax: (604) 806-8076 1) D. Landsberg, 2) W. Gourlay, 3) L. DeLuca, 4) Immuno Lab-VGH, 5) H. Cyr	56	69	76	968
Vancouver Hosp, c/o British Columbia Transp Sc, 3th Flr W Tower, 555 W 12th Ave, Vancouver, BC V5Z 3X7 Ph: (604) 877-2240 Fax: (604) 877-2111 1) Mr B. Barrable, 2) M.G. McLoughlin, J. Wright, M. Nigro, W. Gourlay, 3) D.N. Landsberg, J. Shapiro, P.A. Keown, L. Deluc, G. Nusbaumera, 4) B. Draney, 5) S. Duncan, J. Ritchie, H. Cyr	32	61	56	1151
Univ of Calgary Foothills Med Ctr, Div of Tx, Dept of Surg, RmG33, 1403 29th St NW, Calgary, Alberta, T2N 2T9 Ph: (403) 670-4266 Fax: (403) 270-8431 Email: serdar.yilmaz@crha-health.ab.ca 1,2) S. Yilmaz, 2) A. Barama, D. Sigalet, 3) F. Sepandj, J. Klassen, L. Tibbles, K. McLaughlin, J. Midgley, 4) R. McKenna, 5) S. Buckle, M. Miller, J. Costa	71	76	64	818
Health Sci Ctr, Transp Prog, GE441-820 Sherbrook St, Winnipeg, MB R3A 1R9 Ph: (204) 787-7001 Fax: (204) 787-3326 Email: john_jeffery@umanitoba.ca 1,2) J.R. Jeffery, 2) E. Ramsey, H. Fong, 3) D.N. Rush, P. Nickerson, P. Birk, 4) I. Dembinski, D. Pochino, 5) S. Beghin, K. Farstad, K. Peters, T. Wilson, S. Stokoloff	26	31	46	909
Ste Justine Hosp, Dept of Peds, 3175 Cote St Catherine, Montreal, PQ H3T 1C5 Ph: (514) 345-4737 Fax: (514) 345-4838 Email: mj.clermont@sympatico.ca 1) M.J. Clermont, 2) S. Yazbeck, A.L. Bensoussan, M. Lallier, S. Busque, 3) P. Robitaille, A. Merouani, 4) Institut Armand Frappier, 5) M.S. Ouellette	1	8	6	251
Queen Elizabeth II Health Sci Ctr, Victoria General Site, Kidney Transplant Program, 1278 Tower Road, Halifax,Nova Scotia, NS B3H 2Y9 Ph: (902) 473-6877/4026 Fax: (902) 492-2437 1,2) J.G. Lawen, 1,3) B.A. Kiberd, 2) P. Belitsky, A.S. MacDonald, H. Bitter-Suermann, V. McAllister, 3) K. Jindal, M. West, K. West, C. Clase, 4) K. West, 5) R. Leblanc, J. Cruickshank	81	107	132	2058
St Joseph's Hosp-McMaster Univ, Dept of Neph, 50 Charlton Ave E, Hamilton, ON L8N 4A6 Ph: (416) 521-6049 Fax: (416) 521-6088 1,3) D. Arlen, 1,2) P. Whelan, 2) S. Tsai, K. Piercy, A. Kapoon, 3) D. Ludwin, D. Russell, 4) D.P. Singal, 5) F. Fyfe, T. Hamilton, S. Upson	72	51	57	1030
Kingston Gen Hosp, Dept of Med, 2058-Etherington Hall, Queen's Univ, Kingston, ON K7L 3N6 Ph: (613) 533-6983 Fax: (613) 548-0686 Email: dh9@post.queensu.ca 1) D.C. Holland, 2) J. Heaton, A. MacNeilly, 3) E.B. Toffelmire, A.R. Morton, E.A. Iliescu, M.A. Singer, S. Iqbal, 4) L. Shepherd, 5) S. Scott-Seary	11	8		263
LHSC, University Campus, 339 Windemere Rd, London, ON N6A 5A5 Ph: (519) 663-3688 Fax: (519) 663-8808 1,3) A. Jevnikar, 2) J. Sharpe, J. Chin, 3) N. Muirhead, D. Hollomby, 4) S. Leckie, 5) M.A. Henry,	74	50	78	1390
Ottawa Civic Hosp, Dept of Neph, 1053 Carling Ave, Ottawa, ON K1Y 4E9 Ph: (613) 761-4752 Fax: (613) 761-5368 1,3) S.L. Jindal, 2) P. Barron, A. Thijssen, 4) D.P.S. Sengar, 5) D. Dumont	5			485

1)=Director, 2)=Tx Surgeons, 3)=Physicians, 4)=Tissue Typers, 5)=TxCoords	1998	1999	2000	Total
Toronto General Hosp, Multi-Organ Transp Prog, 200 Elizabeth St, NU 10-158, Toronto, ON M5G 2C4 Ph: (416) 340-4669 Fax: (416) 340-3492 Email: edward.cole@uhn.on.ca 1) E. Cole, 2) M. Robinette, M. Cattral, D. Grant, P. Greig, 3) D. Cattran, S.S. Fenton, C.J. Cardella, 4) J. Wade, 5) T. McKnight, L. Cotter, L. Lamb, D. Gordon, J. Ly	98	98	94	1119
Univ of Toronto, St Michael's Hosp, Transp Office, 30 Bond St, Toronto, ON M5B 1W8 Ph: (416) 867-3665 Fax: (416) 867-3709 Email: jeffrey.zaltzman@utoronto.ca 1,3) J. Zaltzman, 2) J. Honey, R. Stewart, 3) R. Prasad, 4) J. Wade, 5) M. Connelly, F. Shamy, G. Meliton, J. Huckle	77	52	77	1222
Hosp Maisonneuve-Rosemont, Dept of Neph, 5415 Boul de L'Assomption, Montreal, PQ H1T 2M4 Ph: (514) 252-3489 Fax: (514) 255-3026 1,3) R. Dandavino, 2) E. Bastien, R. Girard, M. Morin, 3) A. Boucher, C. Beaudry, 4) C. Perreault, 5) P. Brunet, S. Bureau	41	37	45	784
Hosp Notre Dame, Montreal, Dept of Transp Surg, 1560 Sherbrooke Est, Montreal, PQ H2L 4M1 Ph: (514) 281-6000 x6605 Fax: (514) 896-4736 Email: pierre.daloze.chum@ssss.gouv.qc.ca 1,2) P. Daloze, 2) C. Smeesters, S. Busque, 3) G. St-Louis, 4) Inst Armand Frappier, Montreal, 5) Quebec Transp	44	59	69	943
Royal Victoria Hosp, Medicine & Surgery, 687 Pine Ave W, Montreal, PQ H3A 1A1 Ph: (514) 843-1649 Fax: (514) 843-1708 Email: rloert@po-box.mcgill.ca 1,3) R. Loertscher, 1,2) P. Metrakos, 2) J. Tchervenkov, 3) M. Lipman, R. Mangel, D. Baran, 4) P. Imperial, C. McIntyre, L. Nong, 5) L. Peters, M. Fortier, Z. Aalamian, K. O'Mcara	48	54	36	959
L'Hotel-Dieu de Quebec, Dept of Neph, 11 Cote du Palais, Quebec, PQ G1R 2J6 Ph: (418) 691-5474 Fax: (418) 691-5253 1) J.G. Lachance, 2) A. Naud, Y. Fradet, G. Bedard, R. Charrois, M. Gregoire, L. Lacombe, 3) R. Noel, I. Houde, 4) R. Roy, 5) F. Quevillon, C. Le Beau, L. Otis	47	49	62	996
Royal Univ Hosp, Saskatoon, Saskatchewan Transp Prog, Box 86, Saskatoon, SK S7N0W8 Ph: (306)655-1054 Fax: (306)655-1046 1,2) A. Shoker, 2) Lawlor, Ulmer, Duval, Barrett, Gonor, Taranger, Fentie, Weckworth, 3) M. Baltzan, R. Dyck, 4) D. Sheridan, 5) Sask Transplant Program	62	51	28	813

CHILE

	1998	1999	2000	Total
Barros Luco Trudeau, Dept of Neph, Av Jose Miguel Carrera 3204, Santiago Ph: (56)2 551 0897 Fax: (56)2 551 2404 1,2) A. Mocarquer, 1,3) J. Pefaur, 2) J. Aguilo, J. Gaete, O. Rodriguez, I. Galleguillos, 3) James, Salinas, Valderrama, Panace, Chea, Montana, Fiabane, 4) S. Elgueta, E. Wegmann, 5) R. Ponce, Veloso	48			663
Unidad de Trasplantes, Clinica las Condes, Lo Fontecilla 441, Santiago Ph: (56)2 2105005 Fax: (56)2 2172998 1,2) E.G. Buckel, 2) M. Uribe, J. Aguilo, R. Rosenfeld, 3) J. Morales, A. Vususic, A. Fierro, J. Brahm, G. Silva, S. Ceresa, 5) C. Herzog, T. Santander	13	12		70
Universidad Catolica De Chile, Urologia-Unidad Trasplante, Marcoleta 367-3rd Piso, Santiago, 6510260 Ph: (562) 632-3462 Fax: (562) 632-9620 Email: tprenal@med.puc.cl 1,2) P. Troncoso, 2) C.Trucco.A. Velasco, P. Baquedano, 3) F. Cavaguaro, A. Jara, M. Ortiz, 4) L. Rodriguez, 5) M. Acuna	8	8	12	350
Hosp Base Valdivia, Dept of Neph, Bueras 850, PO Box 8-D, Valdivia Ph: (56)63 215890 Fax: (56)63 297023 Email: smezzano@uach.cl 1) S.A. Mezzano, 2) D. Corti, A. Foneron, L. Troncoso, 3) L. Ardiles, Arriagada, C. Flores, C. Aros, 4) A. Droguett, P. Alruiz, 5) S. Elgueta, V. Jerez	18	24	18	195
Carlos Van Buren Hosp, Dept ofNeph/Dial/Transp, San Ignacio 725, Casilla 4129, Valparaiso Ph: (56)32 699 373 Fax: (56)32 237 229 Email: centrosermedial@entelchile.net 1) H.L. Poblete-Badal, 2) G. MacMillan Soto, C. Carmona Soto, D. Jara Valenzuela, 3) J.W. Toro Cornejo, V. Nicovani Hermosilla, 4) Inst de Salud Publica de Chile (Santiago), 5) J.W. Toro Cornejo	11	7	12	125

CHINA, P.R.

	1998	1999	2000	Total
Beijing Friendship Hosp, Dept of Uro, 95 Yong An Rd, Beijing, 100050 Ph: (86)10 6301 4411 Fax: (86)10 6302 3261 1,2) Y.H. Zhang, 2) Y. Tian, 3) L. Ma, 4) Z.X. Li, 5) P. Yang	197	201	256	2362

KIDNEY

1)=Director, 2)=Tx Surgeons, 3)=Physicians, 4)=Tissue Typers, 5)=TxCoords	1998	1999	2000	Total
Affiliated First Hosp, Sun Yat-sun Med Univ, 58 Zhongahan Rd, Guangzhou, PR 510080 Ph: (86)208 7766335 Fax: (86)208 7775030 1,2) K.I. Zheng, 2) P.P. Dai, C.X. Wang, 3) L.Y. Zhu, S.G. Zhang, Q.R. Shen, P.G. Wu, 4) X.B. Wang, J. Bi	156	160	230	1739
Tongji Med Univ, Tongji Hosp, Inst of Organ Transp, 13 Hangkong Rd, Wuhan, Hubei, 430030 Ph: (86)27 83611175 Fax: (86)27 83611175 Email: iot@tjh.tjmu.edu.cn 1) S.S. Xia, 2) F.Q. Zhen, Z.S. Chen, Z.Y. Wen, 3) Z.P. Ling, 4) Z.S. Chen, 5) H.Y. Jiang	157	167	195	1361
Shanghai First People's Hosp, Uro Inst, Transp Ctr, 85 Wujin Rd, Shanghai, 200080 Ph: (86)21 6324 0090 Fax: (86)21 6324 0825 1,2) X.D. Tang, 1.3) J.X. Qin, 2) D. Xu, G. Ling, X. Wang, X.Y. Zhang, 3) Z. Lu, 4) Y. Ding, P. Qiu, 5) Nephro & Uro Staff	76	116	141	1638
Taiping People's Hosp, Transpl Center, 34 Jiefang St, HuMen DongGuan, DongGuan, 511761 Ph: (86) 769-5505268 Fax: (86) 20 84420813 1) S.T. Deng, 1) S.Z. Ma, 2) W. Gao, J. Lee, W.H. Xu, Z.Z. Guo, 3) W. Gao, J.H. Xu, 4) S. Jang, L.Y. Li	149	163	171	1048
Shanghai Long March Hosp, Dept of Urology, 415 Fengyang Rd, Shanghai, 200003 Ph: (86)21 6327-5997 Fax: (86)21 63724488 Email: urologyb@online.sh.cn 1,2) Z.L. Min	181	187		1945

COLOMBIA

	1998	1999	2000	Total
Fundocion Santa Fe de Bogota, Surg, Div of Transpl, Calle 116, #9-02, Bogota Ph: (57)1 2148607 Fax: (57)1 6122486 1,2) J.D. Arenas, 2) E. Figueredo, A. Cortes, J.M. Valdez, 3) E. Carrizosa, D. Garcia, M. Nieto, 4) N. Merino, 5) A.M. Alfonso, O. Florez	24			24
Hosp San Vincente De Paul, Univ of Antioquia, Dept of Neph, Calle 64 x Carrera 51D, Medellin-Antioquia Ph: (57)4 2639191 Fax: (57)4 2631002 1,2) A. Velasquez, 2) F. Cano, J.I. Gutierrez, 3) M. Arbelaez, J.L. Arango, J.E. Henao, G. Mejia, A. Garcia, I. Arroyave, 4) L.F. Garcia, 5) E. Duque, J. Duque	192	226	236	2093

CROATIA

	1998	1999	2000	Total
Univ Clin Hosp-Rebro Zagreb, Nat'l Referral Organ Transp &, Tissue Typ Ctr - Dept of Uro, 12 Kispaticeva, Zagreb, HR-10000 Ph: (385)1 233 3235 Fax: (385)1 212 684 Email: andrija.kastelan@zg.tel.hr 1,2) A. Kastelan, 2) Z. Marekovic, J. Pasini, 3) Z. Puretic, L.J. Bubic, 4) V. Kerhin-Brkljacic, R. Zunec, 5) Z. Kastelan, V. Vegar	31	38	18	388

CYPRUS

	1998	1999	2000	Total
Surg & Transp Found, Dept of Surgery, 4A Char Mouskos Str, PO Box 24307, Nicosia, 1102 Ph: (357)2 672323 Fax: (357)2 668980 Email: gkyriakides@transplant.com.cy 1,2) G.K. Kyriakides, 2) P. Nicolaou, 3) M. Hadjigaviriel, 4) A. Nicolaides, 5) M. Kyriakides	27	41	39	451

CZECH REPUBLIC

	1998	1999	2000	Total
Chrales Univ, Hradec Kralove, Dept of Uro, Transp Ctr, Teaching Hosp Med Fac, Hradec Kralove, 50036 Bohemia Ph: (42)49 583 3564 Fax: (42)49 583 3431 1,2) P. Navratil, 2) Z. Veselsky, I. Novak, 3) P. Fixa, R. Stilec, 4) B. Jilkova, 5) M. Grofova	33	41	47	640
Fakultni Nemocnice, 1 Chir Klin, I P Pavlova 6, 775 20 Olomouc, Olomouc Ph: (42)68 541 7609 Fax: (42)68 541 7609 Email: petr.bachleda@fhol.cz 1,2) P. Bachleda, 2) P. Utikal, V. Kral, 3) J. Zadrazil, 4) M. Petrek, 5) Z. Petrova	40	26	46	419
Univ Hosp Pilsen, Dept of Surg, Dr E Benese 13, Pilsen, 30599 Ph: (420)19 273336 Fax: (420)19 273336 1) V. Treska, 2) M. Cechura, J. Krizan, J. Klecka, B. Certik, 3) M. Rouda, T. Reischig, 4) J. Fikerlova, 5) D. Hasman	20	23	24	454
Inst for Clin and Exper Med, Transp Ctr, Dept of Surg/Neph, Videnska 800, 14000 Prague 4 Ph: (420)2 613-64103 Fax: (420)2 613-63113 Email: stvi@medicon.cz 1) S. Vitko, 2) M. AdAmec, 3) V. Teplan, J. Lacha, 4) E. Ivaskova, 5) E. Pokorna, E. Laszikova, V. Charova, M. Skachova	162	137	151	2308

1)=Director, 2)=Tx Surgeons, 3)=Physicians, 4)=Tissue Typers, 5)=TxCoords	1998	1999	2000	Total
Univ Hosp Motol & 2nd Med Faculty, Transp Ctr, Charles Univ Prague, V Uvalu 84, Prague 5, 15006 Ph: (420)2 5722 1056 Fax: (420)2 5722 1056 Email: jaroslav.spatenka@lfmotol.cuni.cz 1,2) J. Spatenka, 2) L. Zeman, J. Moravek, 3) J. Feber, J. Janda, J. Dusek, E. Simkova, J. Kreisinger, 4) Inst of Exp Med Prague-Krc, 5) I. Cesalova, A. Habrmanova	10	11	7	104

DENMARK

Skejby Hosp, Univ Aarhus, Nephrology C, Brenstrupgaardvej, Aarhus, DK 8200 Ph: (45)89 495704 Fax: (45)89 496003 1,3) S. Madsen, 2) S. Ellebaek, 3) K.A. Jorgensen, H.E. Hansen, 4) L. Fugger, 5) D, Mathiassen, P. Lauenborg	45	60		1625
Rigshospitalet, Dept of Surg, D 2112, 9 Blegdamsvej, DK-2100 Copenhagen Ph: (45) 3545 2110 Fax: (45) 3545 2158 1,2) J.K. Kristensen, 3) J. Ladefoged, K. Olgaard, 4) A. Svejgaard, 5) I. Palfeldt	45	55	51	1556
Univ of Copenhagen-Herlev, Dept of Surg H/Med Dept B, Herlev Ringvej, Herlev, DK-2730 Ph: (45)9 4488 3632 Fax: (45)9 4488 4615 1) H.E. Jorgensen, 2) F. Rasmussen, 3) H. Lokkegaard, 4) A. Svejgaard, 5) H. Lokkegaard	22	25	16	904
Odense Univ Hosp, Dept of Neph, DK-5000 Odense Fax: (45)65 906413 1,3) S.A. Birkeland, 2) N. Rohr, 4) Aarhus Histo Lab	31	28	29	911

EGYPT

Cairo Kidney Ctr, Dept of Renal Transp, PO Box 91, Bab-El-Louk, Cairo 11513 Ph: (20)2 578 0821 Fax: (20)2 769749 1) R.S. Barsoum, 2) A. Morsi, A. Nassef, 3) R.M. Botros, R.R. Faltas, M.T. Tadros, H. Mohey, S.A. Soliman, 4) I. Iskander, 5) M. Mehanny, T. Fayad	22	26	21	327

FINLAND

Children's Hosp, Univ of Helsinki, Dept of Ped Surg, Stenbackinkatu 11, Helsinki 29, SF 00029 Ph: (90)358 471 72730 Fax: (90)358 47174705 1,2) M. Leijala, 2) H. Sairanen, I. Mattila, M. Kaarne, 3) C. Holmberg, H. Jalanko, 4) S. Koskimies	7	13		97
Helsinki Univ Ctr Hosp, IV Dept of Surg, Div of Transp, Kasarmikatu 11-13, SF-00130 Helsinki Ph: (358)9 174942 Fax: (358)9 174975 Email: kaija.salmela@hus.fi 1) K. Salmela, 2) Eklund, Hockerstedt, Isoniemi, Kyllonen, Makisalo, Halme, 4) J. Partanen, 5) E. Hartikka, A.K. Mattila, M-L. Heikkila, L. Toivonen	187	163	194	4051

FRANCE

Univ Hosp of Bicetre, Dept of Neph, 78 Ave du General Leclerc, Kremlin-Bicetre, 94275 Ph: (33)1 4521 2722 Fax: (33)1 4521 2116 1,3) B. Charpentier, 2) G. Benoit, J. Bellamy, P. Blanchet, 3) C. Hiesse, A. Durrbach, F. Kriaa, 4) C. Raffoux, D. Charron, 5) L. Joseph, J. Decaris	80	61	70	2042
G Montpied Hosp, Dept of Neph/Uro, BP 69, Clermont-Ferrand, 63003 Ph: (33)4 7375 1425 Fax: (33)4 7375 1551 1,3,5) P.M. Deteix, 2) J.P. Boiteux, L. Guy, 3) N. Gazuy, L. Escaravage, C.H. Brandely, A.E. Heng, 4) C. Coussediere, Ph. Gallon, B. Lamy, 5) N. Mathieu	33	39	33	358
Ctr Hosp Lyon Sud, Lyon Univ, Div of Neph, Pav 2F, 69310 Pierre Benite, Lyon Ph: (33)478 861309 Fax: (33)478 861941 1) M. Labeeuw, 2) P. Perrin, M. Devonec, 3) R. Cahen, P. Trolliet, C. Pouteil Noble, C. Lorriaux, C. Boudray, 4) H. Betuel, L. Gebuhrer, 5) J.J. Colpart	31			289
Hosp Edouard Herriot, Ped Renal Unit, Pavillon S, Pl d'Arsonval, 69437 Lyon Ph: (33)472 110346 Fax: (33)472 110343 Email: cochat@univ-lyon1.fr 1,3) P. Cochat, 2) X. Martin, M. Dawahra, 3) B. Parchoux, M.H. Said, B. Ranchin, 4) L. Gebuhrer, 5) J.J. Colpart	9	7	17	180
Lapeyronie Hosp, Dept of Neph, 555 Rte de Ganges, Montpellier Cedex, 34059 Ph: (33)67 338475 Fax: (33)67 412599 1,3) G. Mourad, 2) J. Guiter, F.J. Iborra, 3) G. Chong, 4) J. Seignalet, 5) A. Boularan	80	60	84	1254

KIDNEY

1)=Director, 2)=Tx Surgeons, 3)=Physicians, 4)=Tissue Typers, 5)=TxCoords	1998	1999	2000	Total
Ctr Hosp Reg et Univ-Nancy, Hosp de Brabois, Dept of Neph, 54511 Vandoeuvre, Nancy Cedex Ph: (33)83 153163 Fax: (33)83 153531 1,3) M. Kessler, 2) Ph. Mangin, 3) E. Renoult, 4) P. Perrier, 5) F. Jacob	78	62	72	1122
Hotel Dieu-Univ Nantes, Dept of Neph/Clin Immun, 1 Pl Alexis Ricordeau, Nantes Cedex 01, 44035 Ph: (33)240 083303 Fax: (33)240 083312 1) J.P. Soulillou, 2) G. Karam, O. Bouchot, P. Glemain, L. Lenormand, 3) M. Hourmant, D. Cantarovich, J. Dantal, M. Giral, G. Blancho, 4) J.M. Bignon, 5) J.N. LeSant, C. LeNormand	126	111	149	2527
Hosp Necker, Dept of Transp, 161 Rue de Sevres, Paris Cedex 15, 75015 Ph: (33)1 44495432 Fax: (33)1 44495430 1,2) H. Kreis, 2) M. Lacombe, Y. Chretien, A. Mejean, 3) M.N. Peraldi, M.F. Mamzer-Brun, E. Morelon, N. Chkoff, 4) S. Zuckman, 5) S. Premel, C. Fournier	53	41	51	1785
Hosp Necker Enfants Malades, Dept of Ped Neph, 149 Rue de Sevres, 75743 Paris Cedex 15 Ph: (33)1 4449-4462 Fax: (33)1 4449-4460 1,3) P. Niaudet, 2) D. Beurton, Y. Revillon, D. Jan, 3) M.F. Gagnadoux, G. Guest, 4) St Louis Hosp(Paris)	21	19	22	1044
Hosp Saint-Louis, Serv De Neph, Lavande 3, 1 Av Claude Vellefaux, Cedex 10, Paris, 75475 Ph: (33)1 42 499608 Fax: (33)1 42 499606 1) Ch. Legendre, 2) A. LeDuc, P. Teillac, F. Desgranchamps, 3) J. Bedrossian, E. Thervet, F. Martinez, 4) C. Suberbielle, 5) F. Roussin	76	51	71	808
La Pitie Salpetriere, Dept of Surg, 83 Blvd de L'Hopital, Paris, 75013 Ph: (33)1 4217-7111 Fax: (33)1 4217-7112 1) F. Richard, 2) M.O. Bitker, B. Barrou, 3) Mouquet, Benalia, Ourhama, 4) C. Suberbielle, 5) M. Tallier, S. Jehan, N. Cornillot	60	55	68	1497
Tenon Hosp, Dept of Neph/Uro, 4 Rue de la Chine, Paris, 75020 Ph: (33)1 403 06502 Fax: (33)1 403 07968 1) J.D. Sraer, 2) P. Thibault, Nussaume, 3) E. Rondeau, Kanfer, Peraldi, 4) C. Raffoux, Hosp St. Louis, 5) M.S.C. Marlin, NS.M. Andrieux	27	19		938
CHU Reims, Hosp Maison Blanche, Hosp Robert Debre, Dept Uro/Neph, Reims Cedex, 51092 Ph: (33)326 787181 Fax: (33)326 788482 Email: jchanard@chu-reims.fr 1,3) J. Chanard, 2) B. Lardennois, 3) O. Toupance, S. Lavaud, A. Wynckel, J.P. Melin, 4) J.H.M. Cohen, 5) V. Reiter Chenel	35	38	42	427
Hosp Nord, CHU de Saint Etienne, Dept of Neph/Dial/Transp, Ave Albert Raimond, 42055 St Etienne Cedex 2 Ph: (33)477 930785 Fax: (33)477 828357 1,3) F.C. Berthoux, 2) X. Barral, 3) E. Alamartine, 4) J.C. LePetit, 5) A. Gignoux, R. Riffard	46	38	40	961
Ctr Hosp, Univ Hautepierre, Transp Unit, Ave Moliere, Strasbourg, 67098 Ph: (33)388 127279 Fax: (33)388 127286 1,2) P. Wolf, 2) C. Meyer, M. Audet, J. Cinqualbre, 3) M.L. Woehl-Jaegle, B. Ellero, 4) M.M. Tongio, 5) V. Fuss, C. Becker	84	74	72	1090
Hosp Toulouse, Serv of Neph, CHU Rangueil Chemin du Vallon, Toulouse Cedex, F31400 Ph: (33)501 322671 Fax: (33)501 322864 1) D. Durand, 2) J.P. Sarramon, P. Rischmann, B. Malavaud, 3) L. Rostaing, 4) M. Abbal, 5) F. Boudet	58	96	79	1386

GERMANY

	1998	1999	2000	Total
Univ Hosp Aachen, Dept of Intern MedII/Uro, Pauwelsstr 30, D-52057 Aachen Ph: (49)241 808 8555 Fax: (49)241 874 139 1) J. Floege, 2) G. Jakse, 3) A. Homburg, 4) R. Lutticken, 5) D. Wilhelms	24	19	14	294
Charite Humboldt-Univ of Berlin, Clin of Uro, Schumannstr 20-21, 10117 Berlin Ph: (49)30 2802 5710 Fax: (49)30 2802 5615 1) Loening, 2) Schoenberger, Schnorr, Turk, 3) Fritsche, Budde, Neumayer, Querfeld, 4) Schonemann, 5) Giessing	42	57	54	548
Univ Klin Benjamin Franklin, Dept of Transp, Hindenburgdamm 30, 12200 Berlin Ph: (49)30 8445-2379 Fax: (49)30 834-7591 Email: transplantation@medizin.fu-berlin.de 1) Miller, 1,3) Offermann, 2) Fiedler, Heicapell, Sauter, Steiner, Muller, 4) Thiel, Buente, 5) E. Mueller	81	66	57	1601

1)=Director, 2)=Tx Surgeons, 3)=Physicians, 4)=Tissue Typers, 5)=TxCoords	1998	1999	2000	Total
University Hospital Bochum, Knappschafts-Krankenhaus, Dept of Surgery, In Der Schornau 23-25, Bochum-NRW, 44892 Ph: (49)234-299-3260 Fax: (49)234-299-3269 1) W.O. Bechstein, 2) K. Kohlhaw, R. Schwarz, 4) H. Grosse-Wilde, 5) A. Deiss	83	51	21	385
Zentralkrankenhaus St Jurgen, Dept of Uro/Neph & Transp, St Jurgen Strasse, Bremen, 28205 Ph: (49)421 497-5723 Fax: (49)421 447738 1,2) K. Dreikorn, 3) A. Lison, 4) Blasczyk	48	51	35	462
Transplantation Zentrum Koeln, Klinikum Koeln-Merheim, Ostmerheimer Str 200, Cologne 51109 Ph: (49)221 2907-3200 Fax: (49)221 89073335 Email: wolfgang.arns@uni-koeln.de 1) M. Weber, H. Troidl, C.A. Baldamus, A.H. Hoelscher 2) A. Paul, T. Beckurts, 3) W. Arns, M. Pollok,4) R. Doerner, 5) Deutsche Stiftung Organtransplantation	90	111	104	1837
Univ Hosp Duesseldorf, Dept of Neph/Vasc Surg/Transp, Moorenstr 5, Duesseldorf, D40225 Ph: (49)211 311 8627 Fax: (49)211 312085 1,3) B. Grabensee, 1,2) W.Sandmann, 2) Grabitz, Luther, Huber, Muller, Pfeiffer, 3) Plum, Hetzel, Brause, Ivens, Veicullsen, 4) R. Dorner, 5) B. Schaepers, S. Hinkel	66	62	79	1286
Transp Erlangen-Nurnberg, Uro Klin Erlangen, Krankenhausstr 12, D91054 Erlangen Ph: (49)131 853282 Fax: (49)131 854851 1,2) K.M. Schrott, 2) G. Schott, R. Kuehn, 3) R.B. Sterzel, 4) R.J. Kalden, 5) I. Hauser	70	66	88	1790
Univ Clin Essen, Dept of Gen Surg, Hufeland strasse 55, Essen, 45122 Ph: (49)201 723-1140 Fax: (49)201 723-5946 1,2) C.E. Broelsch, 2) M. Malago, G. Testa, H. Janssen, M. Hertl, S. Nadlain, 3) T. Philipp, 4) H. Grosse-Wilde	74	96	73	1981
Univ Hosp Frankfurt am Main, Dept of Neph, Theodor Stern Kai 7, Frankfurt, D60596 Ph: (49)69 6301 5645 Fax: (49)69 638 682 1) E.H. Scheuermann, 2) D. Jonas, W. Kramer, 3) Gossmann, 4) S. Seidl, 5) N.N. , H.J. Schoeppl	67	53	59	1590
Univ Hosp Freiburg, Dept of Surg, Organ Transp, Hugstetter Strass 55, Freiburg, G-79106 Ph: (49)761 270 2732 Fax: (49)761 278 970 Email: bluemke@cu11.ukl.uni-freiburg.de 1,2) G. Kirste, 2) P. Pisarski, 3) G. Walz, 4) H. Lang, 5) M. Blumke	99	99	84	2093
Georg-August Univ Gottingen, Klin fur Transp Chir, Robert-Koch Str 40, 37075 Gottingen Ph: (49)551 36866 Fax: (49)551 374862 Email: tx-plant@med.uni-goettingen.de 1,2) B. Ringe, 2) T. Lorf, R. Canelo, 3) G.A. Mueller, 4) H. Neumeyer, C. Krome-Cesar, 5) E. Schmidt	37	24	21	822
Martin Luther Univ, Halle-Wittenberg, Uro Klin, Nieren Transp, Magdeburger Str 16, PF 302, 06097 Halle Ph: (49)345 557-1210 Fax: (49)345 202 9632 1,2) P. Fornara, 2) A. Hamza, 3) O. Rettkowski, 4) H.K.G. Machulla	56	43	38	1150
Univ Hosp Eppendorf-Hamburg, Dept of Urology, Martinistr. 52, Hamburg, 20246 Ph: (49)40 47173446 Fax: (49)40 47174662 1,2) H. Huland, 2) S. Fernandez, S. Conrad, P. Hammerer, J. Noldus, H. Heinzer, 3) W. Tenschert, L. Cremaschi, B. Pfalzer, S. Marendza, 4) P. Kuhnl, C. Loliger, 5) C. Clausen	53	66	49	1388
Univ Klin des Saarlandes, Dept of Med, Kirrberger Strasse, Homburg/Saar, D-66421 Ph: (49)6841 163520 Fax: (49)6841 163516 1,3) H. Kohler, 2) M. Stoeckle, 3) M. Girndt, 4) B. Thiele, Kasierslautern, 5) K. Nehammer	24	29	22	305
Neph Ctr Niedersachsen, Dept of Uro/Renal Transp, Vogelsang 105, D-34346 Hann-Muenden Ph: (49)5541 996326 Fax: (49)5541 996391 1,2) W.R. Schott, 2) J. Kuester, V. Fenner, M. Warnecke, 3) Kliem, 4) R. Blasczyk, 5) G. Schaefer	70	59	67	1121
Med Hochschule Hannover, Dept of Visceral/Transp Surg, Carl-Neuberg-Str. 1, 30625 Hannover Ph: (49)511 532 6534 Fax: (49)511 532 2265 1) J. Klempnauer, 2) B. Nashan, R. Luck, T. Becker, 3) H. Haller, A. Schwarz, G. Offner, J. Strehlau, 4) R. Blascyk, 5) G. Gubernatis, S. Tietze, G. Oelmann	212	183	180	3726
Transp Jena, Dept of Urol, Klilin der Friedrich Schiller Univ, Lessingstra 1, 07740 Jena Ph: (49)3641 450943 Fax: (49)3641 449710 Email: rudolf.boerner@dso.de 1,2) J. Schubert, 2) W. Werner, 3) H. Sperschneider, 4) Machulla, 5) Borner	92	71	76	471
Westpfalz Klinikum, Med Klin III, Hellmut-Hartert-Str.1, Kaiserslautern, 67655 Ph: (49)631 2031256 Fax: (49)631 2031412 1) F.W Albert, 1) Albert, U., 2) W. Seybold-Epting, 3) U. Schmidt, 4) B. Thiele	20	19	26	584

KIDNEY

1)=Director, 2)=Tx Surgeons, 3)=Physicians, 4)=Tissue Typers, 5)=TxCoords	1998	1999	2000	Total
Transp Central Kiel, Dept of Surg, Arnold-Heller Str 7, 24105 Kiel Ph: (49)431 597-4341 Fax: (49)431 597-4586 1) B. Kremer, 2) D. Henne-Bruns, 3) A. Proppe, 4) E. Westphal, 5) G.R. Schuett, N. Robien	18	16	18	516
Univ of Leipzig, Clin of Abdom/Vasc/Transp Surg, Liebigstr 20a, Leipzig, 04103 Ph: (49)341 9717200 Fax: (49)341 9717209 1) J. Hauss, 2) P. Lamesch, U. Jost, H. Witzigmann, H. Fangmann, I. Geisler, 3) U. Achenbach, 4) Halle/Saale Tissue Typ Lab, 5) T. Weisskirchen	46	37	65	259
Med Univ of Luebeck, Dept of Surg & Internal Med, Ratzeburger Allee 160, Luebeck, 23538 Ph: (49)451 503637 Fax: (49)451 505451 Email: hoyer@medinf,mu-luebeck.de 1,3) L. Fricke, 1,2) M. Strik, 2) M. Strik, U. Markert, C. Franke, 3) J. Steinhoff, 4) H. Kirchner, M. Muller-Steinhardt, 5) N.N.	61	51	73	972
Johnanes-Gutenberg Univ of Med, Dept of Neph, Transp Ctr-Mainz, Langenbeck Str 1, 55131Mainz Ph: (49)6131 222572 Fax: (49)6131 231021 1,3) E. Wandel, 2) R. Hohenfellner, 4) W. Hitzler, 5) K. Strathmann	23	28	29	275
Klin Mannheim, Univ of Heidelberg, Dept of Surg, V. Med Klinik, Theodor Kutzer Ufer 1-3, Mannheim, 68135 Ph: (49)62 383-2674 Fax: (49)62 383-3804 1) F.J. van de Woude, 1) S.Post, 2) S. Post, J. Sturm, 3) P. Schnuelle, 4) G. Opelz, 5) Ch. Krenzel	15	25	19	205
Univ Hosp of Marburg, Dept of Neph, Ctr Int Med, Baldinger StrBe, 35033 Marburg Ph: (49)6421 286 6480 Fax: (49)6421 2866365 Email: transpea@mailer.uni-marburg.de 1,2) H. Lange, 2) M. Rothmund, A. Hellinger, J. Geks, A. Zielke, 3) H. Ebel, U. Kuhlmann, 4) E. Wollmer, A. Gorski, 5) U. Heck, M. Bauer, S. Moos	20	31	25	627
Klin Grosshadern, Univ of Munich, Div of Transp Surg, Marchioninistr 15, Munich, 81377 Ph: (49)89 7095 2706 Fax: (49)89 700 4160 Email: walterland@aol.com 1,2) W. Land, 2) W.D. Illner, J. Theodorakis, H. Arbogast, 4) E.D. Albert, S. Scholz, 5) C. Schulz	173	159	121	3388
Tech Univ Munchen-Klin Rechts Isar, Dept of Surg, Ismaninger Str 22, Munich, 81675 Ph: (49)89 4140 2011 Fax: (49)89 478917 1,3) J.R. Siewert, 2) M. Stangl, 4) E. Albert, 5) W. Eberhardt	45	52	39	721
Univ of Rostock Med Faculty, Clin of Uro, Ernst-Heydemann Str 06, Rostock, D-18057 Ph: (49)381 494 7801 Fax: (49)381 494 7802 1,2) H. Seiter, 2) R. Bast, 3) M. Burde, 4) H. Kiefel, 5) F.P. Nitschke	47	57	29	1074
Katherine Hosp, Dept of Neph, Kriegsbergstr 60, 70174 Stuttgart Ph: (49)711 278 4150 Fax: (49)711 226 8554 Email: jnfo@nierentransplantation.de 1) C.J. Olbricht, 2) Kruger, Teschner, Wellinger, Dimitrijevic, 3) Hornberger, Hasche, Stokenmaier, 4) HLA-Labor Heidelberg, 5) M. Kalus	50	66	64	567
Univ of Tuebingen, Dept of Surg, Hoppe Seyler Str 3, Transp Ctr, Tuebingen, 72076 Ph: (49)70 712986600 Fax: (49)70 714 4532 1) H.D. Becker, 2) R. Viebahn, P. Petersen, K. Dietrich, 3) T. Risler, N. Braun, 4) Northoff, Wernet, 5) Fischer-Frohlich	30	33	39	1065
Univ Ulm Klinikum, Dept of Surg II, Steinhovelstr 9, D-89075 Ulm Ph: (49)731 502 6985 Fax: (49)731 23167 1,2) D. Abendroth, 4) S.F. Goldmann, 5) A. Michels	42	42	64	1080
Univ of Wuerzburg Med Sch, Dept of Transp, Josef-Schneider Str 2, D-97080 Wuerzburg Ph: (49)931 24047 Fax: (49)931 286750 Email: monika@zwirner@exc.dso-online.de 1,2) H. Riedmiller, 2) K. Weingartner, R. Bonfig, G. Ohnheiser, 3) C. Wanner, 4) Labor fur Gewebetypisierung, 5) M. Zwirner	36	24	33	494

GREECE

	1998	1999	2000	Total
Laikos Gen Hosp, Transp Ctr, 17 Agiou Thoma Str Goudi, Athens 11527 Ph: (30)1 770 9274 Fax: (30)1 778 2634 1,2) A. Kostakis, 2) S.T. Kyriakides, C. Diles, J. Bokos, 3) G. Vosnides, J. Boletis, 4) K. Stavropoulou-Gioka, 5) C. Anagnostopoulou	87	77	53	1053

1)=Director, 2)=Tx Surgeons, 3)=Physicians, 4)=Tissue Typers, 5)=TxCoords	1998	1999	2000	Total
HUNGARY				
Semmelweis Med Univ, Transp & Surg Clin, Baross u.23, Budapest, 1082 Ph: (36)1 266-0815 Fax: (36)1 117-0964 Email: borka@medscape.com 1,2) F. Perner, 2) F. Alfoldy, J. Jaray, A. Toth, D. Gorog, H. Podder, L. Kobora, A. Peter, 3) A. Remport, K. Foldes, J. Jansen, I. Sasvary, Sz. Torok, 4) G. Petranyi, E. Gyodi, 5) T. Feszt, Zs. Roczko, E. Tornai, P. Borka	141	116	140	1898
Med Univ Sch of Debrecen, 1st Dept of Surg, Nagyerdei krt 98, POB 27, H-4012 Debrecen Ph: (36)52 315517 Fax: (36)52 316098 1) Gy. Balazs, 2) L. Asztalos, L. Varga, F. Juhasz, Z. Kincses, C. Berczi, 3) L. Locsey, 4) V. Stenszky, 5) E. Uray	24	37	40	354
Pecs Univ, Faculty of Medicine, Dept of Surgery, Ifjusag u. 13, Pecs, H-7624 Ph: (36) 72 53 6128 Fax: (36) 72 53 6128 Email: kalmar@iseb.pote.hu 1,2) K. Kalmar-Nagy, 2) P. Szakaly, A. Papp, 3) M. Molnar, 4) M. Paal Uherkovichne, 5) K. Kalmar, I. Kovats	32	28	30	206
Albert Szent-Gyorgyi Med Univ, Dept of Surg, PO Box 464, Pecsi u.4, H-6701 Szeged Ph: (36)62-321-643 Fax: (36)62-321-643 1,2) P. Szenohradsky, 2) F. Marofka, J. Marton, L. Varga, E. Szederkenyi, R. Vangel, 4) G.I. Kajser, I. Petri, F. Toldi	44	43	39	710
INDIA				
All-India Inst of Med Sci, Dept of Surg/Kidney Transp, Ansari Nagar, New Delhi, 110029 Ph: (91)11 686 4851x3206 Fax: (91)11 686 2663 1,2) S.N. Mehta, 2) S. Guleria, 3) S.C. Dash, S.C. Tiwari, S. Aggarwal, 4) N.K. Mehra	47	53		555
INDONESIA				
CIKINI-RSCM Hosp, Dept of Neph/Hypertension, Jalan Raden Saleh 40, Jakarta 10330 Ph: (62)21 336569 Fax: (62)21 3107793 1) T.D. Situmorang, 2) D. Manuputty, D. Rahardjo, 3) Suhardjono, Endang Susalit, T.D. Situmorang, P. Wiguno, 4) E. Sutjahjo, 5) I. Sukadis	11	6	8	250
IRAN, ISLAMIC REPUBLIC				
Shahid Labbafi Nejad Med Ctr, Dept of Uro, Transp Unit, Boustan 9, Pasdaran Ave, Tehran Ph: (98)21-244913 Fax: (98)21-249039 1,2) N. Simforoosh, 2) A. Bassiri, 3) Behzad-Einollahi, A. Firoozan, 4) M. Kamgoian, 5) Sodubeh-Farhangi	116	153		1228
IRAQ				
Univ of Baghdad, Med City Hosp, Kidney Transp Unit, PO Box 8083, Baghdad Ph: (964)1 541 4436 Fax: (964)1 541 4436 1,2,5) U.N. Rifat, 2) R. Abdusatar, U. Aljumaily, 3) S. Wandawi, A. Husain, A. Thirib, H.M. Ali, 4) I. Alobeidi	28	28	28	276
ISRAEL				
Beilinson Med Ctr, Dept of Organ Transp, Zabotinski 66, Petach Tikva, 49100 Ph: (972)3 922 4285 Fax: (972)3 924 9680 1) Z. Shapira, 2) A. Yussim, N.B. Nathan, E. Shaharabani, E. Mor, 3) S. Lustig, 4) T. Klein, 5) R. Michowiz	150	105	93	1706
ITALY				
Ospedale Regionale, "Ospedali Riuniti di Bergamo", Dept of Neph, Largo Barozzi 1, Bergamo, BG 241000 Ph: (39)035 259272 Fax: (39)035 269692 1,3) G. Remuzzi, 1,2) G. Locatelli, 3) E. Gotti, P. Ruggenenti, M. Perico, 4) G. Sirchia	42	36	35	374
St Orsola Univ Hosp, Dept of Clin Surg, Via Massarenti, 9, Bologna, 40138 Ph: (39)051 341700 Fax: (39)051 397661 1) A. Cavallari, 2) A. Faenza, B. Nardo, 3) V. Bonomini, S. Stefoni, P. Scolari, B. Liviano, D. Arcangelo, 5) A. Buscaroli	63	63	70	1061

KIDNEY

1)=Director, 2)=Tx Surgeons, 3)=Physicians, 4)=Tissue Typers, 5)=TxCoords	1998	1999	2000	Total
San Michele Hosp, Dept of Uro/Neph, Via Peretti, 09125 Cagliari Ph: (39)070 543333 Fax: (39)070 530814 1,5) F. Meloni, 1) V.Storelli, 2) M. Frongia, S. Lilliu, 3) P. Altieri, G. Piredda, 4) L. Contu, M. Bajorek	18	21	25	367
Azienda Ospedale San Martino, Dept of Transp, Largo Rosanna Benzi, 10, Genova, 16132 Ph: (39)010 5553862 Fax: (39)010 5556772 Email: itc@transplant.smartino.ge.it 1) U. Valente, 2) V. Arcuri, M. Beatini, M. Bertocchi, I. Fontana, G.V. Tommasi, 3) Cannella, Messa, Paoletti, Ginevri, Perfumo, Viscoli, Dodi, Siani, 4) G. Sirchia, A. Nocera, 5) C. Pizzi, A. Gianelli Castiglione, S. Pisanu, M. Tognoni, I. Cirelli	86	64	69	844
G.Gaslini Children's Hosp, Nephrology, Largo G Gaslini 5, 16148 Genova Ph: (39)010 3740231 Fax: (39)010 395214 1,3) F. Perfumo, 2) U. Valente, 3) G. Basile, F. Ginevri, 4) A. Nocera, 5) Castiglione	29	15	24	235
Inst Sci " San Raffaele", Univ of Milano, Dept of Med, Via Olgettina 60, 20132 Milano Ph: (39)02 2643 2805 Fax: (39)02 2643 2752 1,2) G. Pozza, 2) V. Di Carlo, 3) G. Bianchi, A. Secchi, 4) G. Sirchia, 5) A. Secchi	11	14	11	85
Policlinico Univ Hosp, Dept of Surgery, Via F Sforza 35, 20122 Milano Ph: (39)02 5503 5653 Fax: (39)02 5503 5650 Email: luisa.berardinelli@unimi.it 1,2) L. Berardinelli, 2) C. Beretta, E. Pozzoli, 3) C. Ponticelli, V. Sereni, A. Tarantino, 4) G. Sirchia, 5) C. Pizzi	80	92	78	2247
Hosp of Padova, Depts of Uro/Peds, via Giustiniani 2, Padova PD, 35128 Ph: (39)49 821 2720 Fax: (39)49 821 2721 1,2) F. Pagano, 2) G. Passerini, G.F. Zanon, 3) G. Zacchello, G. Montini, 4) NIT Milano, 5) G. Zacchello	16			154
Univ di Padova, 1st di Chir Generale II, Ospedale Giustinianeo, Via Giustinianeo, 2, 35128 Padova Ph: (39)49 8213151 Fax: (39)49 750919 Email: traprepa@uxl.unipd.it 1,2) E. Ancona, 2) P. Rigotti, 3) F. Marchini, 4) V. Fagiolo, G. Sirchia, 5) NIT (Nord Italia Transp)	51	68	59	451
Univ di Padova, Dept of Ped Surg, Ospedale Giustinianeo, Via Giustinianeo, 2, 35128 Padova Ph: (39)49 8213500 Fax: (39)49 8213502 1,3) F. Zacchello, 1,2) F.Pagano, 4) V. Fagiolo, G. Sirchia, 5) NIT (Nord Italia Transp)	16	17	17	189
ISMETT, Piazza Sett'Angeli, 10, Palermo, 90134 Ph: (39) 091 6661111 Fax: (39) 091 6668136 Email: mail@ismett.edu 1,2) I.R. Marino, 2) C. Doria, C. ScottiFoglieni, 3) H. Doyle, M. Magnone, U. Palazzo, D. Paterson, V. Scott, 4) A. Salerno, 5) M. Castellese, S. Guercio, R. DiGaudio		3	14	17
Univ of Pisa, Osp di Cisanello, Inst of Gen Surg, Via Paradisa 2, 56124 Pisa Ph: (39)50 596820 Fax: (39)50 543692 Email: uboggi@patchir.med.unipi.it 1,2,5) F. Mosca, 2) U. Boggi, 3) P. Rindi, R. Palla, 4) G. Rizzo	47	80	58	595
Policlinico "Umberto 1", Univ "La Sapienza", Dept of Surg II, Viale del Policlinico, 00161 Rome Ph: (39)6 445 6296 Fax: (39)6 446 3667 1,2) R. Cortesini, 1) P. Berloco, 2) M. Rossi, M. Iappelli, 3) R. Pretagostini, 4) E. Renna-Molajoni, A. Bachetoni, 5) S. Venettoni	64	45	33	1383
Univ Cattolica del Sacro Cuore, Policlin Gemelli, Dept of Surg, Transp Ctr, Largo Gemelli 8, 00168 Rome Ph: (39)6 301 4300 Fax: (39)6 301 0019 1,2) M. Castagneto, 2) Agnes, Citterio, Magalini, Avolio, Foco, Nanni, 4) G. Luciani, 5) T. Borzi	34	44	27	523
Treviso Gen Hosp, Transplant Ctr, Piazza Ospedale, 31100 Treviso Ph: (39)0422 322634 Fax: (39)0422 322657 Email: avianello@ulss.tv.it 1,3) G. Calconi, 1,2) G. DiFalco, 2) G.F. Mora, C. Caldato, 3) M.C. Maresca, A. Vianello, 4) M. Mordacchini, L. Moro, 5) D. Milani	53	55		641
Ospedale Reg "Civile Maggiore", Div of Clin Gen Surg, Piazz Stefani, Verona, VR 37126 Ph: (39)45 807 2520 Fax: (39)45 807 2006 1,2) G. Ancona, 2) Muolo, Galvani, Dean, Galante, Gulino, Zampieri, Firpo, Prati, 3) Muolo, Galvani, Dean, Galante, Gulino, Zampieri, Firpo, Boschiero, 4) C. Zanuso, 5) F. Procaccio	45	43	48	1030
Ospedale Civ di San Bortolo, Unita di Transp Renal, Chir 2, Via MONS. Rodolfi 4, 36100 Vicenza VI Ph: (39)444 993803 Fax: (39)444 993803 1) F Favretti, 2) D. Zuccarotto, 3) S. Chiaramonte, 4) G. Sirchia, M. Belloni, 5) S. Barbacini	26	22	32	303

1)=Director, 2)=Tx Surgeons, 3)=Physicians, 4)=Tissue Typers, 5)=TxCoords	1998	1999	2000	Total
JAPAN				
Nagoya Daini Red Cross Hospital, Dept of Transp Surg, 2-9 Myoken-cho, Showa-ku, Nagoya, Aichi 466 Ph: (81)652 832-1121 Fax: (81)652 831-0149 1) K. Uchida, 2) Y. Tominaga, T. Haba, K. Yamada, A. Katayama, Y. Hibi, T. Sato, 3) A. Yoshida, A. Takeda, M. Fukuta, O. Uemura, M. Shimizu, K. Morozumi, 4) H. Kamura, S. Kohara, E. Nagao, 5) M. Otsuka	34			532
Oyokyo Kidney Rsrch Inst, Dept of Uro, 90 Yamazaki, Kozawa, Hirosaki City, Aomori 036 Ph: (81)172 87 1221 Fax: (81)172 87 1228 1) T. Funyu, 2) Takakashi, Suzuki, Momose, Oh, Kajihara, 3) H. Yamabe, H. Osawa, 4) K. Kabasawa, A. Iwasaki, 5) W. Uematsu	4	2	1	68
Ehime Univ Sch of Med, Dept of Uro, Shigenobu Onsen-gun, Ehime 791-02 Ph: (81)899 60 5356 Fax: (81)899 60 5358 1) M. Yokoyama, 2) H. Ohoka, 4) H. Inoue, 5) N. Kan	15	10	17	158
Hokkaido Univ Sch of Med, Dept of Uro, Kita-15 jyo, Nishi 7, Kitaku, Sapporo 060-8638, Hokkaido Ph: (81)11-716-1161 Fax: (81)11-706-7853 Email: watarai@med.hokudai.ac.jp 1) T. Koyanagi, 2) K. Nonomura, Y. Watarai, J. Shindo, T. Usuki, 3) T. Koike, 4) T. Sasaki, 5) H. Osuda	5	8	8	126
Sapporo City Gen Hosp, Dept of Renal Transp, North 11, West 13, Chuoku, Sapporo, HK 060-8604 Ph: (81)11 726 2211 Fax: (81)11 726 9564 1,2) T. Hirano, 2) T. Seki, T. Harada, M. Togashi, 3) T. Sakurai, T. Ueda, 4) T. Sasaki, N. Kameishi, 5) K. Ohsuda, M. Nishimura	14	11	26	181
Hyogo Coll of Med, Dept of Uro, 1-1 Mukogawa-cho, Nishinomiya, Hyogo, 663 Ph: (81)79 845-6366 Fax: (81)79 845-6368 1,2) H. Shima, 2) M. Nojima, T. Yoshimoto, 3) Y. Takamitsu, 4) M. Hashimoto, 5) T. Fukunishi, A. Soga	5	7	7	137
Hyogo Pref Nishinomiya Hosp, Uro/Kid Transp Ctr, 13-9 Rokutanji-cho, Nishinomiya City, Hyogo 662 Ph: (81)798 34-5151 Fax: (81)798 36-3745 1,5) T. Fukunishi, 2) Y. Ichikawa, T. Hanafusa, S. Nagano, 4) M. Hashimoto, T. Kinoshita, Y. Taniguchi	7	14	12	335
Kanazawa Med Univ Hosp, Dept of Uro/Neph, Uchinada, Ishikawa, 920-0293 Ph: (81)76-286-2211 Fax: (81)76-286-5516 1,2) K. Suzuki, 2) R. Ikeda, T. Tanaka, K. Miyazawa, K. Kawamura, 3) I. Ishikawa, T. Yuri, N. Tomosugi, M. Asaka, 4) Y. Tanaka, M. Sakuma, 5) M. Ogawa, S. Tamura, Y. Sugimoto	9	8	4	242
Kakegawa City Gen Hosp, Dept of Transp Surg, 721 Sugiya, Kakegawa 436, Shizuoka Ph: (81)537-22-6211 Fax: (81)537-24-2539 1) A. Orihara, 2) M. Numano, 3) K. Goshima	3	1	2	29
Kitasato Univ Hosp, Dept of Uro/Surg, 1-15-1, Kitasato, Sagamihara, Kanagawa, 228-8555 Ph: (81)427 778-9091 Fax: (81)427 78-9374 1,2) T. Endo, 1) A. Kakita, 2) K. Yoshida, K. Satoh, 3) K. Kamata, 4) K. Watanabe, 5) T. Nomura	2	10	6	370
Nagasaki Univ Sch of Med, Dept of Uro, 7-1 Sakamoto-Cho, Nagasaki City 852, Nagasaki Ph: (81)95 849-7340 Fax: (81)95 849-7343 1) H. Kanetake, 2) S. Koga, M. Nishikido, 3) K. Harada, 4) M. Nagatomo, 5) N. Nishida	2	2	1	129
Nagoya Univ Hosp, Dept of Surg II, 65 Tsuruma-cho, Showa-ku, Nagoya, 466-8550 Ph: (81)52 744-2248 Fax: (81)52 744-2255 1,2) I. Yokoyama, 2) S. Hayashi, T. Kobayashi, T. Tokoro, 3) T. Kato	2	1	1	51
Osaka University Medical School, Dept of Uro, 2-2 Yamada-oka, Suita-City, Osaka 565-0871 Ph: (81)6 6879 3531 Fax: (81)6 6879 3539 1,2) S. Takahara, 2) T. Hanafusa, K. Yazawa, K. Toki, 4) Osaka Prefectural Gen Hosp	14	14	15	499
Osaka Prefectural Gen Hosp, Dept of Uro, 3-1-56 Bandai-Higashi, Sumiyoshi-ku, Osaka 558-8558 Ph: (81)66 692-1201 Fax: (81)66 606-7030 Email: sonoda@gh.pref.osaka.jp 1) T. Sonoda, 2) S. Sagawa, K. Ito, N. Fujimoto, 3) Y. Tsubakihara, 4) R. Yasunami, M. Tada, 5) T. Konaka	10	7	6	136
Osaka Med Coll, Dept of Uro, 2-7 Daigaku-machi, Takatsuki, Osaka, 569-8686 Ph: (81)6 726 831221 Fax: (81)6 726 846546 Email: uro009@poh.osaka-med.ac.jp 1) Y. Katsuoka, 2) H. Ueda, M. Kusaka, Y. Iwamoto, H. Noumi, 3) N. Shibahara, 5) L. Arike	0	2	1	46

1)=Director, 2)=Tx Surgeons, 3)=Physicians, 4)=Tissue Typers, 5)=TxCoords	1998	1999	2000	Total
Saga Pref Hosp-Kohseikan, Dept of Surg and Urol, Kohseikan, Mizugae 1-12-9, Saga City, Saga 840 Ph: (81)952 24-2171 Fax: (81)952 25-6102 1,2) T. Kayajima, 2) T. Hayashi, N. Oka, T. Yayama, T. Shiramizu, 4) S. Yoshitake, 5) K. Hujimoto	1			82
Nat'l Defense Med Coll Hosp, Dept of Uro, 3-2 Namiki, Tokorozawa, Saitama, 359 Ph: (81)429 95-1511 Fax: (81)429-96-5210 1) M. Hayakawa, 2) T. Asano, 3) N. Yoshizawa, 4) M. Atoh, 5) R. Muguruma	2	4		38
Hamamatsu Univ Hosp, Dept of Uro, Handa-cho 3600, Hamamatsu, Shizuoka, 431-3192 Ph: (81)53 435-2306 Fax: (81)53 435-2305 1) K. Fujita, 2) K. Suzuki, 3) A. Ishikawa, 4) S. Nakatsuji, 5) T. Suzuki	11	7	13	247
Tokyo Women's Medical University, Kidney Ctr, Dept of Third Surg, 8-1 Kawada-cho, Shinjuku-ku, Tokyo, 162-8666 Ph: (81)3 3353-8111 Fax: (81)3 3356-0293 1,2) H. Toma, 2) S. Fuchinoue, I. Nakajima, K. Tanabe, 3) H. Nihei, T. Babazono, 4) M. Yasuo	80	92	116	1636
Hosp of the Inst of Med Sci, Univ of Tokyo, 4-6-1, Shirokanedai, Minato-ku, Tokyo 108 Ph: (81)3 3443-8111 Fax: (81)3 3446-2459 1,2) H. Uchida, 2) S. Tomikawa, , 4) S. Nakayama, T. Takahashi, 5) H. Kimura	6	10	3	335
Toho Univ, Ohmori Hosp, Dept of Neph, 6-11-1, Ohmori-Nishi, Ota-ku, Tokyo 143, 143-0015 Ph: (81)3 3762-4151 Fax: (81)3 5471-3056 1,2) A. Hasegawa, 2) T. Ohara, N. Hirayama, A. Aikawa, 3) S. Mizuiri, T. Fushemi, K. Sakai, 4) M. Okuda, M. Kato, T. Kanai	17	24	26	303
Keio Univ Hosp, Dept of Uro, 35 Shinanomachi, Shinjuku-ku, Tokyo, 160-8582 Ph: (81)3 3353-1211 Fax: (81)3 3225-1985 1,2) M. Murai, 2) M. Tachibana, H. Asakura, 3) T. Saruta, M. Hayashi, 4) S. Watanabe	2	1		52
Univ of Tsukuba, Dept of Surg/Uro, 1-1-1 Tennoudai, Tsukuba, Ibaraki-Ken, 305-8575 Ph: (81)298 53-3210 Fax: (81)298 53-3222 Email: kfukao@md.tsukuba.ac.jp 1) K. Fukao, 2) M. Otsuka, K. Yuzawa, Y. Takada, 3) A. Koyama, 4) Y. Jinzenji	7	12	9	127

KOREA

	1998	1999	2000	Total
Chonbuk National Univ Hosp, Dept of Surg/Int Med, 634-18 Keumam-dong,Dukjin-gu, Chonju, 561-712 Ph: (82)652 2501579 Fax: (82)652 2716197 Email: chobh@moak.chonbuk.ac.kr 1,2) B.H. Cho, 2) H.C. Yu, Y.G. Kim, 3) S.K. Kang, S.K. Park, 4) S.I. Choi, D.S. Kim, 5) H.S. Min	16	14	11	159
Hanyang Univ Hosp, HYU Transp Unit, 17 Haengdang-Dong, Sungdong-Ku, Seoul, 133-792 Ph: (82)2 290-8865 Fax: (82)2 295-4576 Email: hyorgan@hanmail.net 1,2) J.Y. Kwak, 2) H.Y. Park, O.J. Kwon, 3) C.M. Kang, C.H. Park, H.J.Kim.S.M. Kim, 4) T.Y. Kim, 5) W.H. Lee	58	41	23	695
Kang Nam St Mary's Hosp, Dept of Surg, Catholic Univ Med Coll, 505 Ban Po Dong, Seo cho ku, Seoul 137-040 Ph: (82)2 590-1436 Fax: (82)2 595-2992 1,2) Y.B. Koh, 2) T.G. Whang, I.S. Moon, J.C. Kim, Y.G. Kim, 3) B.K. Bang, Y.S. Kim, C.W. Yang, 4) B.K. Kim, 5) H.O. Chun	59	43	43	1275
Seoul Nat'l Univ Hosp, Coll of Med, Dept of Gen Surg, 28 Yongon-Dong, Chongno-gu, Seoul, 110-744 Ph: (82)2 760-2318 Fax: (82)2 3672-4947 1,2) S.J. Kim, 2) J. Ha, 3) J.S. Lee, S.K. Kim, C.R. Ahn, 4) M.H. Park, 5) J.S. Kim	40	36		677
Soon Chun Hyang Univ Hosp, Kidney Ctr, 657 Hannam-dong, Yongsan-koo, Seoul, 140-743 Ph: (82)2 792-6657 Fax: (82)2 792-5812 Email: sd7hwang@hosp.sch.ac.kr 1,3) D.C. Han, 2) C. Moon, Y.S. Song, 3) H.B. Lee, M.S. Park, 4) M.H. Kim, 5) S.J. Ahn	11	8	2	247
Yonsei Univ Coll of Med, Severance Hosp, Dept of Surg, 134 Shinchon-Dong, Sudaemoon-ku, Seoul 120-752 Ph: (82)2 361-5545 Fax: (82)2 365-3069 Email: transplant@yumc.yonsei.ac.kr 1,2) K. Park, 2) Y.S. Kim, S.I. Kim, 3) D.S. Han, H.Y. Lee, K.H. Choi, S.W. Kang, 4) H.J. Kim, 5) K.O. Cheon, H.J. Kim	108	116	93	1972

LUXEMBOURG

	1998	1999	2000	Total
Ctr Hosp de Luxembourg, Dept of Neph, 4 rue Barble, L 1210 Luxembourg Ph: (352) 4411 2022 Fax: (352) 441324 1,3) P. Duhoux, 2) St. Lamy, 4) F. Hentges, 5) E. Tasch, J. DeSousa	6	6	8	115

1)=Director, 2)=Tx Surgeons, 3)=Physicians, 4)=Tissue Typers, 5)=TxCoords	1998	1999	2000	Total
MEXICO				
Hosp Miguel Hildalgo, Dept of Surg, Galeana Sur 465, Centro, Aguascalientes, CP 20000 Ph: (52)49 185054 Fax: (52)49 128748 Email: sancosme@acnet.net 1,2) R. Reyes Acevedo, 2) I. Romo-Franco, S. Lupercio, E. Gil, 3) O. Ron-Torres, A. Chew, 4) R. Ceballos, 5) I. Davila-Vazquez	30	46	63	264
Hosp General de Culiacan, Dept of Transp, Aldama y Nayarit S/N, Col. Rasales, Culican, Sinaloa, 80000 Ph: (52)67 16 97 91 Fax: (52)67 16 98 51 1,3) R. Gaxiola Borrego, 2) A. Aguilar Montoya, H.E. Gomez Ponce, G. Gaxiola Mexa, 5) R.B. Gaxiola	7	6	10	124
Centro Medico Nacional "20 de Nov", Transplant Services, Av Felix Cuevas 540, Col Del Valle CP 03229 D.F., Ciudad de Mexico, DF 03229 Ph: (52)5 5725050 Fax: (52)5 3930866 Email: bmartinez@starnet.net.mx 1,2) B. Martinez-Navarrete, 2) A. Munoz, L. Avila, B. Perez-Ascencio, 3) M. Manrique-Najera, 4) L. Diaz, R.A. Escalante, 5) E. Cabrera, A. Montoya	48	32	48	619
Hosp Civil de Guadalajara, Prog de Transp, Hosp 278, Guadalajara, Jal, 44280 Ph: (52)3 614-7456 Fax: (52)3 817-3514 Email: janssens@prodigy.net.mx 1,3) G. Garcia-Garcia, 2) A. Castellanos, F. Garcia, L.C. Rodriguez, R. Gonzalez, 3) M. Ibarra, 4) J. Peregrina, 5) R. Garcia	19	12		60
Hosp Ctr Med Nacional de Occidente, IMSS - Dept of Neph/Transp, Sierra Morena y Belisario, Dominguez Col Ind, Colomos 2110, Guadalajara, Jal, 44349 Ph: (52)3 617-0060 Fax: (52)3 817-3514 Email: eitg@prodigy.net.mx 1) F.J. Monteon, 2) C. Valdespino, M. Sandoval, F. Mendoza, F. Gutierrez, 3) J.L. Camarena, M.D.G. Rosales, S. Chavez, A. Flores, B. Gomez, 4) C. Rosas, F. Chatro, 5) G. Paredes, B. Bonilla, C. Delgadillo, L. Gallardo	107	125	176	963
Hosp de Pediatria, Unidad de Trasplantes, IMSS, Belisaro Dominquez #1000, Guadalajara, Jal, 44340 Ph: (52)3 618-8618 Fax: (52)3 617-0264 Email: ernestogh@megared.net.mx 1) M. Castillero Manzano, 2) E. Gomez-Hernandez, 3) S.A. Ojeda-Duran, 4) QFB L. Luquin-Martinez, 5) S.A. Ojeda-Duran, E. Gomez-Hernandez	45	44	76	340
Hosp Mexico Americano, Unit of Neph/Transp, Colomos 2110, Guadalajara, Jal, 44610 Ph: (52)3 642-6093 Fax: (52)3 817-3514 Email: janssens@prodigy.net.mx 1,3) G. Garcia-Garcia, 2) A. Castellanos, L.C. Rodriguez, F. Gutierrez, A. Muhoz, F. Garcia, 3) F. Monteon, 4) J. Peregrina, C. Rosas, 5) A.M. Anaya	5	7		23
Hosp San Javier, S.A.De C.V., Unidad de Trasplantes, Av. Pablo Casals No. 640, Col. Prados Providencia, Guadalajara, Jalisco, 44670 Ph: (52)3 669-0222 Fax: (52)3 669-0222 Email: ernestogh@megared.net.mx 1) N. Leon-Quintero, 2) E. Gomez-Hernandez, 3) S. Ojeda-Duran, 4) QFB M.M. Garcia-Lorea, 5) E. Gomez-Hernandez, S. Ojeda-Duran	16	8	10	62
Hosp de Pediatria Centro Med, Unidad de Trasplantes, Inst Mexicano del Seguro Social, Belisario Dominquez #1000, Jalisco, Guadalajara, 44340 Ph: (52)3 6188618 Fax: (52)3 6170264 1) P. Arenas-Arechiga, 2) E. Gomez-Hernandez, 3) S. Ojeda-Duran, 4) QFB M.M. Garcia-Lorea, 5) S. Ojeda-Duran, E. Gomez-Hernandez	45			220
Ped Centromedico Nat'l "Siglo XXI", Transplant, Avenida Cuauntemol 330, Col Doltores, Mexico, DF Ph: 52-5627-6900 x3502 Fax: 52-5627-6900 1,2) J.T. Bellido, 2) A.Y. Nagano, 3) M.E. Pamagoa, 4) N.J. Sjarez	41	42	18	231
Especialidades C.M.N. Siglo XXI, Transp Unit, Zacatecas 36-113 Col. Roma, Mexico City, DF 06720 Ph: (52)5 538 4747 Fax: (52)5 264 8711 Email: jlmelchoro@compuserve.com.mx 1) C. Gracida, 2) A. Lopez, J. Cancino, M.A. Sanmartin, R. Espinoza, 3) J.L. Melchor, A. Ibarra, 4) E. Romano	110	107	107	1232
Inst Nacional de Cardiologia, "Ignacio Chavez", Nephrology, Juan Badiano No.1, Colonia Seccion XVI, Mexico City, CP 14080 Ph: (52)5 5732911 x354 Fax: (52)5 5737716 1,2) E. Mancilla Urrea, 2) S. Aburto M, A. Mendoza V, 3) J. Herrera Acosta, H. Perez Grovas, F. Rodriguez, 4) C. deLeo, N. Castelan, M. Lopez, N. Gonzalez, 5) I. Diaz, S. Aburto	41	49	43	491
Hosp Gen Ctr Med "La Raza", IMSS, Dept of Transp, Ave. Jacarandas y Vallego s/n, Col La Raza, Mexico City, DF, 02990 Ph: (52)5 583-6369 Fax: (52)5 583-6418 Email: aholm@prodigy.net.mx 1,3) A. Holm, 2) M. Hernandez, A. Jimenez, J. Sanchez, 3) J. Laguna, A. Camarena, 4) J.A. Vega, 5) A. Soberanes	65	70	75	555

1)=Director, 2)=Tx Surgeons, 3)=Physicians, 4)=Tissue Typers, 5)=TxCoords	1998	1999	2000	Total
Hosp Infant de Mexico, Federico Gomes, Dept of Neph, Dr Marquez 162, Mexico City, DF, 06720 Ph: (52)5 228-9917x1156 Fax: (52)5 761-8974 1,3) R. Munoz-Arizpe, 2) R. Valdez-Gonzalez, 3) B. Romero-Navarro, M. Medeiros-Domingo, S. Valverde-Rosas	25	34	34	291
Inst Nacional De La Nutricion, Dept of Transp, Vasco de Quiroga No 15 Tlalpan, Mexico City, DF, 14000 Ph: (52)5 655-9471 Fax: (52)5 655-1076 1,2) J. Alberu Gomez, 2) F. Gabilondo, 3) E. Correa-Rotter, 4) C. de Leo, N. Castelan, M. Lopez. N. Gonzalez, 5) L. Ostos	35	32	34	574
Ctr Med del Potosi S A De CV, Dept of Int Med Int/Neph, Antonio Aguilar #155, Col Morales, San Luis Potosi, SLP, 78200 Ph: (52)91 48 134311 Fax: (52)91 48 131377 1) C. Barcena-Jannet, 2) F. Moncada, F. Garcia, 3) J. Isordia, 4) R. Ceballos, 5) J. Isordia	6	3	10	82
Hosp de Especialidades 71, Torreon, Inst Mexicano del Seguro Soc, Transp Unit-Dept of Surg, Torreon, Coahuila, 27000 Ph: (52)17 290800 Fax: (52)17 132679 1,2) F.J. Juarez de la Cruz, 2) Y. Barrios, M. Benavides, A. Gomez, A. Villarreal, 3) L. Cano, R. Camacho, E. Chavez, J. Martinez, E. Lopez, E. Fernandez, 4) M. Limones, C. Adalid, 5) L. Peniche, I. Espino	121	126	130	743

NETHERLANDS

1)=Director, 2)=Tx Surgeons, 3)=Physicians, 4)=Tissue Typers, 5)=TxCoords	1998	1999	2000	Total
Academic Med Ctr, Renal Transp Unit-F4-215, Meibergdreef 9, 1105 Az Amsterdam Ph: (31)20 566 5990 Fax: (31)20 691 4904 1) S. Surachno, 2) C. Kox, T.M. v Gulik, D.A. Legemate, M.J. Lubbers, 3) R.J.M. ten Berge, F.J. Bemelman, 4) N. Lardy, 5) J.L. Popma, D.B.J. Naafs	64	53		1270
Univ Hosp Groningen, Dept of Surg, Hanzeplein 1, 9700 RB Groningen Ph: (31)50 361 2896 Fax: (31)50 361 4873 Email: b.s.g.makkes@chir.azg.nl 1,2) R.J. Ploeg, 1,3) A.Tegzess, 2) TenCate Hoedemaker, Hofker, deJong, Peeters, Porte, Wijffels, 3) W. Van Son, J. Homan, V.D. Heide, 4) S. Lems, B.G. Hepkema, 5) M. ElMoumni, A. Schuur, C.W. Graveland	67	89	100	1722
Leiden Univ Med Ctr (LUMC), Dept of Neph, PO Box 9600, 2300 RC Leiden Ph: (31)71 526 2148 Fax: (31)71 524 8118 Email: l.c.paul@nephrology.medfac.leidenuniv.nl 1) L.C. Paul, 2) J. Ringers, 3) J.W. DeFyter, 4) F.H.J. Claas, 5) M.E.G. van Gurp	76	73	71	1760
Univ Hosp Maastricht, Dept of Surg, P.Debyelaan, PO Box 5800, 6202 AZ Maastricht Ph: (31)43 3877478 Fax: (31)43 3875473 1,2) G. Kootstra, 1,3) J.P. van Hooff, 2) J. Tordoir, P. Kitslaar, 4) E. van den Berg-Loonen, 5) O. Stroosma	63	42		699
St Radboud Hosp, Div of Neph, P.O. Box 9101, 6500 HB Nymegen Ph: (31)24-3614761 Fax: (31)24-3540022 Email: ahoitsma@neho.asn.nl 1) R.A.P. Koene, 2) F.H.M. Buskens, D. van der Vliet, 3) A.J. Hoitsma, 4) W. Allebes, 5) W. Hordyk	97	91	102	2307
Univ Hosp "Dijkzigt", Dept of Surg, Dr Molewaterplein 40, 3015 GD Rotterdam, Rotterdam Ph: (31)10 463 3733 Fax: (31)10 463 5307 1) J.N.M. Ijzermans, 2) H.J. Bonjer, C.H.J. VanEyck, W.R. Schouten, H.W. Tilanus, N.A. DuBois, 3) W. Weimar, 4) Eurotransplant, 5) P. Pasma	83			1243
Univ Hosp Utrecht, Dept of Neph, Rm F03-226, PO Box 85500, 3508 Ga Utrecht Ph: (31)30 506222 Fax: (31)30 541822 1,3) R.J. Hene, 2) R.H. van Reedt Dortland, 3) J. Ligtenberg, P. Vos, 4) H. Otten, 5) P. Batavier	56	54		693

NORWAY

1)=Director, 2)=Tx Surgeons, 3)=Physicians, 4)=Tissue Typers, 5)=TxCoords	1998	1999	2000	Total
Rikshosp-The Nat'l Hosp, Dept of Ped/Surg/Med, Oslo, NO-0027 Ph: (47)2307 00 00 Fax: (47)2307 05 10 1) A. Bergan, 2) I. Brekke, O. Bentdal, P. Pfeffer, B. Lien, B. Husberg, O. Oyen, 3) P. Fauchald, K. Nordal, E. Monn, 4) E. Thorsby, T. Leivestad, 5) S. Foss, P.A. Bakkan, P.E. Vatsaas, K. Meyer	196	194	199	4109

PHILIPPINES

1)=Director, 2)=Tx Surgeons, 3)=Physicians, 4)=Tissue Typers, 5)=TxCoords	1998	1999	2000	Total
Nat'l Kidney & Transp Inst, Dept of Surg, East Ave, Quezon City, 1100 Ph: (63)2 924-0135 Fax: (63)2 922-5608 1,2) E.T. Ona, 2) R.M. Liquete, B.V. Purugganan, A. Amante, A.P. Siquijor, C.B. Ramirez, 3) Paraiso, Ingles, Tanseco, Anonuevo, Lloren, Tempongko, Bayog, Mora, 4) F. Tumangli, M. Canlas, F. Padua, 5) R.M. Aranas, A.A. Yusi, M.L. Garcia	85	135		1627

1)=Director, 2)=Tx Surgeons, 3)=Physicians, 4)=Tissue Typers, 5)=TxCoords	1998	1999	2000	Total
POLAND				
Children's Memorial Hlth Institue, Organ Transplants, Al. Dzieci Polskich, Warsaw - Mledzylesle, 04-736 Ph: (48)22 815 1935 Fax: (48)22 815 2871 1,2) P. Kalicinski, 1,3) R. Grenda, 2) A. Kaminski, A. Prokurat, 3) Prokurat, Jobs, Baczkowska, Latoszynska, Smirska, Rubik, 4) B. Piatosa, J. Gdowska, B. Paluchow, 5) E. Danielewska	24	30	38	312
Childrens Health Ctr Memorial Insti, Nephrology & Kidney Transp, Al.Dzicci Polskich 20, Warsaw-Miedzylesie, 04-736 Ph: (48)22 815 1935 Fax: (48)22 815 2871 1,2) R. Grenda, 2) P. Kalicinski, A. Kaminski, M. Szymczak, H. Ismail, T. Drewniak, 3) S. Prokurat, K. Jobs, E. Smirska, A. Baczkowska, J. Latosynska, Rubik, 4) B. Piatosa, J. Gdowska, B. Juraczko, 5) E. Danielewska	24	30	38	310
PORTUGAL				
Univ Hosp de Coimbra, Dept of Uro-Renal Transp, Praceta Prof Pinto, 3000 Coimbra Ph: (351)239 403939 Fax: (351)239 400475 Email: urologichuc@mail.telepac.po 1,2) L. Furtado, 2) A. Mota, C. Bastos, F. Rolo, A. Roseiro, V. Dias, A. Figueiredo, 3) Borges, Gomes, Pratas, Alves, Freitas, Patricio, H. Sa, F. Macario, 4) F. Regaterio, A. Martinno, P. Santos, A. Paiva, 5) A.M. Calvao	89	82	85	1001
Cruz Vermelha Portuguesa Hosp, Unidade de Transp, Rua Duarte Galvao No 54, 1510 Lisbon Ph: (351)21 7781159 Fax: (351)21 7781159 1,2) J.R. Pena, 3) M.J. Sampaio, 4) H. Trindade, 5) M.O. Ribeiro	32			1088
H.C.L. (Curry Cabral), Transp Unit, Rua da Beneficencia, 8, 1069-166 Lisbon Ph: (351)21 797 5361 Fax: (351)21 797 5361 1,2) J.R. Pena, 2) E. Barroso, J.R. Andrade, A. Martins, 3) F. Nolasco, 4) H. Trindade, 5) C. DaCamara	38	50		419
Hosp Santa Maria, Dept of Renal Transp, Av Prof Egas Monis, Lisbon, 1699 Ph: (351)21 795 7472 Fax: (351)21 795 7471 1,2) M. Vale, 2) C. Coelho, F. Aldeia, L. Batista, R. Maio, M. Goncalves, 3) M. Prata, J. Guerra, A. Santana, 4) H. Trindade, 5) T. Afonso, I. Ramalhosa	24	31	29	251
Hosp de St Joao, Gabinete de Coordenacac de Tx, Alam. Prof Hernani Monteiro, 4200 Porto Ph: (351)917558706 Fax: (351)22 5507086 1) A. Braga, 2) F. Viana, E. Silva, J. Tenreiro, J. Teixeira, P. Roncon, Albuquerque, 3) J. Fernandes, 4) A. Mendes, 5) J. Teixeira, C. Fiuza, J. Cruz, R. Aravjo, J. Fonseca	29	33	40	405
Hosp Geral de Santo Antonio, Dept of Organ Transp, Largo Prof Abel Salazar, 4000 Porto Ph: (351)2 3325541 Fax: (351)2 3325541 Email: dto@hgsa.min-saude.pt 1,2) M. Caetano-Pereira, 2) J. Mergulhao-Mendonca, A. Moreira, A. Matos, J. Tavares, R. Almeida, 3) A. Sarmento, C. Henriques, 4) A. Mendes, P. Xavier, H. Alves, 5) R. Pereira, M. Valente	72	78	81	1035
PUERTO RICO				
Auxilio Mutuo Hosp, Transp Office, Box 1227, Hato Rey, PR 00919-1227 Ph: (787) 758-2000 Fax: (787) 765-7650 1) E.A. Santiago Delpin, 2) Z.A. Gonzalez, L.A. Morales Otero, 3) N. Cruz, C. Guerra, F. Torre, 4) A. Rodriguez Trinidad, S. de Echegaray, 5) J. Dominguez, E. Zayas, S. Calderon, H. Perez, N. Correa	71	56	68	803
SAUDI ARABIA				
King Fahad National Guard Hosp, Dept of Surg, P.O.Box 22490, Riyadh 11426 Ph: (966)1 252-0088 Fax: (966)1 252-0121 1,2) W. Al-Khudair, 2) A. Al-Abdulkareem, 3) S. Huraib, M. Quadri, G. Gormullah, A. Flaiw, 4) M. Hajali, A. Ballow, K. Al-Owiais, 5) H.A. Al-Hoshy, H. Selim	17	18	18	272
King Faisal Spec Hosp & Research Ctr, Dept of Renal Transp, PO Box 3354, Riyadh 11211 Ph: (966)1 442-3693 Fax: (966)1 442-3846 Email: shaibani@kfshrc.edu.sa 1,2) K. Al-Shaibani, 2) A. Chaballout, I. Ahmadi, S. Raza, K. Mohan, 3) Alfurayh, Al-Meshari, Taher, Al-Lehbi, Pall, Al-Sabban, Abbad, 4) A. Tbakhi, M. Al-Harthy, 5) T. Achanzar, A.M. Marfil	41	45	44	620
Riyadh Armed Forces Hosp, Dept of Uro, PO Box 7897, Riyadh, 11159 Ph: (966)1 4777714 Fax: (966)1 4769250 1,2) M.S. Abomelha, 2) Jawdat, Al Otaibi, Orkubi, Said, 3) Al-Khader, Suliman, 5) M. Jondeby	40	28	20	677

1)=Director, 2)=Tx Surgeons, 3)=Physicians, 4)=Tissue Typers, 5)=TxCoords	1998	1999	2000	Total
SINGAPORE				
Singapore Gen Hosp, Dept of Renal Med, Outram Rd, Singapore, 169608 Ph: (65) 321 4436 Fax: (65) 220 2308 Email: grmtsa@sgh.com.sg 1,3) K.T. Woo, 2) M.K. Li, C. Cheng, 3) A. Vathsala, 4) P. Tan, 5) S. Seah, S. Kong, Kykoh	42	38	35	829
SLOVAKIA				
Comenius Univ Sch of Med, Derer's Hosp, Dept of Uro, Transp Ctr, Limbova St 5, 83305 Bratislava Ph: (421)75 9544579 Fax: (421)75 9543578 1) J. Reznicek, 2) P. Bujdak, J. Breza, 3) V. Pribylincova, 4) M. Chrenova	37	25	29	661
SOUTH AFRICA				
Groote Schuur Hosp, Dept of Surg, Med Sch, Observatory 7925, Cape Town Ph: (27)21 404 3318 Fax: (27)21 448 6461 1,2) D. Kahn, 2) A.R. Pontin, 3) M. Pascoe, 4) E.D. DuToit, 5) F. McCurdie, E. Schmidt	92	66	85	1810
Tygerberg Hosp, Renal Unit, Ward A7, P.O.Box 19161, Tygerberg, Cape Town, 7505 Ph: (27)21 938 5791 Fax: (27)21 938 5555 Email: rmm@maties.sun.oc.za 1,3) M.R. Moosa, 2) A. Schmidt, C. Heyns, P. LeRoux, 3) M.R. Davids, 4) E. DuToit, 5) R. Presence, A. Theunissen	28	25	49	686
Addington Hosp, Renal Unit, PO Box 977, Durban, 4000 Ph: (27)31 3322111 x305 Fax: (27)31 3375755 Email: naickers17@med.und.ac.za 1,3) S. Naicker, 1,2) A.A. Haffejee, 2) N.G. Naidoo, 3) K. Msolwa, N. Madala, 4) M.G. Hammond, 5) M. Azor, N. Cadle	22	18		401
Univ Witwatersrand Med Sch, Johannesburg Hosp, Dept of Surg, York Rd, Parktown, Johannesburg, 2193 Ph: (27)11 488-3829 Fax: (27)11 488-3927 1,2) J.R. Botha, 2) R. Britz, P. Beale, G. Fetter, G. Pitcher, 3) L.P. Margolius, H. Viljoen, 4) S African Bld Transf Serv, 5) B. Rossi, M. Seyffert	89	126	102	2124
Pretoria Academic Hospital, Dept of Surg, PO Box 667, Pretoria 0001 Ph: (27)12 354 2104 Fax: (27)12 329 4589 1) C.J. Mieny, 2) V.O.L. Karusseit, 3) C.D. Potgieter, 4) R. Anderson, 5) L. Botes	23	21	23	537
SPAIN				
Infanta Cristina, Dept of Neph, Avda de Elvas s/n, Badajoz, 06080 Ph: (34)24 218117 Fax: (34)24 218110 1) J.J. Cubero Gomez, 2) Villafana, Asuar, 4) E. Doblare, 5) J.F. Esparrago, J. del Viejo	25	39	42	264
Son Dureta Gen Hosp, Dept Neph/Uro/Immun, Andrea Doria St, 55, Palma de Mallorca, Baleaves, 07014 Ph: (34)971 175000 Fax: (34)971 175151 1) J.E. Marco-Franco, 2) M. Ozonas, P. Piza, E. Sala, V. Riera, 3) Alarcon, Morey, Munarz, 4) J. Mila, N. Matamros, 5) P. Marce, J. Velasco	10	34	40	236
Hosp Cruces, Dept of Neph, Plaza de Cruces, s/n 48903 Cruces, Baracaldo Ph: (34)9 460-06000 Fax: (34)9 460-06074 1) Gonzalez, 2) D.C. Pertusa, 3) I. Lampreabe, 4) D. Garcia, 5) F. Corral, P. Elomieta	142	149	129	1404
Fundacio Puigvert, Dept of Neph, Cartagena 340, Barcelona, 08025 Ph: (34)3 4169700 Fax: (34)3 4504422 1) R. Sola, 2) J. Caparros, 3) L.L. Guirado, 4) I. Martorell, 5) A. Lopez	71	77	70	794
Gen Vall D'Hebron, Dept of Neph, Paseo de la Vall D'Hebron, 119-129, 08035 Barcelona Ph: (34)93 274-6079 Fax: (34)93 274-6204 1) L. Piera, 2) E. Tremps, A. Fakiani, M.A. Lopez-Pacios, J. Morote, A. Montesinos, 3) L. Capdevila, C. Cantarell, 4) J. Martorell R, 5) Deulofeu, T. Pont, R. Gracia	30	36	30	718
Hosp de Bellvitge, Dept of Neph, L'Hosp de Llobregat, Feixa Llarga, Barcelona, s/n 08907 Ph: (34)3 335 61111 Fax: (34)3 263 156118 1) J. Alsina, 2) N. Serrallach, 3) J.M. Grino, 4) J. Martorell, 5) C. Gonzalez	80	73	78	1260
Hosp Del Mar, Dept of Neph, Transp Sect, Passeig Maritim, 25-29, Barcelona, 08003 Ph: (34)93 221 1010 Fax: (34)93 221 0541 Email: 88316@imas.imim.es 1) J. Lloveras, 2) J.J. Ballesteros, 3) A. Orfila, 4) J. Martorell, 5) J.M. Puig	29	22	11	480

1)=Director, 2)=Tx Surgeons, 3)=Physicians, 4)=Tissue Typers, 5)=TxCoords	1998	1999	2000	Total
Hosp Materno-Infantil Vall d'Hebron, Dept of Neph Infantil, Vall d'Hebron s/n, 08035, Barcelona Ph: (34)3 4272000 Fax: (34)3 4282171 1) L. Callis, 2) J. Martin, C. Piro, 3) A. Via, 4) J. Martorell	8	9		164
Univ of Barcelona Hosp Clinico, Dept of Urol, Villarroel 170, Barcelona 08036 Ph: (34)3 227 5423 Fax: (34)3 227 5498 1,2) J. Alcover, 2) Vijande, Gutierrez, Alcover, Alcaraz, Franco, Luque, Corral, 3) Oppenheimer, Ricart, Campistol, Cofan, Torregrosa, Inigo, Vila, 4) J. Vives, J. Martorell, A. Gaya, 5) M. Manalich, C. Cabre, D. Paredes	136	120	126	1959
Univ "Puerta Del Mar", Cadiz, Serv de Neph, ANA de Viya 21, Cadiz, 11009 Ph: (34)56 242849 Fax: (34)56 242323 1,3) M. Rivero, 2) J. Flores, M. Romero Tenorio, 4) J.A. Brieva, 5) A.S. Rodriguez, L. Benitez	50	58		430
University Hosp "Reina Sofia", Dept of Neph, Avd Menendez Pidal 1, 14004 Cordoba Ph: (34)57 217229 Fax: (34)57 202542 1) P. Aljama, 2) M.J. Reguena, 3) R. Perez, D. Castillo, 4) J. Pena Martinez, 5) E. Riohlees	69	66		627
"Clin de San Carlos" Hosp, c/Prof Martin Lagos s/n, Dept of Immun, Ctna Andalucia km 5,4, Madrid, 28041 Ph: (34)91 3303000 Fax: (34)91 3303216 Email: antonio.arnaiz@inm.h12o.es 1,4,5) A. Arnaiz-Villena, 4) J. Martinez-Laso, 5) J. Alvarez-Rodriguez, R. Del Barrio-Yesa	86	94	67	800
"Doce de Octubre" Hosp Univ, Dept of Neph, Ctra. Andalucia, Madrid, 28041 Ph: (34)91 3908315 Fax: (34)91 3908399 Email: antonio.arnaiz@inm.h12o.es 1) A. Arnaiz-Villena, 3) J. Morales, 4) A. Arnaiz-Villena, J. Martinez-Laso, 5) A. Andres, J.I. Rodicio	130	136	123	1590
"La Paz" Hosp, C/O Hosp 12 de Octubre, Dept of Immun, Ctra Andulcia km 5,4, 28041 Madrid Ph: (34)91 390 8315 Fax: (34)91 390 8399 Email: antonio.arnaiz@inm.h12o.es 1,4,5) A. Arnaiz-Villena, 4) J. Matinez-Laso, 5) L. Sanchez-Sicillia, A. Ballesteros	49	76	41	464
Fundacion Jimenez Diaz, Dept of Surg, Av Reyes Catolicos 2, 28040 Madrid Ph: (34)1 549 2971 Fax: (34)1 549 4764 1) F.M. Calderin, 2) R. Vela, 3) S. Casado, 4) M. Kreisler, 5) J.J. Plaza	17	21	21	678
Hosp Gen Gregorio Maranon, Dept of Neph, Dr Esquerdo 46, Madrid, 28007 Ph: (34)91 586 8319 Fax: (34)91 586 8018 1) F. Valderrabano, 2) C. Hernandez, 3) M. Rengel, F. Anaya, 4) M. Kreisler, 5) J.L. Escalante	26	31	29	759
Infantil "La Paz" Hosp, Dept of Neph, Poseo de la Castellana #261, Madrid, 28046 Ph: (34)91 7293041 Fax: (34)91 3582545 1) M. Navarro, 2) E. Jaureguizar, M.J. Urrutia, P. Lopez Peretra, 3) C. Garcia Meseguer, A. Alonso, 4) A. Arnaiz Villena	18	20		176
Puerta de Hierro, Dept of Neph, S Martin Porres 4, Madrid, E-28035 Ph: (34)1 316 2240 Fax: (34)1 373 0535 1,3) J. Botella, 2) J. Carballido, 3) J. Fernandez, 4) M. Kreisler	23			467
Ramon y Cajal Hosp, Dept of Neph, Ctra de Colmenar,Km.9,100, Madrid, 28034 Ph: (34)91 336-8018 Fax: (34)91 336-8800 Email: jortuno@hrc.insalud.es 1) J. Ortuno, 2) F.J. Burgos, E. Fernandez, J.M. Rodriguez, 3) C. Quereda, R. Marcen, J. Pascual, 4) A. Bootello, 5) S. Arevalillo, C. Mosacula, A. Candela	42	38	49	826
Regional "Carlos Haya, Coordination de Transp, Avda Carlos Haya, C Antequera s/n, Malaga, 29010 Ph: (34)95 261 1842 Fax: (34)95 261 1842 1,2) V. Baena, 2) J. Ramos, 3) M. Gonzalez-Molina, 4) A. Alonso, 5) M.A. Frutos	74			1134
Clin Univ de Navarra, Dept of Uro, Pio XII Ave, Aptdo 4209, Pamplona, Navarra, 31080 Ph: (34)48 296500 Fax: (34)48 172294 Email: jberian@unav.es 1,2) J.M. Berian, 2) J.E. Robles, J.J. Zudaire, D. Rosell, 3) A. Purroy, P. Errasti, 4) M.L. Subira, A. Sanchez-Ibarrola, 5) P. Errasti	27	31	23	567
Central De Asturias(Hosp Covadonga), Medicina (Nefrologia), Celestino Villamil S/N, Oviedo, 33006 Ph: (34)8 5108000 Fax: (34)8 5108015 1,3) J.A. Grande, 2) A.S. Trilla, M.A. Suarez Hevia, 3) E.G. Huertas, F.O. Suarez, 4) C. Lopez-Larrea, L.T. Aizpun, 5) J.O. Hernandez, E.G. Gonzalez	47	42	58	632
Univ Hosp Valdecilla, Dept of Neph, Div of Nephrologia, Santander Ph: (34)42 202738 Fax: (34)42 320415 1) M. Arias, 2) Portillo, Valle, Gutierrez, Correas, Roca, Martino, Herrera, 3) J.G. Cotorruelo, A. de Francisco, J.A. Zubimendi, P. Morales, S. Sanz, 4) J.M. Pastor, 5) J.G. Cotorruelo	62	76	53	1243

KIDNEY

1)=Director, 2)=Tx Surgeons, 3)=Physicians, 4)=Tissue Typers, 5)=TxCoords	1998	1999	2000	Total
Hosp Xeral de Galicia, Unidad de Trasplantes, C/Galeras s/n, Santiago de Compotel, 15705 Ph: (34)9 81 540218 Fax: (34)9 81 570102 1,2) E. Varo, 2) Bustamante, Conde, Martinez, Paredes, Segade, Punal, Blanco, 3) D.S. Guisande, R. Romero, X.M. Lens, 4) M. Vega, 5) A. Marino, A. Vazquez	38			348
Infantil Virgen Del Rocio, Dept of Ped Neph, Avda Manuel Siurot s/n, 41013 Sevilla Email: govantes@cica.es 1,3) J. Martin Govantes, 2) P. Montanez, F. Torrubia, 3) R. Bedyar, 4) A. Nunez, 5) J. Ruano	7	12	4	125
Hosp Infantil La Fe, Ped Neph Unit, Av Campanar 21, 46009 Valencia Ph: (34)96 386-8777 Fax: (34)96 386-8700 1) J.M. Simon, 2) F. Garcia-Ibarra, F. Estornell, M. Matinez-Verduch, 3) I. Zamora, D. Mendizabal, 4) J. Montoro, 5) P. Genoves	12	43	14	261
Universitario, Nefrologia, Avda Ramony Cajal 3, Valladolid, 47011 Ph: (983) 420000-121 Fax: (983) 257511 Email: bustaman@med.uva.sp 1) J. Bustamante, 2) E. Fernandes de Busto, 3) A. Mendiluce, 4) M. Nocito, 5) P. Ucio	15	16	28	67

SULTANATE OF OMAN

	1998	1999	2000	Total
Sultan Qaboos Univ Hosp, Royal Hosp, Dept of Surg, P O Box 35, Al-Khod,Muscat, 123 Ph: (968) 515119 Fax: (968) 513419 1,2) A.S. Daar, 2) Q. Busaidi, 3) H. Marhubi, N. Mohsin, 4) H. Al Riyami, S. Al Hashmi, M. Varghese, 5) A. Ismaily	43	52	39	620

SWEDEN

	1998	1999	2000	Total
Sahlgrenska Univ Hosp, Transpl and Liver Surg, Su/Sahlgrenska, FACK3, S-41345 Gothenburg Ph: (46)31 3421000 Fax: (46)31 820557 1,2) M. Olausson, 2) I. Blohme, S. Friman, L. Mjornstedt, L. Backman, O. Ostraat, L. Wrammer, 3) G. Nyberg, C. Norden, 4) L. Rydberg, 5) Eriksson, Wolfbrandt	146	128	106	3670
Malmo Univ Hosp, Lund Univ, Dept of Neph and Transp, Transp Unit, S Forstadsgatan 101, Malmo, S-20502 Ph: (46)40 33 1000 Fax: (46)40 33 6211 Email: nils.persson@kir.mas.lu.se 1,2) N.H. Persson, 2) H. Ekberg, R. Kallen, 3) G. Sterner, B. Oqvist, 4) D. Bucin, 5) M. Omnell Persson, K. Karud, M. Lundell, A. Waldner	53	63	45	1476
Huddinge Univ Hosp, Dept of Transp Surg, stockholm, SE-14186 Ph: (46)8 58580000 Fax: (46)8 7743191 1,2) A. Tibell, 2) G. Tyden, J. Sandberg, 3) P. Barany, 4) E. Moller, 5) B. Blom	82	59	66	2154
Univ Hosp Uppsala, Dept of Transp Surg, Unit 70TD, S-75185 Uppsala Ph: (46)18 664669 Fax: (46)18 559468 1,2) J. Wahlberg, 2) J. Wadstrom, G.Tufveson.K. Claesson, F. Duraj, 3) B. Fellstrom, 4) O. Sjoberg, M. Bengtsson, 5) E. Bjorklund, I. Skarp, C. Moller	76	51	66	1565

SWITZERLAND

	1998	1999	2000	Total
Kantonsspital Basel, Univ of Basel, Dept of Surg/Med, Petersgraben 4, CH-4031 Basel Ph: (41)61 265 4407 Fax: (41)61 265 2410 1,3) J. Steiger, 2) Th. Gasser, D. Oertli, L. Gurke, 3) M. Dickenmann, 4) F. Brunner, 5) T. Voegele	59	70	73	1316
Inselspital Bern, Visceral Surg/Transp/Med Polik, Freiburgstr 10, CH-3010 Bern Ph: (41)31 632 3144 Fax: (41)31 632 4789 1,3) M.W. Buchler, 2) C. Seiler, M. Schilling, 3) H.U. Marti, 4) C. Dahinden, 5) P. Bischoff	41	28	41	796
Univ Hosp Geneva, Dept of Surg, 24 Rue Micheli du Crest, 1211 Geneva 14 Ph: (41)22 372 7702 Fax: (41)22 372 7755 1) P.Y. Martin, 1,2,) Ph. Morel, 2) J. Oberholzer, J.F. Bolle, 3) F. Moser	19	30	31	574
Ctr Hosp Univ Vaudois, Dept of Med, Div of Neph, Ch-1011 Lausanne Ph: (41)21 314-1130 Fax: (41)21 314-1139 Email: jean-pierre.wauters@chuv.hospvd.ch 1,3) J.P. Wauters, 2) F. Mosimann, 3) G. Halabi, 4) V. Aubert, 5) C. Gachet, G. Eschenmoser, L. Imperatori	25	34	31	525
Kantonsspital St Gallen, Dept of Med/Surg, Rorschacherstrasse 95, CH-9007 St Gallen Ph: (41)71 494 1111 Fax: (41)71 494 2877 1,3) R.P. Wuthrich, 2) D. Sege, 3) D. Garzoni, 4) M. Disler, 5) U. Elfrich	21	18	21	376

1)=Director, 2)=Tx Surgeons, 3)=Physicians, 4)=Tissue Typers, 5)=TxCoords	1998	1999	2000	Total
Univ Hosp Zurich, Dept of Surg, Ramistr 100, Zurich, CH-8091 Ph: (41)1 255 3300 Fax: (41)1 255 4449 Email: clavien@chir.unizh.ch 1) P.A. Clavien, 2) M. Weber, N. Demartines, Z. Kadry, 3) U. Binswanger, 4) M. Weber, 5) P. Seeburger, T. Reh, M. Struker	98	80	65	2070

TAIWAN

	1998	1999	2000	Total
Chang Gung Mem Hosp, Dept of Surg/Uro, 199 Tung Hwa North Rd, Taipei 105 Ph: (886)3 328 1200 Fax: (886)3 328 5818 1) S.H. Chu, 2) C.K. Chuang, H.W. Chen, C.S. Chen, C.C. Chou, Y.J. Chiang, 3) C.C. Huang, C.Y. Huang, 4) C.C. Huang, 5) G.F. Yeh, J.C. Liou	32	32	33	499

THAILAND

	1998	1999	2000	Total
Praram 9 Hosp, Renal Transpl Unit, 99 Soi Praram 9 Hosp, Rama IX Rd, Huaykhwang, Bangkok, 10320 Ph: (662) 248-8020 Fax: (662) 248-8018 1) K. Danviriyasup, 2) S. Jirasiritham, 3) V. Mavichak, 4) P. Chiewsilp, 5) P. Ngorsakun	16	19	21	171
Ramathibodi Hosp Med Sch, Dept of Surg, 270 Rama VI Rd, Bangkok, 10400 Ph: (662) 2011576 Fax: (662) 2011316 Email: soponj@hotmail.com 1) P. Gojaseni, 2) S. Jirasiritham, 3) V. Sumlthkul, 4) P. Chiewsilp, 5) S. Jirasiritham	80	80		598

TURKEY

	1998	1999	2000	Total
Baskent Univ Hosp, Dept of Gen Surg, I Cadde, No 77, Kat 4 Bahcelievler, Ankara, 06500 Ph: (90)312 212 6868 Fax: (90)312 215 0835 Email: melekk@baskent-ank.edu.tr 1,2) M. Haberal, 2) N. Bilgin, H. Karakayali, 3) F. Nurhan Ozdemir, 4) M. Turan, 5) H. Akkoc	45	62	59	1333
Akdeniz Univ Med Sch Hosp, Dept of General Surgery, Dumlupinar Bulvari-Kampus, Antalya, 07060 Ph: (90)532 277 1485 Fax: (90)242 227 8837 1) T. Karpuzoglu, 2) N. Oygur, S. Aktan, K. Emek, A. Demirbas, 3) G. Suleymanlar, F. Isitan, F. Ersoy, I. Suleymanlar, 4) O. Yegin, M. Coskun, 5) N. Kececioglu	18	18		332
Ege Univ Med Sch, Organ Transp & Rsrch Ctr, Level 3, Bornova, Izmir Ph: (90)232 339-8838 Fax: (90)232 339 8838 1,2) H. Kaplan, 2) C. Hoscoskun, Y. Tokat, M. Sozbilen, 3) A. Basci, E. Ok, S. Mir, 4) A. Keskinoglu, 5) A. Boreklar	53	37	36	458

UNITED KINGDOM

	1998	1999	2000	Total
Queen Elizabeth Hosp, Renal Unit, Edgebaston, Birmingham, B15 2TH Ph: (44)121 472-1311 Fax: (44)121 627-2527 1,3) N.T. Richards, 2) L. Buist, A. Ready, H. Krishnan, 3) D. Adu, C. Savage, D. Wheeler, L. Lipkin, P. Cockwell, 4) D. Briggs, 5) A. Hooker, F. Wellington, D. McPake, N. Jain, M. Gordon	101	107		2589
Addenbrooke's Hosp, Transplant, Box No. 210, Hills Road, Cambridge, CB2 2QQ Ph: (441) 223-245151 Fax: (441) 223 217825 1,2) A.Bradley, 2) A. Bradley, N. Jamieson, P. Gibbs, C. Watson,L.Delriviere 3) J. Firth, K. Smith, J. Bradley, 4) C. Taylor, 5) P. Jones, A.Wray	75	54	59	1759
Derriford Hosp, Renal Unit, Derriford Rd, Plymouth, Devon, PL6 8DH Ph: (44)752 792258 Fax: (44)752 774651 1,3) P.A. Rowe, 2) D. Wilkins, J.F.L. Shaw, J. Akoh, 3) R. McGonigle, W. Tse, 4) N. Hurlock, E. Kaminski, K. Poole, 5) R. Stoddard-Murden, J. Spencer, B. Bishop, S. Preston	49	41	45	492
Leicester Gen Hosp, Univ Dept of Surg, Gwendolen Rd, Leicester, LE5 4PW Ph: (44)116 249 0490 Fax: (44)116 258 4666 1,2) M.L. Nicholson, 2) P. Veitch, P.R.F. Bell, T. Doughman, 3) J. Walls, J. Feehally, K. Harris, G. Warwick, S. Carr, N. Brunskill, 4) T. Horsburgh, N. Mistry, S. Weston, I. Underwood, A. Lycett, 5) R. Elwell, R. Taylor, A. Cummings, J. Bailey	44	49	63	907
Royal Liverpool & Broadgreen Univ, Hosp Trust-Renal Transp Unit, Link Unit 9C, Prescot St, Liverpool, L7 8XP Ph: (44)151 708 0163 Fax: (44)151 706 5819 1,2) A.Q. Hammad, 2) A. Bakran, R.A. Sells, 3) J.M. Bone, 4) P. Beals, 5) J. Godfrey, T. Rhodes, E. Linacre	52	71	83	1645

1)=Director, 2)=Tx Surgeons, 3)=Physicians, 4)=Tissue Typers, 5)=TxCoords	1998	1999	2000	Total
Dulwich Hosp, King's Coll Hosp, Renal Admin, E Dulwich Grove, London, SE22 8PT Ph: (44)171 346-6256 Fax: (44)171 346-6472 1) H. Cairns, 2) N. Heaton, P. Gibbs, M. Rela, 3) H. Cairns, I. MacDougall, 4) D. Bevan, 5) H. Mandefield	26	28		1474
Hammersmith Hosp & Royal Postgrad, Med Sch, Dept of Surg, Ducane Rd, London, W12 0HS Ph: (44)181 383 3218 Fax: (44)181 383 3443 1,2) G. Williams, 2) S. Ararwal, 3) E. Clutterbuck, R. Lechler, C. Gaskin, E. Lightstone, A. Wassens, 4) R. Lechler, 5) A. Cromie, J. Nichols, J. Griffiths	41			985
St Mary's Hosp, Transp Unit, Praed St, Paddington, London, W2 1NY Ph: (44)171 886 1852 Fax: (44)171 886 1707 1,2) N.S. Hakim, 1,3) D. Taube, 2) V. Papalois, 3) A. Palmer, T. Cairns, 4) M. Van Dam, N. Browning, 5) J. Griffiths, P. Keenan, V. Morgan	45	50	28	1035
Royal Infirm Hosp, Renal Transp Unit, Oxford Rd, Manchester, M13 9WL Ph: (44)161 276-4413 Fax: (44)161 276-8020 1,2) H.N. Riad, 2) N.R. Parrott, R.C. Pearson, T. Augustin, 3) R. Gokal, C. Short, A.J. Hutchison, F. Qasim, 4) P. Dyer, S. Martin, 5) S. Clark, S. Frew, D. Lee	145	143	156	2758
Belfast City Hosp, Dept of Neph/Transp, Lisburn Rd, Belfast, North Ireland, BT9 7AB Ph: (44)1232 329241 Fax: (44)1232 263535 1,3) C.C. Doherty, 2) R.A. Donaldson, P. Keane, J. Connolly, 3) J.F. Douglas, W.E. Nelson, P.T. McNamee, A.P. Maxwell, J.D. Woods, 4) D. Middleton, 5) E. Donaghy, A. McCook, D. Elliott	27	40	42	1084
Oxford Radcliffe Hosp, Oxford Transp Ctr, The Churchhill, Oxford, OX3 7LJ Ph: (44)865 226092 Fax: (44)865 225616 1,2) P. Friend, 2) D. Gray, C. Darby, P.J. Morris, C. Russell, 3) P. Ratcliffe, P. Mason, P. Altman, 4) S. Fuggle, M. Barnado, 5) M. Jackson	64	88	102	1769
West Glasgow Hosps, Univ NHS Trust, Renal Transp Unit, Western Infirmary, Dumbarton Rd, Glasgow, Scotland, G11 6NT Ph: (44)141 211 2177 Fax: (44)141 211 1711 Email: jindalr@aol.com 1,2) R.M. Jindal, 2) D.M. Hamilton, B. Jaques, K. Kyle, 3) J.D. Briggs, B.J.R. Junor, R.S.C. Rodger, M.A. McMillan, C. Geddes, 4) N. Henderson, A. Farrell, 5) D. Walsh, K. Brown, L. Thomson	83	96	94	1838
Northern Gen Hosp, Renal Unit, Herries Road, Sheffield, S5 7AU Ph: (44)114 243 4343 Fax: (44)114 256 2514 1) A.T. Raftery, 2) M.S. Karim, 3) C.B. Brown, A.M. El Nahas, P.J. Moorhead, M.E. Wilkie, D. Throssell, 4) D. Ashton, J. Goodwin, 5) V. Lennon, S. Siddall	38	35	28	954

URUGUAY

	1998	1999	2000	Total
Hospital Americano, Isabelino Bosh 2466, Montevideo Ph: (598)7 086041 Fax: (598)7 094231 1) E. Nesse, 2) C. Gomez Fossati, F. Scivoli, 3) S. Bonetti, 4) BNOT, I. Alvarez, R. Toledo, M. Bengochea, E. Carreto, 5) R. Mizraji, A. Brun, P. RealdeAzua, M. Canepa, A. Castro, Cagarbado	5	2	2	9
Hospital de Clinicas, Universidad de la Republica, Av. Italia s/n Piso 14, Montevideo Ph: (598)4 809850 Fax: (598)4 809850 1) F. Gonzalez, 1) L. Rodriguez, 2) C. Gomez Fossati, L. Garcia Guido, 3) S. Orihuela, 4) BNOT, I. Alvarez, R. Toledo, M. Bengochea, E. Carreto, 5) R. Mizraji, A. Brun, P. RealdeAzua, M. Canepa, A. Castro, C. Agarbado			1	31
Hospital Evangelico, Mateo Vidal 3392, Montevideo Ph: (598)4 872319x319/321 Fax: (598)4 872334 1) N. Dibelo, 2) C. Gomez Fossati, D. Lopez, H. Puente, 3) I. Wibher, 4) BNOT, I. Alvarez, R. Toledo, M. Bengochea, E. Carreto, 5) R. Mizraji, A. Brun, P. RealdeAzua, M. Canepa, A. Castro, C. Agarbado			2	2
Instituto de Nefrologia y Urologia, Jaime Cibils 2824 bis, Montevideo Ph: (598)4 871114 Fax: (598)4 879183 1) F. Gonzalez, 1) L. Rodriguez, 2) O. Balboa, L. Garcia Guido, J. Zeballos, D. Portos, 3) S. Orihuela, L. Curi, N. Nunez, G. Gonzalez, 4) BNOT, I. Alvarez, R. Toledo, M. Bengochea, E. Carreto, 5) R. Miraji, A. Brun, P. RealdeAzua, M. Canepa, A. Castro, C. Agarbado	58	39	52	529

1)=Director, 2)=Tx Surgeons, 3)=Physicians, 4)=Tissue Typers, 5)=TxCoords	1998	1999	2000	Total
VENEZUELA				
Hosp Univ de Caracas, Serv de Neph/Renal Transp, Apartado Postal 47365, Caracas, 1010 Ph: (58)2 986 9354 Fax: (58)2 661 4031 1) J.R. Weisinger, 2) C. Bernal, G. Rosito, E. Bercowsky, M. Garcia, 3) C.L. Milanes, P. Clesca, A. Arminio, 4) G. Perez-Rojas, 5) E. Hernandez	13	25		469
Hosp Univ de Maracaibo, Dept of Neph, Apartado Postal 1430, Maracaibo, Estado Zulia, 4001-A Ph: (58)61 519610 Fax: (58)61 524838 1) B. Rodriguez-Iturbe, 2) N. Teran, G. Vera, 3) R. Garcia, Salgado, Rubio, Henriquez, Marin, Herrera, Parra, Colic, 4) G. Parra, C. Portillo, 5) O. Salgado	27	38	24	648

KIDNEY Transplants

	1998	1999	2000	Total
United States	12,454	12,849	13,538	222,785
Foreign	14,975	14,982	13,886	277,760
Total	27,429	27,831	27,424	500,545

KIDNEY Transplant Centers

United States	238
Foreign	350
Total	588

KIDNEY

WORLDWIDE TRANSPLANT CENTER DIRECTORY
KIDNEY/PANCREAS TRANSPLANTS

1)=Director, 2)=Tx Surgeons, 3)=Physicians, 4)=Tissue Typers, 5)=TxCoords	1998	1999	2000	Total

UNITED STATES

ALABAMA

Univ of Alabama at Birmingham, Dept of Surg, 619 S 19th St, Birmingham, AL 35294
Ph: (205) 934-5200 Fax: (205) 934-0952
1,2) M. Deierhoi, 1,2) C. Young, 2) J.S. Bynon, M.H. Gallichio, M. Sellers, 3) J. Curtis, B. Julian, R. Gaston, 4) R. Acton, 5) J. Hardin, C. Huey, T. Allan, Mayes, D. Brasfield — 14 11 21* 111

ARIZONA

Good Samaritan Reg Med Ctr, Samaritan Transp Serv, 1410 N 3rd St, Phoenix, AZ 85004-1608
Ph: (602) 251-2700 Fax: (602) 251-2750
1,2) A.J. Fabrega, 1,3) E. Polito, 2) L.J. Koep, 3) Petrides, Smith, Bailey, Yee, Chang, Guerra, Hyde, 4) T. Vyvial, DNA HLA, 5) J. Bell, A. Moore, M. Ruocco, K. Helzer, K. Fitzpatrick — 11 12 16* 43

ARKANSAS

The Univ Hosp of Arkansas, Dept of Surg, 4301 W Markham, Box 520, Little Rock, AR 72205
Ph: (501) 686-6644 Fax: (501) 686-5725
1,2) B. Ketel, 2) G. Barone, 3) M. Bunke, 4) V. Smith, P. Treadway, 5) S. Turton-Weeks, L. Lingo, K. Conery-Reed — 2 5 9* 73

CALIFORNIA

Loma Linda Univ Med Ctr, Transp Inst, 11234 Anderson St, Ste 1405, Loma Linda, CA 92354
Ph: (909) 558-4252 Fax: (909) 558-0112
1,2) W. Concepcion, 2) O. Ojogho, P. Baron, 3) S. Teichman, 4) S. Nehlsen-Cannarella, L. Buckert, 5) R. Custodio, C. Maas, J. Vickers — 13 15 15 100

St. Vincent Medical Center, Dept Of Transplant, 2200 W. 3rd Street, Suite 500, Los Angeles, CA 90057 Ph: (213)484-6307 Fax: (213)413-0190
1,2) U. Khetan, 2) P. Asai, R. Mendez, R.G. Mendez, H. Shidban, R. Naraghi, T. Bogaard, 3) M. Spira, E. Feinstein, R. Minansian, 4) Y. Iwaki, J. Cicciarelli, 5) Uleman, Lozada, Warkentien, Luellen, Norfles, Razo, Felty — 19 17 11* 108

Stanford Univ Med Ctr, Kidney-Pancreas Program, 750 Welch Rd., Suite 200, Palo Alto, CA 94304-1509 Ph: (650) 725-9891 Fax: (650) 723-3997
1,2) C. Esquivel, 2) M. Millan, 3) J.D. Scandling, 4) C. Grumet, 5) Waskerwitz, Knoppel, Salvatierra, Law, Wong — 14 9 0* 97

Univ of Calif, Davis Med Ctr, Transplant Program, 2315 Stockton Blvd, Housestaff facility, Room 1018, Sacramento, CA 95817 Ph: (916) 734-2111 Fax: (916) 456-2407
1,2) R.V. Perez, 2) J. McVicar, 3) S. Gandhi, 4) P. Holland, 5) M.E. Friend, D.B. Higgs, M. Sturges, D. Lehe — 8 5 6* 76

Univ Calif-San Diego Med Ctr, Kidney/Pancreas Transp, 200 W Arbor Dr, San Diego, CA 92103-8745 Ph: (619) 294-6257 Fax: (619) 296-1852
1,2) J. Dunn, 3) R. Steiner, 4) M. Garovoy, L. Lebeck, 5) L. Conley, K. Hall — 8 10 6* 51

Calif Pacific Med Ctr, Transp Serv, PO Box 7999, 2340 Clay St, Ste 417, San Francisco, CA 94115 Ph: (415) 923-3450 Fax: (415) 923-3836
1,2) W. Bry, 3) B. Levin, 4) S. Steen, 5) H. Hei — 9 11 6* 59

Univ Calif-San Francisco, Transp Serv, Moffitt Hosp, Box 0116, Rm 884, San Francisco, CA 94143 Ph: (415) 353-1551 Fax: (415) 353-8708
1,2) P.G. Stock, 2) C. Freise, R. Hirose, S. Feng, 3) W. Amend, S. Tomlanovich, F. Vincenti, D. Adey, 4) L. Baxter-Lowe, 5) Garrick, Del Grosso, Moczkowski, Sabatte, Torres, Driscoll — 15 14 21* 196

* Preliminary UNOS data

1)=Director, 2)=Tx Surgeons, 3)=Physicians, 4)=Tissue Typers, 5)=TxCoords	1998	1999	2000	Total
COLORADO				
Centura Porter Adventist Hosp, Transp Serv, 2535 S Downing St, #380, Denver, CO 80210 Ph: (303) 778-5797 Fax: (303) 778-5205 1,2) W.B. Vernon, 2) W. Kortz, E. Kortz, 3) C. Kuruvila, M. Dillingham, M. Yanover, D. Gillum, S. Osa, J. Scott, 4) Laboratories at Bonfils, 5) D. Long, M. Luedtke, G. Lewis, K. Bramley, T. Sandoval	9	5	9	46
Presbyterian/St Luke's Med Ctr, Transp Program, 1719 E 19th Ave, 1C, Denver, CO 80218 Ph: (303) 869-2155 Fax: (303) 869-2106 1,3) K. Fitting, 2) I. Kam, M. Wachs, T. Bak, 3) A. Cooper, 4) IAD, 5) B. Guyon, R. Otto, K. O'Dea, I. Sansoucy	1	2	2	37
Univ of Colorado Hosp, Dept of Transp Surg, 4200 E Ninth Ave, Box C-318, Denver, CO 80262 Ph: (303) 372-8750 Fax: (303) 372-8737 1,2) M. Wachs, 2) T. Bak, 3) L. Chan, A. Wiseman, A. Jani, 4) UCHSC-Clin Immun & Histo Lab, 5) B. Britz	8	5	4	90
CONNECTICUT				
Yale New haven Hosp, Dept of Surg, Div of Organ Tx, 333 Cedar St, FMB 112, New Haven, CT 06510 Ph: (203) 785-2565 Fax: (203) 785-7162 Email: kathy.lorber@yale.edu 1,2) G.P. Basadonna, 2) M.I. Lorber, A.L. Friedman, 3) M.J. Bia, A.S. Kliger, 4) M.I. Lorber, M. Marcarelli, 5) M. Corrigan, J. Albert, N. Sowers, J. Bates	4	4	4	35
DISTRICT OF COLUMBIA				
Georgetown Univ Med Ctr, Dept of Surg, Kid/Panc Transp, 4 PHC, 3800 Reservoir Rd NW, Washington, DC 20007 Ph: (202) 784-3700 Fax: (202) 687-3004 1,2) L.B. Johnson, 2) P.C. Kuo, A. Lu, 3) J. Conin, 4) S. Rosen-Bronson, 5) A. Cribbs, C. Story, W. Sachau, N. Lawson	2	1	1	42
Walter Reed Army Med Ctr, Organ Transp Serv, WD 48, WRAMC, 6825 Georgia Ave,NW, Washington, DC 20307 Ph: (202) 782-6462 Fax: (202) 782-4313 1,2) S.J. Swanson III, 2) D.S. Batty, A. Kirk, 3) S. Polly, 4) W. Nelson, H. Dinh, J. Gaffney, J. Carr, 5) J. Burke, B. Reinmuth, S. Carson, B. Barros, M. Gooden	7	3	3*	26
Washington Hosp Ctr, Transp Serv, Rm 3B1, 110 Irving St NW, Washington, DC 20010 Ph: (202) 877-6029 Fax: (202) 877-6581 1,2) J. Light, 2) C. Currier, T. Sasaki, 3) J. Moore, J. Veis, 4) W. Ward, 5) J. Flores, J. Trollinger, J. Stein, W. Cascon, D. Lepley	15	4	8	143
FLORIDA				
Shands at the Univ of Florida, Transplant Center, Box 100251, 1600 SW Archer Road, Gainesville, FL 32610-0251 Ph: (352)395-0130 Fax: (352)395-0108 1,2) W.J. VanderWerf, 2) A. Reed, R.J. Howard, A. Hemming, 3) T.R. Srinivaz, 4) J. Scornik, 5) J. Lloyd-Turner	6	10	13	42
Mayo Clinic Jacksonville/St. Luke's, Renal & Pancreatic Transp, 4203 Belford Rd, Suite 204, Jacksonville, FL 32216 Ph: (904) 296-9075 Fax: (904) 296-5874 1,2) J.L. Steers, 2) J. Nguyen, C. Hughes, V. Gopalan, 3) J.R. Spivey, R.C. Dickson, D.M. Harnois, 4) P. Genco, 5) D. Boyum	0	0	6	6
Univ of Miami-Jackson Mem Med Ctr, Dept of Surg, Transp Div, PO Box 012440, Miami, FL 33101 Ph: (305) 355-5000 Fax: (305) 355-5063 1,2) J. Miller, 1,2) A. Tzakis, 2) G.W. Burke III, G. Ciancio, 3) R. Alejandro, 4) V. Esquenazi, 5) J. Colona, D. Balboa-Jorge, G. Jefferson	25	22	28*	192
GEORGIA				
Emory Univ, Dept of Surg, 1364 Clifton Rd NE, H-124, Atlanta, GA 30322 Ph: (404) 727-0717 Fax: (404) 727-8972 1,2) C.P. Larsen, 1,2) T.C. Pearson, 2) P. Tso, 3) S. Gebhart, C. Zayas, 4) R. Bray, 5) G. McGrath, C. Johnson, M. Jeffrey, T. Ofenloch, B. Begley, W. Wilson	23	14	22	146
ILLINOIS				
Northwestern Mem Hosp, Div of Organ Transp, 675 North St Clair Street, Galter 17-200, Chicago, IL 60611 Ph: (312) 695-8900 Fax: (312) 695-9194 1,2) D. Kaufman, 2) J. Leventhal, J. Fryer, M. Abecassis, F. Stuart, 3) D. Batlle, L. Gallon, 4) M. Buckingham, 5) P. Gierut, D. Penrod, E. DeMayo, B. Olszewski	24	36	37	189

1)=Director, 2)=Tx Surgeons, 3)=Physicians, 4)=Tissue Typers, 5)=TxCoords	1998	1999	2000	Total
Rush Presbyterian St Luke's Med Ctr, Organ & Tissue Transp Serv, 1653 W Congress Prkwy, 201 Jones, Chicago, IL 60612 Ph: (312) 942-4252 Fax: (312) 942-3055 Email: dmital@rush.edu 1,2) D. Mital, 2) S. Jensik, H. Sankary, 3) Orlowski, Mazzone, Saltzberg, Baldwin, 4) H. Gebel, M. Prod, 5) T. Partida, L. Cowan, D. Ding, E. Blicharski, I. Alonso, S. Vasquez	11	6	4	51
Univ of Chicago Med Ctr, Dept of Transp Surg, 5841 S Maryland, m/c 5026, Chicago, IL 60637 Ph: (773) 702-6338 Fax: (773) 702-2126 1,2) D.S. Bruce, 2) J.R. Thistlethwaite, J. Millis, K.A. Newell, D.C. Cronin, 3) M.A. Josephson, M. Cavaghan, 4) V. Lazda, 5) S. Pellar	35	29	14*	232
Univ of Illinois Hosp & Clins, Dept of Surg, Div of Transp, 801 S Paulina, Rm 411, m/c 960, Chicago, IL 60612-7213 Ph: (312) 996-6771 Fax: (312) 413-3483 1,2) E. Benedetti, 2) L. Cicalese, 3) J. Arruda, I. Brodsky, 4) V.A. Lazda, 5) F. Pascual, O. Woghiren, X. Lopez	2	4	4*	38
So Univ Illinois School Of Medicine, Memorial Medical Center, Transplant Service, 701 N 1st, Springfield, IL 62781-0001 Ph: (217)788-3441 Fax: (217)788-4610 Email: toconnor@siumed.edu 1,2) T.P. O'Connor, 3) Khardori, Mitra, 4) P. McConnachie, 5) T. Beauchamp, D. Daily, B. Grantham	4	5	3	20

INDIANA

	1998	1999	2000	Total
Indiana Univ Med Ctr, Dept of Surg/Organ Transp, 550 N University Blvd, Rm UH 4258, Indianapolis, IN 46202 Ph: (317) 274 4370 Fax: (317) 274 3084 1,2) R.S. Filo, 2) S.B. Leapman, M.D. Pescovitz, M.L. Milgrom, 3) K. Bodziak, T. Butaih, 4) Z. Brahmi, 5) P. Martin, M.L. Tolin, M. Judge	5	13	8*	84

IOWA

	1998	1999	2000	Total
Univ of Iowa Hosps & Clins, Dept of Surg/Transp Serv, University Hospitals, Iowa City, IA 52242 Ph: (319) 356-3585 Fax: (319) 356-1556 1,2) S.C. Rayhill, 2) A. Bozorgzadeh, 3) L.G. Hunsicker, M. Flanigan, J.A. Bertalotus, C. Thomas, Golconda, 4) N.E. Goeken, E. Fields, 5) B. Schanbacher, P. Zehr, L. Reynolds, A. Satterly, D. Cox, M. Schulz	14	14	8*	179
Univ of Iowa Hosps & Clins, Dept of Surg/Transp Serv, University Hospitals, Iowa City, IA 52242 Ph: (319) 356-1334 Fax: (319) 356-1556 1,2) Y. Wu, 2) S. Rayhill, A. Bozorgzadeh, D. Katz, 3) L.G. Hunsicker, J.A. Bertalotus, C. Thomas, Kalil, 4) N.E. Goeken, E. Fields, 5) B. Schanbacher, L. Reynolds, A. Satterly, D. Cox, M. Schulz	0	0	8	8

KANSAS

	1998	1999	2000	Total
Univ of Kansas Med Ctr, Div of Neph, 3901 Rainbow Blvd, Kansas City, KS 66160-7382 Ph: (913) 588-6074 Fax: (913) 588-3867 1,2) G. Pierce, 2) D. Murillo, 3) A. Chonko, B. Cowley, J. Grantham, F. Winklhofer, 4) Midwest Organ Bank, 5) J. Greathouse, D. Todd, P. Hunt		13	11*	24

KENTUCKY

	1998	1999	2000	Total
Univ of Kentucky Med Ctr, Dept of Surg, 800 Rose St, Lexington, KY 40536 Ph: (859) 323-4661 Fax: (859) 323-3644 1,2) D. Ranjan, 2) T. Johnston, S. Reddy, 3) T. Waid, W. McKeown, D. Karounos, E. Jackson, 4) T. Eichorn, J. Byrne, J.S. Thompson, D. Jennings, F. Lower, 5) S. Salyer, T. Miller, M. Blevins	9	14	14	44
Jewish Hosp, Transp Serv, 217 E Chestnut St, Louisville, KY 40202 Ph: (502) 587-4358 Fax: (502) 587-4879 1,2) J. Jones, 2) F.R. Bentley, D. Granger, 3) R. Ouseph, D. Woo, 4) J. Ogle, P. Laudrum, R. Pound, J. Cassin, M. Steele, 5) C. Mattingly, P. Kaiser, N. Bellis, L. Adcock-Oliver, C. Schuhmann	5	7	6*	82

LOUISIANA

	1998	1999	2000	Total
Memorial Medical Center (LSUNO), Transplant Inst, 3535 Bienville, Suite 225 East, New Orleans, LA 70119 Ph: (504) 488-8121 Fax: (504) 488-9672 1,2) J.P. Boudreaux, 2) D.J. Frey, J. Jerius, 3) F. Gonzales, 4) P. Kumar, 5) P. Ryan, C. Stechmann, C. Schrader, D. Radcliff	3	3	2	14

1)=Director, 2)=Tx Surgeons, 3)=Physicians, 4)=Tissue Typers, 5)=TxCoords	1998	1999	2000	Total
Ochsner Foundation Hospital, Multi-Organ Transp Program, 1514 Jefferson Hwy, BH309, New Orleans, LA 70121 Ph: (504) 842-3925 Fax: (504) 842-5746 1,2) J. Eason, 2) G. Loss, 3) J.B. Copley, C.G. Staffeld, 4) G. Stewart, S. Herbert, E.S. Cooper, 5) Bailey, Bouvette, White, Guillera, Stevenson, McNeil	2	4	5	36
Tulane Univ Hosp & Clin, Dept of Surg, SL 22, 1430 Tulane Ave, New Orleans, LA 70112 Ph: (504) 588-5344 Fax: (504) 587-7510 Email: scheng@mailhost.tcs.tulane.edu 1,2) S. Cheng, 2) D. Slakey, 3) T. Hammond, V. Fonseca, 4) K.A. Sullivan, 5) M. White, L. Larmeu, J. Hahn	6	10	9*	75

MARYLAND

	1998	1999	2000	Total
Univ of Maryland Med Sys, Dept of Surg, Organ Transp, 29 S Greene St, Ste 200, Baltimore, MD 21201 Ph: (410) 328-5408 Fax: (410) 328-3837 1) S.T. Bartlett, 2) E. Schweitzer, A. Farney, B. Philosophe, J. Colonna, C. Foster, 3) D. Klassen, M. Weir, P. Light, E. Ramos, L. Cangro, J. Fink, R. Wali, 4) American Red Cross Natl Histo Lab at Univ of Maryland, 5) Evans, Stern, Wilson, Young, Ford, Roberts, Aiken, Lee, Hopkins, Mann	23	14	20	225

MASSACHUSETTS

	1998	1999	2000	Total
Beth Israel Deaconess Med Center, Div Transp, 1 Deaconess Rd, Boston, MA 02215 Ph: (617) 632-9700 Fax: (617) 632-9775 1,2) A.P. Monaco, 2) D. Shaffer, 3) Strom, Brown, Steinman, Kuhlik, Cautley, Derman, Solomon, Williams, 4) New England Organ Bank, 5) M. Hoar, E. Chizan	6	2	0	32
Massachusetts Gen Hosp, Dept of Surg, 32 Fruit St, Boston, MA 02114 Ph: (617) 726-8418 Fax: (617) 726-8137 1,2) H. Auchincloss, 2) A.B. Cosimi, F.L. Delmonico, S. Feng, D. Ko, 3) D. Nathan, 4) D. Fitzpatrick, S. Saidman, 5) S. Noska	3	2	0	47
Univ of Massachusetts Med Ctr, Transplantation, 55 Lake Ave N, S3-709, Worcester, MA 01655 Ph: (508) 856-6202 Fax: (508) 856-3920 1,2) R. Harland, 2) P. Alyvazian, R. Chari, 3) J. Stoff, M. Thompson, P.Y. Fan, D. Mandelbrot, 4) New England Organ Bank, 5) T. Lovewell, P. Bigwood, J. Lane	0	2	1	10

MICHIGAN

	1998	1999	2000	Total
Univ of Michigan Med Ctr, Dept of Gen Surg,Div of Transp, 2926 Taubman Ctr, Box 0331, 1500 E Medical Ctr Dr, Ann Arbor, MI 48109-0331 Ph: (734) 936-5816 Fax: (734) 763-3187 Email: janco@umich.edu 1,2) J.C. Magee, 2) D.A. Campbell, Jr, R. Merion, J.D. Punch, S.M. Rudich, J. Arenas, 3) A. Leichtman, A. Ojo, D. Cibrik, B. Kaplan, H. Meier-Kriesche, 4) J. Baker, 5) M. Fox, S. Hutmacher, A. Moloney, J. Novak	15	9	4	128
St John Hosp Med Ctr, Transp Surg, Prof Bldg II, Ste 174, 22101 Moross, Detroit, MI 48236 Ph: (313) 343-3048 Fax: (313) 343-7349 1,2) H.K. Oh, 3) R. Provenzano, 4) D. Levin, 5) N. Satmary, K. Heckman, C. McQuerry	3	2	1	29

MINNESOTA

	1998	1999	2000	Total
Fairview Univ Med Ctr, The Transp Ctr, 516 Delaware St SE, MMC 482 Mayo, Minneapolis, MN 55455 Ph: (612) 625-5115 Fax: (612) 625-2190 1,2) D.E.R. Sutherland, 2) A. Humar, R. Kandaswamy, R. Gruessner, 3) Hering, Daniels, Manske, Rosenberg, 4) H. Noreen, D. McKinley, N. Hendrickson, 5) C. Garvey, P. Halvorsen, C. Trettin, M. Drangstveit, E. Norris	44	54	45	528
Mayo Clinic-Rochester Methodist Hosp, Transplant Center, 200 1st St, SW, Rochester, MN 55905 Ph: (507) 266-8731 Fax: (507) 266-2810 1,2) M.D. Stegall, 2) S. Sterioff, S. Nyberg, M. Prieto, M. Ishitani, 3) Gloor, Larson, Schwab, Torres, Velosa, Griffin, 4) S.B. Moore, S. DeGoey, 5) L. Fix, M. Kreps, D. Dicke-Henslin, C. Bauer, M. Murphy	4	11	25	113

MISSOURI

	1998	1999	2000	Total
St Louis Univ Hosp, Abdom Organ Transp, 3635 Vista Ave at Grand, PO Box 15250, St Louis, MO 63110-0250 Ph: (314) 577-8867 Fax: (314) 268-5133 1,2) P.J. Garvin, 2) H. Soloman, C. Varma, 3) B. Bastani, 4) K. Riordan, 5) Hoff, Carter, Kirkpatrick, Aridge, Lindsey, Johns, Maxfield, Nagel	10	7	12	160

1)=Director, 2)=Tx Surgeons, 3)=Physicians, 4)=Tissue Typers, 5)=TxCoords	1998	1999	2000	Total
NEBRASKA				
Nebraska Health Systems, Clarkson Hosp-Univ Hosp, Kidney/Pancreas Transpl Office, 987555 Nebraska Med Center, Omaha, NE 68198-7555 Ph: (402) 552-2440 Fax: (402) 552-3052 2) R. Taylor, A. Langnas, B. Shaw, D. Sudan, K. Iyer, 3) Hammeke, Groggel, Ranga, Guirguis, 4) J. Wisecarver, R. Rubocki, S. Shepard, 5) S. Miller, T. Baker, M.E. Krobot, C. Lykke, K. McAnally, Frisbie, Livers	16	9	14	184
NEVADA				
NVUM-Univ Med Ctr, Transp Serv, 1800 W Charleston Blvd, Las Vegas, NV 89102 Ph: (702) 383-2224 Fax: (702) 383-3035 1,2) G. Shen, 3) J. Snyder, 4) C. Lively, 5) L. Scott, P. Hess	3	0	1	10
NEW JERSEY				
St Barnabas Med Ctr, Renal Transp Dept, E Wing-Ste 303, Old Short Hills Rd, Livingston, NJ 07039 Ph: (973) 322-5938 Fax: (973) 322-8465 1,3) S. Mulgaonkar, 2) S. Geffner, 3) L. Bonomini, G. Friedman, P. DeFranco, N. Lyman, M.G. Jacobs, N. Shah, 4) C. Pancoska, 5) P. Lipere, L. Bogert	7	10	9*	48
NEW YORK				
Albany Med College, Sectn of Transp, A-61-GE, 47 New Scotland Ave, Albany, NY 12208 Ph: (518) 262-5614 Fax: (518) 262-5571 1,2) D. Conti, 2) T. Singh, G. Shen, 3) D. McGoldrick, 4) D. Constantino, A. Hahn, 5) F. Taft	5	3	2*	28
Mt Sinai Med Ctr, Recanati/Miller Transp Insti, Box 1104, One Gustave Levy Pl, New York, NY 10029 Ph: (212) 241-8086 Fax: (212) 426-2015 1) J. Bromberg, 2) R. Sung, S. Ames, 3) B. Murphy, E. Akalin, V. Sehgal, 4) M. Fotino, 5) L. Daly, K. McKeough, C. Derrien, R. Ifrah, M. Gonzalez	9	11	10	53
New York Hosp,Cornell Med Ctr, Dept Of Surgery, 525 E 68th Street, Room M204, New York, NY 10021 Ph: (212)517-3099 Fax: (212)517-4762 Email: mkinkhab@surgery.med.cornell.edu 1,2) M. Kinkhabwala, 2) W. Stubenbord, S. Kapur, 3) D. Serur, 4) M. Suthanthiran, M. Fotino, 5) R. Billman, L. Johnson, E. Carey, J. Hambleton, M. Charlton	17	12	5*	53
Strong Mem Hosp, Dept of Surg/Med, 601 Elmwood Ave, Rochester, NY 14642 Ph: (716) 275-5875 Fax: (716) 271-3394 1,2) L. Mieles, 3) R. Pabico, 4) M. Coppage, 5) B. Byer, J. Yaeger, M. Kramer, L. Boccardo	7	6	5*	47
SUNY Upstate Med Univ, Dept of Surg, 750 E Adams St, Syracuse, NY 13210 Ph: (315) 464-4550 Fax: (315) 464-6250 1) D.S. Kittur, 2) F.S. Szmalc, 3) Schroeder, Scheinman, Knudson, Izquierdo, Leggat, Narsipur, 4) C. Hubbell, J.B. Henry Sr, 5) M. Leaf, A. Roman, J.B. Henry Jr	2	0	3*	24
NORTH CAROLINA				
Univ of North Carolina Hospitals, Comprehensive Transplant Ctr, 3306 West Wing, 101 Manning Drive, Chapel Hill, NC 27514 Ph: (888) 263-5293 Fax: (919) 966-5697 Email: transplant@unch.unc.edu 1,2) M. Johnson, 2) J. Fair, D. Gerber, K. Andreoni, 3) W. Finn, 4) J. Crawford, J. Schmitz, 5) L. McCoy, L. Friedman, B. Rodegast, L. Scott	8	2	3	27
Duke Univ Med Ctr, Dept of Surgery, Box 3522, Erwin Rd, Durham, NC 27710 Ph: (919) 668-1856 Fax: (919) 681-7508 Email: kuo00004@mc.duke.edu 1,2) P.C. Kuo, 2) J. Tuttle-Newhall, B. Collins, R. Bollinger, 3) M. Feinglos, S. Smith, P. Conlon, D, Butterly, 4) F. Ward, N. Reinsmoen, 5) J. Thompson, L. Hicks, C. Boone	16	17	15	162
OHIO				
Univ of Cincinnati Coll of Med, Dept of Medicine, 231 Bethesda Ave, Cincinnati, OH 45267-0585 Ph: (513) 584-7001 Fax: (513) 584-5571 Email: zavalaey@healthall.com 1,2) E.S. Woodle, 2) J.W. Alexander, R. Munda, J. Buell, M. Hanaway, 3) M.R. First, R. Peddi, P. Roy-Chaudhury, 4) L. Whitacre, D. Eckels, 5) S. Brown	8	9	6	131

1)=Director, 2)=Tx Surgeons, 3)=Physicians, 4)=Tissue Typers, 5)=TxCoords	1998	1999	2000	Total
Cleveland Clin Fnd, A110 Transplant Center, 9500 Euclid Ave, Cleveland, OH 44195 Ph: (216) 444-4600 Fax: (216) 445-7088 1,2) V. Krishnamurthi, 3) B. Hoogwerf, V. Dennis, 4) D. Cook, 5) M. Lard	11	7	8	56
Univ Hosps of Cleveland, Dept of Surg, 11100 Euclid Ave, Cleveland, OH 44106 Ph: (216) 844-3689 Fax: (216) 844-7764 1,2) J.A. Schulak, 2) D.S. Seaman, C.T. Siegel, 3) D. Hricik, T. Knauss, 4) N. Greenspan, 5) M. Bartucci, J. Arnovitz, H. Dorsey	15	11	12	162
The Ohio State Univ Hosps, Dept of Surg, Div of Transp, 363 Means Hall, 1654 Upham Dr, Columbus, OH 43210 Ph: (614) 293-8545 Fax: (614) 293-4541 1,2) R.M. Ferguson, 2) M.L. Henry, E. Elkhammas, E. Davies, G. Bumgardner, R. Pelletier, 3) Bay, Hebert, Cosio, Middendorf, Nahman, Falkenhain, Pesevento, 4) P. Adams, 5) B. Miller, L. McDonnell	35	32	35*	491

OREGON

	1998	1999	2000	Total
Oregon Health Sci Univ/PVAMC, Sec of Liver/Pancreas Transp, 3181 SW Sam Jackson Park Rd, L 590, Portland, OR 97201-3098 Ph: (503) 494-7810 Fax: (503) 494-5292 1,2) J. Rabkin, 2) S. Orloff, 3) L. Loriaux, A. Demattos, 4) D.J. Norman, 5) L. Hanson	8	9	4*	66

PENNSYLVANIA

	1998	1999	2000	Total
Univ Hosp Penn State Coll, Milton S.Hershey Med Ctr, Sec of Transp, Dept of Surg, 500 University Dr, Hershey, PA 17033 Ph: (717) 531-5852 Fax: (717) 531-6579 1,2) H.C. Yang, 2) M. Holman, J.D. Arenas, 3) J. Cheung, J. Diamond, N. Ahsan, M. Waybill, Groff, 4) P.J. Romano, 5) Scouten, Norton, Bollinger, Kratzer, Farrell, Nafziger-Eberly, Ulsh	0	8	13*	50
Albert Einstein Med Ctr, Sec of Kidney/Pancreas Transpl, 5401 Old York Rd, Klein 505, Philadelphia, PA 19141 Ph: (215) 456-6933 Fax: (215) 456-6716 1) F. Badosa, 2) S.L. Yang, 3) R. Raja, 4) R. McAlack, 5) L. Lerner, K. Austin, C. Morrison	5	2	2	84
Hahnemann Univ Hosp Tenet, Dept of Surg, Div of Transp, Broad & Vine Sts, MS 417, Philadelphia, PA 19102 Ph: (215) 762-1857 Fax: (215) 762-1621 1,2) M.S.A. Kumar, 3) J. Brezin, P. Lyons, 4) M. McCreary, 5) M. McSorley, K. Phillips	2	4	1*	43
Hosp of the Univ of Pennsylvania, The Penn Transplant Center, 3400 Spruce St, Philadephia, PA 19104 Ph: (215) 662-6200 Fax: (215) 349-5096 Email: diane.jakobowski@uphs.upenn.edu 1,2) C. Barker, 2) A. Naji, K. Brayman, J. Markmann, 3) R.A. Grossman, R. Bloom, K. Mange, 4) M. Kamoun, J. Kearns, 5) T. Holland, C. Hooper, J. Eyer, M. Palanjian, K. Kilgarriff, C. Naus	13	10	16	146
Temple Univ Hosp, Transplant Surg, 3401 N Broad St, PP4, Philadelphia, PA 19140 Ph: (215) 707-8889 Fax: (215) 707-8894 1,2) S. Guy, 3) C. Bastl, P. Silva, 4) S. Leech, 5) G. Libetti, P. Sellers, M. McSorley, K. Wuest	4	3	1	8
Allegheny Gen Hosp, Dept of Surg, Transp Serv, 320 E North Ave, Pittsburgh, PA 15212 Ph: (412) 359-6800 Fax: (412) 359-4721 1,2) D.D. Nghiem, 3) B.J. Carpenter, R. Marcus, 4) S. Hsia, 5) B.A. Kijanka, M.A. Breckenridge, K. Kinter	7	6	8*	71
UPMC-Presbyterian, Starzl Transplantation Inst, 4 Falk Clinic, 3601 Fifth Ave, Pittsburgh, PA 15213 Ph: (412) 648-3200 Fax: (412) 648-3085 1,2) T.E. Starzl, 1,2) J.J. Fung, 2) R. Corry, R. Shapiro, V. Scantlebury, T. Hakala, M. Jordan, C. Vivas, 3) S. Kusne, J. McCauley, 4) R. Duquesnoy, A. Zeevi, 5) D. Good, H. Woods, J. Lignoski	32	35	19	164

SOUTH CAROLINA

	1998	1999	2000	Total
Med Univ of South Carolina, Dept of Surg, 171 Ashley Ave, Charleston, SC 29425 Ph: (803) 792-3553 Fax: (803) 792-8596 1,2) P.R. Rajagopalan, 2) P. Baliga, K. Chavin, J. Rogers, 3) M. Budisavljevic, 4) J. Jakubek, 5) T. Sill, G. Magwood, L. Hildebrand, E. Thurman, J. Dawson, R. Hogarth	9	16	17*	96

TENNESSEE

	1998	1999	2000	Total
Johnson City Med Ctr Hosp, Dept of Transp, 408 State at Franklin Rd, Ste 46, Johnson City, TN 37604 Ph: (423) 431-6164 Fax: (423) 928-6795 1,2) R.M. Weingart, 2) P.N. Joshi, 3) C.F. Wiegand, F. Montenegro, L. Panus, 4) University of Tenn-Knoxville, 5) L. Walker, K. Kelley, J. Hawkins	5	6	4	23

1)=Director, 2)=Tx Surgeons, 3)=Physicians, 4)=Tissue Typers, 5)=TxCoords	1998	1999	2000	Total
TEXAS				
Baylor Univ Med Ctr, Transp Serv, Dept of Surg, 3500 Gaston Ave, Dallas, TX 75246 Ph: (214) 820-2050 Fax: (214) 820-4527 1,2) G. Klintmalm, 2) R. Goldstein, M. Levy, E. Molmenti, C. Fasola, 3) T. Gonwa, M. Mai, L. Melton, 4) D. Smith, 5) R. Manley, C. Johnson, P. Fertig, K. Roman, S. Hashim	5	12	8*	34
Methodist Med Ctr, Transp Serv, PO Box 655999, 1441 N Beckley, Dallas, TX 75265-5999 Ph: (214) 947-1800 Fax: (214) 941-8061 1,3) P. Vergne-Marini, 2) G. Trevino, R.M. Dickerman, 3) K. Brinker, D. Nesser, R. Velez, 4) G. Land, 5) A. Louzau, R. Bunton, J. McDonald, C. Cannon	7	13	9	103
Parkland Memorial Hosp, Transp Clin, 5201 Harry Hines Blvd, Dallas, TX 75235-7747 Ph: (214) 590-5656 Fax: (214) 590-6929 1,2) S. Li, 2) B. Nibhanupudy, 3) P. Raskin, C. Lu, 4) P. Stastny, 5) B. Martin, L. Coorpender, D. Sexton, J. Grammer	7	3	1*	53
Univ of Texas Med Branch, Dept of Surg, 301 University Blvd, Route 0533, Galveston, TX 77551-0533 Ph: (409) 772-2412 Fax: (409) 747-7364 Email: kris.gugliuzza@utmb.edu 1,2) K.K. Gugliuzza, 2) J.A. Daller, 3) J. Rice, T.J. Ahuja, R. Remmers, R. Beach, 4) S. Vaidya, 5) M. Byrd, J. Boughton, D. Devine, Armendariz, Medina, Upchurch, Parhan	8	12	10*	121
Baylor Coll of Med, Methodist Hosp, Multi-Organ Transp Ctr, 6565 Fannin-SM 447, Houston, TX 77030 Ph: (713) 790-2501 Fax: (713) 793-1335 1,2) W.G. Guerriero, 2) W.R. Rosenberg, 3) R. Johnson, 4) G. Rodey, 5) L. Coomes-Hill, C, Matula	0	3	5*	45
Univ of Texas-Hermann Hosp, Dept of Surg-Organ Transp, 6411 Fannin, Houston, TX 77030 Ph: (713) 500-7415 Fax: (713) 704-6195 1,2) R. Knight, 2) S. Katz, 3) N. Rahman, K. Finkel, 4) R.H. Kerman, 5) S. Zela	7	6	4	21
Methodist Specialty & Transp Hosp, Renal/Pancreas Prog, 8026 Floyd Curl Dr, San Antonio, TX 78229 Ph: (210) 575-8400 Fax: (210) 575-8420 1,2) F.H. Wright Jr, 2) M. Schultz, 3) S. Rosenblatt, 4) Southwest Immuno, 5) McFarlin, Farias, Leonhardt, Richardson, McNeill, Hudson, Galliardt	1	2	4	8
Univ of Texas HSC, Med Ctr Hosp, Organ Transp Prog, 7703 Floyd Curl Dr, San Antonio, TX 78229-3900 Ph: (210) 567-5777 Fax: (210) 567-6608 1,2) R. Esterl Jr, 2) G.A. Halff, K. Washburn, F. Ciqarroa, 3) D. Riley, B. Kashinath, 4) P. Blackwell, K. Rocha, 5) A. Lopez, L. Nichols, M. Buecher, C. Castillo, A. Vasquez	4	8	6	25
UTAH				
LDS Hosp, Dept of Transp, 8th Ave & C St, Salt Lake City, UT 84143 Ph: (801) 408-3090 Fax: (801) 408-3098 1,2) L.P. Belnap, 2) J. Sorensen, M.H. Stevens, 3) R.C. Lambert, J.B. Stinson, E. Thor, R. Cline, G. Rabetoy, M. McAnulty, 4) T. Fuller, 5) J. Arata, K. Baker, G. Martin	6	10	8*	123
VIRGINIA				
Univ of Virginia HSC, Transp Ctr, Box 265-Univ Station, Charlottesville, VA 22908 Ph: (804) 924-8604 Fax: (804) 982-0099 1,2) T. Pruett, 2) R.G. Sawyer, H. Sanfey, 3) P.L. Lobo, R. Isaacs, 4) C. Spencer, J. Guan, C. Davis, 5) B. Shephard, W. Simmons	3	4	6	64
Transp Ctr of Fairfax Hosp, Dept of Surg, 3300 Gallows Rd, Falls Church, VA 22046 Ph: (703) 698-2986 Fax: (703) 698-2797 Email: johann.jonsson@inova.com 1,2) J. Jonsson, 2) T. Shaver, D. Kelly, 3) R. Mackow, 4) W. Ward, 5) P. Disanto, Hicks, B. Erikson, E. Skipper, V. Charity	7	8		40
WASHINGTON				
Swedish Medical Center, Organ Transplant Program, 1120 Cherry St, Ste 400, Seattle, WA 98104 Ph: (206) 386-3660 Fax: (206) 386-3644 1,2) W.H. Marks, 2) L.S. Florence, 3) B. O'Neill, D. Perkinson, 4) Puget Sound Blood Ctr, K. Nelson, 5) S. Canniff, D. Gould, K. Ross, A. Alering, M. Kurtz	2	1	3	10
Univ of Washington Med Ctr, Transp Services, 1959 N.E. Pacific St, Box 356174, Seattle, WA 98195 Ph: (206) 598-6700 Fax: (206) 598-6706 Email: cmarsh@u.washington.edu 1,2) C.L. Marsh, 2) J.D. Perkins, B. Stevens, P. Healey, L. Wrenshall, A. Levy, C. Kuhr, 3) Davis, Hirsch, Couser, Bomsztyk, Ahmad, Muczynski, Shankland, 4) K. Nelson (Puget Sound Blood Ctr), 5) P. Forg, C. Arp, C. Conover, D. Mullenix	21	17	14	205

KIDNEY/PANCREAS

1)=Director, 2)=Tx Surgeons, 3)=Physicians, 4)=Tissue Typers, 5)=TxCoords	1998	1999	2000	Total
Virginia Mason Med Ctr, Div of Renal/Pancreas Transp, 1100 9th Ave, C7-Neph, Seattle, WA 98111 Ph: (206) 341-0925 Fax: (206) 341-0886 1,3) R.L. Wilburn, 2) T.R. Hefty, F. Govier, T. Pritchett, R. Weissman, 3) C. Thompson, C. Cryst, M. Cooper, 4) K. Nelson, 5) M. Cressman, J. Buck, W. Ryan	7	6	8*	53

WISCONSIN

Univ of Wisconsin-Madison, Transp Ofc H4/785, Clin Sci Ctr, 600 Highland Ave, Madison, WI 53792 Ph: (608) 263-1385 Fax: (608) 262-5624 1,2,4) H. Sollinger, 2) A. D'Alessandro, S. Knechtle, J. Odorico, Y. Becker, 3) J. Pirsch, B. Becker, 5) Groshek, Armbrust, Nelson, Jaeger, Schappe, Shanahan, Miller	51	55	52*	673
Froedtert Mem Lutheran Hosp, Med Coll of Wisconsin, Dept of Transp Surg, 9200 W Wisconsin Ave, Milwaukee, WI 53226 Ph: (414) 456-6920 Fax: (414) 456-6222 1,2) C.P. Johnson, 2) M.B. Adams, A.M. Roza, 3) G. Sonnenberg, 4) D. Eckels, Blood Center of S.E. Wisconsin, 5) P. Walczak, C. Weickert, L. Venturi, S, Klennr, D. Pierce	15	16	13	161

ARGENTINA

Hosp Italiano de Buenos Aires, Dept of Surg, Gascon 450, Arregui 4111, Buenos Aires 1181 Ph: (54)1 981-1537 Fax: (54)1 958-2200 Email: pargiba@hitalba.edu.ar 1) P.F. Argibay, 2) J. Pekolj, C. Giudice, A. Domenech, S.H. Hyon, 3) R. Groppa, S. Algranatti, 4) N. Prigoshin, 5) L. Walsh	1	9	6	27

AUSTRALIA

Westmead Hosp, Dept of Surg, Westmead, NSW, 2145 Ph: (61)29 845 6962 Fax: (61)29 633 9351 Email: paul-robertson@wsahs.nsw.gov.au 1,2) R.D.M. Allen, 2) H.M.H. Lau, 3) J.R. Chapman, P. O'Connell, B. Nankivell, 4) Red Cross Tissue Typ Serv, 5) P.R. Robertson	14	12	18	130

AUSTRIA

Univ Hosp, Dept of Transp Surg, Anichstrasse 35, Innsbruck, 6020 Ph: (43)512 504-2603 Fax: (43)512 504-2605 1,2) R. Margreiter, 2) A. Koenigsrainer, B. Spechtenhauser, W. Steurer, 4) D. Schoenitzer, 5) H. Fetz, P. Schobel	24	26	30	221
Allegemeines Hosp, Univ of Vienna, Dept of Surg, Transp Ctr, Wahringer Gurtel 18-20, 1090 Vienna Ph: (43)1 40400 4000 Fax: (43)1 40400 6872 1,2) F. Muhlbacher, 2) R. Steininger, 3) J. Kovarik, 4) W. Mayr, 5) M. Bodingbauel, R. Asari	5	1	0	23

BELGIUM

Clin Univ Saint Luc, Dept of Transp, 10 Ave Hippocrate, 1200 Brussels Ph: (32)2 7642207 Fax: (32)2 7707858 Email: squifflet@chir.ucl.ac.be 1,2) J.P. Squifflet, 2) M. Mourad, J. Malaise, 3) Y. Pirson, B. Vandeleen, 4) D. Latinne, 5) C. Lecomte, V. Dumont, P. van Ormelingen	3	5	1	67
Ctr Hosp Univ-Liege, Dept of Surg/Transp, Domaine Univ du Sart-Tilman-B35, B-4000 Liege Ph: (32)43 667206 Fax: (32)43 667517 1,2) M. Meurisse, 2) P. Honore, O. Detry, A. DeRoover, 3) M. Beaujean, 4) C. Bouillenne, 5) M.H. Delbouille, M.F. Hans	0	3	0	13

BRAZIL

Beneficencia Portuguese Hosp, Hepato-Hepatology & Organ Tx, Rua Maestro Carsim 377,cj 75, Rua Maestro Carsim 769,Bloco V,2 SS, Sao Paulo, 01323-001 Ph: 55-11-2831450 Fax: 55-11-37714769 Email: marcelo-perosa@uol.com.br 1,2) M. Perosa, 1,2) T. Genzini, 2) P. Rodrigues, A. Gil, 3) I. Noronha, H. Abensur, M.R. Araujo, J.D.Romno Jr. , 5) F.L. Pandullo	0	5	28	43
Santa Casa De Porto Alegre, Serv De Transp (Enf 2), Praca Dom Feliciano S/N, Porto Alegre, RS 90020-160 Ph: (55)51 226-0848 Fax: (55)51 228-0496 1,2) V.D. Garcia, 2) G. Cantisani, P. Vitola, 3) J.J. Bianchini, J.C. Goldani, A.E. Bittar, E. Keitel, 4) J. Neumann, 5) N. Hoefelmann	1	0	1	11

1)=Director, 2)=Tx Surgeons, 3)=Physicians, 4)=Tissue Typers, 5)=TxCoords	1998	1999	2000	Total
CANADA				
Vancouver Hosp, c/o British Columbia Transp Sc, 3th Flr W Tower, 555 W 12th Ave, Vancouver, BC V5Z 3X7 Ph: (604) 877-2240 Fax: (604) 877-2111 1) Mr B. Barrable, 2) R.M. Meloche, M. Nigro, 3) J. Shapiro, 4) B. Draney, 5) J. Ritchie	8	7	8	60
Univ of Calgary Foothills Med Ctr, Div of Tx, Dept of Surg, G33, 1403 29th St NW, Calgary, Alberta, T2N 2T9 Ph: (403) 670-4266 Fax: (403) 270-8431 Email: serdar.yilmaz@crha-health.ab.ca 1,2) S. Yilmaz, 2) A. Barama, 3) F. Sepandj, J. Klassen, L. Tibbles, K. McLaughlin, 4) R. McKenna, 5) S. Buckle, M. Miller	7	11	7	25
Royal Victoria Hospital, Surgery, 687 Pine Avenue West, Montreal, QC H3A 1A1 Ph: (514) 842-1231 Fax: (514) 843-1503 1,2) P. Metrakos, 3) M. Cantarovich, R. Mangel, 4) P. Imperial, R. Schreier, C. McIntyre, 5) M. Poloni, M. Fortier	3	4		8
Queen Elizabeth II Health Sci Cnt, Multi Organ Transp Prog, 1278 Tower Rd, Halifax, NS B3H 2Y9 Ph: (902) 473-5500 Fax: (902) 473-4423 1,2) A.S. MacDonald, 2) H. Bitter-Suermann, V. McAlister, P. Belitsky, J.G. Lawen, 3) K. Jindal, M. West, K. West, B. Kiberd, 4) S. Eastwood, M. Decoste, K. West, 5) R. Leblanc, J. Cruickshank	4	4	7	30
Hosp Notre Dame, Dept of Transp Surg, 1560 Sherbrooke Est, Montreal, PQ H2L 4M1 Ph: (514) 281-6000 x6605 Fax: (514) 896-4736 Email: pierre.daloze.chum@ssss.gouv.qc.ca 1,2) P. Daloze, 2) C. Smeesters, S. Busque, 3) H. Beauregard, 4) Inst Armand Frappier, Montreal, 5) Quebec Transp	0	3	2	27
CZECH REPUBLIC				
Inst for Clin and Exper Med, Transp Ctr, Dept of Surg, Videnska 800, 14000 Prague 4 Ph: 420 2 425-8237 Fax: 420 2 472-2255 1) S. Vitko, 2) M. Adamec, 3) F. Saudek, 4) E. Ivaskova, 5) E. Pokorna, E. Laszikova, V. Charova, M. Skachova	20	19	18	157
FRANCE				
Univ Hosp of Bicetre, Dept of Neph/Uro, 78 Av du General Leclerc, Kremlin-Bicetre Ced, 94275 Ph: (33)1 4521 2722 Fax: (33)1 4521 2116 1,2) B. Charpentier, 1,3) G. Benoit, 2) J. Bellamy, P. Blanchet, 3) C. Hiesse, A. Durrbach, F. Kriaa, 4) C. Raffoux, D. Charron, 5) L. Joseph, J. Decaris	4	1		43
Lapeyronie Hosp, Dept of Neph, 555 Rte de Ganges, Montpellier Cedex, 34059 Ph: (33)67 338475 Fax: (33)67 412599 1,3) G. Mourad, 2) J.P. Carabalona, 4) J. Seignalet, 5) A. Boularan	0	2	1	24
Ctr Hosp Reg et Univ-Nancy, Hosp de Brabois, Dept of Neph, 54511 Vandoeuvre, Nancy Cedex Ph: (33)83 153163 Fax: (33)83 153531 1,3) M. Kessler, 2) Ph. Mangin, P. Boissel, 3) E. Renoult, 4) P. Perrier, 5) F. Jacob	1	4	2	18
Hotel Dieu-Univ Nantes, Dept of Neph/Clin Immun, 1 Pl Alexis Ricordeau, Nantes Cedex, 44035 Ph: (33)240 083303 Fax: (33)240 084649 1) J.P. Soulillou, 2) G. Karam, C. Glemain, 3) D. Cantarovich, 4) J.M. Bignon, 5) J.N. LeSant	18	13	16	191
Hosp Saint-Louis, Serv De Neph, Lavande 3, 1 Av Claude Vellefaux, Paris, 75010 Ph: (33)1 424 99631 Fax: (33)1 424 99606 1) Ch. Legendre, 2) A. LeDuc, P. Teillac, F. Deseranchamps, 3) J. Bedrossian, E. Thervet, F. Martinez, 4) C. Suberbielle, 5) F. Roussin	5	4	5	14
La Pitie Salpetriere, Dept of Uro, 83 Bd de l'Hopital, Paris Cedex 13, 75013 Ph: (33)1 42 177111 Fax: (33)1 42 177112 1) F. Richard, 2) M.O. Bitker, B. Barrou, 3) Mouquet, Benalia, Ourhama, 4) C. Suberbielle, 5) M. Tallier, S. Jehan, N. Cornillot	6	6	5	59
Ctr Hosp Hautepierre, Transp Unit, Ave Moliere, Strasbourg, 67098 Ph: (33)88 127289 Fax: (33)88 127286 1,2) P. Wolf, 2) C. Meyer, M. Audet, 3) B. Ellero, M.L. Jaegle, 4) M.M. Tongio, 5) C. Becker, V. Fuss	2	5	3	60

1)=Director, 2)=Tx Surgeons, 3)=Physicians, 4)=Tissue Typers, 5)=TxCoords	1998	1999	2000	Total
GERMANY				
University Hospital Bochum, Knappschafts-Krankenhaus, Dept of Surgery, In Der Schornau 23-25, Bochum-NRW, 44892 Ph: (49)234-299-3260 Fax: (49)234-299-3269 1) W.O. Bechstein, 2) K. Kohlhaw, R. Schwarz, 4) H. Grosse-Wilde, 5) A. Deiss	27	22	13	166
University Med Sch Hosp, Dept of Surg, Sigmund-Freud Str 25, Bonn, 53105 Ph: (49)228 287-5109 Fax: (49)228 287-4856 1) A. Hirner, 1) T. Scuerbouch, 2) J. Kalff, M. Wolff, 3) H.U. Klehr, 5) E. Backhaus, B. Salz, T. Uhr	9	8	3	20
Transplantation Zentrum Koeln, Klinikum Koeln-Merheim, Ostmerheimer Str 200, Cologne 51109 Ph: (49)221 8907-3200 Fax: (49)221 89073335 Email: wolfgang.arns@uni-koeln.de 1) M. Weber, H.Troidl,C.A.Baldamus, A.H. Hoelscher 2) A. Paul, T. Beckurts, 3) W. Arns, M. Pollok, 4) R. Doerner, 5) Deutsche Stiftung Organtransplantation	13	11	19	53
Univ Clin Essen, Dept of Gen Surg, Hufelandstr 55, Essen, 45122 Ph: (49)201 723-1140 Fax: (49)201 723-5946 1,2) C.E. Broelsch, 2) M. Malago, G. Testa, K. Albrechi, 3) T. Philipp, G. Gerken, 4) H. Grosse-Wilde, 5) F. Weber	3			20
Univ Hosp Freiburg, Dept of Surg, Organ Transp, Hugstetter Strabe 55, Freiburg, G-79106 Ph: (49)761 270-2732 Fax: (49)761 278-970 Email: bluemke@cu11.ukl.uni-freiburg.de 1,2) G. Kirste, 2) P. Pisarki, 3) G. Walz, 4) H. Lang, 5) M. Blumke	7	13	18	46
Univ Clin Eppendorf-Hamburg, Dept of Surg, Martinistr 52, 2000 Hamburg 20 Ph: (49)40 4717 6136 Fax: (49)40 4717 3431 1,2) X. Rogiers, 2) M. Gundlach, D. Broring, 3) F. Rinninger, R.A.K. Stahl, 4) P. Kuhnl, C. Lolinger, Wenzel, 5) T. Karbe, R. Kutemeier, S. Wannoff, C. Clausen	0	5	3	13
Med Hochschule Hannover, Dept of Abdom/Transp Surg, Konstanty Gutschow Str 8, W-3000 Hannover 61 Ph: (49)511 532 6534 Fax: (49)511 532 4010 1,2) J. Klempnauer, 2) R. Luck, B. Nashan, Th. Becker, 3) H. Haller, A. Schwarz, G. Offner, J. Strehlau, 4) R. Blascyk, 5) G. Guernatis, S. Tietze, G. Oelmann	0	10	21	57
Klin Mannheim, Univ of Heidelberg, Dept of Surg, V. Med Ctr, Theodor Kutzer Ufer 1-3, Mannheim, 68135 Ph: (49)62 383-2674 Fax: (49)62 383-3804 1) F.J. van de Woude, 1) S.Post, 2) S. Post, J. Sturm, 3) P. Schnuelle, 4) G. Opelz, 5) Ch. Krenzel		1	2	3
Univ Hosp of Marburg, Dept of Int Med, Baldinger Str, 35033 Marburg Ph: (49)6421 286 6480 Fax: (49)6421 2866365 Email: transpla@mailer.uni-marburg.de 1,2) H. Lange, 2) M. Rothmund, A. Hellinger, J. Geks, A. Zielke, 3) H. Ebel, U. Kuhlmann, 4) E. Wollmer, A. Gorski, 5) U. Heck, M. Bauer, S. Moos	2	5	7	34
Klin Grosshadern Univ of Munich, Div of Transp Surg, Marchioninistr 15, Munich, 81377 Ph: (49)89 7095 2706 Fax: (49)89 700 4160 Email: walterland@aol.com 1,2) W. Land, 2) W.D. Illner, J. Theodorakis, H. Arbogast, 3) R. Landgraf, 4) E.A. Albert, S. Scholz, 5) C. Schulz	31	22	31	317
Univ of Rostock Med Faculty, Clin of Surgery, Schillingallee, Rostock, D-18057 Ph: (49)381 494 6000 Fax: (49)381 494 6002 1) U. Hopt, 2) W. Schareck, 3) R. Schmidt, 4) R. Barz, 5) F.P. Nitschke	19	20	19	76
Univ of Tuebingen, Dept of Surg, Hoppe-Seyler Str 3, Transp Ctr, Tuebingen, 72076 Ph: (49)70 7129 86600 Fax: (49)70 714 4532 1) H.D. Becker, 2) R. Viebahn, K. Dietrich, 3) R. Schmulling, T. Risler, G. Overkamp, 4) Northoff, Wernet, 5) Fischer-Frohlich	7	10	9	150
HUNGARY				
Pecs Univ, Faculty of Medicine, Dept of Surgery, Ifjusag u.13, PECS, H 7624 Ph: (36) 72 53 6128 Fax: (36) 72 53 6128 Email: kalmar@iseb.pote.hu 1,2) K. Kalmar-Nagy, 2) P. Szakaly, A. Papp, 3) I. Wittmann, J. Baumann, 4) M. Paal Uherkovichne, 5) K. Kalmar, I. Kovats	2	2	7	11
ISRAEL				
Beilinson Med Ctr, Dept of Organ Transp, Zabotinski 66, Petach Tikva, 49100 Ph: (972)3 922-4285 Fax: (972)3 924-9680 1) Z. Shapira, 2) A. Yussim, E. Sharabani, N. Natan, E. Mor, 3) S. Lustig, 4) T. Klein, 5) R. Michowiz	1	1	1	16

1)=Director, 2)=Tx Surgeons, 3)=Physicians, 4)=Tissue Typers, 5)=TxCoords	1998	1999	2000	Total
ITALY				
Azienda Ospedale San Martino, Dept of Transp, Largo Rosanna Benzi, 10, Genova, 16132 Ph: (39)010 5553862 Fax: (39)010 5556772 Email: itc@transplant.smartino.ge.it 1) U. Valente, 2) V. Arcuri, M. Beatini, M. Bertocchi, I. Fontana, G.V. Tommasi, 3) Cannella, DeFerrari, Traverso, Viviani, Messa, Siani, Ardizzone, 4) G. Sirchia, A. Nocera, 5) C. Pizzi, A. Gianelli Castiglione, S. Pisanu, M. Tognoni, C. Gualeni	5	2	0	38
Inst San Raffaele Hosp, Univ of Milano, Dept of Med, Via Olgettina 60, Milano, 20132 Ph: (39)02 2643 2805 Fax: (39)02 2643 7788 1,2) G. Pozza, 2) V. DiCarlo, 3) A. Secchi, 4) G. Sirchia, 5) A. Secchi	17	9	13	142
Univ di Padova, 1st di Chir Generale II, Ospedale Guistinianeo, Via Guistinianeo, 2, 35128 Padova Ph: (39)49 821 3151 Fax: (39)49 750919 Email: traprepa@uxl.umipd.it 1) E. Ancona, 2) P. Rigotti, 3) F. Marchini, 4) V. Fagiolo, 5) NIT (Nord Italia Transp)	8	4	7	38
Univ of Pisa, Osp di Cisanello, Inst of Gen Surg, Via Paradisa 2, 56124 Pisa Ph: (39)50 596820 Fax: (39)50 543692 Email: uboggi@patchir.med.unipi.it 1,2,5) F. Mosca, 2) U. Boggi, 3) G. Rizzo, 4) G. Rizzo	7	7	14	30
Treviso General Hosp, Transplant Ctr, Piazza Ospedale, 31100 Treviso Ph: (39)0422 322727 Fax: (39)0422 322657 Email: avianello@ulss.tv.it 1,3) G. Calconi, 1.2) G. DiFalco, 2) G. Caldato, G.F. Mora, 3) Scaldaferri, M.C. Maresca, A. Vianello, 4) M. Mordacchini, L. Moro, 5) D. Milani	1	0		8
KOREA				
Yonsei Univ Coll of Med, Severance Hosp, Dept of Surg, 134 Shinchon-Dong, Sudaemoon-ku, Seoul 120-752 Ph: (82)2 361-5545 Fax: (82)2 365-3069 1,2) K. Park, 2) S.I. Kim, 3) D.S. Han, H.Y. Lee, K.H. Choi, S.W. Kang, K. Huh, H. Lee, S. Lim, Y. Song, 4) H.J. Kim, 5) K.O. Cheon, H.J. Kim	2	2	1	6
MEXICO				
Especialidades C.M.N. Siglo XXI, Transp Unit, Av Cuauhtemoc 330 Col Doctores, Heriberto Frias 112-8 CP 03020, Mexico City, DF 06720 Ph: (52) 5 538 4747 Fax: (52) 5 264 8711 Email: jlmelchoro@compuserve.com.mx 1) H. Aguirre-Gas, 2) C. Gracida, A. Lopez, J. Cancino, M. Sanmartin, 3) J.L. Melchor, A. Ibarra, 4) E. Romano	0	1		9
NETHERLANDS				
Univ Hosp Groningen, Dept of Surg, Hanzeplein 1, 9713 GZ Groningen Ph: (31)50 361 6161 Fax: (31)50 361 4873 Email: b.s.g.makkes@chir.azg.nl 1) R.J. Ploeg, 2) Van Schilfgaarde, Porte, Hofker, 3) Van Son, J. Homan, V.D. Heide, 4) S.P.M. Lems, 5) M. ElMoumni, A. Schuur, C.W. Graveland	4	6	6	37
Univ Hosp Leiden, Dept of Surg, PO Box 9600, Leiden, 2300 RC Ph: (31)71 526 4005 Fax: (31)71 526 6746 Email: terpstra@lumc.nl 1) O.T. Terpstra, 2) J. Ringers, A. Baranski, 3) J.S. van der Pijl, J.W. de Fijter, 4) F.H.J. Claas, 5) M.E.G. van Gurp, R. Dam	9	13		121
Univ Hosp Maastricht, Dept of Surg, P Debyelaan 5, PO Box 5800, 6202 AZ Maastricht Ph: (31)43 3877478 Fax: (31)43 3875473 1,2) G. Kootstra, 1,3) J.P. van Hooff, 2) J. Tordoir, P. Kitslaar, 4) E. van den Berg-Loonen, 5) A. Omen, A. Nederskigt		1		31
NORWAY				
Rikshosp-The Nat'l Hosp, Dept of Surg/Med, Oslo, NO-0027 Ph: (47)2307 00 00 Fax: (47)2307 05 10 1) A. Bergan, 2) I. Brekke, P. Pfeffer, 3) P. Fauchald, K. Nordal, 4) E. Thorsby, T. Leivestad, 5) S. Foss, P.A. Bakkan, P.E. Vatsaas, K. Meyer	6	10	7	125

KIDNEY/PANCREAS

1)=Director, 2)=Tx Surgeons, 3)=Physicians, 4)=Tissue Typers, 5)=TxCoords	1998	1999	2000	Total
SWEDEN				
Sahlgrenska Univ Hosp, Dept of Transpl and Liver Surg, su/Sahlgrenska, 41345 Gothenburg Ph: (46)31 3421000 Fax: (46)31 820557 1,2) M. Olausson, 2) L. Mjornstedt, L. Wrammer, O. Ostraat, J. Blomme, 3) G. Nyberg, G. Norden, 4) L. Rydberg, 5) Eriksson, Wolfbrandt	2	1	3	107
Univ Hosp Uppsala, Dept of Transp Surg, Unit 70TD, S-75185 Uppsala Ph: (46)18 664669 Fax: (46)18 559468 1,2) J. Wahlberg, 2) J. Wadstrom, G. Tufveson, F. Duraj, 3) B. Fellstrom, C. Berne, 4) O. Sjoberg, M. Bengtsson, 5) E. Bjorklund, I. Skarp, C. Moller	3	3	4	68
SWITZERLAND				
Univ Hosp Geneva, Dept of Surg, Transp Unit, 24 rue Micheli-du-Crest, 1211 Geneva 14 Ph: (41)22 372-7702 Fax: (41)22 372-7755 1,2) Ph. Morel, 2) J. Oberholzer, J.F. Bolle, 3) M. Leski, N. Von der Weid, J. Philippe, 4) C. Goumaz, 5) F. Roch, N. Decarpentry	0	3	1	15
Univ Hosp Zurich, Dept of Surg, Ramistr 100, Zurich, CH-8091 Ph: (41)1 255 3300 Fax: (41)1 255 4449 Email: clavien@chir.unizh.ch 1) P.A. Clavien, 2) M. Weber, N. Demabines, Z. Kadry, 3) U. Binswanger, 4) M. Weber, 5) P. Seeburger, T. Reh, M. Struker	3	0	4	134
TURKEY				
Akdeniz Univ Med Sch Hosp, Dept of General Surgery, Dumlupinar Bulvari-Kampus, Antalya, 07060 Ph: (90)532 277 1485 Fax: (90)242 227 8837 1) T. Karpuzoglu, 2) N. Oygur, S. Aktan, A. Demirbas, 3) G. Suleymanlar, U. Karayalcin, F. Isitan, I. Suleymanlar, 4) O. Yegin, M. Coskun, 5) N. Kececioglu	1	0		1
UNITED KINGDOM				
Royal Liverpool & Broadgreen Univ, Hosp Trust-Renal Transp Unit, Link Unit 9C, Prescot St, Liverpool, L7 8XP Ph: (44)151 708 0163 Fax: (44)151 706 5819 1,2) R.A. Sells, 2) A. Bakran, M. Brown, 3) J.M. Bone, 4) P. Beals, 5) T. Rhodes, J. Godfrey, E. Linacre	1	1	4	61
St Mary's Hosp, Transp Unit, Praed St, Paddington, London, W2 1NY Ph: (44)171 886 6726 Fax: (44)171 886 1707 1,2) N.S. Hakim, 2) V. Papalois, 3) A. Palmer, D. Taube, T. Cairns, 4) M. Van Dam, N. Browning, 5) J. Griffiths, P. Keenan, V. Morgan	5	13	7	51

KIDNEY/PANCREAS Transplants

	1998	1999	2000	Total
United States	836	844	816	8,135
Foreign	321	350	382	3,406
Total	1,157	1,194	1,198	11,541

KIDNEY/PANCREAS Transplant Centers

United States	89
Foreign	69
Total	158

WORLDWIDE TRANSPLANT CENTER DIRECTORY
PANCREAS TRANSPLANTS

1)=Director, 2)=Tx Surgeons, 3)=Physicians, 4)=Tissue Typers, 5)=TxCoords	1998	1999	2000	Total

UNITED STATES

ARIZONA

Good Samaritan Reg Med Ctr, Samaritan Transp Serv, 1410 N 3rd St, Phoenix, AZ 85004-1608 Ph: (602) 251-2700 Fax: (602) 251-2750 1,2) A.J. Fabrega, 1,3) E. Polito, 2) L.J. Koep, 3) Petrides, Smith, Bailey, Yee, Chang, Guerra, Hyde, 4) T. Vyvial, DNA HLA, 5) J. Bell, A. Moore, M. Ruocco, K. Helzer, K. Fitzpatrick		1	1*	2
Univ of Arizona Med Ctr, Dept of Transp Serv, 1501 N Campbell Ave, P.O.Box 245145, Tucson, AZ 85724 Ph: (520) 694-4984 Fax: (520) 694-4983 1,2) J.U. Zamora, 1) II, 2) P. Nakazato, 3) H. Lein, S. James, 4) C. Spier, 5) L. Maselli, N. Stubbs, S. Anderson, C. Gebremariam	0	0	3*	6

CALIFORNIA

Scripps Green Hosp, Ctr for Organ & Cell Transp, 10666 N Torrey Pines Rd, 200-N, La Jolla, CA 92037 Ph: (858) 554-4310 Fax: (858) 554-4311 Email: ahassoun@scippsclinic.com 1,2) A. Hassoun, 2) M. Brunson, 3) D. Salomon, S. Bhaduri, 4) UCSD HLA Lab, 5) J. Henry, K. Bounds, K. Thorson, L. Biermann		2	8	10
St Vincent Med Ctr, Dept of Transp, 2100 W 3rd St #500, Los Angeles, CA 90057 Ph: (213) 483-6830 Fax: (213) 484-2947 1,2) R. Mendez, 2) R.G. Mendez, T. Bogaard, U. Khetan, P. Asai, H. Shidban, K. McEvoy, 3) M. Spira, 4) Y. Iwaki, J. Cicciarelli, 5) Workentain, Tolcher, Park, Webb, Lozada, Uleman, Delannoy, Luelleni	19	0	3*	83
Univ Calif-Los Angeles Med Ctr, Renal Transp Serv Dept of Neph, 10833 LeConte Ave, Rm BH-427 CHS, Los Angeles, CA 90095-1796 Ph: (310) 825-6836 Fax: (310) 206-0564 1,2) C.V. Smith, 2) H.A. Gritsch, 3) G.M. Danovitch, A.H. Wilkinson, 4) UCLA Immunogenetics Center, 5) Harris, Kaufman, Henderson, Dutton, Butenschoen, Foley, Sanford	15	23	2*	82
Sutter Mem Hosp, Sutter Transp Serv, 5151 F St, Sacramento, CA 95819-3295 Ph: (916) 733-8133 Fax: (916) 733-1967 1,2) R.E. Ward, 2) C. Brownridge, 3) J. O'Green-Koenig, P. Lim, M.S. Mezger, 4) Sacramento Med Foundation Bld Ctr, 5) K. Guerrero, R. Vrchoticky, M. Basten	2	3	3	20
Univ of Calif, Davis Med Ctr, Transplant Program, 2315 Stockton Blvd, Housestaff faculty, Room 1018, Sacramento, CA 95817 Ph: (916) 734-2111 Fax: (916) 734-0432 1,2) R.V. Perez, 2) J. McVicar, 3) S. Gandhi, 4) P. Holland, 5) M.E. Friend, D.B. Higgs, M. Sturges, D. Lehe	0	1	1*	12

CONNECTICUT

Yale New Haven Hosp, Dept of Surg, Div of Organ Tx, 33 Cedar St, FMB112, New Haven, CT 06510 Ph: (203) 785-2565 Fax: (203) 785-7162 Email: kathy.lorber@yale.edu 1,2) G.P. Basadonna, 2) M.I. Lorber, A.L. Friedman, 3) A. Kliger, M.J. Bia, 4) M.I. Lorber, 5) M. Corrigan, J. Albert, N. Sowers, J. Bates	4	8	5	41

FLORIDA

Shands Hosp-Univ of Florida, Dept of Surg, 1600 SW Archer Rd, Rm 6142, PO Box 100286, Gainesville, FL 32610-0286 Ph: (352) 265-0130 Fax: (352) 265-0108 1,3) T.R. Srinivaz, 1,2) W.J. Vanderwerf, 4) J. Scornik, 5) J. Lloyd-Turner	0	0	7	8
Mayo Clinic Jacksonville/St Luke's, Renal & Pancreatic Transp, 4203 Belfort Rd, Suite 204, Jacksonville, FL 32216 Ph: (904) 296-9075 Fax: (904) 296-5874 1,2) J.L. Steers, 2) J. Nguyen, C. Hughes, V. Gopalan, 3) J.R. Spivey, R.C. Dickson, D.M. Harnois, 4) P. Genco, 5) D. Boyum	0	0	1	1

* Preliminary UNOS data

1)=Director, 2)=Tx Surgeons, 3)=Physicians, 4)=Tissue Typers, 5)=TxCoords	1998	1999	2000	Total
GEORGIA				
Emory Univ, Dept of Surg, 1364 Clifton Rd NE, H-124, Atlanta, GA 30322 Ph: (404) 727-0717 Fax: (404) 727-8972 1,2) C.P. Larsen, 1,2) T.C. Pearson, 2) P. Tso, 3) S. Gebhart, C. Zayas, 4) R. Bray, 5) G. McGrath, M. Jeffrey, C. Johnson, T. Ofenloch, B. Begley, W. Wilson	2	1	1	5
HAWAII				
St Francis Med Ctr, Transplant Inst, 2230 Liliha St, Honolulu, HI 96817 Ph: (808) 547-6228 Fax: (808) 547-6750 1,2) A. Cheung, 2) W. Limm, L.L. Wong, F.L. Fan, H. Noguchi, 3) J. Sugihara, J. Musgrave, R. Ng, 4) Y.K. Paik, C. Hamerick, 5) P. Bouhan, J. Nekoba, C. Bailey	1	1	2	12
ILLINOIS				
Northwestern Mem Hosp, Div of Organ Transp, 675 North St. Clair Street, Galter 17-200, Chicago, IL 60611 Ph: (312) 695-8900 Fax: (312) 695-9194 1,2) D. Kaufman, 2) J. Leventhal, J. Fryer, M. Abecassis, 3) D. Batlle, 4) M. Buckingham, 5) P. Gierut, D. Penrod, E. DeMayo, B. Olszewski	4	1	6	19
Univ of Chicago Med Ctr, Dept of Transp Surg, 5841 S Maryland, m/c 5027, Chicago, IL 60637 Ph: (773) 702-6338 Fax: (773) 702-2126 1,2) D.S. Bruce, 2) J.R. Thistlewaite, E.S. Woodle, J.B. Piper, J.M. Millis, D.S. Bruce, 3) K. Polonski, 4) V. Lazda, 5) E. Huss	1		2*	14
Univ of Illinois Hosp & Clins, Dept of Surg, Div of Transp, 801 S Paulina, Rm 411, m/c 960, Chicago, IL 60680-7213 Ph: (312) 996-6771 Fax: (312) 413-3483 1,2) E. Benedetti, 2) L. Cicalese, 3) J. Arruda, S.C. Kukreja, J.P. Lash, K.J. Pursell, 4) V.A. Lazda, 5) F. Pascual, O. Woghiren, X. Lopez	2	2	2*	13
IOWA				
Univ of Iowa Hosps & Clins, Dept of Surg/Transp Serv, University Hospitals, Iowa City, IA 52242 Ph: (319) 356-1334 Fax: (319) 356-1556 1,2) Y. Wu, 2) S. Rayhill, A. Bozorgzadeh, D. Katz, 3) L.G. Hunsicker, J.A. Bertalotus, C. Thomas, Kalil, 4) N.E. Goeken, E. Fields, 5) B. Schanbacher, L. Reynolds, A. Satterly, D. Cox, M. Schulz	1	1	4	54
KANSAS				
Via Christi Regional Med Ctr, Dept of Renal Transp, 929 N St Francis, Wichita, KS 67214 Ph: (316) 268-5890 Fax: (316) 291-7727 1,2) J.L. Smith, 2) C.F. Shield, 4) E. Thien, T. Hughes, 5) M. Blackmore, J. Lemon, K. Zecha, J. Wenz	0	2	2	19
KENTUCKY				
Univ of Kentucky Med Ctr, Dept of Surg, 800 Rose St, Lexington, KY 40536 Ph: (859) 323-4661 Fax: (859) 323-3644 1,2) D. Ranjan, 2) T. Johnston, S. Reddy, 3) T. Waid, W. McKeown, D. Karounos, E. Jackson, 4) T. Eichorn, J. Byrne, J.S. Thompson, D. Jennings, F. Lower, 5) S. Salyer, T. Miller, M. Blevins	0	1	4	6
LOUISIANA				
Memorial Medical Ctr (LSUNO), Transplant Institute, 3535 Bienville St, Suite 225, New Orleans, LA 70119 Ph: (504) 488-8121 Fax: (504) 488-9672 1,2) J.P. Boudreaux, 2) D.J. Frey, J. Jerius, 3) F. Gonzales, S. Andrews, 4) P. Kumar, 5) P. Ryan, C. Stechmann, C. Schrader, D. Radcliff	1	1	6	8
Tulane Univ Hosp & Clin, Dept of Surg, SL 22, 1430 Tulane Ave, New Orleans, LA 70112 Ph: (504) 588-5344 Fax: (504) 587-7510 Email: scheng@mailhost,tes.tulane.edu 1,2) S. Cheng, 2) D. Slakey, 3) V. Fonseca, 4) K.A. Sullivan, 5) M. White, L. Larmeu, J. Hahn	6	13	3*	76
Willis Knighton Med Ctr, Dept of Surg, 2600 Greenwood Rd, Shreveport, LA 71130 Ph: (318) 632-4676 Fax: (318) 632-2425 1,2) G.B. Zibari, 2) R. McMillan, D. Aultman, J.C. McDonald, 3) Work, Abreo, Paulson, Pervez, Gadallah, White, Lynn, 4) T. Roggero, D. Michell, K. Horton, W. Blackburn, R. Jones, 5) N. Noles, E. Kilpatrick	8	1	0*	18

1)=Director, 2)=Tx Surgeons, 3)=Physicians, 4)=Tissue Typers, 5)=TxCoords	1998	1999	2000	Total
MARYLAND				
The Johns Hopkins Hosp, Dept of Surg, Harvey 611, 600 N Wolfe St, Baltimore, MD 21287-8611 Ph: (410) 955-1532 Fax: (410) 614-2079 1,2) J. Markowitz, 2) Klein, Ratner, Montomery, Burdick, 3) P. Scheel, M. Choi, W. Briggs, T. Watnick, E. Kraus, M. Sananiego, 4) J. Hart, 5) Barshick, Burrell, Refugia, Kusel, Kahan, Dane, Mascari, Donovan	12	18	9	91
Univ of Maryland Med Systems, Dept of Surg, Organ Transp, 29 S Greene St, Ste 200, Baltimore, MD 21201 Ph: (410) 328-5408 Fax: (410) 328-3837 1) S.T. Bartlett, 2) E. Schweitzer, A. Farney, B. Philosophe, J. Colonna, C. Foster, 3) D. Klassen, M. Weir, P. Light, E. Ramos, C. Cangro, J. Fink, R. Wali, 4) American Red Cross Natl Histo Lab at Univ of Maryland Med Ctr, 5) Evans, Stern, Wilson, Young, Ford, Roberts, Aiken, Lee, Hopkins, Mann	38	67	50	282
MASSACHUSETTS				
Beth Israel Deaconess Med Ctr, Div of Organ Transp, One Deaconess Rd, Boston, MA 02215 Ph: (617) 632-8549 Fax: (617) 632-9929 1,2) A.P. Monaco, 2) P. Madras, A. Sahyoun, D. Shaffer, 3) A. Kaldany, P. Silva, M. William, Solomon, Stanton, D'Elia, 4) T. Maki, 5) M. Hoar, E. Chrzan	2	2	0	61
Univ of Massachusetts Med Ctr, Dept of Transp Surg, 55 Lake Ave N, 53-709, Worcester, MA 01655 Ph: (508) 856-6202 Fax: (508) 856-3920 1,2) R.C. Harland, 2) P. Ayvazian, R. Chari, 3) M. Thompson, P.Y. Fan, J.S. Staff, D. Mandelbrot, 4) New England Organ Bank, 5) T. Lovewel, P. Bigwood, J. Lane	0	2	13*	15
MICHIGAN				
Univ of Michigan Med Ctr, Dept Gen Surg, Div of Transp, 2926 Taubman Ctr-Box 0331, 1500 E Medical Ctr Dr, Ann Arbor, MI 48109-0331 Ph: (734) 936-5816 Fax: (734) 763-3187 Email: janco@umich.edu 1,2) J.C. Magee, 2) D.A. Campbell, Jr, J.D. Punch, S.M. Rudich, R.M. Merion, J. Arenas, 3) A. Leichtman, A. Ojo, B. Kaplan, D. Cibrik, H. Meier-Kriesche, 4) J. Baker, 5) M. Fox, S. Hutmacher, A. Maloney, J. Novak	6	8	8	45
St John Hosp and Med Ctr, Transp Surg, Prof Bldg II, Ste 174, 22101 Moross, Detroit, MI 48236 Ph: (313) 343-3048 Fax: (313) 343-7349 1,2) H.K. Oh, 3) R. Provenzano, 4) D. Levin, 5) N. Satmary, K. Heckman, C. McQuerry	0	1	1	13
MINNESOTA				
Fairview Univ Med Ctr, The Transplant Center, 516 Delaware St SE, MMC 482 Mayo, Minneapolis, MN 55455 Ph: (612) 625-5115 Fax: (612) 625-2190 1,2) D.E.R. Sutherland, 2) A. Humar, R. Kandaswamy, R. Gruessner, 3) B. Hering, Daniels, Rosenberg, Manske, 4) H. Noreen, D. McKinley, N. Hendrickson, 5) C. Garvey, P. Halvorsen, C. Trettin, M. Drangstveit, E. Norris	70	97	107	782
Mayo Clinic-Rochester Methodist Hosp, Transp Surg, 201 W Center St, Rochester, MN 55902 Ph: (507) 266-8731 Fax: (507) 266-1069 1) M.D. Stegall, 2) S. Sterioff, S. Nyberg, M. Prieto, M. Ishitani, 3) Gloor, Larson, Milliner, Morgenstern, Nath, Schwab, Torres, Velosa, 4) S.B. Moore, S. DeGoey, 5) L. Fix, M. Kreps, D. Dicke-Henslin, C. Bauer	12	17	17*	52
NEBRASKA				
Nebraska Health System, Dept of Surg-Sec of Transplant, 687400 Nebraska Med Ctr, Omaha, NE 68198-7400 Ph: (402) 552-2440 Fax: (402) 552-3052 1,2) A.N. Langnas, 2) R. Taylor, D. Sudan, J. Leone, 3) Hammeke, Duckworth, Larsen, Groggel, Shipman, Anderson, 4) S. Shepherd, A. Larsen, 5) L. Williams, S. Miller, K. Prisbe	9	1	4*	60
Nebraska Health Systems, Clarkson Hosp-Univ Hosp, Kidney/Pancreas Transpl Office, 987555 Nebraska Medical Center, Omaha, NE 68198-7555 Ph: (402) 552-2440 Fax: (402) 552-3052 2) R. Taylor, A. Langnas, B. Shaw, D. Sudan, K. Iyer, 3) Hammeke, Groggel, Ranga, Guirguis, 4) J. Wisecarver, R. Rubocki, S. Shepherd, 5) S. Miller, T. Baker, M.E. Krobot, C. Lykke, K. Frisbie, McAnally, Livers	7	5	4	68

PANCREAS

1)=Director, 2)=Tx Surgeons, 3)=Physicians, 4)=Tissue Typers, 5)=TxCoords	1998	1999	2000	Total
NEW JERSEY				
Our Lady of Lourdes Med Ctr, Dept of Surg, Ambulatory Care Center, 1601 Haddon Ave, Camden, NJ 08103-3117 Ph: (856) 757-3840 Fax: (856) 757-3519 1,3) J. Capelli, 2) N. Youssef, R. Santos, 3) S.M. Chen, M.A. Torres, P.S. Panebianco, B.E. Michel, 4) G. Kirshnan, S. Borrero, A. Biehl, 5) J.F. Dennis, S. Lay-Martino, M. Naurath	8	5	0	35
NEW YORK				
Mt Sinai Med Ctr, Recanati/Miller Transp Insti, Box 1104, One Gustave Levy Pl, New York, NY 10029 Ph: (212) 241-8086 Fax: (212) 426-2015 1) J. Bromberg, 2) Sung, S. Ames, 3) B. Murphy, E. Akalin, V. Sehal, 4) M. Fotino, 5) L. Daly, K. McKeough, C. Derrien, R. Ifrah, M. Gonzalez	2	1	7	10
NYU Medical Center, Dept of Surg, 403 E. 34th St, 3rd floor, New York, NY 10016 Ph: (212) 263-8134 Fax: (212) 263-8157 Email: devon.john@med.nyu.edu 1,2) D. John, 2) L. Teperman, G. Morgan, T. Diflo, 3) J. Weisstuch, J. Benstein, B. Soberman, T. Seltzer, 4) Rogosin Institute, 5) L. Irwin, D. Campbell, L. Johnson	4	3	3*	15
NORTH CAROLINA				
Carolinas Med Ctr, Dept Surg, PO Box 32861, 1000 Blythe Blvd, Charlotte, NC 28232 Ph: (704) 355-6649 Fax: (704) 355-7616 1,2) P. Gores, 2) D. Hayes, L. Eskind, 3) P. Walker, G. Hart, C. Fotiadis, 4) S. Bruner, S. Mallory, B. Ranson, J. Blankenship, 5) B. Thrasher, R. Jones, R. Hogarth, D. O'Brien, T. Pierce, M. Zebedis	10	2	2*	47
Duke Univ Med Ctr, Dept of Surgery, Box 3522, Erwin Rd, Durham, NC 27710 Ph: (919) 668-1856 Fax: (919) 681-7508 Email: kuo00004@mc.duke.edu 1,2) P.C. Kuo, 2) J. Tuttle-Newhall, B. Collins, R. Bollinger, 3) M. Feinglos, S. Smith, P. Conlon, D, Butterly, 4) F. Ward, 5) J. Thompson, L. Hicks	2	4	7*	17
OHIO				
Univ of Cincinnati Coll of Med, Dept of Medicine, 231 Bethesda Ave, Cincinnati, OH 45267-0585 Ph: (513) 584-7001 Fax: (513) 584-5571 Email: zavalaey@healthall.com 1,2) E.S. Woodle, 2) J.W. Alexander, R. Munda, J. Buell, M. Hanaway, 3) M.R. First, R. Peddi, P. Roy-Chaudhury, 4) L. Whitacre, D. Eckels, 5) S. Brown	1	2	0	19
Cleveland Clin Fnd, A110 Transplant Center, 9500 Euclid Ave, Cleveland, OH 44195 Ph: (216) 444-4600 Fax: (216) 445-7088 1,2) V. Krishnamurthi, 3) B.J. Hoogwerf, V.W. Dennis, 4) D. Cook, 5) M. Lard	11	7	13	60
Univ Hospitals of Cleveland, Department of Surgery, 11100 Euclid Ave, Cleveland, OH 44106 Ph: (216)844-3689 Fax: (216)844-7764 1,2) J.A. Schulak, 2) D.S. Seaman, C.T. Siegel, 3) D. Hricik, T. Knauss, 4) N. Greenspan, 5) M. Bartucci, J. Arnovitz, H. Dorsey	1	3	7	17
Ohio State Univ Hosp, Div of Transp, 363 Means Hall, 1654 Upham Dr, Columbus, OH 43210 Ph: (614) 293-8545 Fax: (614) 293-4541 1,2) R.M. Ferguson, 2) M. Henry, E.A. Elkhammas, G. Bumgardner, R. Pelletier, 3) Bay, Hebert, Cosio, Middendorf, Nahman, Fallkenhain, Pesevento, 4) P. Adams, 5) I. Osis, B. Miller, L. McDonnell	1	4	8*	53
OKLAHOMA				
Integris Baptist Med Ctr, Oklahoma Transp Inst, Dept of Pancreas Transp, 3300 NW Expressway, Oklahoma City, OK 73112-4481 Ph: (405) 949-3349 Fax: (405) 945-5467 1,2) B.M. Nour, 2) W.J. Miller, 3) B. Matter, H. Wright, 4) D. Smith, 5) M. Lancaster	1	1	0*	10
Univ Hosp, Transp Svc, Rm 5E190, 800 NE 13th St, Oklahoma City, OK 73104 Ph: (405) 271-7498 Fax: (405) 271-1772 1,2) L. Pennington, 2) R. Squires, 3) L. Olansky, 4) J. Baker, 5) E. Grubbs	2	0	0*	8
OREGON				
Oregon Hlth Sci Univ, Sec of Liver/Pancreas Transp, 3181 SW Sam Jackson Park Rd, L590, Portland, OR 97201-3098 Ph: (503) 494-7810 Fax: (503) 494-5292 1,2) J. Rabkin, 2) S. Orloff, 3) L. Loriaux, A. Demattos, 4) D.J. Norman, 5) L. Hanson	0	1	0*	6

1)=Director, 2)=Tx Surgeons, 3)=Physicians, 4)=Tissue Typers, 5)=TxCoords	1998	1999	2000	Total
PENNSYLVANIA				
Hosp of the Univ of Pennsylvania, The Penn Transp Ctr, 3400 Spruce St, Philadelphia, PA 19104 Ph: (215) 662-6200 Fax: (215) 349-5096 Email: diane.jarobowski@uphs.upenn.edu 1,2) K. Brayman, 2) A. Naji, J. Markmann, C. Barker, 3) R. Grossman, R. Bloom, K. Mange, 4) C. Zmijewski, M.K. Antonio, M. Kamoun, 5) T. Holland, C. Hooper, M. Palanjian, J. Eyer, K. Kilgarriff, C. Naus	2	1	3	73
UPMC-Presbyterian, Starzl Transplantation Inst, 4 Falk Clinic, 3601 Fifth Ave, Pittsburgh, PA 15213 Ph: (412) 648-3200 Fax: (412) 648-3085 1,2) T.E. Starzl, 1,2) J.J. Fung, 2) R. Corry, R. Shapiro, 3) S. Kusne, J. McCauley, 4) R. Duquesnoy, A. Zeevi, 5) D. Good, H. Woods	6	9	37	112
NEW YORK				
SUNY Upstate Med Univ, Dept Of Surgery, 750 E Adams St, Syracuse, NY 13210 Ph: (315)464-4550 Fax: (315)464-6250 1) D.S. Kittur, 2) F.S. Szmalc, 3) Schroeder, Scheinman, Knudson, Izquierdo, Narsipur, Leggat, 4) C. Hubbell, J.B. Henry Sr, 5) M. Leaf, A. Roman, J.B. Henry Jr	2	0		3
TENNESSEE				
Johnson City Med Ctr Hosp, Dept of Transp, 408 State at Franklin Rd, Ste 46, Johnson City, TN 37604 Ph: (423) 431-6164 Fax: (423) 928-6795 1,2) R.M. Weingart, 2) P.N. Joshi, 3) C.F. Wiegand, F. Montenegro, L. Panus, 4) University Of Tenn-Knoxville, 5) L. Walker, K. Kelley, J. Hawkins	2	0	2	4
William F Bowld Hosp, Univ of Tenn, Dept of Surg, 956 Court Ave, Room A202, Memphis, TN 38163 Ph: (901) 448-5924 Fax: (901) 448-7208 1,2) A.O. Gaber, 2) R. Stratta, H. Shokouh-Amiri, S. Vera, H. Grewal, 3) J. Fisher, H. Sacks, A. Kitabchi, T. Hughes, M.F. Egidi, 4) B. Loehman, 5) B. Culbreath, N. O'Keefe, R. Vincent	33	34	45*	267
TEXAS				
Medical City Dallas Hosp, Transplant Center, 7777 Forest Lane, A-14th Floor, Dallas, TX 75230 Ph: (800) 348-4318 Fax: (972) 566-4872 1,2) S. Seitz, 2) D. Ogden, M. Mack, T. Dewey, M. McGee, R. Bowman, I. Davidsons, S. Reeder, 3) J.E. Rosenthal, M. Lerman, J. Hunt, A. Shulkin, K. Hoang, A. Anderson, 4) A. Nikaein, 5) M. Covin, T. McMellon, D. Stevenson, C. Cava-Bartsch, A. Kuhnel	0	0	1	1
Univ of Texas Med Branch, Dept of Surg, 301 University Blvd, Route 0533, Galveston, TX 77551-0533 Ph: (409) 772-2412 Fax: (409) 747-7364 1,2) K.K. Gugliuzza, 2) J.A. Daller, 3) J. Rice, T.J. Ahuja, R. Remmers, R. Beach, 4) S. Vaidya, 5) M. Byrd, J. Boughton, D. Devine, Armendariz, Medina, Upchurch, Parhan	0	0	1*	5
Univ of Texas-Hermann Hosp, Dept of Surg-Organ Transp, 6411 Fannin, Houston, TX 77030 Ph: (713) 500-7415 Fax: (713) 704-6195 1,2) R. Knight, 2) S. Katz, 3) P. Orlander, 4) R.H. Kerman, 5) S. Zela	8	6	3	23
Methodist Specialty & Transplant Hosp, 8026 Floyd Curl Dr, San Antonio, TX 78229 Ph: (210) 692-8250 Fax: (210) 692-8154 1,2) F.H. Wright, Jr, 3) S. Diamond, C. Hura, M. Isbell, H. Reineck, M. Schultz, S. Schwartz, 4) J. Morrisey, 5) Farias, Galliardt, Hudson, Leonhardt, Martinez, McNeil, Rhoden, Richardson	0	0	1*	1
UTAH				
LDS Hosp, Dept of Transp, 8th Ave & C St, Salt Lake City, UT 84143 Ph: (801) 321-3090 Fax: (801) 321-3098 1,2) L.P. Belnap, 2) J. Sorensen, M. Stevens, 3) R. Bond, R.C. Lambert, J.B. Stinson, 4) T. Fuller, 5) J. Arata, G.M. Reid, K. Baker	0	0	1*	4
VIRGINIA				
Univ of Virginia Health Science Ctr, Transp CTR, Box 265, Lee Street, Charlottesville, VA 22908 Ph: (800) 543-8814 Fax: (804) 982-0099 1,2) T. Pruett, 2) R.G. Sawyer, H. Sanfey, 3) P.L. Lobo, R. Isaacs, 4) C. Spencer, J. Guan, C. Davis, 5) B. Shephard, W. Simmons	1	2	1	14

PANCREAS

1)=Director, 2)=Tx Surgeons, 3)=Physicians, 4)=Tissue Typers, 5)=TxCoords	1998	1999	2000	Total
WASHINGTON				
Univ of Washington Med Ctr, Transplant Services, 1959 N.E. Pacific St, Box 356174, Seattle, WA 98195 Ph: (206) 598-6700 Fax: (206) 598-6706 Email: cmarsh@u.washington.edu 1,2) C.L. Marsh, 2) J.D. Perkins, P. Healey, L. Wrenshall, B. Steven, A. Levy, C. Kuhr, 3) C. Davis, I. Hirsch, K. Muczynski, 4) K. Nelson (Puget Sound Blood Ctr), 5) P. Forg, C. Arp, C. Conover, D. Mullenix	4	9	4	35
Virginia Mason Med Ctr, Div of Renal/Pancreas Transp, 1100 9th Ave, C7-Neph, Seattle, WA 98111 Ph: (206) 341-0925 Fax: (206) 341-0886 1,3) R.L. Wilburn, 2) F. Govier, T.R. Hefty, T. Pritchett, R. Weissman, 3) C. Thompson, C. Cryst, M. Cooper, 4) K. Nelson, 5) M. Cressman, W. Ryan, J. Buck	0	1	1*	11
AUSTRIA				
Univ Hosp, Dept of Transp Surg, Anichstrasse 35, Innsbruck, 6020 Ph: (43)512 504-2603 Fax: (43)512 504-2605 1,2) R. Margreiter, 2) A. Koenigsrainer, B. Spechtenhauser, W. Steurer, 4) D. Schoenitzer, 5) H. Fetz, P. Schobel	1	3	0	22
BELGIUM				
Clin Univ Saint Luc, Dept of Transp, 10 Ave Hippocrate, 1200 Brussels Ph: (32)2 7642207 Fax: (32)2 7707858 Email: squifflet@chir.ucl.ac.be 1,2) J.P. Squifflet, 2) M. Mourad, J. Malaise, 3) Y. Pirson, B. Vandeleen, 4) D. Latinne, 5) C. Lecomte, V. Dumont, P. van Ormelingen	1	1	0	2
Erasme-Clin Univ de Bruxelles, Dept of Neph/Dial/Transp, 808 Rte de Lennik, B-1070 Brussels Ph: (32)2 555 3334 Fax: (32)2 555 6499 Email: ludepauw@ulb.ac.be 1,2) L. De Pauw, 3) F. Fery, D. Abramowicz, 4) E. Dupont, M. Andrien, 5) E. Angenon, R. Carpintero, A. Menu, I. Senepart	1	6	4	38
CANADA				
Univ of Alberta Hosp, Surgery, 2D4.37 Walter Mackenzie Center, Edmonton, AB T6G 2B7 Ph: (403) 407-7330 Fax: (403) 407-7374 1,2) D.L. Bigam, 2) N.M. Kneteman, A.N.J. Shapiro, 3) S. Cockfeld, P. Halloran, A. Murray, P. Campbell, 4) A. Halpin, 5) S. Riaka	3	4	5	12
Univ of Calgary Foothills Med Ctr, Div of Tx, Dept of Surg, RmG33, 1403 29th St NW, Calgary, Alberta, T2N 2T9 Ph: (403) 670-4266 Fax: (403) 270-8431 Email: serdar.yilmaz@crha-health.ab.ca 1,2) S. Yilmaz, 2) A. Barama, 3) F. Sepandj, J. Klassen, L. Tibbles, K. McLaughlin, 4) R. McKenna, 5) S. Buckle, M. Miller, J. Costa		1	0	1
Royal Victoria Hospital, Surgery, 687 Pine Avenue West, Montreal, QC H3A 1A1 Ph: (514) 842-1231 Fax: (514) 843-1503 1,2) P. Metrakos, 3) M. Cantarovich, R. Mangel, 4) P. Imperial, R. Schreier, C. McIntyre, 5) M. Poloni, M. Fortier	6	8		17
Hosp Notre Dame, Dept of Transp Surg, 1560 Sherbrooke Est, Montreal, PQ H2L 4M1 Ph: (514) 281-6000 x6605 Fax: (514) 896-4736 Email: pierre.dalozechum@ssss.gouv.qc.ca 1,2) P. Daloze, 2) C. Smeesters, S. Busque, 3) H. Beauregard, 4) Inst Armand Frappier, Montreal, 5) Quebec Transp	3	3	11	31
CZECH REPUBLIC				
Inst for Clin/Exper Med/Transp Ctr, Transp Ctr, Dept of Diabetol. Exp. The, Videnska 800, 14000 Prague 4 Ph: (42)02 61364103 Fax: (42)02 61363117 1,3) S. Vitko, 2) M. Adamec, 3) F. Saudek, 4) E. Ivaskova, 5) E. Pokorna, V. Charova, M. Skachova, A. Prazanova	0	4	4	9
GERMANY				
Charite-Campus Virchow Klinkum, Dept of Surg, Augustenburger Platz 1, Berlin, 13353 Ph: (49)30 450-52001 Fax: (49)30 450-52902 Email: chirurgie@charite.de 1,2) P. Neuhaus, 2) A.R. Mueller, U. Settmacher, A.R. Mulles, 3) U. Frei, 4) A. Salama, C. Schoenemann, 5) D.F. Horch	22	37	22	110

1)=Director, 2)=Tx Surgeons, 3)=Physicians, 4)=Tissue Typers, 5)=TxCoords	1998	1999	2000	Total
Med Sch Hannover, Dept of Abdom/Transp Surg, Konstanty-Gutschow Str 8, W-3000 Hannover 61 Ph: (49)511 532 2290 Fax: (49)511 55 6747 1,2) J. Klempnauer, 2) B. Nashan, R. Luck, T. Becker, 4) D. Mueller, Muenz, 5) Vogelsang	0	0	2	5
Univ of Rostock Med Faculty, Clin of Surgery, Schillingallee, Rostock, D-18057 Ph: (49)381 494 6000 Fax: (49)381 494 6002 1) U. Hopt, 2) W. Schareck, 3) R. Schmidt, 4) R. Barz, 5) F.P. Nitschke	3	4	0	12
Univ Ulm Klinikum, Dept of Surg II, Steinhovelstr 9, 89075 Ulm Ph: (49)731 502 6985 Fax: (49)731 23167 1,2) D. Abendroth, 3) G. Adler, 4) S. Goldmann, 5) S. Seegmuller, S. Rettenberger	7			38

ITALY

	1998	1999	2000	Total
Univ of Pisa, Osp di Cisanello, Inst of Gen Surg, Via Paradisa 2, 56124 Pisa, Pisa Ph: (39)50 596820 Fax: (39)50 543692 Email: uboggi@patchir.med.unipi.it 1,2,5) F. Mosca, 2) U. Boggi, 3) G. Rizzo, 4) G. Rizzo	0	0	1	1

NORWAY

	1998	1999	2000	Total
Rikshosp-The Nat'l Hosp, Dept of Surg/Med, Oslo, NO-0027 Ph: (47)2307 00 00 Fax: (47)2307 05 10 1) A. Bergan, 2) I. Brekke, P. Pfeffer, 3) P. Fauchald, K. Nordal, 4) E. Thorsby, T. Leivestad, 5) S. Foss, P.A. Bakkan, P.E. Vatsaas, K. Meyer	0	1	1	13

SWEDEN

	1998	1999	2000	Total
Huddinge Univ Hosp, Dept of Transp Surg, Stockholm, SE-14186 Ph: (46)8 58580000 Fax: (46)8 7743191 1,2) A. Tibell, 2) G. Tyden, 3) J. Bolinder, 4) E. Moller, 5) M. Larsson, B. Blom	5	3	3	172

SWITZERLAND

	1998	1999	2000	Total
Univ Hosp Zurich, Dept of Surg, Ramistr 100, Zurich, CH-8091 Ph: (41)1 255 3300 Fax: (41)1 255 4449 Email: clavien@chir.unizh.ch 1) P.A. Clavien, 2) N. Demartines, M. Weber, Z. Kadry, 3) U. Binswanger, 4) M. Weber, 5) P. Seeburger, T. Reh, M. Struker	4	0	5	144

PANCREAS

PANCREAS Transplants

	1998	1999	2000	Total
United States	323	375	426	2,848
Foreign	56	75	58	736
Total	379	450	484	3,584

PANCREAS Transplant Centers

United States	61
Foreign	33
Total	94

WORLDWIDE TRANSPLANT CENTER DIRECTORY
ISLET TRANSPLANTS

1)=Director, 2)=Tx Surgeons, 3)=Physicians, 4)=Tissue Typers, 5)=TxCoords	1998	1999	2000	Total

UNITED STATES

FLORIDA

Univ of Miami, Jackson Mem Hosp, Dept of Surg/Transp, PO Box 012440, Miami, FL 33101 Ph: (305) 355-5100 Fax: (305) 355-5134 1,2) J. Miller, 1,2) A.Tzakis, 2) J. Nery, G. Burke III, F. Kahn, G. Ciancio, 3) R. Alejandro, 4) V. Esquenazi, 5) J. Colona	2	3		31

MINNESOTA

Fairview Univ Med Ctr, Transp Ctr, 516 Delaware St SE, Box 482, Minneapolis, MN 55455 Ph: (612) 625-5115 Fax: (612) 625-2190 1,3) B. Hering, 2) D. Sutherland, 3) B. Hering, 4) H. Noreen, D. McKinley, N. Henrickson, 5) K. Duderstadt, K. Jacobsen, C. Gibson	0	0	3	59

AUSTRIA

Univ Hospital, Dept of Transplant Surgery, Anichstrasse 35, Innsbruck, 6020 Ph: (43)512 504-2603 Fax: (43)512 504-2605 1,2) R. Margreiter, 2) A. Koenigsrainer, 3) W. Steurer, 4) D. Schoenitzer, 5) H. Fetz, P. Schobel	0	1	1	4

CANADA

Univ of Alberta Hosp, Surgery, 2D4.37 Walter Mackenzie Center, Edmonton, AB T6G 2B7 Ph: (780) 407-7330 Fax: (780) 407-7374 1,2) A.M.J. Shapiro, 2) N.M. Kneteman, D. Bigam, E. Ryan, 3) R.V. Rajotte, J.R.T. Lakey, G. Korbutt, G.L. Woneck, 4) A. Halpin, 5) I. Larsen, T. Davyduke	0	5	10	22

ITALY

Inst San Raffaele, Univ of Milano, Dept of Med, Via Olgettina 60, Milano, 20132 Ph: (39)02 2643 2805 Fax: (39)02 2643 2752 1,2) G. Pozza, 2) V. DiCarlo, C. Socci, 3) A. Secchi, L. Falqui, P. Maffi, 4) G. Sirchia, 5) A. Secchi	5	5	12	46

SWITZERLAND

Univ Hosp Geneva, Dept of Surg, Transp Unit, 24 rue Micheli-du-Crest, 1211 Geneva 14 Ph: (41)22 372 7702 Fax: (41)22 372 7755 1,2) Ph. Morel, 2) J. Oberholzer, 4) C. Goumaz, 5) N. Decarpentry	4	5	6	22

UNITED KINGDOM

Oxford Radcliffe Hosp, Oxford Transp Ctr, The Churchill, Oxford, OX3 7LJ Ph: (44)865 226092 Fax: (44)865 225616 1) P. Friend, 2) D. Gray, C. Darby, P.J. Morris, 3) P. Mason, P.A. Hamann, 4) S. Fuggle, M. Barnado, 5) M. Jackson	1	1	0	10

WORLDWIDE TRANSPLANT CENTER DIRECTORY
HEART TRANSPLANTS

1)=Director, 2)=Tx Surgeons, 3)=Physicians, 4)=Tissue Typers, 5)=TxCoords	1998	1999	2000	Total

UNITED STATES

ALABAMA

| Univ of Alabama at Birmingham, Dept of Surg, 701 S 19th St, Birmingham, AL 35294
Ph: (205) 934-3368 Fax: (205) 934-5261
1,2) J.K. Kirklin, 2) W.L. Holman, G.L. Zorn, D. McGiffin, 3) R.C. Bourge, B. Rayburn, R. Benza,
B. Foley, M. Aaron, 4) R. Senkbeil, 5) C. White-Williams, M. Hubbard, T. Smith, M. Arndt | 35 | 29 | 38* | 610 |

ARIZONA

| Univ Med Cent, Dept of Cardio/Thor Surg, Rm 4604, 1501 N Campbell Ave, Tucson, AZ 85724
Ph: (520) 694-6299 Fax: (520) 694-2692
1,2) J.G. Copeland, 2) G. Sethi, F. Arabia, D. Arzouman, V. Paramesh, S. Sharma, R. Bose,
3) S. Butman, C. Lui, S. Knoper, 5) N. Edling, J. Wild, N. Harrington, D. Allen, S. Mullarkey | 34 | 28 | 27 | 587 |

ARKANSAS

| Arkansas Children's Hosp, Dept of Cardio/Vasc Surg, Slot #835, 800 Marshall St, Little Rock, AR
72202-3591 Ph: (501) 320-1479 Fax: (501) 320-3667 Email: frazierelizabeth@uams.edu
1,3) E.A. Frazier, 2) J.E. Harrell, Jr, 3) M.R. Morrow, E.E. Fontenot, P.M. Seib, 4) V. Smith,
5) K.A. Ainley | 9 | 14 | 6* | 89 |

| Baptist Med Ctr, Transp Services, 9601 Interstate 630, Medical Towers, Little Rock, AR 72205
Ph: (501) 202-2635 Fax: (501) 202-1357
1,2) S.W. Hutchins, 1,2) J. Ransom, 2) W. Hearnsberger, T. Hoffmann, 3) J. Kizziar, S. Hutchins,
4) V. Smith, 5) B. Wilson | 5 | 5 | 5* | 84 |

CALIFORNIA

| Loma Linda Univ Med Ctr, Cardiac Transp Unit, Ste 7700H, 11234 Anderson St, Loma Linda, CA
92354 Ph: (909) 558-4201 Fax: (909) 558-4142
1,2) L. Bailey, 2) S. Gundry, A. Razzouk, M. del Rio, 3) R. Chinnock, M. Baum, T. Heywood,
D. Cutler, 4) S. Nehlsen-Cannarella, 5) Robie, Thomas, Stout, Griffin, Chatigny, Messenger,
DeAmaya | 29 | 21 | 25 | 481 |

| Cedars-Sinai Med Ctr, Dept of Cardio/Thor Surg, 8700 Beverly Blvd, Suite 6215, Los Angeles,CA
90048 Ph: (310) 423-3851 Fax: (310) 423-0851
1,2) A. Trento, 2) C. Blanche, E. Kass, 3) L.S.C. Czer, 4) S.C. Jordan, D. Tyan
5) P. Nusser, D. Harasty | 21 | 26 | 25 | 300 |

| Children's Hosp Los Angeles, Dept of Cardio/Thor Transp, 4650 Sunset Blvd MS #66,
Los Angeles, CA 90027 Ph: (323) 669-5965 Fax: (323) 668-7979
1,2) V.A. Starnes, 2) R.G. Cohen, 3) M.L. Barr, J. Szmuszkovicz, 5) M. Horn | 7 | 2 | 4 | 33 |

| St Vincent Med Ctr, Dept of Thor/Cardio/Vasc Surg, Cardiac Transp Prog, 2200 West 3rd St.#300
Los Angeles, CA 90057 Ph: (213) 484-7676 Fax: (213) 413-0553
1,2) A. Gheissari, 1,2) T. Yokoyama, 2) E. Capouya, R.G. Cohen, V.A. Starnes, 3) J. Hendel,
J. Katz, 4) Y. Iwaki, J. Cicciarelli, 5) J. Fuentes | 9 | 10 | 13* | 126 |

| Univ Calif-Los Angeles Med Ctr, Dept of Surg, Div of Cardio/Thor Surg, 10833 Le Conte Ave,
Los Angeles, CA 90095 Ph: (310) 825-6068 Fax: (310) 206-6301
1,2) H. Laks, 2) F. Esmalian, A. Ardehali, D. Marelli, M. Plunkett, 3) Kobashigawa, Moriguchi,
Kawata, Hamilton, Hage, Fonarow, Alejos, 4) UCLA Immunogenetics Center,
5) C. Burch, R. Camara, Velleca, Mark, Lackey, Brown | 95 | 89 | 102 | 1083 |

| Univ of Southern Calif Univ Hosp, Dept of Thor/Cardio/Vasc Surg, Cardiac Transp Prog,
1500 San Pablo St, Los Angeles, CA 90033 Ph: (323) 442-8419 Fax: (323) 442-6201
1,2) V.A. Starnes, 2) R.G. Cohen, 3) M.L. Barr, 4) Y. Iwaki, J. Cicciarelli,
5) F. Schenkel, D. Lake, J. Onga | 11 | 10 | 14 | 65 |

* Preliminary UNOS data

1)=Director, 2)=Tx Surgeons, 3)=Physicians, 4)=Tissue Typers, 5)=TxCoords	1998	1999	2000	Total
Stanford Univ Med Ctr, Dept of Cardio Surg, Falk Bldg, MC 5407, Palo Alto, CA 94305 Ph: (650) 723-5771 Fax: (650) 725-3846 1,2) R. Robbins, 2) P. Oyer, B. Reitz, 3) Hunt, Valantine, Fowler, Schroeder, Bernstein, Vagelos, Perlroth, 4) C. Grumet, 5) P. Gamberg, J. Miller, L. Levine, M. Merlo	36	36	37	1051
Sutter Mem Hosp, Dept of Heart Transp, Sutter Transp Ctr, 1 South, 5151 F St, Sacramento, CA 95819 Ph: (916) 733-8133 Fax: (916) 733-1967 1,3) J. Chin, 2) M.T. Ingram, D. Schuch, J. Longoria, 3) M. Winchester, 4) Sacramento Med Found Blood Ctr, 5) P. Hoffman	3	8	5	80
Sharp Mem Hosp, Cardiac Transp, 7901 Frost St, San Diego, CA 92123 Ph: (858) 541-3831 Fax: (858) 541-4547 1,2) R.M. Adamson, 2) P. Daily, W. Dembitsky, A. Klijian, 3) B. Jaski, P. Hoagland, J. Gordon, 4) J. Cicciarelli, L. Lebeck, 5) J. King, J. Andrews	13	10	13*	222
Univ of Calif-San Diego, Div of Cardio/Thor Surg, 200 W Arbor Dr, San Diego, CA 92103-8892 Ph: (619) 543-7777 Fax: (619) 543-2652 Email: jkriett@ucsd.edu 1,2) S.W. Jamieson, 2) J.M. Kriett, D. Kapelanski, P. Thistlethwaite, 3) R. Shabatai, D. Herman, A. Rothman, B. Greenberg, 4) M. Garavoy, L. Lebeck, 5) D. Garcia, S. Osborne, L. Gayhart, D. Glasser	13	10	5*	126
Calif Pacific Med Ctr, Dept Cardiac Surg, 2100 Webster St, Ste 512, San Francisco, CA 94115 Ph: (415) 923-3014 Fax: (415) 885-8665 1,2) J.D. Hill, 2) G.J. Avery, 3) E.A. Haeusslein, B.S. Levin, 4) S. Steen, 5) D. Miniaci, J. Murphy	11	9	17*	320
Univ of Calif-San Francisco, Dept of Cardio/Thor Surg, 505 Parnassus, Box 1267, San Francisco, CA 94143-1267 Ph: (415) 476-3503 Fax: (415) 502-5316 1,2) F. Keith, 2) T. Hall, M. Ratcliffe, 3) T. DeMarco, 5) C. Rifkin, A. Fukano	14	7	3	128

COLORADO

	1998	1999	2000	Total
The Children's Hosp-Denver, Dept of Cardio/Vasc Surg, Univ Colorado Sch of Med, 1056 E 19th Ave, B100, Denver, CO 80218 Ph: (303) 861-6821 Fax: (303) 837-2595 1,2) D.N. Campbell, 2) M.B. Mitchell, 3) M. Boucek, H. Sondheimer, B. Pietra, D. Ivy, E. Shaffer, 4) IAD, 5) T. Dean, D. Ripe, C. Mashborn, D. Johnson	24	17	21*	179
Univ of Colorado Hlth Sci Ctr, Dept of Cardio/Thor Surg, Div of Cardio, 4200 E 9th Ave, Denver, CO 80262 Ph: (303) 372-0618 Fax: (303) 372-0669 1,2) D.N. Campbell, 2) F.L. Grover, S. Aziz, J. Manlt, M. Mitchell, 3) E. Woffel, M. Bristow, B. Lowes, S. Shakar, M. Mestroni, 4) Univ of Colorado Hlth Sci Ctr, 5) K. Keller, N. Ireland, L. Rohrbough	29	24	16*	241

CONNECTICUT

	1998	1999	2000	Total
Hartford Hosp, Transp Program, 85 Seymour St, Suite 321, Hartford, CT 06106 Ph: (860) 545-4132 Fax: (860) 545-4208 1,3) J.E. Dougherty, 1,2) H.B.C. Low, 2) J. Hammond, P. Preissler, D. Underhill, 3) Nino, Bartus, Lawrence, Rossi, Brown, 4) L. Bow, T. Alberghini, 5) N. Moody, J. McNabl	8	15	10	216
Yale New Haven Hosp, Dept of Cardio/Thor/Surg, 333 Cedar St, FMB 121, New Haven, CT 06510 Ph: (203) 785-2700 Fax: (203) 785-3346 Email: eddygl@ynhh.com 1,2) G. Tellides, 2) G. Kopf, G. Hammond, J.A. Elefteriades, 3) F. Lee, 4) M. Lorber, 5) G.L. Eddy, K. Nystrom	17	13	12*	170

DISTRICT OF COLUMBIA

	1998	1999	2000	Total
Washington Hosp Ctr, Washington Heart Transp Dept, 110 Irving St NW, Rm 1E-21, Washington, DC 20010 Ph: (202) 877-3220 Fax: (202) 877-7521 1,2) S. Boyce, 3) R. Cooke, 4) W. Ward, 5) S. Cupples	9	8	8	159
Children's National Med Ctr, Dept of Cardio Surg, 111 Michigan Ave NW, Washington, DC 20010 Ph: (202) 884-2137 Fax: (202) 884-5572 1,2) J. Sell, 2) F.M. Midgley, 3) G.R. Martin, E.S. Quivers, 4) Medlantic Histo Lab	3	2	1*	26

FLORIDA

	1998	1999	2000	Total
Shands at the Univ of Florida, Transplant Center, Box 100251, 1600 SW Archer Rd, Gainesville, FL 32610-0251 Ph: (352) 265-0130 Fax: (352) 265-0108 1,2) E.D. Staples, 1,3 1,3) J.A.Hill,K.Schowengerdt, 2) D. Knauf, T. Martin, T. Beaver, 3) J.M. Aranda, R.S. Schofield, F.J. Fricker, 4) J. Scornik, 5) McGinn, Walker, Harker, Cleeton, Learn, Holder	40	34	40	466

1)=Director, 2)=Tx Surgeons, 3)=Physicians, 4)=Tissue Typers, 5)=TxCoords	1998	1999	2000	Total
Univ of Miami Sch of Med, Dept of Thor/Cardio/Vasc Surg, Jackson Mem Hosp, PO Box 016960 (R-114), Miami, FL 33101 Ph: (305) 355-5135 Fax: (305) 355-5207 1,2) S. Pham, 2) H. Bolooki, R. Kaplon, K. Katariya, E. Rosenkrantz, 3) J. Bauerlein, S. Mallon, R. Sequrira, P. Rusconi, A. Galindo, R. Munoz, 4) V. Esquenazi, 5) B. Bednar, L. Futterman, D. Bennett, S. Gerity, C. Ortega, A. Loo	33	31	20	249
All Children's Hosp, Transplant Adm #6630, 801 6th St So, St Petersburg, FL 33701 Ph: (727) 892-8298 Fax: (727) 892-4803 Email: smithda@allkids.org 1,3) R. Boucek, 2) J. Quintessenza, H. vanGelder, J. Jacobs, 3) J. McCormack, A. Asante-Korang, 4) Y. Chang, L. Desal, 5) S. DiSano, S. Sharf, D. Smith	8	7	7	38
Tallahassee Memorial Hosp, Heart Surg Ctr, 1401 Centerville Rd, Ste 508, Tallahassee, FL 32312 Ph: (850) 878-6164 Fax: (850) 656-5575 1,2) T. Bixler II, 2) D. Saint, J. Hurt, 3) Allee, Williams, Gredier, Tedrick, Smith, Cox, Katapodis, Burgett, 4) D. Craig, 5) D. Guthrie	4	9	10*	123
Tampa General Hosp, Transp Serv, Divis Island, Tampa, FL 33606 Ph: (813) 251-7137 Fax: (813) 253-4016 1,2) K. Sommers, 2) T.M. Beaver, D. Novitsky, N.S. Satry, 3) Canedo, Cintron, Garcia, Spoto Jr, Mester, Weston, Hoffman, Bugni, 4) W. LeFor, 5) S. Mabbott, R. Brauner, L. Dichiara, H. Smith, L. Anderson	47	33	24*	446

GEORGIA

	1998	1999	2000	Total
Egleston Children's Hosp at Emory U, Dept of Cardio/Thor Sur, 1365 Clifton Rd NE, Box 7, Atlanta, GA 30322 Ph: (404) 778-5288 Fax: (404) 778-4346 1,2) K. Kanter, 2) V. Tam, D. Vega, J. Puskas, 3) A. Smith, J. Lutz, R. Vincent, 4) A. Love, 5) C. D'Amico, A. Berg, N. Chestnut	39	37	11*	506
St Joseph's Hosp of Atlanta, Transp Serv, 5665 Peachtree Dunwoody Rd, Atlanta, GA 30342 Ph: (404) 851-5757 Fax: (404) 851-7746 1,3) D.E. Jansen, 2) Murphy, Mayfield, Carabajal, Thomas, Kauten, Wolfe, Langford, 3) V.E. Corrigan, W.D. Knopf, 4) R. Bray, 5) P. Arnold, J. Freniere, S. Leighty	16	13	7*	316

HAWAII

	1998	1999	2000	Total
St Francis Med Ctr, Dept of Transp, 2230 Liliha St, Honolulu, HI 96817 Ph: (808) 547-6385 Fax: (808) 547-6750 1,2) C. Moreno-Cabral, 3) R. Hong, C. Wong, S. Matsumoto, 4) Y.K. Paik, 5) D. Pacheco	2	2	2*	35

ILLINOIS

	1998	1999	2000	Total
Children's Mem Hosp, Siragusa Transplant Center, 2300 Children's Plaza, Box 57, Chicago, IL 60614 Ph: (773) 880-3027 Fax: (773) 880-3054 Email: siragusatx@childrensmemorial.org 1,2) C. Mavroudis, 2) C.L. Backer, 3) E. Pahl, D. Wax, 5) S. Rodgers	5	8	8	86
Rush-Presbyterian-St Luke's Med Ctr, Rush Cardiac Transp Prog, 1725 West Harrison, Professional Bldg, Ste 439, Chicago, IL 60612 Ph: (312) 563-2121 Fax: (312) 850-0913 1) M.R. Costanzo, 2) W. Piccione, R. March, V. DiSesa, E. Savase, V. Disesa, 3) W. Kao, E. Winkel, A. Heroux, M. Saltzberg, J. Barron, S. Pamboukian, 5) Burke, Sitt, Ertman, Grady, Rummel, Phillip, Hayes	9	8	9	130
Univ of Chicago Hosps, Sec of Cardiac Surg, Box MC 5040, 5841 S Maryland Ave, Chicago, IL 60637 Ph: (773) 702-2500 Fax: (773) 702-4187 1,2) V. Jeevanandam, 2) M.K. Ferguson, 3) A. Anderson, 4) Reg Organ Bank of Ill, 5) C. Murks	9	11	23*	97
Univ of Illinois Hosp and Clinics, Sec of Cardiothoracic Surg, Box 6998, Rm 920, m/c 787, Chicago, IL 60680-6998 Ph: (312) 996-6215 Fax: (312) 996-2013 1,2) M.G. Massad, 2) A. Geha, 3) S. Dunlap, G. Kondos, R. Candipan, 4) V.A. Lazda, 5) J. Herman, D. Fontana	2	5	2	39
Loyola Univ Med Ctr, Dept of Thor/Cardio/Vasc Surg, 2160 S 1st Ave, Bldg 110 Rm 6296, Maywood, IL 60153 Ph: (708) 327-2736 Fax: (708) 327-2770 1,2) B.K. Foy, 1,3) G.M. Mullen, 2) M. Stout, 3) B. Pisani, J. Mendez, 4) B. Susskind, 5) L. Dusek, M. Laff	26	27	24	484
OSF St Francis Med Ctr, Transp Serv-Heart, 530 NE Glen Oak Ave, Peoria, IL 61637 Ph: (800) 635-1440 Fax: (309) 655-2597 1,2) R.C. Gomez, 2) J.R. Munns, D.M. Geiss, D. Mueller, 3) D. Best, B.S. Clemson, R.P. McRae, 4) ROBI, 5) C. Linett, S. Faulkner, D. Joseph	14	13	11*	165

1)=Director, 2)=Tx Surgeons, 3)=Physicians, 4)=Tissue Typers, 5)=TxCoords	1998	1999	2000	Total
INDIANA				
Northern Indiana Heart Inst, Lutheran Hosp of Indiana, Cardio/Pulm Transp/Implant Dept, 7950 W Jefferson Blvd, Fort Wayne, IN 46804 Ph: (219) 435-7434 Fax: (219) 435-7615 1,2) R. Scheeringa, 2) J.S. Ladowski, A. Peterson, W. Deschner, C. Danby, B. Hook, D. Herlan, 3) J. Gilbert, S. Reed, M. O'Shaughnessy, 4) Indiana Reg, 5) M. Scatena, L. Beatty, M. Phillips	6	4	10	173
Indiana Univ Med Ctr, Dept of Cardiac Transp, 550 N University Blvd, Rm 4546, Indianapolis, IN 46202-5250 Ph: (317) 274 8387 Fax: (317) 274 3084 1,2) J.W. Brown, 2) O. Mohamed, K. Kesler, M. Turrentine, 3) R.A. Caldwell, R. Darragh, J. O'Donnell, 4) Z. Brahmi, 5) A. Darroca, L. Hiles	8	12	10*	191
Methodist Hosp, Transp Ctr, I 65 at 21st St, PO Box 1367, Indianapolis, IN 46202-1367 Ph: (317) 929-8677 Fax: (317) 929-5768 1,2) H. Halbrook, 2) J. Fehrenbacher, D. Beckman, D. Hormuth, T. Wozniak, A. Coffey, 3) D. Pitts, R. Schumacher, P. Kirlin, R. Valentine, H. Genovely, 4) J. McIntyre, N. Higgins, 5) S. Mitchell, A. Currin	19	9	12	292
St Vincents Hosp, Health Care Ctr, Dept of Cardio/Vasc Surg, 2001 W 86th St, Indianapolis, IN 46260 Ph: (317) 338-9157 Fax: (317) 338-9081 1) J.M. Paris, 2) R.J. Robison, R.J. Matheny, 3) M.L. See, J.H. Adlam, E.T.A. Fry, M.N. Walsh, 4) Ctr Indiana Reg Bld Ctr, 5) J. Bogdon, C. Kartman	11	10	14*	169
IOWA				
Mercy Hosp Med Ctr, Transp Serv, 400 University Ave., Des Moines, IA 50314 Ph: (515) 247-4261 Fax: (515) 247-8870 1,2) S.J. Phillips, 1,3) W.Wickemeyer, 2) R. Zeff, 3) K.P. Anderson, 4) S. Dhannavada, 5) K. Carlberg, P. Freeman, K. Reha	1	0	0	86
Univ of Iowa Hosp & Clin, Dept of Cardio/Thor Surg, 200 Hawkins Dr, 1601 JCP, Iowa City, IA 52242-1062 Ph: (319) 384-8268 Fax: (319) 353-7773 1,2) W.E. Richenbacher, 2) D.M. Behrendt, J.E. Everett, 3) R. Oren, L. Cadaret, E. Edens, 4) N.E. Goeken, 5) S. Vance, C. Laxson, B. Crane	11	16	6	166
KANSAS				
St Francis-Via Christi, Dept of Cardiac Transp, 929 N St Francis, Wichita, KS 67214 Ph: (316) 268-5891 Fax: (316) 291-7890 1,2) T.H. Estep, 2) G.S. Benton, R.H. Fleming, 5) C. Hagerty, M. Richardson	8	10	7	138
KENTUCKY				
Jewish Hosp, Transp Serv, 217 E Chestnut St, Louisville, KY 40202 Ph: (502) 587-4939 Fax: (502) 587-4184 1,2) G. Bhat, 2) L. Gray, S. Etoch, R. Dowling, 3) G. Bhat, K. Erbeck, G. Aronoff, 4) P. Landrum, R. Pound, J. Cassin, M. Steele, 5) J. Brohm, D. Strunk, A. Fish, D. Harris	17	14	21	272
Univ of Kentucky Med Ctr, Dept of Cardio/Thor Surg, Transplant Center, 800 Rose St C-430, Lexington, KY 40536 Ph: (859) 323-6497 Fax: (859) 323-1700 1,2) R.M. Mentzer JR, 2) T. Mullett, S. Jahania, 3) T. Waid, 4) F. Lower, W. O'Conner, 5) J. Leigh, A. Hartman, J. Patrick	22	12	13	154
LOUISIANA				
Ochsner Foundation Hospital, Multi-Organ Transplant Program, 1514 Jefferson Hwy, New Orleans, LA 70121 Ph: (504) 842-5630 Fax: (504) 842-4184 Email: mmehra@ochsner.org 1,3) M.R. Mehra, 2) J. Ochsner, M. McFadden, C.H. VanMeter, J. Davis, 3) R.L. Scott, M.H. Park, 4) G. Stewart, S. Herbert, D. Nordman, 5) Cassidy, DumasHicks, Stevenson, Bordelon, Bourgeois	41	35	30	529
Tulane Univ Med Ctr, Dept of Surg, SL 22, 1430 Tulane Ave, New Orleans, LA 70112 Ph: (504) 582-7998 Fax: (504) 587-2141 1,3) F.W. Smart, 2) J.D. Pigott, 3) A. Pickoff, A. Buda, 4) K.A. Sullivan, 5) D. Storey, S. Israel	8	13	8*	59
MARYLAND				
The Johns Hopkins Hosp, Dept of Cardio Surg, Blalock Bldg #618, 600 N Wolfe St, Baltimore,MD 21287-4618 Ph: (410) 955-1753 Fax: (410) 955-3809 1,3) E. Kasper, 1,2) J.V. Conte, 2) W.A. Baumgartner, D. Cameron, R. Stuart, P. Greene, 3) E. Kasper, K. Baughman, J. Hare, I. Wittstern, D. Judge, 4) J. Hart, 5) K. Shagna, D. Carter, S. Kelby, S. Metler, J. Stanik-Hutt	19	22	25*	327

1)=Director, 2)=Tx Surgeons, 3)=Physicians, 4)=Tissue Typers, 5)=TxCoords	1998	1999	2000	Total
Univ of Maryland Med Ctr, Dept of Surgery, Thoracic Tx, N4W94, 22 S Greene St, Baltimore, MD 21201 Ph: (410) 328-2737 Fax: (410) 328-2750 1) J. Brown, 2) J. Sonett, S. Downing, Z. Gamliel, 3) R. Freudenberger, 4) American Red Cross, 5) R. Anzeck	6	4	2	59

MASSACHUSETTS

	1998	1999	2000	Total
Brigham & Women's Hosp, Dept of Med, Cardio Div, 75 Francis St, Boston, MA 02115 Ph: (617) 732-7141 Fax: (617) 278-6931 1,3) G. Mudge, 1,2) G. Couper, 2) D. Adams, J. Byrne, L. Aklog, 3) J. Jarcho, P. Johnson, L.W. Stevensen, J. Fang, W. Johnson, 4) NEOB, 5) C. Flavell, C. Smith, L. James23	23	30	19*	421
Children's Hosp Boston, Dept of Cardio/Vasc Surg, 300 Longwood Ave, Boston, MA 02115 Ph: (617) 335-3629 Fax: (617) 734-9930 1,2) J.E. Mayer Jr, 2) P. del Nido, 3) S. Perry, L. Smoot, E. Blume, 4) New England Organ Bank, 5) P. O'Brien, H. Bastardi	14	8	12	104
Massachusetts Gen Hosp, Cardiac Div, 55 Fruit St, Bigelow 645, Boston, MA 02114 Ph: (617) 724-1400 Fax: (617) 726-4105 1) G.W. Dec Jr, 2) G. Vlahakes, D. Torchiana, J. Madsen, T. MacGillirray, A.K. Agnihotri, 3) M. Semigran, T. DiSalvo, R. Hajjar, 4) J. Gougan, 5) S. Keck, K. Gonczarek	21	10	15	207
New England Med Ctr, Div of Cardio/Thor Surg, Box 104, 750 Washington St, Boston, MA 02111 Ph: (617) 636-5593 Fax: (617) 636-7616 1,3) M.A. Konstam, 2) R. Bojar, H. Rastegae, K. Warner, 3) J. Udelson, J. Smith, 4) E. Milford, 5) A. Turbett	2	11	12*	104

MICHIGAN

	1998	1999	2000	Total
Univ of Michigan Med Ctr, Section of Cardiac Surgeons, Box 0348, 2120 Taubman Ctr, 1500 E Medical Center Dr, Ann Arbor, MI 48109 Ph: (734) 647-2894 Fax: (734) 764-2255 1,2) F.D. Pagani, 2) G.M. Deeb, S.F. Bolling, 3) K. Aaronson, R. Cody, T. Koelling, J. Nicklas, 4) J. Baker, 5) A. Richardson, J. Below, J. Edwards	38	40	202*	616
Henry Ford Hosp, Dept of Cardio/Thor Surg, 2799 W Grand Blvd, Detroit, MI 48202 Ph: (313) 876-2695 Fax: (313) 916-2687 1) Bernabei, 2) N. Silveman, R. Brewer, 3) B. Czerska, 4) D. Kukuruga, 5) C. Drost, G. Franklin, D. Rickard, C. Nelson	23	10	32	275

MINNESOTA

	1998	1999	2000	Total
Abbott Northwestern Hosp/, Minneapolis Heart Inst, Cardio/Thoracic Transpl, 800 E 28th St, Ste G004, Minneapolis, MN 55407 Ph: (612) 863-5638 Fax: (612) 863-3194 1,2) R.W. Emery, 2) Eales, Kshettry, Joyce, King, Lillehei, Nicoloff, Heck, Burdine, 3) M.R. Pritzker, M.T. Olivari, D. Burns, 4) Univ of Minnesota, 5) F. Hoffman, N. Siemers, J. Price, K. Gilkerson	19	10	10*	260
Fairview-University Med Ctr, Thoracic Transplant Program, Box 398, 420 Delaware St SE, Minneapolis, MN 55455 Ph: (612) 625-9922 Fax: (612) 626-6968 1,2) S. Shumway, 1) L. Miller, 2) R.M. Bolman, E. Molina, S. Park, C. Harrinton, 3) A. Bank, 4) H. Noreen, 5) Ormaza, Monson, Steen, Locher	17	16	19*	410
Mayo Clin, St Mary's Hosp, Dept of Cardio/Thor Surg, 6-716 St Mary's Hosp, Rochester, MN 55905 Ph: (507) 255-6038 Fax: (507) 255-4500 1,2) C.G.A. McGregor, 2) R. Daly, J. Dearani, 3) R. Rodeheffer, L.J. Olson, B.S. Edwards, R.P. Frantz, S.S. Kushwaha, 4) S.B. Moore, 5) S. Carlson, J. Hanson, J. Meyer, K. Sandstrom	21	21	15	188

MISSISSIPPI

	1998	1999	2000	Total
Univ of Mississippi Med Ctr, Transp Prog, Heart Station/UMC, 2500 N State St, Jackson, MS 39216-4505 Ph: (601) 984-2634 Fax: (601) 984-2631 1,3) C. Moore, 2) G. Aru, 3) T. Skelton, 4) J. Cruse, R. Lewis, 5) T. Thomas	14	13	13*	118

MISSOURI

	1998	1999	2000	Total
Univ Hosp & Clin, Cardio/Transp Dept, One Hospital Dr, Columbia, MO 65212 Ph: (573) 882-8763 Fax: (573) 884-4237 1,2) J. Curtis, 2) T. Demmy, 3) H.K. Reddy, 4) Red Cross Lab, 5) M. Misplay, C. Russell	9	13	8	103

HEART

1)=Director, 2)=Tx Surgeons, 3)=Physicians, 4)=Tissue Typers, 5)=TxCoords	1998	1999	2000	Total
Mid America Heart Inst of St Lukes, Cardiac Transp Prog, 4401 Wornall Rd, Kansas City, MO 64111 Ph: (816) 932-3264 Fax: (816) 932-5645 1,2) G.F. Muellebach, 2) M. Gorton, A.M. Borkon, , 3) D.R. Bresnahan Jr, A. Magalski, T.L. Stevens, 4) Midwest Transplant Network, 5) E.H. Russell, K. St Clair, P.J. Arnold	18	17	20	224
Barnes-Jewish Hosp, Washington Univ, Heart Failure/Heart Transp, Suite 4455 N Campus, 216 S. Kingshighway, St Louis, MO 63110 Ph: (314) 454-7687 Fax: (314) 454-8364 1,2) T.M. Sundt, 1,3) J.G. Rogers, 2) M.K. Pasque, M.R. Moon, 3) E.M. Geltman, G. Ewald, 4) T. Mohanakumar, D. Phelan, 5) C. Pasque, S. Moorhead, P. Solon, J. Casstevens, L. Crawford, J. Klein	20	15	15	395
Cardinal Glennon Childrens Hospital, Dept of Ped Cardio/Thor Surg, 1465 S Grand, St Louis, MO 63104 Ph: (314) 577-5674 Fax: (314) 268-4141 1,3) I. Balfour, 2) L. McBride, A. Fiore, 3) S. Nouri, 4) St. Louis University, 5) B. Friedman, R. Freeze, L. Sosa	3	1	2*	31
St Louis Children's Hosp, Med Ctr, Dept Cardio/Thor Surg, 400 S Kings Hwy, Ste 5W24, St Louis, MO 63110 Ph: (314) 454-6095 Fax: (314) 454-2561 1,3) C.E. Canter, 1,2) C.B. Huddleston, 2) E.N. Mendeloff, 3) C.E. Canter, 4) D. Phelan, 5) P. Murphy, S. Basile, N. Hagin	14	16	14*	168
St Louis Univ Hlth Sci Ctr, Cardiology Div, 3635 Vista Ave, PO Box 15250, St Louis, MO 63110 Ph: (314) 577-8896 Fax: (314) 268-5138 1,3) P.I. Hauptman, 2) L.R. McBride, G. Lowdermilk, 3) D. Yip, A. Betkowski, T. Wolford, 4) K. Riordan, B. Hoover, L. Santiago, 5) L. Horn, C. Zirges	15	17	9*	340
NEBRASKA				
Bryan LGH Med Center East, Transp Serv, 1600 S 48th St, Lincoln, NE 68506-1299 Ph: (402) 481-3911 Fax: (402) 481-3918 1,2) D. Gangahar, 2) E. Raines, J. Wudel, 3) S. Liggett, 4) Univ of Nebraska Med Ctr, 5) N. Steckelberg	4	4	6*	111
Nebraska Health System, Dept of Surg, Sec of Cardio/Thor Surg, 982315 Nebraska Med Ctr, Omaha, NE 68198-2315 Ph: (402) 559-4424 Fax: (402) 559-6913 1,2) T.A. Galbraith, 1,3) G.C.Groggel, 2) K. Franco, T.A. Galbraith, 3) J. Rogers, 4) S. Radio	2	1	0*	29
NEW JERSEY				
Newark Beth Israel Med Ctr, Dept of Cardiothoracic Transp, 201 Lyons Ave, ACC 4, Newark, NJ 07112 Ph: (973) 926-7205 Fax: (973) 923-8993 Email: mzucker@sbhcs.com 1,3) M.J. Zucker, 2) D. Goldstein, T. Prendergast, S. Shah, 3) H.S. Ribner, L. Arroyo, D. Petrowsky, 4) C. Pancoska, 5) L. Mele, S. Pardi, T. Martin, S. Bausback-Aballo, S. Garber	20	30	28	242
NEW MEXICO				
Presbyterian Hosp Ctr, Transp Serv, 1100 Central SE, PO Box 26666, Albuquerque, NM 87106 Ph: (505) 841-1434 Fax: (505) 222-2149 1,2) C. Wehr, 2) D. Sansonetti, W. Dean, R. Geretey, J. Storey, C. Lagerstrom, 3) J. Heilman, 5) C. Moore, K. McEvoy	8	6	4*	149
NEW YORK				
State Univ of New York at Buffalo, Buffalo Gen/VA/Chldrns Hosps, Dept of Surg, 100 High St, Buffalo, NY 14203 Ph: (716) 859-2230 Fax: (716) 859-2885 1,2) J.N. Bhayana, 2) J. Bergland, S. Raza, 3) J. Schwartz, S. Graham, 4) T. Shanahan, 5) M.A. Schnapp, C. Schaff	0	4	0*	118
Columbia Presbyterian Med Ctr, Dept of Surg/Cardio Transp, PH 14 West, 622 W 168th St, New York, NY 10032 Ph: (212) 305-7600 Fax: (212) 305-8304 1) N.M. Edwards, 2) E.A. Rose, C.R. Smith, M.C. Oz, Y. Naka, 3) Mancini, Drusin, Blood, Ravelli, Maybaum, Restaino, 4) N. Suciu-Foca, 5) H. Hauff, J. Guzy, K. Ryan	104	84	93*	1249
Mount Sinai Med Ctr, Cardio/Thor Div, Box 1028, 1 Gustave Levy Place, New York, NY 10029 Ph: (212) 241-8181 Fax: (212) 534-3357 1,2) S. Lansman, 2) S. Lansman, R. Griepp, M.A. Ergin, J. McCullough, D. Spielvogel, 3) iA. Gass, M. Kukin, D. Baran, 4) Rogosin Inst, 5) M. Courtney, D. Correa	27	27	29*	270

1)=Director, 2)=Tx Surgeons, 3)=Physicians, 4)=Tissue Typers, 5)=TxCoords	1998	1999	2000	Total
NORTH CAROLINA				
Univ of North Carolina Hosp, Div of Cardio/Thor Surg, Dept of Surg, CB 7065, 108 Burnett-Womack Bldg, Chapel Hill, NC 27599-7065 Ph: (888) 263-5293 Fax: (919) 966-3475 Email: mrm@med.unc.edu 1,2) M.R. Mill, 2) T.M. Egan, F.C. Detterbeck, 3) K.F. Adams Jr, C.A. Sueta, E. Frantz, S. Kushwaha, 4) J. Schmitz, J. Thomas, 5) S. Kowalczyk, M. Grady	12	15	17	172
Carolinas Med Ctr, Dept of Transp, PO Box 32861, Charlotte, NC 28232-2861 Ph: (704) 355-4725 Fax: (704) 355-7616 1,3) A.M. Thomley, 1,2) E. Skipper, 2) P. Hess, J. Cook, M. Stiegel, J. Selle, 3) R. Haber, R.T. Smith, 4) S. Bruner, 5) J. Boger, D. Watkins, S. DeLuca	16	22	15*	273
Duke Univ Med Ctr, Dept of Surg, Box 3235, DUMC, Durham, NC 27710 Ph: (919) 684-2651 Fax: (919) 681-8860 1,2) R.D. Davis, 2) C. Milano, K. Landolfo, J. Jaggers, 3) M. Higginbotham, S. Russell, 4) F. Ward, N. Reinsmoen, 5) L. Blue, B. Everton	21	24	52*	283
North Carolina Baptist Hosp, Dept of Cardio/Thor Surg, Medical Ctr Blvd, Winston Salem, NC 27157-1096 Ph: (800) 277-7654 Fax: (336) 716-3348 1,2) T.E. Oaks, 2) J. Hammon, N. Kon, M. Hines, G. Pennington, 3) B.K. Rayburn, T. Wannenburg, 4) E. Heise, 5) S. Close	4	13	4*	74
OHIO				
Children's Hosp Med Ctr, Cardiac Surg, 3333 Burnet Ave, Cincinnati, OH 45229-3039 Ph: (513) 636-4200 Fax: (513) 636-3952 1,2) J.M. Pearl, 1,3) R.Spicer, 2) P. Manning, 3) L. Wagner, 4) Hoxworth Bld Center, 5) K. Uzork, S. Rykman	0	5	4	26
Univ of Cincinnati Coll of Med, Dept of Int Med, Div of Cardio, 231 Bethesda Ave, ML 542, Cincinnati, OH 45267-0542 Ph: (513) 558-3487 Fax: (513) 558-3116 Email: wagonele@ucmail.uc.edu 1,3) L. Wagoner, 1,3) S.G. Menon, 2) T.D. Ivey, T. Axford, 3) J. Nickelson, L. Wagoner, 4) L. Whitacre, D. Eckels, 5) R. Giesting, B. Bell, S. Dudikis	26	22	17	298
Cleveland Clin Foundation, A110 Transplant Center, 9500 Euclid Ave, Cleveland, OH 44195 Ph: (216) 444-8351 Fax: (216) 444-0777 1,3) J.B. Young, 1,2) P.M. McCarthy, 2) R. Mee, N. Smedira, J. Navia, M. Banbury, 3) Hobbs, Rincon, Bott-Silverman, James, Starling, Kichuk, Lutton, 4) D.J. Cook, 5) D. Pelegrin, R. Courey, R. Bennett, K. Kiefer, P. Colosimo, S. Haliowell	113	77	76	859
Ohio State Univ Hosp, Dept of Cardio/Thor Surg, 410 W 10th Ave, 825 E Doan Hall, Columbus, OH 43210 Ph: (614) 293-3787 Fax: (614) 293-4726 Email: ballinger_2@medctr.osu.edu 1) R. Michler, 2) P. Ross, D. Brown, A. Goldstein, R. Michler, 3) C.V. Leier, P.F. Binkley, R. Alvarez, 4) C. Orosz, 5) M. Ballinger, J. Mueller, S. Wissman	23	31	12*	229
Medical College Hospitals, Dept of Med, Div of Cardio, PO Box 10008, 3000 Arlington Ave, Toledo, OH 43699 Ph: (419) 381-3500 Fax: (419) 382-5728 1,3) T. Walsh, 2) D.S. Durzinsky, X. Mousset, W. Wilson, 3) J. Hennesey, B. Grubbs, G. Ansel, 4) A. Blair, 5) J.M. Dickenson	5	7	8*	93
OKLAHOMA				
Integris Baptist Med Ctr, Nazih Zuhdi Transpl Inst, 3300 NW Expressway, Oklahoma City, OK 73112 Ph: (405) 949-3349 Fax: (405) 945-5467 1) B.M. Nour, 2) J. Chaffin, D. Vanhooser, C. Elkins, 3) D. Nelson, 4) S. Oleinick, 5) C. Smith, S. Kesinger, L. French	17	17	22*	312
Univ Hosp, Transp Serv, Rm 5E 190, 800 NE 13th St, Oklahoma City, OK 73104 Ph: (405) 271-7498 Fax: (405) 271-1772 1) L.R. Pennington, 2) R. Elkins, J. Randolph, C. Knott-Craig, E. Howell, 3) J.A. Pederson, 4) J. Baker, 5) T. Greenfield	1	1	0*	57
OREGON				
Oregon Univ Hosp, Div of Cardio Surg, 3181 SW Sam Jackson Pk Rd, Portland, OR 97201 Ph: (503) 494-7820 Fax: (503) 494-7829 1) H. Storm Floten, 2) J. Blizzard, P. Ravichandran, I. Shen, A. Furnary, 3) R. Hershberger, K. Crispell, M. Vossler, 4) D.J. Norman, 5) D. Penk, J. Caster, Cummings	16	22	23*	375

1)=Director, 2)=Tx Surgeons, 3)=Physicians, 4)=Tissue Typers, 5)=TxCoords	1998	1999	2000	Total
PENNSYLVANIA				
Milton S Hershey Med Ctr, Surg, Section Cardio/Thor, PO Box 850, Hershey, PA 17033 Ph: (717) 531-8329 Fax: (717) 531-3664 1,2) B. Sun, 2) D.B. Campbell, J.L. Myers, W.E. Pae Jr, 3) D. Davis, J. Boehmer, D. Silber, L. Sinoway, S. Mehta, 4) P.J. Romano, 5) J. Burg, F.A. Hrenko, P. Frazier, P. Coe, K. Newman	29	16	23	283
Hahnemann Univ Hosp, Heart Failure/Transp Ctr, Broad & Vine, MS 115, Philadelphia, PA 19102 Ph: (215) 762-4444 Fax: (215) 762-4953 1,3) J.M. Fitzpatrick, 2) L. Samuels, A. Guerraty, 3) J. Narula, D. Wood, 4) E. Tecza, 5) H. Jones, C. Dogonniuk	18	20	15*	241
Temple Univ School of Med, Cardiology Section, 3401 N Broad St, Suite 920, Philadelphia, PA 19140 Ph: (215) 707-1503 Fax: (215) 707-4521 1,3) H.J. Eisen, 2) S. Furukawa, J. Garcia, J.B. McClurken, W. Spotnitz, 3) K. Margulies, P. Mather, S. Rubin, G. Berman, J. Wald, 4) S. Leach, 5) T. Rourke, E. Hobson, B. Ebert, P. Pavelchak, T. Rowe, S. Fontana	56	51	54	809
The Children's Hosp of Philadelphia, Thoracic Organ Transp Program, 34th St & Civic Ctr Blvd, Philadelphia, PA 19104 Ph: (215) 590-6051 Fax: (213) 590-1340 1,2) T.L. Spray, 2) J.W. Gaynor, W.M. DeCampli, T.R. Karl, 3) B.J. Clark, N.D. Bridges, R.M. Donner, B.D. Hanna, T. Hoffman, 4) D. Monos, 5) M. Sowa, J. Menendez	8	11	15	91
Univ of Pennsylvania Med Ctr, Cardio Div, 6 Penn Tower, 3400 Spruce St, Philadelphia, PA 19104 Ph: (215) 662-6838 Fax: (215) 615-0828 1,2) M. Acker, 1,3) E. Loh, 2) B. Rosengard, A. Pochettino, R. Morris, R. Garman, 3) A. Kao, L. Goldber, S. Brazena, M. Jessup, 4) M. Kamoun, 5) C. Dorozinsky, S. Roan, D. Chojurwski, S. Chambers, C. Taomey	48	59	50*	386
Allegheny Gen Hosp, Dept of Surg, Transp Serv, 320 E North Ave, Pittsburgh, PA 15212 Ph: (412) 359-6800 Fax: (412) 359-4721 1,2) G.M. Magovern Jr, 2) G. Marrone, G. Sydlowski, J. Uddi-coat, 3) M.A. Mathier, 4) S. Hsia, 5) C.L. Paul, T. Ryan	9	9	5	138
Children's Hosp of Pittsburgh, Dept of Cardiology, 3705 Fifth Ave, One Children's Place, Pittsburgh, PA 15213 Ph: (412) 692-5541 Fax: (412) 692-6991 Email: webbers@heart.chp.edu 1,2) S. Webber, 2) F. Pigula, 3) J. Boyle, S. Miller, Y. Law, 4) A. Zeevi, 5) D. Dorsey, B. Stinner	14	10	14	163
Univ of Pittsburgh-Presbyterian Hosp, Dept of Cardio/Thor Surg, C-700 Presbyterian Univ Hosp, 200 Lothrop St, Pittsburgh, PA 15213-2582 Ph: (412) 648-1963 Fax: (412) 648-1029 Email: ristichj@msx.upmc.edu 1,2) R. Kormos, 2) B. Griffith, R. Kormos, K. McCurry, M. Zenati, B. Hattler, 3) S. Murali, D. McNamara, W. Rosenblum, 4) A. Zeevi, 5) A. Lee, S. Zomak, T. Tokarczyk, C. Cornell	34	31	32	839
SOUTH CAROLINA				
Med Univ of South Carolina, Div of Cardio/ThorSurg, 150 Ashley Ave, PO Box 250586, Charleston, SC 29425 Ph: (843) 792-9259 Fax: (843) 792-1729 1,2) A.J. Crumbley III, 2) J.M. Kratz, J. Zellner, 3) A.B. VanBakel, G.H. Hendrix, H.B. Wiles, N. Periera, 4) S. Self, 5) S. Odom, B. Ryan, B. Dority, D. York	26	24	26*	231
TENNESSEE				
Baptist Memorial Hosp, Thoracic Transp Serv, 930 Madison Ave, Ste 456, Memphis, TN 38103 Ph: (901) 227-6106 Fax: (901) 227-6196 1,2) H.E. Garrett Jr, 2) J. Gooch, D. Weiman, R. Carter, 3) K. Newman, G. Murray, S. Himmelstein, T. Edwards, 4) C. Miller, B. Loehmann, Y. Cao, L. Marek, 5) D. Combs, D. DuVall-Seaman, R. Suggs	17	16	11*	157
Le Bonheur Childrens Med Ctr, The Heart Center, 50 N Dunlap, Memphis, TN 38103 Ph: (901) 572-5438 Fax: (901) 572-5052 1,3) S. Birnbaum, 2) E. Garrett Jr, N. Novick, 3) M. Salim, 4) C. Miller, B. Loehman, R. Fletcher, 5) J. Ammons, S. Powell	4	1	0*	21
Methodist Hosp of Memphis, Dept of Cardio Surg, 1325 Eastmoreland #220, Memphis, TN 38104 Ph: (901) 725-9450 Fax: (901) 274-0741 1,2) G.P. Schoettle Jr, 2) O.B. Harrington, E. Owen Jr, E.J. Chauvin, 3) M. Gelfand, 4) Diaclin Lab, 5) C. Simmons	0	14		87

1)=Director, 2)=Tx Surgeons, 3)=Physicians, 4)=Tissue Typers, 5)=TxCoords	1998	1999	2000	Total
St Thomas Hosp, Dept of Transp, 1st Floor, 105-A West, 4230 Harding Rd, Nashville, TN 37205 Ph: (615) 222-6618 Fax: (615) 222-6074 1,3) M. Wigger, 2) Glassford Jr, Lea IV, Shuman, Coltharp, Ball, Pirolo, 3) J. Fields, 4) DCI, 5) E. Weaver, M. Dubuque, V. Barnes-Eubank, H. Marshall	15	18	20	226
Vanderbilt Univ Med Ctr, The Vanderbilt Transp Ctr, Heart Transp Program, 908 Oxford House, Nashville, TN 37232-4734 Ph: (615) 936-3500 Fax: (615) 936-0396 1,2) D. Drinkwater, 2) W.H. Merrill, R.N. Pierson III, K.J. Christian, 3) S. Davis, D. Chomsky, J. Butler, 4) DCI Labs, 5) T. Donaldson, R. Howser, B. Davidson	31	32	29	384

TEXAS

	1998	1999	2000	Total
Seton Med Ctr, Seton Heart Center, 1301 W 38th St, Suite 700, Austin, TX 78705-105 Ph: (512) 324-1374 Fax: (512) 324-1300 1,3) M.B. Cishek, 1,2) M. Mueller, 2) E. Dilling, S. Dewan, L. King, M. Felger, A. Hume, W. Kessler, J.D. Oswalt, 3) D. Morris, J. Dieck, P. Roach, K. Thompson, 4) Southwest Immunodiagnostics, 5) B. Richards, R. Koneski, D. Johnson, S. Younger	14	27	17	197
Baylor Univ Med Ctr, Roberts Hosp, Cardio/Thoracic Transp, 4 Roberts, 3500 Gaston Ave, Dallas, TX 75246 Ph: (214) 820-6856 Fax: (214) 820-4527 1,2) W.S. Ring, 2) J. Capehart, D. Meyer, M. Wait, M. Jessen, M. DiMaio, 3) C. Yancy, S. Hall, J. Escobar, J. Kuiper, 4) J. McCormack, 5) R. Kauffman, A. Boronow, S. Moore, J. West, A. Dierlam, A. Sonnen	19	22	15	256
Children's Med Ctr of Dallas, Dept of Thor Surg, 1935 Motor Street, Dallas, TX 75235-8879 Ph: (214) 648-4589 Fax: (214) 648-2465 1,2) W.S. Ring, 2) D. Meyer, H. Nikaidoh, M. Wait, 3) D. Fixler, K. Rotondo, D. Stromberg, 4) P. Stastny, 5) J. Wells, M. Drury, K. Srokoscz	4	3	3*	45
Medical City Dallas Hosp, Transplant Center, 7777 Forest Lane, A-14th Floor, Dallas, TX 75230 Ph: (800) 348-4318 Fax: (972) 566-4872 1,2) S. Seitz, 2) D. Ogden, M. Mack, T. Dewey, M. McGee, R. Bowman, I. Davidsons, S. Reeder, 3) J.E. Rosenthal, M. Lerman, J. Hunt, A. Shulkin, K. Hoang, A. Anderson, 4) Texas Med Specialty Inc.(A. Nikaein), 5) M. Covin, T. McMellon, D. Stevenson, C. Cava-Bartsch, A. Kuhnel	29	23	22	187
Methodist Med Ctr, Heart Ctr, PO Box 655999, 1441 N Beckley, Dallas, TX 75265-5999 Ph: (214) 947-2757 Fax: (214) 941-8061 1,2) R. Dickerman, 1,3) K.Brinker, 2) L. Whiddon, 3) P. Vergne-Marini, D. Nesser, R. Velez, 4) G. Land, 5) R. Bunton, J. McDonald, A. Louzau, C. Cannon	1	0	0	76
St Paul Med Ctr, Univ of Texas Southwstern, Transp office, Ste 623, 5939 Harry Hines Blvd, Dallas, TX 75235 Ph: (214) 648-8811 Fax: (214) 879-6209 1,2) W.S. Ring, 2) D. Meyer, C. Moncrief, M. Jessen, M. Wait, M. DeMaio, 3) C. Yancy, B. Baldwin, V. Horn, D. Dries, J. Boehrer, M. Drazner, D. Garry, 4) P. Stastny, 5) P. Kaiser, K. Weber, M. Stenstrom, K. Rozelle, K. Bush	24	21	21*	262
Brooke Army Med Ctr, Dept of Cardio, 3851 Roger Brooke Dr, Bldg 3600, Fort Sam Houston, TX 78234-6200 Ph: (210) 916-4193 Fax: (210) 916-3051 1,2) D.J. Cohen, 2) C. Moore, 3) M. Kwan, 4) Wilford Hall Air Force Med Ctr HLA Lab, 5) N.A. Khan	2	3	3*	23
Univ of Texas Med Branch-Galveston, Dept of Cardio/Thor Surg, 301 University Blvd, Rte 05-28, Galveston, TX 77555-0528 Ph: (409) 772-1203 Fax: (409) 772-1421 1,2) S.D. Lick, 2) V. Conti, P.S. Brown, E. MacInerney Jr, A. Bankar, J. Zwishchenberger, 3) B. Uretsky, 4) S. Vaidya, 5) S. Johnson	6	10	7*	79
Baylor Coll of Medicine, The Methodist Hosp, Multi-Organ Transp Ctr, 6565 Fannin-SM 447, Houston, TX 77030 Ph: (713) 790-2501 Fax: (713) 793-1335 1,2) G.P. Noon, 2) S. Scheinin, J. Lafuente, 3) G. Torre-Amione, M. Koerner, 4) G.E. Rodey, 5) L. Johnson, J. Zener, S. Zylicz	30	27	31*	461
Texas Heart Inst, St Luke's Episcopal Hosp, Transp Serv 2-114, PO Box 20269, Houston, TX 77225 Ph: (713) 791-2285 Fax: (713) 794-6696 Email: ppowers@sleh.com 1,2) O.H. Frazier, 2) G. Noon, S. Scheinen, I. Gregoric, 3) E.K. Massin, T. Khan, 4) R. Kerman, 5) P. Powers, P. Odegaard, T. Isom, A. Riley, M. Norman, G. Martinson	35	35	46	821

1)=Director, 2)=Tx Surgeons, 3)=Physicians, 4)=Tissue Typers, 5)=TxCoords	1998	1999	2000	Total
Methodist Specialty & Transp Hosp, Dept of Cardio Transp, 8026 Floyd Curl, San Antonio, TX 78229 Ph: (210) 692-8250 Fax: (210) 692-8154 1,2) C. Moore, 1) L.Zorvilla, 2) L. Hamner, C. Christian, 3) J. Mulgrow, R. Bogaev, 4) J. Morrisey, 5) L. McFarlin, L. Parker, D. Smith, K. Cunningham	11	10	12	195
UTHSCSA, Dept of Surg, Organ Transpl, Mail code 7858, 7703 Floyd Curl Dr, San Antonio, TX 78284 Ph: (210) 567-5777 Fax: (210) 567-5122 Email: sako@uthscsa.edu 1,2) E. Sako, 1,3) D.Murray, 2) J. Calhoon, L. Miller, S. Johnson, 3) D. Murray, S. Bailey, 4) P. Blackwell, K. Rocha, G. Bruun, 5) L. Nichols, T. Cronin	5	5		131
UTAH				
Primary Children's Med Ctr, Dept of Pediatric Cardio, 100 N Medical Dr, Salt Lake City, UT 84113-1100 Ph: (801) 588-2600 Fax: (801) 588-2612 1,3) R.E. Shaddy, 2) J. Hawkins, E.C. McGough, 3) L.Y. Tani, G.S. Orsmond, 4) T. Fuller, 5) E.A. Bullock	1	3	6	51
LDS Hosp, Dept of Cardio, 8th Ave & C St, Salt Lake City, UT 84143 Ph: (801) 408-8162 Fax: (801) 408-8162 1) D.G. Renlund, 2) K.W. Jones, D. Doty, R. Millar, J. Long, 3) Lappe, Sorensen, Crandall, Osborn, Burke, Horton, Walsh, Taylor, 4) T. Fuller, 5) S. Swanson-Schmitz, P. Grizzell	7	7	9*	273
Univ of Utah Hosp, Dept of Cardio Transp, Div of Cardiology - 4A100, 50 N Medical Dr, Salt Lake City, UT 84132 Ph: (801) 585-3693 Fax: (801) 585-5685 1) D.G. Renlund, 2) S.V. Karwande, J. Stringham, D. Bull, 3) D.O. Taylor, A. Kfoury, 4) T. Fuller, 5) B. Carpenter, C. Huff	8	10	13*	263
Veteran's Admin Med Ctr, Dept of Cardio Transp, 500 Foothill Blvd, Salt Lake City, UT 84132 Ph: (801) 582-1565 x4544 Fax: (801) 524-1251 1) D.G. Renlund, 2) S.V. Karwande, D. Bull, 3) D.O. Taylor, 4) T. Fuller, 5) M.B. Hagan, T.L. Cobb	5	4		194
VIRGINIA				
Univ of Virginia Health Science Ctr, Cardio/Pulm Transp Ctr, Box 191, Lee Street, Charlottesville, VA 22908 Ph: (800) 257-0757 Fax: (804) 924-2359 1,3) J. Bergin, 2) I. Kron, C.G. Tribble, 3) N. Lewis, 4) C. Spencer, T. Prichett, C. Paschall, 5) C. Ballew, K. Walker-Cooke, T. Broccoli	12	16	15*	227
Inova Fairfax Hosp, Transp Ctr, Dept of Heart/Lung, 3300 Gallows Rd, Falls Church, VA 22042-3300 Ph: (703) 698-2986 Fax: (703) 698-2797 1,2) N. Burton, 2) P. Massimiano, E. Lefrak, A. Coffey, A. Speir, 3) A. Keller, S. Nathan, 4) Transp/Immun Lab, Washington, D.C. , 5) D. Campbell, A. Klem, L. Geisen	15	13	10*	176
Sentara Norfolk Gen Hosp, Dept of Cardiac Surg, 600 Gresham Dr, Norfolk, VA 23507 Ph: (757) 622-2677 Fax: (757) 623-2707 1,2) G.R. Barnhart, 2) J. Rich, S. Szenpetery, R. Hagberg, M. McGrath, 3) J. Herre, D. Eich, W. Old, 4) K. Keatly, T. McRacken, 5) P. Bradshaw, D. Milteer, L. Rettig, B. Smith, B. Morrill	19	17	11*	175
Henrico Doctors' Hosp, Virginia Transp Ctr, 1602 Shipwith Rd, Richmond, VA 23229 Ph: (804) 289-4700 Fax: (804) 285-5148 1,2) M. Katz, 1,3) J.A. Thompson, 2) J.J. Zocco, T.C. Wolfgang, 4) C. Breitenbach, C. Duvall, K. Pepeliaev, 5) M. Currier, S. Maguire	8	8	11*	121
McGuire Veteran Affairs Med Ctr, Transp Office (111H), 1201 Broad Rock Blvd, Richmond, VA 23249 Ph: (804) 230-6827 Fax: (804) 230-6921 1) McHarty, 2) R. Higgins, D. Salter, Cohen, 4) MCV Tissue Typ Lab, 5) J.S. Hanrahan, P. Joyner	5	2	5*	270
Med Coll of Virginia, Dept of Cardio/Pulm Transp, Box 980204-MCV Station, Richmond, VA 23298 Ph: (804) 828-4571 Fax: (804) 828-7710 1,2) R. Higgins, 2) D. Salter, N. Cohen, I. Mehta, V. Kasirajin, 3) M. Hess, 4) C. Rhodes, P. Kimble, 5) M. Flattery	1	1	6	328
WASHINGTON				
Children's Hosp Med Ctr, Dept of Surg, Cardio Transp Unit, 4800 Sand Point Way, NE, Seattle, WA 98105 Ph: (206) 526-2039 Fax: (206) 527-3925 1,2) E.D. Verrier, 2) M. Allen, M. Lupinetti, 3) D. Fishbein, J. French, M.L. Hall, P. Herndon, 4) Puget Sound Bld Ctr, 5) A. Kruse		1	1*	11

1)=Director, 2)=Tx Surgeons, 3)=Physicians, 4)=Tissue Typers, 5)=TxCoords	1998	1999	2000	Total
Univ Washington Med Ctr, Dept of Surg, Div Cardio/Thor Surg Box 356310, 1959 NE Pacific St, Seattle, WA 98195 Ph: (206) 543-8065 Fax: (206) 543-0325 1,2) E.D. Verrier, 2) W.E. Curtis, 3) D.P. Fishbein, W.C. Levy, K. O'Brien, 4) K. Nelson, 5) S. Kruse, V. Hines	26	32	32	306
Sacred Heart Med Ctr, Dept Thor Organ Transp, W 101 8th Ave, P.O.Box 2555, Spokane, WA 99220-2555 Ph: (509) 474-2041 Fax: (509) 474-4906 1,2) T.B. Icenogle, 2) D. Sandler, 3) R.D. Hill, 4) Inland Nowest Bld Ctr, 5) P. Hester, C. Sparks, P. Kaley	8	8	10	129

WISCONSIN

	1998	1999	2000	Total
Univ of Wisconsin Hosp & Clin, Div of Cardio/Thor Surg, 600 Highland Ave, H4-370, Madison, WI 53792-3236 Ph: (608) 263-7832 Fax: (608) 263-0597 1,2) R.B. Love, 2) R.P. Cochran, D. Woolley, 3) C. Van der Ark, P. Rahko, 4) D. Lorentzen, 5) E. Golz, L. Wick	34	33	20*	449
Children's Hosp of Wisconsin, MS 600-Cardio/Thor Transp Surg, 9000 W Wisconsin Ave, PO Box 1997, Milwaukee, WI 53201 Ph: (414) 266-3360 Fax: (414) 266-2109 1,2) J.T. Tweddell, 2) J. Crouch, B. Litwin, 3) S. Berger, P. Havens, T. Rice, K. Sagar, 4) Bld Ctr of SE Wisconsin, 5) M.K. Hintermeyer	0	2	3*	10
Froedtert Hospital, Med Coll of Wisconsin, Dept of Cardio/Thor Surg, 9200 W Wisconsin Ave, Milwaukee, WI 53226 Ph: (414) 456-6756 Fax: (414) 456-6203 Email: nicolosi@mcw.edu 1,2) J. Tweddell, 2) A. Nicolosi, 3) R. Siegel, M. Cinquegrani, J. Hosenpud, 4) Bld Ctr of SE Wisconsin, 5) J. Schweiger, J. Janusz	4	4	4	92
St Luke's Med Ctr, Transplant Program, 2900 W. Oklahoma Ave, Milwaukee, WI 53201-2901 Ph: (414) 649-7734 Fax: (414) 649-5414 1,2) A.J. Tector, 2) Downey, Kress, Schmahl, Barragry, Crouch, Auer, Seifert, O'Hair, 3) T. Gronski, J. Hosenpud, 4) M. Oaks, 5) J. Heimler, L. Halverson, J. Keepers, K. Meunier	42	36	32*	425

ARGENTINA

	1998	1999	2000	Total
ICYCC-Favaloro Foundation, Cardio/Vasc Surg, Transp Div, Av Belgrano 1746, Buenos Aires, C1093AAS Ph: (5411) 4378-1350 Fax: (5411) 4378-1311 Email: rfavaloro@ffavaloro.org 1,2) R.R. Favaloro, 2) J. Abud, H. Raffaelli, M. Favaloro, H. Machain, 3) S.V. Perrone, C. Gomez, L. Favaloro, M. Sultan, F. Klein, 4) E. Hass, E. Raimondi, 5) C. Presa, C. Gomez	12	27	25	190

AUSTRALIA

	1998	1999	2000	Total
Alfred Hosp, Heart & Lung Replacement Serv, Commercial Rd, Prahran, Melbourne,Victoria,3181 Ph: (613)9 276-2862 Fax: (613)9 276-2317 1,2) D.S. Esmore, 2) J. Smith, 3) P. Bergin, M. Richardson, D. Kaye, 4) B. Tait, L. Holder, 5) A. Griffiths, W. Moule, K. Waters	23	25	22	346
Royal Children's Hosp, Dept of Cardiac Surg, Flemington Rd, Parkville, Melbourne, Victoria, 3052 Ph: (61)3 9345 5717 Fax: (61)3 9345 6001 1,2) C. Bizad, 1,3) J.L. Wilkinson, 2) A. Cochrane, 3) R.G. Weintraub, 4) B. Tait, 5) A.T. Shipp	4	3		52

AUSTRIA

	1998	1999	2000	Total
Univ Klin fur Chir, Dept of Transp Surg, Auenbruggerplatz 29, A-8036 Graz Ph: (43)316 385-2707 Fax: (43)316 385-4446 1,2) K.H. Tscheliessnigg, 3) W. Klein, 4) G. Lanzer, 5) R. Resch	21	15		180
Univ Hosp, Dept of Transp Surg, Anichstrasse 35, Innsbruck, 6020 Ph: (43)512 504-2603 Fax: (43)512 504-2605 1,2) R. Margreiter, 1,2) G. Laufer, 2) H. Antretter, 3) O. Pachinger, G. Poelzl, 4) D. Schoenitzer, 5) H. Fetz, P. Schobel	22	20	21	155
Allgemeines Krankenhaus Wien, Univ Klinik Fuer Chirurgie, ABT.Herz-Thoraxchir, Waehringer Guertel 18-20, A 1090 Vienna Ph: (43)140400 5643 Fax: (43)140400 5642 1,2) M. Grimm, 2) E. Wolner, A. Zuckermann, G. Wieselthaler, 3) R. Pacher, 4) A. Hajek-Rosenmayr, 5) H. Koller	54	50	53	852

1)=Director, 2)=Tx Surgeons, 3)=Physicians, 4)=Tissue Typers, 5)=TxCoords	1998	1999	2000	Total

BELGIUM

	1998	1999	2000	Total
Onze Lieve Vrouw Hosp, Dept of Cardio Surg, Moorselbaan 164, B-9300 Aalst Ph: (32)53 72-4111 Fax: (32)53 72-4585 1) F. Wellens, 2) H. Vanermen, R. De Geest, Y. Degrieck, F. van Praet, 3) M. Goethals, J. Bartunek, 5) T. Gooris, W. Tack	10	15	10	217
Clin Univ St Luc, Dept of Cardio/Thor Surg, 10, Ave Hippocrate, Brussels, 1200 Ph: (32)2 764 6109 Fax: (32)2 764-8938 1,3) M. Goenen, 2) Noirhomme, Dion, Verhelst, Khoury, D'Udekern, d'Acoz, Rubay, Elkhour, 3) L. Jacquet, M. DeKock, 4) M. de Bruyere, D. Latinne, 5) P. van Drmelingen, T. Timmerman	18	17	14	288
Erasmus Hosp, Dept of Cardiac Surg, Rte de Lennick, 808, B-1070 Brussels Ph: (32)2 555-3817 Fax: (32)2 555-4405 1,2) J.L. LeClerc, 2) M. Antoine, 3) J.L. Vachiery, 4) E. Dupont, Erasmus Hosp, 5) B. van Haelewyck	15	14	8	391
Univ Hosp Antwerpen, Dept of Cardio Surg, Wilrijkstr 10, Edegem, B2650 Ph: (32)3 821 3129 Fax: (32)3 830 2099 1,2) A.C. Moulijn, 2) I. Rodrigus, B. Stockman, 3) V. Conraads, B.J. Amsel, A. Vorlat, 4) L. Muylle, 5) G. van Beeumen, W. van Donink	7	3	4	36
Univ Hosp Ghent, Dept of Cardiac Surg, De Pintelaan 185, B-9000 Ghent Ph: (32)91 40-4700 Fax: (32)91 40-3882 1,2) G. van Nooten, 2) F. Caes, K. Francois, 3) Y. Taeymans, M. DePauw, 4) E. Noens, 5) M. van der Vennet, F. De Somer	10	8	6	75
Univ Hosp Gasthuisberg, Dept of Cardiology, Herestraat 49, Leuven, B-3000 Ph: (32)16 344235 Fax: (32)16 344240 Email: johan.vanhaecke@uz.kuleuven.ac.be 1,2) W. Daenen, 1,3) J.Vanhaecke, 2) W. Flameng, P. Sergeant, B. Meyns, 3) J. van Cleemput, W. Droogne, 5) F. van Gelder, D. van Hees, S. Kimpen	20	17	26	304
Ctr Hosp Univ-Liege, Dept of Surg/Transp, Domaine Univ du Sart-Tilman-B35, B-4000 Liege Ph: (32)41 667206 Fax: (32)41 667517 1,2) M. Meurisse, 1,2) Limet, 2) Limet and collegues, 3) J.C. Demoulin, 4) C. Bouillenne, 5) M.H. Delbouille, M.F. Hans	16	16	16	243

BRAZIL

	1998	1999	2000	Total
Hosp Santa Casa-Curitiba-Brazil, Dept of Cardiac Surg, Praca Rui Barbosa, Curitiba, PR 80010-030 Ph: (55)41 232 0990 Fax: (55)41 232 0990 Email: icosta@mps.com.br 1,2) I.A. Da Costa, 2) F.D.A. Da Costa, 3) G.T.F. Martins, A.L. Brasil, 5) G.T.F. Martins	0	5		14
Instituto de Cardiologia, Fundacao Univ de Cardiologia, Av. Princesa Isabel 395, Porto Alegre, RS 90620.001 Ph: (55)51 223-4050 Fax: (55)51 217-1358 Email: nesralla@cardnet.tche.br 1,2) I. Nesralla, 3) S. Bordignon, 4) L.F. Jobim, 5) L.L. Lima	8	8	7	98

CANADA

	1998	1999	2000	Total
Univ of Alberta Hosp, Dept of Cardio/Vasc/Thor Surg, 40 Hope Prog, 8440 112 St, Edmonton, AB T6G 2B7 Ph: (780) 407-8411 Fax: (780) 407-3056 1,2) D. Modry, 2) A. Koshal, J.C. Mullen, S.H. Wang, I.M. Rebeyka, 3) J. Burton, W. Tymchak, D. Lien, J. Crockett, J. Preiksaitis, 4) J. Schlaut, 5) A. Tchoryk, S. Sukalak, K. Young, K. Jackson, S. Chorney	32	29	41	322
St. Paul's Hosp, Heart Transplant Program, Rm 5051 5C Providence Wing, 1081 Burrard St, Vancouver, BC V5Z 3X7 Ph: (604) 806-8602 Fax: (604) 806-8763 1,3) A. Ignaszewski, 1,2) J. Abel, 2) S. Cheung, S. Litchenstein, 3) L. Straatman, 4) B. Draney, 5) S. Mortimer	14	16	11	173
Queen Elizabeth II Health Sci Center, Multi-Organ Transp Prog, 4th Halifax Infirmary Rm 4627, P.O.Box 9000, Halifax, NS B3H 3A7 Ph: (902) 473-5511 Fax: (902) 473-8598 1,3) H. Haddad, 1,2) G. Hirsch, 2) Id. Ali, D. Ross, J. Sullivan, K. Stewart, Im. Ali, J. Wood, 3) B. O'Neill, J. Howlett, R. Crowell, C. Kells, 4) S. Eastwood, 5) R. LeBlanc, J. Cruckshank, K. Storm, D. Murray	9	9	12	123
London Hlth Sci Ctr/Univ Campus, Dept of Transp, 339 Windermere Rd, PO Box 5339, London, ON N6A 5A5 Ph: (519) 663-3762 Fax: (519) 663-3100 Email: alan.menkis@lhsc.on.ca 1) A.H. Menkis, 2) F.N. McKenzie, R. Novick, D. Boyd, M. Quantz, J. Lee, 3) W. Kostuk,P. Pflugfelder, 4) B. Howson, 5) C.A. Smith, S. Williams, M. Bloch, C. Weernick, J. Drew, M. Mohamed	16	18	16	477

1)=Director, 2)=Tx Surgeons, 3)=Physicians, 4)=Tissue Typers, 5)=TxCoords	1998	1999	2000	Total
Univ of Ottawa Heart Inst, Dept of Surg, c/o Roy Masters, 40 Ruskin St, Ottawa, ON K1Y 4W7 Ph: (613) 761-4233 Fax: (613) 761-5323 1) W. Keon, 2) R. Masters, P. Hendry, 3) R.A. Davies, S. Smith, 4) The Ottawa Hosp Tissue Typing Lab, 5) C. Struthers	19			292
Inst de Cardio de Montreal, Dept of Surg, 5000 Belanger St, East, Montreal, PQ H1T 1C8 Ph: (514) 376-3330 Fax: (514) 376-4766 1,2) M. Carrier, 2) L. Perrault, M. Pellerin, D. Bouchard, 3) J.B. Pelletier, M. White, N. Raeinc, 4) I.A. Frappier, 5) D. Normandin, C. Dupre, J. Vizina	14	11	19	244
Royal Victoria Hosp, McGill Heart Failure & Transp, 687 Pine Ave W, E341, Montreal, H3A 1A1 Ph: (514) 842-1231 Fax: (514) 843-1689 1,2) R. Cecere, 2) B. DeVarennes, P. Ergina, K. Lachapelle, 3) M. Cantarovich, Gianneth, 4) P. Imperial, C. McIntyre, 5) R. Chartier, E. Cyr	14	15	17	293
Ste Justine Hosp, Dept of Cardio/Vasc Surg, 3175 Cote Ste Catherine, Montreal, PQ H3T 1C5 Ph: (514) 345-4676 Fax: (514) 345-4804 1) C. Chartrand, 2) S. Vobecky, 3) J.C. Fourron, 4) A. Frappier, 5) S. Chartrand	1	5	1	44

COLOMBIA

Clinica Cardiovascular Santa Maria, Thor and Cadrio Surg, Calle 78B No.75-21, Medellin-Antioquia Ph: (574) 442 2200 Fax: (574) 441 7869 Email: cardiovascular@congregacionmariana.org.co 1,2) A. Villegas, 2) Duran, Gonzalez, Montoya, Jaramillo, Zapata, 3) E. Escorcia, C. Tanorio, D. Fernandez, 4) L.F. Garcia, 5) D. Fernandez	23	3	11	144

CROATIA

Univ Clin Hosp-Rebro Zagreb, Nat'l Referral Organ Transp &, Tissue Typ Ctr, 12 Kispaticeva, Zagreb, HR-10000 Ph: (385)1 233-3235 Fax: (385)1 212-684 Email: andrija.kastelan@zg.tel.hr 1,2) A. Kastelan, 2) I. Jelic, Z. Sutlic, 3) D. Milicic, D. Planinc, 4) V. Kerhin-Brkljacic, R. Zunec, 5) V. Vegar	9	6	3	55

CZECH REPUBLIC

Inst for Klin & Exper Med (IKEM), Transp Ctr, Dept of Cardio Surg, Videnska 800, 14000 Prague 4 Ph: (420) 24723245 Fax: (420) 24721362 Email: japx@medicon.cz 1,2) J. Pirk, 2) J. Pirk, P. Pavel, V. Rohn, I. Skalsky, S. Cerny, 3) V. Stanek, I. Malek, 4) E. Ivaskova, 5) E. Pokorna, R. Schrotterova, E. Laszikova, V. Charova	35	45	37	417

DENMARK

Skejby Hosp, Dept of Cardio, DK 8200 Aarhus N Ph: (45)89 49 6109 Fax: (45)89 49 6025 Email: skejks@au.dk 1) H. Eiskjaer, 2) H. Allermand, 3) H. Egeblad, H. Molgard, J.E. Kudsk-Nielsen, 5) E.M. Tram	14	10		97

FINLAND

Children's Hosp, Univ of Helsinki, Dept of Ped Surg, Stenbackinkatu 11, Helsinki, SF 00029 Ph: (358)9 471 72730 Fax: (358)9 471 74705 1,2) M. Leijala, 2) H. Sairanen, I. Mattila, M. Kaarne, 3) C. Holmberg, H. Jalanko, 4) S. Koskimies	3	0		30
Helsinki Univ Ctr Hosp, Dept of Thor/Cardio Surg, Haartmaninkatu 4, Helsinki, SF-00290 Ph: (358)9 471 72290 Fax: (358)9 471 74006 1,2) S. Matilla, 2) Staff Members of Cardio/Vasc Surgery, 3) M. Nieminen, 4) Finnish Red Cross Lab, 5) M. Lindstrom, M.L. Hellstedt	15			240

FRANCE

Univ Paris XII-Hosp Henri Mondor, Dept of Thor/Cardi/Vasc Surg, 51 av Marechal Delattre, Creteil, 94010 Ph: (33)1-4981-2151 Fax: (33)1-4981-2152 1,2) D. Loisance, 2) M.L. Hillion, R. Mouel, 3) E. Vermes, 4) Hosp St Louis, 5) F. Bonnet	19	14		319
Louis Pradel Hosp, Dept of Cardio/Vasc, PAM de Transp et Chir Cardio, 28 Ar du Doyen Lepine, Lyon Cedex 03, 69394 Ph: (33)472 357994 Fax: (33)472 357395 1) D. Dureau, 2) O. Jegaden, D'Chuzel, J.F. Obadia, 3) P. Boissonnat, J.R. Gare, L. Sebbag, 4) H. Betuel, M. Gebuhrer, 5) Colpart	25	21	20	708

1)=Director, 2)=Tx Surgeons, 3)=Physicians, 4)=Tissue Typers, 5)=TxCoords	1998	1999	2000	Total
Laennec Hosp, Dept of CTCV, BP 1005, Nantes Cedex, 44035 Ph: (33)40 165084 Fax: (33)40 165133 1,2) J.L. Michaud, 2) P. Despins, D. Duveau, 3) T. Petit, M. Treilhaud, J.N. Trochu, 4) J. Bignon, 5) N. LeSant	22	24		382
Groupe Hosp Pitie Salpetriere, Dept Cardio/Vasc Surg, 83 Blvd de L'Hospital, Paris, 75013 Ph: (33)1 4217 7001 Fax: (33)1 4217 7656 Email: monique.tallier@psl.ap.hop-paris.fr 1,2) I. Gandjbakhch, 2) A. Pavie, V. Bors, 3) R. Dorent, P. Leger, E. Vaissier, J.P. Levasseur, 4) C. Raffoux, 5) F. Maillet, M. Tallier	46	37	46	1265
Pontchaillou Hosp, Dept of Cardio/Vasc/Thor Surg, CHU Rennes, 35033 Rennes Ph: (33)99 284273 Fax: (33)99 284129 1,2) A. Leguerrier, 2) C. Rioux, T. Langanay, H. Corbineau, 3) B. Lelong, H. LeCouls, 4) R. Fauchet, M.A. LeGall, 5) D. Noury	14	11	16	232
CHUR Strasbourg, Hosp Ctr, Dept of Cardio/Vasc Surg, RP 426, Strasbourg Cedex, 67091 Ph: (33)388 116244 Fax: (33)388 116342 1,2) B. Eisenmann, 2) J.G. Kretz, A. Charpentie, J.P. Mazzucotelli, N. Chakfe, 3) F. Levy, B. Mettauer, J. Thiranos, E. Epailly, 4) Tongio, Belloco, 5) E. Epailly	12	8	16	191

GERMANY

	1998	1999	2000	Total
Kerckhoff Klin GmbH, Dept of Heart Surg, Cardio/Vasc Surg, Beneke Str 2-8, 61231 Bad Nauheim Ph: (49)6032-9962501 Fax: (49)6032-9962567 1,2) W. Kloevekorn, 3) Haberbosch, 4) Eurotransplant-Leiden, 5) Bauer	5	4		77
Heart Ctr North Rhine Westfalia, Ruhr-Univ of Bochum, Dept of Thor/Cardio/Vasc Surg, Georgstrasse 11, Bad Oeynhausen, 32545 Ph: (49)5731 97 1331 Fax: (49)5731 97 1820 1,2) R. Koerfer, 2) Minami, Seifert, Breymann, Arusoglu, Kleikamp, Bairaktaris, Hansky, 3) G. Tenderich, 4) G.W. Prohaska, C. Wolf, 5) S. Wlost, B. Heistermann-Linstaedt	77	70	68	1098
German Heart Inst, Dept of Thor/Cardio/Vasc Surg, Augustenburger Platz 1, Berlin, D-13353 Ph: (49)30 4593 2000 Fax: (49)30 4505 4047 1) R. Hetzer, 2) Weng, Loebe, Alexi, Pasic, Zurbrugg, Knorig, 3) M. Hummel, P.E. Lange, R. Ewert, 4) Salama, 5) H. Kriegler	77	59		1152
Fulda Med Ctr, Dept of Thor/Cardio/Vasc Surg, Pacelliallee 4, Fulda, D-36043 Ph: (49)661 84-5652 Fax: (49)661 84-5653 1,2) T. Stegmann, 2) H.U. Gunther, L. Konig, W. Schlurmann, B. Rosada, 3) T. Bonzel, G. Strupp, 4) H. Kruepe, 5) R. Werner	8	7	1	125
Univ Hosp Gottingen, Dept Thor/Cardio/Vasc Surg, Robert-Koch Str 40, Gottingen, 37075 Ph: (49)551 39 6001 Fax: (49)551 39 6002 1) H.G.J. Dalichau, 2) M.M. Baryalei, 3) F. Reitmer, D. Zenker, I. Aleksic, C. Hahnke, O. Rode, A. Rastau, 4) H. Neumeyer, C. Krome-Cesar	8	7		80
Univ Hosp Eppendorf-Hamburg, Dept of Thor/Cardio/Vasc Surg, Martinistr 52, Hamburg 20, 20246 Ph: (49)40 4717-3471 Fax: (49)40 4717-4591 1,2) N. Tsilimingas, 1,2) V.Doering, 3) W. Roediger, H. Naegele, 4) Kuehnl, 5) C. Clausen, B. Hollenrieder	13			138
Univ Klin des Saarlandes, Dept of Thoracic Surg, Oscar-Orth—Strabe, Hamburg/Saar, D-66421 Ph: (49)6841 163520 Fax: (49)6841 163516 1,3) H.J. Schafers, 2) T. Graeter, O. Wendler, 3) H.J. Schieffer, B. Schwaab, 4) B. Thiele, Kasierslautern, 5) C. Friedrichsohn	7	4	2	26
Hannover Med Sch, Dept of Surg, Div Thor/Cardio/Vasc Surg, Carl-Neuberg-STR.1, 30625 Hannover Ph: (49)511 532-6581 Fax: (49)511 532-5404 1,2) A. Haverich, 2) W. Harringer, M. Strueber, 3) K. Pethig, 4) Robin-Winn, Pastucha, 5) G. Gubernatis	34	31	26	679
Westpfalz-Klinikum, Dept Cardio Surg, HTG, Hellmut-Hartert Str 1, Kaiserslautern, 67653 Ph: (49)0631 2031426 Fax: (49)0631 2031727 Email: w.seyblod-epting@t-online.de 1,2) W. Seybold-Epting, 3) G.Heim.D.Suitor.F. Sutter, H. Kuttler, B. Haaff, G. Glunz, 4) B. Thiele, 5) H. Kuerwitz-Hof, D. Sutor	5	3	3	55
Transplant Ctr Kiel, Dept of Cardio/Vasc Chir, Univ Kiel Hosp, Arnold-Heller Strasse 7, 24105 Kiel Ph: (49)431 5974341 Fax: (49)431 5972235 Email: shirt@hielheart.uni-kiel.de 1) Cremer, 2) S.W. Hirt, 4) E. Westphal, 5) G.R. Schuett, N. Robien	16	35	11	380

1)=Director, 2)=Tx Surgeons, 3)=Physicians, 4)=Tissue Typers, 5)=TxCoords	1998	1999	2000	Total
Clin Grosshadern, Dept of Cardiac Surg, Marchioninstr. 15, 81377 Munich Ph: (49)89 7095 3460 Fax: (49)89 7095 3465 Email: bruno.meiser@hch.med.uni-muenchen.de 1) B. Reichart, 2) Uberfuhr, Kreuzer, Reichenspurner, Meiser, 3) B. Meiser, 4) E.D. Albert, 5) Transp Grosshadern	40	37	36	697
German Heart Ctr-Munich, Dept of Cardio/Vasc Surg, Lazarett Str 36, Munich, 80636 Ph: (49)89 1218 4111 Fax: (49)89 1218 4113 Email: chinfo@dhm.mhn.de 1,2) R. Lange, 2) M. Overbeck, 3) B. Permanetter, 4) E. Albert, 5) C. Schulz	14	14	8	152
Univ Hosp Munster, Dept of Thor/Cardio/Vasc Surg, Munster, 48129 Ph: (49)251 83-47401 Fax: (49)251 83-48316 1) H.H. Scheld, 2) D. Hammel, M. Wilhelm, C. Schmid, B. Asfour, 3) G. Breithardt, 4) H. Gross-Wilde, Sibrowski, 5) Kley	23	23	27	265
Univ of Tuebingen, Dept of Surg, Hoppe-Seyler Str 3, Transp Ctr, Tuebingen, 72076 Ph: (49)7071 2986600 Fax: (49)7071 294047 1,2) Ziemer, 2) Aebert, Steger, 3) Kuhlkamp, 4) Northoff, Wernet, 5) Fischer-Frohlich	5	3		13

IRELAND

	1998	1999	2000	Total
Mater Misericardiac Hosp-Dublin 7, Cardiac Transp Unit, Eccles St, Dublin 7 Ph: (353)1 80 32164 Fax: (353)1 80 34773 1,2) M.C. Neligan, 2) A.E. Wood, J. Hurley, 3) C. McCarthy, D. Sugrue, 5) L. Costello, K. Clapperton	17	9		166

ITALY

	1998	1999	2000	Total
Hosp San Michele, Dept of Cardio Surg, Via Peretti, 09126 Cagliari Ph: (39)070 543333 Fax: (39)070 530814 1,5) F. Meloni, 1,5) M. Spissu, 2) V. Martelli, A. Ricchi, 3) D. Mereu, A. Sanna, 4) L. Contu, M. Arnone	7	7	7	87
Hosp Ca' Granda Niguarda-Milano, Dept of Cardio Surg, "A De Gasperis", Piazza Ospedale Maggiore 3, 20162 Milano Ph: (39)02 64442566 Fax: (39)02 6438631 1,2) E. Vitali, 2) E. Vitali, 3) M. Frigerio, 4) G. Sirchia	50	50	31	575
Univ Hosp Med Sch. Padova, Dept of Cardio/Vasc Surg, Via Giustiniani 2, 35128 Padova Ph: (39)49 821 2410 Fax: (39)49 821 1895 1,2) D. Casarotto, 2) A. Gambino, L. Testolin, 3) A.L.P. Caforio, 4) G. Sirchia, 5) V. Bressan	37	29	23	521
San Matteo Hosp/Univ of Pavia, Div of Cardiac Surg, Piazzale Golgi 2, Pavia, 27100 Ph: (39)0382 503515 Fax: (39)0382 503059 Email: darmini@smatteo.pv.it 1,2) M. Vigano, 2) M. Rinaldi, A.M. D'Armini, C. Goggi, 4) G. Sirchia	39	48	34	620
Ospedale Ped "Bambino Gesu", Dept Med Chir di Cardio Ped, Piazza S Onofrio 4, Rome, 00165 Ph: (39)06 6859 2611 Fax: (39)06 6859 2200 Email: parisi@opbg.net 1,2) R. DiDonato, 2) C. Squitieri, A. Carotti, 3) F. Parisi, P. D'Argenio, 4) D. Adorno, 5) F. Parisi	6	5	5	86
S Maria Della Misericordia, Div of Cardio/Thor Surg, Pza Santa Maria Della Misericordia, Udine, 33100 Ph: (39)432 552430 Fax: (39)432 552967 1,2) U. Livi, 2) R. Frassani, A. Morelli, L. Porreca, R. Nucifora, P. DaCol, R. Lumini, 3) M.C. Albanese, D. Miani, 4) P. Sirchia(Milano), F. Biffoni, V. Miotti, 5) E. Valle, R. Cocconi, M. Delendi	12	21	25	202

KOREA

	1998	1999	2000	Total
Seoul Nat'l Univ Hosp, Coll of Med, Dept of Gen Surg, 28 Yongon-Dong, Chongno-gu, Seoul, 110-744 Ph: (82)2 760-2316 Fax: (82)2 3672-4947 1,2) S.J. Kim, 2) J.R. Rho, K.B. Kim, J.R. Lee, K.H. Kim, 3) B.H. Oh, I.H. Chae, J.I. Rho, 5) J.S. Kim	4	5		27

MEXICO

	1998	1999	2000	Total
Centro Medico-Nacional "20 de Nov", Transplant Services, Av Felix Culvas 540, Col Del Valle CP 03229, Ciudad de Mexico, DF 03229 Ph: (52)5 5725050 Fax: (52)5 3930866 Email: bmartinez@starnet.net.mx 1,2) B. Martinez-Navarrette, 2) A. Archundia-Garcia, E. Gonzalez, 3) D. Hurtado, 4) R.A. Escalante, L. Diaz, 5) E. Cabrera, A. Montoya	2	2	3	14

1)=Director, 2)=Tx Surgeons, 3)=Physicians, 4)=Tissue Typers, 5)=TxCoords	1998	1999	2000	Total
Hosp de Especialidades 71, Torreon, Inst Mexicano del Seguro Soc, Transp Unit-Dept of Surg, Torreon, Coahuila, 27000 Ph: (52)17 290800 Fax: (52)17 132679 1,2) F.J. Juarez de la Cruz, 2) Y. Barrios, M. Benavides, A. Gomez, A. Villarreal, 3) L. Cano, E. Chavez, R. Camacho, J. Martinez, E. Lopez, E. Fernandez, 4) M. Limones, C. Adalid, 5) L. Peniche, I. Espino	0	1	0	1

NETHERLANDS

Univ Hosp Rotterdam "Dijkzigt", Dept of Cardiothoracic Surg, Dr Molewaterplein 40, P.O. Box 2040, 3000 CA Rotterdam Ph: (31)10 463-5412 Fax: (31)10 463-3993 1,2) A.Y.Y.C. Bogers, 2) L.A. van Herwerden, A.J. Bogers, A.P. Maat, J.A. Bekkers, P.L. deJong, 3) M.L. Simoons, A.H.M.M. Balk, W. Weimar, 4) F.H.J. Claas, 5) M. van Gurp, P. Pasma, M. Kruyswyk	18	24	19	389
Univ Hosp Utrecht, Dept of Cardio, Rm F03-411, PO Box 85500, 3508 Ga Utrecht Ph: (31)30 2507273 Fax: (31)30 2505423 1,2) N. de Jonge, 1,2) J.R.Lahpor, 2) E.W.L. Jansen, G.B.W. Bennink, 3) C. Klopping, J.H. Kirkel, 4) H. Otten, 5) P. Batavier	23	20	19	273

NEW ZEALAND

Green Lane Hosp, Cardio/Thor Surg Unit, Green Lane West, Auckland 3 Ph: (64)9 638-9909 Fax: (64)9 631-0768 1,2) D.A. Haydock, 2) A. Kerr, K.J. Graham, F.P. Milson, 3) H.A. Coverdale, T.M. Agnew, J. Garrett, K. Whyte, P. Ruygrok, 4) K. Figgins, M. Roberts, Auck Reg Bld Ctr, 5) H. Gibbs, D. Reddy	10	10	13	122

NORWAY

Rikshosp Nat'l Hosp, Dept Thoracic & Cardiovase, Sognsvannsveien 20, Oslo, 0027 Ph: (47)23 073735 Fax: (47)23 073741 Email: odd.geiran@rikshospitalet.no 1) O. Geiran, 2) H. Lindberg, E. Seem, S. Birkeland, A. Fiane, 3) S. Simonsen, A. Andreassen, 4) E. Thorsby, T. Leivestad, 5) P.A. Bakkan, S. Foss, P.E. Vatsaas, K. Meyer	33	32	25	374

POLAND

Silesian Univ Ctr for Heart Disease, Dept of Cardio Surg, ul Szpitalna 2, Zabrze, 41-800 Ph: (48) 32 2715266 Fax: (48) 32 2732682 Email: transpl@poczta.onet.pl 1,2) M. Zembala, 2) R. Przybylski, J. Kaperczak, B. Ryfinski, F. Pacholewicz, Borzymowski, 3) M. Zakliczynski, J. Foremny, D. Puszczewicz, B. Chodor, 4) R. Wojnicz, 5) A. Dmitrowicz, K. Tkocz	51	57	55	459

PUERTO RICO

Cardiovascular Ctr of Puerto Rico, and the Caribbean/Transp Serv, P.O. Box 366528, San Juan, 00936-6528 Ph: (787) 754-8500x2280 Fax: (787) 765-8471 1,2) I.F. Gonzalez Cancel, 2) C. Quintana, 3) H. Banchs Pieretti, J.A. Castillo Lugo, 4) C. Climent, 5) V. Gonzalez, E. Padilla		6	12	18

SINGAPORE

Singapore Gen Hosp, National Heart Centre, Dept of Cardio/Thor Surg, 17 Third Hospital Ave, 168752 Ph: (65) 436-7598 Fax: (65) 224-3632 1,2) M.C. Tong, 2) C. Sivathasan, Y. Seng, Y.S. Tan, Y.L. Chua, 3) C.Y. Lee, B. Kwok, 4) Nat'l Bld Ctr, 5) J. Ang, S.M. Liew, L.C. Yeo, S.L. Hou	1	4		18

SOUTH AFRICA

Univ of Cape Town, Groote Schuur Hosp, Dept of Cardio/Thor Surg, Private Bag Observatory, Cape Town, 7925 Ph: (27)21 404-5019 Fax: (27)21 448-1145 1,2) J. Brink, 2) J. Hewitson, 3) K. Moore, K. Seele, 4) F. DuToit, 5) F. McGurdie, C. Broomberg	20	9	11	449

SPAIN

"Doce de Octubre" Hosp Univ, Dept of Cardio Transp, Ctra de Andalucia km 5.4, Madrid, 28041 Ph: (34)91 390 8289 Fax: (34)91 390 8669 Email: mangomez@retemail.es 1) J.J. Rufilanchas, 2) J.E. Rodriguez, T.J. Cortina, E. Perez de Lasota, L. Maroto, 3) M.A. Gomez-Sanchez, J. Delgado, P. Escribano, 4) A. Arnaiz, J. Martinez-Laso, 5) A. de Andres, M.P. Cebrian, M. Vereda, S. Vazquez	29	30	22	261

1)=Director, 2)=Tx Surgeons, 3)=Physicians, 4)=Tissue Typers, 5)=TxCoords	1998	1999	2000	Total
Clin Univ de Navarra, Cardio/Vasc/Thor Surg, PIO XII (s/n), 31080 Pamplona, Navarra Ph: (34)948 255400 Fax: (34)948 274550 1,2) G. Rabago, 2) A.M. Trenor, Lopez-Coronado, 3) E. Alegria, J.D. Saenz de Buruaga, D. Coma, 4) M.L. Subira, A. Sanchez-Ibarrola	7			162

SWEDEN

	1998	1999	2000	Total
Sahlgrenska Hosp, Dept of Cardio/Thor Surg, Transp Unit, Gothenburg, S 41345 Ph: (46)31 601000 Fax: (46)31 417991 1,2) S.E. Svensson, 2) F. Nilsson, 3) C. HakanBergh, 4) L. Sandberg, L. Rydberg, 5) U. Lorentzon, U. Nysrom	23	21	14	287
Univ Hosp of Lund, Dept of Cardio/Thor Surg, Getingev 4, Lund, S-221 85 Ph: (46)46 171683 Fax: (46)46 158635 1,2) B. Koul, 2) S. Steen, C. Luhrs, P. Johnsson, M. Dobre, 3) L. Eriksson, B. Kornhall, 4) U. Johnsson, 5) A.K. Morin, K. Wallentin, A. Klitthammar, M. Zepeda, K. Henriksson	13	13	6	104

SWITZERLAND

	1998	1999	2000	Total
Ctr Hosp Univ Vaudois, CHUV, Dept of Surg Cardio/Vasc, Rue de Bugnon 46, Lausanne, CH-1011 Ph: (41)21 314 2279 Fax: (41)21 314 2278 1) L.K. Von Segesser, 2) F. Stumpe, X. Mueller, 3) J.J. Goy, 4) V. Aubert, 5) C.H. Seydoux	13	12	7	135
Univ Hosp Zurich, Dept of Surg, Clin Cardio/Vasc/Surg, Ramistr 100, Zurich, CH-8091 Ph: (41)1 255 3298 Fax: (41)1 255 4446 1,2) M. Turina, 2) Kunzli, Rohn-Schonbeck, Genoni, Lachat, Kunz, Pretre, Zund, 3) W. Kiowski, 4) R. Schlumpf, 5) P. Seeburger	16	11	7	281

TAIWAN

	1998	1999	2000	Total
Nat'l Taiwan Univ Hosp, Dept of Surg, 7 Chang-Shan South Rd, Taipei 100 Ph: (886)2 2341-0240 Fax: (886)2 2341-0933 1) S.H. Chu, 2) S.S. Wang, 3) Y.T. Lee, W.P. Lien, C.S. Lian, 4) R.F. Hsieh, 5) H.I. Lin	23	23		127

TURKEY

	1998	1999	2000	Total
Ege Univ Med Sch, Organ Transp, Cardio/Surg Dept, Bornova,Izmir Ph: (90)232 388-2866 Fax: (90)232 339-0002 1) M. Ozbaran, 1) A. Hamulu	4	3	6	13

UNITED KINGDOM

	1998	1999	2000	Total
Queen Elizabeth Hosp, Dept Transp, Cardio/Thor Surg, Edgbaston, Birmingham, B15 2TH Ph: (44)121 627-2544 Fax: (44)121 627-2542 1,2) R.S. Bonser, 2) I.C. Wilson, 3) J.N. Townend, 4) P. Macintosh, 5) S.A. Beer	27	27	24	258
Papworth Hospital, Transp Unit, Papworth Hosp, Cambridge, CB3 8RE Ph: (44)480 830541 Fax: (44)480 364610 1,2) J. Wallwork, 2) S.R. Large, F.C. Wells, S.A.M. Nashef, J. Dunning, A. Ritchie, S. Tsui, 3) J. Parameshwar, K. McNeil, 4) C. Taylor, 5) Smith, Baines, Ryan, Woods, Castle, Lockhurst, Wiggins	51	36	42	885
St George's Hosp, Cardiac Dept of Med, Blackshaw Rd, Tooting, London, SW17 0QT Ph: (44)181 725-3565 Fax: (44)181 725-2049 1,2) A.J. Murday, 2) J. Gaer, V. Gandra, 3) B.P. Madden, 4) D. Sage, 5) L. Backhouse, L. Reynolds, J. Barros	23	24	8	371
Wythenshawe Hosp, Reg Cardio/Thor Ctr, Southmoor Rd, Manchester, M23 9LT Ph: (44)161 998-7070 Fax: (44)161 291-2091 1,2) A.K. Deiraniya, 2) C. Campbell, N. Yonan, T. Hooper, M.T. Jones, 3) N. Brooks, R. Levy, 4) P.A. Dyer, S. Sheldon, 5) H. Pyatt, J. Nuttall, J. Stewart	20	17	24	326
Harefield Hosp, Dept of Cardio/Thor Surg, Harefield, Middlesex, UB9 6JH Ph: (44)1 895 823737 Fax: (44)1 895 824983 1) M. Yacoub, 2) A. Khaghani, J. Pepper, 3) A. Mitchell, N. Banner, R. Radley-Smith, M. Hodson, 4) M. Rose, 5) P. Baldock, H. Blair, T. Jackson	53	40		1482

1)=Director, 2)=Tx Surgeons, 3)=Physicians, 4)=Tissue Typers, 5)=TxCoords	1998	1999	2000	Total

URUGUAY

Casa de Galicia, Heart Transp, Av.Millan 4480, Montevideo
Ph: (598) 3041666 3042095 Fax: (598) 3 042098
1) J.L. Filgueira, 2) D. Bigalli, 3) N. Russo, 4) BNOT, I. Alvarez, R. Toledo, M. Bengochea, E. Carreto,
5) R. Mizraji, A. Brun, P. RealdeAzua, M. Canepa, A. Castro, C. Agarbado

	1998	1999	2000	Total
	2	3	6	12

Hospital Italiano, Instituto de Cardiologia, Bvar.Artigas 1632 Piso 2, Montevideo
Ph: (598)4 870416 Fax: (598)4 875767
1) J. Nozar, 2) R. Leone, D. Picarelli, R. Anzibar, 3) B. Cerutti, D. Chafes, 4) BNOT, I. Alvarez,
R. Toledo, M. Bengochea, E. Carreto, 5) R. Miraji, A. Brun, P. RealdeAzua, M. Canepa,
A. Castro, C. Agarbado

	1998	1999	2000	Total
	3	6	8	18

HEART Transplants

	1998	1999	2000	Total
United States	2,254	2,162	2,266	31,947
Foreign	1,551	1,412	1,099	25,096
Total	3,805	3,574	3,365	57,043

HEART Transplant Centers

United States	130
Foreign	99
Total	229

WORLDWIDE TRANSPLANT CENTER DIRECTORY
HEART/LUNG TRANSPLANTS

1)=Director, 2)=Tx Surgeons, 3)=Physicians, 4)=Tissue Typers, 5)=TxCoords	1998	1999	2000	Total

UNITED STATES

ALABAMA

Univ of Alabama Birmingham Med Ctr, Dept of Surg/Med, 701 S 19th St, Birmingham, AL 35294 Ph: (205) 934-3368 Fax: (205) 934-5261 1,2) J.K. Kirklin, 2) W.L. Holman, G.L. Zorn, D. McGiffin, 3) R.C. Bourge, B. Rayburn, R. Benza, M. Aaron, B. Foley, K. Young, D. Weill, 4) R. Senkbeil, 5) C. White-Williams, M. Hubbard, T. Smith, M. Arndt	2	2	5*	24

ARIZONA

Univ Med Ctr, Dept of Cardio/Thor Surg, 1501 N Campbell Ave, Rm 4604, Tucson, AZ 85724 Ph: (520) 694-6299 Fax: (520) 694-2692 1,2) J.G. Copeland, 2) G. Sethi, V. Paramesh, F. Arabia, D. Arzouman, S. Sharma, R. Bose, 3) S. Butman, C. Lui, S. Knoper, 5) N. Edling, J. Wild, N. Harrington, D. Allen, S. Mullarkey	3	0	4	47

CALIFORNIA

Children's Hosp of Los Angeles, Dept of Cardio/Thor Transp, 4650 Sunset Blvd, Los Angeles, CA 90027 Ph: (323) 669-5965 Fax: (323) 668-7979 1,2) V.A. Starnes, 2) R.G. Cohen, 3) P. Wong, E. MacLaughlin, M. Woo, 5) M. Horn	0	1	1*	12
Univ California-Los Angeles, Dept of Heart-Lung Transp, Div of Cardio Surg, 10833 Le Conte Ave, Los Angeles, CA 90095 Ph: (310) 825-6068 Fax: (310) 206-6301 1,2) H. Laks, 3) Moriguchi, Kobashigawa, Levine, Hamilton, Perloff, Shpiner, Ross, 4) UCLA Immunogenetics Center, 5) C. Burch, R. Camara, Velleca, Mark, Lackey, Brown	0	1	0	4
Stanford Univ Med Ctr, Dept of Cardio, Falk Bldg, MC 5407, Palo Alto, CA 94305 Ph: (650) 723-5771 Fax: (650) 725-3846 1,2) R. Robbins, 2) J.I. Fann, P.E. Oyer, B.A. Reitz, 3) J. Theodore, R. Doyle, 4) C. Grumet, 5) P. Gamberg, J. Miller, L. Levine, M. Merlo	6	7	11	179
Univ California-San Diego, Div of Cardio/Thor Surg, 200 W Arbor Dr, San Diego, CA 92103-8892 Ph: (619) 543-7777 Fax: (619) 543-2652 Email: jkriett@ucsd.edu 1,2) S.W. Jamieson, 2) J.M. Kriett, D. Kapelanski, P. Thistlethwaite, 3) M. Light, P. Stillwell, G. Yung, 4) M. Garavoy, L. Lebeck, 5) D. Garcia, S. Osborne, L. Gayhart, D. Glasser	0	2	1*	14

MARYLAND

The Johns Hopkins Hosp, Dept of Cardiac Surg, Blalock Bldg,#618, 600 N Wolfe St, Baltimore, MD 21287-4618 Ph: (410) 955-7935 Fax: (410) 955-3809 1,2) S. Yang, 2) D. Cameron, J. Laschinger, P. Greene, 3) T. Traill, S. Walden, P. Becker, 4) J. Hart, 5) S. Augustine, D. Carter	0	0	1*	20

MASSACHUSETTS

Children's Hosp Boston, Dept of Cardio/Vasc Surg, 300 Longwood Ave, Boston, MA 02115 Ph: (617) 735-6215 Fax: (617) 735-0310 1,2) J.E. Mayer Jr, 3) C. Lillchei, 4) New England Organ Bank, 5) P. O'Brien	1	0	0	4

MICHIGAN

Univ of Michigan Med Ctr, Dept of Thor Surg, Box 0344, 1500 E Medical Ctr Dr, Ann Arbor, MI 48109 Ph: (734) 763-7418 Fax: (734) 615-2656 1,2) M. Iannettoni, 2) M. Orringer, J. Yee, 3) J. Lynch, F. Martinez, T. Ojo, K. Flaherty, S. Gay, 4) J. Baker, 5) R. Florn, J. Berry	1	1	0	13

* Preliminary UNOS data

1)=Director, 2)=Tx Surgeons, 3)=Physicians, 4)=Tissue Typers, 5)=TxCoords	1998	1999	2000	Total
MINNESOTA				
Fairview Univ Med Ctr, Thoracic Transp Prog, Box 398, 420 Delaware St SE, Minneapolis, MN 55455 Ph: (612) 625-9922 Fax: (612) 626-6968 1,2) S. Park, 1,3) M. Hertz, 2) S. Shumway, H. Bittner, C. Herrington, R. Kelly, R. Bolman, 3) M. King, J. Dunitz, M. Hertz, C. Wendt, L. Miller, 4) H. Noreen, 5) Rosenthal, Ormaza, Munson, Elmajri, Gibson, Dunbar	3	0	1	45
MISSOURI				
Barnes Hosp, Washington Univ Med Ctr, Dept of Cardio/Thor Surg, One Barnes Plaza, West Pavilion, Lower Level, St Louis, MO 63110 Ph: (314) 454-7687 Fax: (314) 454-8364 1,2) T.M. Sundt, 1,3) J.G. Rogers, 2) M.K. Pasque, M.R. Moon, 3) J. Rogers, E.M. Geltman, G. Ewald, 4) T. Mohanakumar, D. Phelan, 5) C. Pasque, J. Vassolo, S. Moorehead	0	1	1	4
St Louis Children's Hosp, Med Ctr, Dept Cardio/Thor Surg, 1 Childrens Place, St Louis, MO 63110 Ph: (314) 454-6165 Fax: (314) 454-2381 1,3) C.E. Canter, 1,2) C.B. Huddleston, 2) E.N. Mendeloff, 3) C.E. Canter, D. Balzer, 4) D. Phelan, 5) P. Shaner, D. Springhart, D. Watkins, G. McBride	0	0	2	12
St Louis Univ Hlth Sci Ctr, Dept of Thor Transp, 3635 Vista Ave, P.O.Box 15250, St Louis, MO 63110 Ph: (314) 268-5421 Fax: (314) 268-8315 1,2) L.R. McBride, 3) C.A. Keller, T, Donohue, T. Wolford, P. Hauptman, 4) K. Riordan, 5) P. Haselhorst, L. Horn, C. Zirgus, S. Paulson	3	2	1*	19
NEW YORK				
Columbia Presbyterian Med Ctr, Dept of Surg/Cardio Transp, PH 14 West, 622 W 168th St, New York, NY 10032 Ph: (212) 305-7600 Fax: (212) 305-8304 1,2) N.M. Edwards, 2) C.R. Smith, 3) C. McGregor, L. Schulman, 4) N. Sucia-Foca, 5) B. Jorgensen, R. Geron-Smith	7	2	0*	38
Mount Sinai Med Ctr, Cardio/Thor Div, Box 1028, 1 Gustave Levy Place, New York, NY 10029 Ph: (212) 241-8181 Fax: (212) 534-3357 1,2) S. Lansman, 2) R. Griepp, S. Lansman, J. McCullough, 3) A. Gass, M. Padilla, G. Schilero, 4) Rogosin Inst, 5) M. Courtney, D. Correa	0	0	1*	8
NORTH CAROLINA				
Univ of North Carolina Hosp, Div of Cardio/Thor Surg, Dept of Surg, CB 7065, 108 Burnett-Womack Bldg, Chapel Hill, NC 27599-7065 Ph: (919) 966-3381 Fax: (919) 966-3475 Email: mrm@med.unc.edu 1,2) M.R. Mill, 2) T. Egan, F.C. Detterbeck, 3) C.A. Sueta, S. Kushwaha, 4) J. Crawford, 5) M. Grady, S. Kowalczyk	1	0	2	9
Duke Univ Med Ctr, Dept of Surg, Box 3235, DUMC, Durham, NC 27710 Ph: (919) 684-2651 Fax: (919) 681-8860 1,2) R.D. Davis, 1) K.P.Landolfo, 2) R. Messier, J. Jaggers, T. D'Amico, 3) S. Palmer, V. Tapson, D. Hadjiliadis, W. Mariencheck, 4) N. Reinsmoen, F. Ward, 5) C. Lawrence, A. Miralles, L. Blue, B. Ross, A. Petersen, D. Gibson	4	2	2*	17
OHIO				
Cleveland Clin Fnd, A110 Transplant Center, 9500 Euclid Ave, Cleveland, OH 44195-5066 Ph: (216) 445-1115 Fax: (216) 445-3127 1,2) N. Smedira, 2) P. McCarthy, G. Pettersson, M. DeCamp, 3) A. Mehta, R. Schilz, K. James, M. Kichuk, 4) D. Cook, L. Klingman, 5) H. Blazey, T. Evans-Walker, J. Foertch, Nassman	0	0	1	6
OREGON				
Oregon Univ Hosp, Div of Cardio Surg, 3181 SW Sam Jackson Pk Rd, Portland, OR 97201 Ph: (503) 494-7820 Fax: (503) 494-7829 1,2) A. Cobanoglu, 2) G. Ott, 3) M. Meyer, R. Ratkovic, 4) D.J. Norman, 5) J.A. Nussbaum	0	0	1*	3

1)=Director, 2)=Tx Surgeons, 3)=Physicians, 4)=Tissue Typers, 5)=TxCoords	1998	1999	2000	Total
PENNSYLVANIA				
Temple Univ Hosp, Dept of Cardio/Thor Surg, Broad & Tioga Sts, 9th Flr, 320 Parkinson Pavilion, Philadelphia, PA 19140 Ph: (215) 707-3782 Fax: (215) 707-8191 1,3) H.J. Eisen, 2) J.B. McClurken, S. Furukawa, T. Pendergrast, 3) Bove, Pina, Margulies, Mather, Robin, Berman, Criher, O'Brien, 4) S. Leach, 5) A. Kuzma, L. Ohler, R. Washington, T. Rourke, D. McCarthy, E. Hobson	3	1	1*	12
The Children's Hosp of Philadelphia, Thoracic Organ Transp Program, 34th St & Civic Ctr Blvd, Philadelphia, PA 19104 Ph: (215) 590-6051 Fax: (215) 590-1340 1,2) T.L. Spray, 2) J.W. Gaynor, W.M. DeCampli, T.R. Karl, 3) B.J. Clark, N.D. Bridges, R.M. Donner, B.D. Hanna, T. Hoffman, 4) D. Monos, 5) M. Sowa, J. Menendez	6	7	1	21
Children's Hosp of Pittsburgh, Dept of Cardio/Thor Surg, 3705 Fifth Ave, One Children's Place, Pittsburgh, PA 15213 Ph: (412) 692-5541 Fax: (412) 692-6991 Email: webbers@heart.chp.edu 1,2) S. Webber, 2) F. Pigula, 4) A. Zeevi, 5) D. Dorsey, B. Stinner	1	5	1	36
Univ of Pittsburgh Sch of Med, Dept of Cardio/Thor Surg, C-700 Presbyterian Univ Hosp, 200 Lothrop St, Pittsburgh, PA 15213-2582 Ph: (412) 648-1963 Fax: (412) 648-1029 Email: ristichj@msx.upmc.edu 1,2) K. McCurry, 2) R. Kormos, B. Hattler, B.P. Griffith, M. Zenati, 3) J. Dauber, A. Iacono, J. Pilewski, 4) A. Zeevi, 5) A. Lee, J. Manzetti, G. Bouldof, J. Vensak, S. Zomak, C. Cornell	2	2	1	99
TENNESSEE				
Vanderbilt Univ Med Ctr, The Vanderbilt Transp Ctr, Dept of Heart/Lung Transp, 908 Oxford House, Nashville, TN 37232-4734 Ph: (615) 936-0393 Fax: (615) 936-0396 1,2) R.N. Pierson III, 2) W.H. Merrill, K.J. Richey, J.R. Roberts, D. Drinkwater, 3) J.E. Loyd, S. Dummer, J. Wilson, S. Davis, G. Miller, A. Milstone, 4) DCI Labs, 5) A. Goodwin, S. England	0	2	1	13
TEXAS				
Medical City Dallas Hosp, Transplant Center, 7777 Forest Lane, A-14th Floor, Dallas, TX 75230 Ph: (800)348-4318 Fax: (972)566-4872 1,2) S. Seitz, 2) D. Ogden, M. Mack, T. Dewey, M. McGee, 3) J.E. Rosenthal, M. Lerman, J. Hunt, D. Weill, 4) Baylor Immunology, 5) M. Covin, T. McMellon, C. Goheen, D. Stevenson	1	0	0	1
Texas Heart Inst, St Luke's Episcopal Hosp, Transp Serv 2-114, PO Box 20269, Houston, TX 77225 Ph: (713) 791-3952 Fax: (713) 794-6696 Email: kneylor@sleh.com 1,2) O.H. Frazier, 2) G. Noon, S. Scheinen, 3) A. Frost, I. Nizami, 4) R. Kerman, 5) K. Neylor	0	1	0	2
Methodist Specialty & Transplant Hosp, Dept of Cardiac Transp, 8026 Floyd Curl Dr, San Antonio, TX 78229 Ph: (210) 692-8272 Fax: (210) 692-8154 1,2) C. Moore, 1) L.Zorvilla, 2) L. Hamner, C. Christian, 3) W. Craig, D. Kramer, N. Sanderson, R. Schnitzler, 4) J. Morrisey, 5) K. Cunningham, V. Martinez, D. Richardson	0	1		7
WASHINGTON				
Sacred Heart Med Ctr, Thor Organ Transp, W 101 8th Ave, P.O.Box 2555, Spokane, WA 99220-2555 Ph: (509) 474-2041 Fax: (509) 474-4906 1,2) T.B. Icenogle, 2) D. Sandler, 3) S. Joseph, 4) Inland Nowest Bld Ctr, 5) P. Hester, C. Sparks, P. Kaley	0	1	0	18
WISCONSIN				
Univ of Wisconsin Hosp & Clin, Div of Cardio/Thor Surg, 600 Highland Ave, H4-370, Madison, WI 53792-3236 Ph: (608) 263-7832 Fax: (608) 263-0597 1,2) R.B. Love, 2) J.R. Pellett, R.P. Cochran, D. Woolley, 3) K. Meyer, R. Cornwell, 4) D. Lorentzen, 5) D. Welter, A. Hoffman	0	2	0	8
ARGENTINA				
ICYCC-Favaloro Foundation, Cardio/Vasc Surg-Transp Div, Av Belgrano 1746, Buenos Aires, C1093AAS Ph: (5411) 4378-1350 Fax: (5411) 4378-1311 Email: rfavaloro@ffavaloro.org 1,2) R.R. Favaloro, 2) J. Abud, 3) S. Perrone, C. Gomez, F. Klein, L. Favaloro, M. Sultan, 4) E. Hass, E. Raimondi, 5) C. Presa, C. Gomez	3	3	3	21

638

1)=Director, 2)=Tx Surgeons, 3)=Physicians, 4)=Tissue Typers, 5)=TxCoords	1998	1999	2000	Total

AUSTRALIA

Alfred Hosp, Heart/Lung Replacement Serv, Commercial Rd, Prahran 3181, Melbourne, Victoria Ph: (613)9 276-2862 Fax: (613)9 276-2317 1,2) D.S. Esmore, 2) M. Rabinov, J. Smith, A. Pick, 3) T. Williams, G. Snell, T. Kotsimbos, 4) B. Tait, L. Holder, 5) A. Griffiths, W. Moule, K. Waters	0	1	0	49

AUSTRIA

Univ Hosp, Dept of Transp Surg, Anichstrasse 35, Innsbruck, 6020 Ph: (43)512 504-2603 Fax: (43)512 504-2605 1,2) R. Margreiter, 1,2) G. Laufer, 2) L. Mueller, H. Antretter, 3) C. Prior, O. Pachinger, G. Poelzl, 4) D. Schoenitzer, 5) H. Fetz, P. Schobel	1	0	0	10

BELGIUM

Erasmus Hosp, Dept of Cardio Surg, Rte de Lennick, 808, B-1070 Brussels Ph: (32)2 555-3817 Fax: (32)2 555-6652 Email: masntoin@ulb.ac.be 1,2) J.L. LeClerc, 2) M. Antoine, 3) M. Estenne, 4) E. Dupont, 5) B. van Haelewyck	2	5	2	88
Univ Hosp Gasthuisberg, Dept of Cardiology, Herestr 49, Leuven, B-3000 Ph: (32)16 344235 Fax: (32)16 344240 Email: johan.vanhaeche@uz.kuleuven.ac.be 1,2) W. Daenen, 1,3) J. Vanhaecke, M. Demedts, 2) W. Flameng, P. Sergeant, D. van Raemdonck, 3) G. Verleden, 5) F. van Gelder, D. van Hees, S. Kimpen	3	0	3	25

CANADA

Univ of Alberta Hosp, Dept of Cardio/Vasc/Thor Surg, 40 Hope Prog, 8440 112 St, Edmonton, AB T6G 2B7 Ph: (780) 407-8411 Fax: (780) 407-3056 1,2) D. Modry, 2) A. Koshal, J.C. Mullen, 3) J. Burton, W. Tymchak, D. Lien, J. Crockett, J. Preiksaitis, 4) J. Schlaut, 5) A. Tchoryk, S. Shukalak, K. Young, K. Jackson, C. Chorney	3	0	2	18
Univ Hosp, Div of Cardio/Vasc/Thor Surg, 339 Windermere Rd, PO Box 5339, London, ON N6A 5A5 Ph: (519) 663-3159 Fax: (519) 663-3858 1,2) R.J. Novick, 2) N. McKenzie, D. Boyd, M. Quantz, A.H. Menkis, 3) D. Ahmad, 4) S. Leckie, 5) M. Bloch, C. Weernick, J. Drew, M. Mohamed, C.A. Smith	1	1	0	46
Royal Victoria Hosp, McGill Ctr Clin Immun/Transp, 687 Pine Ave W, Montreal, PQ H3A 1A1 Ph: (514) 842-1231 Fax: (514) 843-1689 1,2) R. Cecere, 2) P. Ergina, K. Lachapelle, 3) M. Cantarovich, N. Giannetti, 4) P. Imperial, C. McIntyre, 5) C. Magnan, R. Chartier, E. Cyr	1	1	0	28

FINLAND

Helsinki Univ Ctrl Hosp, Dept of Thor/Cardio/Vasc Surg, Haartmaninkatu 4, Helsinki, SF-00290 Ph: (358)9 471 2290 Fax: (358)9 471 4006 1,2) S. Mattila, 2) Staff Members of Cardio/Thor/Vasc Surgery, 3) M. Nieminen, 4) Finnish Red Cross Typ Lab, 5) M. Lindstrom, M.L. Hellstedt	1			19

FRANCE

Laennec Hosp, Dept of CTVC, BP 1005, Nantes Cedex, 44035 Ph: (33)40 165084 Fax: (33)40 165133 1,2) J.L. Michaud, 2) P. Despins, D. Duveau, 3) A. Haloun, M. Treilhaud, 4) Bignon, Cesbron, 5) N. LeSant	3	7		74
Groupe Hosp Pitie Salpetriere, Dept of Cardio/Vasc Surg, 83 Blvd de L'Hospital, Paris, 75013 Ph: (33)1 4217 7001 Fax: (33)1 4217 7656 Email: monique.tallier@psl.ap.hop-paris.fr 1,3) I. Gandjbakhch, 2) A. Pavie, V. Bors, 3) R. Dorent, P. Leger, E. Vaissier, J.P. Levasseur, 4) C. Raffoux, 5) F. Maillet, M. Tallier	2	2	2	156

GERMANY

Heart Ctr North Rhine Westfalia, Ruhr-Univ of Bochum, Dept of Thor/Cardio/Vasc Surg, Georgstrasse 11, Bad Oeynhausen, 32545 Ph: (49)5731 97 1331 Fax: (49)5731 97 1820 1,2) R. Koerfer, 2) K. Minami, B. Hansky, 3) G. Tenderich, 4) W. Prohaska, C. Wolf, 5) S. Wlost, B. Heistermann-Linstaedt	1	1	2	17

1)=Director, 2)=Tx Surgeons, 3)=Physicians, 4)=Tissue Typers, 5)=TxCoords	1998	1999	2000	Total
German Heart Inst, Dept of Thor/Cardio/Vasc Surg, Augustenburger Platz 1, Berlin, D-13353 Ph: (49)30 4593 2000 Fax: (49)30 4593 2100 1,2) R. Hetzer, 2) Y. Weng, et, al. , 3) M. Hummel, P. Lange, R. Ewert, 4) Salama, 5) H. Kriegler	6	5		76
Hannover Med Sch, Dept of Surg, Div Thor/Cardio/Vasc/Surg, Carl-Neuberg-STR.1, 30625 Hannover Ph: (49)511 532-6581 Fax: (49)511 532-5404 1,2) A. Haverich, 2) W. Harringer, M. Strueber, 3) J. Niedermeyer, 4) Robin-Win, Pastucha, 5) G. Gubernatis	2	4	2	52
Clin Grosshadern, Dept of Cardiac Surg, Marchionini str 15, 81377 Munich Ph: (49)89 7095 3450 Fax: (49)89 7095 3465 Email: hcr@hch.med.uni-muenchen.de 1) B. Reichart, 2) Reichenspurner, 3) B. Meiser, 4) E.A. Albert, 5) Transp Grosshadern	3	8	4	50
Univ Hosp Munster, Dept of Thor/Cardio/Vasc Surg, Munster, 48129 Ph: (49)251 83-47401 Fax: (49)251 83-48316 1) H.H. Scheld, 2) D. Hammel, M. Weyand, 3) M.C. Deng, 4) H. Gross-Wilde, S. Browski, 5) Kley	2	0		5

ITALY

Ospedale Ped "Bambino Gesu", Dept Med Chir di Cardio Ped, Piazza S Onofrio 4, Rome, 00165 Ph: (39)06 6859 2611 Fax: (39)06 6859 2200 Email: parisi@opbg.net 1,2) R. DiDonato, 2) C. Squitieri, A. Carotti, 3) F. Parisi, A. Turchetta, V. Lucidi, 4) D. Adorno, 5) F. Parisi	2	4	5	25

NORWAY

Rikshosp Nat'l Hosp, Dept Thoracic & Cardiovasc, Sognsvannsveien 20, Oslo, 0027 Ph: (47)23 073735 Fax: (47)23 073741 Email: odd.geiran@rikshospitalet.no 1) O. Geiran, 2) H. Lindberg, E. Seem, 3) S. Simonsen, O. Bjortuft, 4) E. Thorsby, T. Leivestad, 5) P.A. Bakkan, S. Foss, P.E. Vatsas, K. Meyer	3	0	2	17

SWEDEN

Sahlgrenska Hosp, Dept Cardio/Thor Surg, Transp Unit, Gothenburg, S 41345 Ph: (46)31-601000 Fax: (46)31-417991 1,2) S.E. Svensson, 2) F. Nilsson, , 3) G. Martensson, 4) L. Sandberg, Lennart, Rydberg, 5) U. Lorentzon, U. Nystrom	0	2	1	32

UNITED KINGDOM

Papworth Hosp, Transp Unit, Papworth Everard, Cambridge, CB3 8RE Ph: (44)480 830541 Fax: (44)480 364610 1,2) J. Wallwork, 2) S.R. Large, F.C. Wells, S.A.M. Nashef, J. Dunning, A. Ritchie, S. Tsui, 3) J. Parameshwar, K. McNeil, 4) C. Taylor, 5) Baines, Smith, Ryan, Woods, Castle, Lockhurst, Wiggins	23	23	17	288
Wythenshawe Hosp, Dept of Cardio/Thor Surg, Southmoor Rd, Manchester, M23 9LT Ph: (44)161 998 7070 Fax: (44)161 291 2091 1,2) A.K. Deiraniya, 2) C.S. Campbell, N. Yonan, T. Hooper, M.T. Jones, 3) N. Brooks, R. Levy, K. Carroll, C.T. Leonard, 4) P. Dyer, S. Sheldon, 5) H. Pyatt, J. Nuttall, J. Stewart	1	0	1	39
Harefield Hosp, Dept of Cardio/Thor Surg, Harefield, Middlesex, UB9 6JH Ph: (44)1 895 287551 Fax: (44)1 895 824983 1) M. Yacoub, 2) A. Khaghani, J. Pepper, 3) A. Mitchell, N. Banner, R. Radley-Smith, M. Hodson, 4) M. Rose, 5) P. Baldoc, H. Blair, T. Jackson	21	13		471

HEART/LUNG Transplants

	1998	1999	2000	Total
United States	44	43	40	777
Foreign	84	80	46	1,820
Total	128	123	86	2,597

HEART/LUNG Transplant Centers

United States	40
Foreign	32
Total	72

WORLDWIDE TRANSPLANT CENTER DIRECTORY
LUNG TRANSPLANTS

1)=Director, 2)=Tx Surgeons, 3)=Physicians, 4)=Tissue Typers, 5)=TxCoords	1998	1999	2000	Total

UNITED STATES

ALABAMA

| Univ of Alabama Birmingham Med Ctr, Dept of Surg/Med, 701 S 19th St, 739 Zeigler Research Bldg, Birmingham, AL 35294 Ph: (205) 975-8615 Fax: (205) 975-9792 1,2) D.C. McGiffin, 2) W.L. Holman, G.L. Zorn, J.K. Kirklin, 3) K.R. Young, D. Weill, 4) R. Senkbeil, C. Mink, 5) C. White-Williams, M. Hubbard, M. Arndt, T. Smith | 30 | 31 | 39* | 231 |

ARIZONA

| Univ Med Ctr, Dept of Cardio/Thor Surg, 1501 N Campbell Ave, Rm 4604, Tucson, AZ 85724 Ph: (520) 694-6299 Fax: (520) 694-2692 1,2) F.A. Arabia, 2) G. Sethi, J.G. Copeland, V. Paramesh, D. Arzouman, S. Sharma, 3) S. Butman, C. Lui, S. Knoper, 5) N. Edling, J. Wild, N. Harrington, D. Allen, S. Mullarkey | 4 | 0 | 4 | 52 |

CALIFORNIA

Cedars-Sinai Med Ctr, Cardio Surg-Lung Transp Prog, 8700 Beverly Blvd, Suite 6215, Los Angeles, CA 90048 Ph: (310) 423-3851 Fax: (310) 967-0127 1,2) R. Kass, 2) A. Trento, C. Blanche, S. Raissi, W. Cheng, G. Fontana, K. Magliato, 3) M. Biring, G. Chaux, 4) S. Jordan, D. Tyan, 5) B. Kearney	1	3	3	82
Children's Hosp of Los Angeles, Dept of Cardio/Thor Transp, 4650 Sunset Blvd MS#66, Los Angeles, CA 90027 Ph: (323) 669-5965 Fax: (323) 668-7979 1,2) V.A. Starnes, 2) R.G. Cohen, 3) M.L. Barr, K.C. Kocis, E. MacLaughlin, M. Woo, 5) M. Horn	1	6	5*	38
Univ Calif-Los Angeles Med Ctr, Dept of Surg, Div of Cardio Surg, 10833 Le Conte Ave, 62-182A CHS, Los Angeles, CA 90095 Ph: (310) 825-6068 Fax: (310) 206-6301 1,2) H. Laks, 2) A. Ardehali, 3) M. Levine, R. Shipner, D. Ross, 4) UCLA Immunogenetics Center, 5) M. Brown	14	10	8	118
Univ of Southern Calif Univ Hosp, Dept of Thor/Cardio/Vasc Surg, Cardiac Transp Prog, 1500 San Pablo St, Los Angeles, CA 90033 Ph: (323) 442-8419 Fax: (323) 442-6201 1,2) V.A. Starnes, 2) R.G. Cohen, 3) R.G. Barbers, M.L. Barr, 4) Y. Iwaki, J. Cicciarelli, 5) F. Schenkel, J. Onga, D. Lake	15	22	23*	128
Stanford Univ Med Ctr, Dept of Cardio, Falk Bldg, MC 5407, Palo Alto, CA 94305 Ph: (650) 723-5771 Fax: (650) 725-3846 1,2) R.C. Robbins, 2) T.A. Burdon, P.E. Oyer, B.A. Reitz, 3) R.L. Doyle, J. Theodore, 4) C. Grumet, 5) P. Gamberg, J. Miller, L. Levine, M. Merlo	22	9	21	152
Univ Calif-Davis Med Ctr, Transp Admin, 2315 Stockton Blvd, Housestaff Facility, Room 1018, Sacramento, CA 95817 Ph: (916) 734-2111 Fax: (916) 734-0432 1,3) T.E. Albertson, 2) H.A. Berkoff, D.M. Follette, 3) R.P. Allen, S.H. Cohen, 4) P. Holland, 5) D. Smith, A. Hoso	8	13	1	56
Univ California-San Diego, Div of Cardio/Thor Surg, 200 W Arbor Dr, San Diego, CA 92103-8892 Ph: (619) 543-7777 Fax: (619) 543-2652 Email: jkriett@ucsd.edu 1,2) S.W. Jamieson, 2) J.M. Kriett, D. Kapelanski, P. Thisthethwaite, 3) M. Light, P. Stillwell, G. Yung, 4) M. Garavoy, L. Lebeck, 5) D. Garcia, S. Osborne, L. Gayhart, D. Glasser	19	16	18*	180
Univ of Calif-San Francisco, Dept of Cardio/Thor Surg, 505 Parnassus, Box 1267, San Francisco, CA 94143 Ph: (415) 476-3503 Fax: (415) 502-5316 1,2) F. Keith, 2) T. Hall, M. Block, D. Jablons, 3) J. Golden, 5) C. Rifkin, A. Fukano	10	6	8	79

COLORADO

| Univ of Colorado Hlth Sci Ctr, Dept of Cardio/Thor Surg, Div of Cardio, 4200 E 9th Ave, Denver, CO 80262 Ph: (303) 270-4409 Fax: (303) 270-3065 1,2) F.L. Grover, 2) D.N. Campbell, J.E. mault, 3) J. Lindenfeld, E. Woffel, M. Bristow, W. Abraham, 4) IAD, 5) K. Keller, A. Hornbaker, P. Parmalee | 15 | 22 | 29* | 126 |

LUNG

* Preliminary UNOS data

642

1)=Director, 2)=Tx Surgeons, 3)=Physicians, 4)=Tissue Typers, 5)=TxCoords	1998	1999	2000	Total
FLORIDA				
Shands at the Univ of Florida, Transplant Center, Box 100251, 1600 SW Archer Rd, Gainesville, FL 32610-0251 Ph: (352) 265-0130 Fax: (352) 265-0108 1,2) E.D. Staples, 1,3) M.A.Baz, G.A.Visner, 2) D. Knauf, T. Beaver, 3) E.M. Harmon, 4) J. Scornik, 5) L. McGinn, K. Harker, W. Swafford, B. Williams	27	19	19	148
GEORGIA				
Egleston Children's Hosp at Emory U, Dept of Cardio/Thor Sur, 1365 Clifton Rd NE, Box 7, Atlanta, GA 30322 Ph: (404) 315-6394 Fax: (404) 315-2277 1,2) K. Kanter, 2) K. Kanter, D. Vega, J. Puskas, 3) C. Lawrence, 4) A. Love, 5) C. Martindele	12	9	0	59
ILLINOIS				
Univ of Illinois Hosp, Chicago, Sec of Cardiothoracic Surg, 1740 W Taylor St, Chicago, IL 60680-6998 Ph: (312) 996-6215 Fax: (312) 996-2013 1,2) M.G. Massad, 2) A.S. Geha, N. Snow, 3) A. Jaffe, 4) V.A. Lazda, 5) S. Steinhiser, D. Fontana	3	3	4	37
Loyola Univ Med Ctr, Lung Transp Prog, 2160 S First Ave, Blg 110, Rm 6271, Maywood, IL 60153 Ph: (708) 327-5864 Fax: (708) 327-2424 1,3) E.R. Garrity Jr, 1,2) W. Vigneswaran, 2) T. Hinkamp, M. Bakhos, J. Schwartz, 3) C. Alex, K. Simpson, S. Bhorade, A. Khurshid, 4) B. Susskind, 5) M. McCabe, W. Williams, K. Martin, P. Kelly, R. Ghusein	20	33	33	303
INDIANA				
Methodist Hosp, Transp Ctr, I-65 at 21st St, PO Box 1367, Indianapolis, IN 46206-1367 Ph: (317) 929-8677 Fax: (317) 929-7192 Email: wjjohnson@clarian.com 1,2) J.W. Fehrenbacher, 1,3) M.R. Niemeier, 2) D. Beckman, D. Hormuth, H. Halbrook, T. Wozniak, A. Coffey, 3) M.F. Busk, K.M. Wolf, 4) N. Higgins, Z. Brahmi, 5) S. Houck, W. Johnson, L. Kempf, K. Fox, D. Gooch	21	16	32	164
KENTUCKY				
Jewish Hosp, Transp Serv, 217 E Chestnut St, Louisville, KY 40202 Ph: (502) 587-4939 Fax: (502) 587-4184 1) M. Bousamra, 2) L. Gray, S. Etoch, R. Dowling, 3) W. McConnell, R. Karman, 4) P. Landrum, R. Pound, J. Cassin, M. Steele, 5) J. Brohm, P. Buckley, A. Fish, D. Carter, D. Harris	10	14	9	84
Univ of Kentucky Med Ctr, Dept of Cardio/Thor Surg, 800 Rose St,C428, Lexington, KY 40536-0293 Ph: (859) 257-5188 Fax: (859) 323-1700 1,2) T.W. Mullett, 2) J. Sanchez, D. Mandapati, 3) T. Waid, 4) F. Lower, W. O'Conner, 5) J. Leigh, A. Hartman, J. Patrick	6	18	13*	106
LOUISIANA				
Ochsner Foundation Hospital, Multi-Organ Transplant Center, 1514 Jefferson Hwy, New Orleans, LA 70121 Ph: (504) 842-3925 Fax: (504) 842-6228 Email: dfuchs@ochsner.org 1,2) P.M. McFadden, 1,3) V.G. Valentine, 2) C. Van Meter, J.L. Ochsner, 3) S.P. Kantrow, 4) E.S. Cooper, G. Stewart, S. Herbert, 5) D. Fuchs, M. Ripoll, B. Stevenson, W. Black	18	19	23	135
MARYLAND				
The Johns Hopkins Hosp, JHH Lung & Heart/Lung Transp, Blalock 147, 600 N Wolfe St, Baltimore, MD 21287-5674 Ph: (410) 614-4898 Fax: (410) 614-7008 1,2) S. Yang, 2) J. Conte, R. Stuart, M. Sussman, 3) J. Orens, P. Becker, C. Weiner, A. Polito, R. Girgis, 4) J. Hart, 5) D. Carter, K. Shagena, S. Kelley, J. Stanik-Hutt, M. Jordan, S. Miller	18	30	21	95
Univ of Maryland Med Ctr, Dept of Surgery, Thoracic Tx, N4E35, 22 S Greene St, Baltimore, MD 21201 Ph: (410) 328-2737 Fax: (410) 328-1311 1,2) J. Sonett, 2) Z. Gamliel, M. Krasna, 3) E.J. Britt, 4) American Red Cross, 5) R. Anzeck	11	4	5	65
MASSACHUSETTS				
Brigham & Women's Hosp, Div of Thor Surg, 75 Francis St, Boston, MA 02115 Ph: (617) 732-6824 Fax: (617) 732-3441 Email: www.chestsurg.org 1,2) S.J. Swanson, 2) S.J. Mentzer, M.T. Jaklitsch, R. Bueno, J.M. Lukanich, D.J. Sugarbaker, 3) J.J. Reilly, E.P. Ingenito, A. Deykin, A. Fohlbrigge, C. Donovan, 4) J. Goguen, 5) G.P. Fagan, K.A. Boyle, D. Mindilk	12	18	18	153

1)=Director, 2)=Tx Surgeons, 3)=Physicians, 4)=Tissue Typers, 5)=TxCoords	1998	1999	2000	Total
Children's Hospital-Boston, Dept of Pediatrics, Pulm Med/Gen Surg, 300 Longwood Ave, Boston, MA 02115 Ph: (617) 335-6681 Fax: (617) 566-7810 1,2) C. Lillehei, 3) D. Waltz, W. Robinson, 4) Brigham Women's Tissue Typ Lab, 5) L. Skinder, Gourville	2	3	4*	29
Massachusetts Gen Hosp, Dept of Thor Surg, Blake 1570, 32 Fruit St, Boston, MA 02114 Ph: (617) 726-5200 Fax: (617) 726-7667 1,2) J.C. Wain, 1,3) L.C. Ginns, 2) D.P. Ryan, C. Wright, D. Donahuei, J. Allen, 5) S. Zorb	8	9	25*	107

MICHIGAN

	1998	1999	2000	Total
Univ of Michigan Med Ctr, Dept of Thor Surg, Box 0344, 1500 E Medical Ctr Dr, Ann Arbor, MI 48109 Ph: (734) 763-7418 Fax: (734) 615-2656 1,2) M. Iannettoni, 2) M. Orringer, J. Yee, 3) J. Lynch, F. Martinez, T. Ojo, K. Flaherty, S. Gay, 4) J. Baker, 5) R. Florn, J. Berry	27	25	40	214
Henry Ford Hosp, Dept of Cardio/Thor Surg, 2799 W Grand Blvd, Detroit, MI 48202 Ph: (313) 876-2695 Fax: (313) 916-2687 1) Bernabei, 2) N. Silveman, G. Paone, 3) L. Allenspach, K. Chan, 4) D. Kukuruga, 5) L. Wilcocks	7	6	7	52

MINNESOTA

	1998	1999	2000	Total
Fairview Univ Med Ctr, Thoracic Transp Ctr, Box 398, 420 Delaware St SE, Minneapolis, MN 55455 Ph: (612) 625-9922 Fax: (612) 626-6968 1,2) S. Park, 1,3) M. Hertz, 2) S. Shumway, H. Bittner, C. Herrington, R. Kelly, R. Bolman, 3) M. Hertz, M. King, J. Dunitz, C. Wendt, 4) H. Noreen, 5) Elmajri, Gibson, Zirbes, Rosenthal, Dunbar	28	39	31	309
Mayo Clin, St Mary's Hosp, Dept of Cardio/Thor Surg, 6-716 St Mary's Hosp, Rochester, MN 55905 Ph: (507) 255-6038 Fax: (507) 255-4500 1,2) C.G.A. McGregor, 2) R.C. Daly, J. Dearani, 3) J.C. McDougall, S.G. Peters, J.P. Scott, W.M. Brutinel, M.E. Wylam, 4) S.B. Moore, 5) S. Carlson, J. Hanson, J. Meyer, K. Sandstrom	3	2	3	42

MISSOURI

	1998	1999	2000	Total
Barnes-Jewish Hosp, Dept of Thor/Cardio Surg, Ste 3108 Queeny Tower, One Barnes Hosp Plaza, St Louis, MO 63110 Ph: (314) 362-5378 Fax: (314) 362-9272 1,2) G.A. Patterson, 2) J.D. Cooper, B. Meyers, 3) E.P. Trulock, 4) D. Phelan, 5) S. Waxman, K. Sander, L. Peterson, J. Fassler, M. Scavuzzo	54	48	53*	553
St Louis Children's Hosp, at Washington Univ Med Ctr, Dept of Cardio/Thor Surg, 1 Children's Pl, St Louis, MO 63110 Ph: (314) 454-6165 Fax: (314) 454-2381 1,2) C.B. Huddleston, 2) E. Mendeloff, 3) S. Sweet, S. Shapiro, M. de la Morina, P. Schuller, 4) D. Phelan, 5) D. Watkins, P. Shaner, D. Springhart, G. McBride, C. Driver	33	19	19	225
St Louis Univ Hosp, Dept of Thor Transp, 3635 Vista Ave, PO Box 15250, St Louis, MO 63110 Ph: (314) 577-5421 Fax: (314) 577-8867 1,2) L.R. McBride, 3) C.A. Keller, 4) K. Riordan, 5) P. Haselhorst	4	2	3*	46

NEBRASKA

	1998	1999	2000	Total
BryanLGH Med Center East, Transp Serv, 1600 S 48th St, Lincoln, NE 68506-1299 Ph: (402) 481-3911 Fax: (402) 481-3918 1,2) D. Gangahar, 2) E. Raines, 3) A. Chakraborty, 4) Univ of Nebraska Med Ctr, 5) N. Steckelberg, B. Markey	0	1	3*	17
Nebraska Health System, Dept of Surg, Sec of Cardio/Thor Surg, 982315 Nebraska Med Ctr, Omaha, NE 68198-2315 Ph: (402) 559-4424 Fax: (402) 559-6913 1,2) T.A. Galbraith, 2) K. Franco, 3) A.B. Thompson, P.H. Sammut, C.A. Piquette, 4) J.L. Wisecarver, S. Shepherd	2	0	0*	21

NEW YORK

	1998	1999	2000	Total
Columbia Presbyterian Med Ctr, Dept of Surg/Cardio Transp, PH 14 West, 622 W 168th St, New York, NY 10032 Ph: (212) 305-7600 Fax: (212) 305-8304 1,2) M. Galantowiez, 2) C.R. Smith, M. Ginsburg, L. Gorenstein, 3) C. McGregor, L. Schulman, 4) N. Sucia-Foca, 5) B. Jorgensen, R. Gerow-Smith	14	21	18*	232

1)=Director, 2)=Tx Surgeons, 3)=Physicians, 4)=Tissue Typers, 5)=TxCoords	1998	1999	2000	Total
Mount Sinai Med Ctr, Cardio/Thor Div, Box 1028, 1 Gustave Levy Place, New York, NY 10029 Ph: (212) 241-8181 Fax: (212) 534-3357 1,2) S. Lansman, 2) R. Griepp, S. Lansman, J. McCullough, 3) A. Gass, M. Padilla, G. Schilero, 4) Rogosin Inst, 5) M. Courtney, D. Correa	0	0	3*	12
NYU Medical Center, Dept of Surg, Faculty Practice Offices, 530 First Ave, Ste 6D, New York, NY 10016 Ph: (212) 263-7461 Fax: (212) 263-2042 1,2) L. Glassman, 1,2) G. Ribakove, 3) J. Lowy, G. Haralambou, 4) Rogosin Inst, 5) J. Stecher	1	3	0	5
NORTH CAROLINA				
Univ of North Carolina Hosp, Comprehensive Transp Ctr, 3306 West Wing, Chapel Hill, NC 27514 Ph: (888) 263-5293 Fax: (919) 966-7564 Email: transplant@unch.unc.edu 1,2) T.M. Egan, 2) F.C. Detterbeck, M.R. Mill, 3) L.J. Paradowski, R. Aris, 4) J. Schmitz, J. Thomas, 5) J. McSweeney, E. Cairns, B. Mueller	12	17	13*	198
Duke Univ Med Ctr, Dept of Transp, Box 31175, DUMC, Durham, NC 27710 Ph: (800) 249-LUNG Fax: (919) 681-7502 1,2) R.D. Davis, 2) R. Messier, J. Jaggers, T. D'Amico, 3) S. Palmer, V. Tapson, D. Hadjiliadis, W. Mariencheck, 4) N. Reinsmoen, F. Ward, 5) C. Lawrence, A. Miralles, A. Petersen, J. Rea, D. Gibson	35	52	53*	311
OHIO				
Cleveland Clin Fnd, A110 Transplant Center, 9500 Euclid Ave, Cleveland, OH 44195 Ph: (216) 445-1115 Fax: (216) 445-3127 1,2) J. Maurer, 1,2) M.DeCamp, 2) N. Smedira, G. Pettersson, S. Murthy, 3) A. Mehta, O. Minai, R. Schilz, J. Chapman, 4) D. Cook, L. Klingman, 5) T. Evans-Walker, J. Foertch, H. Blazey	29	32	46	229
OKLAHOMA				
Integris Baptist Med Ctr, Nazih Zuhdi Transpl Inst, 3300 NW Expressway, Oklahoma City, OK 73112 Ph: (405) 949-3349 Fax: (405) 945-5467 1) B.M. Nour, 2) J. Chaffin, D. Vanhooser, C. Elkins, 3) D. Nelson, I. Paradis, 4) S. Oleinick, 5) J. Wood	4	6	9*	49
OREGON				
Oregon Health Sci Univ Hosp, Div of Cardio Surg, 3181 SW Sam Jackson Pk Rd, Portland, OR 97201 Ph: (503) 494-7820 Fax: (503) 494-7829 1,2) I. Shen, 2) V. Reddy, 3) M. Meyer, M. Chesnutt, 4) D.J. Norman, 5) J.A. Nussbaum	2	1	2*	19
PENNSYLVANIA				
Temple Univ Hosp, Dept of Cardio/Thor Surg, Broad & Tioga Sts, 9th Flr, 320 Parkinson Pavilion, Philadelphia, PA 19140 Ph: (215) 707-1722 Fax: (215) 707-6867 1,2) S. Furukawa, 1,3) G. O'Brien, 2) J.B. McClurken, V.P. Addonizio, V. Jeevanandam, 3) C. Criner, 4) S. Leach, 5) A.K. Kuzma	9	9	5*	82
The Children's Hosp of Philadelphia, Thoracic Organ Transp Program, 34th St & Civic Ctr Blvd, Philadelphia, PA 19104 Ph: (215) 590-6051 Fax: (213) 590-1340 1,2) T.L. Spray, 2) J.W. Gaynor, W.M. DeCampli, T.R. Karl, 3) B.J. Clark, N.D. Bridges, B.D. Hanna, R. Zinman, T. Hoffman, 4) D. Monos, 5) M. Sowa, J. Menendez	8	3	6	43
Univ of Pennsylvania Med Ctr, Lung Transp Program, 3400 Spruce St, Grnd Flr Rhoads Pavilion, Philadelphia, PA 19104 Ph: (215) 662-2365 Fax: (215) 349-8235 Email: kotloff@mail.med.upenn.edu 1,2) J. Bavaria, 1,3) R. Kotloff, 2) A. Pochettino, B. Rosengard, J. Golman, R. Gorman, 3) H. Palevsky, S. Arcasoy, D. Zisman, 4) M. Kamoun, 5) N.P. Blumenthal, R.A. Price, M.E. Carr	23	25	31*	250
Children's Hosp of Pittsburgh, Dept of Cardio/Thor Surg, 3705 Fifth Ave, One Children's Place, Pittsburgh, PA 15213 Ph: (412) 692-5541 Fax: (412) 692-6991 Email: webbers@heart.chp.edu 1,2) F. Pigula, 1,3) S. Webber, 2) B.P. Griffith, 3) G. Kurland, 4) A. Zeevi, 5) B. Stinner, D. Dorsey	7	0	6	48
Univ of Pittsburgh Sch of Med, Dept of Cardio/Thor Surg, C-700 Presbyterian Univ Hosp, 200 Lothrop St, Pittsburgh, PA 15213-2582 Ph: (412) 648-1963 Fax: (412) 648-1029 Email: ristichj@msx.upmc.edu 1,2) K. McCurry, 2) B. Hattler, B. Griffith, M. Zenati, K. McCurry, 3) J. Dauber, A. Iacono, J. Pilewski, 4) A. Zeevi, 5) A. Lee, J. Vensak, J. Manzetti, S. Zomak, C. Cornell	33	34	38	472

1)=Director, 2)=Tx Surgeons, 3)=Physicians, 4)=Tissue Typers, 5)=TxCoords	1998	1999	2000	Total
TENNESSEE				
Baptist Mem Hosp, Thoracic Transp Serv, 930 Madison Ave, Ste 456, Memphis, TN 38103 Ph: (901) 227-6106 Fax: (901) 227-6196 1,2) H.E. Garrett Jr, 2) J. Gooch, R. Carter, 3) E. Golden, S. Headley, T. Edwards, K. Newman, 4) C. Miller, B Loehmann, Y. Cao, L. Marek, 5) D. Combs, D. DuVall-Seaman, R. Suggs	3	1	0	24
Vanderbilt Univ Med Ctr, The Vanderbilt Transp Ctr, Dept of Heart/Lung Transp, 908 Oxford House, Nashville, TN 37232-4734 Ph: (615) 936-0393 Fax: (615) 936-0396 1,2) R.N. Pierson III, 2) W.H. Merrill, J.R. Roberts, , 3) J.E. Loyd, S. Dummer, G. Miller, A. Milstone, 4) DCI Lab, 5) A. Goodwin, S. England	15	19	16	140
TEXAS				
Baylor Univ Med Ctr, Dept of Cardio/Thoracic TX, 4 Roberts, 3500 Gaston Ave, Dallas, TX 75246 Ph: (214) 820-6856 Fax: (214) 820-4527 1,2) W.S. Ring, 2) J. Capehart, D. Meyer, M. Wait, M. DiMaio, M. Jessen, 3) K. Ausloos, D. Luterman, 4) J. McCormack, 5) R. Kauffman, A. Boronow, S. Moore, J. West, A. Dierlam, A. Sonnen	14	11	9	110
Medical City Dallas Hosp, Heart Lung Center, 7777 Forest Lane, A-14th Floor, Dallas, TX 75230 Ph: (800) 348-4318 Fax: (972) 566-4872 1,2) S. Seitz, 2) D. Ogden, M. Mack, T. Dewey, M. McGee, R. Bowman, I. Davidsons, S. Reeder, 3) E. Rosenthal, J. Hunt, M. Lerman, A. Shulkin, K. Hoang, A. Anderson, 4) Texas Med Specialty Inc (A. Nikaein), 5) M. Covin, T. McMellon, D. Stevenson, A. Kuhnel	12	4	2	37
St Paul Med Ctr, Univ of Texas Southwstrn, Transp Ofc, Ste 623, 5939 Harry Hines Blvd, Dallas, TX 75235 Ph: (214) 648-8811 Fax: (214) 879-6209 1,2) W.S. Ring, 2) D. Meyer, M. Jessen, C. Moncrief, M. Wait, M. DeMaio, 3) R. Rosenblatt, O. Utset, F. Torres, 4) P. Stastny, 5) P. Kaiser, K. Weber, M. Stenstrom, K. Rozelle, K. Bush	11	9	8*	61
St Luke's Episcopal Hosp, Transp Serv 2-114, PO Box 20269, Houston, TX 77225 Ph: (713) 791-3952 Fax: (713) 794-6696 Email: kneylor@sleh.com 1,2) O.H. Frazier, 2) G. Noon, S. Scheinen, 3) A. Frost, I. Nizami, 4) R. Kerman, 5) K. Neylor	8	7	9	37
Baylor Coll of Med, The Methodist Hosp, Multi-Organ Transp Ctr, 6565 Fannin-SM 491, Houston, TX 77030 Ph: (713) 790-2501 Fax: (713) 793-1335 1,3) A.E. Frost, 2) R. Espada, G.P. Noon, J. Lafuente, 3) I. Nizami, 4) M. Pollack, 5) N. Eisenhour, A. Brown	8	10	16*	152
UTHSCSA, Dept of Surg, Organ Transpl, Mail code 7858, 7703 Floyd Curl Dr, San Antonio, TX 78229-3900 Ph: (210) 567-5777 Fax: (210) 567-5122 Email: sako@uthscsa.edu 1,2) E. Sako, 1) S.Levine, 2) J. Calhoon, O.L. Miller, S. Johnson, 3) A. Anzueto, S. Levine, J. Peters, C. Bryan, S. Im, 4) P. Blackwell, K. Rocha, G. Bruun, 5) L. Nichols, T. Cronin	12	11		146
UTAH				
Univ of Utah Hosp, Lung Transpl Program, 50 N Medical Dr, Salt Lake City, UT 84132 Ph: (801) 581-7806 Fax: (801) 585-5685 1,2) S.V. Karwande, 2) J. Stringham, D. Bull, 3) B. Cahill, B. Marshall, W. Samuelson, M. Elstad, 4) T. Fuller, 5) M. O'Rourke, S. Parker	9	12	9*	56
VIRGINIA				
Univ of Virginia Health Science Ctr, Cardio/Pulm Transp Ctr, Box 191, Lee Street, Charlottesville, VA 22908 Ph: (800) 257-0757 Fax: (804) 924-2359 1,3) M. Robbins, 2) I. Kron, C.G. Tribble, 3) J. Bergin, 4) C. Spencer, C. Paschall, J. Guan, 5) M. Ball, T. Broccoli, V. Reel	7	16	22*	150
Inova Fairfax Hosp, Dept of Heart/Lung Transp, 3300 Gallows Rd, Falls Church, VA 22042-3300 Ph: (703) 698-2986 Fax: (703) 698-2797 1,2) N. Burton, 2) P. Massimiano, E. Lefrak, 3) S. Nathan, 4) Transp/Immun Lab, Washington, D.C., 5) P. Roberts, O. Evoemon	10	16	19*	65
Sentara Norfolk Gen Hosp, Transp Ctr, 600 Greshham Dr, Norfolk, VA 23507 Ph: (804) 668-2831 Fax: (804) 668-2814 1,2) J.B. Rich, 2) S. Szentpetery, R. Hagberg, 3) J. Tomlinson, R. Garnett, A.J. Quaranta, 4) A. Arnold, K. Wall, K. Keatley, V. Buxton, T. McRacken, J. Ahuett, F. Peed, 5) P. Bradshaw, D. Milteer, B. Smith, B. Morrill, S. Walton	2	0	3*	24

1)=Director, 2)=Tx Surgeons, 3)=Physicians, 4)=Tissue Typers, 5)=TxCoords	1998	1999	2000	Total
McGuire Veteran Affairs Med Ctr, Transp Srv 111-H, 1201 Broadrock Blvd, Richmond, VA 23249 Ph: (804) 675-5442 Fax: (804) 675-5420 1) McHarty, 2) R. Higgins, D. Salter, Cohen, 3) L. Moses, P. Fairman, 4) MCV Tissue Typ Lab, 5) J. Hanrahan, P. Joyner	4	2	4	25
Medical College of Virginia, Dept of Pulmonology/Thor Surg, PO Box 980204 MCV STATION, Richmond, VA 23298 Ph: (804) 828-4571 Fax: (804) 828-7710 1,2) N.M. Cohen, 2) R. Higgins, D. Salter, A. Deanda, V. Kasirajan, 3) P. Fairman, L. Moses, 4) C. Rhodes, P. Kimble, 5) M. Flattery, P. Joyner, J. Hanrahan	0	0	3*	29

WASHINGTON

Univ Washington Med Ctr, Dept of Surg, Div Cardio/Thor Surg, Box 356310, 1959 NE Pacific St, Seattle, WA 98195-6310 Ph: (206) 543-3093 Fax: (206) 543-0325 1,2) M.S. Mulligan, 2) M. Allen, R. Anderson, D. Wood, E. Vallieres, 3) J. Benditt, M. Aitken, G. Raghu, 4) K. Nelson, 5) K. Hoffman	12	20	26*	135

WISCONSIN

Univ of Wisconsin Hosp & Clin, Div of Cardio/Thor Surg, 600 Highland Ave, H4-370, Madison, WI 53792-3236 Ph: (608) 263-7832 Fax: (608) 263-0597 1,2) R.B. Love, 2) J.R. Pellett, R.P. Cochran, D. Woolley, 3) L. Chosy, K. Meyer, R. Cornwell, 4) D. Lorentzen, 5) D. Welter, A. Hoffman	23	35	20*	179
Children's Hosp of Wisconsin, Lung Transpl/Pulmonary, 9000 W Wisconsin Ave, Ste 211, Milwaukee, WI 53226 Ph: (414) 266-6458 Fax: (414) 266-6742 Email: mhintermeyer@chw.org 1,3) T. Rice, 2) J. Tweddell, G. Haasler, 3) J. Biller, W. Gersham, K. Presberg, L. Rusakow, 4) Bld Ctr of SE Wisconsin, 5) M. Hintermeyer	2	2	3*	17
St Luke's Med Ctr, Transplant Program, 2900 W. Oklahoma Ave, Milwaukee, WI 53201-2901 Ph: (414) 649-7734 Fax: (414) 649-5071 1,2) A.J. Tector, 2) Downey, Kress, Schmahl, Barragry, Crouch, Seifert, 3) T. Gronski, J. Hosenpud, 4) M. Oaks, 5) J. Heimler, L. Halverson, J. Keepers, K. Meunier	1	2	3*	21

ARGENTINA

Hosp Italiano de Buenos Aires, Dept of Surg, Gascon 450, CP181 Buenos Aires Ph: (54)1 981 1537 Fax: (54)1 981 3881 1) B.C. Vassallo, 2) C. Ruiz, E. Beveraggi, 3) A. de la Canal, J. Perscerutti, G. Svetliza, 4) L. Dalurzo, 5) P. Alvarez	3	1	3	22
ICYCC-Favaloro Foundation, Cardio/Vasc Surg, Transp Div, Av Belgrano 1746, Buenos Aires, C1093AAS Ph: (5411) 4378-1350 Fax: (5411) 4378-1311 Email: rfavaloro@ffavaloro.org 1,2) R.R. Favaloro, 2) A. Abud, 3) S. Perrone, C. Gomez, F. Klein, L. Favaloro, M. Sultan, 4) E. Hass, E. Raimondi, 5) C. Presa, C. Gomez	2	11	14	50

AUSTRALIA

Alfred Hosp, Heart/Lung Replacement Serv, Commercial Rd, Prahran, Melbourne, Victoria, 3181 Ph: (613)9 276-2862 Fax: (613)9 276-2317 1,2) D.S. Esmore, 2) M. Rabinov, J. Smith, A. Pick, 3) G. Snell, T. Williams, T. Kotsimbos, 4) B. Tait, L. Holder, W. Dandy, 5) A. Griffiths, W. Moule, K. Waters	41	33	41	308

AUSTRIA

Univ Hosp, Dept of Transp Surg, Anichstrasse 35, Innsbruck, 6020 Ph: (43)512 504-2603 Fax: (43)512 504-2605 1,2) R. Margreiter, 1,2) G. Laufer, 2) L. Mueller, 3) C. Prior, C. Geltner, C. Kaehler, 4) D. Schoenitzer, 5) H. Fetz, P. Schobel	6	10	12	55

BELGIUM

Erasmus Hosp, Dept of Cardio Surg, Rte de Lennick, 808, B-1070 Brussels Ph: (32)2 555-3817 Fax: (32)2 555-6652 Email: masntoin@ulb.ac.be 1) J.L. LeClerc, 1) P.Rocmans, 2) P. de Francquen, M. Antoine, 3) M. Estenne, 4) E. Dupont, 5) B. van Haelewyck	13	9	11	73

1)=Director, 2)=Tx Surgeons, 3)=Physicians, 4)=Tissue Typers, 5)=TxCoords	1998	1999	2000	Total
Univ Hosp Antwerpen, Dept Of Pulmonary Medicine, Wilrijkstraat 10, Edegem, B2650 Ph: (32)3 821-3000 Fax: (32)3 829-0520 1,2) P. van Schil, 2) F. van den Brande, I. Rodrigus, A. Moulijn, 3) P. Vermeire, R. De Paep, 4) L. Muylle, 5) W. van Donink, G. van Beeumen	2	2	0	5
Univ Hosp Gasthuisberg, Dept of Pneumology, Herestr 49, B-3000 Leuven Ph: (32)16 346800 Fax: (32)16 346803 1,2) T. Lerut, 1,3) G. Verleden, 2) W. Coosemans, D. van Raemdonck, P. Deleyn, T. Lerut, 3) G. Verleden, M. Deccroix, L. Dupont, 4) M.P. Emonds, 5) F. van Gelder	10	12	16	92
CANADA				
Univ of Alberta Hosp, Dept of Cardio/Vasc/Thor Surg, 40 Hope Prog, 8440 112 St, Edmonton, AB T6G 2B7 Ph: (780) 407-8411 Fax: (780) 407-3056 1,2) D. Modry, 2) J.C. Mullen, C. McNamee, T. Winton, 3) J. Burton, W. Tymchack, D. Lien, J. Crockett, Preiksaitis, 4) J. Schlaut, 5) A. Tchoryk, S. Shukalak, K. Young, K. Jackson, S. Chorney	12	14	21	100
British Columbia Transpl Society, West Tower, 3rd Floor, 555 W 12th Ave, Vancouver, BC V5Z 3X7 Ph: (604) 877-2240 Fax: (604) 877-2111 1) B. Barrable, 2) G. Fradet, 3) R. Levy, 4) B. Draney, 5) C. Storseth	7	3	6	76
Univ British Columbia, Dept of Surg/Med, Lung Transp, British Columbia Transp Soc, Ste 620,W 8th Ave, Vancouver 575, BC V5Z 166 Ph: (604) 875-8298 Fax: (604) 877-0977 1,2) G. Fradet, 2) K. Evans, R. Finley, 3) D. Ostrow, R. Levy, 4) P.A. Keown, 5) C. Storseth	7	3	6	91
Hlth Sci Ctr, Respiratory Dept, Rm RS103, 820 Sherbrook St, Winnipeg, MB R3A 1R9 Ph: (204) 787-2377 Fax: (204) 787-2420 1,2) H. Unruh, 1,3) W. Kepron, 2) L. Tan, 3) Z. Bhouty, 4) P. Nickerson, 5) A. Szabo	5	6	10	57
Univ Hosp, Div of Cardio/Vasc/Thor Surg, 339 Windermere Rd, PO Box 5339, London, ON N6A 5A5 Ph: (519) 663-3159 Fax: (519) 663-3858 1,2) R. Novick, 1) N. Quantz, 2) A. Menkis, N. McKenzie, 3) D. Ahmad, 4) S. Leckie, 5) M. Bloch, C. Wernick, J. Drew, M. Mohammed	4	5	4	47
The Toronto Hosp-Toronto Gen Div, Multiorgan Transplants, 200 Elizabeth St 10EN-224, Toronto, ON M5G 2C4 Ph: (416) 340-4010 Fax: (416) 340-3478 1,2) S. Keshavjee, 2) T. Waddell, 3) C. Chan, M. Hutcheon, G. Downey, J. Granton, C. Chaparro, 4) J. Wade, 5) M.C. Ghattas, C. Whythead, M. Siefert-Hansen	32	39	50	396
COLOMBIA				
Clinica Cardiovascular Santa Maria, Universidad De Antioquia, Hospital San Vincente De Paul, Medellin Ph: (574) 442 2200 Fax: (574) 441 7869 Email: cardiovascular@congregacionmariana.org.co 1,2) A. Villegas, 2) Jaramillo, Montoya, Zapata, Duran, Gonzalez, Saldarriaga, 3) A. Porras, E. Escorcia, C. Tenorio, D. Fernandez, J. Ortega, 4) L.F. Garcia, 5) D. Fernandez	3	2	0	6
CZECH REPUBLIC				
Univ Hosp Motol & 2nd Med Faculty, Transp Ctr, Charles Univ Prague, V Uvalu 84, Prague 5, 15006 Ph: (420)2 5722 1056 Fax: (420)2 5722 1056 Email: jaroslav.spatenka@lfmotol.cuni.cz 1,2) J. Spatenka, 2) P. Pafko, J. Schutzner, 3) M. Marel, 4) Inst of Exp Med Prague-Krc, 5) I. Cesalova, A. Habrmanova, R. Lischke, J. Simonek	8	14	7	30
FINLAND				
Helsinki Univ Ctrl Hosp, Dept of Thor/Cardio/Vasc Surg, Haartmanikatu 4, Helsinki, SF-00290 Ph: (358)9 471 2290 Fax: (358)9 471 4006 1,2) S. Mattila, 2) Staff Members of Cardio/Thor/Vasc Surgery, 3) M. Nieminen, 4) Finnish Red Cross Lab, 5) M. Lindstrom, M.L. Hellstedt	1			40
FRANCE				
Laennec Hosp, Dept of CTVC, BP 1005, Nantes Cedex, 44035 Ph: (33)40 165084 Fax: (33)40 165133 1,2) J.L. Michaud, 2) P. Despins, D. Duveau, 3) A. Haloun, M. Treilhaud, 4) Bignon, 5) N. LeSant	5	2		33

648

1)=Director, 2)=Tx Surgeons, 3)=Physicians, 4)=Tissue Typers, 5)=TxCoords	1998	1999	2000	Total
Groupe Hosp Pitie Salpetriere, Dept of Cardio/Vasc Surg, 83 Blvd de l'Hopital, Paris, 75013 Ph: (33)1 4217 7001 Fax: (33)1 4217 7656 Email: monique.tallier@psl.ap-hop.paris.fr 1,2) I. Gandjbakhch, 2) A. Pavie, V. Bors, 3) R. Dorent, P. Leger, E. Vaissier, J.P. Levasseur, 4) C. Raffoux, 5) F. Maillet, M. Tallier	2	2	0	44

GERMANY

	1998	1999	2000	Total
Heart Ctr Northrhine Westfalia, Ruhr-Univ of Bochum, Dept of Thor/Cardio/Vasc Surg, Georgstrasse 11, Bad Oeynhausen, 32545 Ph: (49)5731 97 1331 Fax: (49)5731 97 1820 1,2) R. Koerfer, 2) K. Minami, B. Hansky, 3) G. Tenderich, 4) W. Prohaska, C. Wolf, 5) S. Wlost, B. Heistermann-Linstaedt	3	2	2	7
German Heart Inst, Dept of Thor/Cardio/Vasc Surg, Augustenburger Platz 1, Berlin, D-13353 Ph: (49)30 4593 2000 Fax: (49)30 4593 2100 1,2) R. Hetzer, 2) Y. Weng, et al. , 3) M. Hummel, P.E. Lange, R. Ewert, 4) Salama, 5) H. Kriegler	15	19	19	139
Essen Univ Med Sch, Dept of Thor/Cardio/Vasc Surg, Hufelandstr 55, D-45122 Essen Ph: (49)201 723-3454 Fax: (49)201 723-5931 1) H.G. Jakob, 2) J. Piotrowski, 3) R. Erbel, St. Sack, 4) H. Grosse-Wilde, 5) H.J. Pietsch	12	8	9	114
Fulda Med Ctr, Dept of Thor/Cardio/Vasc Surg, Pacelliallee 4, Fulda, D-36043 Ph: (49)661 84-5652 Fax: (49)661 84-5653 1,2) T. Stegmann, 2) H.U. Gunther, L. Konig, W. Schlumann, B. Rosada, 3) T. Bonzel, G. Strupp, 4) H. Krupe, 5) R. Wernes	0	1	0	7
Univ Klin des Saarlandes, Dept of Thoracic Surg, Oscar-Orth—Strabe, Hamburg/Saar, D-66421 Ph: (49)6841 163520 Fax: (49)6841 163516 1,3) H.J. Schafers, 2) O. Wendler, T. Graeter, 3) G. Sybrecht, H. Wilkens, 4) B. Thiele, Kasierslautern, 5) C. Friedrichsohn	14	10	10	47
Hannover Med Sch, Dept of Surg, Div of Thor/Cardio/Vasc Surg, Carl-Neuberg-Str.1, 30625 Hannover Ph: (49)511 532-6581 Fax: (49)511 532-5404 1,2) A. Haverich, 2) W. Harringe, M. Strueber, 3) J. Niedermeyer, 4) Robin-Winn, Pastucha, 5) G. Gubernatis	40	50	49	344
Clin Grosshadern, Univ of Munich, Dept of Surg, Marchioninistr 15, Munich, 81377 Ph: (49)89 7095 3511 Fax: (49)89 7095 3508 1) F.W. Schildberg, 2) H. Fuerst, C. Muller, 3) C. Vogelmeier, 4) E. Albert, 5) C. Schultz	15	14	23	133
Clin Grosshadern, Dept of Cardiac Surg, Marchionini Str 15, 81377 Munich Ph: (49)89 7095 3450 Fax: (49)89 7095 3465 Email: hcr@hch.med.uni-muenchen.de 1) B. Reichart, 2) Reichenspurner, Fuerst, 3) C. Vogelmeier, B. Meiser, 4) E.D. Albert, 5) Transp Grosshadern	19	14	23	201
Univ Hosp Munster, Dept of Thor/Cardio/Vasc Surg, Munster, 48129 Ph: (49)251 83-47401 Fax: (49)251 83-48316 1) H.H. Scheld, 2) D. Hammel, M. Weyand, 3) M.C. Deng, 4) H. Gross-Wilde, S. Browski, 5) Kley	0	1		2

ITALY

	1998	1999	2000	Total
San Matteo Hosp/Univ of Pavia, Div Di Cardiac Surg, Piazzale Golgi 2, Pavia, 27100 Ph: (39)0382 503515 Fax: (39)0382 503059 Email: darmini@smatteo.pv.it 1,2) M. Vigano, 2) M. Rinaldi, A.M. D'Armini, C. Goggi, 4) G. Sirchia	20	34	13	148
Policlinico "Umberto I", Univ "La Sapienza", Dept of Surg II, Viale del Policlinico, 00161 Rome Ph: (39)6 445 6296 Fax: (39)6 446 3667 1,2) R. Cortesini, 1,2) C.Ricci, G.F.Coloni, 2) E. Rendina, F. Venuta, T. DeGiacomo, 3) D. Vizza, S. Quattrucci, 4) E. Renna-Molajoni, A. Bachetoni, 5) M. Caricato, S. Venettoni	16	22	13	87

NETHERLANDS

	1998	1999	2000	Total
Academic Hosp Groningen, Thorax Ctr, Oostersingel 59, Groningen Ph: (31)50 3614932 Fax: (31)50 3613151 Email: m.e.erasmus@thorax.azg.nl 1,2) M.E. Erasmus, 3) Von Bij, 5) Stel, Nieboer	17	19	17	160

1)=Director, 2)=Tx Surgeons, 3)=Physicians, 4)=Tissue Typers, 5)=TxCoords	1998	1999	2000	Total
NEW ZEALAND				
Green Lane Hosp, Cardio/Thor Surg Unit, Green Lane West, Auckland 3 Ph: (64)9 638-9909 Fax: (64)9 631-0768 1,2) D.A. Haydock, 2) A. Kerr, K.J. Graham, F.P. Milson, 3) H.A. Coverdale, T.M. Agnew, J. Garrett, K. Whyte, P. Ruygrok, 4) K. Figgins, M. Roberts, Auck Reg Bld Ctr, 5) H. Gibbs, D. Reddy	5	7	12	43
NORWAY				
Rikshosp Nat'l Hosp, Dept Thoracic & Cardiovasc, Sognvannsveien 20, Oslo, 0027 Ph: (47)23 073735 Fax: (47)23 073741 Email: odd.geiran@rikshospitalet.no 1) O. Geiran, 2) H. Lindberg, E. Seem, S. Almdahl, S. Birkeland, 3) O. Bjortuft, A. Nalsund, 4) E. Thorsby, T. Leivestad, 5) P.A. Bakkan, S. Foss, P.E. Vatsaas, K. Meyer	9	11	13	107
SWEDEN				
Sahlgrenska Hosp, Dept of Cardio/Thor Surg, Transp Unit, Gothenburg, S 41345 Ph: (46)31 601000 Fax: (46)31-417991 1) S.E. Svensson, 2) F. Nilsson, 3) G. Martensson, 4) L. Sandberg, L. Rydberg, 5) U. Lorentzon, U. Nystrom	23	15	14	140
Univ Hosp of Lund, Dept of Cardio/Thor Surg, Lund, S-221 85 Ph: (46)46 171685 Fax: (46)46 158635 1,2) B. Koul, 2) C. Luhrs, P. Johnsson, M. Dobre, 3) L. Eriksson, B. Kornhall, 4) U. Johnsson, 5) A.K. Morin, K. Wallentin, A. Klitthammar, M. Zepeda, K. Henriksson	10	11	11	82
SWITZERLAND				
Univ Hosp Geneva, Dept of Pneumology, 24 Rue Micheli du Crest, 1211 Geneva 14, Geneva Ph: (41)22 3729901 Fax: (41)22 3729929 1,3) L.P. Nicod, 2) A. Spiliopoulos, 3) T. Rochat, 4) M. Jeannet, C. Goumaz, 5) F. Roch	11	10	4	59
Univ Hosp Zurich, Dept of Surg, Ramistr 100, Zurich, CH-8091 Ph: (41)1 255 8801 Fax: (41)1 255 8805 1,2) W. Weder, 3) A. Bochler, 4) M. Weber, 5) P. Seeburger	16	16	15	103
UNITED KINGDOM				
Papworth Hosp, Transp Unit, Papworth Everard, Cambridge, CB3 8RE Ph: (44)480 830541 Fax: (44)480 364610 1,2) J. Wallwork, 2) F.C. Wells, S.R. Large, S.A.M. Nashef, J. Dunning, A. Ritchie, S. Tsui, 3) J. Parameshwar, K. McNeil, 4) C. Taylor, 5) Baines, Smith, Ryan, Woods, Castle, Lockhurst, Wiggins	14	27	20	197
St George's Hosp, Cardiac Dept of Med, Blackshaw Rd, Tooting, London, SW17 0QT Ph: (44)181 725-3565 Fax: (44)181 725-2049 1,2) A.J. Murday, 2) J. Gaer, R. Sayer, 3) B.P. Madden, 4) D. Sage, 5) L. Backhouse, L. Reynolds, J. Barros	10	10	2	51
Wythenshawe Hosp, Dept of Cardio/Thor Surg, Southmoor Rd, Manchester, M23 9LT Ph: (44)161 998 7070 Fax: (44)161 291 2091 1) A.K. Deiraniya, 2) C.S. Campbell, N. Yonan, T. Hooper, M.T. Jones, 3) N. Brooks, R. Levy, K. Carroll, C.T. Leonard, 4) P. Dyer, S. Sheldon, 5) H. Pyatt, J. Nuttall, J. Stewart	13	15	12	134
Harefield Hosp, Dept of Cardio/Thor Surg, Harefield, Middlesex, UB9 6JH Ph: (44)1 895 823737 Fax: (44)1 895 824983 1) M. Yacoub, 2) A. Khaghani, J. Pepper, 3) A. Mitchell, N. Banner, R. Radley-Smith, M. Hodson, 4) M. Rose, 5) P. Baldock, H. Blair, T. Jackson	17	16		361

LUNG

LUNG Transplants

	1998	1999	2000	Total
United States	795	855	926	7,673
Foreign	462	500	482	4,403
Total	1,257	1,355	1,408	12,076

LUNG Transplant Centers

United States	72
Foreign	47
Total	119

WORLDWIDE TRANSPLANT CENTER DIRECTORY
LIVER TRANSPLANTS

1)=Director, 2)=Tx Surgeons, 3)=Physicians, 4)=Tissue Typers, 5)=TxCoords	1998	1999	2000	Total

UNITED STATES

ALABAMA

| Univ of Alabama-Birmingham, Dept of Surg-LHR748, 701 S 19th St, Birmingham, AL 35294
Ph: (205) 934-7714 Fax: (205) 934-8378
1,2) J.S. Bynon Jr, 2) M. Sellers, D. Eckhoff, 3) J. Bloomer, G. Abrams, M. Fallon, B. McGuire,
D. VanLeeuwen, 4) J. Thomas, 5) C. Ingram, P. Wilson, C. Jones, B. Maharrey, B. Campbell | 110 | 93 | 98 | 764 |

ARIZONA

| Mayo Clinic Hosp, Div of Trnaspl Med, 5777 East Mayo Blvd, Phoenix, AZ 85054
Ph: (480) 342-0514 Fax: (480) 342-2324 Email: rakela.jorge@mayo.edu
1,3) J. Rakela, 1,2) D.C. Mulligan, 2) A.A. Moss, 3) M.E. Harrison III, V. Balan, D.D. Douglas,
4) Donor Network of AZ, 5) K.L. Hansen, L. Nelson, J. Ortiz | | 24 | 26 | 50 |
| Univ of Arizona Med Ctr, Dept of Transp Serv, 1501 N Campbell Ave, P.O. Box 245145, Tucson,
AZ 85724 Ph: (520) 694-4984 Fax: (520) 694-4983
1,2) P.Z. Nakazato, 3) T. Boyer, U. Blecker, 4) C. Spier, 5) L. Maselli, N. Stubbs | 25 | 13 | 21 | 160 |

CALIFORNIA

Scripps Green Hosp, Ctr for Organ & Cell Transp, 10666 N Torrey Pines Rd, 200-N, La Jolla, CA 92037 Ph: (858) 554-4310 Fax: (619) 554-4311 1,2) A. Hassoun, 2) M. Brunson, 3) J.G. McHutchison, P. Pockros, L. Nyberg, 4) UCSD HLA Lab, 5) L.A. Biermann, J. Henry, K. Bounds, K. Thorson	18	23	26	247
Loma Linda Univ Med Ctr, Transp Inst, 11234 Anderson St, Ste 1405, Loma Linda, CA 92354 Ph: (909) 558-4252 Fax: (909) 558-0112 1,2) W. Concepcion, 2) O. Ojogho, P. Baron, 3) B. Runyon, D. Hillebrand, M. Walter, J. McCracken, 4) S. Nehlsen-Cannarella, L. Buckert, 5) J. Joseph, B. Elhazin	22	13	27	138
Cedars-Sinai Med Ctr, Ctr for Liver & Kidney Transp, 8635 W 3rd St, Ste 590W, Los Angeles, CA 90048 Ph: (310) 423-2641 Fax: (310) 423-0234 1,2) C. Shackleton, 2) S. Colquhoun, W. Arnaout, 3) J. Vierling, T. Fong, P. Martin, A.A. Demetriou, F. Watanabe, 4) S. Jordan, D. Tyan, 5) Grubic, Clarke-Platt, Jung, Schienger	48	46	39	629
Univ of Calif-Los Angeles, Dumont-UCLA Transp Ctr, Dept of Surg, Rm 77-132 CHS, 10833 LeConte Ave, Los Angeles, CA 90024 Ph: (310) 825-8138 Fax: (310) 206-7760 1,2) R.W. Busuttil, 2) A. Shaked, C. Schackleton, O. Jurim, D. Imagawa, 3) L. Goldstein, M. Ament, S. McDiarmid, P. Martin, J. Vargas, 4) UCLA Immunogenetics Center, 5) B. Nuesse, K. Butenschoen, Maxfield, Prior, Duncan, Tooley, Ponthieux	214	204	202*	2985
Univ Southern Calif Hosp, Dept of Transp, 1500 San Pablo, Los Angeles, CA 90033 Ph: (213) 484-5551 Fax: (213) 484-2947 1,2) R. Mendez, 2) R.G. Mendez, T. Bogaard, Khetan, Asai, Hamid, Shidban, McEvoy, 3) S. Massry, M. El Shawry, 4) Y. Iwaki, J. Cicciarelli, 5) M. Correa	13	20	33*	82
UCI Medical Center, Division Of Transplantation, 101 The City Drive, Bldg.26, Room 1001, Orange, CA 92868 Ph: (714) 456-8441 Fax: (714) 456-8796 1,2) D.K. Imagawa, 2) R.W. Busuttil, J. Ortiz, S. Colquhoun, C. Smith, R. Ghobrial, D. Farmer, 3) N.G.B. Murray, 4) Metic Lab, 5) J.B. Mize, D. Huddleston, L. Gibson, G. Ginther	21	18	15	126
Stanford Univ Med Ctr, Dept of Surg, Division of Liver Transplantation, 750 Welch Rd St 319, Palo Alto, CA 94304-1510 Ph: (650) 498-5689 Fax: (650) 498-5690 1,2) C.O. Esquivel, 2) S.K. So, K. Drazan, M. Millan, 3) E. Keeffe, J. Imperial, G. Garcia, K. Cox, W. Berquist, R. Castillo, 4) C. Grumet, 5) Fizgerald, Salvestrin, Strichartz, Kreisl, Puno, Miller, Heuer	77	66	45*	414
Univ Calif-Davis Med Ctr, Transplant Program, Housestaff facility Room 1018, 2315 Stockton Blvd, Sacramento, CA 95817 Ph: (916) 734-2111 Fax: (916) 734-0432 1,2) J.P. McVicar, 3) M. Zern, C. Bocolus, 4) P. Holland, 5) M. Friend, D. Higgs, M. Sturges, D. Lehe	25	15	18*	105

LIVER

* Preliminary UNOS data

1)=Director, 2)=Tx Surgeons, 3)=Physicians, 4)=Tissue Typers, 5)=TxCoords	1998	1999	2000	Total
Univ Calif-San Diego Med Ctr, Liver Transp Prog, 200 W Arbor Dr, San Diego, CA 92103-8698 Ph: (619) 543-2451 Fax: (619) 543-3353 1,2) M. Hart, 2) E. Wahlstrom, 3) T. Hassanein, 4) M. Garovoy, 5) S. Heisterkamp	24	36	20*	148
Calif Pacific Med Ctr, Dept of Transplant, PO Box 7999, 2340 Clay St-4th Flr, San Francisco, CA 94115 Ph: (415) 923-3450 Fax: (415) 561-1709 Email: millerjl@sutterhealth.org 1,2) R. Gish, 2) J. Roberts, R. Osorio, 3) S. Steady, E. Wakil, 4) S. Inokuchi, 5) K. Devaney, K. Tevis, V. Karp, D. McClone, F. Levy	46	58	88*	948
Univ of Calif-San Francisco, Dept of Surg, PO Box 0780-UCSF, 505 Parnassus Ave, San Francisco, CA 94143-0780 Ph: (415) 353-1888 Fax: (415) 353-8709 1,2) J. Roberts, 2) P. Stock, C. Freise, N. Ascher, R. Hirose, S. Feng, 3) P. Rosenthal, N. Bass, N. Terrault, T. Davern, V. Wu, M. Bissell, 4) L.A. Baxterlowe, 5) Galbraith, Moore, Mudge, Dragovich, Senna, Stritzel, Harris, McKeel	87	89	90*	1213

COLORADO

	1998	1999	2000	Total
Porter Adventist Hosp, Transp Serv, 2535 S Downing St, #380, Denver, CO 80210 Ph: (303) 778-5797 Fax: (303) 778-5205 1) W.B. Vernon, 2) W. Kortz, E. Kortz, 3) C. Kuruvila, M. Dillingham, M. Yanover, D. Gillum, J. Scott, B. Bilir, 4) Laboratories at Bonfils, 5) D. Long, M. Luedtke, G. Lewis, K. Bramley, T. Sandoval	4	6	3	21
The Children's Hosp-Denver, Dept of Transp Surg, 1056 E 19th Ave, Box B-323, Denver, CO 80218 Ph: (303) 861-6571 Fax: (303) 764-8077 1,2) F. Karrer, 2) I. Kam, M. Wachs, T. Bak, 3) R. Sokol, M. Narkewicz, 4) Immun Assoc of Denver, 5) K. Orban-Eller, D. Dovel, M. Christopher	6	3	9	78
Univ of Colorado Hosp, Dept of Transp Surg, 4200 E 9th Ave, Box C-318, Denver, CO 80262 Ph: (303) 373-8750 Fax: (303) 372-8737 1,2) I. Kam, 2) F. Karrer, M. Wachs, T. Bak, 3) G. Everson, T. Trouillot, J. Trotter, M. Kugelmas, 4) Clinical Immunology & Histo Lab (CIHL), 5) T. Steinberg, M. McClure, T. Brackett	68	73	75	821

CONNECTICUT

	1998	1999	2000	Total
Hartford Hosp, Transp Serv, P.O.Box 5037, Hartford, CT 06102-5037 Ph: (860) 545-4132 Fax: (860) 545-4208 1,2) D. Hull, 2) S. Bartus, M. Brown, 3) R. Rosson, J. Hyams, J. Israel, J. Polio, 4) L. Bow, T. Alberghini, 5) D. Palmeri	11	21	29	151
Yale New Haven Hospital, Dept of Surgery, Div of Organ, PO Box 208062, 333 Cedar St, FMB112, New Haven, CT 06520-8062 Ph: (203) 785-2565 Fax: (203) 785-7162 Email: kathy.lorber@yale.edu 1,2,4) M.I. Lorber, 1,2) A.L.Friedman, 2) G.P. Basadonna, 3) S. Moyer, J. Boyer, 4) L.A. Geiselhart, 5) M. Corrigan, J. Albert, N. Sowers, J. Bates	17	12	2	136

DISTRICT OF COLUMBIA

	1998	1999	2000	Total
Georgetown Univ Med Ctr, Dept of Surg, 4 PHC, 3800 Reservoir Rd NW, Washington, DC 20007 Ph: (202) 784-3700 Fax: (202) 687-3004 1,2) L.B. Johnson, 2) P.C. Kuo, A. Lu, 3) V. Rustgi, 4) S. Rosen-Bronson, 5) A. Cribbs, C. Story, W. Sachau, N. Lawson	14	30	37	81

FLORIDA

	1998	1999	2000	Total
Shands at the Univ of Florida, Transplant Center, Box 100251, 1600 SW Archer Road, Gainesville, FL 32610-0251 Ph: (352) 265-0130 Fax: (352) 265-0108 1,2) A. Reed, 1,3) G.L. Davis, 2) R.J. Howard, M.R. Langham, W.J. Van der Werf, A. Hemming, 3) D. Nelson, C. Soldevila-Pico, M. Abdelmalek, R. Gonzalaz, 4) J. Scornik, 5) McDowell, Myers, Venoy, McGinnis, Mackay, Schoonmaker, Kasper	86	105	116	711
Mayo Clinic Jacksonville/St. Luke's, Liver Diseases and Transpl, 4203 Belfort Rd, Suite 204, Jacksonville, FL 32216 Ph: (904) 953-2000 Fax: (904) 296-5874 1,2) J.L. Steers, 2) J. Nguyen, C. Hughes, V. Gopalan, 3) J.R. Spivey, R.C. Dickson, D.M. Harnois, 4) P. Genco, 5) A. DuBois, L. Mitcham, P. McHale, K. Norman, J. Goodrich, B. Handline	54	97	141	292

1)=Director, 2)=Tx Surgeons, 3)=Physicians, 4)=Tissue Typers, 5)=TxCoords	1998	1999	2000	Total
Univ of Miami-Jackson Mem Med Ctr, Dept of Surg-Div of Transp, PO Box 015809(M840), 1801 NW 9th Ave, Suite #511, Miami, FL 33101 Ph: (305) 355-5000 Fax: (305) 355-5161 1,2) A. Tzakis, 2) J. Nery, T. Kato, S. Nishida, J. Madariaga, D. Levi, 3) J. Thompson, G. Neff, N. Mittal, 4) V. Esquenazi, 5) V. Cardenas, L. Kravetz, R. Lavendera, S. Archie, O. Hung, J. Benedict	183	173	177	1352
Tampa General Hosp, Div of Transp Lifelink Tx Inst, 2111 Swann Ave, Tampa, FL 33606 Ph: (813) 251-8017 Fax: (813) 251-0096 1,2) A.E. Alsina, 2) V.D. Bowers, P.L. Tso, 3) K.B. Camacho, D. Pencev, E. Martinez, 4) W. Lefor, 5) D. Wahler, S. Shultz	40	51	52*	179
GEORGIA				
Egleston Children's Hosp at Emory U, Dept of Surg, 1405 Clifton Rd NE, Atlanta, GA 30322 Ph: (404) 315-3886 Fax: (404) 315-2831 Email: thomas_heffron@emory.org 1,2) T.G. Heffron, 3) R. Romero, 4) R. Bray, 5) C. Oneill, J. DePaolo, T. Pillen, S. Henry	25	17	28*	118
Emory Univ, Dept of Surg, 1639 Pierce Dr, Rm 5105 WMB, Atlanta, GA 30322 Ph: (404) 727-3599 Fax: (404) 727-8410 Email: thomas_heffron@emory.org 1,2) T.G. Heffron, 2) A.C. Stieber, M. DeVera, 3) E. Martinez, P. Ricci, 4) R. Bray, 5) R. Adams, R. Chapman	91	68	58*	879
HAWAII				
St Francis Med Ctr, Transplant Inst, 2230 Liliha St, Honolulu, HI 96817 Ph: (808) 547-6228 Fax: (808) 547-6750 1) L.L. Wong, 2) W. Limm, F.L. Fan, A. Cheung, H. Noguchi, 3) N. Tsai, H. Lim, N. Shimeda, S. Buto, 4) Y.K. Paik, 5) D. Pacheco	9	9	11	46
ILLINOIS				
Children's Memorial Hospital, Siragusa Transplant Center, 2300 Children's Plaza, Box 57, Chicago, IL 60614 Ph: (773) 975-8818 Fax: (773) 880-3007 Email: siragusatx@childrensmemorial.org 1) P. Whitington, 2) R. Superina, 3) E. Alonso, 5) J. Lokar, J. Chesterton, B. Stahulak	23	26	27	91
Northwestern Mem Hosp, Div of Organ Transp, 675 North St. Clair Street, Galter 17-200, Chicago, IL 60611 Ph: (312) 695-8900 Fax: (312) 695-9194 1,2) M. Abecassis, 2) F. Stuart, D. Kaufman, J. Fryer, J. Leventhal, 3) A. Blei, S. Flamm, P. Lynch, 4) M. Buckingham, 5) L. Clark, N. Kay, H. Monroe	21	30	44*	175
Rush-Presbyterian-St Luke's Med Ctr, Organ/Tissue Transp Serv, 1653 W Congress Pkwy, 201 Jones, Chicago, IL 60612 Ph: (312) 942-6242 Fax: (312) 563-1529 1,2) J.W. Williams, 2) H. Sankary, P. Foster, L. McChesney, 3) D.M. Jensen, D.J. Rosenblatt, D. Ganger, S. Kaur, S. Cotler, 4) H. Gebel, M. Prod, 5) C. Grant, M. Crissman, J. Strobeck	47	51	27*	743
Univ of Chicago Med Ctr, Dept of Transp Surg, 5841 S Maryland, m/c 5027, Chicago, IL 60637 Ph: (773) 702-6319 Fax: (773) 702-7511 1,2) J.M. Millis, 2) Thistlethwaite, Cronin, Williams, 3) Brady, Faust, Te, Cohen, 4) D. Peace, 5) Dasgupta, Boone, Kelly, Zinnerman, Shortridge, Davis, Solcani	83	74	62	1415
Univ of Illinois at Chicago, Dept of Surg, Div of Transpl, 840 S. Wood Street, Suite 515 CSN, Chicago, IL 60612 Ph: (312) 413-1135 Fax: (312) 996-1320 1,2) R. Pollak, 2) E. Benedetti, 3) T.J. Layden, 4) V.A. Lazda, 5) P. Gaddis	20	29	30	180
INDIANA				
Indiana Univ Med Ctr/Methodist, Dept of Surg/Organ Transp, 550 N University Blvd, Rm UH4258, Indianapolis, IN 46202 Ph: (317) 274-4370 Fax: (317) 274-3084 1,2) R.S. Filo, 2) M.D. Pescovitz, D. Rouch, 3) L. Lumeng, J. Fitzgerald, P. Kwo, N. Chalasani, J. Patel, 4) Z. Brahmi, 5) N. Boyle, M. Schenk, S. Herring, P, Murdock, B. Schwanbeck	35	49	46*	469
IOWA				
Univ of Iowa Hosp & Clin, Dept of Surg, Univ Hosp, Iowa City, IA 52242 Ph: (319) 356-1334 Fax: (319) 356-1556 1,2) Y. Wu, 2) S. Rayhill, A. Bozorgzdeh, D. Katz, 3) LaBrecque, Johlin, Bishop, Voigt, Schmidt, Pashinkar, 4) N.E. Goeken, E. Fields, 5) B.A. Schanbacher, M. Vorhies, S. Abel	41	44	49	363

1)=Director, 2)=Tx Surgeons, 3)=Physicians, 4)=Tissue Typers, 5)=TxCoords	1998	1999	2000	Total
KANSAS				
The Univ of Kansas Med Ctr, Dept of Surg, 3901 Rainbow Blvd, Rm 4950 Murphy Bldg, Kansas City, KS 66160-7309 Ph: (913) 588-6183 Fax: (913) 588-7620 Email: jforster@kumc.edu 1,2) J. Forster, 2) R. Delcore, D. Murillo, 3) S.R.G. Vasa, 4) C.F. Bryan, Midwest Transplant Network, 5) C. Garman, C. Sherman, J. Hoffman	39	39	42	307
KENTUCKY				
Univ of Kentucky Med Ctr, Dept of Surg/Section of Transp, 800 Rose St, Lexington, KY 40536 Ph: (859) 323-4661 Fax: (859) 257-3644 1,2) D. Ranjan, 2) T. Johnston, S. Reddy, 3) D. Hill, 4) T. Eichorn, J. Byrne, J.S. Thompson, D. Jennings, F. Lower, 5) S. Salyer, T. Miller, M. Blevins	26	19	23	118
Jewish Hosp, Transp Serv, 217 East Chestnut St, Louisville, KY 40202 Ph: (502) 587-4939 Fax: (502) 587-4184 1,2) F.R. Bentley, 2) D. Granger, F. Bentley, H. Randall, 3) T. Martin, L. Marsano, C. McClain, 4) P. Landrum, M. McRae, J. Ogle, R. Pound, J. Cassim, 5) P. Kaiser, L. Adcock-Oliver, C. Schuhmann, N. Bellis	27	33	26	239
LOUISIANA				
Memorial Medical Center (LSUNO), Transp Inst of New Orleans, 3535 Bienville, Ste 225 East, New Orleans, LA 70119 Ph: (504) 488-8121 Fax: (504) 488-9672 1,2) J.P. Boudreaux, 2) D.J. Frey, J. Jerius, 3) L. Balart, 4) P. Kumar, 5) D. Seymour, A. Garcia	11	18	15	56
Ochsner Foundation Hosp, Multi-Organ Transp Program, 1514 Jefferson Hwy, BH309, New Orleans, LA 70121 Ph: (504) 842-3925 Fax: (504) 842-5746 1,2) J. Eason, 2) G. Loss, 3) S. Nair, A. Mason, R. Perrillo, 4) E.S. Cooper, G. Stewart, S. Herbert, 5) J. Blazek, D. Dick, B. Stevenson, J. Lipscomb, A. Raspino, D. Kelly	23	49	52	398
Tulane Univ Hosp & Clin, Dept of Surg, SL 22, 1415 Tulane Ave, New Orleans, LA 70112 Ph: (504) 588-5344 Fax: (504) 584-3563 1,2) D. Slakey, 2) S. Cheng, 3) A. Noel, F. Regerstein, P. Goglio, 4) K.A. Sullivan, 5) B. Beck, V. Atkinson, E. Valentino	22	26	20*	89
LSU-Willis Knighton Med Ctr, Dept of Surg, 1501 Kings Hwy, PO Box 33930, Shreveport, LA 71130 Ph: (318) 675-6115 Fax: (318) 675-4243 1,2) J.C. McDonald, 1) H. Gebel, 2) R. McMillan, G. Zibari, D. Altman, 3) C. Paulson, D. Dies, J. Work, A. Poch, Lynn, 4) T. Roggero, D. Michell, K. Horton, W. Blackburn, R. Jones, 5) N. Noles, E. Kilpatrick	11	13	16*	162
MARYLAND				
Johns Hopkins Hosp, Dept of Surg, Harvey 614, 600 N Wolfe St, Baltimore, MD 21287 Ph: (410) 955-5045 Fax: (410) 614-1643 1,2) A.S. Klein, 2) J. Burdick, P. Colombani, H. Lau, J. Markowitz, R. Montgomery, L. Ratner, 3) A.M. Diehl, E. Mezey, P. Thuluvath, R. Rai, F. Poordad, 4) A. Zachary, S. LeFell, 5) D. Burrel-Diggs, J. Darmody, B. Barshick, R. Webb	65	53	47	629
Univ of Maryland Med Ctr, Organ Transp Serv, Dept of Surg, 29 S Greene St-Suite 200, Baltimore, MD 21201 Ph: (410) 328-5408 Fax: (410) 328-3837 1,2) S. Bartlett, 2) Colonna, B. Philisophe, B. Jarrell, 3) C. Howell, J. Lauren, F. Anania, 4) American Red Cross Natl Histo Lab At Univ of Maryland Med Sys, 5) L. Ridge, C. Driscoll	15	23	32	142
MASSACHUSETTS				
Beth Israel Deaconess Med Ctr, Div of Liver Transp/Hepat Surg, 110 Francis St, Ste 8C, Boston, MA 02215 Ph: (617) 632-9779 Fax: (617) 632-7555 1,2) W.D. Lewis, 2) R.L. Jenkins, 3) F.D. Gordon, 4) L. Uhl, E. Pomfret, 5) P. Conway, D. Morin	36	17	0	570
Children's Hosp, Boston, Dept of Surg, Fegan, 300 Longwood Ave, Boston, MA 02115 Ph: (617) 355-8268 Fax: (617) 730-0310 1,2) C. Lillehei, 2) D. Lund, 3) A. Leichtner, E. O'Rourke, M. Jonas, 4) New England Organ Bank, 5) S. Treacy	5	1	2*	108
Massachusetts Gen Hosp, Dept of Surg, 32 Fruit St, Boston, MA 02114 Ph: (617) 726-8256 Fax: (617) 726-8137 1) A.B. Cosimi, 2) F.L. Delmonico, W. Goggins, D.S.C. Ko, T. Kawai, J. Vacanti, 3) J. Dienstag, R. Kleinman, R. Chung, M. Thiem, 4) S. Saidman, 5) S. Noska	32	26	43	392

1)=Director, 2)=Tx Surgeons, 3)=Physicians, 4)=Tissue Typers, 5)=TxCoords	1998	1999	2000	Total
New England Med Ctr, Div of Transp Surg, Box 40, 750 Washington St, Boston, MA 02111 Ph: (617) 636-5592 Fax: (617) 636-8228 1,2) R.J. Rohrer, 2) R.B. Freeman, M. Angelis, 3) D.S. Pratt, 4) A. Rabson, 5) S.E. Fitzmaurice	35	36	44*	492
Lahey Clinic Med Ctr, Div of Liver Transp/Hepat Surg, 41 mall Rd, 4 West, Burlington, MA 01773 Ph: (781) 744-2500 Fax: (781) 744-5743 1,2) W.D. Lewis, 2) R.L. Jenkins, E. Pomfret, J. Pomposelli, 3) F.D. Gordon, 4) K. Heim, 5) P. Conway, D. Morin		23	60	83

MICHIGAN

Univ of Michigan Med Ctr, Dept Surg, 2926 Taubman Ctr,Box 0331, 1500 E Med Ctr Dr, Ann Arbor, MI 48109-0331 Ph: (734) 936-5816 Fax: (734) 763-3187 Email: janco@umich.edu 1,2) J.D. Punch, 2) D.A. Campbell Jr, J.C. Magee, S.M. Rudich, R.M.Merion, J. Arenas, 3) C. Hillemeier, R. Fontana, A. Olson, A. Lok, G. Su, K. Lown, R. Holmes, 4) J. Baker, 5) M. Ingalls, D. Westphal	68	66	60	954
Henry Ford Hosp, Dept of Surg, 2799 W Grand Blvd, Detroit, MI 48202 Ph: (313) 916-2911 Fax: (313) 916-9147 1,2) M. Aboujoud, 2) V. Douzdjian, 3) K. Brown, D. Moonka, L. Shick, 4) D. Kukuruga, 5) N. Hocking, A. Helms, M. Uniewski, L. Philpot	47	30	46*	269

MINNESOTA

Fairview Univ Med Ctr, The Transplant Center, Box 482, 516 Delaware St SE, Minneapolis, MN 55455 Ph: (612) 625-5115 Fax: (612) 625-2190 1,2) W.D. Payne, 1,3) J. Lake, 2) R. Gruessner, A. Humar, R. Kandaswamy, 3) H. Sharp, S. Weisdorf, J. Schwarzenberg, J. Rank, 4) H. Noreen, D. McKinley, N. Henrickson, 5) M. Knaak, K. Strasburg, L. Shriver	16	44	58	558
Rochester Methodist Hosp, Liver Transp Program, Mayo Clinic, 201 W Center SW, Rochester, MN 55905 Ph: (507) 266-7890 Fax: (507) 266-2810 1,2) C.B. Rosen, 2) M.B. Ishitani, R.A.F. Krom, S.L. Nyberg, 3) Hay, Wiesner, Gores, Hay, Poterucha, Charlton, Zein, Brandhagen, Kim, 4) S.B. Moore, S. DeGoey, 5) Pearson, Gaustad, S. Wilson, Bakken, Young, Kirchner, Potter, Miller	96	77	99	1109
St Mary's Hosp, Liver Transp Program, 1216 2nd St SW, Rochester, MN 55905 Ph: (507) 284-2511 Fax: (507) 266-2810 1,2) C.B. Rosen, 2) M.B. Ishitani, S.L. Nyberg, R.A.F. Krom, 3) D. Freese, N. Zein, M. El-Youssef, 4) S.B. Moore, S. DeGoey, 5) L. Pearson, J. Greseth, J. Weckwerth	2	6	10	43

MISSOURI

The Children's Mercy Hosp, Dept of Surgery, 2401 Gillham, Kansas City, MO 64108 Ph: (816) 460-1010 Fax: (816) 460-1012 1,2) W. Andrews, 3) J.S. Sommerauer, J. Daniel, 4) Midwest Organ Bank, 5) V. Fioravanti	2	5	6	26
Barnes-Jewish Hosp, Washington Univ Med Ctr, Transp Serv, Lower Level, One Barnes Hosp Plaza, St Louis, MO 63110 Ph: (314) 362-5376 Fax: (314) 362-5470 1,2) J. Lowell, 2) S. Shenoy, 3) J. Crippin, M. Lisker-Melman, R. Satyanarayana, M. Fallah, 4) D. Phelan, 5) D. Sutter, P. Thurston, P. Reichert, R. Bander, S. Brown, S. Kreutzman	62	41	50*	664
Cardinal Glennon Children's Hosp, Dept of Gastro, 1465 S Grand, St Louis, MO 63104 Ph: (314) 577-5647 Fax: (314) 268-2775 1,3) R. Kane, 2) H. Soloman, R. Varma, 3) T. Foy, 4) J. Cochran, 5) K. Avent, G. Friedman	6	4	4	41
St Louis Children's Hosp, Dial/Transp Unit, One Children's Place, St Louis, MO 63110 Ph: (314) 454-6065 Fax: (314) 454-2762 1,3) D.H. Permutter, 1,3) R. Rothbaum, 2) T. Howard, J. Lowell, 3) J. Molleston, 4) T. Mohanakumar, D. Phelan, 5) M. Nadler, L. Bianchi	10	10	8*	94
St Louis Univ Hosp, Abdom Organ Transp, 3635 Vista Ave at Grand, PO Box 15250, St Louis, MO 63110-0250 Ph: (314) 577-8867 Fax: (314) 268-5133 1,2) P.J. Garvin, 2) H. Solomon, C. Varma, 3) B. Bacon, B, Tetri, B. Luxon, A. Befeler, S. Ramrahkiani, A. DiBisceglie, 4) K. Riordan, 5) Hoff, Carter, Kirkpatrick, Aridge, Lindsey, Johns, Maxfield, Nagel	34	41	37	329

656

1)=Director, 2)=Tx Surgeons, 3)=Physicians, 4)=Tissue Typers, 5)=TxCoords	1998	1999	2000	Total
NEBRASKA				
Nebraska Health System, Dept of Surg, Section of Transplantation, 983285 Nebraska Medical Ctr, Omaha, NE 68198-3285 Ph: (402) 559-4076 Fax: (402) 559-3434 1,2) A.N. Langnas, 2) I.J. Fox, D. Sudan, B.W. Shaw Jr, K. Iyer, 3) Sorrell, Donovan, Zetterman, McCashland, Schafer, Horslen, 4) J. Wisecarver, S. Sheperd, 5) Williams, Rogge, Andersen, Weaver, Brown, Calabro, Mahoney, Sevcik	104	86	123*	1628
NEW JERSEY				
Univ Hosp-New Jersey Med Sch, Dept of Surg-Liver Transp Serv, 65 Bergen St, Rm GA-230, Newark, NJ 07103 Ph: (201) 982-7218 Fax: (201) 982-6227 1,2) B. Koneru, 2) A. Fisher, D. Wilson, 3) C.M. Leevy, 4) C. Pancoska, 5) B. Smith, D. Nolan, M. Higgins, P. Livera	57	82	74*	484
NEW YORK				
SUNY HSC At Brooklyn, Dept Of Surg. Div Transplants, 450 Clarkson Ave, Box 40, Brooklyn, NY 11203-2098 Ph: (718)270-1898 Fax: (718)270-3762 1,2) B.G. Sommer, 2) J.H. Hong, N. Sumrani, D.A. Distant, 3) C. El-Younis, 4) A.J. Norin, 5) A. Dibenedetto, V. Maursky, R. Clayton, L. Neve	11	4	0	19
Mt Sinai Med Ctr, Miller Transp Institute, Box 1104, One Gustave Levy Pl, New York, NY 10029 Ph: (212) 241-8035 Fax: (212) 996-9688 1,2) C. Miller, 1) K.Feifer, 2) M. Schwartz, P. Sheiner, S. Emre, T. Fishbein, 3) H. Bodenheiner, A. Min, L. Kim, M. Schilsky, T. Schiano, 4) Rogosin Inst Lab, 5) O'Rourke, Robinson, David, Arnott, Barton, Rosenthal, Carrera	190	183	186	1968
NYU Med Ctr, Dept of Surg, 403 E 34th St 3rd Flr, New York, NY 10016 Ph: (212) 263-8134 Fax: (212) 263-8157 Email: glyn.morgan@med.nyc.edu 1,2) L.W. Teperman, 1,2) G.R. Morgan, 2) T. Diflo, D. John, 3) A. Goldenberg, H. Tobias, R. Wetherbee, J. Cohen, J. Benstein, 4) Rogosin Inst, 5) L. Irwin, D. Campbell, L. Johnson, H. Park, K. Bognar	71	76	76	512
Strong Mem Hosp, Dept of Surg/Med, 601 Elmwood Ave, Rochester, NY 14642 Ph: (716) 275-5875 Fax: (716) 271-7929 1,2) L. Mieles, 2) O. Bronsther, M. Orloff, 3) M. Brown, W. Chey, R. Pabico, G. Potter, 4) M. Coppage, 5) B. Byer, J. Yaeger, M. Kramer, L. Boccardo	24	40	69*	344
NORTH CAROLINA				
Univ of North Carolina Hospital, Comprehensive Transplant Ctr, 3306 West Wing, 101 Manning Drive, Chapel Hill, NC 27514 Ph: (888) 263-5293 Fax: (919) 966-5697 Email: transplant@unch.unc.edu 1,2) J. Fair, 2) M. Johnson, D. Gerber, K. Andreoni, 3) M. Fried, R. Shrestha, S. Zacks, 4) J. Crawford, J. Schmitz, 5) A. Strzalka, D. Roush, L. Kearns, P. Odell	64	64	73	392
Carolinas Medical Ctr, Transplant Center, PO Box 32861, 1000 Blythe Blvd, Charlotte, NC 28232 Ph: (704) 355-6649 Fax: (704) 355-7616 1,2) L.B. Eskind, 1,3) P. Purdum, 2) P. Gores, D. Hayes, 3) R. Reindollar, 4) S. Bruner, S. Mallory, B. Ranson, J. Blankenship, 5) Thrasher, Jones, Hogarth, O'Brien, Pierce, Zebedis, McKnight, Fowler	32	32	37*	145
Duke Univ Med Ctr, Dept of Surg, Box 3522, Erwin Rd, Durham, NC 27710 Ph: (919) 668-1856 Fax: (919) 681-7508 Email: kuo00004@mc.duke.edu 1,2) P.C. Kuo, 2) B. Tuttle-Newhal, B. Collins, R. Bollinger, 3) P.G. Killenberg, M. Swaim, M. Heneghan, 4) F. Ward, B. Burgess, 5) J. Tart, J. Gentile, D. Phillips	49	25	34	432
OHIO				
Children's Hosp Med Ctr, Dept of Liver Transp, 3333 Burnet Ave, Cincinnati, OH 45229 Ph: (513) 636-4955 Fax: (513) 636-5980 Email: liver@chmcc.org 1,2) F. Ryckman, 1,3) W. Balistreri, 2) M. Alonso, 3) J. Bucuvalas, J. Bezerra, M. Cohen, M. Farrell, J. Heubi, N. Yazigi, 4) D. Eckels, K. Balakrishnan, L. Whitacre, 5) K. Buschle, J. Slusher, C. Cron, B. Andrew, K. Jonson	19	18	29	237
Univ of Cincinnati Coll of Med, Dept of Surg, 231 Albert Sabin Way, Cincinnati, OH 45267-0558 Ph: (513) 558-1846 Fax: (513) 558-3580 Email: hantodw@healthall.com 1,2) D.W. Hanto, 2) J. Buell, M. Hanaway, E.S. Woodle, 3) F. Weber, K. Sherman, S. Martin, J. Aranda-Michel, S. Zucker, 4) L. Whitacre, D. Eckels, 5) M. Bass, P. Auble, K. Rolfes	41	35	41	356

1)=Director, 2)=Tx Surgeons, 3)=Physicians, 4)=Tissue Typers, 5)=TxCoords	1998	1999	2000	Total
Cleveland Clin Fnd, A110 Transplant Center, 9500 Euclid Ave, Cleveland, OH 44195 Ph: (216) 444-8770 Fax: (216) 444-9375 1,2) W. Carey, 1,2) D. Vogt, 2) J. Henderson, 3) D. Barnes, R. Wyllie, V. Hupertz, 4) D. Cook, 5) M. Quinn, P. George, M.L. Farquhar, L. Humphries	51	51	42	550
Univ Hosps of Cleveland, Dept of Surg, 11100 Euclid Ave, Cleveland, OH 44106 Ph: (216) 844-3689 Fax: (216) 844-7764 1,2) J.A. Schulak, 2) D.S. Seaman, C.T. Siegel, 3) A. Post, R. Oshea, S. Czinn, 4) N. Greenspan, 5) M. Penko, D. Tirbaso, M. Denis, M. Gerrick	28	37	30	298
Ohio State Univ Hosp, Div of Transp/Surg, 363 Means Hall, 1654 Upham Dr., Columbus, OH 43210 Ph: (614) 293-8545 Fax: (614) 293-4541 1,2) R.M. Ferguson, 2) M. Henry, E. Elkhammas, G. Bumgardner, R.P. Pelletier, 3) R. Kirkpatrick, C. Mabee, 4) P. Adams, 5) B. Miller, L. McDonnell	37	38	32*	411

OKLAHOMA

	1998	1999	2000	Total
Integris Baptist Med Ctr, Nazih Zuhdi Transpl Inst, 3300 NW Expressway, Oklahoma City, OK 73112 Ph: (405) 949-3349 Fax: (405) 945-5467 1,2) B.M. Nour, 2) A. Sebastian, 3) H. Wright, A. Gurakar, A. Jazzar, 4) D. Smith, 5) J. Carlson, S. Pennington, G. Sigle, J. Duffy	56	49	44*	402

OREGON

	1998	1999	2000	Total
Oregon Hlth Sci Univ/PVAMC, Liver/Pancreas Transp Sec, 3181 SW Sam Jackson Park Rd, L 590, Portland, OR 97201-3098 Ph: (503) 494-7810 Fax: (503) 494-5292 1,2) J. Rabkin, 2) S. Orloff, 3) H. Rosen, 4) D.J. Norman, 5) S. Winters, J. Salsbury, A. Gail, J. Nussbaum	52	52	53	573

PENNSYLVANIA

	1998	1999	2000	Total
Univ Hosp Penn State Coll of Med, Dept of Surg, Sec of Transp, PO Box 850, 500 University Dr, Hershey, PA 17033 Ph: (717) 531-5852 Fax: (717) 531-6579 1,2) H.C. Yang, 2) M. Holman, J.D. Arenas, 3) J. Cheung, J. Diamond, N. Ahsan, M. Waybill, J. Groff, 4) P.J. Romano, 5) E. Norton, J. Nafziger-Eberly	13	22	92*	97
Albert Einstein Med Ctr, Div of Transp Surg, 5401 Old York Road, Klein 509, Philadelphia, PA 19141 Ph: (215) 456-4985 Fax: (215) 456-8058 Email: manzarbe@aehn2.ginstein.edu 1) C. Manzarbeitia, 2) D.J. Reich, J. Ortiz, 3) S. Munoz, K. Rothstein, V. Araya, 4) R. McAlack, 5) E. Bloom, A. Jones, K. McCulley-Little	48	60	46	299
Hosp of the Univ of Pennsylvania &, Childrens Hosp of Philadelphia, Liver Transplant, 3400 Spruce St, Ground Gates, Philadelphia, PA 19104 Ph: (215) 662-6200 Fax: (215) 662-2244 1,2) A. Shaked, 2) K. Olthoff, J. Markmann, 3) M. Lucey, F. Nunes, G. Zeldin, C. Stewart, E. Rand, 4) M. Kamoun, J. Kearns, 5) C. Read, N. Higuchi, V. Shiro, H. Dauter, K. Timmins, C. Goodsell	109	122	101	682
St Christopher's Hosp for Children, Dept of Ped Surg, Erie Ave at Front St, Philadelphia, PA 19134-1095 Ph: (215) 427-5446 Fax: (215) 427-4616 1,2) S.P. Dunn, 2) A.T. Casas, 3) Kevin Kelley, Sheja Abraham, J. DiPalma, J. Malatack, 4) R. Bigler, (Hahnemann Univ), 5) K. Falkenstein, L. Fletcher, K. Freer	16	18	3*	231
Temple Univ Hosp, Abdominal Organ Tx, Broad & Ontario Sts, Philadelphia, PA 19140 Ph: (215) 707-8889 Fax: (215) 707-8894 Email: guysx@tuhs.temple.edu 1,2) S. Guy, 3) M. Black, J. Schwartz, 4) S. Leech, 5) G. Libetti, K. Wuest	6	11	3	20
TJUH Transplant Program, 132 S. 10th Street, Suite 460 Main, Philadelphia, PA 19107 Ph: (215) 955-7625 Fax: (215) 503-2626 1,2) M. Moritz, 2) J. Radomski, V. Armenti, 3) M. Porayko, M. Conn, S. Herrine, 4) Colombe, Lacava, Lynch, vanderHeide, Nguyen, Tecza, Bruneau, 5) U. Hobbs, S. Hozey	33	32	32	396
Children's Hosp of Pittsburgh, Liver Transplant, One Children's Pl, 3705 Fifth Ave, Pittsburgh, PA 15213-2582 Ph: (412) 692-6110 Fax: (412) 692-6116 1,2) J. Reyes, 2) J. Fung, G. Mazariegos, R. Sindhi, 3) M. Green, 4) A. Zeevi, R. Duquesnoy, 5) C. Baird, K. Iurlano, A. Smith	1	26	21*	146

1)=Director, 2)=Tx Surgeons, 3)=Physicians, 4)=Tissue Typers, 5)=TxCoords	1998	1999	2000	Total
UPMC-Presbyterian, Starzl Transplantation Inst, 4 Falk Clinic, 3601 5th Ave, Pittsburgh, PA 15213 Ph: (412) 648-3200 Fax: (412) 648-3085 1,2) T.E. Starzl, 1,2) J.J. Fung, 2) Marsh, Dodson, Mazariegos, Jain, Bonham, Reyes, Geller, Cacciarelli, 3) Carr, Kusne, McCauley, Green, 4) R. Duquesnoy, A. Zeevi, 5) Gadomski, Hartner, Stock, Boig, Nestler, Flynn, Funovits, Yelochan	210	187	148	5788
SPLIT LIVER	3	8	1	57
SOUTH CAROLINA				
Med Univ of South Carolina, Dept of Surg/Sec of Transp, Rm 404-CSB, 171 Ashley Ave, Charleston, SC 29425 Ph: (803) 792-3553 Fax: (803) 792-8596 1,2) P. Baliga, 2) P. Rajalopalan, K. Chavin, J. Rogers, 3) A. Reuben, I. Willner, 4) M. Gautreaux, 5) R. Stockdell, T. Polter, S. Odom	49	66	71*	390
TENNESSEE				
Le Bonheur Children's Med Ctr, Dept of Ped Transp, 50 N Dunlap, Memphis, TN 38103 Ph: (901) 572-5438/5434 Fax: (901) 572-5052 1,2) S. Vera, 2) H. Shakouh-Amiri, A.O. Gaber, H.P. Grewal, 3) L. Lazar, C. Riely, G. Whitington, D. Black, J. Eshun, 4) C. Miller, B. Loehman, T. Northrop, L. Marek, Y. Cao, 5) S. Powell	5	5	2*	69
William F Bowld Hosp, Univ of Tenn, Dept of Surg, Rm A202, 956 Court Ave, Memphis, TN 38163 Ph: (901) 448-5924 Fax: (901) 448-7208 1,2) A.O. Gaber, 2) S. Vera, H. Shokouh-Amiri, R.J. Stratta, H.P. Grewal, 3) J. Fleckenstein, C. Riely, B. Waters, M. Levstik, R. Davila, 4) B. Loehman et al, 5) B. Culbreath, N. O'Keefe, R. Vincent	51	50	46*	450
Vanderbilt Univ Med Ctr, Div Hepat Surg/Liver Transp, Vanderbilt Transp Ctr, 801 Oxford House, Nashville, TN 37232-4753 Ph: (615) 936-0420 Fax: (615) 936-0435 1,2) C.W. Pinson, 2) J.K. Wright, W.C. Chapman, 3) R. Burk, D. Raiford, J. Awad, 4) DCI Labs, 5) J. Payne, A. Kain	45	51	65	341
TEXAS				
Baylor Univ Med Ctr, Dallas Liver Transplant Prog, Dept of Surg, 3500 Gaston Ave, Dallas, TX 75246 Ph: (214) 820-2050 Fax: (214) 820-4527 1,2) G. Klintmalm, 2) R. Goldstein, M. Levy, E. Holmenti, C. Fasola, 3) T. Gonwa, M. Mai, L. Melton, 4) D. Smith, 5) Fertig, Hashim, Roman, Johnson, Manley	128	143	126*	1813
Children's Med Ctr of Dallas, Liver Transp, 1935 Motor St, Dallas, TX 75235 Ph: (800) 846-6768 Fax: (214) 456-8405 1,2) J. Roden, 3) J. Sommerauer, J. Andersen, R. Squires, 4) P. Stastny, 5) W. McPhail, V. Fioravanti	14	15	21*	314
Hermann Hosp Univ of Texas @ Houston, Liver Transp Prog, Div of Immun & Organ Transp, 6431 Fannin MSB 6.246, Houston, TX 77030 Ph: (713) 704-6800 Fax: (713) 704-6616 1,3) V. Ankoma-Sey, 2) J. Goss, C.F. Ozaki, C. Van Buren, P. Wood, 3) R. Ghalib, H. Monsour, 4) R.H. Kerman, 5) L. Baumann	51	59	27*	395
St Luke's Episcopal Hosp, Transp Serv, 6720 Bertner, Ste P-357, Houston, TX 77030 Ph: (713) 791-3787 Fax: (713) 794-6798 1,2) R.P. Wood, 2) C.F. Ozaki, 3) J. Galati, R. Ghalib, 4) R.H. Kerman, 5) R. Euerrero	8	11	17*	75
Texas Children's Hosp, Dept of Transp Serv, 6621 Fannin, Houston, TX 77030 Ph: (713) 770-2577 Fax: (713) 770-2570 1,2) J. Goss, 2) P. Seu, R.P. Wood, C.F. Ozaki, J. Lappin, 3) G.S. Gopalakrishna, B. Reid, G. Ferry, 4) Univ of Texas, 5) S. Doster	3	8	13*	95
The Methodist Hosp, Baylor College of Medicine, 6550 Fannin, Suite 1625, Houston, TX 77030 Ph: (713) 798-8355 Fax: (713) 798-7762 Email: pseu@bcm.tmc.edu 1,2) P. Seu, 2) J. Goss, 3) R.J. Stribling, R. Ghalib, 4) G. Rodey, 5) P. Schock, P. Westergren	9	43	53*	164
Univ of Texas HSC, Med Ctr Hosp, Organ Transp Prog, 7703 Floyd Curl Dr, San Antonio, TX 78284-7842 Ph: (210) 567-5777 Fax: (210) 567-4458 1,2) G.A. Halff, 2) R. Esterl Jr, F. Cigarroa, 4) P. Blackwell, K. Rocha, T. Hoog, L. MacNeish, S. Ament, J. Vargas, Radnik, 5) L. Nichols, J. Silva, G. Bench, D. Carrizales, L. Jackson, I. Infante	81	77	108	374

1)=Director, 2)=Tx Surgeons, 3)=Physicians, 4)=Tissue Typers, 5)=TxCoords	1998	1999	2000	Total
UTAH				
LDS Hosp, Dept of Transp, 8th Ave & C St, Salt Lake City, UT 84143 Ph: (801) 408-3090 Fax: (801) 408-3098 1,2) J. Sorensen, 2) L.P. Belnap, M.H. Stevens, 3) T. Box, J. Bowers, M. Boschert, R. Thomason, W. Hutson, 4) T. Fuller, 5) R. Dilauro, K. Nyman, J. Nielson	38	31	36	348
VIRGINIA				
Univ of Virginia Health Science Ctr, Multi-Organ Transp Prog Div, Box 265, Univ Station, Jefferson Park Ave, Charlottesville, VA 22908 Ph: (800) 543-8814 Fax: (804) 982-0099 1,2) T.L. Pruett, 2) H. Sanfey, R. Sawyer, 3) S. Caldwell, C. Berg, 4) C. Spencer, 5) B. Shepard, T. Golding, N. Carroll	23	23	37	486
Inova Fairfax Hosp, Inova Transp Ctr, 3300 Gallows Rd, Falls Church, VA 22042 Ph: (703) 698-2986 Fax: (703) 698-2797 Email: timothy.shaver@inova.com 1,2) T.R. Shaver, 2) D. Kelly, J. Jonsson, S. Batty, A. Kirk, G. Abrahmian, 3) R. Vinayek, A. Blosser, R. Barkin, P. Scudera, G. Herman, M. Prosky, 4) W. Ward, 5) Erickson, Disanto, Skipper, Stewart, Hicks, Swift, Charity	30	27	19*	237
Med Coll of Virginia, Dept of Surg, Div Transp, MCV Station, Box 980254, Richmond, VA 23298- 0254 Ph: (804) 828-2461 Fax: (804) 828-2462 Email: rafisher@hsc.vcu.edu 1,2) R.A. Fisher, 2) M. Posner, J. Ham, A. Gotterell, S. Dawson, 3) M. Shiffman, A. Sunyal, V. Luketic, R. Sterling, T. Stravitz, 4) P. Kimball, 5) W. Cales, M. Akyeampong, A. Ashworth, J. Myerly, M. Anderson	53	60	45	553
WASHINGTON				
Children's Hosp & Med Ctr, Dept of Surg-CH-78, 4800 Sand Point Way NE, Seattle, WA 98105 Ph: (206) 526-2039 Fax: (206) 527-3925 1,2) P. Healey, 2) R. Sawin, J. Waldhausen, J.D. Perkins, 3) D. Christie, P. Tarr, K. Murray, 4) Puget Sound Bld Ctr, 5) E. Moore	7	13	8	61
Univ of Washington Med Ctr, Transplantation Services, 1959 N.E. Pacific St, Box 356174, Seattle, WA 98195 Ph: (206) 598-6700 Fax: (206) 598-6706 Email: theperk@a.washington.edu 1,2) J.D. Perkins, 2) C.L. Marsh, P. Healey, A. Levy, C. Kuhr, 3) R. Carithers, K. Kowdley, A. Larson, B. Tung, 4) K. Nelson(Puget Sound Blood Ctr), 5) Y. Jo, M. Kester, K. Rimmer, M. Pascual	57	61	86	613
WISCONSIN				
Univ of Wisconsin, Transp Office H4/785, Clin Sci Ctr, 600 Highland, Madison, WI 53792 Ph: (608) 263-1385 Fax: (608) 262-5624 1,2) M. Kalayoglu, 2) A. D'Alessandro, S. Knechtle, J. Odorico, Y. Becker, 3) J. Pirsch, R. Judd, A. Musat, 4) H. Sollinger, 5) M. Armbrust, E. Spaith, M. Douglas, J. Breslow, H. Nelson	71	89	63*	951
Children's Hosp of Wisconsin, Abdominal Organ Transp, 9000 W Wisconsin Ave, PO Box 1997, MS653, Milwaukee, WI 53201 Ph: (414) 266-2000 Fax: (414) 266-2765 1,2) M.B. Adams, 2) C. Johnson, A. Roza, 3) S. Kugathasan, S. Werlin, 4) Bld Ctr of SE Wisconsin, 5) C. Werner	4	4	3	56
Froedtert Mem Lutheran Hosp, Med Coll of Wisconsin, Dept of Transp Surg, 9200 W Wisconsin Ave, Milwaukee, WI 53226 Ph: (414) 456-6920 Fax: (414) 456-6222 1,2) M.B. Adams, 2) C. Johnson, A. Roza, 3) R.R. Varma, J. Franco, K. Saeian, 4) D. Eckels, Blood Center Of S.E. Wisconsin, 5) P. Walczak, L. Venturi, C. Weickardt, S. Klenner, D. Pierce	26	22	27*	321
ARGENTINA				
Hosp Italiano de Buenos Aires, Dept of Surg, Gascon 450, Potosi 4044, Buenos Aires, CPH 81 Ph: (54)1 981-4501 Fax: (54)1 981-4041 Email: edurdod@infostar.com.ar 1,2) E. de Santibanes, 2) M. Ciardullo, J. Sivovi, J. Perkolj, J. Matera, L. McCormack, 3) A. Gadano, 4) G. Gallo, 5) M. Sardo	34	34	41	298
Cosme Argerich, Transplante, Alte Brown 240, Manuel A Rodriguez 1162, Buenos Aires, 1155 Ph: (54)1 362-9884 Fax: (54)1 583-8704 1,2) O. Imventarza, 2) J. Lendoire, G. Bianco, J. Saul, F. Duek, 3) G. Braslavsky, P. Trigo, G. Cueto, 5) M. Zarate	35	37	30	159

LIVER

1)=Director, 2)=Tx Surgeons, 3)=Physicians, 4)=Tissue Typers, 5)=TxCoords	1998	1999	2000	Total
Hosp Garrahan, Transplantation, Combate De Los Pozos 1881, Manuel A Rodriguez 1162 60, Buenos Aires, 1425 Ph: (54)1 941-8812 Fax: (54)1 583-8704 1,2) O. Imventarza, 2) L. Rojas, G. Cervio, G, Bianco, 3) M. Ciocca, M. Cuarterolo, J. Sasbon, 5) M. Labadet	30	52	36	234

AUSTRALIA

	1998	1999	2000	Total
Royal Prince Alfred Hosp, Univ of Sydney, Australian Nat'l Liver Transp Unit, Missenden Rd, Camperdown, Sydney, NSW, 2050 Ph: (61)295153500 Fax: (61)295153512 1,2) P. Pillay, 1,2) J. Thompson, 2) D. Verran, J. Gallagher, G. Stewart, 3) G.W. McCaughan, D. Koorey, S. Strasser, 4) Sydney Red Cross Bld Transf Serv, 5) G. Kyd, N. Koutalistras	52	41	51	575
Queensland Liver Transp Serv, Princess Alexandra Hosp, & Royal Children's Hosp, Ipswich Rd, Woollongabba, Brisbane, QLD 4102 Ph: (61)73240-2111 Fax: (61)73240-2999 Email: s.lynch@uq.net.au 1,2) S. Lynch, 2) T.H. Ong, D. Wall, R. Strong, J. Fawcett, A. Griffin, 3) P. Kerlin, D. Crawford, G. Cleghorn, P. Lewindon, Lee, 5) M. Butler, H. Robinson, K. Beale	51	38	45	669
Austin & Repatriation Med Ctr, Liver Transp Unit, Heidelberg, Melbourne, Victoria, 3084 Ph: (61)3 9496-5353 Fax: (61)3 9496-3487 Email: alice.gleeson@armc.org.au 1,2) R.M. Jones, 2) K. Hardy, I. Michell, B. Wang, R. Berry, M. Fink, 3) P. Angus, 4) B. Tait, 5) A. Gleeson	28	27	31	280

AUSTRIA

	1998	1999	2000	Total
Univ Klin Fur Chir, Dept of Transp Surg, Auenbruggerplatz 29, A-8036 Graz Ph: (43)316 385-2707 Fax: (43)316 385-4446 1,2) K.H. Tscheliessnigg, 3) Stayber, 4) G. Lanzer, 5) F. Iberer	11	10		46
Univ Hosp, Dept of Transp Surg, Anichstrasse 35, Innsbruck, 6020 Ph: (43)512 504-2603 Fax: (43)512 504-2605 1,2) R. Margreiter, 2) A. Koenigsrainer, B. Spechtienhauser, 3) W. Vogel, I. Graziadei, 4) D. Schoenitzer, 5) H. Fetz, P. Schobel	57	62	65	485
Allgemeines Hosp, Univ of Vienna, Dept of Surg, Transp Ctr, Wahringer Gurtel 18-20, Vienna, A-1090 Ph: (43)1 40400 4000 Fax: (43)1 40400 6872 1,2) F. Muhlbacher, 2) R. Steininger, 3) M. Peck-Radosavlevic, 4) W. Mayr, 5) M. Bodingbauel, R. Asari	65	79	72	874

BELGIUM

	1998	1999	2000	Total
Cliniques Univ St Luc, Dept of Transp, 10, Ave Hippocrate, Brussels, 1200 Ph: (32) 2-7641401 Fax: (32) 2-7623680 Email: otte@chex.ucl.ac.be 1,2) J.B. Otte, 2) J. Lerut, R. Reding, 3) A. Geubel, E. Sokal, Y. Horsmans, P. Starkel, 4) M. De Bruyere, D. Latinne, 5) M. Janssen, F. Roggen, P. van Ormelingen	49	59	73	1139
Hosp Erasme, Dept of Digestive Surg, 808 Rte de Lennick, B-1070 Brussels Ph: (32)2 555-3713 Fax: (32)2 555-4905 Email: vdonckie@ulb.ac.be 1,2) M. Gelin, 2) J. Closset, I. El Nakadi, V. Donckier, 3) M. Adler, N. Bourgeois, O. LeMoine, 4) E. Dupont, M. Goldman, 5) B. van Haelewyck	17	31	14	249
Univ Hosp Ghent, Dept of Surg & Liver Transp, De Pintelaan 185, Ghent, 9000 Ph: (32)92 403233 Fax: (32)92 403891 1,2) B. de Hemptinne, 2) P. Pattyn, I. Kerremans, U. Hesse, R. Troisi, W. Ceelen, 3) DeCruyenaere, Robberecht, van Winckel, van Vlierbergh, 4) B. van dekerckhove, 5) M. van der Vennet, L. Colenbie	28	46	45	362
Univ Hosp Gasthuisberg, Dept of Abdominal Tx Surgery, Herestr 49, B-3000 Leuven Ph: (32)16 348727 Fax: (32)16 348743 Email: jacques.pirenne@uz.kuleuven.ac.be 1,2) J. Pirenne, 2) R. Aerts, 3) J. Fevery, F. Nevens, 4) J. Dendievel, M.P. Emonds, 5) F. van Gelder, D. van Hees, S. Kimpen	35	36	57	257
Ctr Hosp Univ-Liege, Dept of Surg Transp, Domaine Univ du Sart-Tilman-B35, B-4000 Liege Ph: (32)43 667206 Fax: (32)43 667517 1,2) M. Meurisse, 2) N. Jacquet, P. Honore, O. Detry, A. DeRoover, 3) P. Honore, 4) C. Bouillenne, 5) M.H. Delbouille, M.F. Hans	22	21	20	193

1)=Director, 2)=Tx Surgeons, 3)=Physicians, 4)=Tissue Typers, 5)=TxCoords	1998	1999	2000	Total
BRAZIL				
Hosp de Clinics, Dept of Cirurgia do Aparelho, Rua General Carneiro, 181, 7 Andar Central, Curitiba, PR 80060-900 Ph: (55)41 262-8406 Fax: (55)41 262-8406 1,2) J. Coelho, 2) A.C.L. Campos, C.Z. Neto, J. Matias, A. Freitas, 3) M. Parolin, M. Parolin, 5) J. Matias	29	38	32	191
Beneficencia Portuguesa Hosp, HEPATO-Hepatology & Organ Tx, Rua Maestro Cardim 377, cj 75, Rua Maestro Cardim 769,Bloco V,2 SS, Sao Paulo, 01323-001 Ph: 55 11 2831450 Fax: 55 11 37714769 Email: marcelo-perosa@uol.com.br 1) M. Perosa, 1) T. Genzini, 2) E.O. Krebsky, S.E.A. Araujo, 3) A. Coppini, F.L. Pandullo, 5) F.L. Pandullo	5	14	20	39
Fac de Med da Univ de Sao Paulo, Dept of Surg, Liver Unit, Av Dr Arnaldo, 455,3 Andar, Sao Paulo, SP CEP.01246 Ph: (55)11 883-3308 Fax: (55)11 881-9418 1,2) S. Mies, 2) P.C.B. Massarollo, A.O.N.G. Femandes, 3) E.L.R. Cancado, A.Q. Farias, 4) J.K. Filho, 5) W.R. Mollo	60	67	79	443
CANADA				
Univ of Alberta Hosp, Dept of Surg, 2D444 Mackenzie Ctr, Edmonton, AB T6G 2B7 Ph: (780) 407-7072 Fax: (780) 407-7374 1,2) N.M. Kneteman, 2) AMJ. Shapiro, D.L. Bigam, 3) V. Bain, M. Ma, K. Gutfreund, W. Wong, 4) P.F. Halloran, 5) B. Pawluk, C. Heekstra, B. Hobson, D. Ogilvie, A. Taskinen	54	69	66	452
British Columbia Transplant Society, West Tower, 3rd Floor, 555 W 12th Ave, Vancouver, BC V5Z 3X7 Ph: (604) 877-2240 Fax: (604) 877-2111 1) B. Barrable, 2) C. Scudamore, S. Chung, 3) S. Erb, E. Yoshida, U. Steinbrecher, R. Schreiber, 4) B. Draney, 5) L. Mori, C. Bannota, J. Waines	24	32	34	269
Queen Elizabeth II Health Sciences, Atlantic Canada Liver Transpl, 1278 Tower Rd, Halifax, NS B3H 2Y9 Ph: (902) 473-7532 Fax: (902) 473-2828 1,2) A.S. MacDonald, 2) H. Bitter-Suermann, 3) K. Peltekian, 4) S. Eastwood, K. West, 5) H. MacKinnon	18	30	25	209
University Hosp, Dept of Transp, 339 Windermere Rd, PO Box 5339, London, ON N6A 5A5 Ph: (519) 663-2940 Fax: (519) 663-3067 1,2) W.J. Wall, 2) D. Quan, 3) C. Ghent, P. Adams, P. Marotta, 4) S. Leckie, 5) M. Bloch, M. Richard-Mohamed, J. Drew, C. Weernick	62	61	64	981
Univ of Toronto Multi-Organ Transp, Toronto Gen Hosp, 200 Elizabeth St, Toronto, ON M5G 2C4 Ph: (416) 340-4252 Fax: (416) 340-3492 1,2) P.D. Greig, 2) M.S. Cattral, A. Fecteau, D.R. Grant, P.D. Grelb, 3) E. Roberts, L. Lilly, G.A. Levy, N. Jonas, 4) J. Wade, 5) Vasco, Freitag, Colpitts, McKillup, DeLuca, Lewis, Bianchi	93	84		996
Hopital Sainte-Justine, Dept of Peds, 3175 Cote Ste Catherine, Montreal, PQ H3T 1C5 Ph: (514) 345-4626 Fax: (514) 345-4999 1,3) F. Alvarez, 2) J.M. Laberge, D. St Vil, M. Lallier, S. Busque, 3) S. Martin, 5) C. Viau	8	22	6	139
Hosp Notre-Dame, Dept of Transp Surg, 1560 Sherbrooke Est, Montreal, PQ H2L 4M1 Ph: (514) 281-6000 x6605 Fax: (514) 896-4736 Email: pierre.daloze.chum@ssss.gouv.qc.ca 1,2) P. Daloze, 2) C. Smeesters, S. Busque, 3) M. Beaudoin, 4) Inst Armand Frappier, Montreal, 5) Quebec Transp	0	0	0	44
Royal Victoria Hosp, McGill Ctr-Clin Immun/Transp, 687 Pine Ave W, Montreal, PQ H3A 1A1 Ph: (514) 842-1231 Fax: (514) 843-1503 1,2) J. Tchervenkov, 2) J. Barkun, P. Metrakos, 3) M. Cantarovich, E. Alpert, M. Deschenes, 4) P. Imperial, R. Schreier, C. McIntyre, 5) M. Poloni, M. Sevapsidis, L. Doyle	43	44	41	321
CHILE				
Clinica Alemana de Santiago S.A., Dept of Surgery, Vitacura, 5951. Vitacura, Santiago Ph: (56)2 2101300 Fax: (56)2 2101400 Email: Jhepp@alemana.cl 1,2) J.K. Hepp, 2) F. Innocenti, H. Rios, L. Suarez, D. Videla, R. Cardenas, R. Humeres, 3) Gonzalez Koch, Valderrama, Zaror, Espinoza, Quiroga, Rodriquez, 4) E. Blackburn, 5) M. Rius	13	11	9	53
Unidad de Trasplantes, Clinica las Condes, Lo Fontecilla 441, Santiago Ph: (56)2 2105005 Fax: (56)2 2105089 1,2,3) E.G. Buckel, 2) M. Uribe, 3) S. Ceresa, J. Zacarias, J. Brahm, G. Silva, J. Cordero, R. Tejias, 4) G. Smock, 5) C. Herzog, T. Santander	20	28		95

1)=Director, 2)=Tx Surgeons, 3)=Physicians, 4)=Tissue Typers, 5)=TxCoords	1998	1999	2000	Total
Universidad Catolica De Chile, Cirugia, Marcoleta 367-3rd Piso, Santiago Ph: (562)632-3462 Fax: (562)632-9620 1,2) C. Fasola, 2) Guzman, Ibanez, Martinez, Herrera, Pimentel, Rossi, Zuniga, S. Zuniga, 3) M. Arrese, J. Chianale, P. Harris, J. Miquel, F. Nervi, 4) L. Rodriguez, 5) R. Giancaspero	3			14
Universidad Catolica De Chile, Cirugia Digestiva, Marcoleta 367, P.O. Box 114-D, Santiago Ph: (562) 686-3462/3870 Fax: (562) 632-9620 Email: cdigest@mcd.puc.cl 1,2) J.A. Martinez, 2) S. Guzman, A. Zuniga, A. Diaz, G. Perez, 3) M. Arrese, J. Chianale, P. Harris, R.M. Perez, C. Perez, A. Dougnac, 4) L. Rodriguez, 5) R. Giancaspero, M. Acuna, M.J. Martinez	2	1	5	22

CHINA, P.R.

	1998	1999	2000	Total
Tongji Med Univ, Tongji Hosp, Inst of Organ Transp, 13 Hangkong Rd, Wuhan, Hubei Prov, 430030 Ph: (86)27 83611175 Fax: (86)27 83611175 Email: iot@tjh.tjmu.edu.cn 1) S.S. Xia, 2) Q.F. Ye, F.Q. Zhen, Z.S. Chen, 3) Z.P. Ling, 4) Z.S. Chen, 5) H.Y. Jiang	5	19	35	84
The Univ of Hong Kong Med Ctr, Liver Transplant Centre, Queen Mary Hosp, 102 Pokfulam Road, Hong Kong Ph: (852) 2855-5800/3634 Fax: (852) 2817-5475 1,2) S.T. Fan, 2) C.M. Lo, C.L. Liu, 3) C.L. Lai, G.K.K. Lau, 4) B.R. Hawkins, 5) B. Lam, A. Leung	23	28	41	155

COLOMBIA

	1998	1999	2000	Total
Fundocion Santa Fe de Bogota, Surg, Div of Transpl, Calle 116, #9-02, Bogota Ph: (57)1 2148607 Fax: (57)1 6122486 Email: rafab@cable.net.co 1,2) J.D. Arenas, 2) E. Figueredo, J.H. Valdez, 3) R.C. Botero, V. Idrobo, 4) N. Merino, 5) A.M. Alfonso, O. Florez	21			21

CZECH REPUBLIC

	1998	1999	2000	Total
Inst for Clin and Exper Med, Transp Ctr, Dept of Surg, Videnska 800, 14000 Prague 4 Ph: 420 2 613-64103 Fax: 420 2 613-63113 Email: stvi@medicon.cz 1) S. Vitko, 2) M. Ryska, F. Belina, 3) J. Spicak, 4) E. Ivaskova, 5) E. Pokorna, E. Laszikova, V. Charova, M. Skachova	42	47	40	198

FINLAND

	1998	1999	2000	Total
Children's Hosp, Univ of Helsinki, Dept of Ped Surg, Stenbackinkatu 11, Helsinki 29, SF 00029 Ph: (90)358 471-72730 Fax: (90)358 47174705 1,2) M. Leijala, 2) H. Sairanen, I. Mattila, M. Kaarne, 3) C. Holmberg, H. Jalanko, 4) S. Koskimies	4	4		61
Helsinki Univ Ctr Hosp, IV Dept of Surg, Transplants and Liver Surgery Unit, Kasarmikatu 11-13, Fin-00130 Helsinki Ph: (358) 9-174942 Fax: (358) 9-174975 1,2) K. Hockerstedt, 2) H. Isoniemi, K. Salmela, H. Makisalo, L. Halme, 4) S. Koskimies, 5) A.K. Mattila, M.L. Heikkila, E. Hartikka, L. Toivonen	39	30		347

FRANCE

	1998	1999	2000	Total
Hosp Jean Minjoz, Ctr Hosp et Univ, Chir Digestive et Vasc, Besancon, 25030 Ph: (33)81 66 8243 Fax: (33)81 66 8366 1,2) G. Mantion, 2) G. Landecy, B. Heyd, P. Mathieu, 3) J.Ph. Miguet, 4) P. Tiberghien, 5) Y. Hudel	27	21		293
Hosp Edouard Herriot, Dept of Transp, Liver Unit, Pavillion, Pl d'Arsonval, 69003 Lyon Ph: (33)472 116291 Fax: (33)472 116264 1,2) O. Boillot, 3) J. Dumortier, 4) L. Gebuhrer	59	51	69	501
L'Archet Hosp, Dept of Digestive Surg/Transp, 151 Route de St Antoine, de Ginestiere, 06202 Nice Ph: (33)493 036041 Fax: (33)493 036198 1) J. Mouiel, 1) J.Gugenheim, 2) M. Dahmann, 3) B. Goubaux, P. Sowska, 4) G. Pommier, 5) M. Genoux	18	24	23	365
Ctr Hosp Hautepierre, Transp Unit, Ave Moliere, Strasbourg, 67098 Ph: (33)88 127258 Fax: (33)88 127286 Email: aniel.jaeck@chru-strasbourg.fr 1) D. Jaeck, 2) P. Wolf, C. Meyer, M. Audet, 3) B. Ellero, M.L. Jaegle, 4) M.M. Tongio, 5) S. Fruh, V. Fuss, C. Becker	47	60	72	732

1)=Director, 2)=Tx Surgeons, 3)=Physicians, 4)=Tissue Typers, 5)=TxCoords	1998	1999	2000	Total
Paul Brousse Hosp, Hepato-Biliary Center, 14 Av P.V. Couturier, Villejuif, 94800 Ph: (33)1 4559 3331 Fax: (33)1 4559 3857 Email: henri.bismuth@pbr.ap-hop-paris.fr 1,2) H. Bismuth, 2) Castaing, Adam, Azoulay, Savier, 3) D. Samuel, F. Saliba, C. Feray, R. Roche, 4) P. Debat, 5) C. Danet, L. Thoraval	86	71	96	1601

GERMANY

	1998	1999	2000	Total
Univ Clinic RWTH, Dept of Surg, Pauwelsstr, Aachen, 52057 Ph: (49)241 808 9500 Fax: (49)241 888 8417 1) V. Schumpelick, 2) R. Kasperk, 3) S. Matern, 5) Homburg	0	0	2	12
Charite-Campus Circhow Klinkum, Dept of Surg, Augustenburger Platz 1, 13353 Berlin Ph: (49)30 450-52001 Fax: (49)30 450-52900 Email: chirurgie@charite.de 1) P. Neuhaus, 2) U. Settmacher, T. Steinmiller, A.R. Mulles, 3) U. Hopf, U. Frei, 4) A. Salama, C. Schoenemann, 5) D.F. Horch	119	91	111	1278
University Med Sch Hosp, Dept of Surg, Sigmund-Freud Str 25, Bonn, 53105 Ph: (49)228 287-5109 Fax: (49)228 287-4856 1) A. Hirner, 2) J. Kalff, M. Wolff, 3) U. Spengler, W. Caselmann, 5) E. Backhaus, B. Salz, T. Uhr	23	19	21	168
Transplantation Zentrum Koeln, Klinikum Koeln-Merheim, Ostmerheimer Str 200, Cologne 51109 Ph: (49)221 8907-3200 Fax: (49)221 89073335 Email: wolfgang.arns@uni-koeln.de 1) M. Weber, H. Troidl, C.A. Baldamus, A. H. Hoelscher 2) A. Paul, T. Beckurts, 3) W. Arns, M. Pollok, 4) R. Doerner, 5) Deutsche Stiftung Organtransplantation	21	22	23	97
Univ Clin Essen, Dept of Gen Surg, Hufeland strasse 55, Essen, 45122 Ph: (49)201 723 1140 Fax: (49)201 723 5946 1,2) C.E. Broelsch, 2) M. Malago, G. Testa, H. Lang, M. Hertl, C. Valentin-Gamazo, 3) T. Philipp, 4) H. Grosse-Wilde	74	97	81	646
Univ Clin Frankfurt am Main, Dept of Gen Surg, Theodor-Stern-kai 7, Frankfurt Am Main, 60590 Ph: (49)69 6301-7642 Fax: (49)69 6301-5984 1) Encke, 2) B.H. Markus, M. Lorenz, V. Paolucci, 3) C. Allers, 5) D. Wilhelm	18	17	15	156
Univ Hosp Freiburg, Dept of Surg, Organ Transp, Hugstetter Strass 55, Freiburg, G-79106 Ph: (49)761 270-2732 Fax: (49)761 278-970 Email: bluemke@cu11.ukl.uni-freiburg.de 1,2) G. Kirste, 2) P. Pisarski, 3) J. Rasenack, 4) H. Lang, 5) M. Blumke	10	24	18	132
Georg-August Univ Gottingen, Klin fur Transp Chir, Robert-Koch Str 40, 37075 Gottingen Ph: (49)551 39-8702 Fax: (49)551 37-4862 Email: tx-plant@med.uni-goettingen.de 1,2) B. Ringe, 2) T. Lorf, R. Canelo, 3) G. Ramadori, 4) H. Neymeyer, C. Krome-Cesar, 5) E. Schmidt	20	14	15	120
Univ Clin Eppendorf-Hamburg, Dept of Hepatobiliary Surg, Martinistr 52, Hamburg, 20246 Ph: (49)40 4717 6136 Fax: (49)40 4717 3431 1,2) X. Rogiers, 2) M. Gundlach, D. Broring, R. Kuhlencordt, 3) M. Burdelski, M. Sterneck, 4) P. Kuhnl, 5) T. Karbe, R. Kutemeier, S. Wannoff	73	81	67	809
Med Sch Hannover, Dept of Visceval/Transp Surg, Carl-Neuberg-Str. 1, 30625 Hannover Ph: (49)511 532 6534 Fax: (49)511 532 2265 1) J. Klempnauer, 2) B. Nashan, R. Luck, T. Becker, 3) M. Manns, M. Melter, 4) R. Blascyk, 5) G. Gubernatis, S. Tietze, G. Oelmann	90	94	121	1586
Transp Central Kiel, Dept of Surg, Arnold-Heller Str 7, 24105 Kiel Ph: (49)431 597-4341 Fax: (49)431 597-4586 1) B. Kremer, 2) D. Henne-Bruns, 3) H. Kraemer-Hansen, 4) E. Westphal, 5) G.R. Schuett	10	16	23	125
Univ of Leipzig, Clin of Abdom/Vasc/Transp Surg, Liebigstr 20, Leipzig, 04103 Ph: (49)341 9717200 Fax: (49)341 9717209 1) J. Hauss, 2) P. Lamesch, K. Kohlhaw, U. Jost, H. Witzigmann, R. Schwarz, H. Fangmann, 3) F. Berr, 4) Halle/Saale Tissue Typ Lab, 5) T. Weisskirchen	26	28		135
Clin Grosshadern, Univ of Munich, Dept of Surg, Marchioninistr 15,, Munich, 81377 Ph: (49)89 7095 3560 Fax: (49)89 7095 8894 1) F.W. Schildberg, 2) H.G. Rau, 3) A. Gerbes, 4) E. Albert, 5) C. Schulz	29	35	36	489
Tech Univ Munchen-Klin Rechts Isar, Dept of Surg, Ismaninger Str 22, Munich, 81675 Ph: (49)89 4140 2011 Fax: (49)89 478917 1,3) J.R. Siewert, 2) M. Stangl, 3) V. Schusdziarra, 4) E. Albert, 5) B. Daldos	11	10	10	167

1)=Director, 2)=Tx Surgeons, 3)=Physicians, 4)=Tissue Typers, 5)=TxCoords	1998	1999	2000	Total
Univ of Rostock Med Faculty, Clin of Surgery, Schillingallee, Rostock, D-18057 Ph: (49)381 494 6000 Fax: (49)381 494 6002 1) U. Hopt, 2) W. Schareck, 3) R. Schmidt, 4) R. Barz, 5) F.P. Nitschke	4	14	10	45
Univ of Tuebingen, Dept of Surg, Hoppe-Seyler Str 3, Transp Ctr, Tuebingen, 72076 Ph: (49)70 7129 86600 Fax: (49)70 714 4532 1) H.D. Becker, 2) R. Viebahn, K. Dietrich, M. Schaffer, 3) Dette, Kreysel, 4) Northoff, Wernet, 5) Fischer-Frohlich	24	23	27	292

HUNGARY

	1998	1999	2000	Total
Pecs Univ, Faculty of Medicine, 1st Dept of Surgery, Ifjusag u.13, PECS, H 7624 Ph: (36) 72 53 6128 Fax: (36) 72 53 6128 Email: kalmar@iseb.pote.hu 1,2) K. Kalmar-Nagy, 2) P. Szakaly, A. Papp, 3) A. Par, J. Baumann, 4) M. Paal Uherkovichne, 5) K. Kalmar		1	0	1

ISRAEL

	1998	1999	2000	Total
Beilinson Med Ctr, Dept of Organ Transp, Zabotinski 66, Petach Tikva, 49100 Ph: (972)3 922 4285 Fax: (972)3 924 9680 1) Z. Shapira, 2) A. Yussim, E. Shaharabani, N. Natan, E. Mor, 3) S. Lustig, 4) T. Klein, 5) R. Michowiz	25	19	28	136

ITALY

	1998	1999	2000	Total
St Orsola Univ Hosp, 2nd Dept of Surg, Via Massarenti, 9, Bologna, 40138 Ph: (39)051 341700 Fax: (39)051 397661 1,2) A. Cavallari, 2) A. Mazziotti, G.L. Grazi, R. Bellusci, B. Nardo, 3) C. Sama, P. Andreone, McMorelli, 4) R. Conte, 5) P. Mazzetti, N. Venturoli	26	95	85	559
Azienda Ospedale San Martino, Dept of Transp, Largo Rosanna Benzi, 10, Genova, 16132 Ph: (39)010 5553862 Fax: (39)010 5556772 Email: itctransplant.smartino.ge.it 1) U. Valente, 2) E. Andorno, A. Antonucci, N. Morelli, G. Bottino, R. Mondello, 3) Picciotto, Gatti, Castellano, Valentini, Testino, Messa, et al, 4) G. Sirchia, F. Celada, A. Nocera, 5) C. Pizzi, A. Gianelli Castiglione, C. Gualeni, M. Tognoni, S. Pisanu	45	47	47	295
Inst Nat'l Tumori, Dept of Surg, Chirurgia Generale I, via Venezian,1, Milano, 20133 Ph: (39)02 2390760 Fax: (39)02 2664584 1,2) V. Mazzaferro, 2) E. Regalia, A. Pulvirenti, M. Schiavo, R. Romito, J. Coppa, G. Torzilli, 3) F. Bonino, M. Colombo, 4) G. Sirchia, 5) T. Bugada, P. Serafin, P. Rota, M. Mitarotonda	20	18	16	164
Osp Maggiore di Milano, Cent Trapianto di Fegato, Inst of Surg Exper Univ Milano, Via F Sforza 35, 20122 Milano Ph: (39)02 5503 5802 Fax: (39)02 5503 5800 1) L.R. Fassati, 2) eG. Rossi, B. Reggiani, U. Maggi, L. Caccamo, S. Gatti, G. Paone, 3) M. Doglia, 4) G. Sirchia, 5) M. Scalamogna	33	43	36	494
Ospedale Niguarda "Ca' Granda", Dept of Surg/Abdom Transp, Pizzamiglio, Via Ospedale Maggiore 3, 20162 Milano Ph: (39)02 6444-2648 Fax: (39)02 6444-2893 1) D. Forti, 2) G.F. Rondinara, L. De Carlis, 3) G. Pimzello, 4) G. Sirchia	40	53	50	525
Univ Hosp Med Sch, Padova, Dept of Gastro Surg, Via Giustiniani 2, 35128 Padova Ph: (39)49 821289 Fax: (39)49 8760820 Email: burra@ux1.unipd.it 1,3) R. Naccarato, 1,2) D. D'Amico, 2) U. Cillo, P. Boccagni, G. Zanus, A. Brolese, 3) P. Burra, S. Fagiuoli, 4) G. Sirchia, 5) G.P. Rupolo	63	59	59	479
ISMETT, Piazza Sett'Angeli, 10, Palermo, 90134 Ph: (39) 091 6661111 Fax: (39) 091 6668136 Email: mail@ismett.edu 1,2) I.R. Marino, 2) C. Doria, C. ScottiFoglieni, 3) H. Doyle, M. Magnone, U. Palazzo, D. Paterson, V. Scott, 4) A. Salerno, 5) M. Castellese, S. Guercio, R. DiGaudio		9	13	22
Univ of Pisa, Osp di Cisanello, Inst of Gen Surg, Via Paradisa 2, Pisa 56124 Ph: (39) 50 996820 Fax: (39) 50 543692 1) F. Mosca, 2) F. Filipponi, 4) G. Rizzo	44	97	71	265
Hosp Policlin Gemelli, Univ Cattolica del Sacro Cuore, Dept of Surg, Transp Ctr, Largo Gemelli 8, 00168 Rome Ph: (39)6 310 54300 Fax: (39)6 310 0019 1,2) M. Castagneto, 2) S. Agnes, G. Nanni, A. Avolio, S. Magalini, Citterio, Foco, 4) G. Luciani, 5) T. Borzi	14	8	9	138

1)=Director, 2)=Tx Surgeons, 3)=Physicians, 4)=Tissue Typers, 5)=TxCoords	1998	1999	2000	Total
Policlinico "Umberto 1", Univ "La Sapienza", Dept of Surg II, Viale del Policlinico, 00161 Rome Ph: (39)6 445 6296 Fax: (39)6 446 3667 1,2) R. Cortesini, 1) P. Berloco, 2) M. Rossi, 3) A. Attili, 4) E. Renna-Molajoni, A. Bachetoni, 5) S. Venettoni	17	29	35	259

JAPAN

	1998	1999	2000	Total
Univ of Tsukuba, Dept of Surg, 1-1-1 Tennoudai, Tsukuba, Ibaraki-Ken, 305-8575 Ph: (81)298 53-3210 Fax: (81)298 53-3222 1) K. Fukao, 2) M. Otsuka, K. Yuzawa, Y. Takada, T. Hori, 3) N. Tanaka, Y. Matsuzaki, 4) Y. Jinzenji	0	1	1	3
Kyoto University Hospital, Dept Of Transp Surg, 54 Kawara-Cho, Shogoin, Sakyo-Ku, Kyoto, 606-8507 Ph: (81)75 751 3660 Fax: (81)75 751 3616 Email: koichi@kuhp.kyoto-u.ac.jp 1,2) K. Tanaka, 2) S. Uemoto, H. Egawa, T. Kiuchi, M. Hayashi, S. Kaihara, F. Oike, 3) M. Nabeshima, 5) N. Iyama	92	95	119	646
Nagoya Univ Hosp, Dept of Surg II, 65 Tsuruma-cho, Showa-ku, Nagoya, 466-8550 Ph: (81)52 744-2248 Fax: (81)52 744-2255 1,2) I. Yokoyama, 2) S. Hayashi, T. Kobayashi, T. Tokoro, 3) T. Kato		1	5	6
Tokyo Women's Medical University, Kidney Ctr, Dept of Third Surg, 8-1 Kawada-cho, Shinjuku-ku, Tokyo, 162-8666 Ph: (81)3 3353-8111 Fax: (81)3 3356-0293 1,2) S. Fuchinoue, 2) K. Takasaki, I. Nakajima, 3) K. Ito, H. Shiraga, 4) M. Yasuo	7	5	10	73

KOREA

	1998	1999	2000	Total
Chonbuk National Univ Hosp, Dept of Surg/Int Med, 634-18 Keumam-dong,Dukjin-gu, Chonju, 561-712 Ph: (82)652 2501579 Fax: (82)652 2716197 Email: chobh@moak.chonbuk.ac.kr 1,2) B.H. Cho, 2) H.C. Yu, 3) D.G. Kim, 4) S.I. Choi, D.S. Kim, 5) H.S. Min	0	2	0	2
Hallym Univ Kangdong, Sacred Heart Hospital, 445 Gil dong, Kangdong-gu, Seoul, 134-701 Ph: (82)2 224-2222 Fax: (82)2 473-8101 1) S.T. Kim, 2) J.S. Kim, Y.C. Lee, M.H. Cho, S. Lee, 3) J.Y. Yoo, C.K. Park, 4) K.W. Lee, 5) M.H. Kim	1	2		10
Kang Nam St Mary's Hosp, Dept of Surg, The Catholic Univ of Korea, 505 Banpo-dong, Seocho-ku, Seoul, 137-040 Ph: (82)2 590-1436 Fax: (82)2 595-2992 1,2) Y.B. Koh, 2) I.C. Kim, S.N. Kim, E.K. Kim, D.G. Kim, M.D. Lee, 3) B.S. Kim, Y.M. Park, C.Y. Choi, S.H. Bae, 4) B.K. Kim, E.S. Chung, 5) H.O. Chun	8	12	7	44
Seoul Nat'l Univ Hosp, Coll of Med, Dept of Gen Surg, 28 Yongon-Dong, Chongno-gu, Seoul, 110-744 Ph: (82)2 760-2316 Fax: (82)2 3672-4947 1,2) S.J. Kim, 2) K.U. Lee, K.W. Park, K.S. Seo, S.E. Jung, 3) H.S. Lee, J.K. Seo, 4) M.H. Park, 5) J.S. Kim	6	29		56
Yonsei Univ Coll of Med, Severance Hosp, Dept of Surg, 134 Shinchon-Dong, Sudaemoon-ku, Seoul 120-752 Ph: (82)2 361-5545 Fax: (82)2 365-3069 1,2) K. Park, 2) Y.S. Kim, S.I. Kim, W.J. Lee, J.S. Choi, K.S. Kim, 3) D.S. Han, H.Y. Lee, K.H. Choi, S.W. Kang, Y.M. Moon, J.Y. Cheon, K.H. Han, 4) E.M. Lee, H.J. Kim, 5) K.O. Cheon, H.J. Kim	2	9	5	17

MEXICO

	1998	1999	2000	Total
Especialidades C.M.N. Siglo XXI, Transp Unit, Av Cuauhtemoc 330 Col Doctores, Zacatecas 36-113 Col Roma, Mexico City, DF 06720 Ph: (52) 5 538 4747 Fax: (52) 5 264 8711 Email: jlmelchoro@compuserve.com.mx 1) H. Aguirre-Gas, 2) C. Gracida, A. Lopez, J. Cancino, M. Sanmartin, 3) J.L. Melchor, A. Ibarra, 4) E. Romano	0	3		3
Hosp de Especialidades 71, Torreon, Inst Mexicano del Seguro Soc, Transp Unit-Dept of Surg, Torreon, Coahuila, 27000 Ph: (52)17 290800 Fax: (52)17 132679 1,2) F.J. Juarez de la Cruz, 2) Y. Barrios, M. Benavides, A. Gomez, A. Villarreal, 3) L. Cano, E. Chavez, R. Camacho, J. Martinez, E. Lopez, E. Fernandez, 4) M. Limones, C. Adalid, 5) L. Peniche, I. Espino	7	1	1	16

1)=Director, 2)=Tx Surgeons, 3)=Physicians, 4)=Tissue Typers, 5)=TxCoords	1998	1999	2000	Total
NETHERLANDS				
Univ Hosp Groningen, Dept of Surg, Hanzeplein 1, 9713 GZ Groningen Ph: (31)050 361 4470 Fax: (31)050 361 4873 Email: m.j.h.slooff@chir.azg.nl 1,2) M.J.H. Slooff, 2) P. Peeters, K.P. deJong, R.J. Porte, 3) I.J. Klompmaker, E. Haagsma, P.L. Jansen, A.P. vandenBerg, R. DeKnegt, 4) S.P.M. Lems, S. Hepkema, 5) E. Graveland, M. ElMoumni, A. Schuur	57	55	60	653
Univ Hosp Leiden, Dept of Surg, PO Box 9600, Leiden, 2300 RC Ph: (31)71 526 4005 Fax: (31)71 526 6746 Email: terpstra@lumc.nl 1,2) O.T. Terpstra, 2) J. Ringers, A. Baranski, 3) B. van Hoek, A. Masclee, R. Veenendaal, 4) F.J. Claas, 5) M.E. van Gurp	15	10		72
Univ Hosp "Dijkzigt", Dept of Surg, Dr Molewaterplein 40, 3015 GD Rotterdam, Rotterdam Ph: (31)10 463 3733 Fax: (31)10 463 5307 1,2) J.N.M. Ijzermans, 2) H.W. Tilanus, 3) H.J. Metselaar, 4) Eurotransp, 5) P. Pasma	27			202
NEW ZEALAND				
Auckland Hospital, New Zealand Liver Transp Unit, Park Road, Private Bag 92-024, Auckland Ph: (64) 9 307-4949 Fax: (64) 9 375-4345 Email: smunn@ahsl.co.nz 1,2) S. Munn, 2) J. McCall, P. Christie, 3) E. Gane, P. Wong, D. Rowbothan, 4) M. Ushakoff, 5) D. Kelly, V. Honeyman	13	27	33	73
NORWAY				
Rikshosp-The Nat'l Hosp, Dept of Ped/Surg/Med, Oslo, NO-0027 Ph: (47)2307 00 00 Fax: (47)2307 05 10 1,2) A. Bergan, 2) I. Brekke, B. Husberg, O. Bentdal, A. Foss, 3) E. Schrumpf, T. Sanengen, 4) E. Thorsby, T. Leivestad, 5) S. Foss, P.A. Bakkan, P.E. Vatsaas, K. Meyer	24	29	30	242
POLAND				
Childrens Health Ctr Memorial Insti, Surgery and Organ Transplant, Al.Dzieci Polskich 20, Warsaw - Miedzylesie, 04-736 Ph: (48)22 815 28 12 Fax: (48)22 815 28 12 1,2,3) P. Kalicinski, 2) A. Kaminski, A. Prokurat, 3) A. Kaminski, A. Prokurat, 4) B. Platosa, J. Gdowska, B. Juraczko-Paluchow, 5) E. Danielewska	10	9		47
PORTUGAL				
Hosp de Univ de Coimbra, Dept of Urol Transp, Praceta Prof Mota Pinto, 3000 Coimbra Ph: (351)239 403939 Fax: (351)239 400475 Email: urologiahuc@mail.telepac.po 1) L. Furtado, 2) F. Oliveira, E. Furtado, J.B. Geraldes, A. Reis, 3) R. Perdigoto, L. Tome, J. Ferrao, O. Mota, I. Goncalves, 4) F. Regateiro, A. Martinno, P. Santos, A. Paiva, 5) A.M. Calvao	62	47	51	370
H.C.L. (Curry Cabral), Transp Unit, Rua da Beneficencia, 8, 1069-166 Lisbon Ph: (351)1 797 5361 Fax: (351)1 797 5361 1,2) J.R. Pena, 2) E. Barroso, J.R. Andrade, A, Martins, 3) E. Monteiro, 4) H. Trindade, 5) C. DaCamara	22	44		148
Hosp Geral de Santo Antonio, Dept of Organ Transp, Largo Prof Abel Salazar, 4000 Porto Ph: (351)2 3325541 Fax: (351)2 3325541 Email: dto@hgsa.min-saude.pt 1,2) M. Caetano-Pereira, 2) V. Ribeiro, M. Teixeira, J. Tavares, R. Almeida, 3) H. Pessegueiro, R. Seca, 4) A. Mendes, P. Xavier, H. Alves, 5) R. Pereira, N. Valente	42	56	53	222
SOUTH AFRICA				
Groote Schuur Hosp Med Sch, Univ of Cape Town, Dept of Surg, Observatory 7925, Cape Town Ph: (27)21 404 3318 Fax: (27)21 448 6461 1,2) D. Kahn, 1,3) W. Spearman, 2) A.J.W. Millar, 4) E. DuToit, 5) F. McCurdie, E. Schmidt	8	4	12	106
SPAIN				
Hosp de Cruces, Unidad Hepato Transpl Hepatico, Plaza Cruces s/n, Baracaldo,Vizcaya, 48903 Ph: (34)94 600 6372 Fax: (34)94 600 6076 1) J. Ortiz-Urbina, 2) A. Valdivieso, M. Campo, L. Perdgo, M. Gastaca, G. Errasti, 3) J. Suarez, M. Testillano, J. Bustamante, M. Montejo, 4) G. Masdevall, 5) I. Lopez, F. Corral, P. Elorrieta	53	74	62	261

1)=Director, 2)=Tx Surgeons, 3)=Physicians, 4)=Tissue Typers, 5)=TxCoords	1998	1999	2000	Total
Hosp Clin I Prov de Barcelona, Dept of Surg, Villarroel 170, na, Barcelona, 08036 Ph: (34)932275711 Fax: (34)93227558 Email: juisa@medicina.ub.es 1) J. Visa i Miracle, 2) J. Garcia-Valdecasas, L. Grande, J. Fuster, A. Lacy, 3) A. Rimola, 4) V. Puiggros, 5) M. Manalich	77	79	73	794
Hosp Princeps D'Espanya, Dept of Surg, L'Hosp de Llobregat, Barcelona, 08907 Ph: (34)3 335 7011 Fax: (34)3 263 1561 Email: jfigueras@csub.scs.es 1,2) E. Jaurrieta, 2) J. Figueras, A. Rafecas, J. Fabregat, J. Torres, E. Ramos, 3) L. Casais, T. Casanovas, X. Xiol, C. Balliellas, J. Castellote, 4) J. Martorell, 5) C. Gonzalez, M. Pascual	65	60	63	620
Vall D'Hebron Hosp, Dept of Surg, Passeig Vall D'Hebron, Barcelona, 08035 Ph: (34)3 2746613 Fax: (34)3 2746112 1) C. Margarit, 2) J.L. Lazaro, E. Murio, R. Charco, 3) R. Esteban, J. Guardia, V. Vargas, 4) J. Martorell, 5) M. Mir, R. Deulofeu	43	55	53	430
University Hosp "Reina Sofia", Dept of Surg-Transp Unit, Avd Menendez Pidal 1, 14004 Cordoba Ph: (34)57 217228 Fax: (34)57 298033 1) C. Pera, 2) Rufian, Solorzano, Lopez-Cillero, Padillo-Ruiz, DiazIglesias, 3) M. Mata, G. Costan, G. Mino, E. Fraga, J.L. Montero, P. Barrera, 4) J. Pena Martinez, E. Munoz, R. Gonzalez, 5) J.C. Robles	39	48	43	451
"Doce de Octubre" Hosp Univ, Dept of Surg, Carr. Andalucia km 5.5, 28041 Madrid Ph: (34)1 3908329 Fax: (34)1 3908523 Email: morenog@mdoc.insalvd.es 1) E. Moreno Gonzalez, 2) I. Garcia, R. Gomez, I. Gonzalez-Pinto, C. Loinaz, C. Jimenez, 4) J. Martinez-Laso, 5) A. Andres, J.I. Rodicio	67	62	59	763
Infantil "La Paz" Hosp, Dept of Ped HepatologyNeph, Paseo de la Castellana #261, 28046 Madrid, 28020 Ph: (34)1 358 2600 Fax: (34)1 358 2545 1,3) P. Jara Vega, 2) M. Gamez, M. Lopez-Santamaria, J. Murcia, 3) M.C. Diaz, C. Cammarena, A. De La Vega, L. Hierro, E. Frauca, 5) A. Ballesteros	22	17	25	291
Puerta De Hierro, Dept of Surg, San Martin De Porres 4, Madrid, 28035 Ph: (34)1 3162240 Fax: (34)1 3737667 1,2) J. Ardaiz, 2) V.S. Turrion, M. Jimenez, L. Alvira, JL. Lucena, 3) V. Cuervas-Mons, C. Barrios, A. Garrido, 4) M. Moreno, 5) M.S. Bachiller, E. Gomez, C. Chamorro	36	34	28	511
Ramon y Cajal Hosp, Liver Transp Unit, Ctra de Colmenar, Km.9.1, Madrid, 28034 Ph: (34)1 336 8719 Fax: (34)1 336 8178 Email: emilvic@bitmailer.net 1,2) E. Vicente-Lopez, 2) J. Nuno, Y. Quijano, P. Lopez-Hervas, 3) L. Arbol, R. Barcena, M. Garcia, F. Garcia-Hoz, 4) A. Bootello, 5) A. Candela, S. Arevalillo, C. Mosacula	49	53	54	335
Virgen Arrixaca, Dept of Surg 3A, El Palmar, Murcia, 30120 Ph: (34)96 836 9677 Fax: (34)96 836 9716 Email: ramirezp@fcu.um.es 1) P. Parrilla, 2) P. Ramirez, R. Robles, Jm. Rodriguez, F. Sanchez-Bueno, J. Lujan, 3) M. Miras, J.A. Pons, 4) A.R. Alvarez, 5) R. Nunez	45	38	44	410
Clin Univ de Navarra, Dept of Gen/Gastro Surg, Pio XII Ave, Aptdo 192, Pamplona, Navarra, 31080 Ph: (34)48 255900 Fax: (34)48 172294 1) J.A. Cienfuegos, 2) F. Pardo, J.L. Hernandez, 3) J. Quiroga, B. Sangro, J.I. Herrero, 4) M.L. Subira	20	15	22	185
Hosp Xeral de Galicia, Unidad de Trasplantes, C/Galeras s/n, Santiago de Composte, 15705 Ph: (34)9 81 540218 Fax: (34)9 81 570102 1,2) E. Varo, 2) Bustamante, Conde, Martinez, Paredes, Segade, Punal, Blanco, 3) A. Brage, S. Tome, E. Otero, 4) M. Vega, 5) A. Marino, A. Vazquez	43			160
Hosp Univ La Fe, Valencia, Dept of Hepatica, Ave Campanar s/n, Valencia, 46009 Ph: (34)6 386-2700 Fax: (34)6 386-8789 Email: mir_jos@gva.es 1,2) J. Mir, 2) M. De Juan, F. San Juan, R. Lopez-Andujar, A. Moya, F. Orbis, J.J. Vila, 3) J. Berenguer, M. Prieto, D. Carrasco, M. Berenguer, 4) J. Montoro, 5) J.L. Vicente	109	106	112	710

SWEDEN

	1998	1999	2000	Total
Sahlgrenska Univ Hosp, Dept of Transpl and Liver Surg, su/Sahlgrenska, 41345 Gothenburg Ph: (46)31 3421000 Fax: (46)31 820557 1,2) M. Olausson, 2) L. Backman, S. Friman, L. Mjornstedt, 3) R. Olsson, M. Castedal, 4) L. Rydberg, 5) Wolfbrandt, Eriksson	58	46	44	508

1)=Director, 2)=Tx Surgeons, 3)=Physicians, 4)=Tissue Typers, 5)=TxCoords	1998	1999	2000	Total
Huddinge Univ Hospital, Dept Of Transplant Surgery, Stockholm, SE-14186 Ph: (46)8 58580000 Fax: (46)8 7743191 1,2) A. Tibell, 2) B.G. Ericson, 3) U. Broome, 4) E. Moller, 5) B. Blom	45	47	58	472
Karolinska Inst, Huddinge Hosp, Dept of Transp Surgery, Stockholm, S-141 86 Ph: (46)8 58580000 Fax: (46)8 774 3191 Email: Bo-Goran.Ericzon@transpl.hs.sll.se 1,2) B.G. Ericzon, 2) G. Soderdahl, 3) U. Broome, A. Oksanen, 4) E. Moller, 5) K. Larsson, M. Asplund	47	47	58	523
Univ Hosp Uppsala, Dept of Transp Surg, Unit 70TD, S-75185 Uppsala Ph: (46)18 664669 Fax: (46)18 559468 1,2) J. Wahlberg, 2) F. Duraj, J. Wadstrom, 3) B. Fellstrom, 4) O. Sjoberg, M. Bengtsson, 5) E. Bjorklund, I. Skarp, C. Moller	2	0	0	51

SWITZERLAND

	1998	1999	2000	Total
Univ Hosp Geneva, Dept of Surg, Transp Unit, 24 rue Micheli-du-Crest, 1211 Geneva 14 Ph: (41)22 372 7702 Fax: (41)22 372 7755 1,2) Ph. Morel, 2) G. Mentha, C. LeCoultre, O. Huber, P. Rajue, 3) D. Belli, E. Giostra, A. Hadengue, 4) C. Goumaz, 5) F. Roch, N. Decarpentry, I. Bohez	30	31	34	242
CHUV Univ Hosp, Dept of Surg, Lausanne, CH-1011 Ph: (41)21 314-1111 Fax: (41)21 314-2411 1,2) M. Gillet, 2) F. Mosimann, 3) J.J. Gonvers, 4) P. Schneider, V. Aubert, 5) G. Couedel, C. Gachet	16	20	15	146
Univ Hosp Zurich, Dept of Surg, Ramistr 100, Zurich, CH-8091 Ph: (41)1 255 3300 Fax: (41)1 255 4449 Email: clavien@chir.unizh.ch 1) P.A. Clavien, 2) Z. Kadry, N. Demartines, M. Weber, 3) E. Renner, 4) M. Weber, 5) P. Seeburger, T. Reh, M. Struker	19	14	13	142

TAIWAN

	1998	1999	2000	Total
Kaohsiung Chang Gung Mem Hosp, Dept of Surg, 123 Ta-Pei Rd, Niao-Sung, Kaohsiung, 83305 Ph: (886)7 731 7123 Fax: (886)7 732 4855 Email: clcltf@ms17.hinet.net 1,2) C.L. Chen, 2) Y.S. Chen, P.P. Liu, C.C. Wang, V.H. de Villa, 4) K.T. Hsu	11	17	31	105

TURKEY

	1998	1999	2000	Total
Baskent Univ Hosp, Dept of Gen Surg, I Cadde, No 77, Kat 4 Bahcelievler, Ankara, 06500 Ph: (90)312 212 6868 Fax: (90)312 215 0835 Email: melekk@baskent-ank.edu.tr 1,2) M. Haberal, 2) N. Bilgin, H. Karakayali, 3) S. Boyacioglu, 4) M. Turan, 5) H. Akkoc	11	8	6	60
Akdeniz Univ Med Sch Hosp, Dept of General Surgery, Dumlupinar Bulvari-Kampus, Antalya, 07060 Ph: (90)532 277 1485 Fax: (90)242 227 8837 1) T. Karpuzoglu, 2) N. Oygur, A. demirbas, K. Emek, 3) F. Isitan, I. Suleymanlar, 4) O. Yegin, M. Coskun, 5) N. Kececioglu	2	1		4
Cerrahpasa Med Faculty, Istanbul Univ, Organ Tranp Ctr (Nakil Merkezi), Dekanligi, Istanbul, 34303 Ph: (90)212 586 3532 Fax: (90)212 632 0050 1,2,5) O.F. Senyuz, 2) M. Sariyar, H. Kalafat, H. Tasci, 3) H. Senturk, A. Sonsuz, 4) E. Yilmaz, N, Celik, H. Baltali	3			19
Ege Univ, Organ Transp & Rsrch Ctr, Level 3, Bornova, Izmir Ph: (90)232 339-8838 Fax: (90)232 339-8838 Email: tokat@med.ege.edu.tr 1,2) H. Kaplan, 2) Y. Tokat, 3) Y. Batur, R. Yagli, U. Akarca, Z. Karasu, S. Aydogdu, 4) A. Keskinoglu, 5) A. Bozoklar	22	16	28	83

UNITED KINGDOM

	1998	1999	2000	Total
Queen Elizabeth Hosp, Liver Transp Unit, Edgbaston, Birmingham, B15 2TH Ph: (44)121 472-1311 Fax: (44)121 627-2412 1,2) P. McMaster, 2) J.A.C. Buckels, A.D. Mayer, D.F. Mirza, D. Candinas, 3) E. Elias, J.M. Neuberger, D.H. Adams, D.J. Mutimer, 5) A. Hooker, F. Wellington, T. Dudley, C. Stanton, M. Perrin, R. Breakweil	163	161	166	1979
Addenbrooke's Hosp, Transplant, Box No. 210, Hills Road, Cambridge, CB2 2QQ Ph: (441) 223-245151 Fax: (441) 223 216111 1,2) A. Bradley, 2) N. Jamieson, P. Gibbs, C. Watson, L. Delriviere, 3) A. Gimson, G. Alexander, 4) C. Taylor, 5) E. Bateman, N. Brown	70	75	57	1600

1)=Director, 2)=Tx Surgeons, 3)=Physicians, 4)=Tissue Typers, 5)=TxCoords	1998	1999	2000	Total
Royal Free Hosp, Dept of Surg, Liver Transp, Pond St, London, NW3 2QG Ph: (44)171 830 2198 Fax: (44)171 830 2198 1,2) K. Rolles, 2) B. Davidson, R. Robles, 3) A.K. Burroughs, D. Patch, 4) J.J. Beo, G. Shirling, 5) L. Selves, L. Davies, G. Amooty, Y. McGarry	61	59		598

LIVER Transplants

	1998	1999	2000	Total
United States	4,373	4,594	4,832	48,743
Foreign	3,829	4,116	3,901	40,435
Total	8,202	8,710	8,733	89,178

LIVER Transplant Centers

United States	103
Foreign	127
Total	230

LIVER

WORLDWIDE TRANSPLANT CENTER DIRECTORY
INTESTINE TRANSPLANTS

1)=Director, 2)=Tx Surgeons, 3)=Physicians, 4)=Tissue Typers, 5)=TxCoords	1998	1999	2000	Total

UNITED STATES

FLORIDA

Univ of Miami Sch of Med, Dept of Surgery Div Liver/GI, 1801 NW 9th Ave, Suite #511, PO Box 015809 (M840), Miami, FL 33136 Ph: (305) 355-5000 Fax: (305) 355-5161
1,2) A. Tzakis, 2) J.R. Nery, T. Kato, S. Nishida, J. Madariaga, D. Levi, 3) J. Thompson, N. Mittal, G. Neff, 4) V. Esquenazi, 5) O. Hung, L. Kravetz, R. Lavendera, S. Archie, J. Benedict, V. Cardenas

| | 2 | 8 | 7 | 26 |

NEBRASKA

Nebraska Health System, Dept of Surg, Transp Serv, 983285 Nebraska Medical Ctr, Omaha, NE 68198-3285 Ph: (402) 559-4076 Fax: (402) 559-3434
1,2) A.N. Langnas, 2) B.W. Shaw, D. Sudan, 3) M.F. Sorrell, J.A. Vanderhoof, S. Horslen, S. Mukherjee, 4) J. Wisecarver, S. Sheperd, 5) Williams, Rogge, Anderson, Zabrocki, Brown, Mahoney, Calabro, Weaver

| | 22 | 13 | 13* | 101 |

PENNSYLVANIA

UPMC-Presbyterian, Starzl Transplantation Inst, 4 Falk Clinic, 3601 5th Ave, Pittsburgh, PA 15213 Ph: (412) 648-3200 Fax: (412) 648-3085
1,2) T.E. Starzl, 1,2) J.J. Fung, 2) K. Abu-Elmagd, Bond, 3) S. Kusne, 4) R. Duquesnoy, A. Zeevi, 5) J. Colangelo

| | 4 | 5 | 14 | 59 |

WISCONSIN

Univ of Wisconsin, Dept of Surg, 600 Highland Ave, Madison, WI 53792
Ph: (608) 263-1385 Fax: (608) 262-5624
1,2) A. D'Alessandro, 2) M. Kalayoglu, S. Knechtle, 3) J. Pirsch, 4) H. Sollinger, 5) M. Armbrust, E. Spaith

| | 0 | 0 | 1* | 2 |

JAPAN

Kyoto University Hospital, Dept Of Transp Surg, 54 Kawara-Cho, Shogoin, Sakyo-Ku, Kyoto, 606-8507 Ph: (81)75 751 3660 Fax: (81)75 751 3616 Email: koichi@kuhp.kyoto-u.ac.jp
1,2) K. Tanaka, 2) S. Uemoto, H. Egawa, T. Kiuchi, M. Hayashi, 3) M. Nabeshima, 5) N. Iyama

| | 1 | 0 | 1 | 3 |

MEXICO

Especialidades C.M.N. Siglo XXI, Transp Unit, Av Cuauhtemoc 330 Col Doctores, Heriberto Frias 112-8 CP 03020, Mexico City, DF 06720 Ph: (52) 5 538 4747 Fax: (52) 5 264 8711 Email: jlmelchoro@compuserve.com.mx
1) H. Aguirre-Gas, 2) C. Gracida, A. Lopez, J. Cancino, M. Sanmartin, 3) J.L. Melchor, A. Ibarra, 4) E. Romano

| | 1 | 0 | | 1 |

Hosp de Especialidades 71, Torreon, Inst Mexicano del Seguro Soc, Transp Unit-Dept of Surg, Blvd Revolucion y Calle 27, Torreon, Coahuila, 27000 Ph: (52)17 322529 Fax: (52)17 322529
1,2) F.J. Juarez de la Cruz, 2) Y. Barrios, M. Benavides, A. Gomez, A. Villarreal, 3) L. Cano, R. Camacho, E. Chavez, E. Lopez, J. Martinez, E. Fernandez, 4) M. Limones, C. Adalid, 5) L. Peniche, I. Espino

| | 0 | 0 | 1 | 2 |

UNITED KINGDOM

Addenbrooke's Hosp, Dept of Surg, Level 9, Hills Rd, Cambridge, CB2 2QQ
Ph: (441)223 336976 Fax: (441)223 410772
1,3) J.A. Bradley, 2) N.V. Jamieson, C. Watson, P. Gibbs, L. Delriviere 3) G. Alexander, A. Gimson, 4) C. Taylor, 5) H. Luckhurst

| | 2 | 0 | 0 | 6 |

* Preliminary UNOS data

WORLDWIDE TRANSPLANT CENTER DIRECTORY
BONE MARROW / PERIPHERAL BLOOD TRANSPLANTS

1)=Director, 2)=Tx Surgeons, 3)=Physicians, 4)=Tissue Typers, 5)=TxCoords	1998	1999	2000	Total

UNITED STATES

ARIZONA

Univ Med Ctr, C Glasby, 1501 N Campbell Ave, Tucson, AZ 85724
Ph: (520) 694-4984 Fax: (520) 694-4983 Email: cglasby@umcaz.edu
1,3) A.F. List, 1,3) M. Graham, 3) C. Taylor, A. Briggs, E. Epner, E. Katsanis, 4) C. Spier,
5) K. Nordorp, N. O'Connor, A. Villela, C. Noirot

	1998	1999	2000	Total
	90	88	82	521

ARKANSAS

Univ Hosp of Arkansas, Arkansas Cancer Rsrch Ctr, Dept of Med/Hem/Onc, 4301 W Markham
Slot 508, Little Rock, AR 72205 Ph: (501) 686-7000 Fax: (501) 686-6442
1,3) S. Jagannath, 3) D.H. Vesole, G. Tricot, D. Siegel, 4) UAMS, 5) N. Copeland, J. Hilton

	1998	1999	2000	Total
		37		226

CALIFORNIA

Alta Bates Med Ctr, Blood and Marrow Tx Program, 2001 Dwight Way, Berkeley, CA 94704
Ph: (510) 204-6401 Fax: (510) 204-6440
1,3) J.L. Wolf, 3) G.R. Cecchi, M. Tracy, D. Irwin, 4) B. Trachtenberg, 5) S. Gooding, C. Ruttan

	1998	1999	2000	Total
	3	1	3	98

City of Hope Nat'l Med Ctr, Hem/Bone Marrow Transp, 1500 E Duarte Rd, Duarte, CA 91010
Ph: (626) 359-8111 Fax: (626) 301-8256
1,3) S.J. Forman, 3) Nademanee, O'Donnell, Snyder, Parker, Stein, Molina, Kashyap, et al,
4) D. Senitzer, 5) Fonbuena, Littrell, Blaylock, Egner, Woo, Stevensen, Krupka

	1998	1999	2000	Total
	173	169	217	1864

Children's Hosp Los Angeles, Rsrch Immun/Bone Marrow Transp, 4650 Sunset Blvd, Box 62,
Los Angeles, CA 90027 Ph: (323) 669-2546 Fax: (323) 660-1904
1,3) R. Parkman, 3) K. Weinberg, D. Kohn, G. Crooks, N. Kapoor, R. Seeger, A. Butturini,
4) A. Jenkins, J. Tagliere, 5) K. Wilson, D. Dellerck

	1998	1999	2000	Total
	31	28	37	471

Kaiser Foundation Hosp, Ped Int Med/Div of BMT, 4700 Sunset Blvd, Los Angeles, CA 90027
Ph: (323) 783-5414 Fax: (323) 783-7266
1,3) P.M. Falk, 1,3) N. Kogut, 3) F. Sahebi, W. Loui, 4) City of Hope, 5) S. Desposito, M. Hurst,
R. Kelble

	1998	1999	2000	Total
	22	20		231

Univ Calif-Los Angeles Med Ctr, Dept of Peds, 10833 LeConte Ave, Los Angeles, CA
90095-1752 Ph: (310) 825-6708 Fax: (310) 206-8089 Email: sfeig@mednet.ucla.edu
1,3) S.A. Feig, 3) C. Denny, K. Sakamoto, S. Dovat, T. Moore, 4) UCLA Immunogenetics Center,
5) S. Brown

	1998	1999	2000	Total
	10	14	11	464

Univ Calif-Los Angeles Med Ctr, Dept of Hem/Onc, 10833 LeConte Ave, Rm 42-121 CHS,
Los Angeles, CA 90095-1678 Ph: (310) 206-5755 Fax: (310) 206-5511
1,3) M. Territo, 3) Schiller, Feig, Paquette, Emmanouilides, Sawyers, Denny, Sakamoto,
4) UCLA Immunogenetics Center, 5) S. Rasti, T. Lambert

	1998	1999	2000	Total
	60	49	48	1445

Children's Hosp of Orange County, Dept of Hem/Onc, BMT, 455 S Main St, Orange, CA 92868
Ph: (714) 532-8884 Fax: (714) 532-8504
1,3) S. Neudorf, 3) Shen, Kempert, Nugent, Young, Kirov, Sender, 4) UCLA Immunogenetics Center,
5) D. Crumly, S. Rhodes, L. Murphy

	1998	1999	2000	Total
	14	30	25	283

Stanford Univ Hosp, Dept of Med, 300 Pasteur Dr, Stanford, CA 94305
Ph: (650) 723-0822 Fax: (650) 725-8950
1,3) R.S. Negrin, 3) K.G. Blume, L.J. Johnson, J.A. Shizuru, K. Stockerl-Goldstein, M. Jain,
4) C. Grumet, 5) S. Moore, S. Lambert, A. Johns, M. Bloom

	1998	1999	2000	Total
	66	81	83	800

Children's Hosp San Diego, Dept of Hem/Onc, 3020 Children's Way, mc/5035, San Diego, CA
92123 Ph: (858) 966-5811 Fax: (858) 495-853 Email: rkadota@chsd.org
1,3) R.P. Kadota, 3) J.B. Allen, W.D. Roberts, D.E. Schiff, M.I. McManus, 4) Scripps Clinic, UCLA

	1998	1999	2000	Total
	6	2	2	92

672

1)=Director, 2)=Tx Surgeons, 3)=Physicians, 4)=Tissue Typers, 5)=TxCoords	1998	1999	2000	Total
Univ Calif-San Francisco, Ped Bone Marrow Transp Div, 505 Parnassus Ave, PO Box 1278, Rm M-659, San Francisco, CA 94143-1278 Ph: (415) 476-2188 Fax: (415) 502-4867 Email: pedibmt@peds.ucsf.edu 1) M.J. Cowan, 3) B. Horn, M. Koerper, W. Mentzer, K. Matthay, 4) L. Baxter-Lowe, 5) L.Z. Abramovitz, D. Norstad	45	37	40	442
Univ Calif-San Francisco, Dept of Med, 400 Parnassus Ave A502, San Francisco, CA 94143 Ph: (415) 476-1220 Fax: (415) 502-0465 1) C. Linker, 3) L. Damon, H. Rugo, C. Ries, 4) L.A. Baxter-Louie, 5) S. Coleman, B. Mazzini, F. Agudello		152		335

COLORADO

	1998	1999	2000	Total
Presbyterian, St Luke's Med Ctr, Bone Marrow Transp Prog, 1719 E 19th Ave, Denver, CO 80218 Ph: (303) 839-6953 Fax: (303) 869-2531 1,3) R. Rifkin, 3) J. Matous, M. Brunvand, 4) Immunological Assoc of Denver, 5) R. Campo, P. Odem.P. Wagner	23	20	33	124
The Children's Hosp-Denver, Dept of Hem/Onc/BMT, B115, Univ Colorado Sch of Med, 1056 E 19th Ave, Denver, CO 80218 Ph: (303) 861-6892 Fax: (303) 864-5158 1,3) R.H. Giller, 3) B. Greffe, A. Hayward, R. Quinones, N. Foreman, B. Garcea, T. Garrington, 4) B. Freed, R. McCalmon, 5) B. Pasut, S. Rottman	40	32	33	206

CONNECTICUT

	1998	1999	2000	Total
John Dempsey Hosp, Univ of Connecticut Hlth Ctr, 263 Farmington Ave, Farmington, CT 06030 Ph: (860) 679-4410 Fax: (860) 679-4491 1,3) P. Tutschka, 3) A. Bilgrami, R. Edwards, J. Feingold, R. Bona, Z. Li, 4) R. Edwards, 5) S. Hensel, M. Gallo	21	19		126
Yale Univ-New Haven Hosp, Dept of Med, 333 Cedar St, #211WWW, New Haven, CT 06520 Ph: (203) 737-5751 Fax: (203) 785-7531 1,3) D. Cooper, 3) J. McGuirk, S. Seropian, 4) Connecticut Red Cross	23			143

DISTRICT OF COLUMBIA

	1998	1999	2000	Total
Children's Hosp Nat'l Med Ctr, Dept of Hem/Onc, 111 Michigan Ave NW, Washington, DC 20010-2970 Ph: (202) 884-2800 Fax: (202) 884-5685 1,3) N. Kamani, 3) P. Dinndorf, E. Perez-Albuerne, 4) Johns Hopkins Univ, 5) K. Ayers, S. Malone	14	28	22	209
Georgetown Univ Hosp, Bone Marrow Transp, 2 East Main Bldg, 3800 Reservoir Rd NW, Washington, DC 20007 Ph: (202) 687-2253 Fax: (202) 784-3655 Email: yanovichs@georgetown.edu 1) S. Yanovich, 3) K. Meehan, 4) S. Rosen-Bronson, 5) J. Dugan	20	9	2	217

FLORIDA

	1998	1999	2000	Total
Shands at the Univ of Florida, Transplant Center, Box 100251, 1600 SW Archer Road, Gainesville, FL 32610-0251 Ph: (352) 265-0130 Fax: (352) 265-0108 1,3) J.R. Wingard, 3) Moreb, Reddy, Graham-Pole, Kedar, Sleasman, Skoda-Smith, Finiewicz, 4) J. Scornik, 5) M. Youngblood, B. Gaa, J. Luzins, M. Doran	54	61	72	627
All Children's Hosp, Dept of Bone Marrow Transp, 801 6th St S Box 6990, St Petersburg, FL 33701 Ph: (727) 892-4235 Fax: (727) 892-8619 1,3) M.R. Klemperer, 3) R.A. Good, H.C. Rossbach, N. Grana, R.A. Cahill, 4) Y. Chang, L. Desai, 5) P. Clark, S. Sharf	13	12	22	215
H Lee Moffitt Cancer Ctr, Bone Marrow Transp Serv, 12902 Magnolia Dr, Tampa, FL 33612 Ph: (813) 979-7202 Fax: (813) 979-3071 1,3) K.K. Fields, 3) Goldstein, Sullivan, Dalton, Djulbegovic, Alsina, Smith, Dalton, 4) K. Benson, 5) K. Daily, A. Davis, B. O'Leary	38	24	38	284

GEORGIA

	1998	1999	2000	Total
Children's Healthcare of Atlanta, Dept of Ped Hem/Onc/BMT, 2040 Ridgewood Dr, NE, Ste #100, Atlanta, GA 30322 Ph: (404) 727-4451 Fax: (404) 727-4455 1,3) A. Yeager, 3) T. Olson, C. Alvavado, M. Briones, 4) R.A. Bray, 5) K. Applegate, C. Brown, M. Lauer, E. Olson	22	19		151

1)=Director, 2)=Tx Surgeons, 3)=Physicians, 4)=Tissue Typers, 5)=TxCoords	1998	1999	2000	Total
Emory Univ Hosp, Bone Marrow & Stem Cell Transp, The Emory Clin, Bldg B-6200, 1365 Clifton Rd NE, Atlanta, GA 30322 Ph: (404) 778-4189 Fax: (404) 778-3904 1,3) E.K. Waller, 3) I. Redei, A, Langston, S. Bucur, 4) R. Bray, 5) P. Smith, V. Bartlett, D. Teagarden	41	71		644

ILLINOIS

	1998	1999	2000	Total
Children's Mem Hosp, Siragusa Transplant Center, 2300 Children's Plaza, Box 57, Chicago, IL 60614 Ph: (773) 975-8643 Fax: (773) 975-3019 Email: siragusatx@childrensmemorial.org 1,3) M. Kietzel, 3) P. Haut, R. Duerst, 5) K. Coyne, K. VanSycle	34	64	74	382
Rush-Presbyterian-St Luke's Med Ctr, Bone Marrow Transp Ctr, 1653 W Congress Pkwy, Chicago, IL 60612 Ph: (312) 942-3047 Fax: (312) 733-1590 1,3) H. Klingemann, 3) T. Rodriguez, R. Meagher, A. Lakahni, E. Robin, 4) H. Gebel, 5) S. Davies, C. Havey	28	27	45	251
Univ of Chicago Children's Hospital, Dept of Ped Hem/Onc, MC-4060, 5841 S Maryland Ave, Chicago, IL 60637 Ph: (773) 702-6808 Fax: (773) 702-9881 1,3,5) C.M. Rubin, 3) J. Nachman, U. Subramanian, R. Rudinsky, E. Beyer, 4) American Red Cross (Milwaukee, WI)	10	2	2	184
Univ of Chicago Med Ctr, Dept of Adult Hem/Onc, MC 2115, 5841 S Maryland Ave, Chicago, IL 60637 Ph: (773) 702-6783 Fax: (773) 702-4889 1,3) R. Larson, 3) C. Daugherty, T. Zimmerman, D. Grinblatt, W. Stock, O. Odenike, 4) Am Red Cross Blood Serv(Madison, WI), 5) B. Weseman, C. Tazic, J. Collins, P. Sibley	28	22	23	382
Loyola Univ Cancer Ctr, Sect of Hem/Onc, 2160 S First Ave, Bldg 112, Rm 240, Maywood, IL 60153 Ph: (708) 327-3148 Fax: (708) 327-3220 1,3) P. Stiff, 3) R. Bayer, D. Malhotra, 4) B. Susskind, 5) P. Schumacker, S. Ingram	25	49	30	308

INDIANA

	1998	1999	2000	Total
Indiana Univ & J Whitcomb Riley Hosp, Bone Marrow Transplant, 1044 West Walnut Street, Room 202/402, Indianapolis, IN 46202 Ph: (317) 274-0843 Fax: (317) 278-2262 1,3) K. Cornetta, 1) F. Smith, 3) R. Abonour, R. Hromas, M. Robertson, K. Robertson, B. Thomson, R. Nelson, 4) Z. Brahmi, 5) J. Baute, K. Stancomb	34	40	39	510
Methodist Hosp of Indiana, Inc, Cancer Ctr, I-65 at 21st St, Indianapolis, IN 46206-1367 Ph: (317) 929-3400 Fax: (317) 929-2908 1,3) J. Jansen, 1,3) L. Akard, J. Thompson, 3) M. Dugan, 4) J. McIntyre, 5) S. Burns, M. Swinney	25	28		222

IOWA

	1998	1999	2000	Total
Univ of Iowa Hosp & Clin, Dept of Int Med, 200 Hawkins Dr, Iowa City, IA 52242 Ph: (319) 356-3425 Fax: (319) 353-8383 1,3) R.D. Gingrich, 3) R. Hohl, C.K. Lee, M. Silverman, J. Buatli, 4) N. Goeken, L. Field, 5) S. Locher, K. Ajram, S. Johannsen, B. Kaufman	47	46	55	994
Univ of Iowa Hosp & Clin, Dept of Ped, 200 Hawkins Dr, 2514 JCP, Iowa City, IA 52242 Ph: (319) 356-7360 Fax: (319) 356-7659 Email: frederick-goldman@uiowa.edu 1,3) F. Goldman, 3) T. Kisker, T. Loew, R. Tannous, S. O'Dorisio, J. DiPaola, 4) E. Field, N. Goeken, 5) J.A. Miller	11	9	9	352

KANSAS

	1998	1999	2000	Total
Univ of Kansas Med Ctr, Div of Hem, 3901 Rainbow Blvd, Kansas City, KS 66160-7233 Ph: (913) 588-6077 Fax: (913) 588-3996 1,3) B. Skikne, 3) J. Cook, D. Bodensteiner, D. Deauna-Limayo, 4) Midwest Organ Bank, 5) M. Boman, S. Fulkerson	10	16	9	264
St Francis-Via Christi, Dept of Onc Serv, Bone Marrow Tx Program, 929 N St Francis, Wichita, KS 67214 Ph: (316) 268-5628 Fax: (316) 291-7855 Email: beverly_randall@via-christi.org 1,3) D. Johnson, 3) D. Moore Jr, B. Mattar, 4) C. Bryan-Midwest Organ Bank, 5) B. Randall, K. Pouch	5	10	13	76

KENTUCKY

	1998	1999	2000	Total
Univ of Kentucky Med Ctr, Markey Cancer Ctr, Dept of Med Div of Hem/Onc, CC 301, 800 Rose St, Lexington, KY 40536 Ph: (859) 323-5768 Fax: (859) 323-8990 1,3) G.L. Phillips, 3) D. Reece, D. Howard, 4) D. Jennings, J. Thompson, F. Lower, 5) Marshall, Bibby, Plummer, Caldwell, Witt, Hargis, Napier, Hidalgo	91	81		816

BONE MARROW / PERIPHERAL BLOOD TRANSPLANTS

674

1)=Director, 2)=Tx Surgeons, 3)=Physicians, 4)=Tissue Typers, 5)=TxCoords	1998	1999	2000	Total
Univ of Louisville Hospital, Blood & Marrow Transplant Prog, Brown Cancer Ctr, Rm 230, 529 S Jackson St, Louisville, KY 40202 Ph: (800) 234-2689 Fax: (502) 562-4374 1,3) R.H. Herzig, 3) G. Goldsmith, D. Fleming, D. Stevens, 4) J. Klein, 5) J. Nix	20	36		247
LOUISIANA				
Children's Hosp, New Orleans, Dept of Ped, Div of Hem/Onc at LSUMC, 200 Henry Clay Ave, New Orleans, LA 70118 Ph: (504) 896-9740 Fax: (504) 896-9758 Email: lyu@lsuhsc.edu 1,3) L.C. Yu, 3) R. Gardner, D. Ode, M. Velez, 5) M. Potter	9	11	10	75
MASSACHUSETTS				
Children's Hosp, Boston, Dana-Farber Cancer Inst., Dept of Hem/Onc, 300 Longwood, Boston, MA 02115 Ph: (617) 632-3961 Fax: (617) 632-1990 1,3) E. Guinan, 3) Guinan, Lehmann, Parsons, Tse, Haining, Irwin, Mueller, Kung, 4) E. Yunis, 5) M. Kearney	42	44	36	524
Dana Farber Cancer Inst, 44 Binney St, Boston, MA 02115 Ph: (617) 632-2525 Fax: (617) 632-5175 1,3) J. Antin, 3) Soiffer, Alyea, Lee, Schlossman, Gilliland, Gribben, Freedman, 4) E. Yunis, E. Milford, 5) M. Tillman, P. DaCosta, T. Harris	115	333	266	1191
Massachusetts Gen Hosp, Dept of Med, 32 Fruit St, Boston, MA 02114 Ph: (617) 724-1124 Fax: (617) 724-1126 1,3) T.R. Spitzer, 3) S. McAfee, R. Sackstein, B. Dey, 4) S. Saidman, 5) C. Campbell, P. Perrino	27	40	27	132
New England Med Ctr, Div of Hem/Onc, Box 542, 750 Washington St, Boston, MA 02111 Ph: (617) 636-6520 Fax: (617) 636-4627 1,3) K. Miller, 3) D. Schenkein, J. Erban, K. Sprague, E. Berkman, 4) A. Rabson, 5) A. Klekar, D. Mogavero	51	44	47	370
MICHIGAN				
Univ of Michigan Med Ctr, Dept of Bone Marrow Transp, Comprehensive Cancer Ctr BI-207, Box 0914, Ann Arbor, MI 48109-0914 Ph: (734) 936-8785 Fax: (734) 936-8788 1) J. Ferrara, 2) R. Hutchinson, J. Uberti, 3) G. Yanik, V. Ratanatharathorn, J. Levine, L. Ayash, K. Cooke, M. Clarke, 5) J. Weick, P. Steele, P. Parker, K. Kyro, S. Anuszkiewicz	113	122	228	844
Detroit Med Ctr-Wayne State Univ, Karmanos Cancr Ins-Harper Hosp, Dept of Hem/Onc-BMT, 3990 John R St-4 Brush South, Detroit, MI 48201-0188 Ph: (313) 993-0205 Fax: (313) 966-8069 1,3) R. Baynes, 2) D. Bouwman, D. Weaver, 3) D. Klein, R. Dansey, E. Abella, C. Hamm, 4) D. Kukuruga, 5) K. McAlpine, M. Flowers, C. Couwlier, D. Jones, D. Monso-Albig	48	56	63	816
MINNESOTA				
Fairview Univ Med Ctr, Dept of Peds/Adult-Div BMT, Box 366 UMHC, 420 Delaware St SE, Minneapolis, MN 55455 Ph: (612) 626-2961 Fax: (612) 626-4074 1,3) N. Ramsay, 1) D. Weisdorf, 3) S. Davies, J. Wagner, P. Orchard, B. Blazar, Kersey, Peters, Krivit, 4) M. Segall, H. Noreen, 5) J. Howard, S. Roell	125	143	152	2330
Mayo Clinic, BMT, CH9, Rm 9-269, 200 1st St SW, Rochester, MN 55905 Ph: (507) 284-4100 Fax: (507) 266-2855 1,3) M.R. Litzow, 3) D.J. Inwards, M.A. Gertz, A. Tefferi, D.A. Gastineau, M.Q. Lacy, 4) S.B. Moore, S. DeGoey, 5) M. Skaar	32	37	61	410
MISSOURI				
St Louis Children's Hosp, Dept of Hem/Onc, One Children's Pl, Box 8116, St Louis, MO 63110 Ph: (314) 454-4240 Fax: (314) 454-2780 1,2) R. Hayashi, 3) Debaun, Jones, Shenoy, Wilson, Kelly, Crawford, 4) B.A. Zehnbauer, 5) C. Ball	12	10	11	70
NEBRASKA				
Univ of Nebraska Med Ctr, Dept of Internal Med-BMT Unit, 987680 Nebraska Med Ctr, Omaha, NE 68198-7680 Ph: (402) 559-5166 Fax: (402) 559-6520 1,3) E. Reed, 3) S. Tarantolo, P. Coccia, S. Pavlectic, J. Vose, P. Bierman, G. Bociek, 4) A. Larsen, 5) K. Grauf, S. Nuss, S. Shannon, K. Maher, C. Heinzen, K. Byar, T. Lee	47	53	3	493

1)=Director, 2)=Tx Surgeons, 3)=Physicians, 4)=Tissue Typers, 5)=TxCoords	1998	1999	2000	Total
Univ of Nebraska Med Ctr-Ped Prog, Dept of Peds, Sec of Onc/Hem, 600 S 42nd St, Omaha, NE 68198-2168 Ph: (402) 559-7257 Fax: (402) 559-6782 1,3) P.F. Coccia, 3) B. Gordon, P. Warkentin, J. Harper, M. Abromowitch, A. Grovas, 4) A. Larsen, J. Wisecarver, R. Rubocki, 5) K. Grauf, S.Nuss.N. Andrews	11	8	6	149
NEW JERSEY				
St Joseph's Hosp & Med Ctr, Dept of Hem/Onc, 703 Main St, Paterson, NJ 07503 Ph: (973) 754-2432 Fax: (973) 754-2444 1,3) A.D. Rubin, 3) G. Rubin, 4) Labcorp, 5) S. Stives	11	21		56
NEW YORK				
Roswell Park Cancer Inst, Dept of Med, Elm & Carlton St, Buffalo, NY 14263-0001 Ph: (716) 845-8707 Fax: (716) 845-3272 1,3) P. McCarthy, 3) Baer, Wetzler, Slack, Czuczman, Bernstein, Bambach, Chandan-Khan, 4) F. Orsini, 5) C. Keesler, B. Anderson, K. Dubel	22	26	37	315
Mem Sloan-Kettering Cancer Ctr, Dept of Ped, 1275 York Ave, New York, NY 10021 Ph: (212) 639-5957 Fax: (212) 717-3447 1,3) R.J. O'Reilly, 3) N. Kernan, E. Papadopoulos, J. Young, T. Small, S. Nimer, F. Boula, 4) B. Dupont, V. Prasad, D. George, 5) P. Walka, C. Landrey	95	87		1712
Mount Sinai Med Ctr, Bone Marrow Transp, Box 1410, 1 Gustave Levy Pl, New York, NY 10029 Ph: (212) 241-6021 Fax: (212) 410-0978 Email: steven_fruchtman@smtplink.mssm.edu 1,3) S. Fruchtman, 3) E. Scigliano, A. Vlachos, L. Isola, 4) Mt Sinai Hosp Bld Bank, 5) G. Ross, A. Rodriguez, L. Leeder	36	25		209
Westchester Cnty Med Ctr, Dept of Onc, NY Med Coll, Munger-Rm 250, Valhalla, NY 10595 Ph: (914) 493-8374 Fax: (914) 594-4420 1,3) T. Ahmed, 3) F. Ozakaynak, K. Seiter, R. Kancherla, D. Liu, A. Mannanchorn, 4) I. Argani, 5) M. Fradkin, L. Kastuk	63	24		347
OHIO				
Cleveland Clin Fnd, Dept of Hem/Onc, 9500 Euclid Ave, Cleveland, OH 44195 Ph: (216) 445-6538 Fax: (216) 445-7444 1,3) B.J. Bolwell, 3) S. Andresen, A. Lichtin, B. Overmoyer, B.L. Pohlman, M. Kalaycioglu, 4) D. Cook, 5) K. Sands, J. Curtis, K. Wise, M. Serafin	50	70	65	601
Univ Hosp of Cleveland, Dept of Hem/Onc, 11100 Euclid Ave, Cleveland, OH 44106 Ph: (216) 844-3629 Fax: (216) 844-5979 1,3) H.M. Lazarus, 3) B. Cooper, S.L. Gerson, M. Nieder, O. Koc, M. Laughlin, 4) N. Greenspan, 5) J. Carlson, S. Erinc	31	30	34	413
A G James Cancer Hosp & Rsrch Inst, Internal Med/Bone Marrow Trans, The OH St Univ Med Ctr,320W 10Th Ave, A437A Starling-Loving Hall, Columbus, OH 43210 Ph: (614) 293-8939 Fax: (614) 293-3074 1,3) S. Farag, 3) B. Avalos, S. Penza, 4) C. Orosz, 5) P. Belt, G. Risley	47	54	46	601
OKLAHOMA				
The Univ Hosp, Bone Marrow Transp Unit, PO Box 26307, Oklahoma City, OK 73126 Ph: (405) 271-4022 Fax: (405) 271-3020 1,3) G. Selby, 3) V. Roy, T. Carter, R. Hassan, 4) Y. Choo, 5) N. Sylvester	38	42	31	384
PENNSYLVANIA				
Children's Hosp of Philadelphia, Dept of Onc/Bone Marrow Transp, 34th & Civic Ctr Blvd, Rm 9097B, Philadelphia, PA 19104 Ph: (215) 590-2141 Fax: (215) 590-4183 1,3) N. Bunin, 3) S. Grupp, K. Nichols, 4) Childrens Hosp of Phila Immunogenetics, 5) D. Artis, A. Kalmus	51	67	79	722
Hahnemann Univ Hosp, Dept of Neoplastic Disease, Broad & Vine St, MS 412, Philadelphia, PA 19102 Ph: (215) 762-7026 Fax: (215) 762-8857 1,3) P. Crilley, 1,2) J.Brodsky 3) D. Topolsky, M. Styler, D. Gladstone, 4) S. Hsu, 5) L. Cathay, C. Dufendach	27	20	10	412

BONE MARROW / PERIPHERAL BLOOD TRANSPLANTS

1)=Director, 2)=Tx Surgeons, 3)=Physicians, 4)=Tissue Typers, 5)=TxCoords	1998	1999	2000	Total
Jeanes Hosp/Temple Univ Health Sys, Fox Chase-Temple Bone Marrow, Friends Hall Physicians Bldg, 7640 Central Ave., Ground Fl., Philadelphia, PA 19111-2442 Ph: (215) 214-3100 Fax: (215) 214-3131 Email: mangank@tuhs.temple.edu 1,3) K.F. Mangan, 3) T.R. Klumpp, P.J. Sabol, J.H. Herman, 4) S. Leech, S. Hsu, 5) C. Miller	18	10	19	157
Univ of Pennsylvania Hosp, Hem/Onc Div, 3400 Spruce St, 6 Penn Tower, Philadelphia, PA 19104 Ph: (215) 662-7909 Fax: (215) 662-4064 Email: stadtman@mail.med.upenn.edu 1,3) E. Stadtmauer, 2) G. Buzby, 3) S. Luger, A. Gewirtz, D. Porter, S. Schuster, G. Laport, 4) M. Kamoun, 5) P. Mangan	21	27	44	123
The Western Pennsylvania Hosp, Cancer Institute, 4800 Friendship Ave, Suite 2303NT, Pittsburgh, PA 15224 Ph: (412) 578-4355 Fax: (412) 578-4391 Email: jlister@wpahs.org 1) J. Lister, 3) Z.R. Zeigler, R.K. Shadduck, J.R. Gryn, J.M. Raymond, 4) Lab Corp of America, UPMC, 5) R.A. Yasko, L.A. Persichetti	37	33	29	288
Univ of Pittsburgh MedCtr/Montefiore, Univ.of Pittsburgh Cancer Inst, Adult Bone Marrow Transp Prog, 200 Lothrop St, Pittsburgh, PA 15213 Ph: (412) 648-6430 Fax: (412) 648-6650 1,3) D. Buchbarker, 3) E. McGuire, 4) A. Zeevi, 5) M. Burgunder, C. Oriss	4	5		37
UPMC/Montefiore, Univ Of Pittsburgh Cancer Inst, Adult Bone Marrow Transplant Prog, 200 Lothrop St, Pittsburgh, PA 15213 Ph: (412) 648-6430 Fax: (412) 648-6650 1) A. Yeager, 3) D. Buchbarker, M. Carroll, M. Aghe, C. Evans, 4) A. Zeevi, 5) M. Burgunder, C. Oriss	3	3	22	249

TENNESSEE

	1998	1999	2000	Total
St.Jude Children's Rsrch Hosp, Dept of Hem/Onc-BMT, 332 N Lauderdale, Memphis, TN 38101 Ph: (901) 495-2529 Fax: (901) 526-7151 1,3) L. Bowman, 3) J. Cunningham, E. Horwitz, E. Benaim, P. Shearer, Woodard, Hale, Leung, 4) V. Turner, 5) S. Richardson, W. Rayburn	65	22		380
Vanderbilt Univ Med Ctr, Bone Marrow Transp Prog, 2617 TVC, Nashville, TN 37232-5505 Ph: (615) 936-1803 Fax: (615) 936-0382 Email friedrich.schuening@ncmail.vanderbilt.edu 1) F. Schuening, 3) R.S. Stein, S. Goodman, D. Morgan, J. Greer, S. Wolff, 4) DCI Labs, 5) V. Welch, E. Benneyworth, A. Galloway, S. Sims	110	117	113	917

TEXAS

	1998	1999	2000	Total
Baylor Univ Med Ctr, Dept of Hem/Onc/BMT, 3409 Worth St, Suite 600, Sammons Tower, Dallas, TX 75246 Ph: (214) 820-2619 Fax: (214) 820-7346 Email: artr@baylordallas.edu 1,3) E.D. Agura, 3) L.A. Pineiro, J.W. Fay, E.A. Vance, 4) O. Smith, 5) L. Brougher, L. Best, B. Reasonover, L. Sanden	71	72		768
Medical City Dallas Hospital, Bldg D400, 7777 Forest Lane, Bldg-A, 12-South, Dallas, TX 75230 Ph: (972)566-6547/5667790 Fax: (972) 566-3897 1,2) C. Rosenfeld, 1,2) C. Lenarsky, 3) Weinthal, S. Goldman, 4) Baylor Immunology Lab, 5) M. Hooker, M. Sutton	24	12	8	93
M D Anderson Cancer Ctr, Dept of BMT, Univ of Texas-Houston, 1515 Holcombe Blvd, Box 24, Houston, TX 77030 Ph: (713) 792-8750 Fax: (713) 794-4902 1,3) R. Champlin, 2) B. Andersson, J. Gajewski, M. Donato, P. Anderlini, 3) Korbling, Chan, Claxton, Giralt, Khouri, Ueno, Braunschweig, 4) H. Fischer, 5) Stone	259	232		2038
Texas Children's Hosp, Dept of Allergy/Immun, 6621 Fannin, MC 1-3291, Houston, TX 77030 Ph: (832) 824-1319 Fax: (832) 825-1260 1,3) W.T. Shearer, 1,3) H.M. Rosenblatt, 3) S.L. Abramson, M.E. Paul, 4) G.E. Rodey, 5) K. Owl	39	2	6	240
Wilford Hall Med Ctr/MMIB, Dept of Hem/Med Onc, 2200 Bergquist Dr, Ste 1, Lackland AFB, TX 78236-5300 Ph: (210) 292-3820/3709 Fax: (210) 292-7686 1,3) D. Ornstein, 3) Ririe, Shaughnessy, 4) E. Menchaca, 5) J. DeChavez, I. Coronado	29	27	35	400
Santa Rosa Childrens Hosp, Univ of Texas HSC, Stem Cell Transplant Program, 519 W. Houston St., 8th floor, San Antonio, TX 78207 Ph: (210) 704-3458 Fax: (210) 704-2396 1) N.R. Kamani, 3) P. Thomas, A.M. Langevin, S. Weitman, J. Kane, 5) L. Worsham	13			130
UTHSCA, Dept of Med, Div of Hem, 7703 Floyd Curl Dr, Mail code 7880, San Antonio, TX 78229-3900 Ph: (210) 617-5268 Fax: (210) 617-5271 1,3) C. Freytes, 2) J.P. Dorman, 3) T. Tsai, N. Callander, J.E. Anderson, 4) M. Pollack, 5) P. Harris, J. Blyle	13	14	19	200

1)=Director, 2)=Tx Surgeons, 3)=Physicians, 4)=Tissue Typers, 5)=TxCoords	1998	1999	2000	Total
VIRGINIA				
Med Coll of Virginia, Dept of Hem/Onc, Box 980157 MCV, 1300 E. Marshall St., Richmond, VA 23298 Ph: (804) 828-4360 Fax: (804) 828-7825 1,2) J. McCarty, 3) H. Chung, G. Ginder, J. Laver, 4) P. Kimball, 5) D. Hudson, A. Buskey, T. Post	35	33	29	324
WASHINGTON				
Fred Hutchinson Cancer Rsrch Ctr, Clin Rsrch Div, 1100 Fairview Ave. N ,D2-100, PO Box 19024, Seattle, WA 98104 Ph: (206) 667-4798 Fax: (206) 667-2147 1,4) P. Martin, 4) J. Hansen, E. Mickelson	296	329	278	7048
VA Puget Sound Health Care System, Marrow Transp Unit, 1660 S Columbian Way, Seattle, WA 98108 Ph: (206) 764-2709 Fax: (206) 764-2851 1,3) T.R. Chauncey, 3) A. Back, R.B. Montgomery, W.H. Schubach, 4) Fred Hutchinson Cancer Rsrch Ctr, 5) B. Porter, L. Cook	26	21	23	448
WISCONSIN				
Univ of Wisconsin Hosp & Clins, Dept of Med & Peds, H4/534 CSC, 600 Highland Ave, Madison, WI 53792-5156 Ph: (608) 263-1836 Fax: (608) 262-1982 1,3) E. Smith, 3) K. DeSantes, W. Longo, M. Juckett, P. Sondel, 4) D. Watkins, 5) B. Flynn, J. McMannes, M. Lisitza	40	34	28	518
Med Coll of Wisconsin, Bone Marrow Transp Prog, 8700 W Wisconsin Ave, Milwaukee, WI 53226 Ph: (414) 805-4646 Fax: (414) 805-4630 1,3) W. Burns, 3) Drobyski, Horowitz, Casper, Margolis, Juckett, Vesole, Rizzo, 4) D. Eckels, 5) J. Bauer, M. Ricco, D. Richards, L. Turney	59	61		904
<div align="center">**ARGENTINA**</div>				
Navy Hosp "Pedro Mallo", Dept of Onc-Hem, IBMTR Ctr 191, Ave Patricias Argentinas 357 Fd Dstr, Buenos Aires, 1405 Ph: (54)114 473-5312 Fax: (54)114 584-7563 Email: anibaljr@fibertel.com.ar 1) A.J. Robinson, 3) M.A. Sorrentino, P. Luchetta, 4) F. Raimondi, 5) H. Longoni, C. Dufour	14	16	12	163
Hosp Privado do Cordoba, Dept of Int Med, Ave Naciones Unidas 346, 5016 Cordoba Ph: (54)351 468 8243 Fax: (54)351 468 8270 1,2) J.J. Garcia, 2) E. Palazzo, 3) A. Berreta, D. Minoldo, 4) C. Giraudo, 5) P. Ablchain	10	27	17	91
<div align="center">**AUSTRALIA**</div>				
St Vincent's Hosp, Dept of Hem, Victoria St, Darlinghurst, NSW, 2010 Ph: (61)2 8382-2381 Fax: (61)2 8382-2645 1,3) A.J. Dodds, 3) D.D.F. Ma, S. Milliken, A. Concannon, P. Presgrave, 4) Bld Transf Serv, 5) I. Nivison-Smith	26	23	26	705
Royal North Shore Hosp, Dept of Hem, Pacific Hywy St Leonards, Sydney, NSW, 2065 Ph: (61)2 9926-7118 Fax: (61)2 9906-1635 1,3,5) C.K. Arthur, 2) R. Scurr, 3) J. Isbister, L. Coyle, R. Ravich, K. Fay, N. Mackinlay, C. Ward, 4) Red Cross Transf Lab-Sydney, 5) Sr.K. Eaton	9	5		79
Royal Prince Alfred Hosp, Hematology Inst, Missenden Rd, Camperdown, Sydney, NSW 2050 Ph: (61)2 9515 8031 Fax: (61)2 9515 8474 1,2) J. Gibson, 3) D. Joshua, H. Kronenberg, G. Young, H. Iland, J. HO, 4) NSW Red Cross Tissue Typing Lab, 5) M. Callochor	12	15	15	138
The Children's Hospital at Westmead, Onc Unit, PO Box 3515, Parramatta, Sydney, 2145 Ph: (61)2 9845-0000 Fax: (61)2 9845-2171 1,3,5) P.J. Shaw, 3) L. Dalla-Pozza, G. McCowage, S.J. Kellie, 5) K. Stephens	13	13	12	152
Westmead Hosp, Inst of Clin Path/Med Rsch, Dept of Hem, Hawkesbury Rd, Westmead, NSW, 2145 Ph: (61)2 9845-7649 Fax: (61)2 9689-2331 1,3) K.F. Bradstock, 3) D. Gottlieb, M. Hertzberg, 4) J. Chapman, NSW Transf Serv, 5) M. McGurgan	41	49	45	301
Hanson Ctr I.M.V.S., Royal Adelaide Hosp, Clin Hem/BMT Transp Unit, Frome Rd, Adelaide, S Aust, 5000 Ph: (61)8 8222 3262 Fax: (61)8 8222 3139 Email: ggower@mail.rah.sa.gov.au 1,3) L.B. To, 3) N. Horvath, G. Dart, T. Hughes, C.H. Hui, P. Bardy, 4) J. McClusky, 5) C. Andary	27	34	27	258

1)=Director, 2)=Tx Surgeons, 3)=Physicians, 4)=Tissue Typers, 5)=TxCoords	1998	1999	2000	Total
Alfred Hosp, Bone Marrow Transp Unit, Commercial Rd, Prahran, Melbourne, Victoria, 3181 Ph: (61)3 9276-3451 Fax: (61)3 9276-2298 Email: a.schwarez@alfred.org.au 1,3) A.P. Schwarer, 3) A. Spencer, 4) B. Tait, R. Holdsworth, 5) N. Kennedy	22	39	44	283
Royal Melbourne Hosp, Dept of Clin Hem/Med Onc, C/O Post Office Royal Melb Hosp, Melbourne, Victoria, 3050 Ph: (61)3 9342 7737 Fax: (61)3 9342 7386 Email: jeffszer@uch.org.au 1,3) J. Szer, 3) A. Grigg, A. Roberts, 4) B. Tait, R. Holdsworth, 5) K. Gray, Y. Panek-Hudson	32	43	41	349
Royal Children's Hosp, Dept of Hem/Onc, Flemington Rd, Parkville, Victoria, 3052 Ph: (61)3 93455656 Fax: (61)3 93456524 1,3) K. Tiedemann, 3) K.D. Waters, H. Ekert, 4) B. Tait, 5) D. Tucker, S. Hanson	22	23	20	230
Royal Perth Hosp, Dept of Hem, Wellington St, Perth, WA, 6000 Ph: (61)9 224 3967 Fax: (61)9 224 3449 1,5) R. Herrmann, 3) P. Cannell, 4) F. Christiansen, 5) S. Buffery	23	23		233
AUSTRIA				
St.Anna Children's Hospital, Transplant Unit, Kinderspitalgasse 6, 1090 Vienna, 431 Ph: (43)1 4017 0292 Fax: (43)1 4017 0759 1,2) H. Gadner, 2) H. Stark, E. Horcher, 3) Ch. Peters, S. Matthes-Martin, R. Ladenstein, 4) A. Hajek-Rosenmayr, 5) C. Peters	39	20	24	298
Karl-Franzens Univ Hosp-Graz, Dept of Ped Hem/Onc, Landeskrankenhaus, Auenbruggerpaltz 30, 8036 Graz Ph: (43)316 385-3485 Fax: (43)316 385-3450 Email: christian.urban@kfunigraz.ac.at 1,3) E.Ch. Urban, 2) W. Schwinger, 3) H. Lackner, 4) G. Lanzer, 5) W. Schwinger	7	6	5	110
Univ Hosp Innsbruck, Dept of Intrn Med, Div Clin Immun, BMT Ctr, Anichstr 35, A-6020 Innsbruck Ph: (43)512 504-3255 Fax: (43)512 504-3338 Email: david.nachbaur@uibk.ac.at 1,3) D. Nachbaur, 4) D. Schonitzer, 5) B. Gritsch	17	20	26	210
Univ of Vienna, Klinik Fuer Innere I, Waehringer Guerter 18-20, Vienna, A-1090 Ph: (43)1 40400 4457 Fax: (43)1 40400 2511 Email: hildegard.greinix@akh-wien.ac.at 1,3) H.T. Greinix, 1,3) P.Kalhs, 3) F. Keil, A. Schulenburg, W. Rabitsch, M. Mitterbauer, 4) G. Fischer, 5) A. Felber	29	43	67	390
BELGIUM				
Antwerp Univ Hosp, Dept Hem, Wilrijkstr 10, B-2650 Edegem, Antwerp Ph: (32)3 821 3198 Fax: (32)3 825 3318 Email: zwi.berneman@uza.uia.ac.be 1,3) Z.N. Berneman, 3) W. Schroyens, J. van Droogenbroeck, A. van de Velde, 4) G. Mertens	10	4	3	75
Academic Hosp, Free Univ Brussels, Dept of Med Onc/Hem, Laarbeeklaan 101, 1090 Brussels Ph: (32)2 477-6211 Fax: (32)2 477-5856 1,3) R. Schots, 3) F. Trullemans, 4) C. Demanet	21	15	12	244
Clin Univ St Luc, Dept of Hem, 10 Ave Hippocrate, 1200 Brussels Ph: (32)2 764 1810 Fax: (32)2 764 8959 Email: ferrrant@sang.ucl.ac.be 1,3) A. Ferrant, 3) N. Straetnans, 4) M. Debruyere, 5) P. van Mulder	14	19	26	295
Univ Hosp Gasthuisberg, Dept of IG Hem, Herestraat 49, B-3000 Leuven Ph: (32)16 346880 Fax: (32)16 346881 Email: marc.boogaerts@uz.kuleuven.ac.be 1,3) M.A. Boogaerts, 2) J. Maertens, 3) J. Maertens, P. Vandenberghe, 4) M.P. Emonds, 5) H. Gilis, M. Cleeren	35	19	38	456
Mont-Godinne Univ Hosp, Dept of Hem, Av Dr Therasse, Yvoir 5530 Ph: (32)81 423831 Fax: (32)81 423832 1,3) A. Bosly, 3) C. Doyen, C. Chatelain, A. Sonet, 4) J.C. Osselaer, B. Chatelain	9	3		65
BRAZIL				
Hosp de Clin-Univ Fed do Parna, Bone Marrow Transp Unit, Rua Gal Carneiro, 181, C Postal 1.920, Curitiba, PR 80001-970 Ph: (55)41 262 6665 Fax: (55)41 264 5472 Email: tmo@hc.ufpr.br 1,3) R. Pasquini, 3) Neto, deMedeiros, Friedrich, Bitencourt, Bonfim, Araujo, 4) M.F. Rodrigues, N.F. Pereira	75	68	81	1112

1)=Director, 2)=Tx Surgeons, 3)=Physicians, 4)=Tissue Typers, 5)=TxCoords	1998	1999	2000	Total
Ctr Nac'l de Transp de Med Ossea, Inst Nac'l de Cancer, Praga Cruz Vermelha, 23-7 andar, Rio De Janeiro, RJ 20230 Ph: (55)21 5066215 Fax: (55)21 5092121 Email: dtabak@inca.org.br 1,3) D.G. Tabak, 4) I. Salatiel, 5) L.F. Bouzas	70	72	92	532
Hosp das Clinicas-FMUSP, Dept of Hem, Av Dr Eneas de Carvalho Aguiar 155, 8 Andar, Sao Paulo, SP 05403-000 Ph: (55)11 3061 5544 Fax: (55)11 853 2290 1) D.A.F. Chamone, 3) R. Saboya, 4) J. Kalil-Filho, 5) F.L. Dulley	49	47	59	533

CANADA

	1998	1999	2000	Total
Alberta Children's Hosp, Dept of Ped Onc Prog, 1820 Richmond Rd, SW, Calgary, AB T2T 5C7 Ph: (403) 229-7396 Fax: (403) 228-9519 1,3) J. Russell, 3) M. Coppes, R. Anderson, J. Wolff, 4) B. Herbut, 5) J. Brooks	7	8	14	107
Foothills Hosp-Tom Baker Cancer Ctr, Dept of Med, 1331 29th St NW, Calgary, AB T2N 4N2 Ph: (403) 670-1706 Fax: (403) 283-1651 Email: jamesrus@cancerboard.ab.ca 1,3) J.A. Russell, 3) C. Brown, D. Ruether, D. Stewart, S. Gluck, D. Morris, 4) B. Herbut, 5) T. Kelly, L. Karlsson	50	57	66	513
British Columbia's Children's Hosp, Dept of Ped, 4480 Oak St, Vancouver, BC V6H 3V4 Ph: (604) 875-2406 Fax: (604) 875-2911 1,3) J.H. Davis, 3) S. Pritchard, K. Schultz, J. Wu, K. Stobart, P. Rogers, C. Strahlendorf, 4) P. Keown, 5) N. Takeuchi	13	10	12	198
Vancouver Hosp, Leuk/Bone Marrow Transp Prog, Dept of Med, 910 W 10th Ave, Vancouver, BC V5Z 4E3 Ph: (604) 875-4863 Fax: (604) 875-4763 1,3) M.J. Barnett, 3) Shepherd, Sutherland, Nantel, Toze, Nevill, Hogge, Conneally, 4) P. Keown, 5) K. Munn, M. Rennie	60	45	49	808
Cancer Care Manitoba, MBMT Program, 675 McDermot Ave, Winnipeg, MB R3E 0V9 Ph: (204) 787-3594 Fax: (204) 787-1345 1,3) M. Rubinger, 3) E. Bow, M. Schroeder, 4) M. Schroeder, 5) D. Britton, T. Robinson	18	24	16	196
McMaster Univ Med Ctr, Hamilton Health Sciences Corp, Dept of Med, 1200 Main St W, Hamilton, ON L8N 3Z5 Ph: (905) 521-2100 Fax: (905) 521-4971 1,3) I.R. Walker, 3) B. Leber, P. Wasi, 4) D. Singal, 5) K. Greene	14	17		226
London Health Sciences Centre, Hematology, 800 Commissioners Rd, London, ON NGA 4G5 Ph: (519) 685-8500 Fax: (519) 685-8477 1,3) K. Howson-Jon, 3) K. Howson-Jon, 4) S. Leckie, 5) M. Christie	22	12	2	182
Hosp for Sick Children, Dept of Hem/Onc, 555 University Ave, Toronto, ON M5G 1X8 Ph: (416) 813-5977 Fax: (416) 813-5327 1,3) J.J. Doyle, 3) E.F. Saunders, 4) J. Wade, 5) K. Yuille, C. Armstrong	52	60	36	531
Ontario Cancer Inst, Princess Margaret Hosp, Dept of Med, 610 University Ave, Ste S-101A, Toronto, ON M5G 2M9 Ph: (416) 946-2268 Fax: (416) 946-6585 1,3) H.A. Messner, 2) J.H.Lipton, 3) Minden, Kiss, Tejpar, Loach, 5) R. MacAskill, J. Killoran	123	117	89	1234
Maisonneuve Rosemont Hosp, Dept of Hem, 5415 Boul l'Assomption, Montreal, PQ H1T 2M4 Ph: (514) 252-3495 Fax: (514) 254-5094 1,3) R. Belanger, 3) Y. Bonny, D.C. Roy, L. Busque, D. Fish, J. Roy, 4) C. Perreault, 5) O. Marchand	90	105		941

CHINA, P.R.

	1998	1999	2000	Total
Queen Mary Hosp, Dept of Med, Marrow Transp, Centre, Queen Mary Hosp, Hong Kong Ph: (852)2 855 4776 Fax: (852)2 974 1165 1,3) R. Liang, 3) A.K.W. Lie, 4) B. Hawkins, 5) W.S. Yuen	40	64	59	488
Bei Tai Ping Lu Hosp, Dept of Hem, 2 Bei Tai Ping Rd, Beijing, 100039 Ph: (86)10 6816-8875 Fax: (86)10 6821-3044 1,3) L.X. Cao, 3) M. Jiang, L.D. Hu, H.L. Liu, B. Wang, 4) F.H. Kun	32	36	35	219
People's Hosp & Inst of Hem, Peking Univ, Bone Marrow Transp Unit, 11 Xizhimen S St, Beijing, 100044 Ph: (86)10 6831-4422 Fax: (86)10 8633-3439 1,3) D.P. Lu, 2) L.P. Xu, H. Chen, Y.Ch. Zhang, K.Y. Liu, X.J. Huang, 3) N.L. Guo, H. Zheng, 4) D. Li, X.R. Liu, 5) N.L. Guo	47	53	78	466
Lanzhou Gen Hosp, Dept of Hem, 58 Xiaoxihuxijei, Qilihe, Lanzhou, Gansu Prov, 730050 Ph: (86)931-235 5486 Fax: (86)931-233 1767 1,3) W.M. Da, 3) J.T. Zhong, X.X. Wu, H. Bai, Y. Liu, C.B. Wang, 4) Y.M. Wei, 5) F. Shi, Z.L. Wei	5			69

BONE MARROW / PERIPHERAL BLOOD TRANSPLANTS

1)=Director, 2)=Tx Surgeons, 3)=Physicians, 4)=Tissue Typers, 5)=TxCoords	1998	1999	2000	Total
COLOMBIA				
Univ de Antioquia, Hosp San Vincent de Paul, Dept of Hem, Calle 64 X Carrera 51 D, Medellin-Antioquia Ph: (57)4 263 7068 Fax: (57)4 263 1002 1,2) A. Velasquez, 3) F. Cuellar, 4) L.F. Garcia	11	12		42
COSTA RICA				
Nat'l Children's Hosp, "Dr. Carlos Saenz Herrera", Dept of Immun, Apartado 1654, 1000 San Jose Ph: (506) 2235125 Fax: (506) 2235125 Email: oporras@hnn.sa.cr 1) O. Porras, 3) A. Baltodano, J.M. Carrillo, A. Fasth, C. Odio, A. Abdelnour, 4) W. Alfaro, 5) O. Arguedas, I. Leiva	3	2		27
CROATIA				
Univ Clin Hosp Rebro-Zagreb, Nat'l Referral Organ Transp &, Tissue Typ Ctr, 12 Kispaticeva, Zagreb, HR-10000 Ph: (385)1 233-3235 Fax: (385)1 212-684 Email: andrija.kastelan@zg.tel.hr 1,3) A. Kastelan, 3) B. Labar, V. Bogdanic, 4) V. Kerhin-Brkljacic, R. Zunec, 5) E. Cecuk-Jelicic	28	25	23	417
CUBA				
Inst of Hem/Immun, Bone Marrow Transp Unit, PO Box 8070, Ciudad de La Habana, Havana 10800 Ph: (53)7 578268 Fax: (53)7 338079 1,3) J.M. Ballester, 3) E. Dorticos, A. Gonzalez, 4) C. Ustariz, 5) E. Dorticos		1		10
CZECH REPUBLIC				
Inst of Hem & Bld Transf, Clin Dept, U Nemocnice 1, Prague 2, 12820 Ph: (42)2 2491 5615 Fax: (42)2 299821 1,3) A. Vitek, 2) R. Gurlich, 3) J. Saidova, J. Hrabanek, 4) P. Korinkova, M. Loudova, E. Matejkova, L. Dolezalova, 5) P. Kobylka	21	24		170
Univ Hosp Motol, Prague 5, 2nd Dept of Ped, V Uvalu 84, Prague 5, 150 06 Ph: (420)2 2443 2201 Fax: (420)2 2443 2220 Email: jan.stary@lfmotol.cuni.cz 1,5) J. Stary, 3) V. Komrska, P. Sedlacek, 4) L. Korinkova, Inst of Exp Med Prague, 5) Inter-Transp Prague	18	21	22	144
DENMARK				
Rigshospitalet, Bone Marrow Transp Unit, Dept of Hem L 4042, Blegdamsvej, 2100 Copenhagen Ph: (45)35 454385 Fax: (45)35 454841 Email: bmtunit@rh.dk 1,3) N. Jacobsen, 3) L. Vindelov, C. Geisler, C. Heilmann, 4) Tissue Typ Lab, Copenhagen, 5) L. Holst	47	39	48	676
EGYPT				
Nat'l Cancer Inst, Cairo Univ, Dept of Med Onc, Clin Path, Kasr Er Aini St, Fum El Khalig, Cairo Ph: (20)2 843 640 Fax: (20)2 364 4720 1,5) H.K. Mahmoud, 3) A. Haddad, 4) A.M. Kamel, N.H. El Shakankiry	63	84	87	396
FINLAND				
Children's Hosp, Univ Helsinki, Div of Hem/Onc, Stenbackinkatu 11, Fin-00290 Helsinki Ph: (358)0 471 2720 Fax: (358)0 471 4702 Email: ulla.pihkala@hus.fi 1,5) U.M. Pihkala, 3) L. Hovi, K. Vettenranta, 4) S. Koskimies	22	18	19	190
Helsinki Univ Central Hosp, Dept of Med, Fin-00029 Hyks, Helsinki Ph: (358)9-471-72338 Fax: (358)9-471-72351 1,5) T. Ruutu, 4) S. Koskimies	55	55	65	550
Turku Univ Hosp, Dept of Med, Kiinamyllynkatu 4-8, 20520 Turku Ph: (358)2 261 1611 Fax: (358)2 261 2030 Email: kari.remes@tyks.fi 1,2,5) K. Remes, 3) T.T. Salmi, A. Rajamaki, M. Itala, 4) Finnish Red Cross, Blood Transfusion Service, 5) K. Remes, M. Itala	11	14	18	132

1)=Director, 2)=Tx Surgeons, 3)=Physicians, 4)=Tissue Typers, 5)=TxCoords	1998	1999	2000	Total
FRANCE				
CHRU d'Angers, Dept of Hem, F 49033 Angers Cedex Ph: (33)241 354472 Fax: (33)241 354582 1,3) M. Boasson, 3) N. Ifrah, C. Foussard, M. Gardembas, S. Francois, 4) B. Coeffic	15	12	12	172
Centre Hospitalo-Universitaire, Hosp Jean Minjoz, Serv Hem/Bld Bank, 1 BD Fleming, 25030 Besancon Ph: (33)381 66-8232 Fax: (33)381 66-8215 1,3) J.Y. Cahn, 1,4) P. Herve, 3) E. Plouvier, E. Deconinck, C.E. Bulabois, 4) J. Chabod, P. Tiberghien	28	25	28	444
Grenoble Hosp A Michallon, Dept of Hem Serv, BP 217X, Grenoble Cedex, 38043 Ph: (33)76 765663 Fax: (33)76 765661 1,3) J.J. Sotto, 3) F. Garban, 4) D. Nasson	16	18	14	244
Claude Huriez, CHR, Maladies Du Sang, Lille Cedex, 59037 Ph: (33)20 44 5551 Fax: (33)20 44 4197 1,3) F. Bauters, 3) J.P. Jouet, 4) F. Dufosse	38	45	44	468
Hosp Edouard Herriot, Dept of Leuk/Bone Marrow/Hem, Pl D'Arsonval, 69437 Lyon Cedex 03 Ph: (33)472 331917 Fax: (33)472 360153 Email: mauricette.michallet@chu-lyon.fr 1,3) D.M. Fiere, 3) M. Michallet, A. Thiebaut, I. Markel, 4) A.M. Freidel, L. Gebuhrer, F. Javaux, 5) M. Michallet	35	39	30	765
Inst Paoli Calnettes, Bone Marrow Transp Unit, 232 Bd de Ste Marguerite, 4, 13273 Marseille Ph: (33)91 22 3354 Fax: (33)91 26 0852 1,3) D. Blaise, 3) C. Faucher, C. Chabannon, N. Vey, Am. Stoppa, 4) D. Reviron, 5) B. Benamo	30	49	28	460
Hotel Dieu-Univ Nantes, Dept of Hem, 1 Pl Alexis Ricordeau, Nantes Cedex 01, 44035 Ph: (332) 40 083271 Fax: (332) 40 083250 1,3) J.L. Harousseau, 3) N. Milpied, P. Moreau, B. Mahe, F. Mechinaud, C. Thomas, 4) J.D. Bignon, A. Cesbron	33	34	39	451
Hosp De L'Archet 1, Dept of Hem, 151 Route De S Antoine De Ginestiere, 06202 Nice Cedex 3 Ph: (33)492 035823 Fax: (33)492 035896 1) J.P. Cassuto, 3) N. Gratecos, 4) G. Bernard, 5) M. Genoud	14	10		106
Hosp Necker, Dept of Adult Hem, 149 Rue de Sevres, 75743 Paris Ph: (33)1-4449 5287 Fax: (33)1-4449 5280 Email: hirsch@necker.fr 1,3) B. Varet, 3) A. Buzyn, C. Belanger, 4) S. Caillat, 5) I. Hirsch	22	28	31	220
Hosp Necker-Enfants Malades, Dept of Ped, 149 Rue de Sevres, Paris 75015 Ph: (33)1-44494823 Fax: (33)1-42732896 Email: fischer@necfan.fr 1,3) A. Fischer, 3) S. Blanche, M. Debre, 4) Ms. Caillat, 5) I. Hirsch	40	50	62	623
Hotel Dieu, Dept of Hem (75), Pl du Parvis Notre Dame, 75181 Paris Cedex 4 Ph: (33)1 4234 8419 Fax: (33)1 4234 8406 Email: hemato.hd@htd.ap-hop-paris.fr 1,3) J.P. Marie, 3) B. Rio, 4) E. Soreau	12	11	19	310
St Louis Hosp, Bone Marrow Transp Unit, 1 Ave Claude Velle Faux, 75475 Paris Cedex 10 Ph: (33)1 4249 9644 Fax: (33)1 4249 9634 1) E. Gluckman, 2) R. Traineau, P. Richard, 3) A. Devergie, H. Esperou, P. Ribaud, G. Socie, 4) D. Charron	82	87	92	1415
Hosp Haut-Leveque, Dept of Gironde, Ave de Magellan, 33604, Pessac Ph: (33)56 55 6511 Fax: (33)56 55 6514 1,3) J. Reiffers, 3) G. Marit, J.M. Boiron, 4) D. Fizet, 5) J.M. Boiron	40	49	40	537
Hosp Jean Bernard, Dept of Hem/Clin Onc, 350 Av Jacques Coeur, La Miletrie, Poitiers 86021 Ph: (33)5 4944 4201 Fax: (33)5 4944 3863 Email: f.guilhot@chu-poitiers.fr 1,3) F. Guilhot, 3) A. Sadoun, E. Randrsamalala, 4) D. Alcalay, M. Bois, 5) C. Giraud	21	9	10	166
CHR Pontchaillou, Dept of Hem, Rue Henri le Guillou, Rennes, 35000 Ph: (33)0299 28-4291 Fax: (33)0299 28-4161 1,3) P.Y. LePrise, 3) C. Dauriac, M. Bernard, T. Lamy, E. LeGall, R. Fauchet, 4) G. Semana, 5) Nourry	15	15	16	200

1)=Director, 2)=Tx Surgeons, 3)=Physicians, 4)=Tissue Typers, 5)=TxCoords	1998	1999	2000	Total
GERMANY				
Charite Virchow-Klinikum, Humboldt Univ, Dept Intrn Med, Div of Hem/Onc, Augustenburger Pl. 1, 13353 Berlin Ph: (49)30 450 53673 Fax: (49)30 450 53925 1,3) W. Siegert, 4) A. Salama	29	32	32	352
Heinrich-Heine Univ Med Ctr, Dept of Ped and Adult Hem/Onc, BMT Prog, Mooren Str 5, Duesseldorf, 40225 Ph: (49)211 811 6783 Fax: (49)211 811 6090 1,3) U. Gobel, 1) R. Haas, 3) D. Dilloo, P. Schneider, H.F. Laws, G. Kobbe, 4) P. Wernet, 5) D. Dilloo, P. Schneider, H.F. Laws	37	48	44	348
Clin fur Kinder und Jugendliche, Univ Erlangen-Nurenberg, Dept of Hem/Onc, Loschgestr 15, Erlangen, 91054 Ph: (49)9131-853118 Fax: (49)9131-853113 1,2) W. Rascher, 1,5) J.D. Beck, 3) J. Greil, T. Langer, D. Stachel, A. Leipold, 4) R. Wasmuth	3	6	4	33
Univ Hosp Essen, Dept of Bone Marrow Transp, Dept of Ped/Immun, Hufelandstr 55, 45122 Essen Ph: (49)201 723-3137 Fax: (49)201 723-5961 1,3) U.W. Schaefer, 3) D.W. Beelen, V. Runde, B. Kremens, 4) H. Grosse-Wilde, 5) H. Ottinger	132	132	134	1365
Univ Hosp of Freiburg, Dept of Hem/Onc, Bone Marrow Transp Unit, Hugstetterstr 55, W79106 Freiburg Ph: (49)761 270-3495 Fax: (49)761 270-3667 1,3) J. Finke, 1,3) R. Mertelsmann, 3) H. Bertz, H. Veelken, 4) H. Lang, 5) E. Lenartz	63	72	91	549
Univ Hosp Eppendorf-Hamburg, Dept of Med-BMT, Martinstr 52, 20246 Hamburg 20 Ph: (49)40 4717-4851 Fax: (49)40 4717-3795 1,3) A.R. Zander, 3) N. Kroger, H. Kabisch, R. Erttmann, W. Kruger, 4) Loeliger, 5) N. Jaburg, G. Amtsfeld	46	78	85	474
Hannover Med Sch, Dept of Hem/Onc, Carl-Neuberg-Str.1, 30623 Hannover Ph: (49)511 532-6394 Fax: (49)511 532-5133 1,2) B. Hertenstein, 1,2) A. Ganser, 2) K.W. Sykora, K. Welte, 4) R. Blasczyk, 5) E. Dammann	114	106	98	760
Clin of BMT/Hem/Onc, Dr Ottmar-Kohler Str 2, Idar-Oberstein, 55743 Ph: (49)6781 661583 Fax: (49)6781 661584 Email: office@bmt-center-io.com 1) A.A. Fauser, 3) 11 Tx physicians, 4) B. Thiele, S. Goldmann, E. Seifried, 5) U. Becker	83	81	62	411
Univ of Jena, Hosp of Peds, Dept of Ped/Hem/Onc, Kochstrasse 2, 07745 Jena Ph: (49)3641 938270 Fax: (49)3641 938470 1,3,5) F. Zintl, 3) J. Hermann, 4) Th. Binder	13	20	17	196
Univ of Kiel-BMT Unit, Dept of Int Med II, Chemnitz Str 33, D 2416 Kiel, Kiel Ph: (49)431 16970 Fax: (49)431 1697202 1,2) N. Schmitz, 4) M. Westphal	12	21	29	95
Univ Leipzig, Ctr of Int Med, Div of Hem/Onc, Philipp-Rosenthal-Strabe 23-25, Leipzig, 04103 Ph: (49)341 97 13050 Fax: (49)341 97 13059 Email: dietger@medizin.uni-leipzig.de 1,3) D. Niederwieser, 2) E. Edel, 3) W. Poenisch, L. Uharek, 4) P. Emmrich, S. Schroeder, 5) R. Krahl	39	73	69	474
Johannes Gutenberg Univ-Mainz, Dept of Int Med/Div of Hem, Langenbeckstr 1, 6500 Mainz Ph: (49)6131 172581 Fax: (49)6131 177252 1,3) D.Ch. Huber, 3) K. Kolbe, G. Derigs, 4) L. Gheleter, 5) E. Alten, C. Schon	36	43	46	207
Kinderklinik d'Univ Munchen-LAF, Dept Hem/Onc-BMT, Lindwurmstr 4, Munich, 80337 Ph: (49)89 5160 2852 Fax: (49)89 5160 4719 1,3) R.J. Haas, 3) I. Schmid, D. Stachel, 4) E.D. Albert, 5) I. Schmid	10	13	8	99
Ludwig-Maximilians Univ Munich, Klinikum Grosshadern, Hematopoietic Cell Transp, Marchioninistr. 15, Munich, D 81377 Ph: (49)89 7095 4241 Fax: (49)89 7095 4242 Email: bmtunit@medo.med.uni-muenchen.de 1,3) H.J. Kolb, 3) C. Bender-Goelze, R.J. Haas, 4) E.D. Albert, W. Mempel	135	169	177	1269
Univ Children's Hosp, Dept of Hem, Hoppe-Seyler-Str.1, 72070 Tuebingen, 72070 Ph: (49)7071 2983781 Fax: (49)7071 294713 1,3) D. Niethammer, 3) T. Klingebiel, 4) C. Mueller	31	37		305
HUNGARY				
Nat'l Inst of Hematology, Dept of BMT, XI Daroczi u.24, PO Box 424, 1519 Budapest Ph: (36)1 209-2311 Fax: (36)1 209-2311 Email: k.paloczi@ohvi.hu 1,3) K. Paloczi, 2) A. Faluhelyi, 3) A. Barta, E. Torbagyi, 4) E. Gyodi	12	14	11	175

1)=Director, 2)=Tx Surgeons, 3)=Physicians, 4)=Tissue Typers, 5)=TxCoords	1998	1999	2000	Total
IRELAND				
St James' Hosp, Dublin, Clin Hem/Onc, James' St, PO Box 580, Dublin 8 Ph: (353)1 4537941 Fax: (353)1 4530557 Email: mcrowley@stjames.ie 1,3) S.R. McCann, 4) A. Finch, 5) J. O'Riordan	38	38		325
ISRAEL				
Hadassah Hebrew Univ Hosp, Dept of Bone Marrow Transp, Kiryat Hadassah Ein Kerem, Jerusalem, 91120 Ph: (972)2 6776561 Fax: (972)2 6422731 1,3) S. Slavin, 3) Or, Nagler, Varadi, Shapira, 4) C. Brautbar, 5) A. Sweed	90	96	89	1100
Schneider Chldrn's Med Ctr of Israel, Dept BMT, Kaplan 14, Petach-Tikva, 49202 Ph: (972)3 925-3604 Fax: (972)3 925-3042 1,3) I. Yaniv, 3) J. Stein, Y. Goshen, 4) T. Klein, 5) N. Ben-Zvi	20	14	17	111
ITALY				
St Orsola Univ Hosp, Inst of Hem, "L & A Seragnoli", Via Massarenti 9, 40138 Bologna Ph: (39)051 390413 Fax: (39)051 398973 1) S. Tura, 3) G. Bandini, G. Rosti, D. Rondelli, 4) R. Conte, 5) G. Bandini	36	41	36	417
Hosp Careggi, BMT Unit- Dept Hem, Viale Morgagni 85, Florence, 50134 Ph: (39)055 427-7726/7067 Fax: (39)055 412098 Email: a.bosi@dfc.unifi.it 1,3) P. Rossi Ferrini, 1) A.Bosi, 3) S. Guidi, R. Saccardi, A.M. Vannucchi, L. Lombardini, S. Ciolli, 4) V. Fossombroni, G. Rombola, 5) G. Tellarini	22	32	39	265
Inst Sci G Gaslini, Unita' TMO, Largo G Gaslini 5, 16148 Genova Ph: (39)010 5636405 Fax: (39)010 3777133 1,3) G. Dini, 3) E. Lanino, S. Dallorso, G. Morreale, M. Faraci, 4) M. Barbanti	19	22	26	199
San Martino Hosp, Dept of Hem II, viale Benedetto XV, Genova, 16035 Ph: (39)010-355469 Fax: (39)010-355583 1,3) A. Bacigalupo, 3) M.T. VanLint, F. Frassoni, D. Occhini, F. Gualandi, T. Lamparelli, 4) M. Barbanti	85	75	76	1126
Ospedale Maggiore-Univ Milano, Dept of Intern Med/Hem, Ctr Trapianti di Midollo, Via F Sforza 35, 20122 Milano Ph: (39)02 55033322 Fax: (39)02 55033341 Email: giorgio.lambertenghi@unimi.it 1,3,5) G. Lambertenghi Deliliers, 3) A. Della Volpe, D. Soligo, C. Annaloro, 4) G. Sirchia	22	19	30	197
Parma Univ Hosp, Dept of Hem, Bone Marrow Transp Ctr, via Gramsci 14, 43100 Parma Ph: (39)521 290787 Fax: (39)521 292765 Email: ematopr@unipr.it 1,3) V. Rizzoli, 3) C. Caramatti, R. Giachetti, 4) M. Savi, 5) L. Mangoni	3	4	5	49
Univ of Perugia, Dept of Hem, Policlinico Montelue via Brunamonti, Perugia 06100 Ph: (39)75 578-3219 Fax: (39)75 578-3691 1,3) M.F. Martelli, 3) F. Aversa, A. Tabilio, A. Terenzi, 4) C. Gambelunghe, 5) F. Aversa	48	62		473
Ospedale Civile/Terapia Intensiva, Dipart Enatologia-Oncologia, Via Fonte Romana 8, Centro Transplants Midollo, Pescara, 65125 Ph: (39)85 425-2689 Fax: (39)85 425-2583 1,3) P. DiBartolomeo, 3) DiGirolamo, Bavaro, Olioso, Papalinetti, 4) D. Adorno, F. Papola, O.C. L'Aquila, 5) P. Di Bartolomeo	32	37	32	583
Policlinico Gemelli, Dept of Hem, Univ Cattolica Del Sacro Cuore, Largo Agostino Gemelli, 00168 Rome Ph: (39)6 3550 3953 Fax: (39)6 3017319 1,3,5) G. Leone, 3) S. Sica, L. Laurenti, N. Piccirillo, P. Chiusolo, F. Sora, 4) Croce Rossa Italiana	10	13	15	92
St Camillo Hosp, Dept of Hem, Circonvallazione Gianicolense 87, 00152 Rome Ph: (39)6 5870-4870 Fax: (39)6 5820-3326 1,3,5) A. DeLaurenzi, 3) L. DeRosa, F. Blandino, 4) C. Ruscio, C. Armentano, 5) N. Petti	5	13		191
Univ Degli Studi "La Sapienza", Inst of Hem, Via Benevento 6, Rome, 00161 Ph: (39)6 857951 Fax: (39)6 4424 1984 1,3) F. Mandelli, 3) W. Arcese, A.P. Iori, C. Guglielmi, A. Mengarelli, 4) G. Girelli, P. Perrone, L. Laurenti, 5) W. Arcese	42	46	51	537
Univ of Turin Hosp, Dept of Ped/Onc, Pzza Polonia 94, 10126 Torino Ph: (39)11 3135566 Fax: (39)11 6635695 1,3,5) E. Madon, 3) E. Vassallo, F. Fagioli, S. Ljoi, 4) A.M. Daulomo, 5) F. Fagioli	10	9	13	119

1)=Director, 2)=Tx Surgeons, 3)=Physicians, 4)=Tissue Typers, 5)=TxCoords	1998	1999	2000	Total
JAPAN				
Japanese Red Cross Nagoya 1st Hosp, Dept of Int Med/Peds, 3-35 Michishita-cho, Nakamura-ku, Nagoya 453, Aichi Ph: (81)562 481-5111 Fax: (81)562 483-3647 1,3) Y. Kodera, 2) Y. Fujiwara, 3) K. Matsuyama, K. Kitaori, M. Kasai, K. Kato, 4) Aichi Bld Ctr, 5) Japan Marrow Program, NMDP, M. Nakamura	67	69	64	763
Nagoya Daini Red Cross Hosp, Dept of Hem, 2-9 Myokencho, Showaku, Nagoya 466, Aichi Ph: (81)52 832-1121 Fax: (81)52 832-1130 1,3) N. Hirabayashi, 3) S. Goto, J. Hiraga, T. Uchida, S. Kayukawa, 4) H. Kamura, 5) Japan Marrow Donor Prog (JMDP)	19	19	21	281
Nagoya Nat'l Hosp, Bld Dis Ctr, 4-1-1 Sannomaru, Naka-ku, Nagoya, Aichi, 460-0001 Ph: (81)52 951-1111 Fax: (81)52 951-0664 1,3) H. Yamada, 3) K. Tsushita, M. Hattori, Y. Kamiya, A. Terasawa, Y. Yamazaki	4	9		57
Nagoya Univ Hosp, Dept of Pediatrics, 65-Tsurumai-cho, Showa-ku, Nagoya 466-8560, Aichi, 466-8560 Ph: (81)52 744-2994 Fax: (81)52 744-2994 1) S. Kojima, 2) H. Ando	4	10	9	96
Akita Univ Sch of Med, 3rd Dept of Int Med, 1-1-1 Hondo, Akita 010 Ph: (81)188 34-1111 Fax: (81)188 36-2613 1,3) A.B. Miura, 3) M. Hirokawa, T. Nimura, 4) SRL, Red Cross Ctr	9	11	8	74
Nat'l Kyushu Cancer Ctr, Dept of Peds/Hemo/Onc, I-1 3 Choume Notame, Minamiku, Fukuoka 815 Ph: (81)92 541-3231 Fax: (81)92 551-4585 1,3) N. Tsukomoto, 3) J. Okamura, Y. Ikuno, Y. Nagatoshi, N. Uike, Y. Yufu, 4) Red Cross, 5) Japan Bone Marrow Donor Prog	16	23	36	260
Hiroshima Red Cross Hosp &, Atomic-bomb Survivors Hosp, 4th Dept of Int Med/Hem, 1-9-6 Senda-machi, Naka-ku, Hiroshima 730 Ph: (81)82 241 3111 Fax: (81)82 246 0676 Email: dohy@wakuwaku.ne.jp 1,3) H. Dohy, 3) T. Kyo, H. Asaoku, K. Iwato, 4) Tatsuno, 5) T. Sueda, N. Matsuhura	15	24	30	237
Sapporo Hokuyu Hosp, Dept of Int Med, Higashisapporo 6-6, Shiroishi-ku, Sapporo 003, Sapporo 003 Ph: (81)11 865-0111 Fax: (81)11 865-9719 1,5) M. Kasai, 3) T. Higa, T. Naohara, Y. Kiyama, 4) N. Yokota, 5) N. Hoshi	22	22	36	163
Hyogo Coll of Med, Dept of Cell Transplantation, 1-1, Mukogawa-cho, Nishinomiya, Hyogo, 663-8501 Ph: (81)798 45 6882 Fax: (81)798 45 6947 1,3) H.E. Hara, 3) S. Kai, M. Misawa, 4) T. Kohriiya, K. Taniwaki	11	11	13	106
Hyogo Coll of Med, 2nd Dept of Int Med, 1-1, Mukogawa-cho, Nishinomiya, Hyogo, 663-8501 Ph: (81)798 45 6592 Fax: (81)798 45 6593 1,3) E. Kakishita, 3) T. Okamoto, Y. Fujimori, 5) K. Hattori	17	16	9	250
Tokai Univ Hosp, Dept of Ped/Int Med, Bohseidai, Isehara, Kanagawa 259-11 Ph: (81)463 93 1121 Fax: (81)463 91 6235 1) S. Kato, 3) H. Yabe, M. Yabe, K. Hattori, M. Matsumoto, Y. Yasuda, T. Hotta, K. Kishi, 4) K. Sato, F. Tsuchida, M. Hagihara, O. Hyodo, 5) M. Takahashi	46	26	43	400
Kanagawa Cancer Ctr, Dept of Hematology, 1-1-2 Nakao, Asahi-ku, Yokohama, 241-0815 Ph: (81)45 391-5761 Fax: (81)45 361-4692 1,3) A. Maruta, 3) E. Yamazaki, A. Mishima, J. Taguchi, 4) Kanagawa Red Cross Bld Ctr	15	11	22	190
Kyoto Univ Hosp, Dept of Pediatrics, Sakyoku, Kyoto 606 Ph: (81)75 751-3298 Fax: (81)75 752-2361 Email: tnakaha@kuhp.kyoto-u.ac.jp 1) T. Nakahata, 3) Y.W. Lin, S. Adachi, K. Watanabe, K. Umeda, 4) H.Saji (HLA lab.), 5) M. Nagase	8	7	8	70
Osaka Med Ctr-Cancer/Cardiovasc Dis., 5th Dept of Int Med, 3 Nakamichi 1-chome, Higashinari-ku, Osaka, 537 Ph: (81)66 9721181 Fax: (81)66 9811531 1,3) A. Hiraoka, 3) H. Nakamura, T. Karasuno, H. Mitsui	16	19	20	51
Kinki Univ Sch of Med, 3rd Dept of Int Med, 377-2 Ohnohigashi, Osakasayama, 589-0014 Ph: (81)723 66 0221 Fax: (81)723 68 3732 Email: ashida@med.kindai.ac.jp 1) A. Kanamaru, 3) T. Ashida, 4) Y. Kanemitsu, 5) T. Ashida	14	8	12	120
Osaka Univ Hosp, Dept of Med III, 2-2, Yamada-Oka, Suita City, Osaka 565 Ph: (81)6 879-3837 Fax: (81)6 879-3839 1,3,5) H. Sugiyama	14			115

1)=Director, 2)=Tx Surgeons, 3)=Physicians, 4)=Tissue Typers, 5)=TxCoords	1998	1999	2000	Total
Hamamatsu Univ Hosp, Dept of Intern Med III, 3600 Handa-cho, Hamamatsu, Shizouka, 431-31 Ph: (81)53 435-2267 Fax: (81)53 434-2910 1,3) R. Ohno, 3) A. Takeshita, K. Naito, 4) SRL Lab	5	3	5	38
Jichi Med Sch Hosp, Dept of Hem/Transf/BMT, Yakushij 3311-1, Minami Kawachi, Machi, Tochigi, 329-0498 Ph: (81)285 442111 Fax: (81)285 445258 1) K. Ozawa, 3) K. Muroi, C. Kawano, 4) K. Muroi	8	8		56
Tokyo Univ Hosp, Cell Therapy & Transplant Med, Hongo 7-3-1, Bunkyo-ku, Tokyo 113, 113-8655 Ph: (81)3 3815 5411 Fax: (81)3 3815 2087 1) H. Hirai, 2) T. Mutoh, 3) S. Chiba, S. Ogawa, 4) R. Machinami, 5) S. Chiba	29	37	37	142
Tokyo Med & Dental Univ, Dept of Pediatrics, 1-5-45, Yushima, Bunkyo-ku, Tokyo, 113-8519 Ph: (81)3 5803 5249 Fax: (81)3 5803 5249 Email: mkajiwara.bldt@tmd.ac.jp 1,3) M. Kajiwara, 3) K. Imai, M. Nagasawa, 4) T. Morio, 5) M. Imai	5	6	3	48
Nat'l Cancer Ctr Hosp, Dept of Med Onc, 1-1, Tsukiji 5-chome, Chuo-ku, Tokyo, 104-0045 Ph: (81)3 3542-2511 Fax: (81)3 3542-3815 Email: ytakaue@mcc.go.jp 1,3) Y. Takaue, 3) Mineishi, Tanosaki, Makimoto, Kanda, 4) M. Goto, 5) R. Tanosaki	20	62	78	204
Nihon Univ Sch of Med, Dept of Pediatrics, 30-1 Oyaguchi, Kamimachi, Itabashi ku, Tokyo 173 Ph: (81)3 3972-8111 Fax: (81)3 3957-6186 1,3) H. Mugishima, 3) C. Chin	15	9		74
Inst of Med Sci, Univ of Tokyo, Div of Molecular Therapy, 4-6-1 Shirokanedai, Minatoku, Tokyo, 108-8639 Ph: (81)3 5449 5540 Fax: (81)3 5449 5429 1,3) S. Asano, 3) T. Iseki, J. Ooi, H. Nagayama, A. Tomonari, A. Tojo, K. Tani, 4) Y. Bessho, T. Takashi, 5) T. Iseki	30	36	31	381
Tokyo Women's Med Coll, Dept of Hem, 8-1 Kawada-cho, Shinjuku-ku, Tokyo 162 Ph: (81)3 3353 8111 Fax: (81)3 3353 8970 1,3) H. Mizoguchi, 3) M. Masuda, 4) H. Fujii	4	4		34

MALAYSIA

	1998	1999	2000	Total
Univ of Malaya Hosp, Dept of Ped, BMT Unit, Kuala Lumpur, 59100 Ph: (603) 750 2065 Fax: (603) 755 6114 1,3) H.P. Lin, 3) L. Lee-Chan, A. Tan, W.A. Ariffin, 4) Inst Med Rsrch-Kuala Lumpur, 5) L.L. Chan	18	19	24	209

NETHERLANDS

	1998	1999	2000	Total
Leiden Univ Med Ctr, Dept of Hem/BMT, Bldg 1:C2-R Rijnsburgerweg 10, P.O.Box 9600, 2300 RC Leiden Ph: (31)71 5262267 Fax: (31)71 5266755 Email: willemze.hematology@lumc.nl 1) R. Willemze, 3) W.E. Fibbe, H.F. Falkenburg, R. Barge, 4) M. Oudshoorn, 5) F. VandeLoo, T. de Vries	23	35	26	411
Leiden Univ Med Ctr, Dept of Ped, Albinus-dreef 2, PO Box 9600, 2300 RC Leiden Ph: (31)71 526 2494 Fax: (31)71 524 8198 Email: j.vossen@leimc.nl 1,3) J.M. Vossen, 3) R. Bredius, M. Egeler, R. tenCate, 4) C.J.M. Melief, (Immuno)Leiden, 5) M. Oudshoorn	35	36	28	509
The Dr Daniel den Hoed Cancer Ctr, Dept of Hem, Groene Hilledijk 301, PO Box 5201, 3008 EA Rotterdam Ph: (31)10 4391367 Fax: (31)10 4391004 1,3) J.J. Cornelissen, 3) B. Lowenberg, M.B. Veer, G.E. de Greef, P.J. Voogt, J.M. Zijlmans, 4) K. Sintnicolaas, 5) T. Landman	36			340
Univ Hosp Utrecht, Dept of Hem-G03.647, PO Box 85500, Heidelberglaan 100, Utrecht, 3584 CX Ph: (31)30 2507230 Fax: (31)30 2511893 1,3,5) L.F. Verdonck, 4) M.G. Otten	45	51	47	409

NEW ZEALAND

	1998	1999	2000	Total
Christchurch Hosp, Dept of Hem, Private Bag 151, Christchurch Ph: (64)3 3640300 Fax: (64)3 3640750 Email: ruths@chchlth.govt.nz 1) R.L. Spearing, 3) D. Heaton, W.N. Patton, S. Gibbons, P. Ganly, 4) D. Delacey, 5) A. Abbott	18	11	11	149

1)=Director, 2)=Tx Surgeons, 3)=Physicians, 4)=Tissue Typers, 5)=TxCoords	1998	1999	2000	Total
POLAND				
K. Dluski Hosp, Inst of Immun & Exper Therapy, BMT Unit, Grabiszynska 105, Weigla 12, Wroclaw, 53-439 Ph: (48)71 3621512 Fax: (48)71 3621512 1,3) A. Lange, 3) M. Sedzimirska, K. Suchnicki, J. Lange, J. Dybuo, 4) K. Bogunia, M. Polak, M. Zawadzka, E. Pietraszek, 5) T. Pacuszko	22	26	35	177
PORTUGAL				
Inst Portugues Onc, Bone Marrow Transp Unit, R Prof Lima Basto, 1093 Lisboa Cedex Ph: (351)1 726 6030 Fax: (351)1 727 5428 1,2) M.M. Abecasis, 2) M. Sousinha, 3) F.L. Costa, A. Guimaraes, 4) P. Carlos, 5) A. Machado	23	24	29	320
SAUDI ARABIA				
King Faisal Spec Hosp & Rsrch Ctr, Dept of Onc, MBC 64, PO Box 3354, Riyadh 11211 Ph: (966)1 464-7272 Fax: (966)1 442-4588 1,2) M. Gyger, 1) M. Ayas, 3) Jurf, Mohareb, Maher, Sullivan, Chaudhri, Shareef, Nasser, Solh, 4) Tbakhi, 5) Reggi, A. Majoub	124	115	122	1032
SINGAPORE				
Singapore Gen Hosp, Dept of Hem, Blk 6, Level 5, Outram Rd, Singapore, 169608 Ph: (65) 321-4625 Fax: (65) 225-0210 1,3) P. Tan, 3) Y.T. Goh, 4) J. Ngai, 5) C.H. Tan	17	28	35	301
SLOVAK REPUBLIC				
Univ Hosp, Dept of Clin Hematology, Partizanska 4, Bratslava, 81103 Ph: (421)7 54412255 Fax: (421)7 54413085 Email: mmistrik@spamba.sk 1,3) M. Mistrik, 3) E. Demeckova, E. Bojtarova, B. Csako, 4) M. Buci, M. Kusikova	15	19	19	134
SLOVENIA				
Univ Med Ctr Ljubljana, Dept of Hem, Zaloska 7, Ljubljana, 1000 Ph: (386)1 432-0330 Fax: (386)1 543-1322 Email: joze.pretnar@kclj.sl 1,3) J. Pretnar, 3) P. Cernelc, U. Mlakar, S. Zver, 4) M. Jeras, B. Vidan	9	11	10	74
SOUTH AFRICA				
Groote Schuur Hosp, Univ of Cape Town, Dept of Hem, Anzio Rd, Observatory 7925, Cape Town Ph: (27)21 404 3073 Fax: (27)21 448-8607 1,3) N. Novitzky, 3) E. Holland, C. duToit, 4) E. DuToit, 5) L. Abrahams	14	21	15	78
Johannesburg Hosp, Univ of Witwatersrand Med Sch, Dept of Med/Cln Hem/Med Onc, 7 York Rd Parktown, 2193, Johannesburg Ph: (27)11 488 3495 Fax: (27)11 642 9949 1,5) W.R. Bezwoda, 3) P. Ruff, D. Moodley, 4) E. Du Toit, 5) M. Colvin	9			163
SPAIN				
Hosp Clin-Univ of Barcelona, Postgr Sch of Hem, Dept of Hem, Villarroel 170, 08036 Barcelona Ph: (34)93 227-5428 Fax: (34)93 227-5428 Email: bmtunit@medicina.ub.es 1,3) E. Montserrat, 1,3) E. Carreras, 3) M. Rovira, A. Urbano-Ispizua, C. Martinez, 4) J. Vives-Puiggros, 5) M. Manalich	37	33	46	669
Hosp Infantil Vall d'Hebron, Dept of Hem/Onc, Paseo Vall d'Hebron - 119, 08035 Barcelona Ph: (34)93 4893093 Fax: (34)93 4893039 1,5) J.J. Ortega, 2) C. Diaz de Heredia, T. Olive, 3) L. Massuet, M. Torrabadella, 5) T. Olive	21	21	32	312
Clin Puerta De Hierro, Dept of Hem, San Martin De Porres 4, Madrid, 28035 Ph: (34)1 316-2240 Fax: (34)1 373-0535 1) M.N. Fernandez, 3) Cabrera, Sanjuan, Fores, Briz, Regidor, Barbolla, Banas, 4) M. Moreno, C. Vilches, 5) G. Bravo	9	15		239
Hosp De La Princessa, Dept of Hem, C/Diego de Leon, 62, Madrid, 28006 Ph: (34)1 520-2316 Fax: (34)1 520-2326 1,3) J. Fernandez-Ranada, 3) R. de la Camara Lanza, A Figuera, F. Tomas, R. Arranz, A. Alegre	37	36	43	506

1)=Director, 2)=Tx Surgeons, 3)=Physicians, 4)=Tissue Typers, 5)=TxCoords	1998	1999	2000	Total
Ramon y Cajal Hosp, Dept of Hem, Rm 9,100, Ctra de Colmenar Viejo s/n, Madrid, 28034 Ph: (34)1 336-8362 Fax: (34)1 336-9016 1) J.L. Navarro, 2) J. Lopez, E. Otheo, M.S. Maldonado, 3) J. Orriozola, A. Munoz, J. Perez de Oteyza, 4) N. Clerici, 5) J. Garcia-Larana	14	18	12	215
Regional "Carlos Haya", Coordination de Transp, Avda Carlos Haya, C Antequera s/n, Malaga, 29010 Ph: (34)5 261 1842 Fax: (34)5 261 1842 1) V. Baena, 3) J. Maldonado, 4) A. Alonso, 5) M.A. Frutos	32			155
Nac'l "Marques de Valdecilla", Dept of Hem, Av Valdecilla s/n, Santander Ph: (34)942 262573 Fax: (34)942 202655 Email: hemala@humv.es 1) A. Zubizarrela, 2) J.S. Cacol, 3) S.C. Garcia, 4) J.M. Pastor, 5) A. Iriondo-Atienza	22	31	21	427
Hosp Univ Virgen Del Rocio, Dept of Hem/BMT, Avda Manuel Siurot s/n, 41013 Sevilla Ph: (34)95 501-3260 Fax: (34)95 501-3265 Email: jrodrigue1@hur.sas.cica.es 1,3) J.M. Rodriguez Fernandez, 3) R. Parody, I. Espigado, M. Carmona, A. Vaquero, 4) A. Nunez Roldan, 5) J.L. Santamaria Mifsut	11	23	16	133
Hosp Clin Univ, Dept Hem/Med Onc, Avd Blasco Ibanez 17, Valencia 46010 Ph: (34)6 386 2625 Fax: (34)6 386 2625 1,3) J. Garcia-Conde, 3) C. Solano, 4) Bone Marrow Allojeneic	15	13		69
Hosp Infantil La Fe, Dept of Onc/Ped, Ave Campanar 21, 46009 Valencia Ph: (34)96 386 2789 Fax: (34)96 386 8700 Email: castel_vic@gva.es 1,3) V. Castel, 3) A. Verdeguer, A. Canete, J.M. Fernandez, 4) N. Puig, 5) A. Picazo	6	3		16
Hosp Univ La Fe, Dept Adult Hem, Ave Campanar 21, 46009 Valencia Ph: (34)96 386 8757 Fax: (34)96 386 8789 Email: sanz_gui@gva.es 1,3) M.A. Sanz, 3) J.A. Martinez, G. Martin, I. Jarque, J. de la Rubia, G. Sanz, C. Jimenez, 4) F. Arriaga, J.A. Montoro, 5) G.F. Sanz	23	32	27	269

SWEDEN

Huddinge Hosp, Ctr for Allo Stem Cell Transpl, Clin Immun, F79, S-14186 Huddinge Ph: (46)8 585-82672 Fax: (46)8 746-6699 Email: olle.ringden@immunlab.ns.sil.se 1) O. Ringden, 2) J. Mattsson, S. Carlens, P. Mentschke, C. Barkholt, 3) J. Aschan, S. Klaesson, J. Suennilsson, 4) U. Persson, T. Dalianis, 5) E. Olsson, A. Franson, S. Omon, BM. Suahn	58	60	88	841
Univ Hosp of Lund, Dept of Int Med, Div of Hem, S-22185 Lund Ph: (46)46 172404 Fax: (46)46 172313 1,3) S. Lenhoff, 3) A. Bekassy, B. Sallerfors, 4) U. Johnson, Z. Kurhus	11	16	19	137
Univ Hosp Uppsala, Dept of Med, Sec of Hem, Akademiska Sjukhuset, S-75185 Uppsala Ph: (46)18-663000 Fax: (46)18-540412 1,3) B. Simonsson, 3) B. Smedmyr, K. Carlsson, M. Hoglund, G. Oberg, G. Lonnerholm, H. Hagberg, 4) T. Totterman, M. Bengtsson, 5) B. Smedmyr, K. Carlsson, M. Hoglund, G. Oberg	52			253

SWITZERLAND

Univ of Basel, Kantonsspital Basel, Dept of Int Med, Div of Hem, Petersgraben 4, CH 4031 Basel Ph: (41)61 265-4277/4259 Fax: (41)61 265-4450 Email: hematology@uhbs.c 1,5) A. Gratwohl, 3) A. Tichelli, J. Passueg, 4) E. Roosnek, J.M. Tiercy	25	40	49	554
Geneva Univ Hosp, Dept of Int Med/Hem, Rue Micheli-du-Crest 24, Geneva 14, Ch-1211 Ph: (41)22 372 3950 Fax: (41)22 372 7288 1,3) B. Chapuis, 3) C. Helg, 4) J.M. Tiercy, 5) C. Helg	19	22	23	258
Univ Children's Hosp, Dept of Immun/Hem/Oncology, Steinwiesstr 75, CH-8032 Zurich Ph: (41)1 266 7311 Fax: (41)1 266 7171 1,5) R. Seger, 3) S. Carbacioglu, S. Ebes, T. Gungos, 4) M. Tiercy, 5) A. Morell	6	8	14	75
Univ Hosp of Zurich, Dept of Int Med, Ramistr 100, 8091 Zurich Ph: (41)1 255 2090 Fax: (41)1 255 4468 1,2) J.P. Gmur, 3) J. Halter, 4) J.M. Tiercy(Geneva)	15	17	27	235

TAIWAN

Veteran's General Hosp, Taipei, Sec Med Onc, Dept of Med, No 201, Sec 2 Shih-Pai Rd, Taipei, 11217 Ph: (886)2 2875-7528 Fax: (886)2 2873-2184 1,3) P.M. Chen, 3) T.J. Chiou, J.H. Liu	21	25	26	350

BONE MARROW / PERIPHERAL BLOOD TRANSPLANTS

1)=Director, 2)=Tx Surgeons, 3)=Physicians, 4)=Tissue Typers, 5)=TxCoords	1998	1999	2000	Total
THAILAND				
Siriraj Hosp, Dept of/Med/Transf/Peds, Faculty of Med Siriraj Hosp, Mahidol Univ, Bangkok 10700 Ph: (66)2 412-1011 Fax: (66)2 412-9783 1,3) S. Issaragrisil, 3) V. Suvatte, S. Visuthisakchai, C. Udomsakdi, 4) D. Chandanayingyong	29	26		212
TURKEY				
Gulhane Military Med Acad, Dept of Med Onc, Adult Bone Marrow Transp Ctr, GATA Med Sch, Ankara, 06018 Ph: (90)312 321 2353 Fax: (90)312 321 7778 Email: onkoloji@obs.gata.edu.tr 1,3) A. Ozet, 1,3) F.Arpaci, 2) A.I. Uzar, 3) S. Komurcu, B. Ozturk, C. Beyan, A.U. Ural, 4) A. Sengul, 5) A. Yalcin, M. Turan	14	19	14	104
UNITED KINGDOM				
Birmingham Heartlands Hosp, Dept of Hematology, Bordesley Green East, Birmingham, B9 5SS Ph: (44)121 766-6611 Fax: (44)121 766-7530 1,3) D. Milligan, 3) C. Fegan, R. Johnson, 4) P. Taylor, 5) S. Chakrabari	13	18	15	94
Leicester Royal Infirmary, Dept of Clin Hem, Sandringham Bldg, Level 2, Leicester, LE1 5WW Ph: (44)116 258 5569 Fax: (44)116 258 5569 1,3) A.E. Hunter, 3) J. Snowden, 4) D. Ashton, 5) L. Stirrup	16	20	17	179
Royal Liverpool Univ Hosp, Dept of Hem-BMT, Prescot St, Liverpool, L7 8XP Ph: (44)151 706 4344 Fax: (44)151 706 5810 1,3) R.E. Clark, 4) P. Beales, 5) E. Ion	14	13	14	176
Great Ormond St Hosp for Child, NHS, Dept of BMT, London, WC1N 3JH Ph: (44)171 405 9200 Fax: (44)171 831 4366 1,3) P. Veys, 3) D. Webb, 4) London Hosp, 5) A. Hassan	50	49	49	660
Imperial College School of Medicine, Hammersmith Hosp, Dept of Hem, Du Cane Rd, London, W12 0NN Ph: (44)20 8383 3238 Fax: (44)20 8740 9679 1,3) J.M. Goldman, 4) R. Lechler	65	66	49	981
Royal Free Hosp, Dept of Hem, Pond St, Hampstead, London, NW3 2QG Ph: (44)171 830 2300 Fax: (44)171 794 0645 1,3) H.G. Prentice, 3) M. Potter, 4) J. O'Shea, A. Nolan, R. Centre, 5) M. Ethel	34	49		581
The Royal London Hosp, Dept of Hem, Whitechapel, London, E1 1BB Ph: (44)171 377 7180 Fax: (44)171 377 7016 1,3) S.M. Kelsey, 3) A.C. Newland, T.A. Lister, A.Z. Rohadnek, 4) D. McCloskey, 5) C. Murrell	14	24		311
Univ Coll London Hospital, Dept of Hematology, Gower St, London, WC1E 6AU Ph: (44)207 387 6424 Fax: (44)207 383 0694 1,3) S. Mackinnor, 3) D.C. Linch, A.H. Goldstone, 4) A.N. Trust, 5) R. Chakraverty	46	62	71	415
Christie Hosp, ALU, Wilmslow Rd, Withington, Manchester, M20 4BX Ph: (44)161 446 3272 Fax: (44)161 446 3300 1,3) R. Chopra, 3) J. Chang, D. Deakin, G.R. Morgenstern, 4) G. Morrell, D.G. Tate, 5) T. Howe, D. Macheta	17	19	30	191
Royal Manchester Children's Hosp, Dept Hem, Bone Marrow Transp, Hospital Rd, Pendlebury, Manchester, M27 1HA Ph: (44)161 794-4696 Fax: (44)161 727-2322 1) A. Will, 3) R.F. Stevens, 4) G. Morrel, 5) S, Crook	26	21	10	229
Royal Victoria Hosp, Dept Of Hem, Grosvenor Rd, Belfast, North Ireland Ph: (44)2890 240503 Fax: (44)2890 325272 1,3) F.G.C. Jones, 3) P. Abram, M.F. McMullin, 4) D. Middleton	7	15	10	117
Nottingham City Hosp, Dept of Hem, Nottingham, NG5 1PB Ph: (44)602 627708 Fax: (44)602 627742 1,3) N.H. Russell, 3) A.P. Haynes, 4) D. Ashton (Sheffield Transf Ctr), 5) H. Hyde, J. Byrne	48			251
Oxford Radcliff Hosp, Dept of Clinical Hem, The John Radcliffe, Headley Way, Headington, Oxford, OX3 9DU Ph: (44)1865 220364 Fax: (44)1865 221778 1,3) T.J. Littlewood, 3) C. Bunch, C. Hatton, 4) M. Bunce, 5) M. Ellis	17	15	14	143
Western General Hospital, Dept of Haematology, Crewe Road, Edinburgh, Scotland, EH4 2XU Ph: (44)31 537-1182 Fax: (44)31 537-1172 1,3) A.C. Parker, 4) P.L. Yap, 5) P. Shepherd	7	14		99

1)=Director, 2)=Tx Surgeons, 3)=Physicians, 4)=Tissue Typers, 5)=TxCoords	1998	1999	2000	Total
Glasgow Royal Infirmary, Dept of Hem, Castle St, Glasgow, Scotland, G4 0SF Ph: (44)141 211-4672 Fax: (44)141 552-8196 1,3) A.N. Parjer, 3) I.G. McQuaker, T.L. Holyocke, I.M. Franklin, 4) N. Henderson, 5) M. Campbell	29	14	34	330
Univ Hosp of Wales, Dept of Hem, Heath Park, Cardiff, South Wales, CF4 4XW Ph: (44)222 744327 Fax: (44)222 745442 1,3) J.A. Whittaker, 3) U. O'Callaghan, C.H. Poynton, A.K. Burnett, S.H. Lim, 4) C. Darke, 5) U. O'Callaghan		16		206

BONE MARROW / PERIPHERAL BLOOD Transplants

	1998	1999	2000	Total
United States	3,487	3,875	2,931	45,589
Foreign	4,913	5,199	4,844	59,093
Total	8,400	9,074	7,775	104,682

BONE MARROW / PERIPHERAL BLOOD Transplant Centers

United States	115
Foreign	255
Total	370

WORLDWIDE ORGAN PROCUREMENT ORGANIZATION DIRECTORY

K=Kidney, P=Pancreas, H=Heart, L=Lung, LV=Liver

Center		2000			
	K	P	H	L	LV

UNITED STATES

ALABAMA

Alabama Organ Center, 301 S 20th St, Suite 1001, Birmingham, AL 35233
Ph: (800) 252-3677 Fax: (205) 731-9250
C.H. Patrick, M.Deierhoi

	K	P	H	L	LV
	200	20	43	54	94

ARKANSAS

Arkansas Regional Organ Rcvry Agency, 1100 N. University, Ste 200, Little Rock, AR
72207 Ph: (501) 224-2623 Fax: (501) 372-6279
M. Manley, C.W. Wagner

	K	P	H	L	LV
	NR	NR	NR	NR	NR

ARIZONA

Donor Network of Arizona, 201 West Coolidge Ave, Phoenix, AZ 85013
Ph: (800) 943-6667 Fax: (602) 222-2202
J. Cremin, S. Davis, C. Wingard

	K	P	H	L	LV
	128	23	24	10	64

CALIFORNIA

So Calif Organ Procurement Center, SCOPC, Data Analyst, 2200 W 3rd St,
Suite 400, Los Angeles, CA 90057 Ph: (213) 413-6219 Fax: (213) 413-5373
Robert Mendez, D. Grieze, S.Geopforth

	K	P	H	L	LV
	459	73	110	43	228

Golden State Donor Services, 1760 Creekside Oaks Dr, Ste 160, Sacramento, CA 95833
Ph: (916) 567-1600 Fax: (916) 567-8300
Janet E. Kappes

	K	P	H	L	LV
	NR	NR	NR	NR	NR

Lifesharing Community Organ Donation, 3465 Caminodel Rio South, Ste 410,
San Diego, CA 92108 Ph: (619) 521-1983 Fax: (619) 521-2833
Rudolph Morgan, S.Shipley

	K	P	H	L	LV
	96	17	22	14	44

Calif Transp Donor Network, 55 Francisco St, Ste 510, San Francisco, CA 94133
Ph: (415) 837-5888 Fax: (415) 837-5880
P.G. Weber, W. Palas, M. Stroube

	K	P	H	L	LV
	NR	NR	NR	NR	NR

COLORADO

Donor Alliance, 3773 Cherry Creek North Dr, Suite 601, Denver, CO 80209
Ph: (303) 329-4747 Fax: (303) 321-1183
Patricia D. Brewster, S. Dunn, K. Fitting

	K	P	H	L	LV
	132	23	34	22	65

CONNECTICUT

NorthEast Organ Proc Organization, Hartford Hospital, 80 Seymour St, P.O. Box 5037,
Hartford, CT 06102-5037 Ph: (860) 545-2256 Fax: (860) 545-4143
D. Savaria, L. Krisiunas

	K	P	H	L	LV
	70	6	21	8	37

FLORIDA

LifeLink of Southwest Florida, 12655 New Brittany Blvd, Building 13, Fort Myers, FL 33907
Ph: (941) 936-2772 Fax: (941) 936-6330
Lawrence Kahana, J. Layne, B. Pierson

	K	P	H	L	LV
	NR	NR	NR	NR	NR

LifeQuest Organ Recovery Services, Ayers Medical Plaza North Tower, Suite 570,
Gainesville, FL 32601 Ph: (352) 338-7133 Fax: (352) 338-7135
Charles J. McCluskey, J. Cardo, R. Howard

	K	P	H	L	LV
	110	15	28	16	73

Univ of Miami OPO, Dept of Surg, 1150 NW 14th ST, Ste 208, Miami, FL 33136
Ph: (305) 243-7622 Fax: (305) 243-7628
L. Olson, S. Henry, L. Cravero

	K	P	H	L	LV
	140	28	26	18	79

OPO

NR=not reported

Center	K	P	2000 H	L	LV
TransLife, Florida Hosp Med Ctr, 2501 N Orange Ave, Ste 40, Orlando, FL 32804 Ph: (407) 303-2474 Fax: (407) 303-2473 R. Metzger, T. Jankiewicz, B. Fetter	133	18	26	14	73
Lifelink of Florida, 409 Bayshore Blvd, Tampa, FL 33606 Ph: (813) 348-6308 Fax: (813) 348-0571 Liz Lehr, J. Layne, B. Pierson	154	7	39	16	80
Lifelink of SW Florida, 12655 New Brittany Blvd., Building 13, Fort Myers, FL 33907-3631 Ph: (813) 348-6308 Fax: (813) 348-0571 Liz Lehr, J. Layne, B. Pierson	52	5	7	7	28

GEORGIA

Center	K	P	H	L	LV
Lifelink of Georgia, 3715 Northside Parkway, Bldg 100, Ste 300, Atlanta, GA 30327 Ph: (404) 266-8884 Fax: (404) 266-0592 Bobbi Beatty, K. Lilly, J. Layne	250	33	53	27	134

HAWAII

| Organ Donor Center of Hawaii, 900 Fort Street Mall, Suite 1140, Honolulu, HI 96813
Ph: (808) 599-7630 Fax: (808) 599-7631
Robyn Kaufman, C. Carroll | 42 | 2 | 8 | 0 | 18 |

ILLINOIS

| Regional Organ Bank of Illinois, ROBI, 800 S Wells, Ste 190, Chicago, IL 60607
Ph: (312) 431-3600 Fax: (312) 803-7643
Jarold A. Anderson, D. Lichtenfeld, R. Raspopovich | 434 | 62 | 82 | 69 | 207 |

IOWA

| Iowa Donor Network, 2732 Northgate Dr, Iowa City, IA 52245
Ph: (800) 831-4131 Fax: (319) 337-6105
S. Conrad, L. Hunsicker, J. Petty | NR | NR | NR | NR | NR |

INDIANA

| Indiana Organ Procur Organization, 429 N. Pennsylvania, Suite 201, Indianapolis, IN 46204 Ph: (317) 685-0389 Fax: (317) 685-1687
L. Driver, R. Spangler, K. Duerden (Data Coord) | NR | NR | NR | NR | NR |

KANSAS

| Midwest Transplant Network, 1900 W 47th Place, Suite 400, Westwood, KS 66205
Ph: (913) 262-1668 Fax: (913) 262-5130
R. Linderer, J. Finn, L. Bruce | 186 | 37 | 43 | 31 | 90 |

KENTUCKY

| Kentucky Organ Donor Affiliates, KODA, 106 E. Broadway, Louisville, KY 40202
Ph: (502) 581-9511 Fax: (502) 589-5157
T. Threlkeld, B. Lucas, R.N. Garrison | NR | NR | NR | NR | NR |

LOUISIANA

| Louisiana Organ Procurement Agency, 3501 N Causeway Blvd, Ste 940, Metairie, LA 70002 Ph: (504) 837-3355 Fax: (504) 837-3587
L. Jacobbi, V. McBride, C. Van Moter | NR | NR | NR | NR | NR |

MARYLAND

| Transplant Resource Cent of Maryland, 1540 Caton Center Dr, Ste R, Baltimore, MD 21227 Ph: (410) 242-7000 Fax: (410) 242-1871
Marion F. Borowiecki, K. Kennedy, R. Kelley | NR | NR | NR | NR | NR |

MASSACHUSETTS

| New England Organ Bank-NEOB, One Gateway Center, Newton, MA 02458
Ph: (617) 244-8000 Fax: (617) 244-8755
R. Luskin, K. O'Connor, F. Delmonico | 267 | 28 | 76 | 61 | 139 |

Center	2000				
	K	P	H	L	LV
MICHIGAN					
Transplantation Society of Michigan, 2203 Platt Rd, Ann Arbor, MI 48104 Ph: (734) 973-1577 Fax: (734) 973-3133 Thomas M. Beyersdorf, R. Pietroski, R. Fortunato	286	37	77	62	140
MINNESOTA					
LifeSource, Upper Midwest OPO, 2550 University Ave West, Ste 315 South, St. Paul, MN 55114-1904 Ph: (651) 603-7800 Fax: (651) 603-7801 S. Gunderson, M. Rogers, R. Wisdorf	257	61	57	36	147
MISSISSIPPI					
Mississippi Organ Recovery Agency, 12 River Bend Place, Jackson, MS 39208 Ph: (601) 933-1000 Fax: (601) 933-1006 K. Stump, S. Schlessinger	72	9	21	6	34
MISSOURI					
Mid-America Transplant Services, 1139 Olivette Executive Pkwy, St Louis, MO 63132 Ph: (314) 991-1661 Fax: (314) 991-2805 Dean F. Kappel, D. Chandler	NR	NR	NR	NR	NR
NEBRASKA					
Nebraska Organ Retrieval System Inc, 5725 'F' St, Omaha, NE 68117 Ph: (402) 733-4000 Fax: (402) 733-9312 K. Risk, M.E. Hook	55	14	9	19	31
NEVADA					
Nevada Donor Network, 4580 S Eastern Ave, Ste 33, Las Vegas, NV 89119 Ph: (702) 796-9600 Fax: (702) 796-4225 K. Richardson, P. Niles	50	2	9	2	21
NEW JERSEY					
New Jersey Organ & Tissue Sharing, Network OPO, 841 Mountain Ave, Springfield, NJ 07081 Ph: (973) 379-4535 Fax: (973) 379-5113 J. Roth, W. Reitsma, G. McKeown	238	36	62	24	106
NEW MEXICO					
New Mexico Donor Services, 2715 Broadbent Pkwy, NE, Suite J, Albuquerque, NM 87107 Ph: (505) 843-7672 Fax: (505) 343-1828 L. Garretson, R. Sikora, K. Huster	45	2	12	2	25
NEW YORK					
Center for Donation and Transplant, 218 Great Oaks Blvd, Albany, NY 12203 Ph: (518) 262-5606 Fax: (518) 262-5427 F.H. Taft, B. McTague	75	5	15	7	41
Upstate New York Transplant Services, 165 Genesee St, Ste 102, Buffalo, NY 14203 Ph: (716) 853-6667 Fax: (716) 853-6674 Mark J. Simon, C. Nordblum, K. Gramlich	74	15	21	10	42
New York Organ Donor Network, 475 Riverside Dr, Ste 1244, New York, NY 10115 Ph: (212) 870-2240 Fax: (212) 870-3299 D. Payne, W. Saunders, J. Liu	NR	NR	NR	NR	NR
Finger Lakes Donor Recovery Network, Corporate Woods of Brighton, Building 130, Ste 220, Rochester, NY 14623 Ph: (716) 272-4930 Fax: (716) 272-4956 R. Morsch, W. Morris	61	9	14	5	30
NORTH CAROLINA					
Lifeshare of the Carolinas, Carolina Medical Center, 101 WT Harris Blvd, Ste 5302, Charlotte, NC 28262 Ph: (800) 932-4483 Fax: (704) 548-6851 Wm. Faircloth, D. Hayes	75	14	23	10	39

Center		2000			
	K	P	H	L	LV
Carolina Donor Services, 205 Plaza Dr, Suite D, Greenville, NC 27858 Ph: (252) 757-0090 Fax: (252) 757-0708 Lloyd H. Jordan Jr, A. Dixon	189	32	57	40	86
OHIO					
Ohio Valley LifeCenter, 2925 Vernon Pl, Suite 300, Cincinnati, OH 45219-2430 Ph: (513) 558-5555 Fax: (513) 558-5556 D. Lewis, T. Tressler, T.K. Craycraft	NR	NR	NR	NR	NR
LifeBank, 20600 Chargin Blvd, Suite 350, Cleveland, OH 44122 Ph: (216) 752-5433 Fax: (216) 751-4204 K. Nelson, J. Mayes	NR	NR	NR	NR	NR
Lifeline of Ohio, LOOP, 770 Kinnear Rd,, Ste 200, Columbus, OH 43212 Ph: (800) 525-5667 Fax: (614) 291-0660 Linda L. Jones, K. Holloway	130	44	30	26	61
Life Connection of Ohio, 1545 Holland Rd, Ste C, Maumee, OH 43537-1694 Ph: (419) 893-4891 Fax: (419) 893-1827 M.G. Phillips, K. Kropp	83	14	20	14	31
OKLAHOMA					
Oklahoma Organ Sharing Network, 5801 N Broadway, Ste 100, Oklahoma City, OK 73118 Ph: (405) 840-5551 Fax: (405) 840-9748 R.T. Turner, T. Herrington, S. Moore	109	9	37	6	51
OREGON					
Pacific Northwest Transp Bank (ORUO), Oregon HSC Univ Hosp & VAMC, 2611 SW Third Ave, Ste 320, Portland, OR 97201 Ph: (503) 494-5560 Fax: (503) 494-4725 John M. Barry, M. Seely	142	18	38	23	69
PENNSYLVANIA					
Gift of Life Donor Program, 2000 Hamilton St, Suite 201, Rodin Place, Philadelphia, PA 19130-3813 Ph: (215) 557-8090 Fax: (215) 557-9359 H. Nathan, R. Hasz, M.J. Moritz	NR	NR	NR	NR	NR
Center for Organ Recovery/Education, 204 Sigma Dr, RIDC Park, Pittsburgh, PA 15238 Ph: (412) 963-3550 Fax: (412) 963-3563 Brian A. Broznick, P.J. Lilnooki	212	40	46	41	120
PUERTO RICO					
LifeLink of Puerto Rico, Digital Plaza/Metro Office Part, Guaynabo, PR 00968 Ph: (787) 277-0900 Fax: (787) 277-0876 M. Saade, J. Layne, B. Pierson	100	4	16	0	28
SOUTH CAROLINA					
So Carolina Organ Procurement Agency, 1064 Gardner Rd, Ste 105, Charleston, SC 29407 Ph: (843) 763-7755 Fax: (843) 763-6393 Nancy A. Kay, P.D. Drake, S. Pitzer	176	30	46	22	87
TENNESSEE					
Mid-South Transplant Foundation, 910 Madison Ave, 10th Floor, Memphis, TN 38103 Ph: (901) 328-4438 Fax: (901) 328-4462 Judy L. Shipman, S.J. Pruitt, L. McGuire	53	8	9	2	21
Tennessee Donor Services, 1600 Hayes Street, Suite 300, Nashville, TN 37203 Ph: (615) 234-5251 Fax: (615) 320-1655 H. Keith Johnson, J. Maxfield, K. Johnson	183	40	60	28	87
TEXAS					
Southwest Transplant Alliance, 3710 Rawlins Suite 1100, Dallas, TX 75219 Ph: (214) 522-0255 Fax: (214) 522-0430 J. Cutler, M.G. White, S. David	259	32	66	25	133

Center		2000			
	K	P	H	L	LV
LifeGift Organ Donation Center, 5615 Kirby Dr, Suite 900, Houston, TX 77005 Ph: (713) 523-4438 Fax: (713) 737-8100 Samuel M. Holtzman, T. Shafer, C. Olivarez, E. Mendoza J. Orlowski	311	23	87	58	137
Texas Organ Sharing Alliance, TXSA, 8122 Datapoint Dr, Ste 1150, San Antonio, TX 78229 Ph: (210) 614-7030 Fax: (210) 614-2129 P. Giordano, G. Halff, A. Roberson	NR	NR	NR	NR	NR
UTAH					
Intermountain Organ Recovery System, 230 S 500 East, Ste 290, Salt Lake City, UT 84102 Ph: (801) 521-1755 Fax: (801) 364-8815 C. Myrick, T. Schmidt, D. McMahan	91	15	21	8	53
VIRGINIA					
Washington Reg Transp Consortium, 8110 Gatehouse Rd, Ste 101 West, Falls Church, VA 22042 Ph: (703) 641-0100 Fax: (703) 641-0211 Lori E. Brigham, P. Schaeffer, T. Webb	NR	NR	NR	NR	NR
LifeNet, 3001 Hungry Spring Rd, Suite F, Richmond, VA 23228 Ph: (800) 847-7839 Fax: (804) 672-8318 Kevin Myer	126	8	42	35	61
Virginias Organ Procurement Agency, 8154 Forest Hill Ave, Suite 4, Richmond, VA 23235 Ph: (804) 330-0800 Fax: (804) 330-0595 Christopher S. McCullough, J.C. Leland	NR	NR	NR	NR	NR
WASHINGTON					
Lifecenter Northwest, 2553 SE 76th Ave, Mercer Island, WA 98040 Ph: (206) 230-5767 Fax: (206) 230-5806 K.K. Denton, C. Blagg, T. Sawyer	NR	NR	NR	NR	NR
WISCONSIN					
UW Organ Prodcurment Organization, Univ Wisconsin Hosp, 600 Highland Ave, F4/316, Madison, WI 53792 Ph: (608) 263-1341 Fax: (608) 262-9099 A. D'Alessandro, H.Nelson	183	53	21	19	66
Wisconsin Donor Network, Froedtert Mem Luthern Hosp, 9200 W. Wisconsin Ave, Milwaukee, WI 53226 Ph: (414) 259-2024 Fax: (414) 259-8059 P. Volek, D. Pierce	90	18	30	19	39
ARGENTINA					
Trasplante Hepatico, Italiano de Buenos Aires, Cirugia General, Gascon 450, 1181, Buenos Aires Ph: (54)1 981-1537 Fax: (54)1 981-3881 E. de Santibanes, J.Mattera, M.A. Ciardullo	NR	NR	NR	NR	NR
AUSTRALIA					
Victorian Liver Transp Unit, Austin Repatration Medical Centre, Liver Transp Unit, Studley Rd., Heidelberg, Melbourne, Vic, 3084 Ph: (61)39 496-5353 Fax: (61)39 496-3487 R. Jones, P. Angus, A.P. Gleeson	0	0	0	0	27
Australian & New Zealand Organ, Donation Registry, The Queen Elizabeth Hospital Bldg, 28 Woodville Rd/Rm 105 Connor, Woodville,S Australi, 5011 Ph: (61) 82226809 Fax: (61) 88459699 Karen Herbertt, L. Excell, J.Raimond	NR	NR	NR	NR	NR
Australia & New Zealand Organ Reg., 10 Pulteney St, PO Box 65, Rundle Mall, Adelaide, SA 5000 Ph: (61)8 82077113 Fax: (61)8 82077102 K. Herbertt, G. Hodgeman, K. Hee	350	1	57	90	149

OPO

Center		2000			
	K	P	H	L	LV
AUSTRIA					
Univ Hosp, Dept of Transp Surg, Anich Strasse 35, 6020 Innsbruck, Innsbruck, A-6020 Ph: (43)512 504-2603 Fax: (43)512 504-2605 R. Margreiter, A. Koenigsrainer, P. Schobel H. Fetz	121	5	18	9	51
Allgemeines Krankenhaus Linz, II Medizinische Abteilung, Krankenhausstrasse 9, A-4020, Linz Ph: (43)732 78066117 Fax: (43)732 78066135 O. Janko, G. Biesenbach	12	0	0	0	0
CANADA					
HOPE Program, Foothills Hosp, Dept of Surgery, 1403 29th St NW, Calgary, AB, T2N 2T9 Ph: (403) 283-2243 Fax: (403) 270-3783 Y. Elmquist, A. Barama, S. Yilmaz	NR	NR	NR	NR	NR
HOPE Prog-Edmonton, Univ of Alberta Hosp, HOPE Program, 8440 112th St, Edmonton, AB, T6G 2B7 Ph: (780) 407-1970 Fax: (780) 407-3058 Paul Shelby, N. Kneteman	46	6	12	11	27
McMaster Univ, St Joseph's Hosp, Dept of Med, 50 Charlton Ave E, Hamilton, ON, L8N 4A6 Ph: (905) 522-4941 Fax: (905) 521-6088 D. Arlen, A. Kapoor, D. Ludwin	57	0	0	0	0
Kingston Gen Hosp, C/O Renal Unit, 76 Stuart St, Kingston, ON, K7L 2V7 Ph: (613) 548-2421 Fax: (613) 548-0686 C. Scott-Seary, D. Holland, J. Heaton	6	0	0	0	0
Quebec Transp, 4200 St Laurent Blvd, Bureau 1111, Montreal, QC, H2W 2R2 Ph: (514) 286-1414 Fax: (514) 286-0615 A. D'Amicantonio, R. Forcione	226	19	44	46	112
Univ of Ottawa Heart Inst, Ottawa Civic Hosp, Dept of Cardio, 40 Ruskin Street, Ottawa, ON, k1Y 4W7 Ph: (613) 761-4233 Fax: (613) 761-5367 W.J. Keon, R. Masters, R. Davies	NR	NR	NR	NR	NR
Saskatchewan Transp Prog, Royal Univ Hosp, Dept of Transp, Box 86, 103 Hospital Dr, Saskatoon, SK, S7N 0X8 Ph: (306) 655-1054 Fax: (306) 655-1046 A. Shoker, B. Boechler	NR	NR	NR	NR	NR
Saskatchewan Transp Prog, Royal Univ Hosp, Dept of Transp, Box 86, 103 Hospital Dr, Saskatoon, SK, S7N OW8 Ph: (306) 655-1054 Fax: (306) 655-1046 A. Shoker, T. Brand	28	0	0	0	0
M.O.R.E., Toronto Region, Lucliff Pl, Suite 2108, 700 Bay St, P.O. Box 152, Toronto, ON, M5G 126 Ph: (416)340-3587 Fax: (416) 340-4539 T. Carr, E. Cole	NR	NR	NR	NR	NR
Queen Elizabeth II health Sci Ctr, V.G. Site, Transpl Services, 5788 University Ave, Mackenzie Building-Rm 43, Halifax, NS B3H 1V7 Ph: (902) 473-5523 Fax: (902) 473-3665 D. Murray, A.S. MacDonald, B. Kiberd	132	7	12	0	25
DENMARK					
Odense Univ Hosp, Dept of Nephrology - Y, DK-5000 Odense C Ph: (45)65 413431 Fax: (45)65 906413 S.A. Birkeland	29	0	0	0	0
Univ Hosp Aarhus, Skejby Hosp, Dept of Med/Neph C, Brendstrupgardsvej, Aarhus N Ph: (45)89 495 566 Fax: (45)89 496 003 M. Madsen	57	0	12	0	0
FRANCE					
Assistance Publique, Pitie Salpetriere, Federation of Transplantation, 83 Bd de l'Hopital, 75651 Paris Cedex 13 Ph: (33)145-702331 Fax: (33)145-702045 M.O. Bitker, B. Riou, M. Tallier	NR	NR	NR	NR	NR

Center	2000				
	K	P	H	L	LV
NICE, L'Archet 2, Dept of Digestive Surg, 151 Rte de St Antoine de Ginestiere, Nice 06202 Ph: (33)492 031656 Fax: (33)492 036198 Mouiel, J. Gugenheim, E. Baldini	32	0	3	0	18

GERMANY

Center	K	P	H	L	LV
Univ Hosp Aachen, Dept of Int Med II/Uro, Pauwelsstr 30, Aachen, D-52057 Ph: (49)241 808 8555 Fax: (49)241 874 139 J. Floege, G. Jakse, A. Homburg	14	0	3	0	0
Kidney Transplant Ctr, Univ of Rostock, Dept of Uro, Ernst-Heydemann StraBe 6, D-18057 Rostock Ph: (49)381 2023300 Fax: (49)381 4923861 H. Seiter, F.P. Nitschke, R. Bast	29	0	0	0	0
Univ Hosp of Marburg, Dept of Nephrology/Internal Med, Baldinger Strabe, D-35033 Marburg Ph: (49)6421 2866480 Fax: (49)6421 2866365 H. Lange, H.Rothmund, Heck	25	7	1	0	0
Tx-Center Fulda, Fulda Medical Ctr, Dept of Thor/Cardio/Vasc Sur, Pacelliallee 4, Fulda, 36043 Ph: (49)661 845652 Fax: (49)661 845653 Th. Stegmann, R. Werner, L. Koenig	14	1	3	1	4

HUNGARY

Center	K	P	H	L	LV
Transp Ctr Debrecen, Med Sch Debrecen, Dept of 1st Surg, 4012 Debrecen, PF 27 Ph: (36)52 318855 Fax: (36)52 316098 L. Asztalos, Z. Kincses, C. Berlzi	40	0	0	0	0

ISRAEL

Center	K	P	H	L	LV
Beilinson Med Ctr, Dept of Organ Transp, Zabotinski St 64, Petah Tikva 49100 Ph: (972)3 922-3343 Fax: (972)3 924-9680 O. Konikoff, D. Shmueli, Z. Shapira	NR	NR	NR	NR	NR

ITALY

Center	K	P	H	L	LV
San Michele Hosp, Rianimazione o Dir Sanitaria, Via Peretti, 09134 Cagliari Ph: (39)70 543333 Fax: (39)70 530814 P. Pettinsao, F. Meloni, P. Altieri	25	0	4	0	4
Univ of Pisa, Ospedale Di Cisanello, Inst of Surg, Gen Esper, Via Paradisa 2, Pisa, 56124 Ph: (39)050 596820 Fax: (39)0.50 543692 V. Boggi, F. Mosca, R. DiStefano	63	15	0	0	71

KOREA

Center	K	P	H	L	LV
Catholic Univ Med Cent, Kang Nam St. Mary's Hosp, Dept of Surg, 505 Banpodong, Seo Cho Ku, Seoul, 137-040 Ph: (82) 2590-1114 Fax: (82) 2595-2992 Y.B. Koh, B.K. Bang, I.S. Moon	NR	NR	NR	NR	NR

NEW ZEALAND

Center	K	P	H	L	LV
Transp Coordination, P.O.Box 99431, Auckland, 1003 Ph: (64)9 638-9909 Fax: (64)9 631-0792 Transp Donor Coord Office	75	3	13	16	34

PHILIPPINES

Center	K	P	H	L	LV
Human Organ Preservation Effort(HOPE), National Kidney and Transpl Inst, Dept of Organ Transplantation, East Ave, Diliman, Quezon City, 1100 Ph: (63)2 924-0680 Fax: (63)2 924-2262 R.M. Aranas, A.A. Yusi, M.L. Garcia	202	0	0	0	0

Center		2000			
	K	P	H	L	LV

SINGAPORE

| Singapore Gen Hosp, Dept of Renal Med, Outram Rd, Singapore, 169608
Ph: (65) 321-4425 Fax: (65) 220-2308
K.T. Woo, A. Vathsala, S. Kong | 40 | 0 | 1 | 1 | 0 |

SOUTH AFRICA

| Groote Schuur Hosp Med Sch, Dept of Surg, Observatory 7925, Cape Town
Ph: (27)21 404 3318 Fax: (27)21 448 6461
D. Kahn, W. Spearman, J. Brink | 85 | 0 | 12 | 0 | 12 |

SPAIN

Bellvitge Hosp, Coord de Transp, Feixa Llarga s/n, Hosp de Llobregat, 08907 Barcelona Ph: (34)3 3356111 Fax: (34)93 2607985 C. Gonzalez, M. Pascual, J. Torras	86	20	0	0	63
Hosp Clinic de Barcelona, Coordinacio de Transplantaments, C/Villarroel, 170, Barcelona, 08036 Ph: (34)93 227-5500 Fax: (34)93 227-5409 M. Manyalich, C.A. Cabrer	126	21	23	0	74
Hosp Univ, "12th De Octobre", Dept of Immunologia, Ctra. Andalucia Km 5,4, Madrid, 28041 Ph: (34)91 390 8315 Fax: (34)91 390 8399 A.A. Arnaiz-Villena	123	2	22	0	53

SWEDEN

| Transp Center, Univ Hosp, Transp Unit 70TD, S-75185 Uppsala
Ph: (46)8 59034139 Fax: (46)8 59034134
Director, J. Waalberg, E. Bjorklund | 48 | 4 | 5 | 3 | 24 |
| Univ Hosp of Lund, Dept of Cardio/thor Surg, Univ Hosp of Lund, 221 85 Lund
Ph: (46)46 171685 Fax: (46)46 158635
B. Koul, S. Steen | NR | NR | NR | NR | NR |

THE NETHERLANDS

| Transp Ctr-Maastricht, Univ Hosp, Dept of Surg, P Debyelaan 25, PO Box 5800, Maastricht,
6202-AZ Ph: (31)43 3877478 Fax: (31)43 3875473
G. Kootstra, J.P. van Hooff | 71 | 1 | 0 | 0 | 0 |

UNITED KINGDOM

Queen Elizabeth Hosp, Transplantation Unit, Dept of Cardio/Thor Surg, Edgbaston, Birmingham, B15 2TH Ph: (44)21 627-2544 Fax: (44)21 627-2542 R.S. Bonser, I.S. Wilson, S.A. Beer	0	0	15	6	0
Papworth Hosp, Transp Unit, Papworth Everard, Cambridge, CB3 8RE Ph: (44)1480 830541 Fax: (44)1480 831114 J. Wallwork, A. Husain	NR	NR	NR	NR	NR
Cardiff Royal Infirmary, Dept of Surg/Transp, Newport Rd, Cardiff, CF2 1SZ Ph: (44)1222 492233 Fax: (44)1222 470620 L. Collar, K. Morgan, L. Coleman	45	1	1	5	23
Newcastle upon Tyne, Freeman Hospital, Dept of Surg, Ward 12 Office, High Heaton, Newcastle Upon Tyne, NE7 7DN Ph: (44)1632 2843111 Fax: (44)1632 2231218 D. Talbot, D. Marras, J. Dark	109	0	44	36	32

Center			**2000**		
	K	P	H	L	LV

WORLDWIDE ORGAN PROCUREMENT ORGANIZATION DIRECTORY

Center	KIDNEY	PANCREAS	HEART	LUNG	LIVER
Total Transplant:					
United States	6,478	985	1,572	959	3,211
Foreign	2,500	120	337	224	862
Total	8,978	1,105	1,909	1,183	4,073
Totals centers: OPO					
United States	61				
Foreign	45				
Total	106				

CUMULATIVE AUTHOR INDEX

Author	vol: pages
Maurer W	86:79
Mayer AD	93:153
Mazariegos G	95:145;98:263
McAlister V	96:231
McBride MA	99:23,71,83; 00:19;85
McBride MM	98:73
McCarthy PM	89:63;99:239
McCashland T	95:177
McCaughan GW	90:145
McCauley J	94:229; 95:199; 99:217
McClelland J	87:415;89:471; 92:405;93:345; 94:407; 95:487
McCune TR	96:129;98:91
McCurry KR	97:209
McDiramid SV	91:127
McGaw LJ	92:119
McGeown MG	89:191;96:265; 00:193
McGlave P	94:283
McGrory CH	97:101;99:111; 00:123
McKenna R	88:159
McKenzie JK	88:159
McMaster P	88:39;93:153; 96:217
McMichael J	98:263
McNamara D	94:121
McNamara P	97:219
McMichael J	95:145
Medina Pestana JO	00:349
Meester JD	96:109
Meharchand JM	99:289
Melchor JL	00:379
Meleason DF	94:213
Melzer JS	87:209
Mendez R	86:61;87:409; 88:375;89:471; 92:405;99:335
Mendez R	92:405
Mercuriali F	86:69
Merion RM	89:153;96:203; 99:139
Merli M	98:315
Messmer K	93:219
Messner HA	99:289
Mestiri T	87:27
Meyer MM	91:153;96:223
Meyer H	92:137; 95:137
Michell I	88:39
Michielsen P	88:91
Michler RE	93:109;96:153
Mickelson EM	93:193; 95:279
Mickey MR	85:1,27,45,205; 86:157,165,231, 367;87:303,325, 467;88:263,409; 89:1,435; 90:385,585
Middleton D	89:191;00:193
Migliori R	87:167
Milano CA	99:273
Milford EL	93:317
Milgrom M	89:215

Author	vol: pages
Millan MT	98:287
Miller CM	94:173;00:247
Miller J	89:215;97:241; 99:159
Miller LW	96:291
Millhollen M	91:153
Millis JM	88:29; 95:187; 99:231
Mimeault RM	88:45
Minami K	92:137; 95:137
Minden MD	99:289
Miranda B	95:111;00:396
Mirza DF	93:153;96:217
Mitchell AG	87:17
Mitchell S	87:141;88:181; 94:229
Mitsuishi Y	91:281,409;92:371
Miwa H	89:275
Mjornstedt L	93:243
Moainie SL	00:411
Mocárquer AM	00:351
Molina A	00:317
Monaco A	98:349
Monge H	98:287
Moon J-I	97:149
Mor E	90:123;94:173
Morales-Otero L	00:390
Moras D	86:47
Moray G	00:404
Morel P	91:141
Moriguchi JD	90:103;93:119; 95:129;98:303; 00:297
Moritz MJ	97:101;99:111; 00:123
Morris CA	90:123
Morris PJ	87:235;93:233 98:107;00:105
Morrissey MP	91:127
Moss A	00:159
Mota A	00:388
Moudry-Munns K	86:7;87:63,109; 88:53;89:19; 90:29;91:31,141; 92:45;93:47
Moulin D	89:143
Mulligan D	93:161
Munda R	91:159
Muneretto C	89:79
Murali S	91:87;94:121
Murase N	98:263
Murphy JB	89:9;90:11; 91:13;92:17
Nademanee A	95:291;00:317
Nagler A	96:281
Naicker S	00:394
Naide Y	98:213
Najarian JS	86:321;87:109,167; 88:79;89:253; 90:217;91:141; 92:227;93:428; 94:203;97:231; 00:159
Naji A	92:215;00:411
Nally JV	95:221
Naparstek E	96:281

Author	vol: pages
Napoli KL	00:145
Naqvi SAA	00:381
Nashan B	99:181
Nataf P	92:129
Naya MT	00:396
Negrin RS	90:157
Nery JR	96:187
Nevins TE	89:253
Newell KA	92:179; 95:187
Ney A	97:119
Neylan JF	93:253;96:249
Nghiem DD	94:213
Nguyen JM	96:257
Nicholls S	93:293
Nicolaidou AV	00:355
Nicolaou P	00:355
Nissen C	89:115
Noble-Jamieson G	95:171
Nocera A	98:133
Nollkemper D	97:183
Nordal K	98:221
Norden G	93:243
Norman DJ	91:153;96:223
Nour B	93:137
Novick AC	95:221
Novick RJ	95:35;96:31;97:29 98:39;99:35;00:31
Nunes FA	99:223
Nyberg G	93:243
O'Brien DP	93:253;96:249
O'Connell JB	92:33
Odorico JS	95:261;97:157; 99:199
Ogura K	90:471;91:245,409; 92:357
Ohashi Y	00:374
Ojo AO	99:139
Olausson M	93:243
Oldhafer KJ	94:181
Oliva F	98:315
Olson AD	96:203
Olson L	89:215;99:159
Olthoff KM	88:29;99:223
Ona ET	00:383
Ong E	98:187
Opelz G	87:239;90:53;91:61
Or R	96:281
Orihuela S	00:408
Orosz CG	87:195
O'Shea JP	99:129
Ossareh S	00:203
Ostman J	90:189
Ota K	88:189;00:374
Otte JB	89:143;00:281
Oyen O	98:221
Oz MC	96:153
Ozawa K	93:179
Ozawa M	96:381
Painter DM	90:145
Palmer SM	98:327
Palumbi MA	94:213
Panzarella A	99:289
Paradis IL	92:149;94:111
Paraiso A	00:383
Park K	92:249;97:149; 00:376

INDEX

---

tx=transplant;   htx=heart tx;   ktx=kidney tx;   ltx=liver tx;   ptx=pancreas tx;   thtx=thoracic tx